evolve

The Latest Evolution in Learning.

Evolve provides online access to free learning resources and activities designed specifically for the textbook you are using in your class. The resources will provide you with information that enhances the material covered in the book and much more.

Visit the web address listed below to start your learning evolution today!

▶▶ *LOGIN:* ***http://evolve.elsevier.com/Nies/***

Evolve Student Learning Resources for Nies/McEwen: *Community Health Nursing,* 3rd edition, offers the following features:

- **WebLinks**
  An exciting resource that lets you link to hundreds of websites carefully chosen to supplement the content of the textbook. The weblinks are regularly updated with new ones added as they develop.

- **Content Updates**
  The latest content updates to keep you current with recent developments in this area of study.

- **Frequently Asked Questions**
  Answers to frequently asked questions about community health nursing issues.

Think outside the book... *evolve.*

Community Health Nursing

Promoting the Health of Populations

THIRD EDITION

Community Health Nursing

PROMOTING THE HEALTH OF POPULATIONS

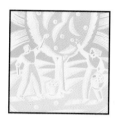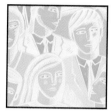
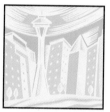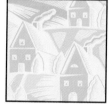

Mary A. Nies, PhD, RN, FAAN
Assistant Dean
Family, Community, and Mental Health
Professor
College of Nursing and Community Medicine
Wayne State University
Detroit, Michigan

Melanie McEwen, PhD, RN, CS
Associate Professor
Louise Herrington School of Nursing
Baylor University
Dallas, Texas

W.B. SAUNDERS COMPANY
A Harcourt Health Sciences Company
Philadelphia   London   Montreal   Sydney   Tokyo   Toronto

SAUNDERS
An Imprint of Elsevier

The Curtis Center
Independence Square West
Philadelphia, Pennsylvania 19106

Vice President and Publishing Director, Nursing: Sally Schrefer
Executive Editor: June D. Thompson
Senior Developmental Editor: Linda Caldwell
Project Manager: Catherine Jackson
Production Editor: Jamie Lyn Thornton
Designer: Judi Lang
Cover Design: Michael Warrell

Library of Congress Cataloging-in-Publication Data

Community health nursing : promoting the health of populations /
[edited by] Mary A. Nies, Melanie McEwen.—3rd ed.

p. ; cm.

Includes bibliographical references and index.

ISBN 0-7216-9161-7

1. Community health nursing.   I. Nies, Mary A. (Mary Albrecht)
   II. McEwen, Melanie.   [DNLM: 1. Community Health
   Nursing. 2. Health Promotion.   WY 106 C73429 2001]

RT98 .S9 2001   610.73'43–dc21

                                                    00-054788

COMMUNITY HEALTH NURSING: Promoting the Health of Populations   ISBN 0-7216-9161-7

Printed in the United States of America.

Last digit is the print number: 9   8   7   6   5   4   3   2

I dedicate this book to Phil Yankovich, my husband, companion, and best friend whose love, caring, and true support are always there for me. He provides me with the energy I need to pursue my dreams.

To Earl and Lois Nies, my parents, for their never-ending encouragement and lifelong support. They helped me develop a foundation for creative thinking and new ideas.

To Kara, my daughter, for whom I wish a happy and healthy life. Her energy, joy, and enthusiasm for life sustained me through my work on this book.

To all my teachers and mentors who have influenced my thinking and vision about community health and taught me the value of critical inquiry and spirited debate.

Mary A. Nies

I dedicate this book to my husband, Scott McEwen, whose love, support, and encouragement have been my foundation for the past quarter of a century.

Melanie McEwen

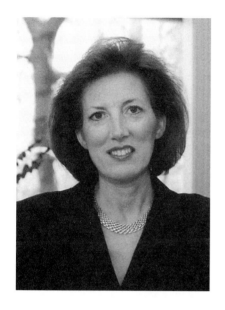

Mary A. Nies

Mary A. Nies, PhD, RN, FAAN, is Professor of Nursing and Community Medicine and Assistant Dean of Family, Community, and Mental Health at Wayne State University. Dr. Nies received her diploma from Bellin School of Nursing in Green Bay, Wisconsin; her BSN from University of Wisconsin, Madison; her MSN from Loyola University, Chicago; and her PhD in Public Health Nursing, Health Services, and Health Promotion Research at the University of Illinois, Chicago. She completed a postdoctoral research fellowship in health promotion and community health with Dr. Nola Pender at the University of Michigan, Ann Arbor. She has been a Fellow of the American Academy of Nursing since 1994. Dr. Nies co-edited *Community Health Nursing: Promoting the Health of Aggregates,* which received the 1993 Book of the Year award from the *American Journal of Nursing.* Her program of research focuses on the outcomes of health promotion interventions for minority and nonminority women and low-income women in the community. Dr. Nies is principal investigator on a research grant funded by the National Institutes of Health, National Institute of Nursing Research. This five-year study tests a nursing intervention targeted at sedentary women in the community to increase their physical activity levels. Her research is involved with energy metabolism particularly in areas of fitness, physical activity, and obesity prevention for populations, especially women. Her work also includes consulting in the areas of public and community health and health promotion education, practice, and research.

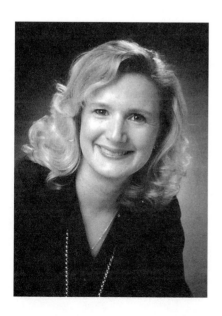

Melanie McEwen

Melanie McEwen, PhD, RN, CS, is an Associate Professor at Louise Herrington School of Nursing, Baylor University. Dr. McEwen received her BSN from the University of Texas School of Nursing in Austin; her Master's in Community and Public Health Nursing from Louisiana State University Medical Center in New Orleans; and her PhD in Nursing at Texas Woman's University. Dr. McEwen wrote *Community-Based Nursing: An Introduction* (Saunders, 1998) and she is currently co-authoring a book on the application of theory in nursing practice, research, education, and administration. In addition, she wrote the instructor's materials for both the first and second editions of *Community Health Nursing: Promoting the Health of Aggregates.*

CONTRIBUTORS

Margaret M. Andrews, PhD, RN
Chairperson and Professor
Department of Nursing
Nazareth College of Rochester
Adjunct Faculty
School of Nursing
University of Rochester
Rochester, New York
Chapter 12, Cultural Diversity and Community Health Nursing

Barbara Artinian, RN, PhD
Professor
School of Nursing
Azusa Pacific University
Azusa, California
Chapter 19, Populations Affected by Disabilities

Joan Bickes, MSN, RN
Lecturer, Community Health Nursing
Wayne State University
Detroit, Michigan
Chapter 32, Community Health Nursing: Making a Difference

Marianne Bond, RN, MS, CIC
Kaiser Permanente Medical Center
Walnut Creek, California
Chapter 25, Communicable Disease and Public Health

Deborah Godfrey Brown, PhD, MS, RN
Undergraduate Director and Assistant Professor
College of Nursing
University of Rhode Island
Kingston, Rhode Island
Chapter 6, Community Health Planning, Implementation, and Evaluation

Patricia M. Burbank, DNSc, RN
Professor
College of Nursing
University of Rhode Island
Kingston, Rhode Island
Chapter 6, Community Health Planning, Implementation, and Evaluation

Patricia G. Butterfield, PhD, RN
Associate Professor
College of Nursing
Montana State University, Bozeman
Missoula, Montana
Chapter 3, Thinking Upstream: Conceptualizing Health from a Population Perspective
Chapter 21, Rural and Migrant Health

Mary Brecht Carpenter, MPH, RN
Project Director and Research Instructor
Georgetown University
Washington, D.C.
Chapter 14, Child and Adolescent Health

Holly Cassells, PhD, RNC, MPH
Professor
University of Incarnate Word
San Antonio, Texas
Chapter 4, Epidemiology
Chapter 5, Community Assessment

Kathleen Chafey, PhD, RN
Professor of Community Health Nursing
College of Nursing
Montana State University, Bozeman
Missoula, Montana
Chapter 21, Rural and Migrant Health

Tom H. Cook, PhD, RN, FNP
Assistant Professor
School of Nursing
Vanderbilt University
Nashville, Tennessee
Chapter 2, Historical Factors: Community Health Nursing in Context

Lucille Davis, PhD, RN, FAAN
Professor and Director of Office of Nursing Research
Southern University School of Nursing
Baton Rouge, Louisiana
Chapter 18, Senior Health

Nellie S. Droes, DNSc, RN, CS
Associate Professor
Department of Community Nursing
School of Nursing
East Carolina University
Greenville, North Carolina
Chapter 20, Homeless Populations

Anita W. Finkelman, MSN, RN
President, Resources for Excellence
Adjunct Associate Professor
Clinical Nursing
University of Cincinnati
Cincinnati, Ohio
Chapter 9, The Health Care System

Susan Rumsey Givens, BSN, RN, C, MPH, LCCE
Childbirth Educator
LCCE Certified Lamaze Instructor
St. Ann's Hospital
Westerville, Ohio
Chapter 14, Child and Adolescent Health

Kathy Lee Dunham Hakala, MARE, MSN, RN, PMHNP, CARN
Senior Lecturer
Louise Herrington School of Nursing
Baylor University
Counselor, Psychotherapy Private Practice
Dallas, Texas
Chapter 23, Violence in the Community

Joanne M. Hall, PhD, RN
Associate Professor
School of Nursing
University of Tennessee, Knoxville
Knoxville, Tennessee
Chapter 13, Environmental Health
Chapter 24, Substance Abuse

Diane C. Hatton, DNSc, RN, CS
Associate Professor
Hahn School of Nursing and Health Science
University of San Diego
San Diego, California
Chapter 20, Homeless Populations

Doris Henson, RN, MS, MPH
Assistant Professor
College of Nursing
Montana State University, Bozeman
Missoula, Montana
Chapter 21, Rural and Migrant Health

Vera Labat, MPH, PNP, PHN, RN
Adjunct Faculty Member
Western Institute for Social Research
Public Health Nurse
Immunization Assistance Program
City of Berkeley, Health and Human Services Department
Berkeley, California
Chapter 25, Communicable Disease and Public Health

Dottie Compton Langthorn, RN, BSN
Immunization Program Coordinator
Contra Costa County Public Health Department
Public Health Nurse Epidemiologist
Martinez, California
Chapter 25, Communicable Disease and Public Health

Jean Cozad Lyon, PhD, FNP, CS, RN
Chief Nurse Executive
Northern Nevada Medical Center
Sparks, Nevada
Chapter 8, Case Management
Chapter 30, Home Health

Erika Madrid, DNSc, RN, CS
Associate Clinical Professor
Department of Community Health Systems
School of Nursing
University of California, San Francisco
San Francisco, California
Chapter 24, Substance Abuse

Melanie McEwen, PhD, RN, CS
Louise Herrington School of Nursing
Baylor University
Dallas, Texas
Chapter 1, Health: A Community View
Chapter 11, Policy, Politics, Legislation, and Community Health Nursing
Chapter 18, Senior Health
Chapter 32, Community Health Nursing: Making a Difference

Cathy D. Meade, PhD, RN
Associate Professor
College of Medicine
University of South Florida, Tampa
Director, Education Program
H. Lee Moffitt Cancer Center and Research Institute
Tampa, Florida
Chapter 7, Community Health Education

Barbara S. Morgan, PhD, RN
Associate Professor
School of Nursing
University of Miami
Miami, Florida
Chapter 6, Community Health Planning, Implementation, and Evaluation

Carrie Morgan, MSN, ARNP
Assistant Professor
Department of Nursing
Western Kentucky University
Bowling Green, Kentucky
Chapter 10, Economics of Health Care
Chapter 16, Men's Health

Mary A. Nies, PhD, RN, FAAN
Assistant Dean
Family, Community, and Mental Health
Professor
College of Nursing and Community Medicine
Wayne State University
Detroit, Michigan
Chapter 1, Health: A Community View
Chapter 30, Home Health
Chapter 32, Community Health Nursing: Making a Difference

Julie Novak, DNSc, RN, CPNP
Professor and Director of Practice and Community Outreach
School of Nursing
Purdue University
West Lafayette, Indiana
Chapter 31, Health in the Global Community

Alice Pappas, RN, PhD
Associate Professor and Associate Dean
Louise Herrington School of Nursing
Baylor University
Dallas, Texas
Chapter 23, Violence in the Community

Cathi A. Pourciau, RN, MSN, FNP-C
School of Nursing
Southern University
Baton Rouge, Louisiana
Chapter 26, School Health

Jill Powell, RN, PhD, CS
College of Nursing
University of Tennessee, Knoxville
Chapter 22, Mental Health
Chapter 28, Correctional Health

Bonnie Rogers, DrPH, COHN-S, FAAN
Director
Occupational Health Nursing Program
School of Public Health
University of North Carolina at Chapel Hill
Chapel Hill, North Carolina
Chapter 27, Occupational Health

Beverly Cook Siegrist, EdD, RN
Associate Professor
Department of Nursing
Western Kentucky University
Bowling Green, Kentucky
Chapter 17, Family Health
Chapter 29, Parish Health

Patricia E. Stevens, PhD, RN, FAAN
Associate Professor
School of Nursing
University of Wisconsin, Milwaukee
Milwaukee, Wisconsin
Chapter 13, Environmental Health

Cecilia M. Tiller, RNC, DSN, WHNP
Abilene Intercollegiate School of Nursing
Abilene, Texas
Chapter 11, Policy, Politics, Legislation, and Community Health Nursing

Patricia Hyland Travers, ScM, MS, RN, COHN-S
Corporate Health Strategies Manager
Corporate Environmental Health, Safety, and Security
Compaq Computer Corporation
Marlboro, Massachusetts
Chapter 27, Occupational Health

Linda L. Treloar, PhD, RN-CS, GNP/ANP-C
Professor
Scottsdale Community College
Fountain Hills, Arizona
Chapter 19, Populations Affected by Disabilities

Elaine C. Vallette, DrPH, RN
Southern University School of Nursing
Baton Rouge, Louisiana
Chapter 26, School Health

Roma D. Williams, PhD, CRNP
Associate Professor, Graduate Studies
Coordinator, MSN/MPH Coordinated Degree Option
School of Nursing
University of Alabama at Birmingham
Birmingham, Alabama
Chapter 15, Women's Health

More money is spent per capita for health care in the United States than in any other country ($3925 in 1997). However, many countries have far better indices of health, including traditional indicators such as infant mortality rates and longevity for both men and women, than does the United States. The United States is the only western country, with the exception of South Africa, that lacks a program of national health services or national health insurance. Although the United States spent 13.5% of its gross domestic product on health care expenditures in 1995—a record high of $1092.4 billion—14.0% of the population had no health care coverage.

The greater the proportion of money put into health care expenditures in the United States, the less money there is to improve education, jobs, housing, and nutrition. Over the years, the greatest improvements in the health of the population have been achieved through advances in public health using organized community efforts, such as improvements in sanitation, immunizations, and food quality and quantity. The greatest determinants of health are still equated with factors in the community, such as education, employment, housing, and nutrition. Although access to health care services and individual behavioral changes are important, they are only components of the larger determinants of health, such as social and physical environments.

UPSTREAM FOCUS

The traditional focus of many health care professionals, known as a *downstream focus*, has been to deliver health care services to ill people and to encourage needed behavioral change at the individual level. The focus of community health nursing has traditionally been on health promotion and illness prevention by working with individuals and families within the community. A shift is needed to an *upstream focus*, which includes working with aggregates and communities in activities such as organizing and setting health policy. This focus will help aggregates and communities work to create options for healthier environments with essential components of health, including adequate education, housing, employment, and nutrition and provide choices that allow people to make behavioral changes, live and work in safe environments, and access equitable and comprehensive health care.

Grounded in the tenets of public health nursing and the practice of public health nurses such as Lillian Wald, this third edition of *Community Health Nursing: Promoting the Health of Populations* builds on the earlier works by highlighting an aggregate focus in addition to the traditional areas of family and community health and thus promotes upstream thinking. The primary focus is on the promotion of the health of aggregates. This approach includes the family as a population and addresses the needs of other aggregates or population subgroups. It conceptualizes the individual as a member of the family and as a member of other aggregates, including organizations and institutions. Furthermore, individuals and families are viewed as a part of a population within an environment (i.e., within a community).

An aggregate is made up of a collective of individuals, be it family or another group that, with others, make up a community. This text emphasizes the aggregate as a unit of focus and how aggregates that make up communities promote their own health. The aggregate is presented within the social context of the community and students are given the opportunity to define and analyze environmental, economic, political, and legal constraints to the health of these populations.

Community health nurses have traditionally addressed the needs of aggregates, such as families and school, work site, clinic, and community groups. However, community health nursing texts have traditionally defined the unit of care of the community health nurse generalist with undergraduate preparation as limited primarily to the individual and family. These texts have defined the unit of care of the specialist with graduate preparation as primarily to other aggregates, the community, or the population. If community health nursing is a synthesis of nursing and public health practice to promote and preserve the health of populations, then all community health nurses carry out this mandate. Diagnosis and treatment of human responses to actual or potential health problems is the nursing component. The ability to prevent disease, prolong life, and promote health through organized community effort is from the public health component.

Community health nursing practice is responsible to the population as a whole. Nursing efforts to promote health and prevent disease are applied to the public, which includes all units in the community, be they individual or collective (e.g., person, family, other aggregate, community, or population). The generalist is competent to practice such at a minimum safe level and the specialist is expected to have expert competence and knowledge through enhanced education and experience and is given a higher level of autonomy and freedom. Community health nurses at generalist and specialist levels of practice need to promote the full synthesis of nursing and public health practice and increase their alliance with public health to promote and preserve the health of populations.

PURPOSE OF THE TEXT

In this text, the student is encouraged to become a student of the community, learn from families and other aggregates in the community how they define and promote their own health, and learn how to become an advocate of the community by working with the community to initiate change. The student is exposed to the complexity and rich diversity of the community and is shown evidence of how the community organizes to meet change.

The use of language or terminology by clients and agencies varies in different parts of the United States and it may vary from that used by government officials. The contributors of this text are a diverse group from various parts of the United States. Their terms vary from chapter to chapter and vary from those in use in local communities. For example, some authors refer to African-Americans, some to blacks, some to Euro-Americans, some to whites. The student must be familiar with a range of terms and, most important, know what is used in his or her local community.

Outstanding features of this third edition include its provocative nature as it raises consciousness regarding the social injustices that exist in the United States and how these injustices, embodied in our market-driven health care system, prevent the realization of health as a right for all. With a focus on social justice, this text emphasizes society's rather than the individual's responsibility for the protection of all human life to ensure that all people have their basic needs met, such as adequate health protection and income. Shifts in reimbursement and the growth of managed care have revitalized the notion of the need for population-focused care, or care that covers all people residing within geographic boundaries, rather than only those populations enrolled in insurance plans. Working toward providing health promotion and population-focused care to all requires a dramatic shift in thinking from individual-focused care for the practitioners of the future. The future paradigm for health care is demanding that the focus of nursing move toward community health promotion if we are to forge toward a health-promoting and wellness-achieving nation.

This text is designed to **stimulate critical thinking and challenge students to question and debate issues**. Complex problems demand complex answers; therefore the student is expected to *synthesize prior biophysical, psychosocial, cultural, and ethical arenas of knowledge*. However, experiential knowledge is also necessary and the student is challenged to *enter new environments within the community* and gain new sensory, cognitive, and affective experiences. The authors of this text have integrated the concept of **upstream thinking**, introduced in the first edition, throughout this third edition as an important conceptual basis for nursing practice of aggregates and the community. The student is introduced to the individual and aggregate roles of community health nurses as they are engaged in a collective and interdisciplinary manner, working **upstream**, to facilitate the community's promotion of its own health. Students using this text will be better prepared to work with aggregates and communities in health promotion and with individuals and families in illness. Students using this text will also be better prepared to see the need to take responsibility for participation in organized community action targeting inequalities in arenas such as education, jobs, and housing and to participate in targeting individual health-behavioral change. These are important shifts in thinking for future practitioners who must be prepared to function in a community-focused health care system.

The text is also designed to increase the **cultural awareness and competency** of future community health nurses as they prepare to address the needs of culturally diverse populations. Students must be prepared to work with these growing populations as participation in the nursing workforce by ethnically and racially diverse people continues to lag. Various models are introduced to help students understand the growing link between social problems and health status, experienced disproportionately by diverse populations in the United States, and understand the methods of assessment and intervention used to meet the special needs of these populations.

The goals of the text are to provide the student with the ability to assess the complex factors in the community that affect individual, family, and other aggregate responses to health states and actual or potential health problems; and to help students use this ability to plan, implement, and evaluate community health nursing interventions to increase contributions to the promotion of the health of populations.

MAJOR THEMES RELATED TO PROMOTING THE HEALTH OF POPULATIONS

This text is built on the following major themes:

- A social justice ethic of health care in contrast to a market justice ethic of health care in keeping with the philosophy of public health as "health for all"
- A population-focused model of community health nursing as necessary to achieve equity in health for the entire population
- Integration of the concept of *upstream thinking* throughout the text and other appropriate theoretical frameworks related to chapter topics
- The use of population-focused and other community data to develop an assessment, or profile of health, and potential and actual health needs and capabilities of aggregates
- The application of all steps in the nursing process at the individual, family, and aggregate levels
- A focus on identification of needs of the aggregate from common interactions with individuals, families, and communities in traditional environments
- An orientation toward the application of all three levels of prevention at the individual, family, and aggregate levels
- The experience of the underserved aggregate, particularly the economically disenfranchised, including cultural and ethnic groups disproportionately at risk of developing health problems

Themes are developed and related to promoting the health of populations in the following ways:

- The commitment of community health nursing is to an equity model; therefore community health nurses work toward the provision of the unmet health needs of populations in a system that allows access to care only for those who can pay (Chapters 1, 2, and 3).
- The development of a population-focused model is necessary to close the gap between unmet health care needs and health resources on a geographical basis to the entire population. The contributions of intervention at the aggregate level work toward the realization of such a model (Chapters 3 and 9).
- Contemporary theories provide frameworks for holistic community health nursing practice that help the students conceptualize the reciprocal influence of various components within the community on the health of aggregates and the population (Chapter 3 and throughout).
- The ability to gather population-focused and other community data in developing an assessment of health is a crucial initial step that precedes the identification of nursing diagnoses and plans to meet aggregate responses to potential and actual health problems (Chapters 5 and 6).
- The nursing process includes, in each step, a focus on the aggregate, assessment of the aggregate, nursing diagnosis of the aggregate, planning for the aggregate, and intervention and evaluation at the aggregate level (Units 2, 3, and 4).
- The text discusses development of the ability to gather clues about the needs of aggregates from complex environments, such as during a home visit, with parents in a waiting room of a well-baby clinic, or with elders receiving hypertension screening, and to promote individual, collective, and political action that addresses the health of aggregates (Units 2, 3, 4, 5, and 6).
- Primary, secondary, and tertiary prevention strategies include a major focus at the aggregate level.
- In addition to offering a chapter on cultural influences in the community, the text includes data on and the experience of underserved aggregates at high risk of developing health problems and who are most often in need of community health nursing services (i.e., low and marginal income, cultural, and ethnic groups) throughout.

ORGANIZATION

The text is divided into seven units. Unit 1 presents an introduction to the concept of health, a perspective of health as evolving and as defined by the community, and the concept of community health nursing as the nursing of aggregates from both historical and contemporary mandates. Health is viewed as an individual and collective right, brought about through individual and collective/political action. The definitions of public health and community health nursing and their foci are presented. Current crises in public health and the medical care system and consequences for the health of the public frame implications for community health nursing. The historical evaluation of public health, the health care system, and community health nursing is presented. The evolution of humans from wanderers and food gatherers to those who live in larger groups is presented. The text also discusses the influence of the group on health, which contrasts with the evolution of a health care system built around the individual person, increasingly fractured into many parts. Community health nurses bring to their practice awareness of the social context; economic, political, and legal constraints from the larger community; and knowledge of the current health care system and its structural constraints and limitations on the care of populations. The theoretical foundations for the text, with a focus on the concept of *upstream thinking*, and the rationale for a population approach to community health nursing are presented.

Unit 2 describes the art and science of community health nursing. The application of the nursing process—assessment, planning, intervention, and evaluation—to aggregates in the community using selected theory bases is presented. The unit addresses the need for a population focus that includes the public health sciences of biostatistics and epidemiology as key in community assessment and the application of the nursing process to aggregates to promote the health of populations. Application of the art and science of community health nursing to meeting the needs of aggregates is evident in chapters that focus on community health planning and evaluation, community health education, and case management.

Unit 3 details factors that influence the health of the community. Beginning with an overview of the health care delivery system, this unit examines the importance of economics and health care financing on the health of individuals, families, and populations. Health policy and legislation are also discussed, focusing on how policy is developed and the effect of past and future legislative changes on how health care is delivered in the United States. Cultural diversity and associated issues are described in detail, showing the importance of consideration of culture when develop-

ing health interventions in the community. The influence of the environment on the health of populations is considered and the reader is lead to recognize the multitude of external factors that influence health.

Unit 4 presents the application of the community health nursing process to aggregates in the community, including children and adolescents, women, men, families, seniors, disabled people, the homeless, and those living in rural areas. The focus is on the major indicators of health (e.g., longevity, mortality, and morbidity), types of common health problems, use of health services, pertinent legislation, health services and resources, selected applications of the community health nursing process to a case study, application of the levels of prevention, selected roles of the community health nurse, and relevant research.

Unit 5 addresses the application of the community health nursing process to the special service needs in community mental health. Chapters include an overview of violence and associated issues and substance abuse. Basic community health nursing strategies are applied to promoting the health of these vulnerable high-risk aggregates.

Unit 6 focuses on special services needs in community health nursing, including communicable disease and public health, school health, rural health, and occupational health. Two new chapters have been added that reflect recognized trends in community health nursing. One new chapter features caring for people in correctional facilities and a second chapter focuses on parish health.

Unit 7 presents an overview of the future of community health nursing. One chapter is dedicated to world health and describes features of the health care systems in developing and developed countries. The final chapter emphasizes the need for community health nursing to show that it "makes a difference," which calls for an accountability-creativity link from community health nurses in all settings.

SPECIAL FEATURES

The following features are presented to enhance student learning:

- Learning objectives: learning objectives set the framework for the content of each chapter.
- Key terms (new to this edition): a list of key terms for each chapter is provided at the beginning of the chapter. The terms are highlighted in bold within the chapter.

- Theoretical frameworks: the use of theoretical frameworks common to nursing and public health will aid the student in application of familiar and new theory bases to problems and challenges in the community.
- *Healthy People 2010*: goals and objectives of *Healthy People 2010* are incorporated throughout the text.
- Upstream thinking: this theoretical construct is integrated into chapters throughout the text.
- Case studies and application of the nursing process at individual, family, and aggregate levels: the use of case studies and anecdotal material throughout the text is designed to ground the theory, concepts, and application of the nursing process in practical and manageable examples for the student.
- Nursing research: the introduction of students to the growing bodies of community health nursing and public health research literature are enhanced by highlighting boxed references to relevant research at the end of each chapter.
- Boxed information: summaries of content by section, examples, research, and other pertinent information are presented as "boxed information" to aid the students' learning by focusing on major points, illustrating concepts, and breaking up sections of "heavy" content.
- Learning activities: selected learning activities are listed at the end of each chapter to enable students to enhance learning about the community and cognitive experiences.
- Photo-novellas: stories in photograph form depicting community health nurses making a home visit to a well family, making a home visit to a family caring for a member with a chronic illness, and giving clinic-based community services to a well family.

NEW CONTENT IN THIS EDITION

- Recognizing the importance of public health and population-based concepts, this edition includes a discrete chapter on **epidemiology**. In the first two editions, this content was included in the chapter on community assessment.
- **Case management** has been added as a chapter in recognition that this area has grown in both acute care and community settings.
- In response to the growing significance of financial issues related to how health care is delivered

and the influence on access for vulnerable people, a separate chapter on **health care economics** has been added.
- As Americans age, a growing segment of the population will have disabling conditions. A chapter on **working with people with disabilities** will assist future community health nurses in understanding the many issues surrounding this aggregate.
- The chapter on rural health has been expanded to include information on **seasonal workers**. The new title of this chapter is Rural and Migrant Health.
- Two new chapters have been added to respond to trends in future employment settings for community health nurses. The chapter on **correctional health** deals with the many issues and problems inherent in this vulnerable and needy aggregate. In addition, **parish health** describes a relatively new and growing opportunity for nurses to influence people in community settings.
- Chapter 31 presents information on **health, illness, and disease patterns and health care delivery systems in countries around the world**. This information will give students and nurses a new perspective on the health of Americans and the advantages and disadvantages provided by the U.S. health care delivery system.

TEACHING AND LEARNING PACKAGE

- Instructor's Electronic Resource CD-ROM: completely on CD, this resource contains key terms, annotated learning objectives, a lecture outline, and teaching strategies for each chapter. It also provides over *150 full-color PowerPoint images* that have been chosen from the text to supplement classroom presentation. Over 300 additional text slides are offered as a Word document that can be downloaded in PowerPoint for any other instructional use. Together these materials complement any teaching presentation. The CD also contains 600 test bank questions.
- Evolve website: the website at http://evolve. elsevier.com/nies/ is devoted exclusively to this text. It provides frequently asked questions, teaching tips, content updates, and WebLinks, which are links to pertinent websites for each chapter in the book.

ACKNOWLEDGEMENTS

Community Health Nursing: Promoting the Health of Populations could not have been written without sharing the experiences, thoughtful critique, and support of many people—individuals, families, groups, and communities. We give special thanks to everyone who made significant contributions to this book.

We are indebted to our contributing authors whose inspiration, untiring hours of work, and persistence have continued to build a new era of community health nursing practice with a focus on the population level. We thank the community health nursing faculty and students who welcomed the first and second editions of the text and responded to our inquiries with comments and suggestions for the third edition. These people have challenged us to stretch, adapt, and continue to learn throughout our years of work. We also thank our colleagues in our respective work settings for their understanding and support during the writing and editing of this edition.

Mary A. Nies
Melanie McEwen

CONTENTS

UNIT 1

Introduction to Community Health Nursing 1

1 **Health: A Community View 3**

Melanie McEwen and Mary A. Nies
Definitions of Health and Community 5
  Health 5
  Community 5
Indicators of Health and Illness 6
Definition and Focus of Public Health and
Community Health 7
Preventive Approach to Health 8
  Health Promotion and Levels of Prevention 8
  Prevention vs. Cure: Is One More Affordable
  than the Other? 10
  Healthy People 2010 11
Definition and Focus of Public and Community
Health Nursing 12
  Public Health Nursing 12
  Community Health Nursing 12
  Community and Public Health Nursing
  Practice 13
  Community Health Nurse Certification 13
Population-Focused Practice 17
  Aggregate-Focused Practice 18
Community Health Nursing and Managed Care 18
Summary 20

2 **Historical Factors: Community Health Nursing in Context 23**

Tom H. Cook
Evolution of Health in Western Populations 23
  Aggregate Impact on Health 24
  Evolution of Early Public Health Efforts 26
Advent of Modern Health Care 30
  Evolution of Modern Nursing 30
  Establishment of Modern Medical Care and
  Public Health Practice 34
  Community Caregiver 36
  Establishment of Public Health Nursing 37
Consequences for the Health of Aggregates 42
  New Causes of Mortality 42
  Hygeia vs. Panacea 42
  Additional Theories of Disease Causation 42
Challenges for Community Health Nursing 44
Summary 45

3 **Thinking Upstream: Conceptualizing Health from a Population Perspective 48**

Patricia G. Butterfield
Thinking Upstream: Looking Beyond
the Individual 49
Historical Perspectives on Nursing Theory 49
Issues of Fit 49
Definitions of Theory 50
How Theory Provides Direction to Nursing 50
Microscopic vs. Macroscopic Approaches to
the Conceptualization of Community Health
Problems 51
Assessing a Theory's Scope in Relation to
Community Health Nursing 52
Review of Theoretical Approaches 52
  The Individual Is the Locus of Change 52
  The Upstream View: Society Is the Locus
  of Change 56
Summary 60

UNIT 2

The Art and Science of Community Health Nursing 63

4 **Epidemiology 65**

Holly Cassells
Use of Epidemiology in Disease Control
and Prevention 66
Calculation of Rates 71
  Morbidity: Incidence and Prevalence Rates 71
  Other Rates 72
Concept of Risk 76
Use of Epidemiology in Disease Prevention 78
  Primary Prevention 78
  Secondary and Tertiary Prevention 78
  Establishing Causality 79
  Screening 80
  Surveillance 81
Use of Epidemiology in Health Services 83
Epidemiological Methods 84
  Descriptive Epidemiology 84
  Analytic Epidemiology 84
Summary 90

5 **Community Assessment 92**

Holly Cassells
The Nature of Community 93
    Aggregate of People 93
    Location in Space and Time 94
    Social System 94
Healthy Communities 95
Assessing the Community: Sources of Data 95
    Census Data 98
    Vital Statistics 99
    Other Sources of Health Data 99
Needs Assessment 100
Application of the Nursing Process 100
    Assessment and Diagnosis 100
    Planning 106
    Intervention 106
    Evaluation 106
Summary 107

6 **Community Health Planning,
    Implementation, and Evaluation 109**

*Deborah Godfrey Brown, Barbara S. Morgan,
and Patricia M. Burbank*
Overview of Health Planning 110
Health Planning Model 113
    Assessment 113
    Planning 116
    Intervention 116
    Evaluation 117
Health Planning Projects 117
    Successful Projects 117
    Unsuccessful Projects 118
    Discussion 120
Health Planning Federal Legislation 121
    Early History 122
    Hill-Burton Act 122
    Regional Medical Programs 122
    Comprehensive Health Planning 122
    Certificate of Need 123
    National Health Planning and Resources
    Development Act 123
    Changing Focus of Health Planning 124
Nursing Implications 125
Summary 127

7 **Community Health Education 129**

Cathy D. Meade
Health Education in the Community 130
Learning Theories, Principles, and Health
Education Models 132
    Learning Theories 132
    Knowles' Assumptions about Adult Learners 134
    Health Education Models 135
    Models of Individual Behavior 137
    Model of Health Education Empowerment 139
    Community Empowerment 141

The Nurse's Role in Health Education 142
    Enhancing Communication 142
Framework for Developing Health
Communications 144
    Stage I: Planning and Strategy Selection 145
    Stage II: Selecting Channels and Materials 145
    Stage III: Developing Materials and
    Pretesting 150
    Stage IV: Implementation 150
    Stage V: Assessing Effectiveness 151
    Stage VI: Feedback to Refine Program 152
Health Education Resources 153
    Assessing the Relevancy of Health
    Materials 155
    Literacy and Health 155
    Assessing Materials: Become a Wise Consumer
    and User 158
Summary 164

8 **Case Management 170**

Jean Cozad Lyon
Overview of Nursing Case Management 171
Origins of Case Management 171
    Public Health 172
    Case Management in Mental Health 172
    Case Management and the Elderly 172
Purpose of Case Management 172
Utilization Review and Managed Care 172
Trends that Influence Case Management 173
Case Manager Education Preparation 173
    Nurse Case Managers 173
Case Manager Services 174
Case Manager Roles and Characteristics 174
Case Identification 174
The Referral Process 175
Case Management Models 175
    Hospital-Based Case Management 175
    Case Management Models Across the Health
    Care Continuum 176
    Community Case Management Models 176
Research in Case Management 177

UNIT 3

**Factors that Influence the Health
of the Community 181**

9 **The Health Care System 183**

Anita W. Finkelman
Major Legislative Actions and the Health Care
System 184
    Federal Legislation 184
    State Legislative Role 187
    Legislation Influencing Managed Care 188
Components of the Health Care System 188

Private Health Care Subsystem 189
Public Health Subsystem 190
Federal Level Subsystem 190
State Level Subsystem 192
Local Health Department Subsystems 192
Health Care Providers 193
Critical Issues in Health Care Delivery 197
Managed Care 197
Quality Care 197
Fraud and Abuse 199
Information Technology 199
Consumerism, Advocacy, and Client Rights 200
Coordination and Access to Health Care 200
Health Care Reform: The Clinton Health
Reform Initiative 200
Future of Public Health and the Health Care
System 201
Summary 201

10 Economics of Health Care 204

Carrie Morgan
Factors Influencing Health Care Costs 207
Historical Perspectives 207
Use of Health Care 207
Health Behaviors 208
Lifestyle 208
Societal Beliefs 208
Technological Advances 208
Public Financing of Health Care 209
Medicare 209
Medicaid 209
Effect of Medicare and Medicaid on Health
Care Economics 209
Private Financing of Health Care 209
Health Insurance Plans 210
Historical Perspective 210
Types of Health Care Plans 210
Reimbursement Mechanisms of Insurance
Plans 211
Covered Services 211
National Health Insurance 212
Access to Health Care 212
Universal Coverage 213
Cost Containment 213
Historical Perspectives of Cost Containment 213
Current Trends in Cost Containment 214
Caring for the Uninsured 214
Historical Perspective 215
Societal Perceptions 215
Ethical Dilemmas 215
Trends in Health Financing 215
Cost Sharing 215
Health Care Alliances 215
Self-Insurance 216
Flexible Spending Accounts 216
Summary 216

**11 Policy, Politics, Legislation, and Community
Health Nursing 218**

Cecilia M. Tiller and Melanie McEwen
Introduction to Health Policy and the Political
Process 219
Definitions 219
Historical Foundations of Health Legislation and
Policy 219
Nurses Who Made a Difference 220
Structure of the Government of the United
States 222
Balance of Powers 222
Overview of Health Policy 224
Public Policy: Blueprint for Governance 224
Policy Formulation: The Ideal 224
Policy Formulation: The Real World 224
Steps in Policy Formulation 225
Government Authority for the Protection of the
Public's Health 226
The Legislative Process 227
How a Bill Becomes a Law 227
Health Policy and the Private Sector 229
Nursing's Involvement in Private Health
Policy 229
Current Health Policy Issues 229
Restructuring of the Health Care Industry 229
Protection of Safety and Quality 231
Accountability 232
Effective Use of Nurses 233
Nurses' Roles in Political Activities 233
Nurses as Change Agents 234
Nurses as Lobbyists 234
Nurses and Political Action Committees 237
Nurses and Coalitions 237
Nurses in Public Office 238
Nurses and Health Policy Development 238
Nurses and Campaigning 239
Nurses and Voting Strength 239
Internet and Political Process 240
Summary 240

**12 Cultural Diversity and Community Health
Nursing 242**

Margaret M. Andrews
Transcultural Perspectives on Community Health
Nursing 243
Population Trends 243
Cultural Perspectives and *Healthy People 2010* 244
Healthy People 2000: Research Overview
and Cultural Issues 244
Historical Perspectives on Cultural Diversity 247
Transcultural Nursing in the Community 248
Overview of Culture 250
Culture and the Formation of Values 250
Culture and the Family 253

xxiv   Contents

Culture and Socioeconomic Factors 254
 Distribution of Resources 254
 Education 256
Culture and Nutrition 256
 Nutrition Assessment of Culturally Diverse
 Groups 256
 Dietary Practices of Selected Cultural
 Groups 257
 Religion and Diet 257
Culture and Religion 257
 Religion and Spirituality 258
 Childhood and Spirituality 259
Culture and Aging 259
Cross-Cultural Communication 259
 Nurse-Client Relationship 260
 Space, Distance, and Intimacy 260
 Overcoming Communication Barriers 260
 Nonverbal Communication 261
 Language 261
 Touch 262
 Gender 263
Health-Related Beliefs and Practices 264
 Health and Culture 264
 Cross-Cultural Perspectives on Causes
 of Illness 264
 Cultural Expressions of Illness 266
 Cultural Espression of Pain 266
 Culture-Bound Syndromes 267
Management of Health Problems: A Cultural
Perspective 267
 Cultural Negotiation 267
Management of Health Problems in Culturally
Diverse Populations 269
 Providing Health Information and
 Education 269
 Delivering and Financing Health Services 270
 Developing Health Professionals from Minority
 Groups 271
 Enhancing Cooperative Efforts with the
 Nonfederal Sector 272
 Improving Methods of Data Development 272
 Promoting a Research Agenda on Minority
 Health Issues 272
Role of the Community Health Nurse in Improving
Health for Culturally Diverse People 274
 Culturological Assessment 274
 Cultural Self-Assessment 277
 Knowledge about Local Cultures 277
 Recognition of Political Issues of Culturally
 Diverse Groups 277
 Provide Culturally Competent Care 278
 Recognition of Culturally Based Health
 Practices 278
Resources for Minority Health 278
 U.S. Department of Health and Human
 Services 278
 Indian Health Service 279
Summary 283

13 Environmental Health 286

Patricia E. Stevens and Joanne M. Hall
A Critical Theory Approach to Environmental
Health 287
Areas of Environmental Health 288
 Living Patterns 289
 Work Risks 292
 Atmospheric Quality 292
 Water Quality 293
 Housing 294
 Food Quality 295
 Waste Control 296
 Radiation Risks 297
 Violence Risks 299
Effects of Environmental Hazards 299
Efforts to Control Environmental Health
Problems 300
Global Environmental Health 302
Approaching Environmental Health at the
Aggregate Level 304
Critical Community Health Nursing Practice 304
 Taking a Stand; Choosing a Side 304
 Asking Critical Questions 305
 Facilitating Community Involvement 306
 Forming Coaltions 306
 Using Collective Strategies 307
Summary 313

UNIT 4

Populations in the Community 319

14 Child and Adolescent Health 321

*Mary Brecht Carpenter
and Susan Rumsey Givens*
Issues of Pregnancy and Infancy 323
 Infant Mortality 323
 Low Birth Weight and Prematurity 325
 Prenatal Care 325
 Prenatal Substance Use 326
Childhood Health Issues 327
 Accidental Injuries 327
 Lead Poisoning 328
 Immunization 328
 Child Abuse and Neglect 328
Adolescent Health Issues 329
 Violence 329
 Adolescent Pregnancy and Childbearing 329
 Sexually Transmitted Diseases 331
 Substance Abuse 331
Factors Affecting Child and Adolescent Health 332
 Poverty 332
 Single Parenting 333
 Parents' Educational Status 333

Health Care Use 333
Health Insurance Coverage 334
Strategies to Improve Child and Adolescent
Health 334
Healthy People 2010 and Child and Adolescent
Health 334
Health Promotion and Disease Prevention 335
Public Health Programs Targeted to Children
and Adolescents 335
Health Care Coverage Programs 337
Direct Health Care Delivery Programs 337
Sharing Responsibility for Improving Child
and Adolescent Health 339
Parents' Role 339
Community's Role 339
Employer's Role 340
Government's Role 340
Community Health Nurse's Role 340
Legal and Ethical Issues in Child and Adolescent
Health 341
Ethical Issues 341
Affecting Outcomes 342
Summary 346

15 Women's Health 349

Roma D. Williams
Major Indicators of Health 351
Life Expectancy 351
Mortality Rate 351
Morbidity Rate 354
Social Factors Affecting Women's Health 356
Health Care Access 356
Education and Work 356
Employment and Wages 356
Working Women and Home Life 357
Family Configuration and Marital Relationship
Status 357
Health Issues for Women 358
Health Promotion Strategies for Women 358
Acute Illness 359
Chronic Illness 360
Reproductive Health 364
Other Issues in Women's Health 367
End-of-Life Issues 368
Major Legislation Affecting Women's Health
Services 368
Public Health Service Act 368
Civil Rights Act 369
Social Security Act 369
Occupational Safety and Health Act 369
Family and Medical Leave Act 370
Health and Social Services to Promote the Health
of Women 370
Women's Health Services 371
Other Community Voluntary Services 371

Levels of Prevention and Women's Health 372
Primary Prevention 372
Secondary Prevention 372
Tertiary Prevention 372
Roles of the Community Health Nurse 373
Direct Care 373
Educator 373
Counselor 373
Research in Women's Health 374
Summary 377

16 Men's Health 382

Carrie Morgan
Men's Health Status 383
Longevity and Mortality in Men 383
Morbidity 385
Use of Medical Care 386
Use of Ambulatory Care 386
Use of Hospital Care 386
Use of Preventive Care 387
Use of Other Health Services 387
Theories that Explain Men's Health 387
Biological Factors 387
Socialization 388
Orientation Toward Illness and Prevention 389
Reporting of Health Behavior 391
Discussion of the Theories of Men's Health 391
Factors that Impede Men's Health 394
Medical Care Patterns 394
Access to Care 394
Lack of Health Promotion 394
Men's Health Care Needs 396
Primary Preventive Measures 397
Health Education 397
Interest Groups in Men and Men's Health 397
Men's Increasing Interest in Physical Fitness
and Lifestyle 398
Policy Related to Men's Health 398
Secondary Preventive Measures 398
Health Services for Men 398
Screening Services for Men 398
Tertiary Preventive Measures 398
Sex-Role and Lifestyle Rehabilitation 398
New Concepts of Community Care 399

17 Family Health 409

Beverly Cook Siegrist
Understanding Family Nursing 411
The Changing Family 412
Definition of Family 412
Characteristics of the Changing Family 413
Approaches to Meeting the Health Needs
of Families 413
Moving from Individual to Family 414
Moving from the Family to the Community 417

Approaches to Family Health 419
   Family Theory 419
   Systems Framework 419
   Structural-Functional Conceptual
   Framework 420
   Developmental Theory 423
Assessment Tools 423
   Genogram 424
   Family Health Tree 425
   Ecomap 429
   Family Health Assessment 429
   Social and Structural Constraints 435
Extending Family Health Intervention to Larger
Aggregates and Social Action 435
   Institutional Context of Family Therapists 435
   Models of Social Class and Health Services 436
   Models of Care for Communities of
   Families 438
Application of the Nursing Process 440
   Home Visit 440
Summary 451

18 Senior Health 457

Melanie McEwen and Lucille Davis
Concepts and Theories of Aging 459
   Concept of Aging 459
   Selected Theories of Aging 459
Demographic Patterns of the Elderly Population
in the United States 460
   Mortality Rate 461
   Morbidity 463
Characteristics of Older Adults 463
   Health Status 464
   Income and Poverty 464
   Literacy and Education 465
   Marital Status, Relationships, and Living
   Arrangements 465
   Religion 465
Health Care Use by Elders 465
   Hospitalization 466
   Ambulatory Health Care 466
   Home Health Care 466
Health Problems of Older Adults 469
   Nutrition 469
   Disability 470
   Accidents 471
   Dental Problems 473
   Hearing Impairment 474
   Vision Impairment 474
   Mental Disorders 475
   Incontinence 477
   Thermal Stress 478
Health Promotion for Older Adults 479
   Clinical Preventive Guidelines 479
   Immunization 479
   Medication Use by Elders 480

Other Issues Related to Care of Older
Adults 481
   Transitions in Later Life 481
   Institutionalization 481
   Family Issues 482
   Death and Bereavement 482
   Elder Abuse 483
   Crime and Older Adults 484
Public Policy and Legislation Affecting
Older Adults 484
   Social Security Act 484
   Older Americans Act 485
   Research on Aging Act 485
   Other Legislation 485
Research on Aging 486
Roles of the Community Health Nurse in Caring
for Older Adults 487
Application of the Nursing Process 488
   Assessment 488
   Planning 488
   Evaluation 488
Summary 493

19 Populations Affected by Disabilities 496

Linda L. Treloar and Barbara Artinian
Self-Assessment: Responses to Disability 497
Definitions and Models for Disability 497
   National Agenda for Prevention of Disabilities
   Model 498
   Quality of Life Issues in Disability 499
Characteristics of Disability 500
   Sources of Disability Data 500
   Prevalence of Disability 501
Costs Associated with Disability 504
   Employment and Earnings 505
   Long-Term Care and Personal Assistance
   Support 505
   Health Insurance 505
Healthy People 2010 and the Health Needs of
People with Disabilities 506
A Historical Context for Disability 507
   Early Attitudes toward People with
   Disabilities 507
   Attitudes toward People with Disabilities
   in the Eighteenth and Nineteenth Centuries 507
   Disability in the Twentieth Century 509
   Contemporary Conceptualizations of People
   with Disabilities 509
Disability and Public Policy 512
   Legislation Affecting People with
   Disabilities 513
Reconceptualizing Health Care for People with
Disabilities 514
The Personal Experience of Disability 516
The Intersystem Model 516

Strategies for the Community Health Nurse in
Caring for People with Disabilities 518
Ethical Issues for People Affected by
Disabilities 522
Summary 523

20 Homeless Populations 526

Nellie S. Droes and Diane C. Hatton
Definitions and Prevalence of Homelessness 527
   Demographic Data 527
Factors that Contribute to Homelessness 530
Health Status of the Homeless 531
   Homeless Men 531
   Homeless Women 532
   Homeless Children 532
   Homeless Adolescents 533
   Homeless Families 534
   Homeless People with Mental Health
   and Substance Abuse Problems 535
Access to Health Care for the Homeless 536
Conceptual Approaches to Health of
the Homeless 538
Research and the Homeless 539
Summary 542

21 Rural and Migrant Health 548

*Doris Henson, Kathleen Chafey,
and Patricia G. Butterfield*
Rural United States 549
   Definitions of Rural Populations 549
Community and Statistical Indicators of Rural
Health Status 550
   Using Statistical Data 550
   Structural and Financial Barriers to Care 551
   Problems Related to Demographic, Personal,
   and Geographical Health Patterns 552
Specific Rural Aggregates 556
   Agricultural Workers 556
   Migrant and Seasonal Farmworkers 558
Application of Relevant Theories and "Thinking
Upstream" Concepts to Rural Health 560
   Attack Community-Based Problems at Their
   Roots 560
   Emphasize the "Doing" Aspects of Health 560
   Maximize the Use of Informal Networks 560
Rural Health Care Delivery System 560
   Health Care Provider Shortages 562
   Community-Wide Health Care Systems 562
   Managed Care in the Rural Environment 563
Community-Based Care 564
   Home Care and Hospice 564
   Faith Communities and Parish Nursing 564
   Informal Care Systems 564
   Rural Public Health Departments 565
   Rural Mental Health Care 565
   Emergency Services 566

Legislation and Programs Affecting Public Health
in Rural Areas 566
   Health Care Programs for Rural Areas 567
   Programs that Augment Health Personnel 568
   Programs that Augment Health Care Facilities
   and Services 568
   Programs that Assist with Health Care Policy,
   Planning, and Research 568
Rural Community Health Nursing 569
   Nursing Roles in Community Health
   Practice 569
   Characteristics of Rural Nursing 570
   Knowledge Base of the Expert Generalist in
   Rural Community Health Nursing 570
Rural Health Research 572
Summary 577

UNIT 5

Special Needs in Community Mental Health 583

22 Mental Health 585

Jill Powell
Overview and History of Community Mental
Health 586
   Age of Confinement 586
   Mental Health Reform 586
   Medicalization of Mental Illness 587
   Community Mental Health
   and Deinstitutionalization 587
   Decade of the Brain 587
Prevalence and Incidence of Mental Illness
in the United States 588
Healthy People 2010 and Mental Health 588
   Suicide Reduction 588
   Increased Accessibility of Mental Health
   Services 589
   Implementation of Assertive Mental
   Health Care 589
Factors Influencing the Mental Health
of Aggregates 590
   Biological Factors 590
   Social Factors 590
   Political Factors 591
Role of the Community Mental Health Nurse 592
Summary 594

23 Violence in the Community 596

Alice Pappas and Kathy Lee Dunham Hakala
Overview of Violence 597
History of Violence 598
Scope and Patterns of Abuse and Violence 598
   Homicide 598
   Suicide 599

Nonhomicide and Nonsuicide Abuse 599
Influence of Firearms 600
Violence and Selected Aggregates 600
Youth-Related Violence 600
Domestic Violence 601
Child Abuse 606
Elder Abuse 607
Violence from a Public Health Perspective 609
Healthy People 2010 and Violence 609
Prevention of Violence 609
Primary Prevention 609
Secondary Prevention 613
Tertiary Prevention 619
Safety of the Health Professional 620
Summary 621

24 **Substance Abuse 624**

Erika Madrid and Joanne M. Hall
Historic Trends in the Use of Alcohol
and Illicit Drugs 625
Prevalence of Substance Abuse 626
Healthy People 2010 Objectives and Substance
Abuse 627
Conceptualizations of Substance Abuse 627
Definitions 628
Etiology of Substance Abuse 630
Sociocultural and Political Aspects of Substance
Abuse 631
Typical Course of Addictive Illness 632
Legal and Ethical Concerns of Substance
Abuse 633
Modes of Intervention 634
Prevention 635
Treatment 635
Pharmacotherapies 637
Other Intervention Approaches 639
Mutual Help Groups 639
Harm Reduction 640
Social Network Involvement 642
Family and Friends 642
Effects on the Family 642
Professional Enablers 643
Vulnerable Aggregates 644
Adolescents 644
Elderly 645
Women 645
Racial and Ethnic Minorities 646
Other Aggregates 647
Nursing Perspective on Substance Abuse 648
Community Health Nurses and Substance
Abusers 648
Attitude toward Substance Abusers 649
Nursing Interventions in the Community 649
Summary 653

UNIT 6

Special Service Needs 657

25 **Communicable Disease and Public
Health 659**

*Marianne Bond, Vera Labat,
and Dottie Compton Langthorn*
Communicable Disease and *Healthy
People 2010* 661
Transmission 661
Immunity 664
Standard/Universal Blood and Body Fluid
Precautions 664
Defining and Reporting Communicable
Diseases 665
Control, Elimination, and Eradication
of Communicable Disease 666
Control 666
Elimination 666
Eradication 666
Prevention and Control of Vaccine-Preventable
Diseases 667
Vaccines 667
Types of Immunization 669
Vaccine Storage, Transport, and Handling 669
Vaccine Administration and Routes 670
Vaccine Dosages 670
Vaccine Spacing 670
Vaccine Hypersensitivity and
Contraindications 670
Vaccine Documentation 671
Vaccine Safety and Reporting Adverse Events
and Vaccine-Related Injuries 671
Vaccine Needs for Special Groups 672
Adolescents and Young Adults 672
Adults and the Elderly 672
Immunosuppressed 672
Pregnancy 672
Vaccine-Preventable Diseases 673
Diptheria 673
Haemophilus Influenzae Type B 674
Hepatitis A, B, and C 674
Influenza Types A, B, and C 676
Lyme Disease 677
Measles (Rubeola) 678
Mumps 679
Pertussis 679
Pneumococcal Disease 679
Polio 680
Rubella 680
Tetanus 681
Varicella (Chickenpox) 681
Vaccines for International Travel 682
Cholera 682

Japanese Encephalitis 683
Meningococcus 683
Plague 684
Rabies 684
Typhoid 685
Yellow Fever 685
Tuberculosis 686
Sexually Transmitted Diseases 687
HIV and AIDS 688
Chlamydia 690
Gonorrhea 691
Herpes Simplex Virus 2 691
Human Papillomavirus 692
Syphilis 692
Prevention of Communicable Diseases 693
Primary Prevention 693
Secondary Prevention 694
Tertiary Prevention 695
Summary 698

26 **School Health 702**

Cathi A. Pourciau and Elaine C. Vallette
History of School Health 703
School Health Services 706
Health Education 706
Health Services 709
Physical Education 709
Nutrition 715
Counseling, Psychological,
and Social Services 717
Healthy School Environment 719
Health Promotion for School Staff 719
Family and Community Involvement 721
School Nursing Practice 722
School-Based Health Centers 722
Summary 727

27 **Occupational Health 730**

Bonnie Rogers and Patricia Hyland Travers
Evolution of Occupational Health Nursing 731
Demographic Trends and Access Issues Related
to Occupational Health Care 732
Occupational Health Nursing Practice
and Professionalism 733
Occupational Health and Prevention Strategies 738
Healthy People 2010 and Occupational
Health 738
Prevention of Exposure to Potential
Hazards 738
Levels of Prevention and Occupational Health
Nursing 738
Skills and Competencies of the Occupational
Health Nurse 747
Competent 747
Proficient 749
Expert 749

Examples of Skills and Competencies
for Occupational Health Nursing 749
Impact of Federal Legislation on Occupational
Health 751
Occupational Safety and Health Act 751
Workers' Compensation Acts 753
Americans with Disabilities Act 753
Legal Issues in Occupational Health 754
Mutidisciplinary Teamwork 754
Summary 758

28 **Correctional Health 761**

Jill Powell
History and Development of Correctional
Environments 762
Issues in Nursing Care in a Correctional
Setting 763
Maintenance of a Safe Environment 763
Prison Culture 763
Patterns of Health Among Incarcerated People 764
Human Immunodeficiency Virus 765
Hepatitis 766
Tuberculosis 766
Special Populations in Correctional Settings 766
Women 766
Adolescents 767
Mental Health Issues in Correctional Settings 767
Legal and Ethical Issues in Correctional
Settings 768
Standards of Nursing Practice in Correctional
Settings 769
Summary 770

29 **Parish Health 772**

Beverly Cook Siegrist
Foundations of Parish Nursing 773
Roles of the Parish Nurse 775
Education of the Parish Nurse 778
The Parish Nurse and Spirituality 778
Issues in Parish Nurse Practice 780
Providing Care to Vulnerable Populations 780
Accountability and Confidentiality 780
Accountability 782
Summary 782

30 **Home Health 784**

Jean Cozad Lyon and Mary A. Nies
Home Health Care 785
Purpose of Home Health Services 785
Types of Home Health Agencies 786
Official Agencies 786
Nonprofit Agencies 786
Proprietary Agencies 786
Chains 786
Hospital-Based Agencies 787

Certified and Noncertified Agencies 787
Special Home Health Programs 787
Reimbursement for Home Care 787
Nursing Standards and Educational Preparation
of Home Health Nurses 788
Documentation of Home Care 790
Formal and Informal Caregivers 790
Hospice Home Care 791
   Caring for the Caregiver 791
   Pain Control and Symptom Management 791
Legal and Ethical Issues in Home Health 792
   Advance Directive 792
   Durable Power of Attorney for Health Care 793
   Living Will 793
Conducting a Home Visit 793
   Visit Preparation 793
   The Referral 793
   Initial Telephone Contact 793
   Environment 795
   Improving Communication 795
   Building Trust 796
Application of the Nursing Process 796
   Assessment 796
   Diagnosis and Planning 796
   Intervention 797
   Evaluation 797
Summary 806

UNIT 7

The Future of Community Health Nursing 809

31 **Health in the Global Community 811**

Julie Novak
Population Characteristics 812
Environmental Factors 812
Patterns of Health and Disease 813

International Organizations 814
International Health Care Delivery Systems 817
   The Role of the Community Health Nurse
   in International Health Care 818
Research in International Health 819
Summary 825

32 **Community Health Nursing: Making
a Difference 827**

*Mary A. Nies, Melanie McEwen,
and Joan Bickes*
Population Variables that Impact Health 828
   Socioeconomic Status 828
   Gender 828
   Age 828
   Race and Ethnicity 829
   Social Interaction 829
   Geography-Politics 829
Public Health: The Past 829
   Impact of Vaccines Universally Recommended
   for Children: United States 830
   Motor Vehicle Safety 830
   Improvements in Workplace Safety 830
   Control of Infectious Diseases 831
   Decline in Deaths from Heart Disease
   and Stroke 831
   Safer and Healthier Food 831
   Healthier Mothers and Babies 831
   Family Planning 832
   Fluoridation of Drinking Water 832
   Tobacco as a Health Hazard 832
Public Health: The Future 833
Community Health Nurses Make a Difference 833
Student Case Examples 835
Summary 835

Introduction to Community Health Nursing

1 Health: A Community View

2 Historical Factors: Community Health Nursing in Context

3 Thinking Upstream: Conceptualizing Health from a Population Perspective

1

Health: A Community View

Melanie McEwen and Mary A. Nies

OBJECTIVES

Upon completion of this chapter, the reader will be able to do the following:

1. Compare and contrast definitions of health.
2. Define and discuss the focus of public health.
3. List the three levels of prevention and give one example of each.
4. Differentiate between the conceptual models of community health nursing as defined by the American Nurses Association and public health nursing as defined by the Public Health Nursing Section of the American Public Health Association.
5. Describe the purpose of *Healthy People 2010* and give examples of the focus areas that encompass national health objectives.
6. Discuss community health nursing practice in terms of public health's core functions and essential services.

KEY TERMS

aggregate
certification
community
community health
community health nursing
core functions of public health
disease prevention
health
health promotion
Healthy People 2010
population-focused nursing
primary prevention
public health
public health nursing
secondary prevention
social justice
tertiary prevention

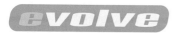

http://evolve.elsevier.com/Nies/

Community health nurses are in a position to assist the U.S. health care system in a transition from a disease-oriented system to a health-oriented system. Costs of caring for the sick account for the majority of escalating health care dollars, which increased from 5.7% of the gross domestic product in 1965 to 13.5% in 1997 (National Center for Health Statistics [NCHS], 1999). National annual health care expenditures reached $1092.4 billion in 1997, or an astonishing $3925 per person.

U.S. health expenditures reflect a focus on the care of the sick. In 1997, $0.34 of each health care dollar supported hospital care and $0.20 supported physician services. Because the majority of these funds provided care for the sick, only $0.03 of every health care dollar backed preventive public health activities (NCHS, 1999). Despite high hospital and physician expenditures, U.S. health indicators rate far below the health indicators of many other countries. This reflects the severe disproportion of funding for preventive services and social and economic opportunities. Furthermore, the health status of the population within the United States varies markedly among areas of the country and among groups (e.g., the economically disadvantaged and many cultural and ethnic groups).

Nurses constitute the largest group of health care workers; therefore they are instrumental in creating a health care delivery system that will meet the health-oriented needs of the people. According to a recent survey of registered nurses (RNs) conducted by the Health Resources and Services Administration (HRSA), about 60% of approximately 2.16 million employed RNs in the United States worked in hospitals during 1996. This survey also found that about 17%, approximately 362,000, of all RNs worked in community, school, or occupational health settings; 8.5% worked in ambulatory care settings; and 8.1% worked in nursing homes or other extended care facilities (US Department of Health and Human Services [USDHHS], HRSA, Bureau of Health Professions [BHP], 1998).

The number of nurses employed by hospitals in 1996 represents a decline of approximately 40,000, or 6.5%, over four years. Hospitals employed 1,270,870 nurses in 1992 and 1,230,717 in 1996. During that same time period, the number of nurses employed in community health experienced a 45% increase, rising from 250,000 to more than 362,000 (USDHHS/HRSA/BHP, 1998). The decline in nurses employed by hospitals and the subsequent increase in nurses employed in community settings indicates a shift in focus from illness and institutional-based care to a focus on health promotion and preventive care. This shift will likely continue and alternative delivery systems will employ more nurses, provide ambulatory care to meet cost-containment mandates, and fulfill a growing proportion of health care needs. Lamm (1998) predicted that between 1988 and 2002, nursing employment in acute care settings will decrease by 4.5% to 15%.

Community health nursing is the synthesis of nursing practice and public health practice. The major goal of community health nursing is to preserve the health of the community and surrounding populations by focusing on health promotion and health maintenance of individuals, families, and groups within the community. Thus community health nursing is associated with health and the identification of populations at risk rather than with an episodical response to patient demand.

The mission of public health is social justice, which entitles all people to basic necessities such as adequate income and health protection and accepts collective burdens to make this possible. Public health, with its egalitarian tradition and vision, conflicts with the predominant U.S. model of justice that only entitles people to what they have gained through individual efforts. Although this market justice respects individual rights, collective action and obligations are minimal. An overinvestment in technology and curative medical services within the market justice system has stifled the evolution of a health system designed to protect and preserve the health of the population.

Current U.S. health policy calls for a change in behavior that may predispose individuals to chronic disease or accident. This policy promotes exercise, healthy eating, and tobacco and alcohol cessation. However, encouraging the individual to overcome the effects of unhealthy social and physical environments negates the collective behavior necessary to change the determinants of health stemming from air and water pollution and workplace hazards. The living environment influences lifestyle and disease; therefore public health policy seeks to elicit lifestyle, social, and environmental changes.

With anticipated changes in the health care system and increased employment in the community setting, there will be greater demands on community health nursing to broaden its public health perspective. When nurses leave the hospital setting, they bring expertise to the community by working with individuals and families and by performing prevention and health promotion via the mandate in the American Nurses Association (ANA) Social Policy Statement (1986). With this move, community health nurses become more responsible for aligning themselves with public health programs to promote and preserve the health of populations.

This chapter establishes a perspective of health from a community viewpoint; therefore it requires a definition of how people identify and describe concepts related to health. The following section explores six major ideas:

1. Definitions of health and community
2. Indicators of health and illness
3. Definition and focus of public health and community health
4. Description of a preventive approach to health
5. Definition and focus of public health nursing and community health nursing
6. Population-focused practice

DEFINITIONS OF HEALTH AND COMMUNITY

Health

The definition of **health** is evolving. The World Health Organization's (WHO) classic definition of health (1958, p. 1) reflects a trend to define health in social terms rather than in medical terms. WHO defines health as "a state of complete physical, mental, and social well-being and not merely the absence of disease or infirmity."

Social health promotes community vitality, hence the need to define health in social terms. *Social* means "of or relating to living together in organized groups or similar close aggregates" (*American Heritage College Dictionary*, 1997, p. 1291). Social refers to units of people in communities who interact with each other. Social health is a result of positive interaction among groups within the community; for example, groups may sponsor food banks in churches and civic organizations. For community groups, interactions that result in poverty, violence, and lack of opportunity negatively affect social health.

In the mid1980s, WHO expanded the definition of health to include the following socialized conceptualization of health:

The extent to which an individual or group is able, on the one hand, to realize aspirations and satisfy needs;

and, on the other hand, to change or cope with the environment. Health is, therefore, seen as a resource for everyday life, not the objective of living; it is a positive concept emphasizing social and personal resources, and physical capacities.

(WHO, 1986, p. 73)

Nursing literature has defined health as the client's "optimal level of functioning" (Archer and Fleshman, 1979); "fitness as a result of individual adaptation to stress" (Leahy, Cobb, and Jones, 1982); "a condition involving a subjective sense of well-being" (Harper and Lambert, 1994); "actualization of inherent and acquired human potential through goal-directed behavior, competent self-care, and satisfying relationships with others" (Pender, 1996); and "a state of a person that is characterized by soundness or wholeness of developed human structures and of bodily and mental functioning" (Orem, 1995).

The variety of meanings illustrates the difficulty in standardizing the definition of health. The major problem herein involves the unit of analysis. Many authors use the individual as the unit of analysis and exclude the community. Others include the concepts of stress, adaptation, and environment in health definitions. Often the authors present the environment as static and requiring human adaptation rather than as changing and enabling human modification.

For many years, nurses have used Dunn's classic concept of wellness (1961), in which family, community, society, and environment are interrelated and have an influence on health. Illness, health, and peak wellness are on a continuum. Health is fluid and changing; therefore the state of health within a social environment depends on the goals, potentials, and performance of individuals, families, communities, and societies.

Community

The definitions of **community** are numerous and variable. Nursing literature has defined community as the following: "a social group determined by geographic boundaries and/or common values and interests" (WHO, 1974); "a social unit in which there is a transaction of a common life among the people making up the unit" (Green and Anderson, 1986); "a group of people who share some type of bond, who interact with each other, and who function collectively regarding common concerns" (Clark, 1999); and "a locality-based entity, composed of systems of formal organizations reflecting society's institutions, informal groups and aggregates" (Shuster and Goeppinger, 2000).

Baldwin and colleagues (1998) noted an evolution in the definition of community in community health nursing texts. The authors observed that before 1996, definitions of community focused on geographical boundaries and combined them with social attributes of people. Through citing several authors from the late 1990s, the authors observed that geographical location became a secondary characteristic in the discussion of what defines a community.

Currently, community is commonly defined as people interacting in social units and sharing common interests. Social units achieve health in many complex ways to meet the demands of rapidly changing conditions. For example, in a social unit of a couple, an elderly woman has become the caregiver of her ill husband. She notices that she had more energy when her husband first became bedfast. Caring for his incontinence takes much of her energy and she withholds a portion of his diuretic to conserve the energy she needs to care for him in other ways.

Other examples of social units include the Sierra Club, whose members lobby for the preservation of natural resource lands, and a group of disabled people who challenge the owners of an office building to obtain equal access to public buildings, education, jobs, and transportation. These social units are striving to realize a level of potential "health" beyond that of past states, which will provide the impetus for future changes.

Communities have a wide range of values. For some, protection of their economic interests is a primary factor in achieving health. For others, human needs and family closeness are primary factors. The community health nurse learns many different definitions and views of health from the rich cultural diversity within a community.

The community health nurse must be able to recognize how the community defines health. The nurse should obtain definitions from families, organizations, various groups, and other **aggregates**, or subgroups, within the community.

INDICATORS OF HEALTH AND ILLNESS

The health status of a community is associated with several factors, such as health care access, economic conditions, social and environmental issues, and cultural practices. A variety of health indicators, such as disease, morbidity, and mortality, measure the health of the community. Health care access contributes to trends in disease, morbidity, and mortality and illustrates changes in the health status of the nation. Local or state health departments, the Centers for Disease Control and Prevention (CDC), and the NCHS provide morbidity, mortality, and other health status-related data.

Indicators of mortality determine the health status of a society because changes in mortality reflect several social, economic, health service, and related trends (Torrens, 1999). These data may be useful in analyzing health patterns over time, comparing communities from different geographical regions, or comparing different aggregates within a community. State and local health departments are responsible for collecting morbidity and mortality data and forwarding the information to the appropriate federal-level agency, which is often the CDC. Some of the more commonly reported indicators are life expectancy, infant mortality, age-adjusted death rates, and cancer incidence rates.

Community health nurses must be aware of health patterns within their practice. Nurses should ask many questions, including the following:

- What are the leading causes of death and disease among various aggregates served?
- How do infant mortality rates and teenage pregnancy rates in their community compare with regional, state, and national rates?
- What are the most serious communicable disease threats?
- What are the most common environmental risks?

The community health nurse may identify areas for further investigation and intervention through an understanding of health, disease, and mortality patterns. For example, if the school nurse learns that the teenage pregnancy rate in her community is higher than regional and state averages, he or she should address the problem with school officials, parents, and students. Likewise, if an occupational health nurse discovers an apparent high rate of chronic lung disease in an industrial facility, he or she should work with company management, employees, and state and federal officials to identify potential harmful sources. If a public health nurse works in a state-sponsored acquired immunodeficiency syndrome (AIDS) clinic and recognizes an increase in the number of women testing positive for human immunodeficiency virus

(HIV), he or she should report all findings to the designated agencies. The nurse should then participate in investigative efforts to determine what is precipitating the increase and work to remedy the identified threats or risks.

DEFINITION AND FOCUS OF PUBLIC HEALTH AND COMMUNITY HEALTH

C.E. Winslow is known for the following classic definition of public health:

> Public health is the Science and Art of (1) preventing disease, (2) prolonging life, and (3) promoting health and efficiency through organized community effort for:
> (a) sanitation of the environment,
> (b) control of communicable infections,
> (c) education of the individual in personal hygiene,
> (d) organization of medical and nursing services for the early diagnosis and preventive treatment of disease, and
> (e) development of the social machinery to ensure everyone a standard of living adequate for the maintenance of health, so organizing these benefits as to enable every citizen to realize his birthright of health and longevity.
>
> (Hanlon, 1960, p. 23)

The key phrase in this definition of public health is "through organized community effort." The term **public health** connotes organized, legislated, and tax-supported efforts that serve all people through health departments or related governmental agencies.

More recently, the Institute of Medicine (1988) identified the following three **core functions of public health**: assessment, assurance, and policy development. Box 1-1 depicts each of the three primary functions and describes them briefly. All nurses working in community settings should develop knowledge and skills related to each of these primary functions.

The term **community health** extends the realm of public health to include organized health efforts at the community level through government and private efforts. Participants include privately funded agencies such as the American Heart Association or the Red Cross. Various private and public structures serve community health efforts.

Public health efforts focus on prevention and promotion of population health at the federal, state, and local levels. These efforts at the federal

---

BOX **1-1**

Core Public Health Functions

Assessment: Regular collection, analysis, and information sharing about health conditions, risks, and resources in a community.

Policy Development: Use of information gathered during assessment to develop local and state health policies and to direct resources toward those policies.

Assurance: Focuses on the availability of necessary health services throughout the community. It includes maintaining the ability of both public health agencies and private providers to manage day-to-day operations and the capacity to respond to critical situations and emergencies.

From Institute of Medicine: *The future of public health,* Washington, DC, 1988, National Academy Press.

---

and state levels concentrate on providing support and advisory services to public health structures at the local level. The local level structures provide direct services to communities through two avenues, which follow:

- Community health services protect the public from hazards such as polluted water and air, tainted food, and unsafe housing.
- Personal health care services such as immunization and family planning services, well-infant care, and sexually transmitted disease (STD) treatment protect the public from disease.

Personal health services are part of the public health effort and target the populations most at risk and in need of services. Public health efforts are multidisciplinary because they require people with many different skills. Community health nurses work with a diverse team of public health professionals, including epidemiologists, local health officers, and health educators. Public health science methods that assess biostatistics and population needs provide a method of measuring characteristics and health indexes within a community.

In 1996, the American Public Health Association (APHA) drafted a list of 10 essential public health services, which the USDHHS (1997) later adopted.

BOX 1-2

Essential Public Health Services

- Monitor health status to identify community health problems.
- Diagnose and investigate health problems and health hazards in the community.
- Inform, educate, and empower people about health issues.
- Mobilize community partnerships to identify and solve health problems.
- Develop policies and plans that support individual and community health efforts.
- Enforce laws and regulations that protect health and ensure safety.
- Link people to needed personal health services and ensure the provision of health care when otherwise unavailable.
- Ensure a competent public health and personal health care workforce.
- Evaluate effectiveness, accessibility, and quality of personal and population-based health services.
- Research for new insights and innovative solutions to health problems.

From US Department of Health and Human Services/ Public Health Service: *The public health workforce: an agenda for the 21st century,* Washington, DC, 1997, The Author.

This list appears in Box 1-2. This chapter describes the specific examples of nursing competencies related to the primary functions of public health, nursing interventions, and essential service activities.

PREVENTIVE APPROACH TO HEALTH

Health Promotion and Levels of Prevention

Public health efforts focus on health promotion and disease prevention. **Health promotion** activities enhance resources directed at improving well-being, whereas **disease prevention** activities protect people from disease and the effects of disease. The following are the three levels of prevention (Leavell and Clark, 1958) (Fig. 1-1 and Table 1-1):

- **Primary prevention** activities prevent a problem before it occurs (e.g., immunizations to prevent disease).
- **Secondary prevention** activities provide early detection and intervention (e.g., screening for STDs).
- **Tertiary prevention** activities correct a disease state and prevent it from further deteriorating (e.g., teaching insulin administration in the home).

Unfortunately, society resists the public funding of preventive health care measures. This resistance emerges out of market justice and the mistaken

FIGURE 1-1

The three levels of prevention.

Level 1.   **Primary Prevention Activities**

Prevention of problems before they occur
Example: Immunization

Level 2.   **Secondary Prevention Activities**

Early detection and intervention
Example: Screening for sexually transmitted disease

Level 3.   **Tertiary Prevention Activities**

Correction and prevention of deterioration of a disease state
Example: Teaching insulin administration in the home

concept of individual responsibility for health (Beauchamp, 1986). Conversely, **social justice** emphasizes societal responsibility for the protection of all human life rather than individual responsibility. This ensures that all people obtain basic needs, such as adequate health protection and income. Market justice rarely considers socially determined preconditions that strongly influence behavior, in particular, those involving health (Beauchamp, 1986).

The private sector contends for more of the health care dollar; employs expensive equipment, supplies, buildings, and pharmaceuticals; and polarizes the domains of prevention and cure. In fact, health services have very minimal involvement with disease prevention and health. Currently, social mandates and legislative appropriations do not emphasize needed resources and services such as education, housing, nutrition, safe work places, and clean air and water.

TABLE 1-1

Examples of Levels of Prevention and Clients Served in the Community

| Definition of Client Served* | Level of Prevention | | |
	Primary (i.e., Health Promotion and Specific Prevention)	Secondary (i.e., Early Diagnosis and Treatment)	Tertiary (i.e., Limitation of Disability and Rehabilitation)
Individual	Dietary teaching during pregnancy Immunizations	HIV testing Screening for cervical cancer	Educating new clients with diabetes to administer insulin Exercise therapy after stroke Skin care for incontinent patient
Family (i.e., two or more individuals bound by kinship, law, or living arrangement and with common emotional ties and obligations [see Chapter 13])	Education regarding smoking, dental care, or nutritional counseling Adequate housing	Dental examinations Tuberculin testing for family at risk	Mental health counseling or referral for family in crisis (e.g., grieving or experiencing a divorce) Dietary instructions and monitoring for family with overweight members
Group or aggregate (i.e., interacting people with a common purpose or purposes)	Birthing classes for pregnant teenage mothers AIDS and other STD education for high school students	Vision screening of first grade class Mammography van for screening of women in a low-income neighborhood Hearing tests at a senior center	Group counseling for grade-school children with asthma Swim therapy for physically disabled elders at a senior center Alcoholics Anonymous and other self-help groups Mental health services for military veterans
Community and populations (i.e., aggregate of people sharing space over time within a social system [see Chapter 5]; population groups or aggregates with power relations and common needs or purposes)	Fluoride water supplementation Environmental sanitation Removal of environmental hazards	Organized screening programs for communities such as health fairs VDRL screening for marriage license applicants in a city Lead screening for children by school district	Shelter and relocation centers for fire or earthquake victims Emergency medical services Community mental health services for chronically mentally ill Home care services for chronically ill

AIDS, acquired immunodeficiency syndrome; HIV, human immunodeficiency virus; VDRL, Venereal Disease Research Laboratories.
*Note that terms are used differently in literature of various disciplines. No clear-cut definitions exist; for example, families may be referred to as an aggregate and a population and subpopulations may exist within a community.

The concepts of prevention and population-focused care figure prominently in a conceptual orientation to nursing practice referred to as "thinking upstream." This orientation is derived from an analogy of patients falling into a river upstream and being rescued downstream by health providers overwhelmed with the struggle of responding to disease and illness. The river as an analogy for the natural history of illness was first coined by McKinlay (1979), with a charge to health providers to refocus their efforts toward preventive and "upstream" activities. In a description of the daily challenges of providers to address health from a preventive versus curative focus, McKinlay contrasts the consequences of illness (*downstream* endeavors) from its precursors (*upstream* endeavors). The author then charges health providers to critically examine the relative weight of their activities toward illness response versus the prevention of illness. Butterfield (1990) adapted McKinlay's upstream analogy to nursing practice by examining preventive health efforts in nursing from a historical and theoretical perspective. In this context, a population-based perspective on health and health determinants is critical to understanding and formulating nursing actions to prevent the development of chronic disease. By examining the origins of disease, nurses identify social, political, environmental, and economic factors that often lead to poor health options for both individuals and populations. The call to refocus the efforts of nurses "upstream, where the real problems lie" (McKinlay, 1979), has been welcomed by community health nurses in a variety of practice settings. For these nurses, this theme provides affirmation of their daily efforts to prevent disease in populations at risk in schools, work sites, and clinics throughout their local communities and in the larger world.

P. Butterfield

Prevention vs. Cure: Is One More Affordable than the Other?

Spending additional dollars for cure in the form of health care services does not improve the health of a population, whereas spending money on prevention does improve health. Lamarche (1995) and others (Evans and Stoddart, 1994; Torrens, 1999), stated that an absence of convincing evidence exists to verify that the amount of money expended for health care improves the health of a population. The real determinants of health are prevention efforts that provide education, housing, food, minimal decent income, and safe social and physical environments. The United States spends nearly one seventh of the nation's wealth on health care or "cure" for individuals, which diverts money from the needed resources and services that *do* determine health (Evans and Stoddart, 1994; NCHS, 1999).

The United States is not committed to improving health outcomes for the poor, vulnerable, and uninsured populations. With a limited health workforce and monetary resources, the United States cannot continue to spend vast amounts on health care services when the investment fails to improve health outcomes. In industrialized countries, life expectancy at birth is not related to the level of health care expenditures; in developing countries, longevity is closely related to the level of economic development and the education of the population (Lamarche, 1995).

A continued overexpansion of the current health care system could be detrimental to the health of a population. This may deter a large investment of the country's wealth in education and other developmental efforts that influence health. Managed care organizations (MCOs) focus on prevention; therefore they have determined that the rate of health care cost increases have slowed among employees of large firms (Shine, 1995; Torrens and Williams, 1999). Prevention programs may help reduce costs for those enrolled in MCOs, but it is unclear who will provide these services for the uninsured, poor, and other vulnerable populations. It is also unclear who will provide adequate schooling, housing, meals, wages, and a safe environment for the disadvantaged. Reductions in health care spending would decrease the effects of economic disparities by allowing investments in sufficient housing, jobs, nutrition, and safe environments.

There is a need for an ethic of social justice for society's responsibility to meet the basic needs of all people rather than the individual's responsibility. There is a need for public funding of prevention to ensure the health of our population.

Healthy People 2010

In 1979, the USDHHS published a national prevention initiative entitled *Healthy People: The Surgeon General's Report on Health Promotion and Disease Prevention.* The 1979 version established goals that would reduce mortality among infants, children, adolescents and young adults, and adults, and increase independence among older adults. In 1990, the mortality of infants, children, and adults declined sufficiently to meet the goal. Adolescent mortality did not reach the 1990 target and data systems were unable to adequately track the target for older adults (USDHHS, 2000).

Published in 1989, *Healthy People 2000* built upon the first Surgeon General's report. *Healthy People 2000* contained the following broad goals:

1. Increase the span of healthy life for Americans.
2. Reduce health disparities among Americans.
3. Achieve access to preventive services for all Americans (USDHHS, 1989).

The purpose of *Healthy People 2000* was to provide direction for individuals wanting to change personal behaviors and to improve health in communities through health promotion policies. The report assimilated the broad approaches of health promotion, health protection, and preventive services and contained more than 300 objectives organized into 22 priority areas. Although many of the objectives fell short of their goal, the initiative was extremely successful in raising provider's awareness of health behaviors and health promotional activities. States, local health departments, and private sector health workers used the objectives to determine the relative health of their community and set goals for the future.

Healthy People 2010 emerged in January 2000. It expands upon the objectives from *Healthy People 2000* through a broadened prevention science base, an improved surveillance and data system, and a heightened awareness and demand for preventive health services. This reflects changes in demographics, science, technology, and disease. ***Healthy People 2010*** lists the following broad goals:

Goal 1. Increase quality and years of healthy life.
Goal 2. Eliminate health disparities.

The first goal moves beyond the idea of increasing life expectancy to incorporate the concept of health-related quality of life (HRQOL). This concept of health includes aspects of physical and mental health and their determinants and measures functional status, participation, and well-being. HRQOL expands the definition of health—beyond simply opposing the negative concepts of disease and death—by integrating mental and physical health concepts (USDHHS, 2000).

In *Healthy People 2010,* some 467 objectives are divided into 28 focus areas. These are listed in Box 1-3. The objectives may help guide work site and health promotion activities and may aid in community-wide initiatives (USDHHS, 2000). All health care practitioners, particularly those working in the community, should review the *Healthy People*

BOX **1-3**

Healthy People 2010 Focus Areas

1. Access to quality health services
2. Arthritis, osteoporosis, and chronic back conditions
3. Cancer
4. Chronic kidney disease
5. Diabetes
6. Disability and secondary conditions
7. Educational and community-based programs
8. Environmental health
9. Family planning
10. Food safety
11. Health communication
12. Heart disease and stroke
13. HIV
14. Immunization and infectious diseases
15. Injury and violence prevention
16. Maternal, infant, and child health
17. Medical product safety
18. Mental health and mental disorders
19. Nutrition and overweight
20. Occupational safety and health
21. Oral health
22. Physical activity and fitness
23. Public health infrastructure
24. Respiratory disease
25. STDs
26. Substance abuse
27. Tobacco use
28. Vision and hearing

From US Department of Health and Human Services: *Healthy people 2010 objectives,* Washington, DC, 2000, The Author.

2010 objectives and focus on the relevant areas in their practice. Practitioners should incorporate these objectives into programs, events, and publications whenever possible and should use them as a framework to promote healthy cities and communities. This book presents and discusses selected relevant objectives to acquaint future community health nurses with the scope of the *Healthy People 2010* initiative and to enhance awareness of current health indicators and national goals.

DEFINITION AND FOCUS OF PUBLIC AND COMMUNITY HEALTH NURSING

The terms public health nursing and community health nursing are often synonymous or interchangeable; however, several nursing authors have attempted to define or differentiate the concepts. The differences are reflected in two definitions that provide similar yet distinctive ideologies, visions, or philosophies of nursing.

Public Health Nursing

Public health nursing is a synthesis of public health and nursing practice. Freeman (1963) provided a classic definition of public health nursing, which follows:

> Public health nursing may be defined as a field of professional practice in nursing and in public health in which technical nursing, interpersonal, analytical, and organizational skills are applied to problems of health as they affect the community. These skills are applied in concert with those of other persons engaged in health care, through comprehensive nursing care of families and other groups and through measures for evaluation or control of threats to health, for health education of the public, and for mobilization of the public for health action (p. 34).

More recently, the APHA Committee on Public Health Nursing (1996) stated the following:

> Public health nursing is the practice of promoting and protecting the health of populations using knowledge from nursing, social, and public health sciences. Public health nursing practice is a systematic process by which:
>
> 1. the health and health care needs of a population are assessed in order to identify subpopulations,

families, and individuals who would benefit from health promotion or who are at risk of illness, injury, disability or premature death;
> 2. a plan for intervention is developed with the community to meet identified needs that takes into account available resources, the range of activities that contribute to health and the prevention of illness, injury, disability, and premature death;
> 3. the plan is implemented effectively, efficiently and equitably;
> 4. evaluations are conducted to determine the extent to which the interventions have an impact on the health status of individuals and the population;
> 5. the results of the process are used to influence and direct the current delivery of care, deployment of health resources, and the development of local, regional, state, and national health policy and research to promote health and prevent disease.

Community Health Nursing

The ANA (1980) uses the term **community health nursing** and gives the following definition:

> Community health nursing is a synthesis of nursing practice and public health practice applied to promoting and preserving the health of populations. The practice is general and comprehensive. It is not limited to a particular age group or diagnosis and is continuing, not episodic. The dominant responsibility is to the population as a whole; nursing directed to individuals, families, or groups contributes to the health of the total population. Health promotion, health maintenance, health education and management, coordination, and continuity of care are utilized in a holistic approach to the management of the health care of individuals, families, and groups in a community (p. 2).

A common theme of these definitions is the provision of nursing service to the community or population as a whole. Muecke (1984) noted that whereas the ANA definition focuses on care to individuals, families, and groups within a community, the APHA definition focuses on care to the community as a whole. The APHA considers the individual or single family *only* as part of a risk group. Both definitions are important for addressing the health of aggregates. In the community, individual health and family health are necessary building blocks to the health of populations, but they represent only one facet of health care provision at the aggregate level.

The public health nursing tradition, begun in the late 1800s by Lillian Wald and her associates, clearly portrays this important distinction (Wald, 1971, see Chapter 2). After moving into the immigrant community to provide care for individuals and families, these nurses saw that neither administering bedside clinical nursing nor teaching family members to deliver care in the home solely combated the true determinants of health. They saw that collective political activity was focused on advancing the health of aggregates by improving social and environmental conditions and addressing the social and environmental determinants of health such as child labor, pollution, and poverty. Wald and her colleagues impacted the health of the community by organizing the community, establishing school nursing, and taking impoverished mothers to testify in Washington, DC (Wald, 1971).

Although important, current interventions with families and individuals in the community are incomplete unless they are extended to intervention at the aggregate level. In an example involving the provision of prenatal care to adolescents, Muecke (1984) clearly made the distinction between actions based on the two definitions. According to Muecke, a nurse subscribing to the ANA definition would focus on each family in the caseload and address the problem of low-birth-weight infants among the population through individual family assessment. The nurse would consider nutritional factors, health education related to nutrition and fetal development, and community resource referrals for nutritional services.

The nurse who subscribes to the APHA definition would focus on the characteristics of the community as a whole. The nurse would determine the proportion of teenagers in the community and the teenage pregnancy rate, intervene at the community level by assessing teenage nutrition sources, and work politically to make nutritious foods available to teenagers by supplying such provisions as food vending machines in schools. Alternatively, the nurse would lobby for a supply of nutritional supplements for the low-income pregnant women in the community. Aggregate care extends the concept of care for the individual and family to care of the population as a whole.

Some nursing authors use community health nursing as a global or umbrella term and public health nursing as a component or subset. Others, as stated, use the terms interchangeably. This book will use the terms interchangeably; however, it is important to note that, although minor, there are distinctive differences in practice parameters and ideology.

Community and Public Health Nursing Practice

The practice of community and public health nurses advocates disease prevention and health promotion. It is important to note that community health nursing practice is collaborative and is based in research and theory. It applies the nursing process to the care of individuals, families, aggregates, and the community. Table 1-2 presents the Standards for Public Health Nursing Practice developed by the Quad Council of Public Health Nursing Organizations. The Quad Council is comprised of representatives from the Association of State and Territorial Directors of Nursing, the Association of Community Health Nursing Educators, the Public Health Nursing Section of the APHA, and the Community Health Nursing Council of the ANA.

Again, the core functions of public health are assessment, policy development, and assurance. In the mid1990s, the Quad Council closely examined these core functions. Following this review, the group outlined a list of related nursing competencies. Future community health nurses and nurses working in community settings should study these competencies (Quad Council, 1993). Table 1-3 lists expected competencies for public and community health nurses for each of these core functions.

Community health practice is unique; therefore nursing interventions in community settings are different from nursing interventions in institutional settings. Table 1-4 shows examples of nursing interventions related to the essential public health services listed in Box 1-2. These interventions focus on assessment of aggregates and populations, recognition of health threats, education of those at risk, and advocacy for the underserved and vulnerable populations.

Community Health Nurse Certification

Certification in a specific area of nursing practice is a voluntary credential that serves to improve nursing practice and promote high-quality health care (The American Nurses Credentialing Center [ANCC], 1999a). The ANCC uses predetermined standards to validate a nurse's knowledge, skills, and abilities in a defined functional or clinical area of nursing. The ANCC provides certification in several areas related to community health, which include the following: Clinical Specialist in Community Health Nursing, Community Health Nurse Generalist, School Nurse, Col-

---

TABLE **1-2**

Standards of Public Health Nursing Practice

Standards of Care	
Standard I. Assessment	The public health nurse assesses the health status of populations using data, community resources identification, input from the population, and professional judgment.
Standard II. Diagnosis	The public health nurse analyzes collected assessment data and partners with the people to attach meaning to those data and determine opportunities and needs.
Standard III. Outcomes Identification	The public health nurse participates with other community partners to identify expected outcomes in the populations and their health status.
Standard IV. Planning	The public health nurse promotes and supports the development of programs, policies, and services that provide interventions that improve the health status of populations.
Standard V. Assurance: Action Component of the Nursing Process for Public Health Nursing	The public health nurse assures access and availability of programs, policies, resources, and services to the population.
Standard VI. Evaluation	The public health nurse evaluates the health status of the population.
Standards of Professional Performance	
Standard I. Quality of Care	The public health nurse systematically evaluates the availability, accessibility, acceptability, quality, and effectiveness of nursing practice for the population.
Standard II. Performance Appraisal	The public health nurse evaluates his or her own nursing practice in relation to professional practice standards and relevant statutes and regulations.
Standard III. Education	The public health nurse acquires and maintains current knowledge and competency in public health nursing practice.
Standard IV. Collegiality	The public health nurse establishes collegial partnerships while interacting with health care practitioners and others and contributes to the professional development of peers, colleagues, and others.
Standard V. Ethics	The public health nurse applies ethical standards in advocating for health and social policy and delivery of public health programs to promote and preserve the health of the population.
Standard VI. Collaboration	The public health nurse collaborates with the representatives of the population and other health and human service professionals and organizations in providing for and promoting the health of the population.
Standard VII. Research	The public health nurse uses research findings in practice.
Standard VIII. Resource Utilization	The public health nurse considers safety, effectiveness, and cost in the planning and delivery of public health services when using available resources to ensure the maximum possible health benefits to the population.

From Quad Council on Public Health/Community Health Nursing: *Scope and standards of public health nursing practice*, Washington, DC, 1999, American Nurses Association.

TABLE 1-3

Core Public Health Functions and Related Community and Public Health Nursing Competencies

Core Function	Community and Public Health Nursing Competencies
Assessment	Evaluate demographic, epidemiological, and biostatistical data to anticipate and identify risks and patterns of morbidity and mortality.
	Evaluate changing health behaviors and patterns that have the potential to place people at risk.
	Determine other indicators to monitor the dimensions of health status valued by the community.
Policy Development	Analyze assessment data to identify potential and actual health problems.
	Work to develop partnerships and strategies to address identified health problems.
	Participate in health policy development as advocates for the needs of children, families, groups, and communities.
Assurance	Assure appropriate service delivery to achieve targeted health care outcomes.
	Monitor health service access, utilization, and appropriateness for the community, including underserved and target populations.
	Participate in developing systems and programs to promote positive health outcomes for the community.
	Work to implement continuous quality improvement for health care systems in the community.
	Provide expert public health nurse consultation to groups and organizations in the community.

From Quad Council; Association of State and Territorial Directors of Nursing; Association of Community Health Nursing Educators; Public Heath Nursing Section/American Public Health Association/and Council of Community; Primary and Long-Term Care/American Nurses Association. Washington, DC, 1993, Quad Council.

lege Health Nurse, Home Health Nurse, and Clinical Specialist in Home Health Nursing. Additionally, the ANCC certifies a number of nurses as Nurse Practitioners (NPs), who generally work in community-based settings.

According to the ANCC (1999a), the Community Health Nurse Generalist synthesizes nursing practice and public health practice to promote and preserve the health of populations. The practice is general, comprehensive, not limited to a particular age group or diagnosis, and continuing rather than episodic. Community health nurses use a holistic approach when managing the health care of individuals, families, and groups in a community. Health promotion, health maintenance, health education, case management, coordination, and continuity of care are essential components of community health nursing practice.

The Clinical Specialist in Community Health Nursing is educated at the graduate level and uses skills to promote the health of an entire community. The specialist possesses substantial clinical experience in community health assessment and proficiency in planning, implementing, and evaluating population-

focused programs. Specialist skills are based on knowledge of epidemiology, demographics, biometrics, environmental health, community structure and organization, community development, management, program evaluation, policy development, and case management. Additionally the specialist engages in research and theory application as relevant to community practice and health policy development (ANCC, 1999a).

Generalist and specialist community health nurses work in ambulatory clinics, private offices, occupational health centers, health departments, schools, health maintenance organizations (HMOs), home health agencies, correctional institutions, camps, and other community-based settings. Table 1-5 lists the credential requirements for the Community Health Nurse Generalist and the Clinical Specialist in Community Health Nursing and outlines the basic content of the specified examination. There are approximately 1800 Community Health Nurse Generalists and 462 Clinical Specialists in Community Health Nursing certified by the ANCC (ANCC, 1999b).

TABLE 1-4

Essential Public Health Services and Community Health Nursing Interventions

Essential Public Health Service	Community Health Nursing Interventions
Monitor health status to identify community health problems.	Participate in community assessment. Identify aggregates at risk for disease and disability. Identify potential environmental hazards.
Diagnose and investigate health problems and health hazards in the community.	Understand and identify determinants of health and disease. Participate in case identification and treatment of people with communicable disease. Recognize multiple causes and factors of health and illness.
Inform, educate, and empower people about health issues.	Develop education plans for individuals and families in multiple settings. Advocate for and with underserved and disadvantaged populations. Develop and implement community-based health education.
Mobilize community partnerships to identify and solve health problems.	Provide leadership to prioritize community problems and development of interventions. Interact regularly with providers and services within each community. Convene groups and providers who share common concerns and interests in special populations.
Develop policies and plans that support individual and community health efforts.	Participate in community and family decision making processes. Advocate for appropriate funding for services. Provide information and advocacy for consideration of the interests of special groups in program development.
Enforce laws and regulations that protect health and ensure safety.	Implement ordinances and laws that protect the environment. Regulate and support safe care and treatment for dependent populations such as children and the elderly. Participate in the development of local regulations that protect communities and the environment from potential hazards and pollution.
Link people to needed personal health services and assure the provision of health care when otherwise unavailable.	Provide clinical preventive services to certain high-risk populations. Establish programs and services to meet special needs. Provide referrals through community links to needed care.
Assure a competent public health and personal health care workforce.	Participate in continuing education and preparation to assure competence. Establish and maintain procedures and protocols for patient care. Establish standards for performance.
Evaluate effectiveness, accessibility, and quality of personal and population-based health services.	Collect data and information related to community interventions. Identify unserved and underserved populations within the community. Review and analyze data on the health status of the community.
Research for new insights and innovative solutions to health problems.	Participate in collecting information and data to improve the surveillance and understanding of special problems. Formulate and use investigative tools to identify and impact care delivery and program planning. Participate in early identification of factors that are detrimental to the community's health.

From Association of State and Territorial Districts of Nursing: *Public health nursing: a partnership for progress,* Washington, DC, 1998, The Association.

TABLE 1-5

ANCC Requirements for Initial Certification: Community Health Nurse Generalist and Clinical Specialist in Community Health Nursing

Requirement/ Examination Topic	Community Health Nurse Generalist	Clinical Specialist in Community Health Nursing
Education	BSN	MSN or higher (specialization in community and public health nursing) or BSN and MPH (specialization in community and public health nursing).
Practice	Practiced as an RN in community health nursing for a minimum of 1500 hours over the past three years and had 30 contact hours of continuing education in the specialty area within the past three years.	Currently practice an average of 12 hours per week in community and public health nursing or have practiced a minimum of 800 hours in community and public health nursing within the past 24 months.
Examination Topics	Public health science Individual and family as client Community as client Areas of practice Public health problems Professional issues	Public health sciences Community assessment Program administration Trends and issues Theory Research Health care delivery systems

From American Nurses Credentialing Center: *Online certification catalog*, 1999a, The Author, www.ana.org.ancc/certify/catalogs/1999.
BSN, Bachelor of Science in Nursing; *MPH,* Master of Public Health; *MSN,* Master of Science in Nursing.

POPULATION-FOCUSED PRACTICE

Community health nurses must use a population-focused approach to move beyond providing direct care to individuals and families. **Population-focused nursing** concentrates on specific groups of people and focuses on health promotion and disease prevention, regardless of geographical location (Baldwin et al., 1998). Although individuals and organizations may be responsible for a specific subpopulation in the community (e.g., a school may be responsible for its pregnant teenagers), population-focused practice is concerned with many distinct and overlapping community subpopulations. The goal of population-focused nursing is to promote healthy communities (Quad Council, 1993).

Population-focused community health nurses would not have exclusive interest in one or two subpopulations, but would focus on the many subpopulations that make up the entire community. A population focus involves concern for those who do,

and for those who do not, receive health services. A population focus also involves a scientific approach to community health nursing; an assessment of the community or population is necessary and basic to planning, intervention, and evaluation for the individual, family, aggregate, and population levels.

The generalist and the specialist apply population focus differently. The generalist community health nurse holds or has a baccalaureate degree and is able to plan and intervene with individual groups, aggregates, and subpopulations. The specialist community health nurse has a master's degree and is able to plan and intervene with multiple and overlapping subpopulations within the community (Fig. 1-2). Regardless of the level of practice, both generalist and specialist community health nurses must be aware of population focus and use it to aid in assessment, planning, intervention, and evaluation with larger units. Nurses need a population focus to plan the required care for groups of individuals and

FIGURE 1-2

Differences in generalist and specialist applications of population focus.

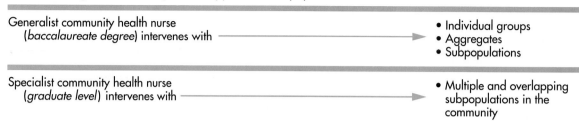

Generalist community health nurse
(*baccalaureate degree*) intervenes with ⟶
- Individual groups
- Aggregates
- Subpopulations

Specialist community health nurse
(*graduate level*) intervenes with ⟶
- Multiple and overlapping subpopulations in the community

groups of families with needs that the community does not address.

According to Williams (2000), a population focus bases assessment and management decisions on the status of a subpopulation. The subpopulation may be made up of a set of individuals (e.g., unmarried, pregnant teenagers), a set of families (e.g., families with high-risk infants younger than one year), or a set of "groups" (e.g., children in several age groups or classes in a school).

Community health nursing practice requires the following types of data for scientific approach and population focus: the epidemiology, or body of knowledge, of a particular problem and its solution, and information about the community. Each type of knowledge and its source appears in Table 1-6. To determine the overall patterns of health in a population, data collection for assessment and management decisions within a community should be ongoing, not episodic.

Aggregate-Focused Practice

Community health nurses focus on the care of individuals and aggregates in many settings including homes, clinics, and schools. In addition to interviewing clients and assessing individual and family health, community health nurses must be able to assess an aggregate's health needs and resources and identify its values. Community health nurses must also work with the community to identify and implement programs that meet health needs and evaluate the effectiveness of programs following implementation. For example, school nurses were once only responsible for running first aid stations. Now they are actively involved in assessing the needs of their population and defining programs to meet those needs through activities such as health screening and group health education and promotion. The activities of school nurses may be as varied as designing health curricula with a school and community advisory group, leading support groups for elementary school children with chronic illness, and monitoring the health status of teenage mothers.

Similarly, occupational health nurses are no longer required to simply maintain an office or dispensary. They are involved in many different types of activities. These activities may include the following: maintaining records of workers exposed to physical or chemical risks, monitoring compliance with Occupational Safety and Health Administration (OSHA) standards, teaching classes on health issues, and leading support group discussions for workers with health-related problems.

Private associations such as the American Diabetes Association employ community health nurses for their organizational abilities and health-related skills. Other community health nurses work with multidisciplinary groups of professionals, serve on boards of voluntary health associations like the American Heart Association, are members of health planning agencies and councils, and work with nursing organizations directed at major public health problems like the Nurses' Environmental Health Watch.

Community health nurses are also involved in the Public Health Nursing Section of the APHA and the Division of Community Health Nursing of the ANA, and perform activities such as updating the definition and role of community health nursing. The community health nurses involved in state nursing associations promote health-related legislation and serve on state task forces that address health issues.

COMMUNITY HEALTH NURSING AND MANAGED CARE

Shifts in reimbursement and the growth of managed care have revitalized the notion of population-based care. MCOs use financial incentives and organiza-

TABLE 1-6

Data Required for Population Focus

| Body of Knowledge About Problem | | Information About the Community | |
Definition	Sources	Definition	Sources
Cause or etiology	Epidemiological research	Demographic data	Demographics such as age, sex, and socioeconomic and racial distributions
Groups at high risk	Community health nursing research	Health status of the sub-populations	Vital statistics such as mortality and morbidity
Treatment methods	Clinical research in nursing and medicine	Services given to various subpopulations	Annual reports of health care organizations Services provided by health planning agencies
Effectiveness of treatment methods	Research in other fields	Measure of effectiveness of services	Computerized information systems for monitoring high-risk populations

From Williams CA: Population-focused practice. In Stanhope M, Lancaster J, editors: *Community health nursing: process and practice for promoting health,* St. Louis, 1984, Mosby.

tional structures to increase efficiency and decrease health care costs. The foundation for managed care is management of health care for an enrolled group of individuals. This group of enrollees becomes the population of interest (Torrens and Williams, 1999).

An understanding of enrolled populations and health care patterns is essential for managing health care services and resources effectively. Most MCOs have become sophisticated in identifying key sub-groups within the population of enrollees at risk for health problems. Typically, managed care systems target subgroups according to characteristics associated with risk or use of expensive services such as selected clinical conditions, functional status, and past service use patterns.

Although comprehensive national health reform has not occurred, the dialogue about health care reform continues. Many experts believe that health care reform is occurring at the state level. Market forces and cost-containment efforts help lead the trend toward managed care (Shi and Singh, 1998). In many states, Medicaid populations are becoming part of managed care plans. A growing number of people are enrolled in HMOs and other types of managed care arrangements and nationally, about 50 million people are part of HMOs. A reformed health care system will include principles of managed care and a population-based approach to public health practice.

The purpose of public health is to improve the health of the public by promoting healthy lifestyles, preventing disease and injury, and protecting the health of communities (Berkowitz, 1995). In the past, shrinking public health resources have supported personal health services over community health. In public health practice, the community is the population of interest. Managed care may consider the served population to be individuals belonging to the HMO and specific HMO client groups. Public health practice continues to focus on public health and community and managed care focuses on service delivery. The personal health care system will be under increasing pressure to provide the services that health departments previously provided. Traditionally served by public health, the most vulnerable populations will pose tremendous challenges to managed care providers. Public health will be responsible for partnering with managed care to provide service to these populations.

Nurses in community and public health have an opportunity to share their expertise regarding population-based approaches to health care for groups of individuals across health care settings. Today, health care practitioners require additional skills in assessment, policy development, and assurance to provide community public health practice and population-based service. A Pew Health Professions

Commission report (1994) states that health care practitioners need key competencies in the year 2005. Competencies pertinent to practitioners in managed care include promoting healthy lifestyles, providing preventive and primary care, expanding and ensuring access to cost-effective and technologically appropriate care, participating in coordinated and interdisciplinary care, and involving patients and families in the decision-making process. Public health nurses must work in partnership with colleagues in managed care settings to improve community health. Partnerships may address information management, cultural values, health care system improvement, and the physical environment roles in health and may require complex negotiations to share data across boundaries. The partners may need to develop new community assessment strategies to augment epidemiological methods that often mask the context or meaning of the human experience of vulnerable populations.

Providing population-focused care requires a dramatic shift in thinking from individual-focused care. Hegyvary (1994) and Greenlick (1991) describe some of the practical demands of population-focused care, which follows:

1. recognition that populations are not homogeneous; therefore it is necessary to address the needs of special subpopulations within populations;
2. identify high-risk and vulnerable subpopulations early in the care delivery cycle;
3. nonusers of services often become high-cost users; therefore it is essential to develop outreach strategies; and
4. quality and cost of all health care services are linked together across the health care continuum.

Health care reform provides rich opportunities for collaboration between service and academia. Health professional schools can take an active leadership role in preparing public health nurses for the twenty-first century and shape the values and directions of the health care system. The reformed health care system will enhance community health if all health professionals, including students, use new skills and knowledge in creating, monitoring, implementing, and evaluating systems of care from a population perspective.

SUMMARY

Specialized knowledge and skills enable community health nurses to work in diverse community settings, ranging from the isolated rural area to the crowded urban ghetto. To meet the health needs of the population, the community health nurse must work with many individuals and groups within the community. The community health nurse must develop sensitivity to these groups and respect the community and its established methods of problem management. This will enable the nurse to become more proficient in helping the community improve overall health.

LEARNING ACTIVITIES

1. Interview several community health nurses and several clients regarding their definitions of health. Share the results with classmates.
2. Interview several community health nurses regarding their opinions on the focus of community health nursing.
3. Ask several neighbors or consumers of health care about their views of the role of public health and community health nursing. Share results with classmates.

REFERENCES

American Heritage College Dictionary, ed 3, New York, 1997, Houghton Mifflin Co.

American Nurses Association: *A conceptual model of community health nursing,* Pub No CH-10, Kansas City, Mo, 1980, The Association.

American Nurses Association: *Social policy statement,* Kansas City, Mo, 1986, The Association.

American Nurses Credentialing Center: *Online certification catalog,* 1999a, The Author, www.ana.org.ancc/certify/catalogs/1999.

American Nurses Credentialing Center: Personal communication, November 16, 1999, 1999b, The Author.

American Public Health Association: *Ad hoc committee on public health nursing: the definition and role of public health nursing practice in the delivery of health care,* Washington, DC, 1996, The Association.

Archer SE, Fleshman EP: *Community health nursing patterns and practice,* ed 2, North Scituate, Mass, 1979, Duxbury Press.

Association of State and Territorial Districts of Nursing: *Public health nursing: a partnership for progress,* Washington, DC, 1998, The Association.

Baldwin JH et al: Population-focused and community-based nursing: moving toward clarification of concepts, *Public Health Nurs* 15(1):12-18, 1998.

Beauchamp DE: Public health as social justice. In Mappes T, Zembaty J, editors: *Biomedical ethics,* ed 2, New York, 1986, McGraw-Hill.

Berkowitz B: Health system reform: a blueprint for the future of public health, *J Public Health Pract* 1:1-6, 1995.

Butterfield PG: Thinking upstream: nurturing a conceptual understanding of the societal context of health behavior, *Adv Nurs Sci* 12:1-8, 1990.

Clark MJ: *Nursing in the community: dimensions of community health nursing,* ed 3, Norwalk, Conn, 1999, Appleton & Lange.

Dunn HL: *High level wellness,* Arlington, Va, 1961, RW Beatty, Ltd.

Evans RG, Stoddart GL: Providing health, consuming health care. In Evans RG, Baver ML, Marmor TR, editors: *Why are some people healthy and others not? the determinants of health of populations,* Hawthorne, NY, 1994, Aldine de Gruyter.

Freeman RB: *Public health nursing practice,* ed 3, Philadelphia, 1963, WB Saunders.

Green LW, Anderson CL: *Community health nursing,* St. Louis, 1986, Mosby.

Greenlick M: Educating physicians for population-based clinical practice, *JAMA* 267:1645-1648, 1991.

Hanlon JJ: *Principles of public health administration,* ed 3, St. Louis, 1960, Mosby.

Harper AC, Lambert LJ: *The health of populations: an introduction,* ed 2, New York, 1994, Springer.

Hegyvary S: The shift in focus from provider processes to population outcomes, *Nurs Admin* Q17:viii-ix, 1994.

Institute of Medicine: *The future of public health,* Washington, DC, 1988, National Academy Press.

Lamarche PA: Our health paradigm in peril, *Public Health Rep* 110:556-560, 1995.

Lamm R: Final report April 1997: National League for Nursing Commission on a workforce for a restructured health care system, *Nurs Health Care Perspect* 19(2): 91-93, 1998.

Leahy KM, Cobb MM, Jones MC: *Community health nursing,* ed 4, New York, 1982, McGraw-Hill.

Leavell HR, Clark EG: *Preventive medicine for the doctor in his community,* New York, 1958, McGraw-Hill.

McKinlay JB: A case for refocusing upstream: the political economy of illness. In Jaco EG, editor: *Patients, physicians, and illness,* ed 3, New York, 1979, The Free Press.

Muecke MA: Community health diagnosis in nursing, *Public Health Nurs* 1:23-35, 1984.

National Center for Health Statistics: *Health: United States, 1999,* Hyattsville, Md, 1999, Public Health Service.

Orem DE: *Nursing: concepts of practice,* ed 5, St. Louis, 1995, Mosby.

Pender NJ: *Health promotion in nursing practice,* ed 3, Stamford, Conn, 1996, Appleton & Lange.

Pew Health Professions Commission: *Current issues in health professions: education and workforce reform,* University of California, San Francisco, 1994, The Author.

Quad Council; Association of State and Territorial Directors of Nursing; Association of Community Health Nursing Educators; Public Heath Nursing Section/ American Public Health Association/and Council of Community; Primary and Long-Term Care/American Nurses Association. Washington, DC, 1993, Quad Council.

Quad Council on Public Health/Community Health Nursing: *Public health nursing in a revitalized health care agenda,* Washington, DC, 1993, American Nurses Association.

Quad Council on Public Health/Community Health Nursing: *Scope and standards of public health nursing practice,* Washington, DC, 1999, American Nurses Association.

Shi L, Singh DA: *Delivering health care in America: a systems approach,* Gaithersburg, Md, 1998, Aspen.

Shine KI: Informed joint decision-making, *Public Health Rep* 110:555, 1995.

Shuster GR, Goeppinger J: Community as client: using the nursing process to promote health. In Stanhope M, Lancaster J, editors: *Community health nursing: process and practice for promoting health,* ed 5, St. Louis, 2000, Mosby.

Torrens PR: Historical evolution and overview of health services in the United States. In Williams SJ, Torrens PR, editors: *Introduction to health services,* ed 5, Albany, NY, 1999, Delmar Publishers.

Torrens PR, Williams SJ: Managed care: restructuring the system. In Williams SJ, Torrens PR, editors: *Introduction to health services,* ed 5, Albany, NY, 1999, Delmar Publishers.

US Department of Health and Human Services: *Healthy people 2000 objectives,* Washington, DC, 1989, The Author.

US Department of Health and Human Services: *Healthy people 2010 objectives,* Washington, DC, 2000, The Author.

US Department of Health and Human Services, Health Resources and Services Administration, Bureau of Health Professions, Division of Nursing: *The registered nurse population: findings from the National*

Sample Survey of Registered Nurses, March, 1996, Rockville, Md, 1998, The Author.

US Department of Health and Human Services/Public Health Service: *The public health workforce: an agenda for the 21st century,* Washington, DC, 1997, The Author.

Wald LD: *The house on Henry Street,* New York, 1971, Dover Publications.

Williams CA: Community-oriented, population-focused practice: the foundation of specialization in public health nursing. In Stanhope M, Lancaster J, editors: *Community health nursing: process and practice for promoting health,* ed 5, St. Louis, 2000, Mosby.

Williams CA: Population-focused practice. In Stanhope M, Lancaster J, editors: *Community health nursing: process and practice for promoting health,* St. Louis, 1984, Mosby.

World Health Organization: A discussion document on the concept and principles of health promotion, *Health Promotion* 1:73-78, 1986.

World Health Organization: *Chronicle of WHO* 1:1-2, 1958.

World Health Organization: *Community health nursing: report of a WHO expert committee,* Rep No 559, Geneva, 1974, The Author.

2

Historical Factors: Community Health Nursing in Context

Tom H. Cook

OBJECTIVES

Upon completion of this chapter, the reader will be able to do the following:

1. Describe the impact of aggregate living on population health.
2. Identify approaches to aggregate health from prehistoric to present times.
3. Understand historical events that have influenced a holistic approach to population health.
4. Compare the application of public health principles to the nation's major health problems at the turn of the twentieth century (i.e., acute disease) with that at the beginning of the twenty-first century (i.e., chronic disease).
5. Describe two leaders in nursing who had a profound impact on addressing aggregate health.
6. Discuss major contemporary issues facing community health nursing and trace the historical roots to the present.

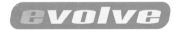

http://evolve.elsevier.com/Nies/

This chapter presents an overview of selected historical factors that have influenced the evolution of community health and explains current health challenges for community health nursing. This text examines the evolving health of Western populations from prehistoric to recent times, the evolution of modern health care and the role of public health nursing, the consequences for the health of aggregates, and the challenges for community health nursing.

EVOLUTION OF HEALTH IN WESTERN POPULATIONS

The study of humankind's evolution has seldom taken into consideration the interrelationship between an individual's health, an individual's environment, and the nature and size of the individual's aggregate. Medical anthropologists use paleontological records and disease descriptions of primitive societies to speculate on the interrelationship of early humans, probable diseases, and environment (Armelagos and Dewey, 1978). Historians have also documented the existence of public health activity (i.e., an organized community effort to prevent disease, prolong life, and promote health) since prehistoric times. The following section describes how aggregates and early public health efforts impact the health of Western populations.

Aggregate Impact on Health

Polgar (1964) defined the following stages in the disease history of humankind: hunting and gathering stage, settled villages stage, preindustrial cities stage, industrial cities stage, and present stage (Fig. 2-1). In these stages, increased population, increased population density, and imbalanced human ecology resulted in changes in cultural adaptation. Humans caused this ecological imbalance by altering their environment to accommodate group living. This imbalance had a marked consequence on health.

Although these stages are associated with the evolution of civilization, it is important to note that the information is limited. For example, the stages depict the evolution of Western civilization from the perspective of the Western world. They consist of overlapping historical time periods, which anthropologists widely debate. However, the stages do provide a frame of reference to aid in determining the relationship among humans, disease, and environment from prehistoric to present day. The stages chronicle the initiation of each stage in the Western world, but it is important to realize that each stage still exists in civilization today. For example, Australian aborigines continue to hunt and gather food and settled villages are common in third world countries.

The community nurse must be aware that populations from each stage represent a great variety of people with distinct cultural traditions and a broad range of health care practices and beliefs. For example, a nurse in an American community may have to plan care for immigrants or refugees from a settled village or a preindustrial city. Community nurses must recognize that the environment, the aggregate's health risks, and the host culture's strengths and contributions affect the health status of each particular aggregate. For example, the Hispanic Health and Nutrition Examination Survey (HHANES) collected data between 1982 and 1984 and found that perinatal outcomes among women born in Mexico worsen in correspondence to the length of time they live in the United States (Guendelman et al., 1990). Whereas Mexico's cultural orientation protects mothers from the risk-associated behaviors of drinking and smoking, Mexican descendants born in the United States are more likely to engage in unhealthy behaviors and practices common to other Americans.

Hunting and Gathering Stage

During the Paleolithic period, or Old Stone Age, nomadic and seminomadic people engaged in hunting and gathering. Generations of small aggregate

FIGURE **2-1**

Stages in the disease history of humankind.

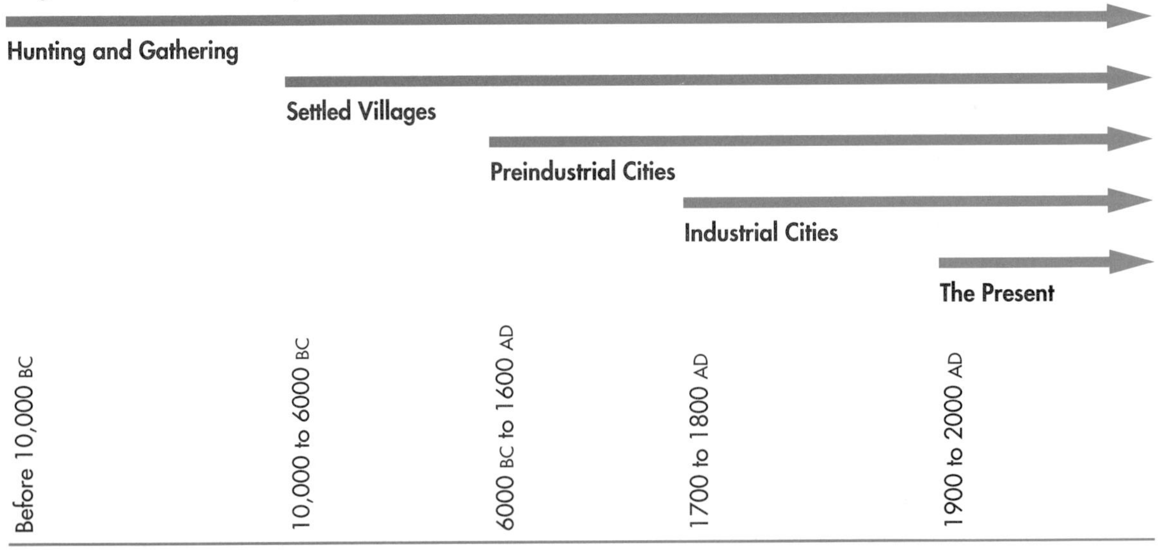

Stages overlap and time periods are widely debated in the field of anthropology. Some form of each stage remains evident in the world today.

groups wandered in search of food for two million years. Armelagos and Dewey (1978) reviewed how their size, density, and relationship to the environment probably affected their health. These groups may have avoided many contagious diseases because the scattered aggregates were small, nomadic, and separated from other aggregates. Under these conditions, disease would not spread between the groups. Evidently the disposal of human feces and waste was not a great problem; the nomadic people most likely abandoned the caves they used for shelter once waste accumulated.

Settled Village Stage

Small settlements were characteristic of the Mesolithic period, or Middle Stone Age, and the Neolithic period, or New Stone Age. Wandering people became sedentary and formed small encampments and villages. The concentration of people in these small areas caused new problems. For example, people began to domesticate animals and live close to their herds, which probably transmitted diseases such as salmonella, anthrax, Q fever, and tuberculosis (TB) (Polgar, 1964). These stationary people also domesticated plants, which may have reduced the range of consumable nutrients and may have led to deficiency disease. They had to secure water and remove wastes, which often resulted in the cross-contamination of the water supply and the spread of waterborne diseases such as dysentery, cholera, typhoid, and hepatitis A.

Preindustrial Cities Stage

In preindustrial times, large urban centers formed to support the expanding population. Populations inhabited smaller areas; therefore preexisting problems increased. For example, the urban population had to resource increased amounts of food and water and remove increased amounts of waste products. Some cultures developed elaborate water systems. For instance, the Aztec king Ahuitzutl had a stone pipeline built to transport spring water to the inhabitants of Mexico City (Duran, 1964). However, waste removal via the water supply led to diseases such as cholera. With the development of towns, rodent infestation increased and facilitated the spread of plague. People had more frequent close contact with each other; therefore the transmission of diseases spread by direct contact increased and diseases such as mumps, measles, influenza, and smallpox became endemic (Polgar, 1964). A population must reach a certain size

to maintain a disease in endemic proportions; for example, approximately one million people are needed to sustain measles at an endemic level (Cockburn, 1967).

Industrial Cities Stage

Industrialization caused urban areas to become denser and more heavily populated. Increased industrial wastes, air and water pollution, and harsh working conditions took a toll on health. During the eighteenth and nineteenth centuries, there was an increase in respiratory diseases such as TB, pneumonia, and bronchitis and in epidemics of infectious diseases such as diphtheria, smallpox, typhoid fever, typhus, measles, malaria, and yellow fever (Armelagos and Dewey, 1978). Furthermore, imperialism spread epidemics to susceptible populations throughout the world because settlers, traders, and soldiers moved from one location to another introducing communicable diseases into native population groups.

DISEASE DEFINITIONS

Endemic: Diseases that are always present in a population (e.g., colds and pneumonia).
Epidemic: Diseases that are not always present in a population but flare up on occasion (e.g., diphtheria and measles).
Pandemic: The existence of disease in a large proportion of the population—a global epidemic (e.g., HIV, AIDS, and annual outbreaks of influenza type A).

Present Stage

Although infectious diseases no longer account for a majority of deaths in the Western world, they continue to cause many deaths in the nonWestern world. They also remain prevalent among low-income populations and some racial and ethnic groups in the West. People from nonindustrial communities rarely develop Western diseases such as cancer, venous disorders, heart disease, obesity, and diabetes. These diseases usually appear when cultures adopt Western customs (Burkitt, 1978). Western diseases also seem to emerge when cultures transition into urban environments. Epidemiological studies suggest that common disease factors are changes in diet (i.e., increases in refined sugar and fats and lack of fiber) and environmental and occupational hazards. An increase in population and population density also increases mental and behavioral disorders (Garn, 1963).

The disease patterns and environmental demands changed when wandering, hunting, and gathering aggregates grew into large populations and became sedentary. Humans had to adapt to an overpopulated, largely urban existence with marked consequences for health; the leading causes of death changed from infectious disease to chronic illnesses.

Evolution of Early Public Health Efforts

Traditionally, historians believed that organized public health efforts were eighteenth and nineteenth century activities associated with the Sanitary Revolution. However, modern historians have shown that organized community health efforts to prevent disease, prolong life, and promote health have existed since prehistoric times.

Public health efforts developed slowly over time. The following sections briefly trace the evolution of organized public health and highlight the periods of prehistoric times (i.e., before 5000 BC), classical times (i.e., 3000 to 200 BC), the Middle Ages (i.e., 500 to 1500 AD), the Renaissance (i.e., fifteenth, sixteenth, and seventeenth centuries), the eighteenth century, and the nineteenth century. However, it is important to note that, like the disease history of humankind, public health efforts exist in various stages of development throughout the world. This brief history encapsulates a Western view of organized public health efforts.

Prehistoric Times

Early nomadic humans became domesticated and tended to live in increasingly larger groups. Aggregates ranging from family to community inevitably shared episodes of life, health, sickness, and death. Whether based on superstition or sanitation, health practices evolved to ensure the survival of many aggregates. For example, primitive societies used elements of medicine (e.g., voodoo), isolation (e.g., banishment), and fumigation (e.g., smoke) to manage disease and thus protect the community for thousands of years (Hanlon and Pickett, 1984).

Classical Times

In the early years of 3000 to 1400 BC, the Minoans devised ways to flush water and construct drainage systems. Circa 1000 BC, the Egyptians constructed elaborate drainage systems, developed pharmaceutical preparations, and embalmed the dead. Pollution is an ancient problem. *Exodus* reported that "all the waters that were in the river stank" and in *Leviticus,* the Hebrews formulated the first written hygiene code. This hygiene code protected water and food by creating laws that governed personal and community hygiene such as contagion, disinfection, and sanitation.

Greece

Greek literature contains accounts of communicable diseases such as diphtheria, mumps, and malaria (Rosen, 1958). The Hippocratic book *Airs, Waters and Places,* a treatise on the balance between humans and their environment, may have been the only volume on this topic until the development of bacteriology in the late nineteenth century (Rosen, 1958). Diseases that were always present in a population, such as colds and pneumonia, were called *endemic.* Diseases that were occasionally present, such as diphtheria and measles, were called *epidemic.* The Greeks emphasized the preservation of health, or good living, which the goddess Hygeia personified, and on curative medicine, which the goddess Panacea personified. Life had to be in balance with environmental demands; therefore the Greeks weighed the importance of exercise, rest, and nutrition according to age, sex, constitution, and climate (Rosen, 1958).

Rome

Although the Romans readily adopted Greek culture, they far surpassed Greek engineering by constructing massive aqueducts, bathhouses, and sewer systems. For example, at the height of the Roman empire, Rome provided its one million inhabitants with 40 gallons of water per person per day, which is comparable with modern consumption rates (Rosen, 1958). However, inhabitants of the overcrowded Roman slums did not share in public health amenities such as sewer systems and latrines.

The Romans also observed and addressed occupational health threats. In particular, they noted the pallor of the miners, the danger of suffocation, and the smell of caustic fumes (Rosen, 1958). For protection, miners devised safeguards by using bags, sacks, and masks made of membranes and bladder skins.

In the early years of the Roman Republic, priests were believed to mediate diseases and often dispensed medicine. Public physicians worked in designated towns and earned money to care for the poor. In addition, they were able to charge wealthier patients a service fee. Much like a modern HMO or group practice, several families paid a set fee for yearly services. Hospitals, surgeries, infirmaries, and nursing homes appeared throughout Rome. In the fourth century, a Christian woman named Fabiola established a hospital for the sick poor. Others repeated this model throughout medieval times.

ROMANS PROVIDED PUBLIC HEALTH SERVICES

The Romans provided public health services that included the following (Rosen, 1958):

- A water board to maintain the aqueducts
- A supervisor of the public baths
- Street cleaners
- Supervision of the sale of food

Middle Ages

The decline of Rome, which occurred circa 500 AD, led to the Middle Ages. Monasteries promoted collective activity to protect public health and the population adopted protective measures such as building wells and fountains, cleaning streets, and disposing of refuse. The commonly occurring communicable diseases were measles, smallpox, diphtheria, leprosy, and bubonic plague. Physicians had little to offer in the management of diseases such as leprosy. The church took over by enforcing the hygienic codes from *Leviticus* and establishing isolation and leper houses, or leprosaria (Rosen, 1958).

A *pandemic* is the existence of disease in a large proportion of the population. One such pandemic, the bubonic plague, ravaged much of the world in the fourteenth century. This plague, or Black Death, claimed close to half the world's population at that time. (Hanlon and Pickett, 1984). For centuries, medicine and science did not recognize that fleas, which were attracted to the large number of rodents that inhabited urban areas, were transmitters of plague. Modern public health practices such as isolation, disinfection, and ship quarantines emerged in response to the bubonic plague.

HUMAN PLAGUE CASE DOCUMENTED IN THE UNITED STATES

Plague is an acute, often fatal bacterium that is endemic and occasionally epidemic in Africa, Asia, and South America. The bite of infectious fleas spread plague and the WHO estimates an average of 1087 cases each year worldwide. Sanitary precautions ensure a low frequency of human plague in the United States. America averages 13 cases of plague each year and approximately 80% of these cases occur in New Mexico, Arizona, and Colorado. In 1996, five reported cases of human plague yielded two fatalities in the United States. Control measures include public education and plague surveillance in rodents and rodent predators. When this surveillance detects plague, local health care providers and the public should receive an alert about possible risks.

From Centers for Disease Control and Prevention: Fatal human plague: Arizona and Colorado, 1996, *MMWR* 46(27):617-620, 1997; Centers for Disease Control and Prevention: Prevention of plague: recommendations of the Advisory Committee on Immunization Practices, *MMWR* 45(RR-14):1-15, 1996.

During the Middle Ages, clergymen acted as physicians and treated kings and noblemen. Monks and nuns provided nursing care in small houses designated as hospitals. Medieval writings contained information on hygiene and addressed such topics as housing, diet, personal cleanliness, and sleep (Rosen, 1958).

LIFE IN AN ENGLISH HOUSEHOLD IN THE SIXTEENTH CENTURY

In the following account, Erasmus described how life in the sixteenth century must have affected health (Hanlon and Pickett, 1984, p. 26):

As to floors, they are usually made with clay, covered with rushes that grow in the fens and which are so seldom removed that the lower parts remain sometimes for twenty years and has in it a collection of spittle, vomit, urine of dogs and humans, beer, scraps of fish and other filthiness not to be named.

Such accounts appeared in literature throughout the nineteenth century.

The Renaissance

Although the cause of infectious disease remained undiscovered, two events important to public health occurred during the Renaissance. In 1546, Girolamo Fracastoro presented a theory that infection was a cause and epidemic was a consequence of the "seeds of disease." Also, in 1676, Anton van Leeuwenhoek described microscopic organisms, but did not associate them with disease (Rosen, 1958).

The Elizabethan Poor Law, enacted in England in 1601, held the parishes responsible for providing relief for the poor. This law governed health care for the poor for more than two centuries and became a prototype for later U.S. laws.

Eighteenth Century

Great Britain

The eighteenth century was marked by imperialism and industrialization. Sanitary conditions remained a great problem. During the Industrial Revolution, a gradual change in industrial productivity occurred. The industrial boom sacrificed many lives for profit. In particular, it forced poor children into labor. Under the Elizabethan Poor Law, parishes established workhouses to employ the poor. Orphaned and poor children were wards of the parish; therefore the parish forced these young children to labor in parish workhouses for long hours (George, 1925). At 12 to 14 years of age, a child became a master's apprentice. Those apprenticed to chimney sweeps reportedly suffered the worst fate because their masters forced them into chimneys at the risk of being burned and suffocated.

Vaccination was a major discovery of the times. In 1796, Edward Jenner observed that people who worked around cattle were less likely to have smallpox. He discovered that immunity to smallpox resulted from an inoculation with the cowpox virus. Jenner's contribution was significant because approximately 95% of the population suffered from smallpox and approximately 10% of the population died from smallpox during the eighteenth century. Frequently, the faces of those who survived the disease were scarred with pockmarks.

Although Europeans like Hume, Voltaire, and Rousseau and Americans like Adams, Jefferson, and Franklin were expounding liberal views on human nature, the Sanitary Revolution's public health reforms were beginning to take place throughout Europe and England. In the eighteenth century, scholars used survey methods to study community-health problems (Rosen, 1958). The survey mapped "medical topographies," which were geographical factors related to regional health and disease. A health education movement provided books and pamphlets on health to the middle and upper classes, but it neglected "economic factors" and was not concerned with the working classes (Rosen, 1958).

Nineteenth Century

Communicable diseases ravaged the population that lived among unsanitary conditions and many lives were lost. For example, in the mid1800s, typhus and typhoid fever claimed two times more lives each year than the battle of Waterloo (Hanlon and Pickett, 1984).

Edwin Chadwick called attention to the consequences of unsanitary conditions that shortened the life span of the laboring class in particular. Chadwick contended that death rates were high in large industrial cities like Liverpool, where more than half of all children born of working class parents died by age five. Laborers lived an average of 16 years. In contrast, tradesmen lived 22 years and the upper classes lived 36 years (Richardson, 1887). In 1842, Chadwick published his famous *Report on an Inquiry into the Sanitary Conditions of the Laboring Population of Great Britain.* The report furthered the establishment of the General Board of Health for England in 1848. Legislation for social reform followed, which concerned child welfare; factory management; education; and care for the elderly, sick, and mentally ill. Clean water, sewers, fireplugs, and sidewalks emerged as a result.

PUBLIC HEALTH INTERVENTIONS USED IN THE THIRD WORLD ARE NEEDED IN THE UNITED STATES

In 1991, the National Council on International Health and the public health organizations in San Francisco, California sponsored a conference that urged public health professionals to consider using technology from the third world to handle the existing third world health conditions in the United States. For example, about 500 infants die of dehydration in the United States each year and about 200,000 are hospitalized for this condition at a cost of approximately $500 million per year. The conference recommended using a United Nations

Children's Fund device to help parents treat dehydration. In addition, the conference suggested shifting funds from sponsoring high-technology interventions to hiring more public health nurses to introduce inexpensive care methods in needy communities.

Data from State studies third world solutions, *Nurseweek* Northern California Edition, March 18, 1991.

In 1849, a pathologist named Rudolf Virchow argued for social action—bettering the lives of the people through improving economic, social, and environmental conditions—to attack the root social causes of disease. He proposed "a theory of epidemic disease as a manifestation of social and cultural maladjustment" (Rosen, 1958, p. 86). He further argued that the public was responsible for the health of the people; social and economic conditions heavily affected health and disease; efforts to promote health and fight disease must be social, economic, and medical; and the study of social and economic determinants of health and disease would yield knowledge to guide appropriate action.

In 1849, these principles were embodied in a public health law submitted to the Berlin Society of Physicians and Surgeons (Rosen, 1958, p. 225).

According to this document, public health has as its objectives (1) the healthy mental and physical development of the citizen; (2) the prevention of all dangers to health; and (3) the control of disease. Public health cares for society as a whole by considering the general physical and social conditions that may adversely affect health and protects each individual by considering those conditions that prevent him from caring for his health.

These "conditions" may fit into one of the following major categories: conditions that give the individual the right to request assistance from the state (e.g., poverty and infirmity) and conditions that give the state the right and obligation to interfere with the personal liberty of the individual (e.g., transmissible diseases and mental illness).

In 1854, an English physician, anesthetist, and epidemiologist named John Snow demonstrated that cholera was transmissible through contaminated wa-

ter. In a large population afflicted with cholera, he shut down the community's water resource by removing the pump handle from a well and carefully documented changes as the number of cholera cases fell dramatically (Rosen, 1958).

United States

In the United States during the nineteenth century, waves of epidemics continued to spread. Diseases such as yellow fever, smallpox, cholera, typhoid fever, and typhus particularly impacted the poor. These illnesses spread because cities grew and the poor crowded into inadequate housing with unsanitary conditions.

Lemuel Shattuck, a Boston bookseller and publisher with an interest in public health, organized the American Statistical Society in 1839 and issued a *Census of Boston* in 1845. The census showed high overall mortality and very high infant and maternal mortality rates. Living conditions for the poor were inadequate and communicable diseases were widely prevalent (Rosen, 1958). Shattuck's 1850 *Report of the Massachusetts Sanitary Commission* outlined the findings and recommended modern public health reforms that included keeping vital statistics and providing environmental, food, drug, and communicable disease control information. Shattuck called for well-infant, well-child, and school-age child health care; mental health care; vaccination; and health education. Unfortunately, the report fell on deaf ears and little was done to improve population health for many years. For example, a state board of health was not formed until 19 years later. Around the same time, the National Institute, a Washington, DC scientific organization, asked the newly formed American Medical Association (AMA) to establish a committee to uniformly collect vital statistics. The AMA began to collect them in 1848.

Early public health efforts evolved further in the midnineteenth century. Administrative efforts, initial legislation, and debate regarding the determinants of health and approaches to health management began to appear on a social, economic, and medical level. The advent of "modern" health care occurred around this time and nursing made a large contribution to the progress of health care. The following sections discuss the evolution of modern nursing, the evolution of modern medical care and public health practice, the evolution of the community caregiver, and the establishment of public health nursing.

ADVENT OF MODERN HEALTH CARE

Evolution of Modern Nursing

Florence Nightingale, the woman credited with establishing "modern nursing," began her work during the midnineteenth century. Historians remember Florence Nightingale for contributing to the health of British soldiers during the Crimean War and establishing nursing education. However, most historians failed to recognize her remarkable use of public health principles and distinguished scientific contributions to health care reform (Cohen, 1984; Grier and Grier, 1978). The following review of Nightingale's work emphasizes her concern for environmental determinants of health; her focus on the aggregate of British soldiers through emphasis on sanitation, community assessment, and analysis; the development of the use of graphically depicted statistics; and the gathering of comparable census data and political advocacy on behalf of the aggregate.

Nightingale was from a wealthy English family, was well educated, and traveled extensively. Her father tutored her in mathematics and many other subjects. Nightingale later studied with Adolphe Quetelet, a Belgian statistician. Quetelet influenced her profoundly and taught her the discipline of social inquiry (Goodnow, 1933). Nightingale also had a passion for hygiene and health. In 1851, at the age of 31 years, she trained in nursing with Pastor Fliedner at Kaiserswerth Hospital in Germany. She later studied the organization and discipline of the Sisters of Charity in Paris. Nightingale wrote extensively and published her analyses of the many nursing systems she studied in France, Austria, Italy, and Germany (Dock and Stewart, 1925).

In 1854, Nightingale responded to distressing accounts of a lack of care for wounded soldiers during the Crimean War. She and 40 other nurses traveled to Scutari, which was part of the Ottoman Empire at the time. Nightingale was accompanied by lay nurses, Roman Catholic sisters, and Anglican sisters. Upon their arrival, they learned that the British army's management method for treating the sick and wounded had created conditions that resulted in extraordinarily high death rates among soldiers. One of Nightingale's greatest achievements was improving the management of ill and wounded soldiers.

Nightingale faced an assignment in The Barrack Hospital, which had been built for 1700 patients. In four miles of beds, she found 3000 to 4000 patients separated by only 18 inches of space (Goodnow, 1933, pp. 55-56).

> The beds were mostly of straw and many were laid directly on the floor. The few sheets to be had were of canvas and so rough that the men begged not to have them used. Practically no laundry was being done; there was no hospital clothing and the patients were still in their uniforms, stiff with blood and covered with filth. There was no soap, no towels, nor basins, very few utensils of any sort. Every place swarmed with vermin. Men ate half-cooked food with their fingers because utensils did not exist.

During the Crimean War, cholera and "contagious fever" were rampant. An equal amount of men died from disease and battlefield injury (Cohen, 1984). Nightingale found that allocated supplies were bound in bureaucratic red tape; for example, supplies were "sent to the wrong ports or were buried under munitions and could not be got" (Goodnow, 1933, p. 86).

Nightingale encountered problems reforming the army's methods for care of the sick because she had to work through eight military affairs departments related to her assignment. She sent reports of the appalling conditions of the hospitals to London and in response immediately set up diet kitchens and a laundry and provided food, clothing, dressings, and laboratory equipment with government money and donated funds (Dock and Stewart, 1925).

Major reforms occurred during the first two months of her assignment. Aware that an interest in keeping social statistics was emerging, Nightingale realized that her most forceful argument would be statistical in nature. She reorganized the methods of keeping statistics and was the first to use shaded and colored Coxcomb graphs of wedges, circles and squares to illustrate the preventable deaths of soldiers. Nightingale compared the deaths of soldiers in hospitals during the Crimean War to the average annual mortality in Manchester and to the deaths of soldiers in military hospitals in and near London at the time (Fig. 2-2). Through her reforms she also showed that, by the end of the war, the death rate among ill soldiers during the Crimean War was no higher than that among well soldiers in Britain (Cohen, 1984). Indeed, Nightingale's careful statistics revealed that the death rate for treated soldiers decreased from 42% to 2%.

FIGURE 2-2

Coxcomb charts by Florence Nightingale (From Nightingale F: *Notes on matters affecting the health, efficiency and hospitalization of the British army,* London, 1858, Harrison and Sons). Photographs of large, fold-out charts from an original preserved at University of Chicago Library (public domain; courtesy University of Chicago Library).   *Continued*

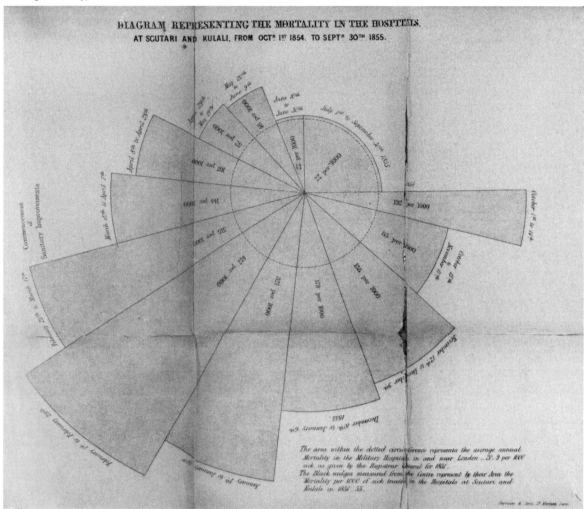

Furthermore, she established community services and activities to improve the quality of life for recovering soldiers. These included rest and recreation facilities, study opportunities, a savings fund, and a post office. She also organized care for the families of the soldiers (Dock and Stewart, 1925).

After returning to London at the close of the war in 1856, Nightingale devoted her efforts to sanitary reform. At home, she surmised that if the sanitary neglect of the soldiers existed in the battle area, it probably existed at home in London. She prepared statistical tables to support her suspicions (Table 2-1).

In one study comparing the mortality of men aged 25 to 35 years in the army barracks of England with that of men the same age in civilian life, Nightingale found the mortality of the soldiers was nearly twice that of the civilians. In one of her reports, she stated that "our soldiers enlist to death in the barracks" (Kopf, 1978, p. 95). Further, she believed that allowing a young soldier to die needlessly from unsanitary conditions was equivalent to taking him out, lining him up, and shooting him (Kopf, 1978). She was very political and did not keep her community assessment and analysis to herself. Nightingale distributed her reports to members of Parliament and to the medical and commanding officers of the army

FIGURE 2-2, cont'd

For legend see previous page.

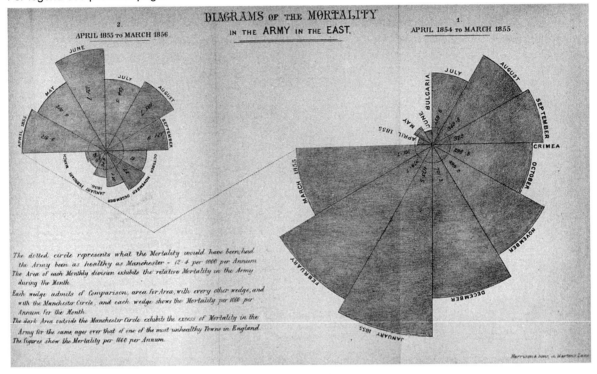

(Kopf, 1978). Prominent male leaders of the time challenged her reports. Undaunted, she rewrote them in greater depth and redistributed them.

In her efforts to compare the hospital systems in European countries, Nightingale discovered that each hospital kept incomparable data and that many hospitals used various names and classifications for diseases. She noted that these differences prevented the collection of similar statistics from larger geographical areas. These statistics would create a regional health-illness profile and allow for comparison with other regions. She printed common statistical forms that some hospitals in London adopted on an experimental basis. A study of the tabulated results revealed the promise of this strategy (Kopf, 1978).

Nightingale continued the development and application of statistical procedures and she won recognition for her efforts. The Royal Statistical Society made her a fellow in 1858 and the American Statistical Association made her an honorary member in 1874 (Kopf, 1978).

NIGHTINGALE USED STATISTICAL METHODS IN COMMUNITY ASSESSMENT

London's Southeastern Railway planned to remove St. Thomas' Hospital to increase the railway's right-of-way between London Bridge and Charing Cross. Nightingale applied her statistical method to the health needs of the community by conducting a *community assessment.* She plotted the cases served by the hospital, analyzed the proportion by distance, and calculated the probable impact on the community if the hospital was relocated to the proposed site. In her view, hospitals were a part of the wider community that served the needs of humanity. Kopf (1978) noted that this method of health planning and matching resources to the needs of the population was visionary and was not reapplied until the twentieth century.

TABLE 2-1

Nightingale's Crimean War Mortality Statistics: Nursing Research that Made a Difference

Year	Deaths That Would Have Occurred in Healthy Districts Among Males of the Soldiers' Ages*	Actual Deaths of Noncommissioned Officers and Men	Excess of Deaths Among Noncommissioned Officers and Men
1839	763	2914	2151
1840	829	3300	2471
1841	857	4167	3310
1842	888	5052	4164
1843	914	5270	4356
1844	920	3867	2947
1845	911	4587	3676
1846	930	5125	4195
1847	981	4232	3251
1848	987	3213	2226
1849	954	4052	3098
1850	919	3119	2200
1851	901	2729	1828
1852	915	3120	2205
1853	920	3392	2472
Total	13,589	58,139	44,550

From Grier B and Grier M: Contributions of the passionate statistician, *Res Nurs Health* 1:103-109, 1978. Copyright © 1978 by John Wiley & Sons, Inc. Reprinted by permission of John Wiley & Sons, Inc.
Number of deaths of noncommissioned officers and men also shows the number of deaths that would have occurred if the mortality were 7.7 per 1000—such as it was among Englishmen of the soldiers' age in healthy districts, in the years 1849 to 1853—which fairly represent the average mortality.
*The exact mortality in the healthy districts is 0.0077122, using the logarithm of 3.8871801.

In 1861, Nightingale lobbied officials to add two areas of data collection to the census. She asked officials to include the number of sick and infirm in the population and data depicting the housing of the population (Kopf, 1978, p. 98). She stated the following:

The connection between the *health* and the *dwellings* of the population is one of the most important that exists. The "diseases" can be approximated also. In all the more important—such as smallpox, fevers, mea-

sles, heart disease, etc., all those which affect the *national* health, there will be very little error. Where there *is* error, in these things, the error is uniform . . . and corrects itself.

Although census officials did not adopt her recommendations linking illness and housing to health, Nightingale's suggestions were visionary. According to Kopf (1978), only a few countries currently gather census data on sickness and housing.

Nightingale also stressed the need to use statistics

at the administrative and political levels to direct health policy. Noting the ignorance of politicians and those who set policy regarding the interpretation and use of statistics, she emphasized the need to teach national leaders to use statistical facts.

In addition to her contributions to nursing and her development of nursing education, Nightingale's credits include the application of statistical information toward an understanding of the total environmental situation (Kopf, 1978). Population-based statistics has marked implications for the development of public health and public health nursing. Grier and Grier (1978) recognized Nightingale's contributions to statistics and stated that "Her name occurs in the index of many texts on the history of probability and statistics . . . in the history of quantitative graphics . . . and in texts on the history of science and mathematics." Specifically, these authors showed that Nightingale's research *preceded* later works, such as the use of correlation in 1880, the *t* test in 1908, and the subsequent development of the chi-square, contingency table analysis, and analysis of variance. In contrast to Nightingale's research, these newer tests aided in judging the relevance of data when the numbers were few and the effects were small.

It is interesting to note that the paradigm for nursing practice and nursing education that evolved through Nightingale's work did not incorporate her emphasis on statistics and a sound research base. It is also curious why nursing education did not consult her writings and stress the importance of determining health's social and environmental determinants until much later.

Establishment of Modern Medical Care and Public Health Practice

To place Nightingale's work in perspective, it is necessary to consider the development of medical care in light of common education and practice during the late nineteenth and early twentieth centuries. Goodnow (1933) called this time a "dark age." Medical sciences were underdeveloped and bacteriology was unknown. Few medical schools existed at the time, so apprenticeship was the path to medical education. The majority of physicians believed in the "spontaneous generation" theory of disease causation, which stated that disease organisms grew from nothing (Najman,

1990). Typical medical treatment included blood-letting, starving, using leeches, and prescribing large doses of metals such as mercury and antimony (Goodnow, 1933).

Nightingale's uniform classification of hospital statistics noted the need to tabulate the classification of diseases in hospital patients and the need to note the diseases patients contracted in the hospital. These diseases, such as gangrene and septicemia, were later called *iatrogenic* diseases (Kopf, 1978). Considering the lack of surgical sanitation in hospitals at the time, it is not surprising that iatrogenic infection was rampant. For example, Goodnow (1933, pp. 471-472) illustrates the following unsanitary operating procedures:

> Before an operation the surgeon turned up the sleeves of his coat to save the coat, and would often not trouble to wash his hands, knowing how soiled they soon would be! The area of the operation would sometimes be washed with soap and water, but not always, for the inevitability of corruption made it seem useless. The silk or thread used for stitches or ligatures was hung over a button of the surgeon's coat, and during the operation a convenient place for the knife to rest was between his lips. Instruments . . . used for . . . lancing abscesses were kept in the vest pocket and often only wiped with a piece of rag as the surgeon went from one patient to another.

During the nineteenth century, the following important scientists were born: Louis Pasteur in 1822, Joseph Lister in 1827, and Robert Koch in 1843. Their research also had a profound impact on health care, medicine, and nursing. Pasteur was a chemist, not a physician. While experimenting with wine production in 1854, he proposed the theory of the existence of germs. Although his colleagues ridiculed him at first, Koch applied his theories and developed his methods for handling and studying bacteria. Subsequently, Pasteur's colleagues gave him acknowledgment for his work.

Lister, whose father perfected the microscope, observed the healing processes of fractures. When the bone was broken but the skin was not, he noted that recovery was uneventful. However, when both the bone and the skin were broken, fever, infection, and even death were frequent. He found the proposed answer to his observation through Pasteur's work. Something outside the body entered the wound through the broken skin causing the infection (Goodnow, 1933). Lister's surgical successes eventually improved when he soaked the dressings and instruments in mixtures of carbolic acid (i.e., phenol) and oil.

In 1882, Koch discovered the causative agent for cholera and the tubercle bacillus. Pasteur discovered immunization in 1881 and the rabies vaccine in 1885. These discoveries were significant to the development of public health and medicine. However, physicians accepted these discoveries slowly (Rosen, 1958). For example, TB was a major cause of death in late nineteenth century America and often plagued its victims with chronic illness and disability. It was a highly stigmatized disease and most physicians thought it was a hereditary, constitutional disease associated with poor environmental conditions. Hospitalization for TB was rare because the stigma caused families to hide their infected relatives. Without treatment, the communicability of the disease increased. Common treatment was a change of climate (Rosen, 1958). Although Koch had announced the discovery of the tubercle bacillus in 1882, it was 10 years before the emergence of the first organized community campaign to stop the spread of the disease.

The case of puerperal (i.e., childbirth) fever illustrates another example of slow innovation stemming from scientific discoveries. Although Pasteur showed that *Streptococcus* caused puerperal fever, it was years before physicians accepted his discovery. However, medical practice eventually changed and physicians no longer delivered infants after performing autopsies on puerperal fever cases without washing their hands (Goodnow, 1933).

Debate over the causes of disease occurred throughout the nineteenth century. Scientists discovered organisms during the latter part of the century, which supported the theory that specific contagious entities caused disease. This discovery challenged the earlier, miasmic theory that environment and atmospheric conditions caused disease (Greifinger and Sidel, 1981). The new scientific discoveries had a major impact on the development of public health and medical practice. The emergence of germ theory of disease focused diagnosis and treatment on the individual organism and the individual disease.

State and local governments felt increasingly responsible for controlling the spread of bacteria and other microorganisms. A community outcry for social reform forced state and local governments to take notice of the deplorable living conditions in the cities. In the New York City riots of 1863, the populace expressed their disgust for overcrowding; filthy streets; lack of provisions for the poor; and lack of adequate food, water, and housing for the people. Local boards of health formed and took responsibility for safeguarding food and water stores and managed the sewage and quarantine operation for victims of contagious diseases (Greifinger and Sidel, 1981).

The New York Metropolitan Board of Health formed in 1866 and state health departments formed shortly thereafter. States built large public hospitals that treated TB and mental disease with rest, diet, and quarantine. In 1889, the New York City Health Department recommended the surveillance of TB and TB health education, but physicians did not welcome either recommendation (Rosen, 1958). Despite their objections, the New York City Health Department required institutions to report cases of TB in 1894 and required physicians to do the same in 1897.

In the later part of the nineteenth century, the National Tuberculosis Association attempted to control TB by "enlisting community support and action through a systematic and organized campaign of public health education" (Rosen, 1958, p. 390). Many voluntary health organizations followed with organized efforts to "further community health through education, demonstrating ways of improving health services, advancing related research or legislation, and guarding and representing the public interest in this field" (Rosen, 1958, p. 384).

In 1883, The Johns Hopkins University Medical School in Baltimore, Maryland formed under the German model that promoted medical education on the principles of scientific discovery. In the United States, the Carnegie Commission appointed Abraham Flexner to evaluate medical schools throughout the country based on the German model. In 1910, the Flexner Report outlined the shortcomings of U.S. medical schools that did not use this model. Within a few years, the report caused philanthropic organizations such as the Rockefeller and Carnegie Foundations to withdraw funding of these schools, which ensured the closure of scientifically "inadequate" medical schools (Greifinger and Sidel, 1981). A "new breed" of physicians emerged who had been taught that germ theory was the "single agent theory" of disease causation (Greifinger and Sidel 1981, p. 132).

The emphasis on the use of scientific theory, or single agent theory, in medical care developed into a focus on disease and symptoms rather than a focus on the prevention of disability and care for the "whole person." The old-fashioned family doctor viewed patients in relation to their families and communities and apparently helped people cope with problems in personal life, family, and society. American medicine adopted science with such vigor that these qualities faded away. Science allowed the physician to deal with tissues and organs, which were much easier to comprehend than the dynamics of human relationships or the complexities of disease prevention. Many physicians made efforts to integrate the various roles, but society was pushing towards academic science.

Philanthropic foundations continued to influence health care efforts. For example, the Rockefeller Sanitary Commission for the Eradication of Hookworm formed in 1909. Hookworm was an occupational hazard among southern workers. The discovery of preventive efforts to eradicate hookworm kept the workers healthy and thus proved to be a great industrial benefit. The model was so successful that the Rockefeller Foundation established the first school of public health, The Johns Hopkins School of Hygiene and Public Health, in 1916. The focus of this institution was the preservation and improvement of individual and community health and the prevention of disease through multidisciplinary efforts. The faculty came from a broad range of sciences including biological, physical, social, and behavioral. Foundations made additional efforts, which led to the formation of the International Health Commission, schools of tropical medicine, and medical research institutes in foreign ports.

HISTORICAL METHODOLOGY FOR NURSING RESEARCH

Historiography is the methodology of historical research. It involves specialized techniques, principles, and theories that pertain to historical matters. Historical research involves interpreting history and contributing to understanding through data synthesis. It relies on existing sources or data and requires the researcher to gain access to sources such as libraries, librarians, and data bases.

Historical research should be descriptive. It should answer the questions of who, what, when, where, how, and the interpretive why. Historians reconstruct an era using primary sources and interpret the story from that perspective. Historical research in nursing will enhance the understanding of current nursing practice and will help prepare for the future.

From Lusk B: Historical methodology for nursing research, *Image J Nurs Sch* 29: 3555-360, 1997.

Community Caregiver

The traditional role of the community caregiver or the traditional healer has nearly vanished. However, medical and nurse anthropologists who have studied primitive and Western cultures are familiar with the community healer and caregiver role (Leininger, 1976; Logan and Hunt, 1978). The traditional healer is common in nonWestern, ancient, and primitive societies (Hughes, 1978). The healer may have taken various forms (e.g., shaman, midwife, herbalist, or priest). Although traditional healers have always existed, professionals and many people throughout industrialized societies may overlook or minimize their role. The role of the healer is often integrated with other institutions of society including religion, medicine, and morality. The notion that one person acts alone in healing may be foreign to many societies; healers can be individuals, kin, or entire societies (Hughes, 1978).

Societies have theories based on disease and the relationship of disease to other aspects of group life. For example, societies often consider disease to be an expression of disharmony with the environment rather than a condition caused by a specific "germ."

Both supernatural and empirical theories of disease exist. Many practices are empirically efficacious by public health standards (e.g., the practice of reheating food that has been left overnight to do away with "coldness" also destroys pathogens) (Hughes, 1978).

Societies retain folk practices because they offer repeated success. Most cultures have a pharmacopoeia and maintain therapeutic and preventive practices. One fourth to one half of folk medicines are empirically effective and many modern drugs are based on the medicines of primitive cultures (e.g., eucalyptus, coca, and opium) (Hughes, 1978).

Folk healing practices may be beneficial to the "patient" and may be socially cohesive; healing rituals and sessions frequently involve the patient and the patient's family and neighbors. When the healer allows the patient to participate in his or her own treatment and to involve his or her family and neighbors, the healer may apply the "treatment" to a whole group, or aggregate (Hughes, 1978).

Since ancient times, cultural practices have affected health. The late nineteenth and early twentieth century practice of midwifery illustrates modern medicine's encroachment over traditional healing in many Western cultures (Ehrenreich and English, 1973; Smith, 1979). For example, traditional midwifery practices made women rise out of bed within 24 hours of delivery to help "clear" the lochia; throughout the mid1900s, modern medicine recommended keeping women in bed (Smith, 1979).

Public health nursing was a holistic approach that developed in the late nineteenth and early twentieth centuries. Public health nursing and community health nursing evolved from home nursing practice, community organizations, and political interventions on behalf of aggregates.

Establishment of Public Health Nursing

England

Public health nursing developed from providing nursing care to the sick poor and providing information and channels of community organization that enable the poor to improve their own health status.

District Nursing

District nursing, which stemmed from the first tradition, developed in England. Between 1854 and 1856, the Epidemiological Society of London developed a plan that trained selected poor women to provide nursing care to the community's sick poor. The society theorized that nurses belonging to their patient's social class would be more effective caregivers and that more nurses would be available in the community (Rosen, 1958).

A similar plan implemented in Liverpool in 1859 was more successful. After experiencing the excellent care a nurse gave his sick wife in his home, William Rathbone, a Quaker, strongly believed that nurses could offer the same care throughout the community.

He developed a plan that divided the community into 18 districts and assigned a nurse and a social worker (SW) to each district. This team met the needs of their communities in nursing, social work, and health education. The community widely accepted the plan. To further strengthen it, Rathbone consulted Nightingale about educating the nurses. She assisted him by providing training for the district nurses, referring to them as "health nurses." The model was successful and eventually voluntary agencies on the national level adopted the plan (Rosen, 1958).

Health Visiting

Health visiting to provide information for improved health is a parallel service based on the district nursing tradition. The Ladies Section of the Manchester and Salford Sanitary Association originated health visiting in Manchester in 1862. Health pamphlets alone had little effect; therefore this service enlisted home visitors to distribute health information to the poor.

In 1893, Nightingale pointed out that the district nurse should be a health teacher and a nurse for the sick in the home. She felt that teachers should educate "health missioners" for this purpose. However, the model charged the district nurse with providing care for the sick in the home and the health visitor with providing health information in the home. Eventually, government agencies sponsored health visitors, medical health officers supervised them, and the municipality paid them. Thus a collaborative model developed between government and voluntary agencies and exists in the United States today.

United States

In the United States, public health nursing also developed from the traditions of district nursing and home nursing. In 1877, the Women's Board of the New York City Mission sent a graduate nurse named Francis Root into homes to provide care for the sick. The innovation spread and nursing associations, later called visiting nurse associations, were implemented in Buffalo in 1885 and in Boston and Philadelphia in 1886.

In 1893, nurses Lillian Wald and Mary Brewster established a district nursing service on the Lower East Side of New York City called the House on Henry Street. This was a crowded area teeming with unemployed and homeless immigrants who needed health care. This organization, later called the Visiting Nurse Association of New York City, played an important role in establishing public health nursing in the United States. Box 2-1 contains Wald's compel-

BOX 2-1

Lillian Wald: The House on Henry Street

The following highlights from *The House on Henry Street,* published in 1915, bring Lillian Wald's experience to life:

A sick woman in a squalid rear tenement, so wretched and so pitiful that, in all the years since, I have not seen anything more appalling, determined me, within half an hour, to live on the East Side.

I had spent two years in a New York training-school for nurses. . . After graduation, I supplemented the theoretical instruction, which was casual and inconsequential in the hospital classes twenty-five years ago, by a period of study at a medical college. It was while at the college that a great opportunity came to me.

While there, the long hours "on duty" and the exhausting demands of the ward work scarcely admitted freedom for keeping informed as to what was happening in the world outside. The nurses had no time for general reading; visits to and from friends were brief; we were out of the current and saw little of life saved as it flowed into the hospital wards. It is not strange, therefore that I should have been ignorant of the various movements which reflected the awakening of the social conscience at the time.

Remembering the families who came to visit patients in the wards, I outlined a course of instruction in home nursing adapted to their needs, and gave it in an old building in Henry Street, then used as a technical school and now part of the settlement. Henry Street then as now was the center of a dense industrial population.

From the schoolroom where I had been giving a lesson in bedmaking, a little girl led me one drizzling March morning. She had told me of her sick mother, and gathering from her incoherent account that a child had been born, I caught up the paraphernalia of the bedmaking lesson and carried it with me.

The child led me over broken roadways—there was no asphalt, although its use was well established in other parts of the city—over dirty mattresses and heaps of refuse—it was before Colonel Waring had shown the possibility of clean streets even in that quarter—between tall, reeking houses whose laden fire-escapes, useless for their appointed purpose, bulged with household goods of every description. The rain added to the dismal appearance of the streets and to the discomfort of the crowds which thronged them, intensifying the odors which assailed me from every side. Through Hester and Division street we went to the end of Ludlow; past odorous fishstands, for the streets were a market-place, unregulated, unsupervised, unclean; past evil-smelling, uncovered garbage-cans; and—perhaps worst of all, where so many little children played—past the trucks brought down from more fastidious quarters and stalled on these already overcrowded streets, lending themselves inevitably to many forms of indecency.

The child led me on through a tenement hallway, across a court where open and unscreened closets were promiscuously used by men and women, up into a rear tenement, by slimy steps whose accumulated dirt was augmented that day by the mud of the streets, and finally into the sickroom.

All the maladjustments of our social and economic relations seemed epitomized in this brief journey and what was found at the end of it. The family to which the child led me was neither criminal nor vicious. Although the husband was a cripple, one of those who stand on street corners exhibiting deformities to enlist compassion, and masking the begging of alms by a pretense at selling; although the family of seven shared their two rooms with boarders—who were literally boarders, since a piece of timber was placed over the floor for them to sleep on—and although the sick woman lay on a wretched, unclean bed, soiled with a hemorrhage two days old, they were not degraded human beings, judged by any measure of moral values.

From Wald L: *The house on Henry Street,* New York, 1971, Dover Publications (original work published 1915, Henry Holt).

BOX 2-1

Lillian Wald: The House on Henry Street—cont'd

In fact, it was very plain that they were sensitive to their condition, and when, at the end of my ministrations, they kissed my hands (those who have undergone similar experiences will, I am sure, understand), it would have been some solace if by any conviction of the moral unworthiness of the family I could have defended myself as a part of a society which permitted such conditions to exist. Indeed, my subsequent acquaintance with them revealed the fact that, miserable as their state was, they were not without ideals for the family life, and for society, of which they were so unloved and unlovely a part.

That morning's experience was a baptism of fire. Deserted were the laboratory and the academic work of the college. I never returned to them. On my way from the sickroom to my comfortable student quarters my mind was intent on my own responsibility. To my inexperience it seemed certain that conditions such as these were allowed because people did not know, and for me there was a challenge to know and to tell. When early morning found me still awake, my naive conviction remained that, if people knew things—and "things" meant everything implied in the condition of this family—such horrors would cease to exist, and I rejoiced that I had had a training in the care of the sick that in itself would give me an organic relationship to the neighborhood in which this awakening had come.

To the first sympathetic friend to whom I poured forth my story, I found myself presenting a plan which had been developing almost without conscious mental direction on my part.

Within a day or two a comrade from the training-school, Mary Brewster, agreed to share in the venture. We were to live in the neighborhood as nurses, identify ourselves with it socially, and, in brief, contribute to it our citizenship.

I should like to make it clear that from the beginning we were most profoundly moved by the wretched industrial conditions which were constantly forced upon us. . . I hope to tell of the constructive programmes that the people them-selves have evolved out of their own hard lives, of the ameliorative measures, ripened out of sympathetic comprehension, and finally, of the social legislation that expresses the new compunction of the community. (pp. 1-9)

ling account of her early exposure to the community where she identified public health nursing needs.

Wald described a range of services that evolved from the house at Henry Street. Nurses provided home visits and patients paid carfare or a cursory fee. Physicians were consultants to Henry Street and families could arrange a visit by calling the nurse directly or a physician could call the nurse on the family's behalf. The nursing service adopted the philosophy of meeting the health needs of aggregates, which included the many evident social, economic, and environmental determinants of health. By necessity, this involved an aggregate approach that empowered people of the community.

Helen Hall, who later directed the House at Henry Street, wrote that the settlement's role was "one of helping people to help themselves" (Wald, 1971) through the development of centers of social

action aimed at meeting the needs of the community and the individual. Community organization led to the formation of a great variety of programs including youth clubs, a juvenile program, sex education for local schoolteachers, and support programs for immigrants. A community studies department carried out systematical community assessments "so that we could tell our neighbors' story where it would do the most good" (Wald, 1971, p. vi). Mothers from the settlement went to Washington, DC and testified about raising children in "decaying tenements." Neighbors of the settlement entered a democratic process that took them from the steps of city hall to the nation's capital to speak out on behalf of the needs of the aggregate. They spoke out for necessities like traffic lights, schools, garbage collection services, unemployment insurance, and health care. The Children's Bureau and the Social Security Act Legislation formed as a result of these efforts. The testimony had an impact on the formation of Medicare in 1963.

Aggregate programs like school nursing were based on individual observations and interventions. Wald reported the following incident that preceded her successful trial of school nursing (1971, pp. 46-47):

> I had been downtown only a short time when I met Louis. An open door in a rear tenement revealed a woman standing over a washtub, a fretting baby on her left arm, while with her right she rubbed at the butcher's aprons which she washed for a living.
>
> "Louis," she explained, "was bad." He did not "cure his head of lice and what would become of him, for they would not take him into the school because of it?" Louis said he had been to the dispensary many times. He knew it was awful for a twelve-year-old boy not to know how to read the names of the streets on the lamp-posts, but "every time I go to school Teacher tells me to go home."
>
> It needed only intelligent application of the dispensary ointments to cure the affected area, and in September, I had the joy of securing the boy's admittance to school for the first time in his life. The next day, at the noon recess, he fairly rushed up our five flights of stairs in the Jefferson Street tenement to spell the elementary words he had acquired that morning.

Overcrowded schools, an uninformed and uninterested public, and an unaware department of health all contributed to this neglect. Wald and the nursing staff at the settlement kept anecdotal notes on the sick children teachers excluded from school. One nurse found a boy in school whose skin was desquamating from scarlet fever and took him to the president of the Department of Health in an attempt to place physicians in schools. A later program had physicians screen children in school for one hour each day; however, this program suffered because it was not comprehensive.

In 1902, Wald convinced Dr. Lederle, Commissioner of Health in New York City, to try a school nursing experiment. Henry Street loaned a public health nurse named Linda Rogers to the New York City Health Department to work in a school (Dock and Stewart, 1925). The experiment was successful and schools adopted nursing on a widespread basis. School nurses performed physical assessments, treated minor infections, and taught health to pupils and parents.

EXAMPLE OF HISTORICAL NURSING RESEARCH

Fairman's (1996) review of 150 fictional novels from 1850 to 1995 revealed how the image of nursing has changed over the past 140 years. The results showed that the image of nursing improved dramatically from the negative perception of the 1850s. Trained nurses became more common in the early 1900s and the novels began to depict strong, independent, female nurses. The positive image continued until the 1960s and 1970s when novels presented the negative image of "bed hopping honeys." Popular literature showed the most negative image of nurses and classics and children's literature showed a more positive image.

From Fairman PL: *Analysis of the image of nursing and nurses as portrayed in fictional literature from 1850 to 1995,* dissertation abstracts, 1996, University of San Francisco.

In 1909, Wald mentioned the efficacy of home nursing to one of the officials of the Metropolitan Life Insurance Company. The company decided to provide home nursing to its industrial policyholders and soon the United States and Canada used the successful program (Wald, 1971).

The increasing demand for public health nursing was hard to satisfy. In 1910, the Department of Nursing and Health formed at the Teachers College of Columbia University in New York City. A course in visiting nursing placed nurses at the Henry Street settlement for fieldwork. In 1912, the newly formed National Organization of Public Health Nursing elected Lillian Wald its first president. This organization was open to public health nurses and to those interested in public health nursing. In 1913, the Los Angeles Department of Health formed the first Bureau of Public Health Nursing (Rosen, 1958). That same year, the PHS appointed its first public health nurse.

At first, many public health nursing programs used nurses in specialized areas such as school nursing, TB nursing, maternal-child health nursing, and communicable disease nursing. In recent years, a more generalized program has become acceptable; a nurse hired by an official agency covers the entire population of one district and, with the exception of occupational health, provides prevention, health pro-

Images of community health nursing in the early and midtwentieth century.

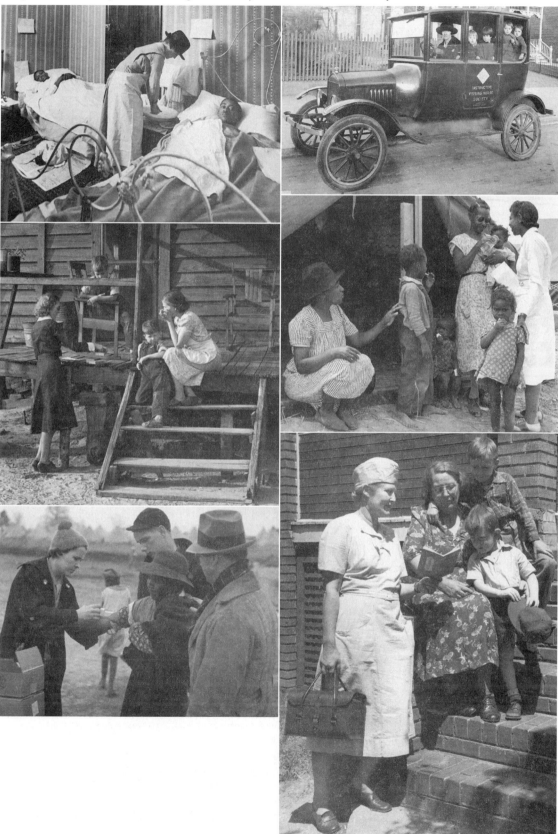

motion, and health maintenance care. Visiting nurses collaborate with voluntary home health agencies such as the Visiting Nurse Association to provide care to the homebound ill through physician referral. Combination agencies providing both services also exist, but these are less available in urban areas.

With the current focus on cost-containment and the provision of health care services under managed care, change is taking place in the traditional models of public health nursing and visiting nursing in voluntary home health agencies. The focus of care is increasing within the community; therefore new models that use nursing in the community to contain costs are appearing with variation among states and areas within a state. For example, some models may focus on providing care to populations that subscribe to HMOs (Graff et al., 1995; Shamansky, 1995), while others focus on specialized areas like communicable diseases.

CONSEQUENCES FOR THE HEALTH OF AGGREGATES

An understanding of the consequences of the health care delivery system's impact on aggregate health is necessary to form conclusions about community health nursing from a historical perspective. Implications for the health of aggregates relate to new causes of mortality (i.e., Hygeia, or good living, vs. Panacea, or curative medicine) and additional theories of disease causation.

New Causes of Mortality

Since the turn of the century, the causes of mortality in Western societies have changed from mostly infectious diseases to chronic diseases. Increased food production and better nutrition during the nineteenth and early twentieth centuries contributed to the decline in infectious disease-related deaths. Other factors include better sanitation through water purification, sewage disposal, improved food handling, and milk pasteurization. According to McKeown (1981) and Evans, Barer, and Marmor (1994), "modern" medicine such as antibiotics and immunization had little effect on health until well into the twentieth century. Indeed, improved vaccination programs began in the 1920s and powerful antibiotics came into use after 1935.

The advent of chronic disease in Western populations puts selected aggregates at risk and those aggregates need health education, screening, and programs to ensure occupational and environmental safety. Too often modern medicine focuses on the single cause of disease (i.e., germ theory) and treating the acutely ill. Therefore health providers have treated the chronically ill with an acute care approach although preventive care, health promotion, and restorative care are necessary to combat escalating rates of chronic disease. This expanded approach may develop under new systems of cost containment.

Hygeia vs. Panacea

The Grecian Hygeia (i.e., healthful living) vs. Panacea (i.e., cure) dichotomy still exists today. Although the change in the nature of health "problems" is certain, the roles of individual and collective activities in the prevention of illness and premature death are slow to evolve. Consequently, "complex life-threatening disorders are better understood; on the other hand, few professionals have been trained to specialize in the treatment of the common, uncomplicated health problems that account for 90 percent of visits to doctors" (Lee et al., 1981, p. 197).

In 1997, about two thirds of the 664,000 active physicians in the United States were specialists (USDHHS/HRSA/BHP, 1999). Medical education is increasingly responsible for training primary care physicians (e.g., internal medicine, obstetrics-gynecology, family medicine, and pediatrics) to meet the growing need for primary care. This need for primary care providers and the phenomenal growth of managed care calls for more NPs in primary care positions. In addition to primary care, Hygeia requires a coordinated system that addresses the problem holistically using multiple approaches and planning outcomes for aggregates and populations. A redistribution of interest and resources to address the major determinants of health, such as food, housing, education, and a healthy social and physical environment, is necessary (Evans, Barer, and Marmor, 1994; Lamarche, 1995) (Box 2-2).

Additional Theories of Disease Causation

The germ theory of disease causation is a unicausal model that evolved in the late nineteenth century. Najman (1990) reviewed the following theories

BOX 2-2

Viewing Immigrants as Assets: A Glimpse into Australia's Public Health History

Like the United States and Canada, Australia is a land of immigration with its own unique public health history. In 1788—eighteen years after Captain Cook claimed the continent for Britain—the British began using Australia as a settlement for England's convicts and continued doing so until 1825. From 1826 to 1850, Australia held England's excess population. After 1850, the living conditions in England improved significantly and caused the level of British immigration to drop dramatically. Populating the Australian colony turned into a public health disaster for England because the journey was a difficult six to eight months at sea.

The first few convict fleets barely survived the journey. By the time the immigrants arrived in Australia, they were plagued with disease and unable to build a settlement. British historical records show that the second English fleet contained 1260 convicts. By the time the fleet reached Australia, 267 convicts perished. Shortly after arriving, 124 of the survivors died in the Sydney hospital. For the next 25 years, the surviving convicts were limited in their ability to help England build a settlement because they were starved and diseased. Overcrowding and reduced food and water rations made the journey difficult to survive. These poor travel conditions were related to the overall negligence and corruption of the private contractors who put priority on valuable cargo.

The British authorities realized that they needed to ensure the convict's safe arrival. William Redfern, the assistant surgeon and former convict of New South Wales, advised Governor Macquarie to regulate the shipping contractors and supervise the convict's health. Redfern recommended placing a convict surgeon aboard each ship to improve traveling conditions. Specifically, he recommended that the surgeons air out passenger cabins and bedding daily, make more drinking water available, provide full rations and articles of comfort, install bathing and cleaning facilities, and regularly fumigate the ship with nitric or muriatic acid. After Macquarie installed these regulations, the death rate among convicts on ships to Australia plummeted between 1788 and 1868; it was much lower in comparison to the passenger deaths on similar private fleets making the shorter trip from Europe to North America.

The Australian government believed that it was even more important that settlers, rather than convicts, arrive healthy and ready to work; therefore these public health standards were extended to ships that carried assisted immigrants. The Australian government prepaid the fares for assisted immigrants. Regulations from London mandated that surgeons and matrons be responsible for the hygiene, medical care, welfare, and discipline of the passengers. This measure, called the Passenger Acts, created a marked improvement in the health of young children and all immigrants by placing a doctor and nurse aboard each ship. The British Board of Trade controlled the health conditions on all passenger ships and made the passage to Australia "so safe that it was looked upon as a holiday by many immigrants, who arrived healthier than when they had left England" (Jupp, 1990).

This glimpse into Australia's immigration policy exemplifies one development in the history of public health. Whether they coerced the convicts or assisted passage for settlers, the Australian government populated its country through the belief that immigrants are assets and proved that the health of immigrants is a public responsibility.

Data from Jupp J: Two hundred years of immigration. In Reid J and Trompf R, editors: *The health of immigrant Australia,* Orlando, 1990, Harcourt Brace & Co.

of disease causation: the multicausal view, which considers the environment multidimensional, and the general susceptibility view, which considers stress and lifestyle factors. Najman contended that each theory accounts for some disease under some conditions, but no single theory accounts for all disease. Other factors such as literacy and nutrition may reduce infectious disease morbidity and mortality to a greater extent than medical interventions alone (Najman, 1990).

CHALLENGES FOR COMMUNITY HEALTH NURSING

Community health nurses face the challenge of promoting the health of populations. They must accomplish this with an "inclusive" understanding of the multiple causes of morbidity and mortality. The specialization of medicine and nursing has affected the delivery of nursing and medical care. Nurses must be aware of the increased technological advances specialization has instigated. These advances resulted in an increase in the number and percentage of advanced practice nurses in the past two decades. In 1996, 6.3% of RNs in the United States were Master's prepared (USDHHS, 1999) and most of these advance practice nurses were specialists. However, the past decade has also seen an increase in the number and percentage of RNs working in community settings. In 1996, approximately 40% of all RNs worked in community settings such as occupational health, public health departments, physician's offices, and schools (USDHHS, 1999).

The community need for a bimodal focus on prevention, health promotion, and home care may become more widespread with the changing patterns of reimbursement. Holistic care requires both dimensions and must have more attention in the future. During the turn of the century, an ethnohistorical study of public health nursing in rural New England examined the cost-benefit ratios of the population-based district nurse (Dreher, 1984). The district nurse provided preventive, curative, and health-maintenance services. Dreher proposed that such a model might better address the nation's health problems.

The need for education in community health nursing calls for a primary care curriculum that would prepare students to meet the needs of aggregates through community strategies. Such a curriculum would move the focus on the individual to a broader population approach. Strategies would promote literacy, nutrition programs, decent housing and income, education, and safe social and physical environments.

Health care services alone cannot solve today's health problems. All health care workers must learn to work with and on behalf of aggregates and help them build a constituency for the consumer issues they face.

A population focus for nursing addresses the health of all in the population through the careful gathering of information and statistics. A population focus will better enable community health nurses to contribute to the ethic of social justice by emphasizing society's responsibility for health (Beauchamp, 1986). Helping aggregates to help themselves will empower the people and create avenues for addressing their concerns.

EXAMPLE OF HISTORICAL NURSING RESEARCH

In response to public health problems, public health and community health nursing evolved in Louisiana between 1835 and 1927. Yellow fever epidemics in the early 1800s provided the early impetus for nursing growth. A nursing service called the Howard Association began in 1833 and provided food, medicine, and nursing care for yellow fever victims. Natural disasters, such as the Mississippi River flood in 1927, also caused the enhancement of accessible public health efforts.

Maternal and child care was another important area for early community and public health nursing efforts. In 1916, the state board of health employed the first public health nurse to reduce infant and maternal mortality, improve the health of preschool and school-aged children, and decrease the mortality and morbidity of communicable diseases.

From Hanggi-Myers LJ: *The origins and history of the first public health/community health nurses in Louisiana: 1935-1927,* dissertation abstracts, New Orleans, 1996, Louisiana State University Medical Center.

A MODEL OF DISTRICT NURSING

In rural New England, an ethnohistorical study of public health nursing's development unexpectedly found a model of population-based nursing that may meet the nation's current and future health concerns (Dreher, 1984). The study collected data from public records, the census, direct observations, and interviews with town residents, public officials, medical care providers, and active and retired public health nurses. The health model of the 1920s used a district nurse, or "town hall" nurse, which exists today. The findings showed that the district nurse provided health education and services to people in four neighboring towns. The district nurse's activities were under local administration and property tax revenues paid for the services; patients and third party reimbursement did not contribute funds. The district nurse provided a full range of community nursing services to people in need, whether or not the patients were able to pay or were covered by insurance. The nurse performed school nursing, health promotion and prevention, and home health care. The district nurse held weekly office hours in the town halls of the four communities, performed blood pressure screening, and gave routine parenteral medications and health counseling. Mobility was not an issue because the district nurse performed home visits for patients confined to their homes. The district nurse conducted routine screening in schools and planned and carried out programs that addressed identified needs. The annual cost per visit from the district nurse was far less than the nurse services from a nearby home health agency. This model exemplifies a way of addressing the nation's health problems through prevention, promotion, and maintenance care.

The history of community health nursing provides insight into the dilemmas faced in contemporary times. Duffus (1938) stated the following about Wald's work:

> The "case" element in these early reports of Wald got less and less emphasis; she instinctively went behind the symptoms to appraise the whole individual, saw that one could not understand the individual without understanding the family, saw that the family was in the grip of larger social and economic forces which it could not control (p. 51).

Health care historians have reconstructed the history of health in Western populations by carefully sifting, weighing, and determining the importance of written fragments of "the facts." The historian's values and theories influence the writing of our past.

Traditionally, historians believed nonphysician healers were inauthentic "amateurs" who were marginal to "the maintenance of the physical health and well-being of society" (Versluysen, 1980, p. 176). This characterization was especially apparent for women healers. However, healers typically practiced in the home until the late nineteenth century. They were invisible, yet represented an extensive system of care delivery. Female historians and feminists are now researching the healer's accounts of home care that

male historians have overlooked, such as diaries, health manuals, and letters (Newbern, 1994).

According to Versluysen (1980), historians also tended to mention a few heroines within typical feminine stereotypes. For example, Nightingale's lifelong intellectual endeavors and marked achievements considerably expanded the profile of this remarkable woman beyond the typical focus on her two years in the Crimea and her role in founding modern nursing education. She was a health statistician, a prolific writer and scientist, a radical environmental sanitarian, and a reformer of both the British Army medical care system and the sanitary policy in India.

In addition, historians have also neglected the social and environmental contexts of health and medical care. These dimensions are necessary to place health care in a broader context. Historians need this broad context to grasp the state of public health and public health efforts during specific periods.

SUMMARY

Western civilization evolved from the Paleolithic Period to the present and people began to live in increasingly closer proximity to each other; therefore they experienced a change in the nature of their health problems.

In the midnineteenth and early twentieth centuries, public health efforts and the precursors of modern and public health nursing began to improve societal health. Nursing pioneers such as Nightingale in England and Wald in the United States focused on the collection and analysis of statistical data, health care reforms, home nursing, community empowerment, and nursing education. They established the groundwork for today's community health nursing.

Modern community health nurses must grapple with an array of philosophical controversies that affect their practice. These controversies include different opinions about what "intervention" means, a focus on both the individual and the aggregate, and the best way to solve the critical problem of runaway health care costs.

LEARNING ACTIVITIES

1. Research the history of the health department or Visiting Nurse Association in the city or county.
2. Find two recent articles about Florence Nightingale. After reading the articles, list Nightingale's

contributions to public health, public health nursing, and community health nursing.

3. Discuss with peers how Lillian Wald's approach to individual and community health care provides an understanding of how to facilitate the empowerment of aggregates in the community.

4. Obtain copies of early articles from nursing journals (*American Journal of Nursing* dates from 1900). Discuss the health problems, medical care, and nursing practice these articles illustrated.

5. Collect copies of early nursing textbooks. Discuss the evolution of thoughts on pathology, illness management, and health promotion.

RECOMMENDED READINGS

Nursing Research

Buhler-Wilkerson K: Bringing care to the people: Lillian Wald's legacy to public health nursing, *Am J Public Health* 83:1778-1786, 1993.

Burgess W: The Great White Plague and other epidemics: lessons from early visiting nursing, *J Home Health Care Pract* 6:12-17, 1993.

Dennis KE and Prescott PA: Florence Nightingale: yesterday, today, and tomorrow, *Adv Nurs Sci* 7:66-81, 1985.

Erickson GP: One hundred years of powerful women: a conversation with Sylvia R. Peabody, *Public Health Nurs* 10:146-150, 1993.

Grier B and Grier M: Contributions of the passionate statistician, *Res Nurs Health* 1:103-109, 1978.

Hawkins JE, Hayes ER and Corliss CP: School nursing in America: 1902-1994: a return to public health nursing, *Public Health Nurs* 11:416-425, 1994.

Lusk B: Historical methodology for nursing research, *Image J Nurs Sch* 29: 3555-360, 1997.

Marchine J and Garland TN: An emerging profession? the case of the nurse practitioner, *Image J Nurs Sch* 29:335-338, 1997.

Mayer SL: Amelia Greenwald: pioneer in international public health nursing, *Nurs Health Care* 15:74-78, 1994.

Mosley M: Jessie Sleet Scales: first black public health nurse, *Asso Black Nurs Faculty J* 5:45-51, 1994.

Newbern VB: Women as caregivers in the South: 1900-1945, *Public Health Nurs* 11:247-254, 1994.

Roberts ER and Reeb RM: Mississippi public health nurses and midwives: a partnership that worked, *Public Health Nurs* 11:57-63, 1994.

Shore HL: Frances Redmond: a pioneer in community health in Vancouver, *Can J Public Health* 84:13, 1993.

Silverstein NG: Lillian Wald at Henry Street: 1893-1895, *Adv Nurs Sci* 7:1-12, 1985.

REFERENCES

Armelagos GK, Dewey JR: Evolutionary response to human infectious diseases. In Logan MH, Hunt EE, editors: *Health and the human condition,* North Scituate, Mass, 1978, Duxbury Press.

Beauchamp DE: Public health as social justice. In Mappes T, Zembaty J, editors: *Biomedical ethics,* ed 2, New York, 1986, McGraw-Hill.

Burkitt DP: Some diseases characteristic of modern western civilization. In Logan MH, Hunt EE, editors: *Health and the human condition,* North Scituate, Mass, 1978, Duxbury Press.

Centers for Disease Control and Prevention: Fatal human plague: Arizona and Colorado, 1996, *Mor Mortal Wkly Rep* 46(27):617-620, 1997.

Centers for Disease Control and Prevention: Prevention of plague: recommendations of the Advisory Committee on Immunization Practices, *Mor Mortal Wkly Rep* 45(RR-14):1-15, 1996.

Cockburn TA: The evolution of human infectious diseases. In Cockburn T, editor: *Infectious diseases: their evolution and eradication,* Springfield, Ill, 1967, Charles C Thomas.

Cohen IB: Florence Nightingale, *Sci Am* 250:128-137, 1984.

Dock LL, Stewart IM: *A short history of nursing: from the earliest times to the present day,* New York, 1925, Putnam.

Dreher M: District nursing: the cost benefits of a population-based practice, *Am J Public Health* 74: 1107-1111, 1984.

Duffus RL: *Lillian Wald: neighbor and crusader,* New York, 1938, Macmillan.

Duran FD: *The Aztecs: the history of the Indies of New Spain,* New York, 1964, Orion Press (Translated, with notes, by Heyden D and Horcasitas F).

Ehrenreich B, English D: *Witches, midwives, and nurses: a history of women healers,* Old Westbury, NY, 1973, The Feminist Press.

Evans RG, Barer ML, Marmor TR: *Why are some people healthy and others not? the determinants of health of populations,* Hawthorne, NY, 1994, Aldine de Gruyter.

Fairman PL: *Analysis of the image of nursing and nurses as portrayed in fictional literature from 1850 to 1995,* dissertation abstracts, 1996, University of San Francisco.

Garn SM: Culture and the direction of human evolution, *Hum Biol* 35:221-236, 1963.

George MD: *London life in the XVIIIth century,* New York, 1925, Knopf.

Goodnow M: *Outlines of nursing history,* Philadelphia, 1933, WB Saunders.

Graff WL et al: Population management in an HMO: new roles for nursing, *Public Health Nurs* 12:213-221, 1995.

Greifinger RB, Sidel VW: American medicine: charity begins at home. In Lee P, Brown N, Red I, editors: *The nation's health,* San Francisco, 1981, Boyd and Fraser.

Grier B, Grier M: Contributions of the passionate statistician, *Res Nurs Health* 1:103-109, 1978.

Guendelman S et al: Generational differences in perinatal health among the Mexican American population: findings from HHANES 1982-84, *Am J Public Health* 80(suppl):61-65, 1990.

Hanggi-Myers LJ: *The origins and history of the first public health/community health nurses in Louisiana: 1935-1927,* dissertation abstracts, New Orleans, 1996, Louisiana State University Medical Center.

Hanlon JJ, Pickett GE: *Public health administration and practice,* ed 8, St. Louis, Mo, 1984, Mosby.

Hughes CC: Medical care: ethnomedicine. In Logan MH, Hunt EE, editors: *Health and the human condition,* North Scituate, Mass, 1978, Duxbury Press.

Jupp J: Two hundred years of immigration. In Reid J, Trompf R, editors: *The health of immigrant Australia,* Orlando, 1990, Harcourt Brace & Co.

Kopf EW: Florence Nightingale as statistician, *Res Nurs Health* 1:93-102, 1978.

Lamarche PA: Our health paradigm in peril, *Public Health Rep* 110:556-560, 1995.

Lee PR, Brown N, Red I, editors: *The nation's health,* San Francisco, 1981, Boyd and Fraser.

Leininger M: *Transcultural health care issues and conditions,* Philadelphia, 1976, FA Davis.

Logan MH, Hunt EE, editors: *Health and the human condition,* North Scituate, Mass, 1978, Duxbury Press.

McKeown T: Determinants of health. In Lee P, Brown N, Red I, editors: *The nation's health,* San Francisco, 1981, Boyd and Fraser.

Najman JM: Theories of disease causation and the concept of a general susceptibility: a review, *Soc Sci Med* 14A:231-237, 1990.

Newbern VB: Women as caregivers in the South: 1900-1945, *Public Health Nurs* 11:247-254, 1994.

Nightingale F: *Notes on matters affecting the health, efficiency and hospitalization of the British army,* London, 1858, Harrison and Sons.

Polgar S: Evolution and the ills of mankind. In Tax S, editor: *Horizons of anthropology,* Chicago, 1964, Aldine.

Richardson BW: *The health of nations: a review of the works of Edwin Chadwick,* vol 2, London, 1887, Longmans, Green.

Rosen G: *A history of public health,* New York, 1958, MD Publications.

Shamansky SL: A longer-than-usual editorial about population-based managed care, *Public Health Nurs* 12:211-212, 1995 (editorial).

Smith FB: *The people's health 1830-1910,* London, 1979, Croom Helm.

State studies third world solutions, *Nurseweek* Northern California Edition, March 18, 1991.

US Department of Health and Human Services, Health Resources and Services Administration, Bureau of Health Professions: *United States health workforce personnel factbook,* Rockville, Md, 1999, The Author.

Versluysen MC: Old wives' tales? women healers in English history. In Davies C, editor: *Rewriting nursing history,* Totowa, NJ, 1980, Barnes and Noble.

Wald L: *The house on Henry Street,* New York, 1971, Dover Publications (original work published 1915, Henry Holt).

Thinking Upstream: Conceptualizing Health from a Population Perspective

Patricia G. Butterfield

OBJECTIVES

Upon completion of this chapter, the reader will be able to do the following:

1. Describe the concept of theoretical scope and its application to the protection and promotion of health in community health nursing.
2. Differentiate between upstream interventions, which are designed to alter the precursors of poor health, and downstream interventions, which are characterized by efforts to modify individuals' perceptions of health.
3. Critique a theory in regard to its relevance in facilitating an understanding of population health dynamics.
4. Explain how theory-based practice achieves the goals of community health nursing by protecting and promoting health in populations.

KEY TERMS

conservative scope of practice
critical social theory
health belief model (HBM)
macroscopic
microscopic
Milio's framework for prevention
Self-care Deficit Theory
theory
upstream thinking

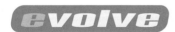

http://evolve.elsevier.com/Nies/

A thorough understanding of the factors contributing to population health is critical to the practice of community health nursing; this fundamental principle differentiates this area of practice from other nursing specialties. For many, the emphasis on population health requires a change in perspective from their original orientation to nursing practice. Novice nurses are frequently acculturated to nursing in a hospital or skilled nursing facility; these settings are designed, for the most part, to intervene on behalf of individuals. The structure of such settings, albeit the important role they play in the health care system, is not conducive to developing an understanding of population health.

This chapter begins with a brief overview of nursing theory followed by a discussion of the scope of community health nursing in addressing population health concerns. Later, the chapter compares several theoretical approaches to demonstrate how different conceptualizations can lead to different conclusions about the range of interventions available to the nurse. The text uses the analogy of upstream vs. downstream thinking to differentiate between population-directed strategies vs. individual-directed strategies.

THINKING UPSTREAM: LOOKING BEYOND THE INDIVIDUAL

In his description of the frustrations in medical practice, McKinlay (1979) used the image of a swiftly flowing river to represent illness. In this analogy, physicians are so busy rescuing victims from the river that they fail to look upstream to see who is pushing patients into the perilous waters. The author used this story to illustrate the ultimate futility of "downstream endeavors," which are characterized by short-term, individual-based interventions, and challenged health care providers to focus more of their energies "upstream, where the real problems lie" (McKinlay, 1979, p. 9). *Upstream* actions focus on modifying economic, political, and environmental factors that are the precursors of poor health throughout the world. Although the story cites medical practice, it is equally fitting to the dilemmas of nursing practice. In addition, although nursing has a rich history of providing preventive and population-based care, the current health system emphasizes episodic- and individual-based care. This system has done little to stem the tide of chronic illness that affects 70% of the American population.

This chapter uses the stream analogy several times to analyze different theories from an upstream, or macroscopic, perspective vs. a downstream perspective. Although these categories are not mutually exclusive, the use of the term *upstream* can provide a point of reference to evaluate a theory's potential for understanding population health.

HISTORICAL PERSPECTIVES ON NURSING THEORY

Many scholars agree that Florence Nightingale was the first nurse to formulate a conceptual foundation for nursing practice. However, in the years after her leadership, nursing practice became largely atheoretical and was based primarily on reacting to the immediacy of patient situations and medical staff. Thus hospital administrative and medical personnel defined nursing's perspective on health and scope of practice. Once nursing leaders saw that others were defining their profession, they began to take proactive action to consolidate their ideas and advance the scientific foundation of nursing practice.

The idea of theoretical orientation to guide nursing practice moved nursing forward. Several of the early nursing theories were extremely myopic and depicted health care situations that involved only one nurse and one patient. Family members and other health professionals were noticeably absent from the context of care. Historically, this characterization may have been an appropriate response to the constraints of nursing practice and the need to emphasize the medically independent activities of the nursing profession.

Although somewhat valuable, theories that address health from a microscopic rather than macroscopic perspective are limited in the current context of community-based nursing. These theories do not incorporate the social and environmental variables that provide a base for community health. More recent advances in nursing theory development address the dynamic nature of health sustaining and/or damaging environments and address the nature of a collective vs. individual client.

ISSUES OF FIT

Sometimes students are not acquainted with a sufficient range of theoretical approaches and select an individual-oriented theory to give them insight into a population-based health problem. A related problem occurs when students prefer a particular theoretical perspective and attempt to use it in all situations regardless of its relevance to the clinical scenario. Nursing is a practice profession; therefore it is important to recognize that the organizing framework for nursing should fit the care situation. The results of a *forced fit* do a disservice to the theory and the student. Understandably, students become perplexed and often frustrated when they begin to practice in the community and learn that their most familiar theoretical approaches offer only limited help in understanding or guiding their practice. Like other professional disciplines, nursing has many theoretical tools of the trade. It is important to know when to pick a hammer when a hammer is required and when to pick a wrench when a wrench is required. A primary goal of this chapter is to enable readers to select theoretical approaches that are compatible with a population perspective on health.

DEFINITIONS OF THEORY

Like other abstract concepts, different nursing authors have defined and interpreted theory in different ways. Listed below are several authors' definitions of **theory**. The lack of uniformity among these definitions reflects the evolution of thought and the individual differences in the understanding of relationships among theory, practice, and research. The definitions also reflect the difficult job of describing complex and diverse theory within the constraints of a single definition. Reading several definitions can foster an appreciation for the richness of theory and help the reader identify one or two particularly meaningful definitions. Within the profession, definitions of theory typically refer to a set of concepts and relational statements and the purpose of the theory. This chapter presents theoretical perspectives that are congruent with a broad interpretation of theory and correspond with the definitions proposed by Dickoff and James (1968), Torres (1986), and Chinn and Kramer (1999).

DEFINITIONS OF THEORY PROPOSED BY NURSING THEORISTS

- "A systematic vision of reality; a set of interrelated concepts that is useful for prediction and control" (Woods and Catanzaro, 1988, p. 568).

- "A conceptual system or framework invented for some purpose; and as the purpose varies so too must the structure and complexity of the system." (Dickoff and James, 1968, p. 19).

- "A creative and rigorous structuring of ideas that projects a tentative, purposeful, and systematic view of phenomena" (Chinn and Kramer, 1999, p. 51).

- "A set of ideas, hunches, or hypotheses that provides some degree of prediction and/or explanation of the world" (Pryjmachuk, 1996, p. 679).

- "Theory organizes the relationships between the complex events that occur in a nursing situation so that we can assist human beings. Simply stated, theory provides a way of thinking about and looking at the world around us" (Torres, 1986, p. 19).

HOW THEORY PROVIDES DIRECTION TO NURSING

The goal of theory is to improve nursing practice. Chinn and Kramer (1999) stated that using theories or parts of theoretical frameworks to guide practice best achieves this goal. Students often find theory intellectually burdensome and cannot see the care benefits of something so seemingly obtuse. Theory-based practice guides data collection and interpretation in a clear and organized manner; therefore it is easier for the nurse to diagnose and address the problems. Through the process of integrating theory and practice, the student can focus on factors that are critical to understanding the situation. Barnum (1990) stated, "A theory is like a map of a territory as opposed to an aerial photograph. The map does not give the full terrain (i.e., the full picture); instead it picks out those parts that are important for its given purpose" (p. 1). Using a theoretical perspective to plan nursing care guides the student in assessing a nursing situation and allows the student "to plan and not get lost in the details or sidetracked in the alleys" (Swanson, 1992).

MICROSCOPIC VS. MACROSCOPIC APPROACHES TO THE CONCEPTUALIZATION OF COMMUNITY HEALTH PROBLEMS

In many ways, each nurse must form a new way of identifying and interpreting the complex forces that shape societies to understand population health. The nurse can best achieve this transformation by integrating population-based practice and theoretical perspectives to conceptualize health from a **macroscopic** vs. **microscopic** perspective. Table 3-1 differentiates between these two approaches to conceptualizing health problems.

It is helpful to use the analogy of a target to understand the concept of microscopic vs. macroscopic. The individual is the bull's eye; this center contains the health problem of interest (e.g., pediatric exposure to lead compounds). In this context, a microscopic approach to assessment would focus exclusively on individual children with lead poisoning. Nursing interventions would focus on the identification and removal of lead sources in the

home. It is critical to remove all children with elevated serum lead levels from all suspect exposure sources immediately. However, the nurse can broaden his or her view of this problem by addressing individual health threats and by examining interpersonal and intercommunity factors that perpetuate lead poisoning on a national scale. This approach would include the bull's eye and the concentric circles that extend from the center of the target. A macroscopic approach to lead exposure may incorporate the following activities: examining trends in the prevalence of lead poisoning over time, estimating the percentage of older homes in a neighborhood that may contain lead pipes or lead-based paint surfaces, and locating industrial sources of lead emissions. These efforts usually involve the collaborative efforts of nurses from school, occupational, and other community settings. Doty (1996) notes that macrolevel perspectives provide nurses with the conceptual tools that empower clients to make health decisions based on their own interests and the interests of the community at large.

One common dilemma in daily community health practice is the tension between working on behalf of individuals and working on behalf of a population. For many nurses, this tension is exemplified by the need to reconcile and prioritize multiple daily tasks. Population-directed actions are often more global than the clear and immediate demands of ill people; therefore they may sink to the bottom of the priority list. A community health nurse or nursing administrator may plan to spend the day on a community project directed at preventive efforts, such as screening programs, updating the surveillance program, or meeting with key community members about a specific preventive program. In reality, the nurse typically spends the day responding to the emergency of the minute, hour, or day, which prevents incremental progress toward "big picture" initiatives and population-based programs. When faced with multiple demands, nurses must be vigilant in devoting a sustained effort toward population-focused projects. Daily pressures can easily distract the nurse from a population-based nursing practice. A strong foundation in upstream thinking and practice can help redirect nursing activities toward promoting health and reducing risk within the community.

A theoretical focus on the individual can preclude understanding of a larger perspective. Dreher (1982)

TABLE 3-1

Microscopic vs. Macroscopic Approaches to the Delineation of Community Health Nursing Problems

Microscopic Approach	Macroscopic Approach
Examines individual, and sometimes family, responses to health and illness.	Examines interfamily and intercommunity themes in health and illness. Delineates factors in the population that perpetuate the development of illness or foster the development of health.
Often emphasizes behavioral responses to individual's illness or lifestyle patterns.	Emphasizes social, economic, and environmental precursors of illness.
Nursing interventions are often aimed at modifying individual's behavior through changing his or her perceptions or belief system.	Nursing interventions may include modifying social or environmental variables (i.e., working to remove care barriers and improving sanitation or living conditions). May involve social or political action.

used the term **conservative scope of practice** in describing frameworks that focus energy exclusively on intrapatient and nurse-patient factors. She stated that such frameworks often adopt psychological explanations of patient behavior. This mode of thinking attributes low compliance, missed appointments, and reluctant participation to problems in patient motivation or attitude. Nurses are responsible for altering patient attitudes toward health rather than altering the system itself "even though such negative attitudes may well be a realistic appraisal of health care" (Dreher, 1982, p. 505). This perspective does not entertain the possibility of altering the system or empowering patients to make changes.

ASSESSING A THEORY'S SCOPE IN RELATION TO COMMUNITY HEALTH NURSING

Theoretical scope is especially important to community health nursing because there are many levels of practice within this specialty area. For example, a home health nurse who is caring for ill people after hospitalization has a very different scope of practice than a nurse epidemiologist or health planner. Although it is important that all nurses practice with an understanding of population health, this understanding is critical for nurses whose practice is founded on interpopulation rather than intrapopulation dynamics. Unless a given theory is broad enough in scope to address health and the determinants of health from a population perspective, the theory will not be very useful to community health nurses. Although the past 25 years yielded many advancements in the development of nursing theory, there continues to be a lack of clarity about community health nursing's theoretical foundation (Batra, 1991). Applying the terms *microscopic* and *macroscopic* to health situations may help nurses fill this void and stimulate theory development in community health nursing.

Although the concept of "macroscopic" is similar to the upstream analogy, the term *macroscopic* refers to a broad scope that incorporates many variables to aid in understanding a health problem. **Upstream thinking** would fall within this domain. Viewing a problem from this perspective emphasizes the variables that precede or play a role in the development of health problems. Macroscopic is the broad concept and upstream is a more specific

concept. These related concepts and their meanings can help nurses develop a critical eye in evaluating a theory's relevance to population health.

REVIEW OF THEORETICAL APPROACHES

The differences among theoretical approaches demonstrate how a nurse may draw very diverse conclusions about the reasons for client behavior and the range of available interventions. The following section uses two theories to exemplify individual *microscopic* approaches to community health nursing problems; one originates within nursing and one is based in social psychology. Two other theories demonstrate the examination of nursing problems from a *macroscopic* perspective; one originates from nursing and another has roots in phenomenology. The format for this review follows:

1. The individual is the locus of change (i.e., microscopic)
   a. Orem's self-care deficit theory of nursing
   b. The health belief model (HBM)
2. Thinking upstream: society is the locus of change (i.e., macroscopic)
   a. Milio's framework for prevention
   b. Critical social theory

The Individual Is the Locus of Change

Orem's Self-Care Deficit Theory of Nursing

Dorothea Orem was a staff and private duty nurse and later worked in the faculty at Catholic University of America. Her combined experience provided the basis for her self-care deficit theory of nursing. In 1958, Orem began to formalize her insights about the purpose of nursing activities and why individuals required nursing care (Eben et al., 1986). The theory is based on the assumption that self-care needs and activities are the primary focus of nursing practice. Orem outlined her general theory of nursing and stated that this general theory is actually a composite of the following related constructs: the theory of self-care deficits, which provides criteria for identifying those who need nursing; the theory of self-care, which explains self-care and why it is necessary; the theory of nursing systems, which specifies nursing's role in the delivery of care and how nursing helps people. The major concepts from Orem's **Self-care**

Deficit Theory (Orem, 1985, p. 31) include the following:

CONCEPTS FROM OREM'S SELF-CARE DEFICIT THEORY

■ Self-care: "The production of actions directed to self or to the environment in order to regulate one's functioning in the interest of one's life, integrated functioning, and well-being."

■ Therapeutic self-care demand: "The measures of care required at moments in time in order to meet existent requisites for regulatory action to maintain life and to maintain or promote health, development, and general well-being."

■ Self-care agency: "The complex capability for action that is activated in the performance of the actions or operations of self-care."

■ Self-care deficit: "A relationship between self-care agency and therapeutic self-care demand in which self-care agency is not adequate to meet the known therapeutic self-care demand."

■ Nursing agency: "The complex capability for action that is activated by nurses in their determination of needs for, design of, and production of nursing for people with a range of types of self-care deficits."

■ Nursing system: "A continuing series of actions produced when nurses link one way or a number of ways of helping to meet their own actions or the actions of people under care that are directed to meet these persons' therapeutic self-care demands or to regulate their self-care agency."

The basic concepts of this theory evolved from observing the chronology of illness in hospitalized patients. The theory is based on the premise that nursing is a response to a sick person's inability to administer self-care. Nursing assumes the role of providing some or all self-care activities on the patient's behalf (Orem, 1985). This focus makes the content and scope of the theory most useful to nurses practicing within an institutionalized setting. Orem briefly specified the role of population-based nursing

in the third edition of her book, *Nursing: Concepts of Practice* (1985). However, the concepts of self-care, self-care deficit, and self-care agency are so embedded in an individual orientation to disease, that applying these concepts to a population can be awkward. In this theory, the process of assessing a patient's abilities supersedes the upstream concepts— environmental, social, and economic—that may explain the development and perpetuation of the community's health problems.

Application of Self-Care Deficit Theory

During a discussion about theory-based initiatives, a British nurse lamented over her nursing supervisors' intention to adopt Orem's self-care deficit theory. It would become the primary theory for her specialty area of occupational health nursing. She was frustrated and argued that much of the model's assumptions seemed incongruous with the realities of her daily practice. Kennedy (1989) maintained that the self-care deficit theory assumes that people are able to exert purposeful control over their environments in the pursuit of health; however, people may have little control over the physical or social aspects of their work environment. On the basis of this thesis, she concluded that the self-care model is incompatible with the practice domain of occupational health nursing.

Kennedy exemplified the dissonance that nurses feel when a particular theory is inappropriately imposed in a work setting. Although it is easy to recognize the importance of Orem's concepts to many arenas of nursing practice, it is also apparent that her perspective would not lend itself well to understanding the diverse health needs of people in a work site. Kennedy clearly articulated this position when she stated that "the many facets of the occupational health nurse's role may 'fit in comfortably with Orem's self-care model.' But will Orem's model fit into the many facets of the occupational health nurse's role? That is the key question we should be asking" (p. 354).

The Health Belief Model

The second theory that focuses on the individual as the locus of change is the **HBM**. The model evolved from the premise that the world of the perceiver determines action. The model had its inceptions during the late 1950s when America was breathing a collective sigh of relief after the development of the polio vaccine. Although a life-saving vaccine finally

FIGURE 3-1

Variables and relationships in the HBM (Redrawn from Rosenstock IM: Historical origins of the health belief model. In Becker MH, editor: *The health belief model and personal health behavior,* Thorofare, NJ, 1974, Charles B. Slack).

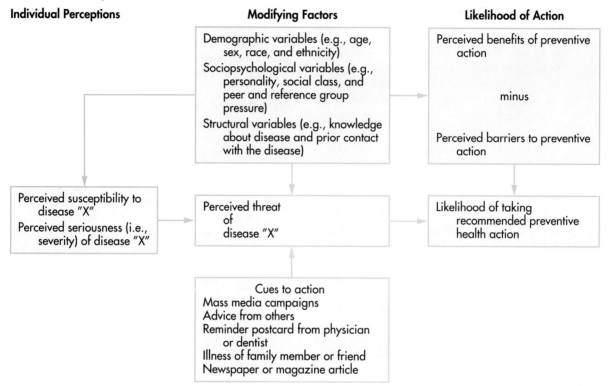

came into existence, health professionals were stymied when some people chose not to bring themselves or their children into clinics for immunization. Social psychologists and other public health workers recognized the need to develop a more complete understanding of factors that influence preventive health behaviors. Their efforts resulted in the HBM.

Kurt Lewin's work lent itself to the model's core dimensions. He proposed that behavior is based on current dynamics confronting an individual rather than prior experiences (Maiman and Becker, 1974). Within this framework, diseases are regions of negative valence, which act to repel the individual. Fig. 3-1 outlines the variables and relationships in the HBM. The model assumes that the major determinant of preventive health behavior is disease avoidance. Major concepts include perceived susceptibility to disease "X," perceived seriousness of disease "X," modifying factors, cues to action, perceived benefits minus barriers of preventive health action, perceived

threat of disease "X," and the likelihood of taking a recommended health action; the arrows specify the direction between concepts. Disease "X" represents a particular disorder that a health action may prevent. Importantly, actions that relate to breast cancer will be different from those relating to measles. For example, in breast cancer, a cue to action may involve a public service advertisement encouraging women to make an appointment for a mammogram. However, for measles, a cue to action may be news of a measles outbreak in a neighboring town.

Application of the Health Belief Model

Over the years, a number of authors have proposed broadening the scope of the HBM to address health promotion and illness behaviors (Kirscht, 1974; Pender, 1987) and to merge its concepts with other theories that describe health behavior (Cummings, Becker, and Malie, 1980). This conceptualization of health and health behaviors represented my first encounter with the power of theory-based practice. The following section contains a brief personal account of my perceptions addressing the strengths and limitations of the model.

My first class in nursing theory followed a format similar to many other courses throughout the country. Each week students considered a new theoretical perspective. Faculty and classmates explored the theorist's background, the theory's assumptions, the theory's concepts and relational statements, and discussed the theory's application to nursing practice. Like many other students, I was experiencing mixed feelings about the class. Most of the content was intellectually interesting, but I found it difficult applying the concepts to patients in neighborhood clinics and those at home. Several weeks into the class, we reviewed the HBM. My interest was immediately piqued; the model captured a perspective on health that was different from any other framework or nursing theory. After the seminar, I went to the library and checked out *The Health Belief Model and Personal Health Behavior* by Marshall Becker (1974) and became absorbed in the book.

The model's focus on compliance was something that many nurses could relate to in their own clinical practice. For the first time, the HBM offered me some insight into patient behavior and helped me organize ideas about why people choose to disregard the instructions of well-intended nurses and doctors. I was intrigued by the way the model interpreted behaviors from the patient's perspective rather than the nurse's perspective. Concepts such as "perceived seriousness," "perceived susceptibility," and "cue to action" afforded new insights into the dynamics of health decision making. The HBM provided answers to problems that many nurses encountered in their everyday clinical practice.

I began to apply the model's concepts to guide my clinical work with some families in the community. One such family had never immunized their 18-month-old son. The father owned a health food store and shunned the use of anything deemed "unnatural." The family believed that childhood immunization for polio, tetanus, measles, and such belonged in the "unnatural" group. In my assessment, I concluded that the family failed to immunize the child because the parents did not perceive the susceptibility and seriousness of childhood illnesses; they belonged to a reference group that disdained most traditional medical practices and favored inaction over action. During the next few weeks, I mapped out a strategy that would focus on raising the parents' perceived susceptibility to childhood illnesses by providing them with information about communicable diseases. During the next three visits, I inundated the family with literature and pictures that graphically demonstrated the sequelae of diphtheria, polio, and pertussis. Eventually the parents took their son to an immunization clinic for his first shot.

Twenty years later, I still have mixed feelings about the means I used to drive this family's compliance to the accepted standard of pediatric health care. For the most part, the family's actions were not based on any true insight into the risks and benefits of childhood immunization; they wanted to please me and avoid further criticism. My training in community health nursing provided me with a very real understanding of the risks incurred when children are not protected against communicable diseases. It is also important to understand that infectious disease prevention is only effective at the population level if the decision to immunize originates within a collective understanding of families within the community. Nurses can be most effective when they work within schools, industries, and civic organizations to provide education and a supportive environment that promotes healthy choices.

In the years since this experience, I have become more skilled in assessing and labeling patient problems and have gained a better appreciation for the strengths and limitations that any theoretical framework imposes on a situation.

Limitations of the Health Belief Model

The HBM places the burden of action exclusively on the client. It assumes that only those clients who have distorted or negative perceptions of the specified disease or recommended health action will fail to act. In practice, this model focuses the nurse's energies on interventions designed to modify the client's distorted perceptions.

True to its historical roots, the model offers an explanation of health behaviors that is similar to a mechanical system. Consulting the HBM, a nurse may induce compliance by using model variables as catalysts to stimulate action. For example, an intervention study based on HBM precepts sought to increase follow-up in hypertensive clients by increasing their perceived susceptibility and seriousness to the dangers of hypertension (Jones, Jones, and Katz, 1987). In addition, the study provided patients with education over the telephone or in the emergency department, which was designed to increase their perception of the benefits of follow-up. According to the authors, the interventions resulted in a dramatic increase in compliance. However, they noted that several patient groups failed to respond to the intervention. In particular, a small group of patients without available child care failed to comply. Although this study demonstrates the predictive power of HBM concepts, it also exemplifies the model's limitations. The HBM may effectively promote behavior change by altering patients' perspectives, but it does not acknowledge the health professional's responsibility to reduce or ameliorate health care barriers.

The HBM is a prototype for the type of theoretical perspective that has dominated nursing education and nursing practice. The narrow scope of the model is its strength and its limitation; the nurse is not drawn outside the scope to the forces that shape the model's characteristics.

The Upstream View: Society is the Locus of Change

Milio's Framework for Prevention

Milio's framework for prevention (1976) provides a thought-provoking complement to the HBM and provides a mechanism for directing attention upstream and examining opportunities for nursing intervention at the population level. Milio outlined six propositions that relate an individual's ability to improve healthful behavior to a society's ability to provide accessible and socially affirming options for healthy choices. Milio used these propositions to move the focus of attention upstream. She conceded that the range of available health choices is critical in shaping a society's overall health status. In addition, she stated that policy decisions in governmental and private organizations shape the range of choices available to individuals. She believed that national-level policy making was the best way to favorably impact the health of most Americans rather than concentrating efforts on imparting information to change individual patterns of behavior.

Milio (1976) proposed that health deficits often result from an imbalance between a population's health needs and its health-sustaining resources. She stated that the diseases associated with excess (i.e., obesity and alcoholism) afflict affluent societies and the diseases that result from inadequate or unsafe food, shelter, and water afflict the poor. Within this context, the poor in affluent societies may experience the least desirable combination of factors. Milio cited the socioeconomic realities that deprive many Americans of a health-sustaining environment despite the fact that "cigarettes, sucrose, pollutants, and tensions are readily available to the poor" (1976, p. 436).

SET OF PROPOSITIONS PROPOSED BY MILIO

- "The health status of populations is the result of deprivation and/or excess of critical health-sustaining resources."
- "Behavior patterns of populations are a result of habitual selection from limited choices and these habits of choice are related to: (a) actual and perceived options available; (b) beliefs and expectations developed and refined over time by socialization, formal learning, and immediate experience."
- "Organizational behavior (decisions or policy-choices made by governmental/nongovernmental, national/nonnational; not-profit/for-profit, formal/nonformal organizations) sets the range of options available to individuals for their personal choice-making."
- "The choice-making of individuals at a given point in time concerning potentially health-promoting or health-damaging selections is affected by their effort to maximize valued resources."
- "Social change may be thought of as changes in patterns of behavior resulting from shifts in the choice-making of significant numbers of people within a population."
- "Health education, as the process of teaching and learning health-supporting information, can have little significantly extensive impact on behavior patterns, that is, on personal choice-making of groups of people, without the easy availability of new, or newly-perceived alternative health-promoting options for investing personal resources."

From Milio N: A framework for prevention: changing health-damaging to health-generating life patterns, *Am J Public Health* 66:435-439, 1976.

Personal and societal resources affect the range of health-promoting or health-damaging choices available to individuals. Personal resources include the individual's awareness, knowledge, beliefs, and the beliefs of the individual's family and friends. Money, time, and the urgency of other priorities are also personal resources. Community and national locale strongly influence societal resources. These resources include the availability and cost of health services, environmental protection, safe shelter, and the penalties or rewards for failure to select the given options.

Milio challenged health education's assumption that knowledge of health-generating behaviors implies an act in accordance with that knowledge. She cited the lifestyles of health professionals to support her argument. She proposed that "most human beings, professional or nonprofessional, provider or consumer, make the easiest choices available to them most of the time" (1976, p. 435). Health-promoting choices must be more readily available and less costly than health-damaging options for individuals to gain health and for society to improve health status. Milio's framework can enable a nurse to reframe this view by understanding the historic play of social forces that have limited the choices available to the parties involved.

Comparison of the Health Belief Model and Milio's Conceptualizations of Health

Milio's health resources bear some resemblance to the concepts in the HBM. The purpose of the HBM is to provide the nurse with an understanding of the dynamics of personal health behaviors. The HBM specifies broader contextual variables, such as the constraints of the health care system, and their influence on the individual's decision-making processes. In contrast, Milio based her framework on an assessment of community resources and their availability to individuals. This differs from the HBM, which may assume that each person has unlimited access to health resources and free will. By assessing such factors up front, the nurse is able to gain a more thorough understanding of the resources people actually have. Milio offered a different set of insights into the health behavior arena by proposing that many low-income individuals are acting within the constraints of their limited resources. Furthermore, she investigated beyond downstream focus and population health by examining the choices of significant numbers of people within a population.

Compared to the HBM, Milio's framework provides for the inclusion of economic, political, and environmental health determinants; therefore the nurse is given broader range in the diagnosis and interpretation of health problems. Whereas the HBM allows only two possible outcomes (i.e., "acts" or "fails to act" according to the recommended health action), Milio's framework encourages the nurse to understand health behaviors in the context of their societal milieu.

Implications of Milio's Framework to the Current Health Delivery Systems

Through its broader scope, Milio's model allows nursing intervention at many levels; for example, nurses may assess the personal and societal resources of individual patients and analyze social and economic factors that may inhibit healthy choices in populations. Population-based interventions may include such diverse activities as mobilizing comprehensive smoking cessation programs in schools and work places and encouraging political activity that calls for an end to federal subsidization of health-damaging industry.

The health care system's current emphasis on efficient care has favored the employment of NPs and advanced practice nurses in settings previously dominated by physician practice. Such settings include managed care and HMOs. Overall, this change is favorable because this type of practice allows a certain level of independence and autonomy. However, the short-term goal of efficient care may preclude broader-based interventions that require significant amounts of nursing time (i.e., individualized patient education and anticipatory guidance). Such care is poorly quantified in billing taxonomies and may not yield immediate results; therefore it may not be cost effective and may be discouraged at the system level. Barnes and colleagues (1995) cautioned that the provision of primary care from a narrow perspective of health determinants leads to nursing's perpetuation of institutionally driven and controlled medical care rather than providing broad-based health care grounded in essential human needs. The authors emphasize the facets of nursing care that address the provision of education and care services through the most direct, simple, and inexpensive means. This type of practice requires a conceptual and operational appreciation of "the larger sociopolitical context within which the health care is delivered and in which health evolves, that is, to the inextricable relationships between health status and levels of poverty, employment, education, quality of life, and general community development" (Barnes et al., 1995, p. 10).

Overall, current health care delivery systems perform best when responding to people with diagnostic-intensive and acute illnesses. Those people who experience chronic debilitation or have less intriguing diagnoses generally fare worse in the health care system despite efforts by community- and home-based care to "fill the gaps." Nurses in both hospital and community-based systems often feel constrained by profound financial and service restrictions imposed by third-party payers. These third parties often terminate nursing care after the resolution of the latest immediate health crisis and fail to cover care aimed toward long-term health improvements. Many health systems use nursing standards and reimbursement mechanisms that originate from a narrow, compartmentalized view of health; therefore it is imperative to practice nursing from a broader understanding of health, illness, and suffering.

Nursing and health service literature often focus on health care access issues. This topic is interesting because tremendous access disparities exist between insured and uninsured people in the United States. Access to care is associated with economic, social, and political factors and, depending on individual and population needs, it can be a primary determinant of health status and survival. Structural variables, such as race-ethnicity, educational status, gender, and income, may be highly predictive of health status. These types of factors, which are also strongly grounded in the sociopolitical and economic milieu, identify risk factors for poor health and opportunities for community-based interventions. Bird and Bauman (1995) used a unique combination of structural variables to explain 65% of the variation in each state's infant mortality. These variables included the percentage of people who graduated from high school, the median earnings ratio between men and women, and the number of times Republican presidential candidates carried each state in the past 20 years. This type of provocative research contained a broad conceptualization of health determinants and succeeded in reestablishing direct associations among demographic, social, and economic variables in infant mortality. Projects like these make more overt links between the precursors of mortality and their effect on individuals and the collective health of a society.

Milio's work focuses on society's opportunities to make healthy choices. In a related article (1981) she elaborated on this theme.

> Personal behavior patterns are not simply "free" choices about "lifestyle" that are isolated from their personal and economic context. Lifestyles are patterns of choices made from available alternatives according to people's socioeconomic circumstances and how easily they are able to choose some over others (Milio, 1981, p. 76).

Critical Social Theory

Milio used societal awareness to aid in the understanding of health behaviors. Similarly, **critical social theory** uses societal awareness to expose social inequalities that keep people from reaching their full potential. This theoretical approach is devised from the belief that social meanings structure life through social domination. Proponents of this theoretical approach maintain that social exchanges that are not distorted from power imbalances will stimulate the evolution of a more just society (Allen, Diekelmann, and Benner, 1986). Critical theory assumes that truth standards are socially determined and that no form of scientific inquiry is value free. Allen and colleagues (1986, p. 34) stated, "One cannot separate theory and value, as the empiricist claims. Every theory is penetrated by value interests."

Application of Critical Social Theory

Application of critical social theory uses the processes of inductive reasoning. Rather than superimposing concepts onto a situation, the nurse discovers relevant concepts through an ongoing process of data collection and analysis. Sources of data may include interviews with critical informants, news articles, and transcripts of governmental proceedings. For example, if the domain of interest involves child care options for employees of a large microcomputer manufacturer, data sources may initially include the age and gender distribution of the workers, a review of work site policies on parental leave, and interviews with both workers and administrative officials. Further into the analysis, the nurse may choose to incorporate additional sources of data, such as interviews with shift workers that address the difficulties in accessing evening and night time child care or statistics on job turnover among child care workers.

The methodological approaches adopted in critical social theory may also differ from those suggested

FIGURE 3-2

Continuum of health behaviors and corresponding intervention foci (From McKinlay JB: A case for refocusing upstream: the political economy of illness. In *Proceedings of an American Heart Association Conference: applying behavioral science to cardiovascular risk,* Seattle, June 17-19, 1979. Reproduced with permission. Copyright © American Heart Association).

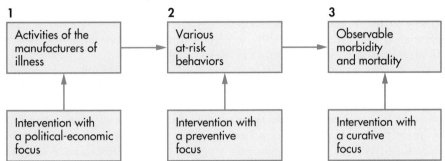

by other nursing theories. The theory does not mandate a specific method of analysis. It chooses methods that are congruent with the focus of study. The dialectic can be a methodological tool; the investigator seeks understanding by examining contradictions within the phenomena of interest. Continuing the previous example, the nurse may examine child care by applying critical social theory. The nurse may contrast an organization's policies with interviews from workers who believe the organization is an impediment to achieving quality child care. Data analysis may also include an examination of the interests of workers and administration in promoting social change vs. maintaining the status quo.

Wild (1993) used critical social theory to analyze the social, political, and economic conditions associated with the cost of prescription analgesics and the corresponding financial burden of clients who require these medications. Wild compared the trends in pharmaceutical pricing with the inflation rates of other commodities. The study stated that pharmaceutical sales techniques, which marketed directly to physicians, distanced the needs of ill clients from the pharmaceutical industry. A critique of this issue from a client perspective revealed limited access to information addressing the extreme variations in cost among different analgesics (e.g., greater than a tenfold difference in cost among similar drug formulations). Wild's analysis specified nursing actions that a downstream analysis would not consider, such as challenging pricing policies on behalf of client groups.

Challenging Assumptions about Preventive Health through Critical Social Theory

The HBM and Milio's prevention model focus on personal health behaviors from a disease avoidance or preventive health perspective; nurses may also analyze this phenomenon using critical social theory. Again, McKinlay's upstream analogy refers to health workers who were so busy fishing sick people out of the river that they did not look upstream to see who was pushing the sick into the water. Later in the same article, McKinlay used his upstream analogy to ask the rhetorical question, "How preventive is prevention?" (1979, p. 22). He used this tactic to critically examine different intervention strategies aimed at enhancing preventive behavior. Fig. 3-2 illustrates McKinlay's model, which contrasts the different modes of prevention. He linked health professionals' curative and lifestyle modification interventions to a downstream conceptualization of health; the majority of alleged preventive actions fail to alter the process of illness at its origin. Political-economic interventions remain the most effective way to address population determinants of health and ameliorate illness at its source.

McKinlay further delineated the activities of the "manufacturers of illness—those individuals, interest groups, and organizations which, in addition to producing material goods and services, also produce, as an inevitable byproduct, widespread morbidity and mortality" (1979, pp. 9-10). The manufacturers of illness embed desired behaviors in the dominant cultural norm and thus foster the habituation of high-risk behavior in the population. Unhealthy consumption patterns are integrated into everyday lives; for example, the American holiday dinner table offers concrete examples of "the binding of at-riskness to culture" (1979, p. 12). The existing health care system devotes its efforts in a misguided attempt to change the products of the illness manufacturers and neglects the processes that create the products.

Waitzkin (1983) continued this theme by asserting that the health care system's emphasis on lifestyle diverts attention from important sources of illness in the capitalist industrial environment and "it also puts the burden of health squarely on the individual rather than seeking collective solutions to health problems" (p. 664). Salmon (1987) supported this position by noting that the basic tenets of Western medicine promote an understanding of individual health and illness factors and obscure the exploration of their social and economic roots. He stated that critical social theory "can aid in uncovering larger dimensions impacting health that are usually unseen or misrepresented by ideological biases. Thus the social reality of health conditions can be both understood and changed" (1987, p. 75).

Nurses in all practice settings face the challenge of understanding and responding to collective health within the context of a health system that allocates resources at the individual level. The Tavistock Group (1999) released a set of ethical principles that summarizes this juxtaposition by noting that "the care of individuals is at the center of health care delivery, but must be viewed and practiced within the overall context of continuing work to generate the greatest possible health gains for groups and populations" (p. 2-3). This perspective is an accurate reflection of Western-oriented thought, which generally gives individual health precedence over collective health. Although nurses can appreciate the concept of individual care at the center of health delivery, they should also consider transposing this principle. This allows the nurse to consider a health care system that places the community in the center of health care and holds the goal of generating health gains for individuals. Fortunately, these worldviews of health delivery systems are not mutually exclusive and nurses can understand the duality of health care needs in individuals and populations.

SUMMARY

Community health nurses have been instrumental in making many of the life-saving advances in sanitation, communicable disease, and environmental con-

ditions that today's society takes for granted. Community health practice helps develop a broad context of nursing practice because community environments are inherently less restrictive than hospital settings. Clarke and colleagues compared the environmental characteristics in community-based settings to those in hospital-based settings. They proposed that the dynamic nature of community settings lends itself best to the education of professional nurses (Clarke and Cody, 1994).

In a discussion addressing the future of community health nursing, Bellack (1998) differentiates between "nursing in the community" and "nursing with the community." This subtle reframing of the nursing role reinforces the notion that the health agenda originates from natural leaders, church members, local officials, parents, children, teens, and other community members. Forming and advancing a shared vision of health can be a formidable challenge for the nurse; like any other complex issue, multiple viewpoints are the norm. Even "naming" health problems can be difficult, because different constituents are likely to see issues differently and pursue different lines of reasoning. However, allowing the genesis of change to occur from within the community is the essential challenge of nursing "with" the community. "Nursing with the community" efforts allow the nurse to create agendas that arise from community members rather than those imposed upon community members. Listening, being patient, providing accurate and scientifically sound information, and respecting the experiences of community members are essential to the success of these efforts.

Many delivery systems restrict the daily activities of nurses who seek to provide individuals and communities with the broadest context of health-sustaining care. This may seem disheartening, but nursing practice is determined by the needs of those served; therefore it is particularly resilient and adaptable to a wide variety of contextual variables.

The nursing profession has advanced and with it the need to develop and disseminate nursing theories to formalize the scientific base of nursing practice. The richness of community health nursing comes from the challenge of conceptualizing and implementing strategies that will enhance the health of many people. Likewise, nurses in this practice area must have access to theoretical perspectives that address the social, political, and environmental determinants of population health. The integration of population-based theory and practice gives nurses the means to favorably impact the health of the global community.

1. Select a theory or conceptual model. Evaluate its potential for understanding health in individuals, families, a population of 400 children in an elementary school, a community of 50,000 residents, and 2000 workers within a corporate setting.

2. Identify one health problem (e.g., substance abuse, domestic violence, or cardiovascular disease) that is prevalent in the community or city. Analyze the problem using two different theories or conceptual models. One should emphasize individual determinants of health and another should emphasize population determinants of health. What are some differences in the way these different perspectives inform nursing practice?

3. Review the ANA's definition of community health nursing practice and the APHA's definition of public health nursing practice, which is listed in Chapter 1. What do these definitions indicate about the theoretical basis of community health nursing? How does the theoretical basis of community health nursing practice differ from that of other nursing specialty areas?

REFERENCES

Allen DG, Diekelmann N, Benner P: Three paradigms for nursing research: methodologic implications. In Chinn P, editor: *Nursing research methodology: issues and implementation,* Rockville, Md, 1986, Aspen Publishers.

Barnes D et al: Primary health care and primary care: a confusion of philosophies, *Nurs Outlook* 43:7-16, 1995.

Barnum BJS: *Nursing theory: analysis, application, evaluation,* Glenview, Ill, 1990, Scott, Foresman/Little, Brown Higher Education.

Batra C: Professional issues: the future of community health nursing. In Cookfair JM, editor: *Nursing process and practice in the community,* St. Louis, 1991, Mosby.

Becker MH, editor: *The health belief model and personal health behavior,* Thorofare, NJ, 1974, Charles B. Slack.

Bellack JP: Community-based nursing practice: necessary but not sufficient, *J Nurs Educ* 37:99-100, 1998 (Guest editorial).

Bird ST, Bauman KE: The relationship between structural and health service variables and state-level infant mortality in the United States, *Am J Public Health* 85:26-29, 1995.

Chinn PL, Kramer MK: *Theory and nursing: integrated knowledge development,* ed 5, St. Louis, 1999, Mosby.

Clarke PN, Cody WK: Nursing theory-based practice in the home and community: the crux of professional nursing education, *Adv Nurs Sci* 17:41-53, 1994.

Cummings KM, Becker MH, Malie MC: Bringing the models together: an empirical approach to combining variables to explain health actions, *J Behav Med* 3:123-145, 1980.

Dickoff J, James P: A theory of theories: a position paper, *Nurs Res* 17:197-203, 1968.

Doty RE: Alternate theoretical perspectives: essential knowledge for the advanced practice nurse in the promotion of rural family health, *Clin Nurs Specialist* 10:217-219, 1996.

Dreher MC: The conflict of conservatism in public health nursing education, *Nurs Outlook* 30:504-509, 1982.

Eben JD et al: Self-care deficit theory of nursing. In Marriner A, editor: *Nursing theorists and their work,* St. Louis, 1986, Mosby.

Jones PK, Jones SL, Katz J: Improving follow-up among hypertensive patients using a health belief model intervention, *Arch Intern Med* 147:1557-1560, 1987.

Kennedy A: How relevant are nursing models? *Occup Health* 41:352-535, 1989.

Kirscht JP: The health belief model and illness behavior. In Becker MH, editor: *The health belief model and personal health behavior,* Thorofare, NJ, 1974, Charles B. Slack.

Maiman LA, Becker MH: The health belief model: origins and correlates in psychological theory. In Becker MH, editor: *The health belief model and personal health behavior,* Thorofare, NJ, 1974, Charles B. Slack.

McKinlay JB: A case for refocusing upstream: the political economy of illness. In *Proceedings of an American Heart Association Conference: applying behavioral science to cardiovascular risk,* Seattle, June 17-19, 1979.

Milio N: A framework for prevention: changing health-damaging to health-generating life patterns, *Am J Public Health* 66:435-439, 1976.

Milio N: *Promoting health through public policy,* Philadelphia, 1981, FA Davis.

Orem DE: *Nursing: concepts of practice,* ed 3, New York, 1985, McGraw-Hill.

Pender NJ: *Health promotion in nursing practice,* ed 2, Norwalk, Conn, 1987, Appleton-Century-Crofts.

Pryjmachuk S: A nursing perspective on the interrelationship between theory, research, and practice, *J Adv Nurs* 23:679-684, 1996.

Rosenstock IM: Historical origins of the health belief model. In Becker MH, editor: *The health belief model and personal health behavior,* Thorofare, NJ, 1974, Charles B. Slack.

Salmon JW: Dilemmas in studying social change versus individual change: considerations from political economy. In Duffy M, Pender NJ, editors: *Conceptual issues in health promotion: a report of proceedings of a Wingspread Conference,* Indianapolis, Ind, 1987, Sigma Theta Tau.

Swanson JM: Personal communication, May 1992.

Tavistock Group: A shared statement of ethical principles for those who shape and give health care: a working draft from the Tavistock Group, *Image J Nurs Sch* 31:2-3, 1999.

Torres G: *Theoretical foundations of nursing,* Norwalk, Conn, 1986, Appleton-Century-Crofts.

Waitzkin H: A Marxist view of health and health care. In Mechanic D, editor: *Handbook of health, health care, and the health professions,* New York, 1983, Free Press.

Wild LR: Caveat emptor: a critical analysis of the costs of drugs used for pain management, *Adv Nurs Sci* 16:52-61, 1993.

Woods NF, Catanzaro M: *Nursing research: theory and practice,* St. Louis, 1988, Mosby.

The Art and Science of Community Health Nursing

4 Epidemiology

5 Community Assessment

6 Community Health Planning, Implementation, and Evaluation

7 Community Health Education

8 Case Management

4

Epidemiology

Holly Cassells

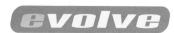

http://evolve.elsevier.com/Nies/

Epidemiology is the study of the distribution and determinants of health and disease in human populations (Harkness, 1995) and is the principal science of community health practice. It entails a body of knowledge derived from epidemiological research and specialized epidemiological methods and approaches to scientific research. Community health nurses use epidemiological concepts to improve the health of population groups by identifying risk factors and optimal approaches that reduce disease risk. Epidemiological methods are important for accurate community assessment and diagnosis, and in planning and evaluating effective community interventions. This chapter discusses the uses of epidemiology and its specialized methodologies.

USE OF EPIDEMIOLOGY IN DISEASE CONTROL AND PREVENTION

Although epidemiology originated in ancient times, formal epidemiological techniques developed in the nineteenth century. Early applications focused on identifying factors associated with infectious diseases and the epidemic spread of disease in the community. Public health practitioners hoped to improve preventive strategies by identifying critical factors in disease development.

Specifically, investigators attempted to identify characteristics of people who suffered from a disease such as cholera or plague and compared them with characteristics of those who remained healthy. These differences might include a broad range of personal factors such as age, socioeconomic status, and health status. Investigators also questioned whether there were differences in the location or living environment of ill people compared with healthy individuals and whether these factors influenced disease development. Finally, researchers examined whether common time factors existed (i.e., when people acquired disease). Use of this **person-place-time model** organized epidemiologists' investigations of the disease pattern in the community. This study of the amount and distribution of disease constitutes *descriptive epidemiology*. Identified patterns frequently indicate possible causes of disease that epidemiologists can examine with more advanced epidemiological methods.

In addition to investigating the person, place, and time factors related to disease, epidemiologists

> **PERSON-PLACE-TIME MODEL**
> Person: "Who" factors such as demographic characteristics, health, and disease status.
> Place: "Where" factors such as geographical location, climate and environmental conditions, and political and social environment.
> Time: "When" factors such as time of day, week, or month and secular trends over months and years.

examine complex relationships among the many determinants of disease. This investigation of the causes of disease, or etiology, is called *analytic epidemiology*.

Even before the identification of bacterial agents, public health practitioners recognized that single factors were insufficient to cause disease. For example, while exploring the cholera epidemics in 1855, Dr. John Snow collected data about social and physical environmental conditions that might favor disease development. He specifically examined the contamination of local water systems. Snow also gathered information about people who became ill; this included their living patterns, their water sources, their socioeconomic characteristics, and their health status. A comprehensive data base helped him develop a theory about the possible cause of the epidemic. Snow suspected that a single biological agent was responsible for the cholera infection, although the organism, *Vibrio cholerae*, was undiscovered. He compared the death rates among individuals using one source of water with those among people using a different water source. This suggested an association between cholera and water quality.

The epidemiologist examines the interrelationships between host and environmental characteristics and uses an organized method of inquiry to derive an explanation of disease. This model of investigation is called the **epidemiological triangle** because the epidemiologist must analyze the following three elements: agent, host, and environment (Fig. 4-1). The development of disease is dependent upon the extent of the host's exposure to an agent, the strength or virulence of the agent, and the host's genetic or immunological susceptibility. Disease is also dependent upon the environmental conditions existing at the time of exposure, which includes the biological, social, political, and physical environment (Table 4-1). The model implies that the rate of disease will change when the balance among these three factors is altered. By examining each of the three elements, a community health nurse can methodically assess a health problem, determine protective factors, and evaluate the factors that make the host vulnerable to disease.

Conditions linked to clearly identifiable agents such as bacteria, chemicals, toxins, and other exposure factors are readily explained by the epidemiological triangle. However, other models that stress the multiplicity of host and environmental interactions have developed and understanding of disease has progressed. The "wheel model" is an example of such a model (Fig. 4-2). The wheel consists of a hub that represents the host and its human characteristics such as genetic make-up, personality, and immunity. The surrounding wheel represents the environment and comprises biological, social, and physical dimensions. The relative size of each component in the wheel depends on the health problem. A relatively large genetic core represents health conditions associated with heredity. Origins of other health conditions may be more dependent on environmental factors (Mausner and Kramer, 1985). This model subscribes to multiple-causation rather than single-causation disease theory; therefore it is more useful for analyzing complex chronic conditions and identifying factors that are amenable to intervention.

FIGURE 4-1

Epidemiological triangle.

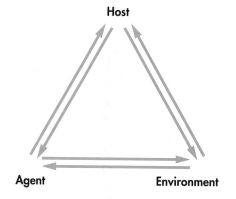

Host

Agent   Environment

AN EXAMPLE OF THE EPIDEMIOLOGICAL APPROACH

An early example of the epidemiological approach is John Snow's investigation of a cholera epidemic in the 1850s. He analyzed the distribution of person, place, and time factors by comparing the death rates among people living in different geographical sectors of London.

TABLE 4-1

A Classification of Agent, Host, and Environmental Factors that Determine the Occurrence of Diseases in Human Populations

Agents of Disease—Etiologic Factors	Examples
A. Nutritive elements	
Excesses	Cholesterol
Deficiencies	Vitamins, proteins
B. Chemical agents	
Poisons	Carbon monoxide, carbon tetrachloride, drugs
Allergens	Ragweed, poison ivy, medications
C. Physical agents	Ionizing radiation, mechanical

Modified from Lilienfeld DE, Stoley PD: *Foundations of epidemiology,* New York, 1994, Oxford University Press.

Continued

T A B L E 4-1—cont'd

A Classification of Agent, Host, and Environmental Factors that Determine the Occurrence of Diseases in Human Populations—cont'd

Agents of Disease—Etiologic Factors	Examples
D. Infectious agents	
Metazoa	Hookworm, schistosomiasis, onchocerciasis
Protozoa	Amoebae, malaria
Bacteria	Rheumatic fever, lobar pneumonia, typhoid, TB, syphilis
Fungi	Histoplasmosis, athlete's foot
Rickettsia	Rocky mountain spotted fever, typhus, Lyme disease
Viruses	Measles, mumps, chicken pox, small pox, poliomyelitis, rabies, yellow fever, HIV

Host Factors (i.e., Intrinsic Factors)—Influence Exposure, Susceptibility, or Response to Agent	Examples
A. Genetic	Cystic fibrosis, Huntington's disease
B. Age	Alzheimer's disease
C. Sex	Rheumatoid arthritis
D. Ethnic group	Tay-Sachs disease, sickle cell disease
E. Physiological state	Fatigue, pregnancy, puberty, stress, nutritional state
F. Prior immunological experience	Hypersensitivity, protection
Active	Prior infection, immunization
Passive	Maternal antibodies, gamma globulin prophylaxis
G. Intercurrent or preexisting disease	
H. Human behavior	Personal hygiene, food handling, diet, interpersonal contact, occupation, recreation, use of health resources, tobacco use

Environmental Factors (i.e., Extrinsic Factors)—Influence Existence of the Agent, Exposure, or Susceptibility to Agent	Examples
A. Physical environment	Geology, climate
B. Biological environment	
Human populations	Density
Flora	Sources of food, influence on vertebrates and arthropods, as a source of agents
Fauna	Food sources, vertebrate hosts, arthropod vectors
C. Socioeconomic environment	
Occupation	Exposure to chemical agents
Urbanization and economic development	Urban crowding, tensions and pressures, cooperative efforts in health and education
Disruption	Wars, floods

Modified from Lilienfeld DE, Stoley PD: *Foundations of epidemiology,* New York, 1994, Oxford University Press.

Snow noted that people using a particular water pump had significantly higher mortality rates resulting from cholera than people using other water sources in the city. Although the cholera organism was yet unidentified, the clustering of disease cases around one neighborhood pump suggested new prevention strategies to public health officials (i.e., that cholera might be reduced in a community by controlling contaminated drinking water sources) (Snow, 1936).

Following the discovery of the causative agents of many infectious diseases, public health interventions that eventually resulted in a decline in widespread epidemic mortality, particularly in developed countries. This caused the focus of public health to shift to chronic diseases such as cancer, coronary heart disease, and diabetes during the past few decades. These chronic diseases tend to have multiple interrelated factors associated with their development rather than a single causative agent.

In studying chronic diseases, epidemiologists use methods that are similar to those used in infectious disease investigation, thereby developing theories about chronic disease control. Risk factor identification is of particular importance to chronic disease reduction. Risk factors are variables that increase the rate of disease in people who have them (e.g., a genetic predisposition) or in those exposed to them (e.g., an infectious agent or a diet high in saturated fat). Therefore their identification is critical to identifying specific prevention and intervention approaches that effectively and efficiently reduce chronic disease morbidity and mortality. For example, the identification of cardiovascular disease risk factors has suggested a number of lifestyle modifications that could reduce the morbidity risk before disease onset. Primary prevention strategies such as dietary saturated fat reduction, smoking cessation, and hypertension control developed in response to previous epidemiological studies that identified these risk factors. The **web of causation** model illustrates the complexity of relationships among causal variables for heart disease (Fig. 4-3).

FIGURE 4-2

Wheel model of human-environment interaction (Redrawn from Mausner JS, Kramer S: *Mausner and Bahn epidemiology: an introductory text,* ed 2, Philadelphia, 1985, WB Saunders).

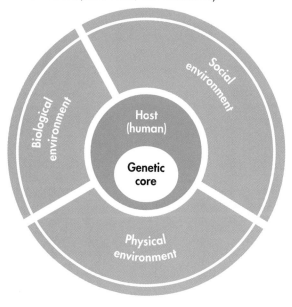

CORONARY HEART DISEASE RISK FACTORS SUPPORTED BY EPIDEMIOLOGICAL DATA

- Age: Male aged 45 years
- Female aged 55 years or premature menopause without estrogen replacement therapy
- Family history of premature coronary heart disease (i.e., definite myocardial infarction or sudden death before age 55 in father, or other first-degree male relative or before age 65 in mother, or other first-degree female relative)
- Current cigarette smoking
- Hypertension (i.e., blood pressure 140/90 mm Hg or prescribed antihypertensive medication)
- Low HDL cholesterol (<35 mg/dL)
- Diabetes mellitus

Data from Summary of the National Cholesterol Education Program (NCEP) expert panel on detection, evaluation, and treatment of high blood cholesterol in adults (adult treatment panel II), *JAMA* 269:3015-3023, 1993.

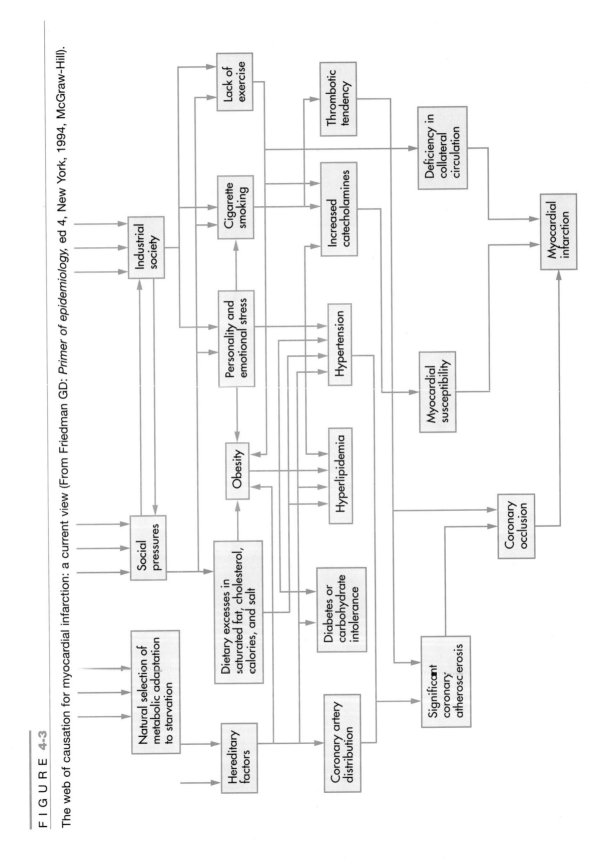

F I G U R E 4-3

The web of causation for myocardial infarction: a current view (From Friedman GD: *Primer of epidemiology*, ed 4, New York, 1994, McGraw-Hill).

CALCULATION OF RATES

The community health nurse must analyze data about the health of the community to determine the pattern of disease in a community. The nurse may collect data by conducting surveys or compiling data from existing records (e.g., data from clinic facilities or vital statistics records). Often assessment data are in the form of counts or simple frequencies of events (e.g., the number of people with a specific health condition). Community health practitioners interpret these raw counts by transforming them into rates.

Rates are arithmetic expressions that help practitioners consider a count of an event relative to the size of the population from which it is extracted (e.g., the population at risk). Rates are population proportions or fractions in which the numerator is the number of events occurring in a specified period of time. The denominator consists of those in the population at the specified time period (e.g., per day, per week, or per year). This proportion is multiplied by a constant *(k)* that is a multiple of 10, such as 1000, 10,000, or 100,000. The constant usually converts the resultant number to a whole number, which is larger and easier to interpret. Thus a rate can be the number of cases of a disease occurring for every 1000, 10,000 or 100,000 people in the population.

$$\text{Rate} = \frac{\text{Numerator}}{\text{Denominator}} = \frac{\text{Number of health events in a specified period}}{\text{Population in same area in same specified period}} \times k$$

When raw counts are converted to rates, the community health nurse can make meaningful comparisons with rates from other districts or states, from the nation, and from previous time periods. These analyses assist the nurse in determining the magnitude of a public health problem in a given area and allow more reliable tracking of trends in the community over time.

USING RATES IN EVERYDAY COMMUNITY HEALTH NURSING PRACTICE

The following school situation exemplifies the value of rates:

A community health nurse screened 500 students for TB in the Southside School and identified 15 students with newly positive tuberculin tests. The proportion of Southside School students affected was 15/500, or 0.03 (3%), or a rate of 30/1000 students at risk for TB. Concurrently, the nurse conducted screening in the Northside School and again identified 15 positive tuberculin tests. However, this school was much larger than the Southside School and had 900 potentially at-risk students. To place the number of affected students in perspective relative to the size of the Northside School, the nurse calculated a proportion of 15/900, or 0.017 (1.7%), or a rate of 17/1000 students at risk.

On the basis of this comparison, the nurse concluded that although both schools had *equal numbers* of tuberculin conversions, Southside School had the *greater rate* of tuberculin test conversions. Based on this information, the nurse could then explore reasons for the difference in these rates.

Sometimes a ratio is used to express a relationship between two variables. A ratio is obtained by dividing one quantity by another and the numerator is not necessarily part of the denominator. For example, a ratio could contrast the number of male births to that of female births. Proportions can describe characteristics of a population. A proportion is often a percentage and it represents the numerator as part of the denominator.

Morbidity: Incidence and Prevalence Rates

The two principal types of **morbidity rates**, or rates of illness, in public health are incidence rates and prevalence rates. **Incidence rates** describe the occurrence of *new* cases of a disease or condition (e.g., teen pregnancy) in a community over a period of time relative to the size of the population at risk for that disease or condition during that same time period. The denominator consists of only those at risk for the disease or condition; therefore known cases or those not susceptible (e.g., those immunized against a disease) are subtracted from the total population.

$$\text{Incidence rate} = \frac{\text{Number of new cases or events occurring in the population in a specified period}}{\text{Population at risk during same specified period}} \times k$$

The incidence rate may be the most sensitive indicator of the changing health of a community because it captures the fluctuations of disease in a population. Although incidence rates are valuable for monitoring trends in chronic disease, they are particularly useful for detecting short-term acute disease changes—such as those that occur with infectious hepatitis or measles—when the duration of the disease is typically short.

If a population is exposed to an infectious disease at a given time and place, the nurse may calculate the **attack rate**, a specialized form of the incidence rate. Attack rates document the number of new cases of a disease in those exposed to the disease. A common example of the application of the attack rate is food poisoning; the denominator is the number of people exposed to a suspect food and the numerator is the number of people who were exposed *and* became ill. The nurse can calculate and compare the attack rates of illness among those exposed to specific foods to identify the critical food sources or exposure variables.

A **prevalence rate** is the number of *all* cases of a specific disease or condition (e.g., deafness) in a population at a given point in time relative to the population at the same point in time.

$$\text{Prevalence rate} = \frac{\substack{\text{Number of existing cases}\\\text{in population at a}\\\text{specified point in time}}}{\substack{\text{Population at same}\\\text{specified point in time}}} \times k$$

When prevalence rates describe the number of people with the disease at a specific point in time, they are sometimes called *point prevalences*. For this reason, cross-sectional studies frequently use them. *Period prevalences* represent the number of existing cases during a specified period or interval of time and include old cases and new cases that develop within the same period of time.

The following factors influence prevalence rates: the number of people who experience a particular condition (i.e., incidence) and the duration of the condition. A nurse can derive the prevalence rate by multiplying incidence by duration ($P = I \times D$). An increase in the incidence rate or the duration of a disease increases the prevalence rate of a disease. With the advent of life-prolonging therapies (e.g., insulin for treatment of type I diabetes mellitus), the prevalence of a disease may increase without a change in the incidence rate. Those who survive a chronic disease without cure remain in the "preva-

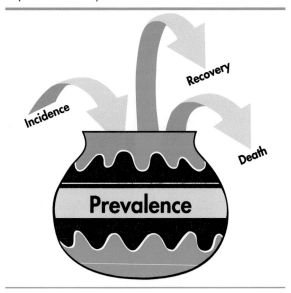

FIGURE 4-4

Prevalence pot: the relationship between incidence and prevalence (Redrawn from Morton RF, Hebel JR, McCarter RJ: *A study guide to epidemiology and biostatistics,* ed 3, Gaithersburg, Md, 1990, Aspen Publishers).

lence pot" (Fig. 4-4). For conditions such as cataracts, surgical removal permits many people to recover and thereby move out of the prevalence pot. Although the incidence has not necessarily changed, the reduced duration of the disease lowers the prevalence rate of cataracts in the population.

Morbidity rates are not available for many conditions because surveillance of many chronic diseases is not widely conducted. Furthermore, morbidity rates may be subject to underreporting when they are available. Routinely collected birth and death rates, or **mortality rates**, are more widely available.

Other Rates

Numerous other rates are useful in characterizing the health of a population. For example, **crude rates** summarize the occurrence of births (i.e., crude birth rate), mortality (i.e., crude death rates), or diseases (i.e., crude disease rates) in the general population. The numerator is the number of events and the denominator is the average population size or the population size at midyear (i.e., usually July 1) multiplied by a constant.

The denominators of crude rates represent the total population and not the population at risk for a given event; therefore these rates are subject to certain biases in interpretation. Crude death rates are sensitive to the number of people at the highest risk for dying. A relatively older population will probably produce a higher crude death rate than a population with a more evenly distributed age range. Conversely, a young population will have a somewhat lower crude death rate. Similar biases can occur for crude birth rates (e.g., higher birth rates in young populations). This distortion occurs because the denominator reflects the entire population and not exclusively the population at risk for giving birth. Age is one of the most common confounding factors that can mask the true distribution of variables. However, many variables such as race and socioeconomic status can also bias the interpretation of biostatistical data. Therefore the nurse may use several approaches for removing the confounding effect of these variables on rates.

Age-specific rates characterize a particular age group in the population and usually consider deaths and births. Determining the rate for specific subgroups of a population and using a denominator that reflects only that subgroup removes age bias.

$$\text{Age-specific rate} = \frac{\begin{array}{c}\text{Number of cases in a specific}\\\text{age category in population}\\\text{at a specified time}\end{array}}{\begin{array}{c}\text{Population in the same age}\\\text{category at the same}\\\text{specified time}\end{array}} \times k$$

To characterize a total population using age-specific rates, rates for each category must be computed because a single summary rate such as a mean is not used to characterize a total population using age-specific rates. Specific rates for other variables can be determined in a similar fashion (e.g., race-specific or gender-specific rates) (Table 4-2).

Age-adjustment or **standardization of rates** is another method of reducing bias when there is a difference between the age distributions of two populations. The nurse uses either the *direct* method or the *indirect standardization* method. The *direct* method selects a standard population, which is often the population distribution of the United States. This method essentially converts age-specific rates for age categories of the two populations to those of the standard population and it calculates a summary age-adjusted rate for each of the two populations of interest. This enables the nurse to compare the two rates as if both had the standard population's age

TABLE 4-2

Comparison of U.S. Mortality Rates—1997

Specific Death Rate	Rate per 100,000—1997
Crude Death Rate	864.7
Age-Adjusted Death Rate	479.1
Age-Specific Death Rates	
Under one year	738.7
1 to 4	35.8
5 to 9	18.5
10 to 14	23.2
15 to 19	74.8
20 to 24	98.6
25 to 29	102.1
30 to 34	126.6
35 to 39	168.7
40 to 44	239.7
45 to 49	352.4
50 to 54	526.2
55 to 59	834.6
60 to 64	1331.2
65 to 69	1995.1
70 to 74	3084.9
75 to 79	4612.5
80 to 84	7425.9
85 and over	15,345.2

From Centers for Disease Control, National Center for Health Statistics: *National vital statistics report: 1997*, vol 47(19), Hyattsville, Md, 1999, US Department of Health and Human Services.

structure (i.e., without the prior problem of age distortion). Tables 4-3, 4-4, and 4-5 give examples of the computations.

The second method, *indirect standardization*, allows the nurse to compare two populations as

TABLE 4-3

Direct Standardization of Mortality Rates by Age for "South Community" and "North Community"

Age (yr)	Size of Population (A)	Percent of Population	Number of Deaths (B)	Age-Specific Death Rate per 1000 (B/A)
South Community*				
<15	5400	30.4	10	1.85/1000
15 to 44	7300	41.1	16	2.19/1000
45 to 64	3400	19.2	38	11.18/1000
>65	1650	9.3	84	50.91/1000
Totals	17,750	100	148	
North Community†				
<15	1030	34.2	2	1.94/1000
15 to 44	1500	49.8	4	2.67/1000
45 to 64	407	13.5	4	9.83/1000
>65	75	2.5	4	53.33/1000
Totals	3012	100	14	

Step 1: Determine age-specific death rates. Divide the number of deaths by the population size for each age category.

*Crude death rate $= \dfrac{148}{17{,}750} = \dfrac{8.34}{1000}$.

†Crude death rate $= \dfrac{14}{3012} = \dfrac{4.64}{1000}$.

TABLE 4-4

Direct Standardization of Mortality Rates

	United States 1990		South Community†		North Community‡	
Age (yr)	Size of Population	Percent of Population (A)*	Age-Specific Death Rate per 1000 (B₁)	Expected No. of Deaths per 1000 (A × B₁)	Age-Specific Death Rate per 1000 (B₂)	Expected No. of Deaths per 1000 (A × B₂)
<15	55,961,000	21.9	1.85	0.405	1.94	0.425
15 to 44	118,490,000	46.5	2.19	1.018	2.67	1.242
45 to 64	48,345,000	19.0	11.18	2.124	9.83	1.868
>65	32,283,000	12.7	50.91	6.466	53.33	6.773
Totals	255,079,000	100		10.013		10.308

Step 2: Compute expected number of deaths by multiplying proportion of U.S. population by age-specific death rates. Sum expected deaths to produce age-adjusted death rate.
*Convert to decimal before computing product **A × B**

*Age-adjusted mortality rate $= \dfrac{10.013}{1000}$ (sum of A = B₁).

‡Age-adjusted mortality rate $= \dfrac{10.308}{1000}$ (sum of A = B₂).

though they possessed similar age distributions (i.e., it removes the effect of age). This is helpful especially when age-specific rates are unknown or, in direct adjustment, when the nurse must compare many strata. Indirect adjustment involves the calculation of a *standardized mortality ratio* (SMR), which is a single age-adjusted death ratio that compares the observed deaths with those that would be expected if the population of interest had the mortality experience of the standard population.

$$SMR = \frac{Total\ observed\ deaths}{Total\ expected\ deaths}$$

A ratio of one indicates that observed deaths and expected deaths were equal. A ratio greater than one indicates that more deaths occurred in the population of interest than expected based on the standard population's rates. A ratio of less than one indicates

that fewer deaths occurred in the population of interest than expected based on the standard population's rates. Standardized rations and rates adjusted using the direct method can be produced for other rates (e.g., birth or morbidity rates) and for other variables (e.g., income or birth weight).

The procedure for calculating a SMR is essentially the reverse of direct standardization (Tables 4-6 and 4-7). First, the nurse applies age-specific rates from a standard population to each age category of the two populations of interest to produce expected deaths for each stratum. The standard population may be the U.S. population, like direct adjustment, or it may be the larger or more stable of the two populations. Second, the nurse divides the actual number of observed deaths by the sum of expected deaths for each population to produce a SMR for each population. Note that age-adjusted rates are actually not "real" death rates; rather they are representations of the experience of populations if their age distributions were similar to the standard population.

The **proportionate mortality ratio** (PMR) method also describes mortality. It represents the percentage of deaths resulting from a specific cause relative to deaths from all causes. It is often helpful in identifying areas in which public health programs might make significant contributions in reducing deaths. In some situations, a high PMR may reflect a low overall mortality or reduced number of deaths resulting from other causes. Therefore the PMR

TABLE 4-5

Summary of Tables 4-3 and 4-4*

Area	Crude Mortality Rate	Age-Adjusted Mortality Rate
South Community	8.34 per 1000	10.013 per 1000
North Community	4.64 per 1000	10.308 per 1000

*When the confounding effect of different age distributions is removed through age adjustment, mortality rates for the two communities are similar.

TABLE 4-6

Indirect Standardization of Mortality Rates

Age (yr)	Age-Specific U.S. Death Rates (A)*	Population Size (B) South Community	North Community	Expected Deaths (A × B)/100,000 South Community	North Community
<15	95.18	5400	1030	5.14	0.98
15 to 44	155.40	7300	1500	11.34	2.33
45 to 64	788.76	3400	407	26.82	3.21
>65	4922.32	1650	75	81.22	3.69

*1991 data from US Bureau of the Census: *Statistical abstract of the United States: 1994*, ed 114, Washington, DC, 1994, The Author.
U.S. age-specific mortality rates are multiplied by population of each community to produce expected deaths. These are then summed and standard mortality ratios are calculated as shown in Table 4-7. Death rates are per 100,000 population.

requires consideration in the context of the mortality experience of the population.

$$PMR = \frac{\text{Number of deaths resulting from a specific cause in a specific time period}}{\text{Total number of deaths in time period}}$$

Table 4-8 summarizes the advantages and disadvantages of crude, specific, and adjusted rates. Numerous other rates assess particular segments of the population. Table 4-9 provides a summary of the major public health rates. A standard epidemiology textbook contains more information.

TABLE 4-7

SMR Based on Data from Tables 4-6 and 4-3

Variable	South Community	North Community
Total expected deaths	124.52	10.21
Total observed deaths (from Table 4-3)	148	14
SMR of deaths (observed to expected)	1.19	1.37

SMRs of greater than one indicate that more deaths were observed in both communities than would be expected based on the mortality experience of the overall U.S. population. When mortality data for the two communities are standardized to a third or standard population, the SMRs indicate a similar mortality experience.

CONCEPT OF RISK

The concepts of risk and risk factor are familiar to community health nurses whose practices focus on disease prevention. **Risk** refers to the probability of an adverse event (i.e., the likelihood that healthy people exposed to a specific factor will acquire a specific disease). **Risk factor** refers to the specific exposure factor such as exposure to cigarette smoke, excessive stress, high noise levels, or environmental chemicals. Frequently, the exposure factor is external to the individual. Risk factors may include fixed characteristics of people such as age, sex, or genetic make-up. Although these intrinsic factors are not alterable, certain lifestyle changes may reduce the effect of the risk factors. For example, positive dietary practices and exercise regimens may modify the effects of the risk factor of aging for certain health conditions. Specifically, calcium and hormonal supplements may reduce the risk of osteoporosis for susceptible women.

Epidemiologists describe disease patterns in aggregates and quantify the effects of exposure to particular factors on the disease rates. To identify specific risk factors, epidemiologists compare rates of disease for those exposed with those nonexposed. One method for comparing two rates is subtracting the rate of nonexposed individuals from the exposed. This measure of risk is called the *attributable risk;* it is the estimate of the disease burden in a population. For example, if the rate of noninsulin-dependent diabetes were 5000 per 100,000 people in the obese population (i.e., those weighing more than 120% of ideal body

TABLE 4-8

Advantages and Disadvantages of Crude, Specific, and Adjusted Rates

Rate	Advantages	Disadvantages
Crude	Actual summary rates Readily calculable for international comparisons (widely used despite limitations)	Populations vary in composition (e.g., age); therefore differences in crude rates are difficult to interpret
Specific	Homogeneous subgroups Detailed rates useful for epidemiological and public health purposes	Cumbersome to compare many subgroups of two or more populations
Adjusted	Summary statements Differences in composition of groups "removed," permitting unbiased comparison	Fictional rates Absolute magnitude dependent on chosen standard population Opposing trends in subgroups masked

Modified from Mausner JS, Kramer S: *Mausner and Bahn epidemiology: an introductory text,* ed 2, Philadelphia, 1985, WB Saunders.

TABLE 4-9

Major Public Health Rates

Rate Denominator	Rates	Usual Factor	Rate for United States, 1997
Total population	Crude birth rate = number of live births during the year/average (midyear) population	Per 1000 population	14.5
	Crude death rate = number of deaths during the year/average (midyear) population	Per 1000 population	8.6
	Age-specific death rate = number of deaths among people of a given age group in one year/average (midyear) population in specified age group	Per 1000 population	0.21 (5 to14 yr)* 4.45 (45 to 54 yr)* 25.34 (65 to74 yr)*
	Cause-specific death rate = number of deaths from a stated cause in one year/average (midyear) population	Per 100,000 population	271.6 (heart diseases) 201.6 (malignant neoplasms)
Women aged 15 to 44	Fertility rate = number of live births during one year/number of women aged 15 to 44 in same year	Per 1000 women aged 15 to 44	65.0
Live births	Infant mortality rate = number of deaths in one year of children younger than one year/number of live births in same year	Per 1000 live births	7.2
	Neonatal mortality rate = number of deaths in one year of children younger than 28 days/number of live births in same year	Per 1000 live births	4.8
	Maternal mortality rate (puerperal) = number of deaths from puerperal causes in one year/number of live births in same year	Per 100,000 live births	7.6*
Live births and fetal deaths	Fetal death rate = number of fetal deaths in one year/number of live births and fetal deaths during same year	Per 1000 live births and fetal deaths	6.8
	Perinatal mortality rate = number of fetal deaths (>28 weeks plus infant deaths <7 days) /number of live births and fetal deaths (>28 weeks during the same year)	Per 1000 live births and fetal deaths	7.3

Table adapted from Mausner JS, Kramer S: *Mausner and Bahn epidemiology: an introductory text,* ed 2, Philadelphia, 1985, WB Saunders.
*Rates are for 1996. Rates from National Center for Health Statistics: *Natl Vital Stat Rep* 47(9), 1999, http://www.cdc.gov/nchs/data.pdf.

weight) and 1000 per 100,000 people in the non-obese population, the attributable risk of noninsulin-dependent diabetes resulting from obesity would be 4000 per 100,000 people (i.e., $\frac{5000}{100,000} - \frac{1000}{100,000}$). This means that 4000 cases per 100,000 people may be attributed to obesity. Thus a prevention program designed to reduce obesity could theoretically eliminate 4000 cases per 100,000 people in the population. Therefore attributable risks are particularly important in describing the potential impact of a public health intervention in a community.

A second measure of the excess risk caused by a factor is the *relative risk ratio*. The relative risk is calculated by dividing the incidence rate of disease in the exposed population by the incidence rate of disease in the nonexposed population. In the prior example, a relative risk of five was obtained by dividing 5000/100,000 by 1000/100,000. This risk ratio suggests that an obese individual has a fivefold greater risk of diabetes than a nonobese individual. In general, a relative risk of one indicates no excessive risk from exposure to a factor; a relative risk of 1.5 indicates a 50% increase in risk; a relative risk of two indicates twice the risk; and a relative risk of less than one suggests a factor may have a protective effect associated with a reduced disease rate.

The relative risk ratio forms the statistical basis for the risk factor concept. Relative risks are valuable indicators of the excess risk incurred by exposure to certain factors. They have been used extensively in identifying the major causal factors of many common diseases and direct public health practitioners' efforts to reduce health risks.

Community health nurses may apply the concept of relative risk to suspected exposure variables to isolate risk factors associated with community health problems. For example, a community health nurse might investigate an outbreak of probable food-borne illness. The nurse may compare the incidence rate among those exposed to potato salad in a school cafeteria with the incidence rate among those unexposed. The relative risk calculated from the ratio of these two incidence rates indicates the amount of excess risk for disease incurred by eating the potato salad. A community health nurse might also determine the relative risks for other suspected foods and compare it with the relative risk for potato salad. *Attack rates* are the calculated incidence rates for foods involved in food-borne illnesses. A food with a markedly higher relative risk than other foods might be the causal agent in a food-borne epidemic. The identification of the causal

agent, or specific food, is critical to the implementation of an effective prevention program such as teaching proper food-handling techniques.

USE OF EPIDEMIOLOGY IN DISEASE PREVENTION

Primary Prevention

The central goals of epidemiology are describing the disease patterns, identifying the etiologic factors in disease development, and taking the most effective preventive measures. When these measures occur before disease development, they are called *primary prevention*. Primary prevention relies on epidemiological information to indicate those behaviors that are protective, or will *not* contribute to an increase in disease, and those that are associated with increased risk.

Two types of activities constitute primary prevention. Those actions that are general in nature and designed to foster healthful lifestyles and a safe environment are called *health promotion*. Actions aimed at reducing the risk of specific diseases are called *specific protection*. Public health practitioners use epidemiological research to understand practices that are likely to reduce or increase disease rates. For example, numerous research studies confirmed that regular exercise is an important health promotion activity that has positive effects on general, physical, and mental health. Immunizations exemplify specific protection measures that reduce the incidence of particular diseases.

Secondary and Tertiary Prevention

Secondary prevention occurs after pathogenesis. Those measures designed to detect disease at its earliest stage, namely screening and physical examinations that are aimed at early diagnosis, are secondary prevention. Interventions that provide for early treatment and cure of disease are also in this category. Again, epidemiological data and clinical trials determining effective treatments are crucial in disease identification. Mammography, guiac testing of feces, and the treatment of infections and dental caries are all examples of secondary prevention. *Tertiary prevention* includes the limitation of disability and the rehabilitation of those with irreversible disease such as diabetes and spinal cord injury. Epidemiological studies suggest optimal strategies in the care of patients with chronic advanced disease.

Establishing Causality

As discussed earlier, a principal goal of classic epidemiology is to identify etiologic factors of diseases to encourage the most effective primary prevention activities and develop treatment modalities. During the last few decades, researchers recognized that many diseases have not one, but multiple causes. Epidemiologists who examine disease rates and conduct population-focused research often find multiple factors associated with health problems. For example, cardiovascular disease rates may vary by location, ethnicity, and smoking status. Even infectious diseases often require not only an organism, but also certain behaviors or conditions to cause exposure. Determining the extent that these correlates represent associative or causal relationships is important for public health practitioners who seek to prevent, diagnose, and treat disease.

The following six criteria establish the existence of a cause and effect relationship:

1. Strength of association: Rates of morbidity or mortality must be higher in the exposed group than in the nonexposed group. Relative risk ratios, or odds ratios, and correlation coefficients indicate whether the relationship between the exposure variable and the outcome is causal. For example, epidemiological studies demonstrated an elevated relative risk for heart disease among smokers compared with nonsmokers (Doll and Hill, 1956).
2. Dose-response relationship: An increased exposure to the risk factor causes a concomitant increase in disease rate. The risk of heart disease mortality is higher for heavy smokers compared with light smokers (Mattson et al., 1987).
3. Temporally correct relationship: Exposure to the causal factor must occur before the effect, or disease. For heart disease, smoking history must precede disease development.
4. Biological plausibility: The data must make biological sense and represent a coherent explanation for the relationship. Nicotine and other tobacco-derived chemicals are toxic to the vascular endothelium. In addition to raising low-density lipoprotein (LDL) and decreasing high-density lipoprotein (HDL) cholesterol levels, cigarette smoking causes arterial vasoconstriction and platelet reactivity, which contributes to platelet thrombus formation.
5. Consistency with other studies: Varying types of studies in other populations must observe similar associations. Numerous studies of different designs have repeatedly supported the relationship between smoking and heart disease.
6. Specificity: The exposure variable must be necessary and sufficient to cause disease; there is only one causal factor. Although specificity may be strong causal evidence, this criterion is less important today. Diseases do not have single causes; they have multifactoral origins.

The exposure variable of smoking is one of several risk factors for heart disease. Few factors are linked to a single condition. Smoking is not specific to heart disease alone. It is a causal factor for other diseases like lung and oral cancers. Further, smoking is not "necessary and sufficient" to the development of heart disease because there are nonsmokers who also experience coronary heart disease. Therefore the causal criteria of specificity pertains to infectious diseases more frequently.

Although these criteria are useful in evaluating epidemiological evidence, it is important to note that causality can never be proven and is always a matter of judgment. In reality, absolute causality is only rarely established. Rather epidemiologists more commonly refer to suggested causal and associated factors. The effect of confounding variables makes it difficult to ascertain true relationships between the exposure and outcome variables. Confounding variables are independently related to *both* the dependent variable and the independent variable. Therefore confounding variables may mask the true relationship between the dependent and independent variables. For example, Buring and Lee (1995) discussed the need to control dietary fat when examining the relationship between physical activity and coronary heart disease. This is necessary because studies have shown that dietary fat is independently related to both physical exercise (Simoes et al., 1995) and heart disease (Willett, 1990) in some populations. The apparent association between physical activity and heart disease may be attributable to the difference in fat intake between those with and without heart disease. Those with heart disease may tend to have a higher fat intake and a decreased activity level than those without heart disease. The outcome is not solely attributable to exercise. On the other hand, Buring and Lee (1995) provided an example in which dietary fat is not a confounding variable despite its relation to physical activity. Dietary fat is not a confounder of the relationship of physical exercise and osteoporosis because dietary fat is not a risk factor for the dependent variable of osteoporosis.

By measuring the confounding variable, the researcher can statistically account for its effect in the analysis (e.g., by using multiple logistical regression analysis or stratification). A biostatistics text contains a discussion of these methods. Alternatively, matching subjects in treatment and control groups with respect to the confounding variable minimizes the effects of the confounder. Again, standardization for variables such as age is another method for managing spurious associations, which makes true relationships more apparent. An understanding of such relationships facilitates the practitioners' interpretation and application of findings.

Screening

Again, a central aim of epidemiology is to describe the course of disease according to person, place, and time. Observations of the disease process may suggest factors that aggravate or ameliorate its progress. This information also assists in determining effective treatment and rehabilitation options (i.e., secondary or tertiary prevention approaches).

The purpose of **screening programs** is to identify risk factors and diseases in their earliest stages. Screening is usually a secondary prevention activity because disease appears *after* a pathological change has occurred, or ideally, early in the disease process. In all forms of secondary and tertiary prevention, the identification of illness prompts the nurse to consider which forms of upstream prevention could have affected disease development.

Community health nurses commonly conduct screening programs. A community health nurse may devote a large portion of his or her work activities to performing physical examinations, promoting client self-examination, or conducting screening programs in schools, clinics, or community settings. Although these secondary prevention activities are important services that provide vital information on community health status, they focus on detecting existing disease. Nurses should contrast secondary prevention activities with primary prevention and anticipatory guidance, which are hallmarks of community health nursing practice.

There are several guidelines community health

nurses should consider for screening programs. First, nurses must plan and execute adequate and appropriate follow-up treatment for patients with disease. Health fairs have been criticized for the lack of consistent follow-up and screening activity. Second, in the planning phase, the nurse should determine if early disease diagnosis constitutes a real benefit to clients, whether in terms of increased life expectancy or quality of life. Third, a critical prerequisite to screening is the existence of acceptable and medically sound treatment and follow-up. In the past decade, public health providers have debated the ethical and practical arguments for implementing HIV screening. Concern exists regarding the potential for stigma and discrimination against those who screen positively for a test; therefore those implementing screening programs should establish procedures for ensuring confidentiality. These procedures, in conjunction with the development of azidothymidine (AZT) and other antiviral treatments, have encouraged earlier identification of HIV-positive individuals.

A screening program's procedures must also be cost effective and acceptable to clients. Although sigmoidoscopy is a common and effective screening procedure for colon cancer, it is not a simple and inexpensive test. Consequently, those who demonstrate a high risk for colon cancer primarily undergo the exam. Finally, a nurse should consider whether or not to screen a population based on the significant costs for screening programs and procedures, follow-up for clients who test positive, and subsequent medical care.

GUIDELINES FOR SCREENING PROGRAMS
1. Screen for conditions in which early detection and treatment can improve disease outcome and quality of life.
2. Screen populations that have risk factors or are more susceptible to the disease.
3. Select a screening method that is simple, safe, inexpensive to administer, acceptable to clients, and has acceptable sensitivity and specificity.
4. Plan for the timely referral and follow-up of positive cases.
5. Identify referral sources that are appropriate, cost-effective, and convenient for clients.

The community health nurse must also evaluate issues specific to the validity of the screening test when developing a screening program. Detecting clients with disease is the purpose of screening and *sensitivity* is the test's ability to do this correctly. Conversely, *specificity* is the extent to which a test can correctly identify those who do not have disease. To obtain estimates of these two dimensions, the nurse must compare screening results with those of some definitive diagnostic procedure (Mausner and Kramer, 1985). For a given test, the sensitivity and specificity tend to be inversely related to each other. When a test is highly sensitive, individuals without disease may be labeled positive. These false-positive tests may cause stress and worry for clients and require further diagnostical testing to confirm a diagnosis. With a highly sensitive test, specificity may be lower and the test may not detect disease in some clients. These false-negative test results mean that some individuals may receive false reassurance and will not receive follow-up care.

Optimally, a screening test should be maximally sensitive *and* specific. To a large extent, this depends on the stringency of the cut-off point established for determining a positive disease case. For example, with an established high blood pressure criterion of 140/90, more people will have high blood pressure than with a cut-off of 150/90. The lower cut-off is more sensitive and will lead to more false positives. The higher criteria may be more specific, and although fewer people will be hypertensive, there will be fewer false-positive cases than with the lower cut-off level. Table 4-10 includes the formula for calculating sensitivity and specificity.

Sensitivity and specificity reflect the *yield* of a screening test, which is the amount of detected disease. One measure of yield is the *positive predic-*tive value* of a test, which is the proportion of true positive results relative to all positive test results. On the basis of Table 4-10, the formula is $\frac{a}{a+b}$. The positive productive value is dependent on the prevalence of undetected disease in a population. Screening for a rare disease like phenylketonuria will yield a lower predictive value and more false-positive results. In phenylketonuria, a low predictive value is acceptable because the false-negative result has such serious consequences. The predictive value is also affected by the nature of the screened population. Screening only the individuals at high risk for a disease will produce a higher predictive value and can be a more efficient way to identify those with health problems. For example, diabetes screening in a Mexican-American or African-American adult population should produce a higher predictive value than screening the general adult population.

Surveillance

In addition to screening, **surveillance** is a mechanism for the ongoing collection of community health information. Monitoring for changes in disease frequency is essential to effective and responsive public health programs. Identifying trends in disease incidence or identifying risk factor status by location and population subgroup over time allows the community health nurse to evaluate the effectiveness of existing programs and implement interventions targeted to high-risk groups. Again, identifying new cases for calculating incidence rates is particularly useful in evaluating morbidity trends. However, this form of surveillance data is more difficult to collect and public health practitioners can only access the data for selected diseases. Prevalence rates, mortality data, risk factor data, and hospital and health service data can help indicate a program's successes or deficiencies.

The PHS coordinates a system of data collection among federal, state, and local agencies. These groups compile numerous sets of data and base some of these data sets on the entire population (e.g., vital statistics data) and other collections on subsamples of the population (e.g., the National Health Interview Survey). The completeness of data reporting is variable because not all diseases are reportable. For example, practitioners are required to report only four STDs (i.e., AIDS, syphilis, gonorrhea, and chlamydia) to local and state health departments. Furthermore, not all practitioners report cases on a regular basis and not all people with STDs actually seek care. Studies have

TABLE **4-10**

Sensitivity and Specificity of a Screening Test

Screening Test	Those With Disease	Those Without Disease
Positive	True positives (a)	False positives (b)
Negative	False negatives (c)	True negatives (d)

$$\text{Sensitivity (in percent)} = \frac{\text{True positives}}{\text{All with disease}} = \frac{(a)}{(a+c)} \times 100$$

$$\text{Specificity (in percent)} = \frac{\text{True negatives}}{\text{All with disease}} = \frac{(d)}{(b+d)} \times 100$$

indicated that practitioners also underreport childhood communicable diseases, such as chicken pox and mumps. The CDC conducts studies that estimate the magnitude of this problem (NCHS, 1995).

Practitioners have a continuing need for comprehensive and systematically collected surveillance data that describe the health status of national and local subgroups. They use this information to evaluate the impact of programs on specific groups in a community. For example, the effectiveness of *Healthy People 2000* and *Healthy People 2010* depends on the availability of reliable baseline and continuing data to characterize health problems and evaluate goal achievement.

Healthy People 2010 (USDHHS, 2000) recognizes the ongoing need to extend the inclusiveness of such surveillance systems. For example, simply documenting children's mortality rates resulting from injury is insufficient for the development of specific methods of injury prevention. Data on the number of injured children and the nature of injury across the nation would increase the usefulness of surveillance information.

Nurses need to describe trends in health and illness by a community's locale, demographics, and risk factor status to intervene effectively on behalf of communities. They must compare the data for their locale with those of a relevant neighboring area (e.g., a census tract, city, county, state, or nation) to gain perspective on the magnitude of a local problem. Ideally, the nurse should have access to surveillance data at several different levels over a period of time. In some instances, community health nurses find it necessary to construct their own surveillance systems that are tailored to specific health conditions or programs in a community. These smaller data collection systems help nurses evaluate programs when the data are readily accessible and compatible with data from large city or statewide surveillance systems.

SURVEILLANCE OF NEURAL TUBE DEFECTS IN TEXAS

In April 1991, a cluster of six neural tube defects (NTDs) occurred in babies born in Brownsville Texas within a span of six weeks. Further investigation in Cameron County indicated a rate of 27.1 cases per 10,000 live births compared to 14.7 for babies conceived from 1986 to 1989 and compared to the U.S. rate of approximately 8 per 10,000. This rate was more than three times the national rate and represented an increased risk in Hispanic women. This increased risk was partially attributable to cultural and environmental factors including lower socioeconomic status and migrant farm work. The investigators implemented a surveillance program that included fetuses of less than 20 weeks gestation, which obtained more accurate population-based data. Additionally, the program implemented folic acid supplementation in Texas counties along the Mexican border. From 1993 to 1996, NTD rates dropped to 13 per 10,000 following supplementation.

Research suggests that 50% to 70% of NTDs may be preventable with folic acid supplementation. This finding supports the fortification of bread and cereal products; in January 1998, the Federal Drug Administration mandated the addition of 140 μ of vitamin B per 100 g of most grain products. Dietary intake alone may be insufficient; therefore the CDC recommends that all women of reproductive age consume 400 μ (0.4 mg) of folic acid daily from a combination of dietary sources such as cereal or grain products, leafy green vegetables, and vitamin supplements.

Data from Centers for Disease Control: Neural tube defects in Texas, *Dis Prev News* 58(2):5-6, 1998; Centers for Disease Control: Neural tube defect surveillance and folic acid intervention: Texas-Mexico border, 1993-1998, *Mor Mortal Wkly Rep* 49(01):1-4, 2000, http://www.cdc.gov/epo/mmwr/preview/mmwr.html.

Again, epidemiologists describe the course of disease over time. These *secular* trends are changes that occur over years or decades, such as the decline in uterine cancer and the increase in breast cancer. Frequently, epidemiologists document the associated patterns of treatment and intervention. In many instances, studies conducted by clinical epidemiologists provide this information. Cancer registries are a form of surveillance that document the prevalence and incidence of cancer in a community and document its course, treatment, and associated survival rates. The Surveillance, Epidemiology, and End Results Program of the National Cancer Institutes compiles national cancer data from the registries of 11 American and Puerto Rican cities (NCHS, 1995).

Public health practitioners need to conduct community surveys of population segments to plan for the sector's health. For example, a survey of the disabled population that assesses prevalence may also evaluate the adequacy of present services and project future needs.

USE OF EPIDEMIOLOGY IN HEALTH SERVICES

Presented epidemiological approaches can be used to describe the distribution of disease and its determinants in populations. However, epidemiological principles are also useful in studying population health care delivery and in describing and evaluating the use of community health services. For example, determining the ratio of health care providers to population size helps assess the system's ability to provide care. The clients' reasons for seeking care, the clients' payment methods, and the clients' satisfaction are also informative. Regardless of whether community health nurses or health services researchers collected these data, the information is essential for those who strive to improve clients' access to quality health care.

HEALTH SERVICES EPIDEMIOLOGY

Health services epidemiology focuses on the population's health care patterns. In particular, public health practitioners are concerned with the accessibility and affordability of services and the barriers that may contribute to excess morbidity in at-risk groups. Traditionally, children are a vulnerable group and they are a particular focus of health services research. Studies examining poverty rates and care access have underscored the need to expand insurance coverage to those who do not have private medical insurance and do not qualify for Medicaid programs.

Community health nurses can use epidemiological studies to evaluate the quality of care. A comparative study of a special geriatric inpatient evaluation ward, which used an interdisciplinary elderly care program, exemplifies this approach (Rubenstein et al., 1984). The study compared the outcomes of interdis-

ciplinary care with the outcomes of typical elderly care in the hospital ward. Patients in the special unit had lower mortality rates, lower morbidity rates, and higher satisfaction levels. Furthermore, clients incurred lower costs on the special unit compared with other units. This important finding suggests another aspect of health service epidemiology, which is evaluating the cost effectiveness of health care and specific interventions or modes of delivery.

Ultimately, nurses must apply epidemiological findings in the practice arena. It is essential that they incorporate study results into prevention programs for communities and at-risk populations. Further, the philosophy of public health and epidemiology dictates that nurses extend its application into major health policy decisions, because the aim of health policy planning is to achieve positive health goals and outcomes for improved societal health.

A goal of policy development is to bring about desirable social changes. Epidemiological factors, history, politics, economics, culture, and technology influence policy development. The complex interaction of these factors may explain the slow application of epidemiological knowledge. Lung disease in the United States exemplifies the incomplete progress in implementing effective health policy. In the early 1950s, studies identified and conclusively linked cigarette smoking to lung cancer and heart disease (Doll and Hill, 1952). Since the 1950s, protective public policies include cigarette taxes, cigarette warning labels, and smoking restrictions in public areas. Nevertheless, until the late 1990s advertising continued to promote cigarette smoking. Indeed, during the 1980s and 1990s there was a proliferation of billboard and media advertisements targeted to vulnerable segments of the population (i.e., adolescents and black and Hispanic males). Community forums vigorously protested and debated this practice and individual states began to hold the tobacco industry legally accountable for cigarette-related disease and death.

In 1976, Milio suggested that public policy also failed to keep pace with epidemiological research findings in other areas. She asserted that consumer health would benefit significantly from a public policy that provides healthier consumer options such as improved work place safeguards, higher environmental standards, higher quality nutritious food, and improved incentives to reduce alcohol consumption. These goals continue to be primary concerns of public health professionals (Milio, 1976).

In summary, there remain many public policies that public health practitioners and epidemiologists have yet to modify in the interest of improved health. Community health nurses should exercise "societal responsibility" in applying epidemiological findings, but this will require the active involvement of the citizen consumer. Community health nurses collaborating with community members can combine epidemiological knowledge and aggregate-level strategies to affect change on the broadest scale.

EPIDEMIOLOGICAL METHODS

Descriptive Epidemiology

Descriptive epidemiology focuses on the amount and distribution of health and health problems within a population. Its purpose is to describe the characteristics of people who are protected from disease and those who have a disease. Factors of particular interest include age, sex, ethnicity or race, socioeconomic status, occupation, and family status. Epidemiologists use morbidity and mortality rates to describe the extent of disease and to determine the risk factors that make certain groups prone to acquiring disease.

In addition to "person" characteristics, the place of occurrence describes disease frequency. For example, certain parasitic diseases such as malaria and schistosomiasis occur in tropical areas. Other diseases may occur in certain geopolitical entities. For example, gastroenteritis outbreaks often occur in communities with lax water quality standards. Time is the third parameter that helps define disease patterns. Epidemiologists may track incidence rates over a period of days or weeks (e.g., epidemics of infectious disease) or over an extended period of years (e.g., secular trends in the cancer death rate).

These person, place, and time factors can form a framework for disease analysis and may suggest variables associated with high vs. low disease rates. Descriptive epidemiology can then generate hypotheses about the cause of disease and analytic epidemiology approaches can test these hypotheses.

AN EXAMPLE OF DESCRIPTIVE EPIDEMIOLOGY

- The **Person-Place-Time Model** is illustrated by an outbreak of TB and its rapid spread in an HIV-infected prison population and into the outside community.

- **Person:** An index case-patient was connected through DNA fingerprinting of *Mycobacterium* TB isolates to TB disease in 14 other inmates and to the spouse who visited the prisoner. Nine prison employees also had skin test conversions. Secondary transmission occurred from the wife of the index case to a young daughter who had no contact with her father.
- **Place:** A 500-person housing unit for HIV-infected inmates at a correctional institution in California.
- **Time:** Initial case entered the prison in May 1995 and was diagnosed with TB in August. Follow-up of contacts occurred from September through April 1996.

From Centers for Disease Control: Tuberculosis outbreaks in prison housing units for HIV-infected inmates: California, 1995-1996, *Mor Mortal Wkly Rep* 48(4): 79-82, 1999, http://www.cdc.gov/epo/mmwr/preview/mmwr.html.

Analytic Epidemiology

Analytic epidemiology investigates the causes of disease by determining why a disease rate is lower in one population group than in another. This method tests hypotheses generated from descriptive data and either accepts or rejects them on the basis of analytic research. The epidemiologist seeks to establish a cause and effect relationship between a preexisting condition or event and the disease. See previous section on causality. To determine this relationship, the epidemiologist may undertake two major types of research studies, which are *observational* and *experimental* studies.

Observational Studies

Epidemiologists frequently use *observational studies* for descriptive purposes, but they also use them to discover the etiology of disease. The investigator can begin to understand the factors that contribute to disease by observing disease rates in groups of people differentiated by experience or exposure. For example, differences in disease rates may occur in the obese compared with the nonobese, in smokers compared with nonsmokers, and in those with high stress levels compared with those with low stress levels. These characteristics (i.e., obesity, smoking, and stress) are called *exposure* variables.

Unlike experimental studies, observational studies do not allow the investigator to manipulate the specific exposure or experience or to control or limit the effects of other extraneous factors that may influence disease development. For example, life stress is related to depression. People with low socioeconomic status also have high depression rates. People with low socioeconomic status frequently experience greater life stresses; therefore the confounding factor of socioeconomic status makes it more difficult to demonstrate the effect of stress on depression. The three major study designs used in observational research are cross-sectional, retrospective, and prospective studies.

Cross-Sectional Studies

Cross-sectional studies, sometimes called *prevalence* or *correlational* studies, examine relationships between potential causal factors and disease at a specific time (Fig. 4-5). Surveys that simultaneously collect information about risk factors and disease exemplify this design. For example, both the National Health and Nutrition Examination Survey (NHANES) and the subsequent HHANES collected cross-sectional data regarding current dietary practices and physical status on people ranging from 1 to 72 years of age

(Delgado et al., 1990). The two surveys detected nutritional deficiencies in the population.

Although a cross-sectional study can identify associations among disease and specific factors, it is impossible to make causal inferences because the study cannot establish the temporal sequence of events (i.e., the cause preceded the effect). For example, the NHANES was unable to determine whether high salt intake preceded hypertension—and thus is the causal factor—or whether the reverse is true. Therefore cross-sectional studies have limitations in discovering etiologic factors of disease. These studies can help identify preliminary relationships that other analytic designs may explore further; therefore they are hypothesis-generating studies.

Retrospective Studies

Retrospective studies compare individuals with a particular condition or disease with those who do not have the disease. These studies determine whether cases, or a diseased group, differ in their exposure to a specific factor or characteristic relative to controls, or a nondiseased group. To make unambiguous comparisons, investigators select the cases according to explicitly defined criteria regarding the type of case and the stage of disease. The investigator also selects

FIGURE **4-5**

Cross-sectional, or prevalence, study.

Time Dimension:

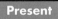

Sample: Subjects sampled from population-at-large at one point in time

Advantages	Disadvantages
Quick to plan and conduct	Cannot calculate relative risk with prevalence data
Relatively inexpensive	Temporal sequence of factor and outcome unknown
May provide preliminary indication of whether an association between a risk factor and disease exists	
Provides prevalence data needed for planning health services	
Hypothesis generating	

a control group from the general population, which is characteristically similar to the cases (Fig. 4-6).

Frequently, people hospitalized for nonstudy diseases become controls if they do not share the exposure or risk factor under study. For example, a researcher may select heart disease patients to be controls in a study of lung cancer patients. However, this may introduce serious bias because these patients often share the risk factor of smoking. The methods of data collection must be the same for both groups to prevent further introduction of bias into the study. Therefore it is desirable for interviewers to remain unaware of which subjects are cases and which are controls.

In retrospective studies, data collection extends back in time to determine previous exposure or risk factors. Investigators analyze study data by comparing the proportion of subjects with disease, or cases, who possess the exposure or risk factors with the corresponding proportion in the control group. A greater proportion of exposed cases than controls suggests a relationship between the disease and the risk factor.

Investigators often use retrospective study designs because they address the question of causality better than cross-sectional studies. Retrospective studies also require fewer resources and less data collection time than prospective studies. Many examples of

---

FIGURE **4-6**

Retrospective, or case-control, study.

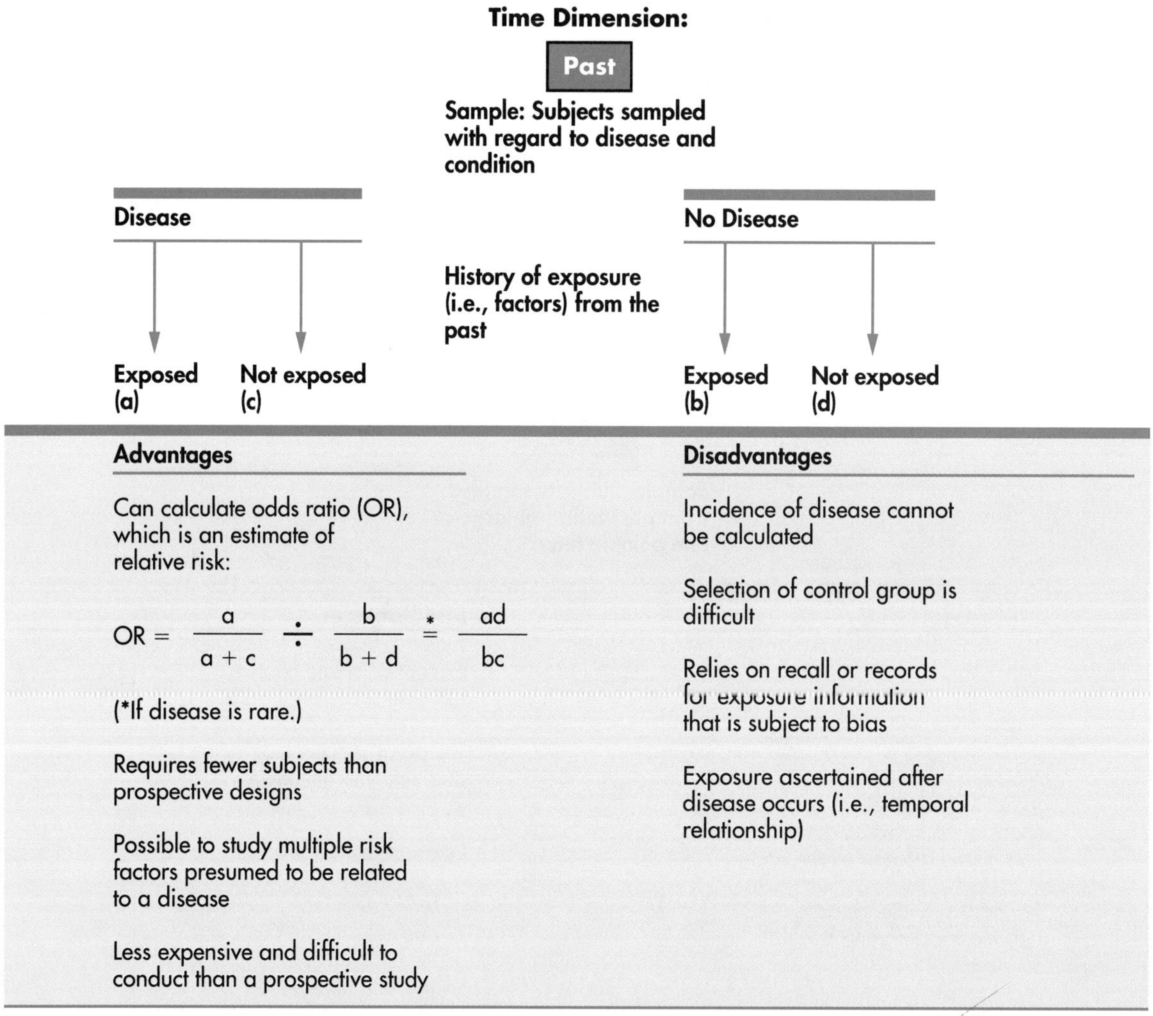

Time Dimension:

Past

Sample: Subjects sampled with regard to disease and condition

Disease

No Disease

History of exposure (i.e., factors) from the past

Exposed (a)   **Not exposed (c)**

Exposed (b)   **Not exposed (d)**

Advantages	Disadvantages
Can calculate odds ratio (OR), which is an estimate of relative risk: $$OR = \frac{a}{a+c} \div \frac{b}{b+d} \stackrel{*}{=} \frac{ad}{bc}$$ (*If disease is rare.)	Incidence of disease cannot be calculated
	Selection of control group is difficult
Requires fewer subjects than prospective designs	Relies on recall or records for exposure information that is subject to bias
Possible to study multiple risk factors presumed to be related to a disease	Exposure ascertained after disease occurs (i.e., temporal relationship)
Less expensive and difficult to conduct than a prospective study	

retrospective, or *case-control,* studies exist in the literature. One classic example is Doll and Hill's (1952) investigation of risk factors for lung cancer. They compared exposure rates for cases diagnosed with lung cancer with those in the control group diagnosed with cancer outside the chest and oral cavity. Doll and Hill recorded detailed smoking histories on all subjects. Compared with the controls, a significantly higher proportion of lung cancer cases smoked. This study yielded the hypothesis that smoking may be etiologically related to lung cancer.

Prospective Studies

Prospective studies monitor a group of disease-free individuals to determine if and when disease occurs (Fig. 4-7). These individuals, or the *cohort,* share a common experience within a defined time period. For example, a birth cohort consists of all people born within a given time period. The study assesses the cohort with respect to an exposure factor associated with the disease and thus classifies it at the beginning of the study. The study then monitors the cohort for disease development. The investigator compares the disease rates for those with a known exposure with rates for those who remain unexposed. The study observes subjects prospectively; therefore it summarizes data collected over time by the incidence rates of new cases. Again, comparing two incidence rates produces a measure of relative risk.

$$\text{Relative risk} = \frac{\text{Incidence rate among exposed}}{\text{Incidence rate among unexposed}}$$

The relative risk indicates the extent of excess risk incurred by exposure relative to nonexposure. A relative risk of one suggests no excess risk resulting from exposure, whereas a relative risk of two suggests twice the risk of experiencing disease from exposure.

Prospective studies, or *longitudinal, cohort,* or *incidence* studies, are advantageous because they

---

F I G U R E **4-7**

Prospective, or cohort, study.

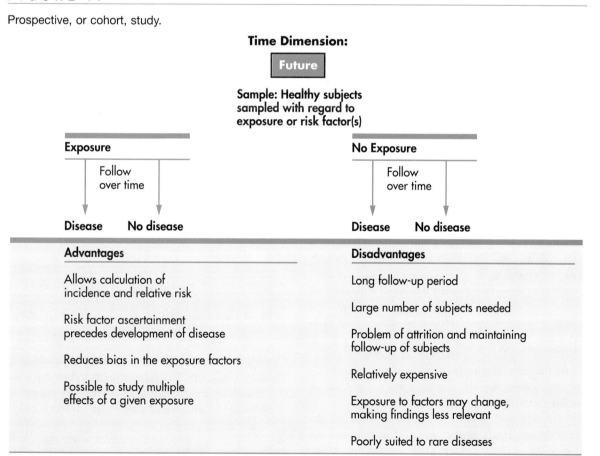

Time Dimension:

Future

Sample: Healthy subjects sampled with regard to exposure or risk factor(s)

Exposure	**No Exposure**
Follow over time	Follow over time
Disease No disease	Disease No disease

Advantages	**Disadvantages**
Allows calculation of incidence and relative risk	Long follow-up period
Risk factor ascertainment precedes development of disease	Large number of subjects needed
Reduces bias in the exposure factors	Problem of attrition and maintaining follow-up of subjects
Possible to study multiple effects of a given exposure	Relatively expensive
	Exposure to factors may change, making findings less relevant
	Poorly suited to rare diseases

obtain more reliable information about the cause of disease than other study methodologies. These studies establish a stronger temporal relationship between the presumed causal factors and the effect than retrospective and cross-sectional studies. Calculations of incidence rates and relative risks provide a valuable indicator of the level of risk that exposure creates.

However, certain disadvantages are inherent in the prospective design. It is costly in terms of resources and staff to monitor a cohort over time and lengthy studies result in subject attrition. Problems arising from the nature of chronic diseases may compound these logistical dilemmas. Frequently, chronic diseases have long latency periods between exposure and symptom manifestation. Furthermore, the onset of chronic conditions may be sufficiently insidious, which makes it extremely difficult to document the incidence of disease. In addition, many diseases do not have a unifactorial cause (i.e., single variable) because many interacting factors influence disease. These problems do not negate the benefits of prospectively designed epidemiological studies; rather they suggest a need to carefully plan and tailor the study specifically to the disease and the study's purpose.

The literature contains numerous prospective studies. In many cases, these studies have been instrumental in substantiating causal links between specific risk factors and disease. A classic example is an early Doll and Hill cohort study of lung cancer deaths (1956). Doll and Hill originally completed questionnaires on a cohort of physicians in Great Britain. Next, they classified the subjects according to several variables, emphasizing the number of cigarettes smoked. In four and a half years, they accessed death certificate data. This data revealed a higher mortality rate resulting from lung cancer and coronary thrombosis among smoking physicians compared with nonsmokers. The death rate for heavy smokers was 166/100,000 vs. 7/100,000 for nonsmokers. Combining these two incidence rates in a measure of excess risk indicated that heavy smokers were 23.7 times more likely to develop lung cancer than nonsmokers (relative risk $= \dfrac{166}{100,000} \div \dfrac{7}{100,000}$, or 23.7). These findings in a prospective study provided strong epidemiological support that smoking is a risk factor for lung cancer.

Another well-known prospective study is the Framingham Heart Study, which has followed an essentially healthy cohort of Framingham, Mass.

residents for almost 45 years. Findings suggest that serum cholesterol level and other risk factors are associated with the future development of cardiovascular disease (Grundy et al., 1998; Kannel et al., 1971). The Framingham Study was one cohort study that formed the basis for later experimental studies aimed at reducing serum cholesterol through diet modification or drug therapy to ultimately lower the incidence rate of coronary heart disease.

Another continuing longitudinal study, The Nurses' Health Study, began to follow female RNs in 1976. This study monitored nurses' changing health status and risk factors and examined factors associated with the development of numerous health conditions such as breast cancer and heart disease. A recent analysis of food-frequency data suggested the protective value of whole grain intake on the development of coronary heart disease (Liu et al., 1999). Another report from The Nurses' Study suggested that women who walk briskly three or more hours a week experience a reduction in coronary events similar to women who perform regular vigorous exercise (Manson et al., 1999).

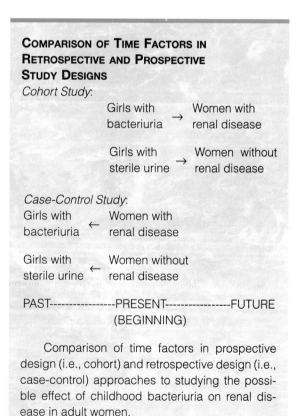

COMPARISON OF TIME FACTORS IN RETROSPECTIVE AND PROSPECTIVE STUDY DESIGNS

Cohort Study:

Girls with bacteriuria → Women with renal disease

Girls with sterile urine → Women without renal disease

Case-Control Study:

Girls with bacteriuria ← Women with renal disease

Girls with sterile urine ← Women without renal disease

PAST----------------PRESENT----------------FUTURE
(BEGINNING)

Comparison of time factors in prospective design (i.e., cohort) and retrospective design (i.e., case-control) approaches to studying the possible effect of childhood bacteriuria on renal disease in adult women.

FIGURE 4-8

Experimental, or clinical trial, study.

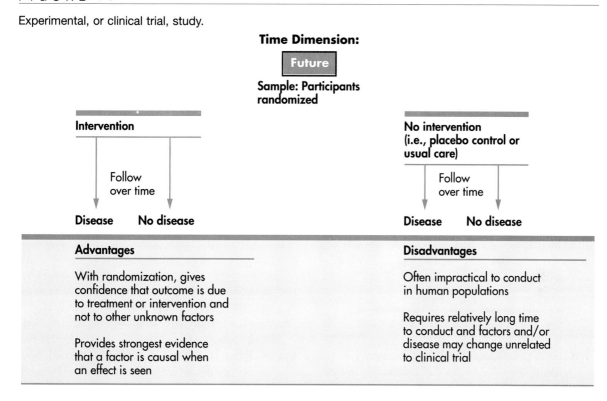

Time Dimension:

Future

Sample: Participants randomized

Intervention		No intervention (i.e., placebo control or usual care)	
Follow over time		Follow over time	
Disease	No disease	Disease	No disease

Advantages	Disadvantages
With randomization, gives confidence that outcome is due to treatment or intervention and not to other unknown factors	Often impractical to conduct in human populations
Provides strongest evidence that a factor is causal when an effect is seen	Requires relatively long time to conduct and factors and/or disease may change unrelated to clinical trial

Experimental Studies

Another type of analytic study is the experimental design (Fig. 4-8). Epidemiological investigations apply experimental methods to test treatment and prevention strategies. The investigator randomly assigns subjects at risk for a particular disease to an experimental or a control group. The investigator observes both groups for the occurrence of disease over time, but only the experimental group receives intervention.

Theoretically, it is possible to introduce an exposure or risk factor as the experimental factor; however, ethical considerations usually prohibit the use of human subjects for these purposes. For example, it is unacceptable to require an experimental group to smoke cigarettes in an experiment; therefore the investigator uses case-control or cohort epidemiological designs. This limitation usually restricts experimental epidemiological studies to prophylactic and therapeutic clinical trials. For example, experimental studies commonly test vaccines and medications for safety and efficacy.

The experimental design is also useful for investigating chronic disease. The Multiple Risk Factor Intervention Trial (MRFIT) tested the following interventions for preventing heart disease: smoking cessation, dietary cholesterol reduction, and hypertension treatment (MRFIT Research Group, 1982).

Also, the Coronary Primary Prevention Trial compared the effects of a cholesterol-lowering drug with those of a placebo in a clinical sample (Lipid Research Clinics Program, 1984). After seven years, the cholesterol-lowering drug reduced the incidence of coronary heart disease by 19%. Thus experimental studies help determine which of many preventive programs to implement. Although these studies are medical, experimental designs may help evaluate community health nursing interventions. For example, they may help determine the effectiveness of a sex education program in preventing high rates of teenage pregnancy or the feasibility of an AIDS prevention program among intravenous drug users. For five years nurses participated in a randomized trial of telephone interventions directed towards high-risk prenatal clients. The trial's findings were the impetus for several community-based programs to reduce the incidence of preterm and low-birth-weight babies (Moore, 1999).

SUMMARY

Epidemiology offers the community health nurse with methods to quantify the extent of health problems in the community and provides a body of knowledge about risk factors and their association with disease. At each step of the nursing process, epidemiological applications support the practice of the community health nurse. Compiling descriptive data from surveys or studies contributes to understanding the community's health level. In assessing community problems, epidemiological rates describe the magnitude of disease and provide support for community diagnoses. Epidemiological studies suggest interventions and their efficacy, which is useful in planning prevention and intervention approaches. Evaluation studies using epidemiological methods, either reported in literature or conducted by community health nurses, are essential for providing optimal research-based care.

LEARNING ACTIVITIES

1. Compile a data base of relevant demographic and epidemiological data for the community by examining census reports, vital statistics reports, city records, and other sources in libraries and agencies.
2. Using numerators from vital statistics and denominators from census data, compute crude death and birth rates for the community.
3. Compare morbidity and mortality rates for the community with those of the state and the nation. Determine whether the community rates are higher or lower and hypothesize about reasons for any disparities.
4. Consult *Healthy People 2010* to find the national goals for selected causes of morbidity and mortality. Identify groups at an increased risk for these selected diseases. What are the approaches suggested by these documents for reducing the rates of disease? How can this information be useful in planning for the community?

REFERENCES

Buring JE, Lee I-M: Annotation: confounding in epidemiologic research, *Am J Public Health* 85:164-165, 1995.

Centers for Disease Control: Neural tube defects in Texas, *Dis Prev News* 58(2):5-6, 1998.

Centers for Disease Control: Neural tube defect surveillance and folic acid intervention: Texas-Mexico border, 1993-1998, *Mor Mortal Wkly Rep* 49(01):1-4, 2000, http://www.cdc.gov/epo/mmwr/preview/mmwr.html.

Centers for Disease Control: Tuberculosis outbreaks in prison housing units for HIV-infected inmates: California, 1995-1996, *Mor Mortal Wkly Rep* 48(4):79-82, 1999, http://www.cdc.gov/epo/mmwr/preview/mmwr.html.

Centers for Disease Control, National Center for Health Statistics: *National vital statistics report: 1997,* vol 47(19), Hyattsville, Md, 1999, US Department of Health and Human Services.

Delgado JL et al: Hispanic Health and Nutrition Examination Survey: methodological considerations, *Am J Public Health* 80(suppl):6-10, 1990.

Doll R, Hill AB: Lung cancer and other causes of death in relation to smoking, *BMJ* 2:1071-1081, 1956.

Doll R, Hill AB: Study of the aetiology of carcinoma of the lung, *BMJ* 2:1271-1285, 1952.

Friedman GD: *Primer of epidemiology,* ed 4, New York, 1994, McGraw-Hill.

Grundy SM et al: Primary prevention of coronary heart disease: guidance from Framingham: a statement for healthcare professionals from the AHA Task Force on Risk Reduction, *Circulation* 97(18):1876-1887, 1998.

Harkness G: *Epidemiology in nursing practice,* St. Louis, 1995, Mosby.

Kannel WB et al: Serum cholesterol, lipoproteins and the risk of coronary heart disease: the Framingham study, *Ann Intern Med* 74:1-12, 1971.

Lilienfeld DE, Stoley PD: *Foundations of epidemiology,* New York, 1994, Oxford University Press.

Lipid Research Clinics Program: The Lipid Research Clinics coronary primary prevention trial results: parts 1 and 2, *JAMA* 251:351-374, 1984.

Liu S et al: Whole-grain consumption and risk of coronary heart disease: results from the nurses' health study, *Am J Clin Nutr* 70:412-419, 1999.

Manson JE et al: A prospective study of walking as compared with vigorous exercise in the prevention of coronary heart disease in women, *New Eng J Med* 341(9):650-658, 1999.

Mattson ME, Pollack ES, Cullen JW: What are the odds that smoking will kill you? *Am J Public Health* 77:425-431, 1987.

Mausner JS, Kramer S: *Mausner and Bahn epidemiology: an introductory text,* ed 2, Philadelphia, 1985, WB Saunders.

Milio N: A framework for prevention: changing health-damaging to health-generating life patterns, *Am J Public Health* 66:435-439, 1976.

Moore ML: From randomized trial to community-focused practice, *Image J Nurs Sch* 31(4):349-354, 1999.

Morton RF, Hebel JR, McCarter RJ: *A study guide to epidemiology and biostatistics,* ed 3, Gaithersburg, Md, 1990, Aspen Publishers.

Multiple Risk Factor Intervention Trial Research Group: Multiple Risk Factor Intervention Trial, *JAMA* 248:1465-1477, 1982.

National Center for Health Statistics: *Health: United States, 1994,* Hyattsville, Md, 1995, Department of Health and Human Services, U.S. Public Health Service.

National Center for Health Statistics: *Natl Vital Stat Rep* 47(9), 1999, http://www.cdc.gov/nchs/data.pdf.

Rubenstein L et al: Effectiveness of a geriatric evaluation unit, *N Engl J Med* 311:1664-1670, 1984.

Simoes EJ et al: The association between leisure-time physical activity and dietary fat in American adults, *Am J Public Health* 85:240-244, 1995.

Snow J: *On the mode of communication of Cholera,* ed 2, London, 1855, Churchill. Reproduced in *Snow on Cholera,* New York, 1936, Commonwealth Fund.

Summary of the National Cholesterol Education Program (NCEP) expert panel on detection, evaluation, and treatment of high blood cholesterol in adults (adult treatment panel II), *JAMA* 269:3015-3023, 1993.

US Bureau of the Census: *Statistical abstract of the United States: 1994,* ed 114, Washington, DC, 1994, The Author.

US Department of Health and Human Services: *Healthy people 2010: conference edition,* Washington DC, 2000, US Government Printing Office.

Willett W: Diet and coronary heart disease. In Willett W, editor: *Nutritional epidemiology,* New York, 1990, Oxford University Press.

CHAPTER

5

Community Assessment

Holly Cassells

OBJECTIVES

Upon completion of this chapter, the reader will be able to do the following:

1. Discuss the major dimensions of a community.
2. Identify sources of information about a community's health.
3. Describe the process of conducting a community assessment.
4. Formulate community and aggregate diagnoses.

KEY TERMS

aggregate
census tracts
community diagnosis
community of solution
Healthy Cities and Healthy Communities
needs assessment
social system
vital statistics
windshield survey

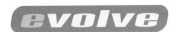

http://evolve.elsevier.com/Nies/

The primary concern of community health nurses is to improve the health of the community. To address this concern, community health nurses use all the principles and skills of nursing and public health practice. This involves using demographic and epidemiological methods to assess the community's health and diagnose its health needs.

Before beginning this process, the community health nurse must define the community. The nurse may wonder how he or she can provide services to such a large and nontraditional "client," but there are smaller and more circumscribed entities that comprise a community than towns and cities. A major aspect of public health practice is the application of approaches and solutions to health problems that ensure the majority of people receive the maximum benefit. To this end, the nurse works to use time and resources efficiently.

Despite the desire to provide services to each individual in a community, the community health nurse recognizes the impracticability of this task. An alternative approach considers the community the unit of service and works with the community using the steps of the nursing process. Therefore the community is not only the context or place where community health nursing occurs; it is the focus of community health nursing care. The nurse partners with community members to identify community problems and develop solutions to ultimately improve the community's health.

Another central goal of public health practitioners is primary prevention, which protects the public's health and prevents disease development. Chapter 3 discussed how these "upstream efforts" are intended to reduce the pain, suffering, and huge expenditures that occur when significant segments of the population essentially "fall into the river" and require downstream resources to resolve their health problems. In a society intolerant of increasingly high health care costs, the need to prevent health problems becomes dire. In addition to reducing the occurrence of disease in individuals, community health nurses must examine the larger aggregate—its structures, environments, and shared health risks—to develop improved upstream prevention programs.

This chapter addresses the first steps in adopting a community- or population-oriented practice. A community health nurse must define a community and describe its characteristics before applying the nursing process. Then the nurse can launch the assessment and diagnosis phase of the nursing process at the aggregate level and incorporate epidemiological approaches. Comprehensive assessment data are essential to directing effective primary prevention interventions within a community.

Gathering this data is one of the core public health functions identified in the Institute of Medicine's (IOM) report on the future of public health (IOM, 1988). The community health nurse participates in assessing the community's health and its ability to deal with health needs. With sound data, the nurse makes a valuable contribution to health policy development (Keppel, 1995).

THE NATURE OF COMMUNITY

Many dimensions describe the nature of community. These include an aggregate of people, a location in space and time, and a social system.

Aggregate of People

An **aggregate** is a community composed of people who share common characteristics. For example, members of a community may share residence in the same city, membership in the same religious organization, or similar demographic characteristics such as age or ethnic background. Communities may consist of overlapping aggregates; therefore some community members may belong to multiple aggregates. Those in senior citizens groups are often all retirees and frequently share common ages, economic pressures, life experiences, interests, and concerns. This group lived through the many societal changes of the past 50 years; therefore they may possess similar perspectives on current issues and trends. Many elderly people share concern for the maintenance of good health, the pursuit of an active lifestyle, and the security of needed services to support a quality life. These shared interests translate into common goals and activities, which are also defining attributes of a community.

Many human factors help delineate a community. Health-related traits, or *risk factors,* are an important group of "people factors." People who have impaired health or a shared predisposition to disease may join together in a group, or community, to learn from and support each other. Parents of disabled infants, people with AIDS (PWA), or those at risk for a second myocardial infarction may consider themselves a community. Even when these individuals are not organized, the nurse may recognize that their unique needs constitute a form of community or aggregate.

A **community of solution** may form when a common problem unites individuals. Although people may have little else in common with each other, their desire to redress problems brings them together. Such problems may include a shared hazard from environmental contamination, a shared health problem arising from a soaring rate of teenage suicide, or a shared political concern about an upcoming city council election. The community of solution often disbands after problem resolution, but it may subsequently identify other common issues.

Each of these shared features may exist among people who are geographically dispersed or in close proximity to each other. However, in many situations proximity facilitates the recognition of commonality and the development of cohesion among members. This active sharing of features fosters a sense of community among individuals.

Location in Space and Time

Regardless of shared features, geographical or physical location may define communities of people. Traditionally, community is an entity delineated by geopolitical boundaries; this view best exemplifies the dimension of location. These boundaries demarcate the periphery of cities, counties, states, and nations. Voting precincts, school districts, water districts, and fire and police protection precincts also set less visible boundary lines.

Census tracts subdivide larger communities. The U.S. Bureau of the Census uses them for data collection and population assessment. Census tracts facilitate the organization of resident information in specific community geographical locales. In densely populated urban areas, the size of tracts tends to be small; therefore data for one or more census tracts frequently describe neighborhood residents. Although residents may not be aware of their census tract's boundaries, census tract data help define and describe neighborhood communities.

The geographical dimension encompasses less formalized types of community that lack official geopolitical boundaries. A geographical landmark may define neighborhoods (e.g., the East Lake section of town or the North Shore area). A particular building style or a common development era may also identify community neighborhoods. Similarly, a dormitory, a communal home, or a summer camp may also be a community because each facility shares a close geographical proximity. Geographical location, including the urban or rural nature of a community, strongly influences the nature of the health problems a community health nurse might find.

Location and the dimension of time define communities. The community's character and health problems evolve over time. Although some communities are very stable, most tend to change with the members' health status and demographics and the larger community's development or decline. For example, the presence of an emerging young workforce may attract new industry, which can alter a neighborhood's health and environment. A community's history illustrates its ability to change and how well it addressed health problems over time.

MAJOR FEATURES OF A COMMUNITY

- Aggregate of people
  The "who": personal characteristics and risks
- Location in space and time
  The "where" and "when": physical location frequently delineated by boundaries and influenced by the passage of time
- Social system
  The "why" and "how": interrelationships of aggregates fulfilling community functions

---

Social System

The third major feature of a community is the relationships that community members form with each other. Community members fulfill the essential functions of community by interacting in groups. These functions provide socialization, role fulfillment, goal achievement, and member support. Therefore a community is a complex **social system** and its interacting members comprise various subsystems within the community. These subsystems are interrelated and interdependent (i.e., the subsystems affect each other and affect various internal and external stimuli). These stimuli consist of a broad range of events, values, conditions, and needs.

A health care system is an example of a complex system that consists of smaller, interrelated subsystems. A health care system can also be a subsystem because it interacts and depends on larger systems like the city government. Changes in the larger system can cause repercussions in many subsystems. For example, when local economic pressures cause a health department to scale back its operations, this affects many subsystems. The health department may eliminate or reduce programs, limit service to other health care providers, reduce access to groups that normally use the system, and deny needed care to families who constitute subsystems in society. Almost every subsystem in the community must react and readjust to such a financial constraint.

EXAMPLE OF SYSTEMS INTERRELATIONSHIPS

Health problems can have a severe impact on multiple systems. For example, the AIDS epidemic has required significant funds for AIDS clients and public AIDS education and prevention. It has made unrelenting demands on many communities that are already strapped for funds to meet its citizens' basic health needs. In San Francisco, the allocation of funds for AIDS programs has reduced funding for other programs such as immunizations, family planning, and well-child care.

HEALTHY COMMUNITIES

Complex community systems receive many varied stimuli. The community's ability to respond effectively to changing dynamics and meet the needs of its members indicates productive functioning. Examining the community's functions and subsystems provides clues to existing and potential health problems. Examples of a community's functions include the provision of accessible and acceptable health services, educational opportunities, and safe, crime-free environments.

The model in Fig. 5-1 suggests assessment dimensions that can help a nurse develop a more complete list of critical community functions. The community health nurse can then prioritize these functions from a particular community's perspective. For example, a study of Americans' views on health and healthy communities conducted for the health care forum suggested that the public is more concerned with quality of life issues than the absence of disease. Fig. 5-2 indicates that the most important determinants of a healthy community are low crime rates and a child-friendly neighborhood environment (The Healthcare Forum, 1994).

A recent movement called **Healthy Cities and Healthy Communities** helps community members

FIGURE 5-1

Diagram of assessment parameters (From Anderson E: *Community as partner: theory and practice in nursing,* ed 3, Philadelphia, 2000, Lippincott).

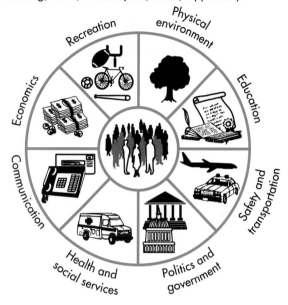

bring about positive health changes. It stresses that interconnectedness among people and among public and private sectors is essential for a community to address the causes of poor health (Flynn, 1992). However, each community and aggregate will presumably have a unique perspective on critical health qualities. Indeed, a community or aggregate may have a divergent definition of health from the community health nurse.

ASSESSING THE COMMUNITY: SOURCES OF DATA

The community health nurse becomes familiar with the community and begins to understand its nature by traveling through the area. The nurse begins to establish certain hunches or hypotheses about the community's health, strengths, and potential health problems through this down-to-earth approach, called "shoe leather epidemiology." The community health nurse must substantiate these initial assessments and impressions with more concrete or defined data before he or she can formulate a community diagnosis and plan.

Community health nurses often perform a community **windshield survey** by driving through an

FIGURE 5-2

What makes a healthy community (From The Healthcare Forum: *What creates health? individuals and communities respond: a national study conducted by DYG, Inc. for the Healthcare Forum,* San Francisco, 1994, The Author).

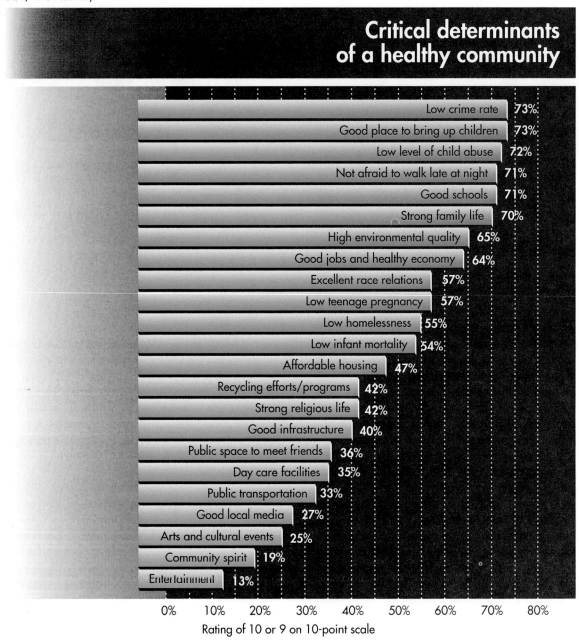

Critical determinants of a healthy community

- Low crime rate — 73%
- Good place to bring up children — 73%
- Low level of child abuse — 72%
- Not afraid to walk late at night — 71%
- Good schools — 71%
- Strong family life — 70%
- High environmental quality — 65%
- Good jobs and healthy economy — 64%
- Excellent race relations — 57%
- Low teenage pregnancy — 57%
- Low homelessness — 55%
- Low infant mortality — 54%
- Affordable housing — 47%
- Recycling efforts/programs — 42%
- Strong religious life — 42%
- Good infrastructure — 40%
- Public space to meet friends — 36%
- Day care facilities — 35%
- Public transportation — 33%
- Good local media — 27%
- Arts and cultural events — 25%
- Community spirit — 19%
- Entertainment — 13%

Rating of 10 or 9 on 10-point scale

area and making organized observations. The nurse can gain an understanding of the environmental layout, including geographical features, the location of agencies, services, businesses, and industries, and can locate possible areas of environmental concern through "sight, sense, and sound." The windshield survey offers the nurse an opportunity to observe people and their role in the community. Box 5-1 provides examples of a windshield survey assessment.

BOX 5-1

Questions to Guide Community Observations During a Windshield Survey

1. Community vitality:
   - Are people visible in the community? What are they doing?
   - Who are the people living in the neighborhood? What is their age range? What is the predominant age (e.g., elderly, preschoolers, young mothers, or school age children)?
   - What ethnicity or race is most common?
   - What is the general appearance of those you observed? Do they appear healthy? Do you notice any obvious disabilities, such as those with walkers or wheelchairs, or those with mental or emotional disabilities? Where do they live?
   - Do you notice residents who are well nourished or malnourished, thin or obese, vigorous or frail, unkempt or scantily dressed, or well dressed and clean?
   - Do you notice tourists or visitors to the community?
   - Do you observe any people who appear to be under the influence of drugs or alcohol?
   - Do you see any pregnant women? Do you see women with strollers and young children?
2. Indicators of social and economic conditions:
   - What is the general condition of the homes you observe? Are these single-family homes or multifamily structures? Is there any evidence of dilapidated housing or of areas undergoing urban renewal?
   - What forms of transportation do people seem to be using? Is there public transit? Were there adequate bus stops with benches and shade? Is transportation available to health care resources?
   - Is there public housing? What is its condition?
   - Are there any indicators of the kinds of work available to residents? Are there job opportunities nearby such as factories, small businesses, or military installations? Are there unemployed people visible such as homeless people?
   - Do you see men congregating in groups on the street? What do they look like and what are they doing?
   - Is this a rural area? Are there farms or agricultural businesses?
   - Do you note any seasonal workers, such as migrant or day laborers?
   - Do you see any women hanging out along the streets? What are they doing?
   - Do you observe any children or adolescents out of school during the daytime?
   - Do you observe any interest in political campaigns or issues such as campaign signs?
   - Do you see any evidence of health education on billboards, advertisements, signs, radio stations, or television stations? Do these methods seem appropriate for the people you observed?
   - What kinds of schools and daycare centers are available?
3. Health resources:
   - Do you notice any hospitals? What kind are they? Where are they located?
   - Are there any clinics? Who do they serve? Are there any family planning services?
   - Are there doctors and dentists offices? Are they specialists or generalists?
   - Do you notice any nursing homes, rehabilitation centers, mental health clinics, alcohol or drug treatment centers, homeless or abused shelters, wellness clinics, health department facilities, family planning services, or pharmacies?
   - Are these resources appropriate and sufficient to address the kinds of problems that exist in this community?
4. Environmental conditions related to health:
   - Do you see evidence of anything that might make you suspicious of ground, water, or air pollutants?
   - What is the sanitary condition of the housing? Is housing overcrowded, dirty, or in need of repair? Are windows screened?

Continued

BOX 5-1—cont'd

Questions to Guide Community Observations During a Windshield Survey—cont'd

- What is the condition of the roads? Are potholes present? Are drainage systems in place? Are there low water crossings and do they have warning signals? Are there adequate traffic lights, signs, sidewalks, and curbs? Are railroad crossings fitted with warnings and barriers? Are streets and parking lots well lit? Is this a heavily trafficked area or are roads rural? Are there curves or features that make the roads hazardous?
- Is there handicapped access to buildings, sidewalks, and streets?
- Do you observe recreational facilities and playgrounds? Are they being used? Is there a YMCA or community center? Are there any daycare facilities or preschools?
- Are children playing in the streets, alleys, yards, or parks?
- Do you see any restaurants?
- Is food sold on the streets? Are people eating in public areas? Are there trash receptacles and places for people to sit? Are public restrooms available?
- What evidence of any nuisances such as ants, flies, mosquitoes, or rodents do you observe?

5. Social functioning:
   - Do you observe any families in the neighborhoods? Can you observe their structure or functioning? Who is caring for the children? What kind of supervision do they have? Is more than one generation present?
   - Are there any identifiable subgroups related to each other either socially or geographically?
   - What evidence of a sense of neighborliness can you observe?
   - What evidence of community cohesiveness can you observe? Are there any group efforts in the neighborhood to improve the living conditions or the neighborhood? Is there a neighborhood watch? Do community groups post signs for neighborhood meetings?
   - How many and what type of churches, synagogues, or places of worship are there?
   - Can you observe anything that would make you suspicious of social problems such as gang activity, juvenile delinquency, drug or alcohol abuse, or adolescent pregnancy?

6. Attitude toward health and health care:
   - Do you observe any evidence of folk medicine practice such as a botanical or herbal medicine shop? Are there any alternative medicine practitioners?
   - Do you observe that health resources are well utilized or underutilized?
   - Is there evidence of preventive or wellness care?
   - Do you observe any efforts to improve the neighborhood's health? Do you notice any health fairs? Do you see advertisements for health-related events, clinics, or lectures?

In addition to direct observational methods, the use of certain public health tools becomes essential to an aggregate-focused nursing practice. The analysis of demographic information and statistical data provides descriptive information about the population. Epidemiology involves the analysis of this data to discover the patterns of health and illness distribution in a population. Epidemiology also involves conducting research to explain the nature of health problems and identify the aggregates at increased risk. The following section provides data sources and describes how the community health nurse can use demographic and epidemiological data to assess the aggregate.

Census Data

Every 10 years, the U.S. Bureau of the Census undertakes a massive survey of all American families. Intermediate surveys collect specific categories of information in addition to this decennial census. These collections of statistical data describe the population characteristics of the nation and progressively smaller geopolitical entities (e.g., states, counties, and census tracts). The census also describes large metropolitan areas that extend beyond formal city boundaries, called metropolitan statistical areas. These areas consist of a central city with more than 50,000 people and include the associated suburban or adjacent counties, which yields a total metropolitan area with over 100,000 people. Cities and their associated counties with a population of one million or more constitute consolidated statistical areas. A census tract is one of the smallest reporting units. It usually consists of 3000 to 6000 people who share similar characteristics such as ethnicity, socioeconomic status, or housing class.

The census is extremely helpful to community health nurses familiarizing themselves with a new community. The census tabulates many demographic variables including population size, socioeconomic status, housing characteristics, and the distribution of age, sex, race, and ethnicity. Variables that describe the community's health are not part of census data. However, census numbers can be denominators for morbidity and mortality rates (see the Calculation of Rates section in Chapter 4). Public and university libraries generally maintain census data and all data following the 1990 census are available on CD-ROM and on the Internet at www.census.gov. Computerization of the data allows the nurse to view several variables in combination (e.g., age and ethnicity) and easily construct a community profile.

The nurse analyzes and interprets data by comparing current and local census data with previous data and information from various locations. The nurse can identify the attributes that make each community unique by comparing data for one census unit, such as a census tract or a city, with those of another community or the entire nation. These attributes provide clues to the community's potential vulnerabilities or health risks. For example, a community health nurse may review census reports and discover that a district has many elderly people. This directs the nurse toward further assessment of the social resources (i.e., housing, transportation, and community centers), health resources (i.e., hospitals, nursing homes, and geriatric clinics), and health problems common to aging people. By identifying the trends in the population over time, the community health nurse can modify public health programs to meet the changing needs of the community.

CENSUS DATA CAN REVEAL "HIDDEN POCKETS" OF NEED

Census data help reveal dominant community features and suggest the existence of small "hidden pockets" of people with special needs. One nurse initially assessed her community in an upper-middle-class bracket. She was surprised to find 20 families living below the poverty level and three living without running water. Therefore deviations from the central trend can determine the community health nurse's priorities in practice.

Vital Statistics

The official registration records of births, deaths, marriages, divorces, and adoptions form the basis of data in **vital statistics**. Every year, city, county, and state health departments aggregate and report these events for the preceding year. When compared with previous years, vital statistics provide indicators of population growth or reduction. In addition to supplying information about the number of births and deaths, registration certificates record the cause of death, which is useful in determining morbidity and mortality trends. Similarly, birth certificates document birth information (e.g., cesarean delivery and teen mothers) and the occurrence of any congenital malformations. This information is also important in assessing the community health status.

Other Sources of Health Data

The U.S. Bureau of the Census conducts numerous surveys on subjects of government interest such as crime, housing, and labor. Results of these surveys, the census reports, and vital statistics reports are usually available through public libraries and on the Internet. The NCHS compiles annual National Health Survey data, which describe health trends in a national sample. The NCHS publishes reports on the prevalence of disability, illness, and other health-related variables. This data is also available on the Internet. See the book's SIMON website to access the site.

In addition to these important sources of information, community health nurses can access a broad range of local, regional, and state government reports that contribute to the comprehensive assessment of a population. Local agencies, chambers of commerce, and health and hospital districts collect invaluable information on their community's health. Local health planning agencies also compile and analyze statistical data during the planning process. The community health nurse can use all of these formal and informal resources in learning about a community or aggregate (Table 5-1). Box 5-2 lists additional information about sources of population health data.

Formal data collection does not exist for all community aspects; therefore many community health nurses must perform additional data collection, compilation, and analysis. For example, school nurses regularly use aggregate data from student records to learn about the demographic composition of their population. They conduct ongoing surveys of classroom attendance and causes of illness, which are essential to an effective school health program. Sometimes the nurse must screen the entire school population to discover the extent of a disease. Thus the school nurse is both a consumer of existent data and a researcher who collects new data for the assessment of the school community.

NEEDS ASSESSMENT

Often the nurse must understand the community's perspective on health status, the services used or required, and concerns. Most official data does not capture this type of information. Data collected directly from an aggregate may be more insightful and accurate; therefore community health nurses sometimes conduct community needs assessments. There are several approaches to gathering subjective data; however, a nurse's careful planning of the process will contribute to its reliability and utility regardless of the method. Box 5-3 presents the required steps in conducting a **needs assessment**.

Selecting a strategy for collecting needs assessment data is dependent upon the size and nature of the aggregate, the purpose for collecting information, and the resources available to the nurse. In some cases, the nurse may survey a small sample of clients to measure their satisfaction with a program. In other situations, a large-scale community needs assessment may determine gaps in service. Although the process of needs assessment can indicate a program's strengths and weaknesses, it can also raise expectations for new services on the part of community members (Timmreck, 1995).

A first approach to gathering data is to *interview key community informants*. These may be knowledgeable residents, elected officials, or health care provid-

ers. It is essential that the community health nurse recognize that the views of these people may not reflect the views of all residents. A second approach is to hold a *community forum* to discuss selected questions. It is important for the nurse to carefully plan the meeting in advance to gain the most useful information. The community health nurse can also mail *surveys* to community members to elicit information from a more diverse group of people who may be unwilling or unable to attend a community forum. *Focus groups* are also effective, particularly for remote and vulnerable segments of a community and for those with underdeveloped opinions (Hildebrandt, 1999). Nurses who conduct focus groups must carefully select participants, formulate questions, and analyze recorded sessions. These sessions can then produce greater interaction and expression of ideas than surveys and may provide more insight into an aggregate's opinions.

APPLICATION OF THE NURSING PROCESS

The second step of the nursing process is synthesizing assessment data into diagnostic statements about the community's health. These statements specify the nature and cause of the actual or potential community health problem and direct the community health nurses' plans to resolve the problem. Muecke (1984) developed a format that assists in writing a **community diagnosis**. The diagnosis consists of four components and identifies the health problem or risk, the affected aggregate or community, the etiologic or causal statement, and the evidence or support for the diagnosis (Fig. 5-3).

Assessment and Diagnosis

The following example demonstrates the process of collecting and analyzing data and deriving community diagnoses. A nurse identified a client health problem during a home visit, which provided the initial impetus for an aggregate health education program. Data collection expanded from the individual client level to a broad range of literature and data about the nature of the problem in populations. The nurse then formulated a community-level diagnosis to direct the ensuing plan.

The Referral

School nurses frequently address student health problems. In the West San Antonio School District, school

Text continued on p. 105

TABLE 5-1

Community Assessment Parameters

Parameter	Importance to CHN*	Sources of Information
Geography Topography Climate (e.g., extreme heat or cold)	Influences nature of health problems and access to health care	Almanac Chamber of Commerce
Population Size Demographic character (e.g., aged or young) Trends Migration Density	Describes population served; suggests their health risks and needs Suggests growth or decline Increases stress; may increase exposure to communicable disease	Census documents Chamber of Commerce Local documents
Environment Water (e.g., source; fluoridated) Sewage and waste disposal Air quality (e.g., ozone; pollutants) Food quality and access Housing (e.g., single-family or multiple family dwellings) Animal control (e.g., exposure to rabies and other zoonotic diseases)	Impacts quality of life and nature of environmental health problems Reflects community resources Suggests socioeconomic issues	Local and state health departments Newspapers Local environmental action group Census documents
Industry Employment levels Manufacturing White vs. blue collar Income levels	Affects social class, access to health care, and resources Influences nature of health problems	Chamber of Commerce Almanac Employment commission Census documents
Education Schools (e.g., physical plant; playground safety) Types of education Literacy rates Special education Health services Sex education School lunch programs (e.g., nutritious diets) After-school programs Day care Access to higher education	Influences socioeconomic status, access to health care, and ability to read and understand health information	Census documents School districts and nurse

*CHN, community health nursing.

Continued

TABLE 5-1—cont'd

Community Assessment Parameters—cont'd

Parameter	Importance to CHN*	Sources of Information
Recreation Parks and playgrounds Libraries Public and private recreation Special facilities	Reflects quality of life, resources available to community, and concern for the young and disadvantaged	Parks and recreation departments Newspapers
Religion Churches and synagogues Denominations Community programs Health-related programs and parish health programs Community organizations	Influences values in community by organizing common interests and concerns Reflects involvement of members, community skills, and resources for community needs	Chamber of Commerce Newspapers Community center newsletters
Communication Newspapers Neighborhood news Radio and television Telephone Hotlines Medical media Public service announcements	Reflects concerns and needs of the community Networks and resources available for health-related use	Local libraries Newspapers Local health department Medical and nursing society
Transportation Intercity and intracity Handicapped Emergency transport	Affects access to services, food, and other resources Reflects resources available to community	Local bus and train service Local hospital emergency service
Public services Fire protection Police protection Emergency medical services Rape treatment centers Utilities	Affects community security Reflects available resources	Local police department
Political organization Structure Methods for filling positions Responsibilities of positions Sources of revenue Voter registration	Reflects level of citizen activism, involvement, values, and concerns Mechanism for nurse activism and lobbying	Newspapers Local political party organization Local board of elections Local representatives
Community development or planning Activities Major issues	Reflects community needs and concerns Affects level of professionals' involvement in issues	Newspapers Local and state planning board Local community organizations

TABLE 5-1—cont'd

Community Assessment Parameters—cont'd

Parameter	Importance to CHN*	Sources of Information
Disaster programs American Red Cross Disaster plans Potential sources of disaster	Offers a level of preparedness, coordination, and available resources Influences resources and plans	Local American Red Cross office Local emergency coordinating council Local fire department
Health statistics Mortality Morbidity Leading causes of death Births	Reflects health problems, trends, and state of community health Affects resources needed and CHN services provided	Local and state health department Health facilities and programs National vital statistics reports NCHS reports *MMWR*
Social problems Mental health Alcoholism and drug abuse Suicide Crime School dropout Unemployment Gangs	Affects health problems and amounts of required services Influences CHN program priorities	Local and state department of social services Local mental health centers Local hotlines Libraries
Health manpower Number of physicians, dentists, and nurses per population	Influences available health resources and nature of CHN practice	Local and state health planning agency Health professional organizations Telephone directory Community service directory
Health professional organizations	Provides support for CHN practice	
Community services (e.g., cost and eligibility, accessibility, and acceptability) Institutional care (e.g., hospitals and nursing homes) Mental health care Ambulatory care Preventive health services Nursing services Welfare services	Reflects available resources	Local United Way organization Local voluntary service directory County hospital Local health department Telephone directory

BOX 5-2

Retrieval of Data

Current data on U.S. population health are stored in many places. Finding the latest statistics at the local, state, or national level can be a challenging experience for a student, community health nurse, graduate student, or nurse researcher. However, statistics provide a necessary comparison in identifying the health status of an aggregate or population in a community. The following guidelines suggest places to begin a search:

Visit the book's SIMON website at *evolve* **http://evolve.elsevier..com/Nies/** to obtain contact information for the specific agencies listed below.

- Reference librarian: The best place to start is in a school or community library or in a large campus' health sciences library. Cultivate a relationship with the reference librarian and learn how to access the literature of interest (e.g., government documents) or how to perform computer-guided literature searches.
- Government documents: Local libraries have a listing of government depository libraries, which house government documents for the public. If the government document is not available at a local library, ask the reference librarian to contact a regional or state library for an interlibrary loan. The Library of Congress in Washington, DC has a Directory of United States Government Depository Libraries.
- *Health: United States, 1999:* This is an annual publication of the NCHS (2000), which reports the latest health statistics for the United States. It presents statistics in areas such as maternal-child health indicators (e.g., prenatal care, low birth weight, and infant mortality), life expectancy, mortality, morbidity (e.g., cancer incidence and survival, AIDS, and diabetes), environmental health indicators (e.g., air pollution and noise exposure), health system use (e.g., national health expenditures, health insurance coverage, physician contacts, and diagnostic and surgical procedures).
- Graphs and tables are easy to read and interpret with accompanying texts. Many statistics include a selected number of years to illustrate trends. Some statistics compare themselves with other countries and U.S. minority populations.
- *Morbidity and Mortality Weekly Report (MMWR):* The CDC in Atlanta, Georgia prepares this publication. State health departments compile weekly reports for the publication, which outline the numbers of cases of notifiable diseases such as AIDS, gonorrhea, hepatitis, measles (rubeola), pertussis, rubella, syphilis, TB, and rabies and reports the deaths in 121 U.S. cities by age. It also reports accounts of interesting cases, environmental hazards, disease outbreaks, or other public health problems. Local and state health departments and many local and health sciences libraries house this weekly publication. A subscription is available on the CDC Internet site.
- CDC: The CDC compiles information on a range of topics including health behavior, educational and community-based programs, unintentional injuries, occupational safety and health, environmental health, oral health, diabetes and chronic disabling conditions, communicable disease, immunizations, clinical preventive services, and surveillance and data systems. Data are reported in several publications and on their website.

BOX 5-3

Steps in the Needs Assessment Process

1. Identify aggregate for assessment.
2. Identify required information.
3. Select method of data gathering.
4. Develop questionnaire or interview questions.
5. Develop procedures for data collection.
6. Train data collectors.
7. Arrange for a sample representative of the aggregate.
8. Conduct needs assessment.
9. Tabulate and analyze data.
10. Identify needs suggested by data.
11. Develop an action plan.

FIGURE 5-3

Format for community health diagnosis (Redrawn from Muecke MA: Community health diagnosis in nursing, *Public Health Nurs* 1:23-35, 1984. Used with permission of Blackwell Scientific Publications).

Increased risk of _____
(disability, disease, etc.)

among _____ related to
(community or population)

_____ as demonstrated
(etiological statement)

in _____ .
(health indicators)

nurses generally reserve several hours a week for home visits.

In a recent case, a teacher expressed concern for a high school junior named "John," whose brother was dying from cancer. In a health class, John shared his personal fears about cancer, which caused his classmates to question their own cancer risks and how they might reduce their risks.

Family Assessment

The school nurse visited John's family and learned that their 25-year-old son had testicular cancer. Since his diagnosis one year earlier, he had undergone a range of therapies that were palliative but not curative; the cancer was advanced at the time of diagnosis. The nurse spent time with the family discussing care, answering questions, and exploring available support for the entire family.

At a school nurse staff meeting, the nurse inquired about her colleagues' experiences with other young clients with this type of cancer. Only one nurse remembered a young man with testicular cancer. The nurses were not familiar with its prevalence, incidence, risk factors, prevention strategies, or early detection approaches. The nurse recognized the high probability that high school students would have similar questions and could benefit from reliable information.

Community Assessment

The school nurse embarked on a community assessment to answer these questions. The nurse first collected information about testicular cancer. Second, the nurse reviewed the nursing and medical literature for key articles discussing client care, diagnosis, and treatment. Epidemiological studies provided additional data regarding testicular cancer's distribution pattern in the population and associated risk factors.

The nurse learned that young men aged 20 to 35 years were at the greatest risk. Other major risk factors were not identified. It was learned that healthy young men do not seek testicular cancer screening and regular health care; they may be apprehensive about conditions affecting sexual function. These factors contribute to delayed detection and treatment. Although only an estimated 6900 new cases of testicular cancer were diagnosed in the United States in 2000, it was one of the most common tumors in young men. Furthermore, this cancer is amenable to treatment with early diagnosis (American Cancer Society, 2000).

Based on these facts, the nurse reasoned that a prevention program would benefit high school students. However, to perform a comprehensive assessment, it was important that the nurse clarify what students did know, how comfortable they were discussing sexual health, and how much the subject interested them. Therefore the nurse approached the junior and senior high school students and administered a questionnaire to elicit this information. The nurse also queried the health teacher about the amount of pertinent cancer and sexual development information the students received in the classroom. The nurse considered the latter an important prerequisite to dealing with the sensitive subject of sexual health. According to the health teacher, the students did receive instruction about physical development and psychosexual issues. Students expressed a strong desire for more classroom instruction on these subjects and more information on cancer prevention. However, they did not have sufficient knowledge of the beneficial health practices related to cancer prevention and early detection.

Community Diagnosis

After collecting a broad range of assessment data, the nurse was able to document that a potential health need existed in the high school community. Next, the nurse analyzed and synthesized the data in a community diagnosis. For this student aggregate, the community diagnosis was the following:

There is an increased risk of undetected testicular cancer among young men related to insufficient knowledge about the disease and the methods for preventing and detecting it at an early stage demonstrated by high rates of late initiation of treatment.

Planning

Clarifying the problem and its cause helped the nurse direct the planning phase of the nursing process. Planning encompassed several activities, including the discovery of recommended health care practices regarding testicular cancer. The nurse also sought to determine the most effective and appropriate educational approaches for male and female high school students. Identifying helpful community agencies was also an essential part of the process. The local chapter of the American Cancer Society provided valuable information, materials, and consultative services. A nearby nursing school's media center and faculty were also very supportive of the program.

After formalizing her objectives, the nurse presented her plan to the high school's teaching coordinator and principal. Their approval was necessary before the nurse could implement the project. After eliciting their enthusiastic support, the nurse proceeded with more detailed plans. She selected and developed classroom instruction methods and activities that would maximize high school students' involvement. The nurse also ordered a film and physical models for demonstrating and practicing testicular self-examination (TSE). She prepared group exercises designed to relax and assist students in being comfortable with the sensitive subject matter.

The nurse scheduled two 40-minute sessions dealing with testicular cancer for the junior-level health class. In a final step of the planning phase, she designed evaluation tools that assessed knowledge levels after each class session and measured the extent students integrated these health practices into their lifestyles at the end of their junior and senior years.

The nurse was now ready to proceed with the implementation of a testicular cancer prevention and screening program. She initiated the assessment phase by identifying an individual client and family with a health need and she extended the assessment to the high school aggregate. Her data collection at the aggregate level, for both the general and local high school populations, assisted in her community diagnosis. The diagnosis directed the development of a community-specific health intervention program and its subsequent implementation and evaluation.

Intervention

The nurse conducted the two sessions in a health education class. At the beginning of the class period, students participated in a group exercise and the nurse asked them about their knowledge of testicular cancer. The nurse showed a film and led a discussion about cancer screening. In the second session, she demonstrated the self-examination procedure using testicular models and supervised the students while they practiced the procedure on the models. The nurse advised the male students about the frequency of self-examination. With the females, she discussed the need for young men to be aware of their increased risk, drawing a parallel to breast self-examination.

Evaluation

After completing the class sessions, the nurse administered the questionnaires she developed for evaluation purposes. Analysis of the questionnaires indicated that knowledge levels were very high immediately after the classes. Students were pleased with the frank discussion, the opportunity to ask questions, and the clear responses to a sensitive subject. Teachers also offered positive feedback. Consequently, the nurse became a knowledgeable health resource in the high school.

Intermediate-term evaluation occurred at the end of the students' junior and senior years. The nurse arranged a 15-minute evaluation during other classes, which assessed the integration of positive health practices and TSEs into the students' lifestyles. At the end of the school year, the prevalence of regular self-assessment was significantly lower than knowledge levels. However, 30% of male students reported regularly practicing self-examinations at the end of one year and 70% reported they had performed a self-examination at least once during the past year.

The compilation of incidence data is ideal for long-term evaluation and it documents the reduction of a community health problem. Testicular cancer is very rare; therefore incidence data are not reliable and may not be feasible to collect. However, for more prevalent conditions, objective statistics help reveal increases and decreases in disease rates, which may be related to the strengths and deficiencies of health programs.

It is evident that epidemiological data and methods are essential to each phase of the nursing process. The community health nurse compiles a range of assessment data that support the nursing diagnosis. Epidemiological studies help plan a program by establishing the effectiveness of certain interventions and their specificity for different aggregates. This information supports the nurse's implementation of tailored intervention strategies. Finally, epidemiological data are important for the community health nurse's documentation of a program's long-term effectiveness.

COMPREHENSIVE PERINATAL PROGRAM IMPROVES BIRTH OUTCOMES IN TEENAGE MEDICAID CLIENTS

A collaborative project among a graduate nursing student, a graduate public health student, and a private, nonprofit, community-based medical center using an epidemiological design (i.e., retrospective and cross-sectional) was carried out to evaluate the effect of enrollment in two special perinatal programs—the Comprehensive Perinatal Services Program (CPSP) and the school-based Comprehensive Teenage Pregnancy and Parenting Program (CTAPPP)—on the occurrence of adverse perinatal outcomes in teenage Medicaid clients who delivered at the medical center. The project was in response to staff nurses' observations of a recurring clinical problem: questionable perinatal outcomes among teenage girls giving birth at the medical center, a clinical problem with implications for the health of the community.

The CPSP program is a comprehensive program that provides perinatal services including medical, nursing, nutritional, psychosocial, childbirth, and parenting educational interventions that must be provided by a physician or a certified nurse midwife, a certified nutritionist, a social worker with a master's degree, and a certified nurse educator, respectively. The CTAPPP offers academic, health, nutrition, perinatal, and parenting education support and case management services to pregnant and parenting teenagers.

Using historic data, pregnancy outcomes were compiled on 312 Medicaid, largely African-American (75.9%) clients, aged 12 to 18 years, who delivered at the medical center between June 1991 and June 1992. Adverse perinatal outcomes including low birth weight, gestational age less than 37 weeks, and admission to neonatal intensive care unit were found in 10.9% of the study sample; 35% received substandard prenatal care. Enrollment in CPSP was associated with reduced adverse perinatal outcomes; however, enrollment in CTAPPP was not. A more comprehensive prenatal program, such as CPSP, may improve birth outcomes in high-risk teenage populations. The project presents a model for linking data on birth outcomes to data on program participation among Medicaid clients to assess the efficacy of existing programs.

From Perkocha VA et al: The efficacy of two comprehensive perinatal programs on reducing adverse perinatal outcomes, *Am J Prev Med* 11(suppl 1):21-29, 1995.

SUMMARY

Communities form for a variety of reasons and can be homogeneous or heterogeneous in their composition. To help assess the nature of a given community, community health nurses study and interpret data from sources such as local government agencies, census reports, morbidity and mortality reports, and vital statistics. Nurses can gather valuable information about the causes and prevalence of health and disease in a community through epidemiological studies. Based on this information, the community health nurse can apply the nursing process, which expands assessment, diagnosis, planning, intervention, and evaluation from the individual client level to a targeted aggregate in the community.

LEARNING ACTIVITIES

1. Walk through a neighborhood and compile a list of variables that are important to describe with demographic and epidemiological data. Write down hunches or preconceived notions about the nature of the community's population. Compare ideas with the collected statistical data.
2. Walk through a neighborhood and describe the sensory information (i.e., smells, sounds, and sights). How do each relate to the community's health?
3. Compile a range of relevant demographic and epidemiological data for the community by examining census reports, vital statistics reports, city records, and other library and agency sources.
4. Using the collected data, identify three community health problems and formulate three community health diagnoses.

REFERENCES

American Cancer Society: *Cancer facts and figures 2000: graphical data,* 2000, The Author, www.cancer.org/statistics/cff2000/data/newCaseSex.html.

Anderson E: *Community as partner: theory and practice in nursing,* ed 3, Philadelphia, 2000, Lippincott.

Flynn BC: Healthy cities: a model of community change, *Fam Com Health* 15(1):13-23, 1992.

Hildebrandt E: Focus groups and vulnerable populations: insight into client strengths and needs in complex community health care environments, *Nurs Health Care Perspect* 20(5):256-259, 1999.

Institute of Medicine: *The future of public health,* Washington, DC, 1988, National Academy Press.

Keppel KG: What is assessment? *J Public Health Management Pract* 1(2):1-7, 1995.

Muecke MA: Community health diagnosis in nursing, *Public Health Nurs* 1:23-35, 1984.

National Center For Health Statistics: *United States: 1999,* Hyattsville Md, 2000, Department of Health and Human Services, U.S. Public Health Service.

Perkocha VA et al: The efficacy of two comprehensive perinatal programs on reducing adverse perinatal outcomes, *Am J Prev Med* 11(suppl 1):21-29, 1995.

The Healthcare Forum: *What creates health? individuals and communities respond: a national study conducted by DYG, Inc. for the Healthcare Forum,* San Francisco, 1994, The Author.

Timmreck TC: *Planning, program development, and evaluation: a handbook for health promotion, aging, and health services,* Boston, 1995, Jones and Bartlett Publishers.

6

Community Health Planning, Implementation, and Evaluation

Deborah Godfrey Brown, Barbara S. Morgan, and Patricia M. Burbank

OBJECTIVES

Upon completion of this chapter, the reader will be able to do the following:

1. Describe the concept "community as client."
2. Apply the nursing process to the larger aggregate within a system's framework.
3. Describe the steps in the health planning model.
4. Identify the appropriate prevention level and system level for nursing interventions in families, groups, aggregates, and communities.
5. Recognize major health planning legislation.
6. Analyze factors that have contributed to the failure of health planning legislation to control health care costs.
7. Describe the community health nurse's role in health planning, implementation, and evaluation.

KEY TERMS

certificate of need (CON)
community as client
health planning
health planning model
Hill-Burton Act
key informant
National Health Planning and Resources Development Act
Partnership for Health Program (PHP)
Regional Medical Programs (RMP)

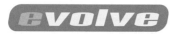

http://evolve.elsevier.com/Nies/

Health planning for and with the community is an essential component of community health nursing practice. The term **health planning** seems simple, but the underlying concept is quite complex. Like many other components of community health nursing, health planning tends to vary at different aggregate levels. Health planning with an individual or a family may focus on direct care needs or self-care responsibilities; at the group level, the primary goal may be health education; and at the community level, health planning may involve population disease prevention or environmental hazard control. The following example illustrates the interaction of community health nursing roles with health planning at a variety of aggregate levels:

Nancy Jones is an RN in a suburban high school. During the course of the school year she noted an increasing incidence of pregnancy-related dropouts. A nurse at the junior high school confirmed a corresponding increase in withdrawal among younger pregnant teenagers. After reviewing information in nursing journals, other professional journals, and the general media, Nancy discovered a national epidemic of unwed pregnant teenagers.

Nancy questioned the reason for the increased pregnancies. Her assessment of the problem included several findings. Sexually active teenagers do not use contraception regularly because they want their actions to seem "spontaneous" and not "planned." Also, a variety of sexual misconceptions led teens to believe they were invulnerable to pregnancy. For example, a typical misconception among female students was "I will not become pregnant if I do not have regular periods or if my boyfriend does not ejaculate inside me." Teenagers also find it difficult or embarrassing to obtain certain contraceptives. The suburb does not have a local family planning clinic and area physicians are reluctant to counsel teenagers or prescribe contraceptives without parental permission. The nurse also discovered that several years earlier, a group of parents stopped an attempt by the local school board to establish sex education in the school system. The parents believed this responsibility belonged in the home.

Nancy considered all of these factors in developing her plan of action. She met with teachers, officials, and parents. Teachers and school officials were willing to deal with this sensitive issue if parents could recognize its validity. In meetings, many parents revealed they were uncomfortable discussing sexuality with their teenaged children and welcomed

assistance. However, they were concerned that teachers might introduce the mechanics of reproduction without giving proper attention to the moral decisions and obligations involved in relationships. The parents expressed their desire to participate in curriculum planning and to meet with the teachers, instead of following a previous plan that required parents to sign a consent form for each teenager. In support of the parents, Nancy asked a nearby metropolitan family planning agency to consider opening a part-time clinic in the suburb. The local school board proposed instituting a home-tutoring program for pregnant teenagers, which would encourage their return to school.

Implementing such a comprehensive plan is time consuming and requires community involvement and resources. The nurse enlisted the aid of school officials and other community professionals. Time will reveal the plan's long-term effectiveness in reducing teen pregnancy.

This example shows how nurses can and should become involved in health planning. Teen pregnancy is a significant health problem and often results in lower education and socioeconomic status (SES), which can lead to further health problems. The nurse's assessment and planned interventions involved individual teenagers, parents and families, the school system, and community resources.

This chapter provides an overview of health planning and evaluation from a nursing perspective. It also describes a model for student involvement in health planning projects and a review of significant health planning legislation.

OVERVIEW OF HEALTH PLANNING

One of the major criticisms of community health nursing practice involves the shift in focus from the community and larger aggregate to family caseload management or agency responsibilities. When focusing on the individual or family, nurses must remember that these clients are members of a larger population group or community and environmental factors influence them. Nurses can identify these factors and plan health interventions by implementing an assessment of the entire aggregate or community. Fig. 6-1 illustrates this process.

The concept of "community as client" is not new. Lillian Wald's work at New York City's Henry Street settlement in the late 1800s exemplifies this concept. At the Henry Street settlement, Miss Wald, Mary

The community as client. Chapter 5, Table 5-1 (pps. 101-103) provides assessment parameters that help identify the client's assets and needs.

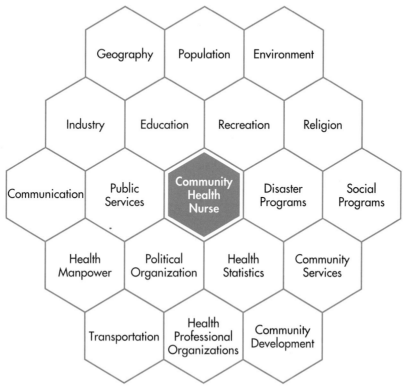

Brewster, and other public health nurses worked with extremely poor immigrants, cared for the homebound ill, and sought large-scale social reform (Kalisch and Kalisch, 1995).

> The "case" element in these early reports of hers [Wald] got less and less emphasis; she instinctively went behind the symptoms to appraise the whole individual, saw that one could not understand the individual without understanding the family, saw that the family was in the grip of larger social and economic forces, which it could not control.
>
> (Duffus, 1938)

The early beginnings of public health nursing incorporated visits to the homebound ill and applied the nursing process to larger aggregates and communities to improve health for the greatest number of people. Wald's goals, and those of other public health nurses, were health promotion and disease prevention for the entire community (Silverstein, 1985). Health planning at the aggregate or community level is necessary to accomplish these goals.

Through the 1950s, public health nursing adopted Wald's nursing concepts, which focused on mobilizing communities to solve local problems, treat the poor, and improve the environmental conditions that fostered disease. During the 1950s, social changes such as suburbanization, increased family mobility, and enhanced government health expenditures updated nursing roles. Since the mid1960s, there has been a shift from public health nursing, which emphasizes community care, to community health nursing, which includes all non-hospital nursing activities. New trends constantly emerge through health care reform debates. It has become more important to use nurses as primary care providers in the health care system. Home health care services are a very significant component of the health care system. A continued shift into the community requires that community health nurses become in-

TABLE 6-1

Levels of Community Health Nursing Practice

Client	Example	Characteristics	Health Assessment	Nursing Involvement
Individual	Lisa McDonald	An individual with various needs	Individual strengths, problems, and needs	Client-nurse interaction
Family	Moniz family	A family system with individual and group needs	Individual and family strengths, problems, and needs	Interactions with individuals and the family group
Group	Boy Scout troop Alzheimer's support group	Common interests, problems, and needs Interdependency	Group dynamics Fulfillment of goals	Group member and leader
Population group	AIDS patients in a given state Pregnant adolescents in a school district	Large, unorganized group with common interests, problems, and needs	Assessment of common problems, needs, and vital statistics	Application of nursing process to identified needs
Organization	A work place A school	Organized group in a common location with shared governance and goals	Relationship of goals, structure, communication, patterns of organization to its strengths, problems, and needs	Consultant and/or employee application of nursing process to identified needs
Community	Italian neighborhood Anytown, USA	An aggregate of people in a common location with organized social systems	Analysis of systems, strengths, characteristics, problems, and needs	Community leader, participant, and health care provider

creasingly visible and vocal leaders of health care reform.

The increased focus on community-based nursing practice yields a greater emphasis on the aggregate becoming the client or care unit. However, the community health nurse should not neglect nursing care at the individual and family levels by focusing on health care only at the aggregate level. Rather, the nurse can use this community information to help understand individual and family health problems and improve their health status. Table 6-1 illustrates the differences in community health nursing practice at the individual, family, and community levels.

However, before nurses can participate in health care planning, they must be knowledgeable about the process and comfortable with the concept of **community as client** or care focus. It is essential that undergraduate and graduate nursing programs integrate these concepts into the curricula. If basic and advanced nursing education includes health planning,

the student becomes aware of the process and the professional involvement opportunities.

Early efforts to provide students with learning experiences in community health investigation included Hegge's use of learning packets for independent study (1973) and Ruybal's opportunities for students to apply epidemiological concepts in community program planning and evaluation (1975). However, neither of these approaches presented a complete model that incorporated the nursing process into a health planning framework. More recently, Ammerman and Parks (1998) stressed that "asset assessment" is an important component of community planning and intervention. Several other authors including Hamilton (1985), Mahon (1991), Shuster and Goeppinger (1996), and Doerr et al. (1998) described the community health planning process. However, none of these models use practical examples for actual student implementation throughout the entire process.

FIGURE 6-2

Health planning model.

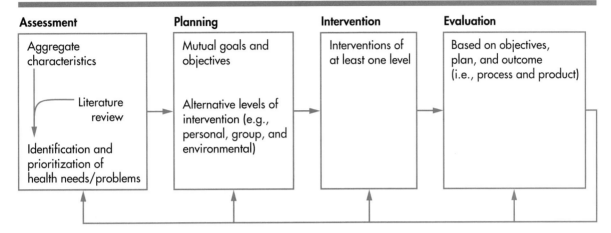

HEALTH PLANNING MODEL

A model based on Hogue's (1985) group intervention model was developed in response to this need for population focus. The **Health Planning Model** aims to improve aggregate health and applies the nursing process to the larger aggregate within a systems framework. Fig. 6-2 depicts this model. Incorporated into a health planning project, the model can help students view larger client aggregates and gain knowledge and experience in the health planning process. Nurses must carefully consider each step in the process using this model. Box 6-1 outlines these steps. In addition, Box 6-2 provides the systems framework premises that nurses should incorporate.

Several considerations affect how nurses choose a specific aggregate for study. The community may have extensive or limited opportunities appropriate for nursing involvement. Additionally, each community offers different possibilities for health intervention. For example, an urban area might have a variety of industrial and business settings that need assistance, whereas a suburban community may offer a choice of family-oriented organizations like boys and girls clubs and parent-teacher associations that would benefit from intervention.

A nurse should also consider personal interests and strengths in selecting an aggregate for intervention. For example, the nurse should consider whether he or she has an interest in teaching health promotion and preventive health or in planning for organizational change; whether his or her communication

skills are better suited to large or small groups; and whether he or she has a preference for working with the elderly or with children. Thoughtful consideration of these and other variables will facilitate assessment and planning.

Assessment

When establishing a professional relationship with the chosen aggregate it is necessary and important for a community health nurse to gain entry into the group. Good communication skills are essential to make a positive first impression. The nurse should make an appointment with the group leaders to set up the first meeting.

The nurse must initially clarify his or her position, organizational affiliation, knowledge, and skills. The nurse should also clarify mutual expectations and available times. Once entry is established, the nurse continues negotiation to maintain a mutually beneficial relationship.

Meeting with the aggregate on a regular basis will allow the nurse to make an in-depth assessment. Determining sociodemographic characteristics (e.g., distribution of age, sex, and race) may help the nurse ascertain health needs and develop appropriate intervention methods. For example, adolescents need information regarding nutrition, abuse of drugs and alcohol, and relationships with the opposite sex. They usually do not enjoy lectures in a classroom environment, but the nurse must possess skills to initiate

BOX **6-1**

Health Planning Project Objectives

I. Assessment
   A. Specify the aggregate level for study (e.g., group, population group, or organization). Identify and provide a general orientation to the aggregate (e.g., characteristics of the aggregate system, suprasystem, and subsystems). Include the reasons for selecting this aggregate and the method for gaining entry.
   B. Describe specific characteristics of the aggregate.
      1. Sociodemographic characteristics: including age, sex, race or ethnic group, religion, educational background and level, occupation, income, and marital status.
      2. Health status: work or school attendance, disease categories, mortality, health care use, and population growth and population pressure measurements (e.g., rates of birth and death, divorce, unemployment, and drug and alcohol abuse). Select indicators appropriate for the chosen aggregate.
      3. Suprasystem influences: existing health services to improve aggregate health and the existing or potential positive and negative impact of other community-level social system variables on the aggregate. Identify the data collection methods.
   C. Provide relevant information from the literature review, especially in terms of the characteristics, problems, or needs within this type of aggregate. Compare the health status of the aggregate with similar aggregates, the community, the state, and the nation.
   D. Identify the specific aggregate's health problems and needs based on comparative data collection analysis and interpretation and literature review. Include input from clients regarding their need perceptions. Give priorities to health problems and needs and indicate how to determine these priorities.
II. Planning
   A. Select one health problem or need and identify the ultimate goal of intervention. Identify specific, measurable objectives as mutually agreed upon by the student and aggregate.
   B. Describe the alternative interventions that are necessary to accomplish the objectives. Consider interventions at each system level where appropriate (e.g., aggregate system, suprasystem, and subsystems). Select and validate the intervention(s) with the highest probability of success. Interventions may use existing resources, or require the development of new resources.
III. Intervention
   A. Implement at least one level of planned intervention when possible.
   B. If intervention was not implemented, provide reasons.
IV. Evaluation
   A. Evaluate the plan, objectives, and outcomes of the intervention(s). Include the aggregate's evaluation of the project. Evaluation should consider the process, product, appropriateness, and effectiveness.
   B. Make recommendations for further action based on the evaluation and communicate these to the appropriate individuals or system levels. Discuss implications for community health nursing.

small-group involvement and participation. An adult group's average educational level will affect the group's knowledge base and their comfort with formal vs. informal learning settings. The nurse may find it more difficult to coordinate time and energy commitments if an organization is the focus group, because the aggregate members may be more diverse.

The nurse may gather information about sociodemographic characteristics from a variety of sources. These sources include observing the aggregate, consulting with other aggregate workers (e.g., the factory or school nurse, a Headstart teacher, or the resident manager of a high-rise senior citizen apartment building), reviewing available records or charts, and

---

BOX **6-2**

Systems Framework Premises

I. Each system is a goal-directed collection of interacting or interdependent parts, or subsystems

II. The whole system is continually interacting with and adapting to the environment, or suprasystem

III. There is a hierarchical structure (suprasystem → system → subsystems)

IV. Each system is characterized by

  A. Structure: arrangement and organization of parts, or subsystems

    1. Organization and configuration (e.g., traditional vs. nontraditional; greater variability [no right or wrong, and no proper vs. improper form])

    2. Boundaries (open vs. closed; regulate input and output)

    3. Territory (spatial and behavioral)

    4. Role allocation

  B. Functions: goals and purpose of system and activities necessary to ensure survival, continuity, and growth of system

    1. General

      a. Physical: food, clothing, shelter, protection from danger, and provision for health and illness care

      b. Affectional: meeting the emotional needs of affection and security

      c. Social: identity, affiliation, socialization, and controls

    2. Specific: each family, group, or aggregate has their own individual agenda regarding values, aspirations, and cultural obligations

  C. Process and dynamics

    1. Adaptation: attempt to establish and maintain equilibrium; balance between stability, differentiation, and growth; self-regulation and adaptation (equilibrium and homeostasis)

      a. Internal: families, groups, or aggregates

      b. External: interaction with suprasystem

    2. Integration: unity and ability to communicate

    3. Decision making: power distribution, consensus, accommodation, and authority

---

interviewing members of the aggregate (i.e., verbally or via a short questionnaire).

In assessing the aggregate's health status, the nurse must consider both the positive and negative factors. Unemployment or the presence of disease may suggest specific health problems, but low rates of absenteeism at work or school may suggest a need to focus more on preventive interventions. The specific aggregate determines the appropriate health status measures. Immunization levels are an important index for children, but nurses rarely collect this information for adults. However, the nurse should consider the need for influenza injections with the elderly. Similarly, the nurse would expect a lower incidence of chronic disease with children, whereas the elderly have higher rates of long-term morbidity and mortality.

The aggregate's suprasystem may facilitate or impede health status. Different organizations and communities provide various resources and services to their members. Some are obviously health related, such as the presence or absence of hospitals, clinics, private practitioners, emergency facilities, health centers, home health agencies, and health departments. Support services and facilities such as group meal sites or Meals on Wheels (MOW) for the elderly and recreational facilities and programs for children, adolescents, and adults are also important. Transportation availability, reimbursement mechanisms or sliding-scale fees, and community-based volunteer groups may determine the use of services. An assessment of these factors requires researching public records (e.g., town halls, telephone directories, and community services directories) and interviewing health professionals, volunteers, and key informants in the community. The nurse should augment existing resources or create a new service rather than duplicating what is already available to the aggregate.

A literature review is an important means of comparing the aggregate with the "norm." For example, children in a Headstart setting, day care center, or elementary school may exhibit a high rate of upper respiratory tract infections during the winter. The nurse should review the pediatric literature and determine the normal incidence for this age range in group environments. Further, the nurse should research potential problems in an especially healthy aggregate (e.g., developmental stresses for adolescents or work or family stresses for adults) or determine whether a factory's experience with work-related injury is within an average range. Comparing the foregoing assessment with research reports, statistics, and health information will help determine and prioritize the aggregate's health problems and needs.

The last phase of the initial assessment is identifying and prioritizing the specific aggregate's health problems and needs. This phase should relate directly to the assessment and the literature review and should include a comparative analysis of the two. Most importantly, this step should reflect the aggregate's perceptions of need. Depending on the aggregate, the nurse may consult the aggregate members directly or interview others who work with the aggregate (e.g., a Headstart teacher). Interventions are seldom successful if the nurse omits or ignores the clients' input.

Finally, the nurse must prioritize the identified problems and needs to create an effective plan. The nurse should consider the following factors when determining priorities:

- Aggregate's preferences
- Number of individuals in the aggregate affected by the health problem
- Severity of the health need or problem
- Availability of potential solutions to the problem
- Practical considerations such as individual skills, time limitations, and available resources

In addition, the nurse may further refine the priorities by applying a framework like Maslow's (1968) hierarchy of needs (i.e., lower level needs have priority over higher level needs) or Leavell and Clark's (1965) levels of prevention (i.e., primary prevention may take priority for children, whereas tertiary prevention may take higher priority for the elderly).

Assessment is ongoing throughout the nurse's relationship with the aggregate. However, the nurse should proceed to the planning stage once the initial assessment is complete. It is particularly important to link the assessment stage with other stages at this step in the process. Planning should stem directly and logically from the assessment and implementation should be realistic.

Planning

Again, the nurse should determine which problems or needs require intervention based on prioritization. Then the nurse must identify the ultimate intervention goal. For example, the nurse should determine whether to increase the aggregate's knowledge level and whether an intervention will cause a change in health behavior. It is important to have specific and measurable goals and objectives. This will facilitate planning the nursing interventions and determining the evaluation process.

Planning interventions is a multistep process. First, the nurse must determine the intervention levels (e.g., subsystem, aggregate system, and/or suprasystem).

Second, the nurse should plan interventions for each system level, which may center on the primary, secondary, or tertiary levels of prevention. These levels apply to aggregates, communities, and individuals. Primary prevention consists of health promotion and activities that protect the client from illness or dysfunction. Secondary prevention includes early diagnosis and treatment to reduce the duration and severity of disease or dysfunction. Tertiary prevention applies to irreversible disability or damage and aims to rehabilitate and restore an optimal level of functioning. Plans should include goals and activities that reflect the identified problem's prevention level.

Third, the nurse should validate the practicality of the planned interventions according to available personal, aggregate, and suprasystem resources. Although teaching is often a major component of community health nursing, the nurse should consider other potential forms of intervention (e.g., personal counseling, game therapy, or community service development). Finally, the nurse should coordinate the planned interventions with the aggregate's input to maximize participation.

Intervention

The intervention stage may be the most enjoyable stage for the nurse and the clients. The nurse's careful preliminary assessment and planning should help ensure the aggregate's positive response to the intervention. Although implementation should follow the initial plan, the nurse should prepare for unexpected problems (e.g., bad weather, transportation problems, poor attendance, or competing events). If the nurse is unable to complete the intervention, the reasons for its failure should be analyzed.

Evaluation

Evaluation is an important component for understanding the success or failure of a project. The evaluation should include the participant's verbal or written feedback and the nurse's detailed analysis. Evaluation includes reflecting on each previous stage to determine the plan's strengths and weaknesses. It is important to evaluate both the positive and negative aspects of each experience honestly and comprehensively. During this stage, the nurse may ask the following questions:

Were plans based on an incomplete assessment?
Did the plan allow adequate client involvement?
Were the interventions realistic or unrealistic in terms of available resources?
Did the plan consider all levels of prevention?
Were the stated goals and objectives accomplished?
Were the participants satisfied with the interventions?
Did the plan advance the knowledge level of the aggregate and the nurse?

The intervention may have limited impact if the nurse fails to communicate follow-up recommendations to the aggregate upon completion of the project. Although follow-up activity is not necessary for every

plan, most require additional interventions within the aggregate using community agencies and resources. A comprehensive health planning project involves a close working relationship with the aggregate and careful consideration of each step.

HEALTH PLANNING PROJECTS

Successful Projects

Student projects have used this health planning model with group, organization, population group, and community aggregates. Table 6-2 describes interventions with these aggregates at the subsystem, aggregate system, and suprasystem levels.

Obese Children

A nursing student and a school nurse identified two obese brothers in a Headstart program. The student made a home visit after contacting the boys' mother and learned that the boys' parents were separated. The children spent time with both parents and the grandparents. Obesity seemed to be a family problem; both parents were obese. The student worked with the boys together and separately, educated the mother and the grandparents, and met once with the boys' father. Both the boys' mother and grandparents participated in the planning. The student created a variety of interventions, which included a food diary, a food collage, and information about low-calorie snacks and menu planning for the adults, and a "Food Land" game for the boys. By the end of the semester, the student noted positive changes in the mother's and boys' dietary patterns. The Headstart nurse tracked the

TABLE 6-2

Interventions by Type of Aggregate and System Level

Project	Type of Aggregate	System Level for Intervention
Obese children	Group	Subsystem and aggregate system
Rehabilitation group	Group	Subsystem and aggregate system
Textile industry	Organization	Aggregate system and suprasystem
Exercise for elderly	Population group	Aggregate system
Bilingual students (case study)	Group, organization, and population group	Aggregate system and suprasystem
Crime watch	Community	Aggregate system and suprasystem

family's progress to continue reinforcement after the student left the situation.

Textile Industry

A nursing student studied a textile plant that had approximately 470 employees and did not have an occupational health nurse. The student collected data and identified three major problems or needs by collaborating with management and union representatives. First, the student observed that the most common, costly, and chronic work-related injury in plant workers was lower back injury. Second, employees had concern about possible undetected hypertension. Third, the first-aid facilities were disorganized and without an accurate inventory system. The student planned and implemented interventions for all three areas.

On the suprasystem level, the student formulated plans with the company's physicians and lobbied management to enact an employee-training program on proper lifting techniques. The student proposed creating specific and concise job descriptions and requirements to facilitate potential employees' medical assessment. In addition, the student organized and clearly labeled the first-aid supplies and developed an inventory system. On the aggregate system level, the student planned and conducted a hypertension screening program. Approximately 85% of the employees underwent screening and 10 people had elevated blood pressure readings. These 10 people were subsequently diagnosed as hypertensive.

As a result of the project, management representatives recognized that a variety of nursing interventions could improve or maintain workers' health. Consequently, management hired the student upon graduation to be the occupational health nurse.

Exercise for the Elderly

Another project involved the residents of a housing complex for the elderly. The nursing student met with 20 women and assessed their needs through a short questionnaire. The answers revealed that the need for exercise was the women's highest priority. The student investigated existing resources and found that the local Young Women's Christian Association's (YWCA) senior exercise class met three times a week at a cost of one dollar per session. The student shared this information with the population group, but members did not consider the program feasible. Instead, the student instituted an aggregate system level intervention, in which it was agreed to have weekly student-directed sessions at the housing complex.

At the close of the study, the participants indicated that they felt better about themselves after exercising and maintaining their range of motion. The student also had a positive experience; she learned more about the elderly and gained skill in applying the nursing process to a larger aggregate in the community.

Crime Watch

Another nursing student was concerned with the rising incidence of crime in a community and organized a crime watch program. The student met periodically with the police and local residents, or aggregate system. Interventions included posting crime watch signs in the neighborhood and establishing more frequent police patrols at the suprasystem level. The program increased the residents' awareness and concern for neighborhood safety.

Rehabilitation Group

After working at a senior citizens' center for a few weeks, a student began a careful assessment of the center's clients. The student interviewed the center's clients and visited its homebound clients served by social workers and the MOW program. Several of the homebound clients identified a need for socialization and rehabilitation. The center had recently purchased a van equipped to transport handicapped people in wheelchairs, which was a necessary factor in fulfilling this need. After the student assessed the clients' health and functional status and determined mutual goals, four of these homebound clients expressed a desire to attend a rehabilitation program at the center. The student and the center's management initiated a weekly program based on the clients' needs, which included van transportation, a coffee hour, a noontime meal, an exercise class, and a craft class. Although some members were initially reluctant to participate and one man withdrew from the group, the group ultimately functioned very well. The student made progress in meeting the goals of increased socialization and rehabilitation.

Unsuccessful Projects

Project failure is usually caused by problems with one or more steps of the nursing process. Usually the student does not discover problems until the evaluation phase. The following unsuccessful projects illustrate failures at different steps in the nursing process. Table 6-3 summarizes the identified problem areas for these examples.

Headstart Program

Periodically, students do not allow sufficient time to follow through with implementation. The difficulty in *gaining entry* may be among the reasons. For example, a student decided to investigate the feasibility of beginning a Headstart program in a low-income community. After calling community leaders for several weeks, she was finally able to locate the appropriate person. However, by the time she finally made contact, the semester was almost complete. Needless to say, she was disappointed at the end result.

This example illustrates the importance of identifying a **key informant** (i.e., someone who is familiar with the community) early in the process. Unfortunately, such people are not always obvious because they may not be "community leaders." For example, the key informant may be the director of a neighborhood health center in one community and it may be the person in charge of a local thrift shop in another community.

Prenatal Clinic

For a few weeks, a nursing student worked in a prenatal clinic serving a low-income population and identified several needs among the clients. Realiz-ing that she needed to gather information regarding the clients' perceived needs, she developed a questionnaire that listed several possible discussion topics and left space for the clients' questions and concerns. The student also included spaces for clients to fill in what times they would be available to attend a health education workshop and whether they had transportation.

After the student collected and tallied the questionnaires for 25 clients, she determined that the clients were most concerned with infant feeding, they did not have a transportation problem, and Tuesday evening was the best time to attend a class. Using this information, the student scheduled her teaching project, made informational posters for the clinic, mailed program descriptions to the clients, and planned her class. The student was extremely disappointed when the clients did not attend the program.

There are many possible reasons for nonattendance. The student deduced that returning to the clinic in the evening was too inconvenient, although the clients wrote it was the most convenient time. Health education may not have been a priority for this group of clients; the questionnaire assumed that education was important and merely asked about interests. Furthermore, the clinic's surrounding neighborhood may have been unsafe during the evening hours.

This example illustrates the importance of careful assessment and the possible results of incomplete assessment. The student recommended communicating health education information to clients during clinic hours and using individual counseling, posters, and other information within the clinic setting.

Group Home for Mentally Retarded Adults

In another unsuccessful project, a nursing student worked with an aggregate of six women living in a group home for mentally retarded citizens. The student observed that the clients were all overweight and she decided to establish a weight reduction program. She proceeded to meet with the women, chart their weight, and discuss their food choices on a weekly basis. After eight weeks, her evaluation revealed that none of the women had lost weight and a few had gained weight. The student failed to consider the women's perceptions of need and priority. The women did not consider their weight a problem and their boyfriends provided positive reinforcement regarding their appearance.

TABLE 6-3

Unsuccessful Projects

Project	Problematic Step of Nursing Process
Headstart program	Assessment (i.e., gaining entry)
Prenatal clinic	Incomplete assessment
Group home for mentally retarded adults	Assessment (i.e., mutual identification of health problems and needs)
Safe Rides program	Planning (i.e., mutual identification of goals and objectives) Evaluation (i.e., recommendations for follow-up)
Manufacturing plant	Implementation

Safe Rides Program

One student assessed a university student community through a questionnaire and identified a drinking and driving problem. Of those she surveyed, 77% admitted to driving under the influence of alcohol and 16.5% stated they were involved in an alcohol-related car accident. After identifying the problem and determining student interest, the student worked with the campus alcohol and drug resource center to plan and implement a program called Safe Rides. In this program, student volunteers would work a hot line and dispatch "on call" drivers to pick up students who are unsafe to drive.

The student resolved many potential complications before implementation (i.e., liability coverage for all participating individuals and expense funds for gasoline). The student formulated a 12-hour training program that lasted three weeks to prepare student volunteers for the Safe Rides program. By the end of the semester, Safe Rides was ready to begin. However, the student graduated at the semester's end and her commitment was the program's prime motivating force. Although others were committed and involved, the student did not arrange for a replacement to coordinate and continue the program upon her departure. The Safe Rides program required ongoing coordination efforts; therefore no one fully implemented the program in the student's absence.

Manufacturing Plant

Even careful planning cannot always eliminate potential obstacles. For example, one student chose to work in an occupational setting involving heavy industry. The occupational health nurse and the nurse's personnel supervisor both approved the student's entry into the organization. After reviewing the literature, working with the nurse for several weeks, and assessing the organization and its employees, the student concluded that back injury risk was a primary problem. She planned to decrease the risk factors involved in back injuries by distributing information about proper body mechanics in a teaching session.

However, the personnel manager resisted this plan. Although he recognized the need for education, he was initially unwilling to allow employees to attend the session on company time. The student and manager reached a compromise by allowing attendance during extended coffee breaks. However, the personnel manager canceled the program before the

---

TABLE 6-4

Level of Prevention for Each Project

Primary Prevention	Secondary Prevention	Tertiary Prevention
Textile industry (first aid and back injury prevention)	Obese children	Rehabilitation group
Exercise for elderly	Textile industry (i.e., blood pressure screening and counseling)	Group home for mentally retarded adults
Crime watch		
Headstart program		
Prenatal clinic		
Safe Rides program		
Manufacturing plant		

---

student could implement the class; negotiations for a new union contract were forming and there was high probability of a strike. This caused management to deny any changes in the usual routine.

The student proceeded appropriately and received clearance from the proper officials, but the student could not anticipate or circumvent union problems. The student could only share her information and concern with the nurse and the personnel manager and encourage them to implement her plan when contract negotiations were complete.

Discussion

Each of these projects attempted to address a particular level of prevention. Most of these examples focused on primary prevention and health promotion because they were student conducted and time limited. Table 6-4 lists these projects and their prevention levels. However, the full-time community health nurse working with an aggregate (e.g., in the occupational health setting) would target interventions for all three levels of prevention at a variety of system levels. It is useful to view nursing interventions with aggregates within a matrix structure to address all intervention opportunities. The matrix in Table 6-5 gives examples of how the occupational health nurse may intervene at all system levels and all prevention levels.

In practice, most interventions occur at the individual level and include all prevention levels.

TABLE 6-5

Occupational Health: Levels of Prevention for System Levels

System Level	Primary Prevention	Secondary Prevention	Tertiary Prevention
Subsystem	Yearly physical examination for each employee	Regular blood pressure monitoring and diet counseling for each employee with elevated blood pressure	Referral for job retraining for employee with a back injury
Aggregate and group system	Incentive program to encourage departments to use safety devices	Weight reduction group for overweight employees	Support group for employees who are recovering from problems with alcohol or drug use
Suprasystem	Health fair open to the community and employees	Counseling and referral of community members with elevated blood pressure or cholesterol on the basis of health fair findings	Media advertising to encourage people with substance abuse problems to seek help and use community resources that provide assistance

Interventions at the aggregate level are usually less frequent. For many occupational health nurses, time does not allow intervention at the suprasystem level. However, industries are integral parts of the community system. Factors that affect community health also affect employee health and vice versa. Some industries take their reciprocal relationship with the surrounding community quite seriously. For nurses in these industries, interventions at the suprasystem level may become a reality and improve the health of the community and the workers. This is a good example of refocusing upstream by addressing the "real" source of problems. Although the chosen example is occupational health nursing, any nurse working with aggregate systems can construct a similar matrix for interventions.

These projects illustrate the variety of available opportunities for aggregate health planning. In addition, they exemplify the application of the nursing process within various aggregate types, at different systems levels, and at each prevention level. These examples demonstrate the vital importance of each step of the nursing process.

1. Aggregate assessments must be thorough. The textile industry project exemplifies this point. Assessments should elicit answers to key questions about the aggregate's health and demo-graphic profile and should compare this information with similar aggregates presented in the literature.

2. The nurse must complete careful planning and set goals that the nurse and the aggregate accept. The exercise for the elderly project and the rehabilitation group project illustrate the importance of mutual planning.

3. Interventions must include aggregate participation and must meet the mutual goals. The Crime Watch project exemplifies this point.

4. Evaluation must include process and product evaluation and aggregate input.

HEALTH PLANNING FEDERAL LEGISLATION

Health planning at the national, state, and local levels is another example of aggregate planning. Planning at any of these levels can be a broader extension of the suprasystem level and impacts the individual, family, group, population, and organization levels. Again, upstream change can occur on these levels; for example, individual consumers and consumer groups have protested some managed care practices at the suprasystem level.

Historically, nurses have influenced health planning only minimally at the community level, but health planning has a tremendous effect on nurses and nursing practice. It is necessary to understand planning on a suprasystem level; therefore the following section contains a review of past health planning efforts with projections for the future.

Early History

Although health planning activities existed in the United States before the 1940s, they usually addressed specific health problems (e.g., services for maternal and child health and provision of health care activities). Furthermore, private, nongovernmental agencies such as the APHA or the American Cancer Society (ACS) usually initiated these activities. The federal government only had limited involvement. For example, in the 1930s, Blue Cross and the United Fund in New York City were responsible for initiating local health planning, and then the Health and Planning Council of New York was formed for implementation. In addition, most of these efforts were provider oriented.

The federal government's involvement in health planning changed at the end of World War II when it turned its attention to issues in the private sector. At this point, there was a general shortage of hospital beds and a lack of coordination among hospitals. In particular, rural areas needed hospital beds and medical personnel (Lee and Benjamin, 1999; Shonick, 1995).

Hill-Burton Act

In 1946, Congress passed the Hospital Survey and Construction Act (Hill-Burton Act, PL 79-725) to address the need for better hospital access. This Act provided federal aid to states for hospital facilities. A state had to submit a plan documenting available resources and need estimates to qualify for hospital construction and modernization funds under the **Hill-Burton Act** (Shonick, 1995). In addition, each state had to designate a single agency for the development and implementation of the hospital construction plan. The Hill-Burton Act caused the expenditure of vast sums of money and resulted in an increase in the number of beds, especially in general hospitals. Although the Act and its amendments focused only on construction, it improved the quality of care in rural areas and introduced systematical statewide planning (Jonas, 1998).

Regional Medical Programs

The Hill-Burton Act provided construction-related planning, but it did not address coordination and care delivery directly. In response to recommendations from Dr. Michael DeBakey's national commission, Heart Disease, Cancer, and Stroke Amendments of 1965 (PL 89-239) were enacted. This legislation was more comprehensive and established regional medical programs.

The **Regional Medical Programs** (RMP) intended to make the latest technology for the diagnosis and treatment of heart disease, cancer, stroke, and related diseases available to community health care providers through the establishment of regional cooperative arrangements among medical schools, research institutions, and hospitals. The goals of these cooperative arrangements were "to improve generally the health manpower and facilities available to the nation and to accomplish these ends without interfering with the patterns, or the methods of financing, or patient care or professional practice, or with the administration of hospitals" (Heart Disease, Cancer and Stroke Amendments of 1965, p. 901).

Although RMPs have been credited with the regionalization of certain services and the introduction of innovative approaches to organization and care delivery, some observers believed the reforms were not comprehensive enough. The RMPs did not partner with the existing federal and state programs; therefore there were gaps and duplication in service delivery, personnel training, and research (Shonick, 1995).

Comprehensive Health Planning

Congress signed the Comprehensive Health Planning and Public Health Services Amendments of 1966 (PL 89-749) into law to broaden the previous legislation's categorical approach to health planning. Combined with the Partnership for Health Amendments of 1967 (PL 90-174), these amendments created the **Partnership for Health Program** (PHP). The PHP provided federal grants to states to establish and administer a local agency program to enact local comprehensive health care planning. The PHP's objectives were promoting and ensuring the highest level of health for every person and not interfering with the existing private practice patterns (Shonick, 1995).

To meet these objectives, the PHP formulated a two-level planning system. Under this system, each state had to designate a single health planning agency, or "A" agency. To play a statewide coordinating role, the "A" agency had to partner with an advisory council, which consisted largely of health care consumers. Meanwhile, the local "B" agencies formulated plans to meet designated local community needs, which could be any public or nonprofit private agency or organization. "A" agencies were to encourage the formation of local, comprehensive, health planning "B" agencies, and federal grants were made available for that purpose (Shonick, 1995).

Although the comprehensive health plans were the first of these programs to mandate consumer involvement, they may have failed in their basic intent. The possible failure may have resulted from funding shortage, conflict avoidance in policy formulation and goal establishment, political absence, and provider opposition (e.g., AMA, American Hospital Association [AHA], and major medical centers). The mission appeared to be a discussion of the shortfalls of health care delivery rather than the provision of mechanisms for action (DeBella et al., 1986; Shonick, 1995).

Certificate of Need

In response to increased capital investments and budgetary pressures, state governments developed the idea of obtaining prior governmental approval for certain projects through the use of a **certificate of need** (CON). New York State passed the first CON law in 1964, which required government approval of hospitals' and nursing homes' major capital investments. Eventually all states supported this CON requirement and it ultimately became a component of health legislation (PL 93-641). In practice, state CON programs differ in structure and goals. These differences include program focus, decision-making levels, review standard scope, and appeals process exemption (Thorpe, 1999).

National Health Planning and Resources Development Act

Given the perceived failure of the comprehensive health planning programs, the federal government focused on a new approach to health planning. The federal government was greatly concerned with the cost of health care, which escalated dramatically following the end of World War II; the uneven distribution of services; the general lack of knowledge of personal health practices; and the emphasis on more costly modalities of care. The **National**

Health Planning and Resources Development Act of 1974 (PL 93-641) combined the strengths of the Hill-Burton Act, RMPs, and the comprehensive health planning program to forge a new system of single-state and area-wide health planning agencies (Shonick, 1995).

The goals and purposes of the new law were an increase in accessibility, acceptability, continuity, and quality of health services; control over the rising costs of health care services; and prevention of unnecessary duplication of health resources. The new law addressed the needs of the underserved and provided quality health care. The provider and consumer were to be involved in planning and improving health services and it placed the system of private practice under scrutiny.

At the center of the program was a network of local health planning agencies, which developed a health systems plan for its geographical service area. The local agencies then submitted these plans to a state health planning and development agency, which integrated the plans into a preliminary state plan. The state agency presented this preliminary plan to a statewide health coordinating council for approval. The law required that the council consist of at least 16 governor-appointed members and that 50% of these members represent health system agencies and 50% represent consumers. One major function of this council was to prepare a state health plan that reflected the goals and purposes of the Act. Once the council formulated a tentative plan, they presented it at public hearings throughout the state for discussion and possible revisions (Shonick, 1995).

Despite careful deliberations by health planners with input from consumers, not all states accepted the health system plan at the grassroots level. For example, federal officials commended Rhode Island's state health plan, which was released to the community in late 1979. The officials considered it a substantial achievement and delivered high praise. However, when the council first presented the plan at seven public hearings throughout the state in early 1980, many of the near 10,000 people in attendance protested two of the recommendations. One recommendation would establish a smaller number of larger hospitals and the second would reduce the number of hospital beds. In Newport, people argued vehemently that if the local hospital closed and women had to deliver their babies in other communities, "native Newporters" would cease to exist. The same recommendations precipitated a candlelight march in the suburban community of Westerly, where protesters chanted "save our hospital" and carried signs that read "don't risk losing your health care services" (Coyle, 1980).

It is difficult to understand why a plan aimed at "promoting quality of care while constraining costs" met such resistance. In retrospect, planners agreed that although they spent an abundance of time and care developing the plan, the public was not prepared for the ambitious recommendations. Furthermore, many believed that the council had more power than it actually held and members of the hospital community attempted to discredit the plan. The council presented a second state health plan in 1983, which substantially modified the two previous recommendations, and the public offered little or no opposition. By this time, the public better understood the council's function and the recommendations were more conservative.

The problems that the recommendations encountered in Rhode Island were symptoms of the legislation's overall failure to affect major change in the health care system. A significant problem was that legislation "grandfathered" the entire health care system (i.e., health care delivery methods did not change). Although legislation mandated consumer involvement in the health system agency, it was often difficult to implement this aspect. In addition, hospitals and other facilities had greater resources to influence the political process. Despite the mandated efforts by CON and required reviews, costs continued to rise and the health care system remained essentially unchanged (Kronenfeld, 1997).

Changing Focus of Health Planning

The Reagan administration encouraged competition within the health care system. During the 1980s, the administration emphasized cost shifting and cost reduction with greater state power, less centralization of functions, and less national control. This approach represented the government's philosophical shift and combined it with a funding cutback from the Omnibus Budget Reconciliation Act in 1981. This combination dealt a deathblow to federal health planning (Mueller, 1993). The cutbacks caused health system agencies to redefine their role and the federal government recommended eliminating these agencies.

A reduction in federal funding and the influence of medical lobbies caused the closure of some health system agencies. Those that remained open experienced a decrease in staff, a resulting decrease in

overall board functioning, and a reordering of priorities. In an effort to compensate for the decrease in federal funding, some health system agencies sought nonfederal funding or built coalitions to provide the necessary power base for change. Although the administration did not renew federal health planning legislation in the 1980s, it used other regulatory approaches to control costs. These included DRGs as method payments to Medicare and, in the 1990s, individual states required their Medicaid recipients to enroll in HMOs.

The Clinton administration's plan for health care reform would have revitalized planning at the national level. The failure of Congress to pass the plan in 1994 gave planning efforts back to state and local agencies. Since the autumn of 1998, 29 states and the District of Columbia were involved in some form of health planning. Of these states, seven states had statewide health plans, local health plans, and some other type of local health planning; two states had statewide and local health plans; six states had statewide health plans and some other local health planning entity; three states had local health plans and some other local health planning entity; eight states and the District of Columbia had statewide health plans exclusively; and three states had some type of local health planning entity (American Health Planning Association [AHPA], 1999).

New York State's Long Term Care Financing and Integration Act of 1997 is an example of state health planning legislation. This piece of legislation allowed New York State's Partnership for Long Term Care to develop continuing care retirement communities and managed long-term care plans. Other examples include the following:

- Louisiana: set a moratorium on nursing home beds in 1996 and extended it until 2001;
- Arkansas: added Act 396 (hospice facility and agency services) and Act 1360 (child health management services clinics); and
- Missouri: passed legislation in 1996 that no longer requires CON review for hospitals, ambulatory surgical centers, and dialysis centers after 2001 (AHPA, 1999).

At the beginning of the twenty-first century, 36 states and the District of Columbia still require CON reviews for selected expenditures that include nursing homes, psychiatric facilities, and expensive equipment. However, within these programs, requirements for approval are more liberal, expedited reviews are conducted, and certain projects are exempted from review, which weakens the CON cost containment mandate. For example, the CON review threshold for capital expenditures in hospitals and nursing homes varies from none in Florida to $4,000,000 in Hawaii. In Nevada, CON review only applies to new construction in rural counties over $2,000,000 (AHPA, 1999).

CON reviews for new equipment are required in 27 states. In these states, the threshold varies from $400,000 in New Hampshire to $3,000,000 in Delaware and New York; however, the mental hygiene threshold is $1,000,000 in New York. Only 12 of the 36 states and District of Columbia require a CON review for all or any new services. The remaining 24 states limit the services CON may review (AHPA, 1999).

Newer high-technology services (i.e., lithotripsy, gamma knives, and position emission tomography) still need CON review in most states. Furthermore, it is anticipated that state CON programs will assume a stronger role because states must increasingly monitor and report the quality, cost, and access to health care that managed care promised (Piper, 1999).

Experts in the health planning area believe there will be a "paradigm shift" from an emphasis on "medical care" to an emphasis on "health care" and local, community-based approaches to health issues. Health planning needs a coordinated approach that combines public and private cooperation with an emphasis on supplies and services to help achieve improved health status. Advances in planning models and the sophistication level of planners will impact future health planning efforts (Thomas, 1999).

Nurses must work collaboratively with health planners to improve aggregate health. Nurses can influence health planning at the local and state, or community level by incorporating current technology with their knowledge of health care needs and skills gained through working with individuals, families, groups, and population groups. This is an example of "upstream interventions"; the nurse presents group needs or concerns to health planning boards. The nurse may become directly involved in the planning process by participating in CON reviews or gaining membership on health planning councils.

NURSING IMPLICATIONS

Increased nursing involvement is one method of strengthening local and national health planning. Nurses can use this health planning model to facilitate a systematic approach to improve aggregate health care. Nurses can assess aggregates from small groups through population groups; identify the group's health needs; and perform planning, intervention, and evaluations by applying this model. The health of individuals, families, and groups would improve if nurses reemphasized the larger aggregate.

CASE STUDY

A bilingual community health nursing student named José Mendez worked with the school system in a community that had a large Portuguese subsystem. His aggregate was the students enrolled in the town's bilingual program. His contacts included the school nurse and the program teachers.

Assessment

José included the specific group of students, the members of the school system's organizational level, and the population group of the town's Portuguese-speaking residents in his assessment of the aggregate's health needs. José identified the subsystem's lack of primary disease prevention, specifically related to hygiene, dental care, nutrition, and lifestyle choices by observing the children, interviewing teachers and community residents, and reviewing the literature. José's continued assessment and prioritization revealed that the problem was related to a lack of knowledge and not a lack of concern.

Diagnosis

Individual

Inadequate preparation at home regarding basic hygiene, dental care, nutrition, and healthy lifestyles   *Continued*

Family
Inadequate knowledge base regarding basic hygiene, dental care, nutrition, and healthy lifestyles

Community
Inadequate resources for communicating basics of hygiene, dental care, nutrition, and healthy lifestyles to the Portuguese community

Planning

The teachers and staff of the bilingual program helped contract and set goals, which reinforced the need for mutuality at this step in the process. A variety of alternative interventions were necessary to accomplish the following goals:

Individual
Long-Term Goal
Students will regularly practice good hygiene, preventive dental care, good nutrition, exercise, and adequate sleep habits.

Short-Term Goal
Students will learn the basics of good hygiene, preventive dental care, good nutrition, exercise, and adequate sleep habits.

Family
Long-Term Goal
Families will regularly practice and teach their children good hygiene, preventive dental care, good nutrition, exercise, and adequate sleep habits.

Short-Term Goal
Families will learn the basics of good hygiene, preventive dental care, good nutrition, exercise, and adequate sleep habits.

Community
Long-Term Goal
Systematic programs will provide families and their children with education and information regarding the basics of good hygiene, preventive dental care, good nutrition, exercise, and adequate sleep habits.

Short-Term Goal
Bilingual personnel will translate information into Portuguese and program teachers will distribute it to families regarding the basics of good hygiene, preventive dental care, good nutrition, exercise, and adequate sleep habits.

Intervention

Sometimes student projects are more limited than the planning stage's "ideal"; in this case, interventions only assessed one grade level.

Individual
The student taught children many healthy lifestyle basics, including nutrition, hygiene, and dental care. Classes presented information in Portuguese and English.

Family
All parents received a summary of the class content in both languages and in pictures.

Community
The local teachers communicated the student's activities to their state-level coordinators and the coordinators incorporated the student's materials into the bilingual program throughout the state.

Evaluation

This community health planning project had an impact on the individuals in the specific aggregate and had broader implications for the family systems and the community suprasystem. The outcomes, or product, were hugely successful. Mutually identified goals and objectives influenced the development of the process and incorporated input from a variety of sources. The student believed the resources and support for the bilingual program were adequate. Although the student only addressed primary prevention, the continuing nature of the project will allow the teachers, the school nurse, and the families to assess problems related to the program's content. Future implementation may address secondary and tertiary prevention.

SUMMARY

Community health nurses are responsible for incorporating health planning into their practice. Nurses' unique talents and skills, augmented by the comprehensive application of the nursing process, can facilitate population health improvement at various aggregate levels. Health planning policy and process constitute part of the knowledge base of the baccalaureate-prepared nurse. Systems theory provides one framework for nursing process application in the community. Interventions are possible at subsystem, system, and suprasystem levels using all three levels of prevention.

LEARNING ACTIVITIES

1. Assess a neighborhood or local community using the following exploratory techniques: drive through the area and identify types of houses, schools, churches, health-related agencies, and businesses; look for potential environmental and safety hazards; interview a town hall clerk, a senior citizen at a meal site or day care center, a newspaper reporter, a visiting nurse, a police officer, a social worker, or a school nurse regarding the community; call the local, county, or state health department for morbidity and mortality statistics; or attend a town council or school committee meeting. Compare and contrast these findings with classmates' findings.
2. Construct a matrix similar to Table 6-5 using interventions from the school nurse setting.
3. In class, identify 10 to 15 questions that will elicit important health information from young adults. Each student must write answers to these questions. Tally the student responses and draw conclusions from this assessment. Identify problems or potential problem areas and construct a plan to solve or prevent these problems.
4. Attend a state or local health planning meeting. Observe the number of health care providers and consumers in attendance. Compare the meeting's issues with the goals of improving care quality and reducing health care costs.
5. Interview a health planner at the state or local level to determine the status of health planning and CON review in the community or state.

REFERENCES

American Health Planning Association: *National directory of health planning, policy, and regulatory agencies,* ed 6, Washington, DC, 1999, The Association.

Ammerman A, Parks C: Preparing students for more effective community interventions: assets assessment, *Fam Commmunity Health* 21(1):32-46, 1998.

Comprehensive Health Planning and Public Health Services Amendments of 1966, Pub No 89-749, 1966.

Coyle P: Music, sirens, voices raised in protest against RI health plan, *The Westerly Sun* January 3, 1980.

DeBella S, Martin L, Siddall S: *Nurses' role in health care planning,* Norwalk, Conn, 1986, Appleton-Century-Crofts.

Doerr B et al: Beyond community assessment into the real world of learning aggregate practice, *Nurs Health Care Perspect* 19(5):214-220, 1998.

Duffus RL: *Lillian Wald: neighbor and crusader,* New York, 1938, Macmillan.

Hamilton PA et al: *Decision making in community health nursing,* Boston, 1985, Little, Brown.

Heart Disease, Cancer, and Stroke Amendments of 1965, Pub No 89-239, 1965.

Hegge ML: Independent study in community health nursing, *Nurs Outlook* 21:652-654, 1973.

Hogue C: An epidemiologic approach to distributive nursing practice. In Hall JE, Weaver BR, editors: *Distributive nursing practice: a systems approach to community health,* ed 2, Philadelphia, 1985, JB Lippincott.

Hospital Survey and Construction Act of 1946 (Hill-Burton Act), Pub No 79-725, 1946.

Jonas S: *An introduction to the U.S. health care system,* ed 4, New York, 1998, Springer Publishing Co.

Kalisch PA, Kalisch BJ: *The advance of American nursing,* Philadelphia, 1995, Lippincott, Co.

Kronenfeld J: *The changing federal role in health care policy,* Westport, Conn, 1997, Praeger Publishers.

Leavell HR, Clark EG: *Preventive medicine for the doctor in his community,* New York, 1965, McGraw-Hill.

Lee P, Benjamin AE: Health policy and the politics of health care. In Williams SJ, Torrens PR, editors: *Introduction to health services,* ed 5, Albany, NY, 1999, Delmar.

Mahon J, McFarlane J, Golden K: De madres a madres: a community partnership for health, *Public Health Nurs* 8:15-19, 1991.

Maslow AH: *Toward a psychology of being,* New York, 1968, Van Nostrand Reinhold.

Mueller K: *Health care policy in the United States,* Lincoln, Neb, 1993, University of Nebraska Press.

National Health Planning and Resources Development Act of 1974, Pub No 93-641, 1974.

Partnership for Health Amendment of 1967, Pub No 90-174, 1967.

Piper T: *CON trends in America: a panorama of change,* The Author, www.aphanet.org/articles.html, 1999.

Ruybal SE, Bauwens E, Fasla MJ: Community assessment: an epidemiological approach, *Nurs Outlook* 23:365-368, 1975.

Shonick W: *Government and health services,* New York, 1995, Oxford University Press.

Shuster GF, Goeppinger J: Community as client: using the nursing process to promote health. In Stanhope M, Lancaster J, editors: Community health nursing: promoting the health of aggregates, families, and individuals, ed 4, St. Louis, 1996, Mosby.

Silverstein NG: Lillian Wald at Henry Street: 1893-1895, *ANS Adv Nurs Sci* 7:1-12, 1985.

Thomas R: *New health planning for the new millennium,* The Author, www.aphanet.org/articles.html, 1999.

Thorpe K: Health care cost containment: reflections and future directions. In Kovner A, Jonas S, editors: *Health care delivery in the Untied States,* ed 6, New York, 1999, Springer Publishing.

Community Health Education

Cathy D. Meade

OBJECTIVES

Upon completion of this chapter, the reader will be able to do the following:

1. Describe the goals of health education within the community setting.
2. Explore the nurse's role in community education within a political and social context.
3. Select a learning theory and describe its application to the individual, family, or aggregate.
4. Examine effective teaching and learning strategies that exemplify client-centered health education for the individual, family, or aggregate.
5. Compare and contrast Freire's approach to health education with an individualistic health education model.
6. Outline a systematic process for creating and delivering health education messages and programs that are culturally, educationally, and linguistically relevant.
7. Identify health education resources and describe their application to an individual, family, or community client.
8. Relate and apply factors that enhance the appropriateness of health materials and media for an intended target group.
9. Prepare an appropriate teaching plan and evaluation criteria for the individual, family, and aggregate.

KEY TERMS

behavioral theory
cognitive theory
community empowerment
culturally competent care
health education
humanistic theory
learner verification
learning
materials and media
problem-solving education
social learning theory

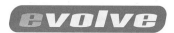

http://evolve.elsevier.com/Nies/

[Health education] is any combination of learning experiences designed to facilitate voluntary actions conducive to health that people can take on their own, individually, or collectively, as citizens looking after their own health or as decision makers looking after the health of others and the common good of the community

(Green et al., 1980).

Nurses may be tempted to ask the following questions:

Why does the patient continue to smoke?

Why does the patient fail to take diabetic medications regularly?

Why do parents fail to immunize their children on schedule?

Why do so few people attend the clinic's free cancer screenings?

Why does this community have an alarming rate of teenage pregnancy?

Although these questions represent the nurse's intense desire to understand the link between health behavior and health education, they do not yield answers or empower individuals. In fact, such questions do not address the root health issues and may be a "blaming the victim" approach (Israel et al., 1994).

The nurse could reframe the previous questions to empower individuals, families, and groups and ask the following:

What life situations or stressors might be occurring while the patient is trying to quit smoking?

What are the learning needs of individuals and families and how can the nurse address them?

What types of barriers prevent families from immunizing their children; what system strategies can decrease these barriers?

What kinds of creative teaching methods or innovative channels can attract more community groups for free cancer screenings?

How can emerging technologies reach community members?

What social, physical, cultural, or structural factors contribute to the high teenage pregnancy rate? How should the nurse consider these factors when planning pregnancy prevention programs?

HEALTH EDUCATION IN THE COMMUNITY

Health education is an integral part of the nurse's role in promoting health and preventing disease in the community setting. Teaching has been a significant nursing responsibility since Florence Nightingale's early work (1859). Gardner (1936) emphasized that health teaching is one of the most fundamental nursing principles and that "a nurse, in even the most obscure position must be a teacher of no mean order." Nurse Practice Acts, professional statements of the ANA (1975), the AHA (1972) Patient's Bill of Rights, and the Joint Commission on Accreditation of Healthcare Organizations (JCAHO) (1995) all support the nurse's involvement in health education.

More health activities and services are occurring outside the hospital walls within a variety of settings such as churches, missions, beauty and barber shops, grocery stores, homeless shelters, community-based clinics, HMO settings, schools, senior centers, mobile health units, Women, Infants, and Children (WIC) sites, and homes. The community is a vital link to health care and provides the nurse with many health education opportunities within neighborhoods.

Health education's goal is to understand health behavior and to translate knowledge into relevant interventions and strategies for health enhancement, disease prevention, and chronic illness management (Glanz et al., 1997; Pender, 1996). In general, health education aims to enhance wellness and decrease disability and attempts to actualize the health potential of individuals, families, communities, and society. Health education does not only provide information, it encompasses activities designed to guide people through a health decision-making process (Duryea, 1983). Steuart and Kark (1962) stated that "health education must achieve its ends through means that leave inviolate the rights of self-determination of the individuals and their community." A major challenge for community health nurse educators is to value the contributions of individuals and address conditions that promote powerlessness (Wallerstein and Bernstein, 1994).

Milio (1981) reminded nurses that individuals often make health choices based on their socioeconomic situation. Health is not necessarily a state or an achievement, but rather an individual's response to the environment. In Chapter 3, Butterfield cogently indicated that most literature focuses on individual relationships that shape a patient's health behaviors. She purported that this downstream thinking seriously restricts a nurse's ability to consider the multitude of external factors that influence behavior (e.g., environment, culture, social roles, and socioeconomics). Upstream endeavors, or a macroscopic perspective, can help nurses gain insight into a more global perspective on behavior and help address the com-

Mr. Kelly often visited the neighborhood senior center to play cards and have lunch. Once a month he participated in the blood pressure clinic offered by the health department. The health department's outreach services provide clinics in community-based centers and an increased number of individuals use the services. Mr. Kelly had limited resources; therefore the clinic provided him with valuable access to health information. On his first visit to the clinic, his blood pressure was 184/92. On his second visit, his reading was 188/94. He stated that the "county hospital" treated him for high blood pressure for over five years and that doctors prescribed several medications six months prior.

The nurse's assessment revealed that Mr. Kelly took his medication only when he did not "feel good." He said his doctor advised him to take his medicines regularly and believed he took them faithfully when he did not feel well. He stated that he remembered receiving literature about his medications, but he found them too confusing and threw them out. The nurse's educational assessment revealed that Mr. Kelly completed only eight years of school, he did not read often, he enjoyed television over print, and he preferred to learn from pictures or the radio. His low reading skills impacted his ability to understand health instruction. He took many health messages literally (e.g., he interpreted "take regularly" to mean take consistently when "I don't feel right" vs. taking the pills on a regular schedule).

To facilitate learning, the nurse established a teaching plan using Mr. Kelly's input. This plan involved communicating health instructions in more relevant ways (e.g., using pictures, drawings, mnemonics, videotapes, or audiotapes). The nurse also established a follow-up plan.

---

plexity of the larger, more powerful systems that influence behavior. Upstream thinking emphasizes variables that precede or play a role in the development of health problems. When nurses view human responses to health and illness within the sociopolitical-economic framework, they can identify and understand power imbalances within the community that prohibit groups from achieving full potential. Butterfield suggested that social critical theory helps nurses explore societal, political, and environmental forces that impact global community health.

Community health education is based on practical, relevant, and scientifically sound methods and widely accessible technology. In the late seventies, Kleinman (1978) described a social and cultural community health care system that related external factors (e.g., economical, political, and epidemiological) to internal factors (e.g., behavioral and communicative). This view of a sociocultural health care system grounds health education activities within sociopolitical structures, especially within local environmental settings, and views the community-as-client (Jezewski, 1993; Lipson, 1999; Travers, 1997).

Nurses cannot set individual, family, or community priorities alone. The lasting effect of cognitive and behavioral changes relies on the learner's active or passive participation. Learners must be involved in determining health needs and health practices to elicit change (Green and Kreuter, 1999). Community health

nurses are in a position to impact community members' health behaviors and practices through a variety of nursing activities and roles. However, nurses must continually refine their skills and knowledge in community-focused practice, especially in providing culturally relevant care (Boyle, 2000; Kuehnert, 1995). The health educator role in nursing is congruent with the year 2010 health objectives for the nation (USDHHS, 1998).

HEALTH EDUCATION ROLES AND ACTIVITIES OF THE NURSE IN THE COMMUNITY

- Advocate
- Caregiver
- Case manager
- Consultant
- Culture broker
- Educator
  - Recognizes dimensions of health choices
  - Promotes self-care and self-efficacy
  - Knows community printed and electronic resources
  - Facilitates health-promoting behaviors

Continued

- Information broker
- Innovator
- Mediator
- Negotiator
- Policy analyst, policy maker, or change agent
- Promoter of collaborative partnerships
- Role
- Sensitizer
- Social activist

Based on data from Clark, 1998; Jezewski, 1993; Rankin and Stallings, 1995; Spellbring, 1991.

LEARNING THEORIES, PRINCIPLES, AND HEALTH EDUCATION MODELS

Learning Theories

Learning theories are helpful in understanding how individuals, families, and groups learn. The psychology field provided the basis for these theories and illustrated how environmental stimuli elicit specific responses. Theories aid in recognizing the mechanisms that potentially modify knowledge, attitude, and behavior. Bigge (1997) asserted that **learning** is an enduring change that may involve the modification of insights, behaviors, perceptions, or motivations. Although psychology textbooks describe learning theories in great detail, the following broad categories relate to the nursing application in a community setting: stimulus-response (S-R) conditioning (i.e., behavioristic), cognitive, humanistic, and social learning. Table 7-1 outlines these learning theories.

The nurse should remember that theories are not completely right or wrong. Different theories work well in different situations. Knowles (1989) related that behaviorists program individuals through S-R mechanisms to behave in a certain fashion. Humanistic theories help an individual develop his or her potential in a self-directing and holistic manner. Cognitive theorists recognize the brain's ability to think, feel, learn, and solve problems and they train the brain to maximize these functions. Although social learning theory is largely a cognitive theory, it also combines elements of behaviorism (Bandura, 1977b). Social learning's premise is based on behavior explaining and enhancing learning through the concepts of efficacy, outcome expectation, and incentives.

Linking Theory to Practice: an Example of Genital Herpes Education

An educational intervention designed to increase self-efficacy among young adults regarding their ability to implement condom use began with the following question: "What is the effect of group psychoeducational interventions (PEI) led by community nurses on sexual health risks (i.e., knowledge, behavior, and disease burden) and psychosocial adaptation (i.e., depression, mood states, and self-efficacy) of young adults with symptomatic genital herpes?" Bandura's Social Cognitive Theory, which used the theoretical tenet of perceived efficacy, was the conceptual basis for this study. A key component of this study was that the client can successfully execute a behavior to achieve the desired outcomes and outcome expectancies. In this case, the desired behavior was condom use to prevent herpes transmission. The study included the following groups: the experimental group, which received the intervention, and the control group, which did not receive the intervention. The experimental group attended three 90-minute sessions that combined a variety of methods including lecturing, discussing, brainstorming, role playing, and skill building. The methods incorporated media such as videos, games, and exercises to influence the variables theoretically important to behavior change and the provision of lists of community resources and health literature. A practice session reinforced safe lubrication and the correct use of condoms and other barriers such as rubber dams, finger cots, and rubber gloves. It is important to note that the control group received the same group intervention following the study's completion.

The study included 252 young adults with symptomatic genital herpes. Three and six months after the intervention, data revealed that the psychoeducational intervention group yielded increased knowledge. The experimental group reported using condoms and spermicides to prevent transmission more often than the control group; however, the PEI and the control group did not differ in their self-efficacy. This may have occurred because participants expressed a lack of control in managing their lives with this stigmatizing disease, which prevented them from having self-efficacy to prevent transmission. In summary, the study supported the hypothesis that psychoeducational intervention provides superior information, support, knowledge, and behavioral skill development for young adults with symptomatic genital herpes to carry out risk reduction efforts.

TABLE 7-1

Learning Theories and Their Relationship to Health Education

Learning Theory	Characteristics	Application to Health Education	Example
Cognitive or Gestalt learning Lewin, Piaget, and Wertheimer (aids in developing high-quality insights)	Learners are active processors of information. The way learners perceive behaviors, the way they represent perceptions, and the relationship of their perception to the past determines behaviors. Learners are influenced by past experiences. A search for underlying meanings, emotions, beliefs, and past influences is considered. Thinking is reflective. Learners interact with their environment on an ongoing basis. Learners make choices based on their own interpretations. Learners may perceive health messages differently in different environments. The environment may not correspond with reality. The whole is more important than individual pieces.	Nurses should recognize that new insights can reorganize perceptions and thoughts. Consider earlier learning experiences. Recognize that the nurses' perceptions may differ vastly from those of individuals, families or groups, and community. Organize learning to match the group's developmental stage or earlier experiences. Organize pieces of information in meaningful ways. Recognize that the environment, individuals, and groups are interacting constantly and perceptions may change.	Student nurse Bill Driver worked with individuals (survivors) whose family members were murder victims. He designed a support group based on their previous experiences, considering their developmental stages and social-family roles. He was aware that such devastating experiences are likely to change the families' perceptions of themselves and their relationships with their family and community. Bill led the support group's discussion to help members gain insight and understanding about the changes and emotions they were experiencing.
Humanistic Maslow and Rogers (focuses on emotions)	Emphasis is placed on the learner's beliefs and emotions and on behavior observations. Emphasizes what is learned in the learning process. Values affective learning and self-expression. Learners are more self-directed when the teacher is warm, accepting, and empathic to the learner's thoughts and emotions. Unconscious thoughts and experiences shape inner nature. The uniqueness of the individual is valuable (learner-centered education). Individuals and groups do what is congruent with their needs. Lower needs must be met before higher needs are realized (i.e. from low to high: physiological, safety-security, love, affection, belongingness, esteem, and self-actualization).	The nurse should consider the hierarchy of needs (for individuals, families, or groups). Recognize that lower order needs should be met first. Assist patients, families, and groups in their learning. Administer warm, compassionate nursing care.	Nursing student Kate Winer conducted a health assessment with a woman seeking care at a homeless shelter. During planning, Kate attempted to enroll the patient in a free cholesterol screening that other students were offering. Although well intentioned, Kate soon realized that her priorities were inconsistent with the woman's priorities. The woman told the student, "I know you want to help me, but I am more worried about my two sick children and getting them food and a warm bed than trying to get here for your screening!" The nursing student's priorities shifted to planning nursing care directed at meeting the lower needs of Maslow's hierarchy.

Based on data from Bandura, 1977b; Bigge, 1997; Lewin, 1938; Maslow, 1970; Pavlov, 1957; Piaget, 1980; Rogers, 1989; Skinner, 1974; Thorndike, 1969; Wertheimer, 1959.

Continued

TABLE **7-1—cont'd**

Learning Theories and Their Relationship to Health Education—cont'd

Learning Theory	Characteristics	Application to Health Education	Example
Behavioral (i.e., S-R) Pavlov, Thorndike, and Skinner (i.e., promotes acquisition of S-R responses)	Patients learn in a structured, systematic way. Learning is based on conditioning or reinforcement. Observable data are most relevant for patients. Learning is enhanced when connections are used to link S-R. Connections are strengthened when patients use them often and weakened when they use them infrequently. Patients are more likely to repeat rewarded actions.	The nurse should create methods to provide immediate feedback to patients and groups. Involve patients in perceptual learning features (i.e., seeing and hearing). Help individuals, families, and groups make connections between ideas. Change or eliminate antecedent events.	Within a community-based nursing center, an interactive video module on nutrition helps mothers learn to select and identify healthy foods and offers tips on economical food preparations. The computerized program provides an organized method of presenting information and providing immediate feedback about the nutritive value of the users' selections.
Social learning Bandura (i.e., aims to explain behavior and facilitate learning)	Four main sources influence learning: 1. personal mastery 2. vicarious experiences 3. persuasion 4. physiological feedback Theory is learner centered. Enhanced self-confidence and self-efficacy can lead to desired behaviors and outcome.	The nurse should provide links for individuals, families, and groups to others with similar health education needs. Offer educational materials and media that convey information or enhance self-confidence (e.g., brochures or audiocassettes). Involve patients in planning. Coach patients in building skills and achieving goals. Provide a role model network. Create interventions that enhance self-confidence.	Based on needs assessment, a group of parish nurses implemented a fitness program for senior men at their church. The educational program provided general fitness information through nurse-led discussion, brochures, and video to gain mastery of the topic. A light snack and conversation period allowed the men to share information about their experiences. A walking program provided 30 minutes of physiological feedback while they gained fitness (e.g., less stiffness, pulse change, and overall vitality).

Based on data from Bandura, 1977b; Bigge, 1997; Lewin, 1938; Maslow, 1970; Pavlov, 1957; Piaget, 1980; Rogers, 1989; Skinner, 1974; Thorndike, 1969; Wertheimer, 1959.

Although continued research is necessary to further validate and refine efficacy enhancing strategies, the study recommended that nurses incorporate theoretical variables in planning, designing, and testing health education interventions (Swanson et al., 1999).

Knowles' Assumptions about Adult Learners

Knowles (1980, 1989) outlined several assumptions about adult learners. He contended that adults, like children, learn better in a facilitative, nonrestrictive, and nonstructured environment. Nurses who are familiar with these assumptions can develop teaching strategies that motivate and interest individuals, families, and groups and encourage active participation in the learning process. Nurses can help create a self-directing, self-empowering learning environment. The following characteristics impact learning: the client's need to know, concept of self, readiness to learn, orientation to learning, experience, and motivation. Table 7-2 and Box 7-1 expand upon these characteristics.

TABLE 7-2

Characteristics of Adult Learners

Characteristics	Application to Health Education
Need to know Adults must know why they need to learn.	The nurse explores why individuals, families, and groups want to learn. The nurse helps individuals recognize their need to learn.
Self-Concept Adults have a self-concept that developed from dependence to independence. It moves from others' direction to self-direction. Adults want to be capable of self-direction.	The nurse acknowledges that individuals, families, and groups are able to make choices and decisions. The nurse creates an environment in which patients can express themselves. The nurse recognizes that individuals, families, and groups can learn from their selected actions and can take self-direction and responsibility for such behaviors.
Experience Adults may draw upon many life experiences. Such experiences are enriching and are powerful learning resources.	The nurse assesses individuals, families, and groups for life experiences related to health issues. The nurse helps facilitate connections between previous and present experiences. The nurse allows individuals, families, and groups to share experiences with others in a supportive manner. Experiential methods, problem solving, case methods, and discussion can help uncover the learner's experiences. The nurse helps clarify previous and present experiences; this is especially helpful with negative or biased experiences.
Readiness to learn Developmental tasks and social roles impact readiness to learn. Timing learning experiences with developmental tasks is important.	The nurse assesses and identifies individual, family, and group roles (e.g., caregivers or single parents) and key developmental tasks. The nurse seeks to understand the impact of roles and tasks on learning. The nurse organizes learning around life application categories. The nurse creates role-modeling experiences.
Orientation to learning Learning is present oriented and "now" based. Learning is directed to the immediate need and is problem centered.	The nurse assesses the learning needs of individuals, families, and groups on the basis of their priority. The nurse recognizes everyday stresses and hassles and addresses them within their learning context. The nurse provides health information, gives responses to their immediate needs, and offers problem-solving skills.
Motivation Internal drives and factors are powerful motivators (e.g., self-esteem, life goals, quality of life, and responsibility).	The nurse determines individual, family, and group motivators. The nurse assesses for barriers that block motivation (e.g., poor self-esteem or lack of resources) and provides appropriate education, counseling, and referrals.

Adapted from Knowles MS: *The making of an adult educator: an autobiographical journey,* San Francisco, 1989, Jossey-Bass and Knowles MS: *The modern practice of adult education: from pedagogy to andragogy,* Chicago, 1980, Association Press/Follett.

Health Education Models

In addition to learning theories, applying education theories and principles to situations involving individuals, families, and groups illustrates how ideas fit together, offers explanations for health behaviors or actions, and helps plan community nursing interventions. Such theoretical elements form the basis of understanding health behavior. Glanz and colleagues (1997) stated that theories give educators the power to assess an intervention's strength and impact and intend to enrich, inform, and comple-

ment practice. Theoretical frameworks offer nurses an intervention blueprint that promotes learning and provides them with an organized approach to explaining concept relationships (Padilla and Bulcavage, 1991).

What the health practitioner needs is not a single theory that would explain all that he or she hears, but rather a framework with meaningful hooks and rubrics on which to hang the new variables and insights offered by different theories. With this customized

B O X **7-1**

Application of Characteristics of Adult Learners to the Development of a Community Support Group

In the 1980s, the author and a colleague began a community support group for individuals with amyotrophic lateral sclerosis (ALS). The support group was also open to family members and friends. ALS is an incurable degenerative neuromuscular disease that affects nerve and muscle function and the brain's ability to control muscle movement. Community members provided feedback and identified the need for education and support for ALS. At that time, Southeast Wisconsin did not have a support group. This initial dialogue provided the organizing framework for the inception of the support group. Based on observations and interactions at the monthly meetings, an illustration of Knowles' assumptions follows:

Need to know: At the support group, the facilitator-nurse introduces topics by describing the reason for the discussion and rationale for the selected subject (e.g., common concerns of patients and family members and informal assessments based on conversations). To prepare for discussion, group members introduce themselves and the nurse asks what they hope to learn from the presentation. In some cases, members are unsure why they desire more information on a given topic, but indicate they want to listen. Progression of the disease is variable; therefore the need to know is facilitated by the nurse and other patients who have already noted the importance of specific learning tasks (e.g., need for assistive walking device, need for financial planning, or need for hospice care).

Self-concept: A comfortable, informal environment allows patients to express emotions and frustrations about this disease. Participants are encouraged to express themselves. Participants cultivate mutual respect and trust and hugs are common. Members understand that others share similar situations and concerns. Group members have an opportunity to speak out about ways to manage their disease (e.g., decisions about life support and feeding tubes). Even if the choices are not congruent with their own, participants recognize and acknowledge these decisions without imposing value judgments. Facilitators and group members are equal partners in the learning process.

Experiences: Some patients and family members have gone through other difficult life experiences (e.g., other illnesses or deaths in the family) and can help others cope with the management of ALS. These patients share the strengths gained from such experiences with other members. Additionally, individuals and family members who are going through varying stages of the disease process are able to share their experiences (e.g., obtaining home care, selecting a computer, and managing breathing difficulties). They share tips and timesaving strategies with each other and newly diagnosed families learn from those previously diagnosed.

Readiness to learn: Family members often assume many roles when someone is ill, especially with a chronic illness such as ALS. The redefinition of roles creates learning opportunities; however, this may also hinder learning if it is too overwhelming. For example, the well spouse may assume the roles of caregiver, parent, and financial supporter. It is helpful to identify resources to help the family cope with new roles (e.g., respite care).

Orientation to learning: Learning a variety of psychomotor skills is necessary to care for the ALS patient (e.g., suctioning, positioning, using a feeding tube, and toileting). The time frame for learning such skills varies depending on the course of illness. Presenting information about such skills too early in the course of the disease may cause fear and anxiety. Families are often unresponsive to learning such tasks until the need is apparent. In some cases, this may be evidenced at a crisis point (e.g., a fall, a choking incident, or severe respiratory distress). However, facilitators introduce these topics slowly by providing information via the support group, newsletter, printed brochures, and personal discussions.

Motivation: Individuals and families experience a shift in life goals when facing ALS. Such shifts may create learning opportunities aimed at enhancing quality of life (QOL) and maintaining self-esteem. For example, a college professor with ALS strove to keep his link to the university. He was highly motivated to continue his research work and supervise his graduate students. To continue his academic work, he learned to manage his breathing by using a ventilator, arranged transportation to the university, obtained nursing care, and created communication methods by using a computer.

metatheory or framework, the practitioner can triage new ideas into categories that have personal utility in his or her practice

(Green, 1998, p. 2).

Models of Individual Behavior

Two models that explain preventive behavior determinants are the Health Belief Model (HBM), which is presented in Table 7-3 (Becker et al., 1977; Hochbaum, 1958; Kegeles et al., 1965; Rosenstock, 1966), and the Health Promotion Model (HPM) (Pender, 1996). Both models are multifactorial, based on value expectancy, and address individual perceptions, modifying factors, and likelihood of action. Glanz and colleagues (1997) conducted an extensive search of the health behavior literature from mid1992 to mid1994 and found that 526 of 1174 relevant articles, or 44.8%, used at least one theory or model. The HBM was the most commonly cited theory.

The HBM is based on social psychology and has undergone much empirical testing to predict compli-

TABLE 7-3

Health Belief Model

Components	Example and Explanation
Perceived susceptibility	Belief that disease state is present or likely to occur
Perceived severity	Perception that disease state or condition is harmful and has serious consequences
Perceived benefits	Belief that health action is of value
Perceived barriers	Belief that health action would be associated with hindrances (e.g., cost)
Self-efficacy	Belief that actions can be performed to achieve the desired outcome
Demographics	Age, sex, and ethnicity
Cues to action	Influencing factors (e.g., billboards and newspapers)

For a more detailed description of the HBM, the reader is directed to Becker (1974).

ance on singular preventive measures. The initial purpose of the HBM was to explain why people did not participate in health education programs to prevent or detect disease, in particular, the failure to participate in TB screening programs (Hochbaum, 1958). Subsequent studies addressed other preventive actions and factors related to adherence to medical regimens (Becker, 1974).

Primarily, the HBM is a value expectancy theory that addresses factors that promote health-enhancing behavior. It is disease specific and focuses on avoidance orientation. The HBM considers perceived susceptibility, perceived severity, perceived benefits, perceived barriers, and other sociopsychological and structural variables. The self-efficacy variable, or the notion that an individual can act successfully on a given behavior to produce the desired outcome, (Bandura, 1977a, 1977b) was also added to the HBM (Rosenstock et al., 1988; Strecher et al., 1986). In review of 46 studies using the HBM, perceived benefits was the most powerful predictive element within the model, whereas perceived severity had the lowest associative value (Janz and Becker, 1984).

Glanz and colleagues (1990) provided an analysis of the HBM and raised several criticisms. In general, the HBM purports that individuals will seek preventive action if they perceive the following: susceptibility to an illness or condition, serious consequences from a given course of action, benefits from a course of action, and benefits that outweigh the barriers. However, the model is focused on individual behavior determinants and less focused on socioenvironmental factors. This view may promote "blaming the victims" for health problems. Additionally, the model is focused on the influence of the individual's health beliefs and values. Although the HBM identifies an array of variables important in explaining individual health, nurses should view these variables within a larger societal perspective. Strecher and Rosenstock (1997) explain that measuring HBM concepts inconsistently and failing to establish reliability and validity before testing are common deficits in HBM research. Also, most studies attempt to establish each of the four major concepts (susceptibility, seriousness, benefits, and barriers) as independent variables rather than as multiplicative variables.

Pender's HPM (1996) modifies the HBM and focuses on predicting health promotion behaviors. Table 7-4 lists the HPM components. The HPM is meant to provide an organizing framework to explain why individuals engage in health actions. Pender

TABLE 7-4

Health Promotion Model Components

Cognitive-Perceptual Factors	Example and Explanation
Importance of health	Perceived value of health to functioning and life
Perceived control of health	Perceived ability to control health (external, internal, or chance)
Perceived self-efficacy	Perceived ability to perform the necessary behaviors to achieve an outcome
Definition of health	Views of what health means for the individual May vary from absence of illness to self-actualization
Perceived health status	Perception of how the individual views health May range from wellness to illness
Perceived benefits of health-promoting behaviors	Perception of positive outcomes that can occur from health-promoting behavior (e.g., feel fit and toned)
Perceived barriers to health-promoting behaviors	Perception of things that obstruct health-promoting behaviors (e.g., money and transportation)

Modifying Factors	Example and Explanation
Demographics	Age, sex, and race
Biological	Weight and body fat
Interpersonal influences	Interactions with family and nurses
Situational factors	Environmental determinants that make health-promoting options available
Behavioral	Previous knowledge or skills
Cues to action	Influencing factors such as internal cues (e.g., good self-image) and external cues (e.g., mass media)

The reader is directed to Pender (1996) for a more comprehensive description and explanation of the HPM.

added the following individual factors: perceived control and perceived health importance. Within the modifying factors, Pender added the variable of interpersonal influence (i.e., interactions with family members and health professionals and expectations of others).

Gillis (1993) reviewed 23 studies conducted between 1983 and 1992 and reported that Pender's HPM was the most common theoretical framework in health promotion studies. Gillis identified that self-efficacy was the strongest determinant of participation in a health-promoting lifestyle, followed by social support, perceived benefits, perceived barriers, and an individual's definition of health education. Locus of control was the least important determinant, although it is the most studied.

The HBM and HPM can assist community health nurses in examining an individual's health choices and decisions. The models offer nurses a cluster of variables that provide important insight into explaining health behavior. These variables are helpful cues; the nurse should consider them in planning and interacting with health education interventions and not try to fit an individual into all the categories. Simply put, models are helpful aids that guide nurses in assessing patients and in developing, selecting, and implementing relevant educational interventions.

In applying the models, a nurse may consider the following questions in relation to his or her own health behavior:

- Are you or is your family susceptible to heart disease or stroke?
- Are you continually striving for improved health?
- Does work, school, or family interfere with your exercise plans?
- Does a family history of cardiovascular disease (CVD) encourage you and your family to exercise?
- Has a family member, friend, or health professional recently reminded you about the benefits of exercise and encouraged you to start exercising?
- Do you believe you can initiate and incorporate an exercise program into your lifestyle, or do you need external reinforcement and cues?
- Does money, safety, and time pose barriers to planning an exercise program?
- In modifying your health behaviors, how important is exercise compared with other health behaviors (e.g., cutting down on fat intake, gaining relief from work and school stresses)?

The nurse should analyze the answers to develop an action plan tailored to *his or her own* needs and capabilities.

Model of Health Education Empowerment

The HBM and HPM focus on individual strategies for achieving optimal health and well-being. Although such approaches may be appropriate in changing individual behaviors, they do not address the complex relationships among social, structural, and physical factors in the environment such as unemployment, racism, lack of social support systems, and inaccessible health services (Israel et al., 1998). Kendall (1992) suggested that nurses stop focusing on adaptation and coping and develop leadership strategies to help emancipate patients from oppressive forces. This includes examining race, gender, and class and recognizing the structural and foundational changes needed to elicit change for socially, politically, and economically disadvantaged groups. This type of thinking may help individuals, who are simply coping with their oppressed situation, fight back. Although information dissemination for behavior change has been the mainstay of traditional health education, Travers (1997) describes this alternative conceptualization as simply "health education for social change." This means people become involved in collective action to create healthy lifestyles and environments.

Features of a new health promotion and education movement embrace a broader health definition that addresses social, political, and economic health aspects (Goodman et al., 1998; Labonte, 1994). Reconceptualizing health beyond the individual to the collective group expands the health education field beyond a narrow lifestyle focus to a focus based on empowerment and community participation (Robertson and Minkler, 1994). Such a theoretical perspective is congruent with community education because it supports learner participation and involvement. The following principles support health education empowerment and social justice: comprehensive education strategies and programming, neighborhood as base, and **community empowerment** (community members gaining mastery over their lives through community participation) (Eisen, 1994). Citizen participation is key for effective and successful health promotion and disease prevention programs (Braithwaite et al., 1994).

Empowerment education evolved from Paulo

Freire's successful literacy work in Brazil in the 1950s. He based his work on a problem-solving approach to education, which contrasts to the *banking education* approach that places the learner in a passive role. **Problem-solving education** allows active participation and ongoing dialogue and encourages learners to be critical and reflective about health issues. Freire suggested that when individuals assume the role of objects, they become powerless and allow the environment to control them. However, when individuals become subjects, they influence environmental factors that affect their lives and community. Community members, or subjects, are the best resources to elicit change (Freire, 1970, 1973).

Freire's approach to health education increases health knowledge through a participatory group process. This process explores the problem's nature and addresses the problem's deeper issues. The nurse, or facilitator-educator, is a resource person and is an equal partner with the other group members. Listening is the first phase and is essential to understanding the issues. The exchange of ideas and concerns creates a problem-posing dialogue and identifies root problems or generative themes. The group discusses and explores the problem's root causes. Finally, group members create relevant action plans that are congruent with their own reality (Freire, 1973).

Information, communication, and health education is at the core of empowerment (WHO, 1994). When nurses involve individuals, families, and groups in their learning, it validates their role and helps ensure the intervention's relevance (Rudd and Comings, 1994; Wallerstein, 1992).

Nurses can use empowerment strategies to help people develop skills in problem solving, networking, negotiating, lobbying, and information seeking to enhance health. Freire's approach may seem similar to health education's emphasis on helping people take responsibility for their health by providing them with information, skills, reinforcement, and support. However, Freire purported that knowledge imparted by the collective group is significantly more powerful than information provided by health educators. Freire's approach attempts to uncover the social and political aspects of problems and encourages group members to define and develop action strategies. Health changes are complex and usually do not have immediate solutions; therefore the term *problem posing,* rather than *problem solving,* may better describe this empowerment process (Bernstein et al., 1994; Travers, 1997; Wallerstein and Bernstein, 1988).

Examples of Empowerment Education

1. **Wang and Burris (1997) described how photo-voice is an empowerment strategy.** Previously called photo novella (Wang and Burris, 1994), this methodology uses photographs or pictures to tell a story or teach literacy. This participatory process integrates empowerment education, feminist theory, and documentary photography to fuel critical consciousness and document a community's strengths and problems directly. Photovoice allows people to identify, represent, and enhance their community through specific photographic techniques. Community members explore issues related to the social, economic, cultural, and biomedical factors that affect them by documenting their everyday lives. The images become educational tools that increase their health status knowledge individually and collectively, empower them to mobilize for social change, and communicate their situation to policy makers. Facilitated group discussions validate concerns about family, self, and community; aid in problem identification; and challenge members to create action strategies.

   Participatory involvement may be a diagnostic tool for readdressing inadequate assumptions. For example, photovoice revealed that the major issues for rural women were the lack of transportation, water, and child care, not a lack of knowledge. Thus empowerment resulted in access to resources and networks and knowledge based on "real needs."

2. **McFarland and Fehir (1994) described how the de Madres a Madres program in Houston's inner-city Hispanic community used the empowerment model in its design and development.** The program intended to increase access to prenatal care and decrease barriers. This program asserted that information is power and women who received culturally relevant social support in combination with community resource information would use the information before they entered the traditional health care system. Key elements of this program were respect and reverence for individual and cultural differences, empowerment of indigenous women through unity, validation of women in key health promoter roles, encouragement of volunteerism, and the belief that community members could identify and address their own health needs. Community members were active decision makers at every level of the program, which further enhanced their leadership skill development and outcome investment.

The group shared responsibility for community decisions and actions. Local channels such as businesses, schools, churches, media, health clinics, elected officials, and social services agencies provided information to pregnant residents. At the end of the 5-year community empowerment process, outcome data revealed that the women's personal strengths were enhanced and their ability to work within the system for improved community health had increased.

3. **Zimmerman and colleagues (1997) described an empowerment approach in an intervention that encouraged preventive HIV and AIDS behavior for homosexual Mexican-American men.** Latino gay and bisexual men may be at the highest risk for HIV infection; intense prevention strategies that address high-risk sexual activities are necessary. This project's hypothesis postulated that an intervention that gives control over content and process could convey AIDS and HIV knowledge effectively and enhance preventive behaviors among this risk group.

   This approach has the following distinct characteristics: it involves the intervention's participants, helps clients become more independent through skill development, and creates a context for clients to work together, solve problems, and make decisions about issues. Personal interviews and focus groups ensured that the content and approach was appropriate for the intended target audience. The program, or intervention, consisted of health education (e.g., HIV testing, self-esteem building, and safer sex training), outreach (e.g., distributing condoms and materials at bars and on the street), and group initiatives (e.g., participant discussions that focused on community change activities). Gay men in the communities were project coordinators and health promoters for outreach activities.

   The 37 individuals in the intervention group reported greater knowledge about HIV and AIDS than the 55 nonparticipants and reported using condoms more often; however, the reported number of partners did not change. The program inspired other collective community activities that were not part of the intervention originally (i.e., fundraising to help PWA, a buddy system for PWAs, and organized drug- and alcohol-free weekly social gatherings).

Robertson and Minkler (1994) indicated that although empowerment education, community participation, and a broader socialized health definition fit the new definition of health promotion, this definition may potentially undervalue individual empowerment. Although this approach provides a socialized conceptualization of health and separates individuals from their health status, it also minimizes the associations between people and their daily difficulties in managing health and illness. This strong push to embrace collective empowerment may negate the value of professionally based direct health services. Rather, Robertson and Minkler suggested an empowerment continuum that acknowledges the value and interdependence of individual and political action strategies aimed at the collective. Labonte (1994) supported this thinking and stated that the community is the engine of health promotion and a vehicle of empowerment.

He described five spheres of an empowerment model, which focus on the following levels of social organization: interpersonal (personal empowerment), intragroup (small group development), intergroup (community), interorganizational (coalition building), and political action. Therefore it seems that both micro- and macro-viewpoints on health education provide nurses with multiple opportunities for intervention across a broad continuum.

Community Empowerment

The nurse must be knowledgeable about key concepts central to community organization to affect change at the community level (Table 7-5). This approach is an effective methodological tool that enables the nurse to

---

TABLE 7-5

Community Organization Practice

Key Concepts	Application to Health Education (Nursing Actions)
Empowerment Help individuals, families, and groups gain insight and mastery over life situations through problem solving and dialogue	The nurse works with community members in identifying and defining issues and creates mechanisms for discussion and problem solving and identification of other factors impacting everyday lives.
Community competence Help the community achieve desired goals through collaboration	The nurse names key leaders and members to work collaboratively to identify and set goals and priorities. The nurse contacts social and political leaders and networks.
Principle of relevancy Know what issues are important to community members (this may differ from the issues important to nurses)	The nurse allows community members to define their own issues and helps them focus on their objectives. The nurse holds town hall meetings and group discussions to allow members to share concerns and important issues. The nurse encourages the community to define issues and enhance their ownership of issues.
Principle of participation Learn by doing	The nurse facilitates community members to make decisions about health programs and messages. The nurse encourages group support. The nurse recognizes that active vs. passive participation results in greater likelihood of attitude and behavior changes.
Issue selection Identify community problems that the community believes are specific, meaningful, and attainable	The nurse uses problem-solving techniques to help group members identify relevant issues vs. troubling problems (e.g., door-to-door surveys and group process activities).
Creation of critical consciousness Encourage relationships of equality and mutual respect among group members and educators to identify root problems and generate appropriate action plans.	The nurse uses problem-posing dialogue (Freire, 1973) to understand root issues and devises creative and innovative methods to transform situations.

Adapted from Minkler M, Wallerstein N: Improving health through community organization and community building. In Glanz K, Lewis K, Rimer BK, editors: *Health behavior and education: theory, research, and practice,* ed 2, San Francisco, 1997, Jossey-Bass.

partner with the community, identify common goals, develop strategies, and mobilize resources to increase community empowerment and community competence. Key concepts inherent in community health education programming are empowerment, community competence, issue selection, principle of relevance, principle of participation, and creation of critical consciousness (Minkler and Wallerstein, 1997).

Keck (1994) indicated that successful community health relies on empowering citizens to make decisions about individual and community health. Empowering citizens causes power to shift from health providers to community members in addressing health priorities. The basic tenets of community empowerment are not new; however, the belief that this framework is valuable and important is new. Collaboration and cooperation among community members, academicians, clinicians, health agencies, and businesses help ensure that scientific advances, community needs, sociopolitical needs, and environmental needs converge in a humanistic manner. The University of Wisconsin-House of Peace Community Nursing Center (UWM-HOPCNC) in Milwaukee illustrates how the basic philosophical tenets of community organization resulted in a nursing center model that brought together members of the university, businesses, health agencies, and most importantly, the community. Box 7-2 describes this program in detail.

THE NURSE'S ROLE IN HEALTH EDUCATION

Although learning theories and health education models provide a useful framework for planning health interventions, the nurse's ability to facilitate the education process and become a partner with individuals and communities is key to the methods' application. At the core of health education is the therapeutic relationship between the nurse and individuals, families, and the community. Nurses hold the process together and are catalysts for change in delivering humanistic care. Nurses can activate ideas, offer appropriate interventions, identify resources, and facilitate group empowerment. Rankin and Stallings (1995) described the following key characteristics of nurses in facilitating the teacher-learner process: confidence, competence, caring, and communication. It is beyond the scope of this chapter to describe communication techniques in detail, but it reminds the reader about the value of delivering inclusion and trust before content.

Enhancing Communication

The critical step of inclusion establishes the base for possible health action; it sets the relationship. The nurse enhances inclusion by greeting individuals, families, and groups in a timely and warm fashion, asking participants about their day, providing comfort, offering refreshments, and attending to immediate concerns or stress. Education does not begin with the first instructional word. Rather, education begins with establishing an atmosphere conducive to learning. If the nurse attends to inclusion, individuals, families, and groups begin to trust the nurse, thereby trusting the health message. This trust is evident through active participation and commitment in the education process. If the content or health message is positive, proactive, and personalized, it is more likely that participants will receive the message.

Community empowerment is reflective of participatory decision making and planning from the bottom up, fosters participant collective action, and is culturally sensitive (Baldwin, 1999; Bernstein et al., 1994; Lugo, 1996). Nurses are essential in creating and delivering appropriate health messages and programs and must address sociopolitical and environmental forces within appropriate cultural and linguistical expressions. Chapter 12 contains a detailed perspective on cultural diversity and community health nursing. Davis and colleagues (1992) outlined the following principles to help nurses become sensitive to cultural diversity and global health care needs:

- Confront personal racism and ethnocentrism.
- Become sensitive to intergroup and intragroup cultural diversity and commonalties in ethnic minority populations.
- Seek knowledge about the dynamics in biculturalism (e.g., how a particular ethnic group may be a synthesis of several cultures).
- Seek understanding of how social and structural factors influence and shape behaviors. Avoid a "blame the victim" ideology.

The nurse should ask the following questions about his or her own practice and respond by noting the frequency (i.e., "very often," "often," "not often," or "rarely"):

Do you interact with people of color on an ongoing basis?

Do you feel comfortable teaching an ethnically diverse group of learners?

BOX 7-2

Example of Community Empowerment-Collaboration-Participation:
UWM-HOPCNC, Milwaukee

In 1991, UWM-HOPCNC, an academic nursing center with vision and innovation, opened in Milwaukee's Near North Side, a core section of Milwaukee. This particular community consists of uninsured, underinsured, and economically challenged families. Plagued by problems that affect many urban communities, this community is challenged by multisocietal problems including drug use, poverty, violence, crime, unemployment, inadequate housing, under education, sickness, and disease. In an effort to respond to these needs and provide greater access to health care, the community nursing center opened and expanded the House of Peace Community Center's successful existing programs, which had been part of the community for 30 years. The House of Peace, originally founded in 1968 by a team of Capuchin Franciscans, offered a variety of social support services such as food and clothing banks and youth and adolescent programs. Building upon the existing infrastructure, advanced practice nurse clinicians, community health nurses, and outreach specialists worked collaboratively with the community to plan and offer a wide range of health services.

The primary goal of the Community Nursing Center (CNC) is to help clients and the community promote, attain, maintain, and restore an optimal, realistic level of physical, social, and mental health. Programs emphasize health education and primary prevention. The CNC provides services through the walk-in clinic, home visits, and collaboration with community agencies within the vicinity of the House of Peace. The CNC is community focused and provides services that are accessible and appropriate culturally and linguistically. Services include the following: wellness and health-risk assessment, case management, crisis intervention, monitoring and follow-up, treatment, counseling, and referral. Mechanisms for ongoing community input and dialogue are an essential component for developing relevant programs and health interventions. The CNC is supported by multiple private and public funds and staffed by a team of advanced practice nurse clinicians, community health nurses, and outreach workers.

Community residents sought health-related assistance during the 1998 to 1999 fiscal year. Using the Omaha Classification System, nurses coded 3334 individual visits and 1884 group visits. Health teaching, guidance, and counseling were the most widely used nursing intervention strategies. Other successful ongoing programs that are part of and have originated from the CNC include the following:

a. Shop Talk: breast cancer awareness program implemented in over 100 African American beauty salons.
b. Wisconsin Women's Cancer Control Program: Hmong and Laotian Initiative: a program designed to provide breast and cervical cancer education and screening to Hmong and Laotian women in a culturally and linguistically relevant manner.
c. Bring Out Your Best: a program designed to remove obstacles that keep women from reaching their goal of economic self-sufficiency. Services include computer training, preemployment physicals, and proper work attire.

Since its inception, the House of Peace and the UMW-HOPCNC have provided a context for community agencies, professional agencies, schools, and churches to combine their resources and talent with community members to enhance the QOL for at-risk populations through partnership and community capacity-building (Nichols, Personal Communication, 2000).

How often do you ask people of color for new ideas on solving problems?

Can you deal with cultural differences positively?

Do you feel comfortable alone in an elevator with a person of color?

Do you have high expectations of people of color?

Are you aware of and confront stereotypical expectations about attitudes, values, communication patterns, or health behaviors based on skin color?

Do you alter your teaching based on situations, individuals, families, or groups?

For questions answered "not often" or "rarely," the nurse should reexamine assumptions that may obstruct effective and relevant health teaching. The nurse should consider ways to modify his or her thinking to include cultural considerations in nursing care. He or she should examine ways to overcome barriers of effective communication (American Management Association, 1993).

According to Meleis (1999), **culturally competent care** exhibits sensitivity to an individual's differences based on his or her vast experiences and responses in accordance with background, sexual orientation, SES, ethnicity, and culture. She also depicts several properties that compose the "essence of the nurse" in delivering culturally competent care. First, the nurse possesses an explanatory system that values diversity (i.e., a system that is not drained by the attempt to interpret symbols, but is energized by the variations). Second, the nurse uses expert assessment skills to discern different and similar response patterns, which helps plan appropriate teaching interventions. Third, the culturally competent nurse is aware of diverse communication patterns and how language and communication influence "trust within the relationship." The culturally competent nurse also recognizes how marginalization may increase health risks for individuals and how using the expertise of insiders in the culture is a highly valued skill. Also, the culturally competent nurse readily acknowledges differences and does not tolerate inequities.

Cultural assessment and cultural negotiation enhance health teaching. Nurses can use these two processes to refine their assessment information (e.g., religion issues, decision-making patterns, and preferred communication styles to plan relevant care) and translate instructions and messages to match individuals, families, or groups (Airhihenbuwa, 1994; Lipson, 1999).

For example, Strickland and colleagues (1999) addressed religion in designing a culturally appropriate cervical health promotion program for Eastern Washington's Yakama Indian women. The investigators conducted personal interviews with spiritual leaders and male and female members of the Wa'Shat Longhouse religion and obtained religious influences by asking questions about life views, communication channels, and leadership. Results showed that program goals must be holistic, teach-ing methods must include circular symbols, and intentions must link to natural communication patterns and involve elders. It was also found that storytelling, talking circles, role models, and multiple sensory modalities were important teaching approaches. For example, the circle symbol of unity connected the people and the earth. The group facilitator was an equal learner who respected the wisdom, experiences, and contributions of each member. Also, time is loosely structured among the Yakama; therefore an educational session may require an entire morning. The investigators also found that, unlike other cultures, the Yakama valued information directly from the elders over the dissemination of prevention information.

Nurses can provide effective community health education through expert knowledge and skill. In her keynote address to the Twentieth Biennial Convention of the National League for Nursing, Shalala (1993, p. 291) stated the following:

> But who will slay the dragon of disadvantage? Who will step in with the wand, the ruby slippers, the handful of magic beans? It will not be one individual, not one profession, not one tower of vision. It must be a consortium of professionals, a combined vision of many different parts and different life stories: corporate leaders, politicians, teachers, leaders of nursing professionals. Yes, very importantly, nurses, whose profession is not just a career, but a lifework. Nurses who have one foot high on the crystal tower of knowledge and theory and one foot in the dust and grit of human need.

FRAMEWORK FOR DEVELOPING HEALTH COMMUNICATIONS

Within the community, the nurse's intended audience may be an individual, family, group, or many segments of the community. Using a systematic approach to the development, design, and delivery of health messages provides the nurse with an organized, user-friendly approach to health message delivery. Although nurses may use a variety of educational models, theoretical frameworks, and teaching and learning principles, the National Cancer Institute suggested using the "Framework for Developing Health Communications" to create a variety of health education messages and programs (USDHHS, 1992) (Fig. 7-1). These six stages depict a circular loop that mirrors the nursing process (assessment, planning, implementation, into every step. See "Launching a Breast Education and Outreach Screening Program," p. 146.

Stage I: Planning and Strategy Selection

The planning stage provides the foundation for the communication program's planning process. Understanding the intended audience's learning needs and targeting the program or message to the audience is key to activating health education. This step reinforces Freire's philosophical tenets of ascertaining the intended audience's needs and creating an open dialogue.

Questions to Ask

- Who is the intended audience?
- What is known about the audience and from what sources?
- What are the objectives and goals?
- What evaluation strategies will the nurse use?
- What is the health issue of interest?

Collaborative Actions to Take

- Review available data from health statistics, local sources, libraries, newspapers, and local or community leaders.
- Obtain new data (i.e., interviews and focus groups with problem-posing dialogue).
- Determine the intended group's needs and perceptions of health problems (i.e., identify audiences).
  - Physical (e.g., sex, age, and health history)
  - Behavioral (e.g., lifestyle characteristics and health-related activities)
  - Demographic (e.g., income, years of schooling, and cultural characteristics)
  - Psychographics (e.g., beliefs, values, and attitudes)
- Identify issues behind the issues.
- Identify existing health knowledge gaps.
- Establish goals and objectives that are specific, attainable, prioritized, and time specific.
- Assess resources (e.g., money, staff, and materials).

Stage II: Selecting Channels and Materials

The nurse's decisions in Stage I can help guide him or her in selecting appropriate communication channels and producing effective and relevant

---

FIGURE 7-1

Framework for developing health communications. The National Cancer Institute suggests using this model to develop health education messages (Data from US Department of Health Human Services: *Making health communication programs work,* NIH Pub No 92-1493, Bethesda, Md, 1992, Office of Cancer Communications, National Cancer Institute).

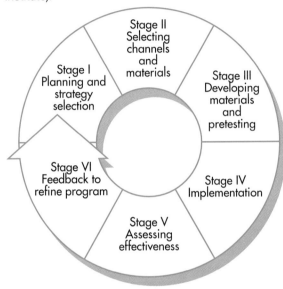

and evaluation) and provide a sequential path for continuous assessment, feedback, and improvement. This model is based on the principles of social marketing, health education, and mass communication theories. This framework relies on target audience assessment to guide the process. It is also congruent with Freire's model of empowerment education, which encourages ongoing dialogue with the potential consumers of health services. Although this model focuses on communication strategies aimed at the programmatic level, the basic elements are applicable to individual, family, and group systems.

The ideas contained in this "Framework for Developing Health Communications" model are a practical schema for planning and implementing health education communications programs. Nurses should use the model as a guide to plan health education messages and programs. The nurse should use an organized and systematic approach rather than attempt to fit his or her health education plan

Launching a Breast Education and Outreach Screening Program

In 1993, H. Lee Moffitt Cancer Center and Research Institute, or Moffitt, formed a partnership with Suncoast Community Health Centers, Inc., or Suncoast, in rural Hillsborough County. The partnership brought breast cancer education and screening services to Hispanic Migrant and Seasonal Farmworkers (MSFW) and low-income rural women via Moffitt's Lifetime Cancer Screening Mobile Unit.

In 1993, a cancer center physician visited Suncoast, which is a federally funded, community-based center located about 30 miles south of Tampa. He was "moved" by the center's services and impressed with the clinic's dedication to reaching medically underserved populations. Suncoast consists of three comprehensive health care clinics in Plant City, Ruskin, and Dover, Florida and offers services to Hillsborough County's low-income rural populations, which includes farmworkers. Suncoast provides a range of medical services, but they do not have mammography facilities. Moffitt was expanding its community outreach initiatives through mobile services. Moffitt is a free-standing, private, nonprofit institution affiliated with and located at the University of South Florida campus in Tampa. Moffitt is the only National Cancer Institute Designated Cancer Center in Florida and is widely known for state-of-the-art treatments, outpatient and ambulatory services, and screening processes. After a series of meetings between Suncoast and Moffitt's Lifetime Cancer Screening Center, the groups formed a partnership from a shared goal. Both parties determined that the *goal* was to develop and offer the community culturally relevant education, accessible mammography service, and follow-up care. This program continues to be a sustainable initiative.

Illustration: Description of Health Issue and Intended Audience

Despite progress in the fight against cancer, many communities continue to bear a disproportionate share of the cancer burden. These communities include racially and culturally diverse populations with low income and education levels, families with inadequate medical insurance, and individuals who experience barriers in differing cultural beliefs and practices or limited literacy or language abilities (ACS, 1999). Cancer is the leading cause of premature death in women and breast cancer accounts for approximately one third of all malignancies, especially in women with low incomes (Fugate Woods, 1995). Low rates of early detection cause treatment delays and poor prognoses in rural women, especially in breast cancer (Frank-Stromborg et al., 1998). Nurses must reach at-risk populations with effective, appropriate, and measurable methods to reduce cancer morbidity and mortality.

The lack of mammography screening and education for rural Hillsborough County's medically underserved women represented a health service gap. In particular, Hispanic MSFW represent a particular subgroup of women (i.e., poor and minority) who face a number of barriers to mammography. These barriers include lack of insurance, limited access to health care, low education and literacy levels, cultural and linguistical differences, and immigrant status. These women need educational interventions and tools that address unique value systems, cultural and linguistical issues, and access problems. These women wanted and needed health information about breast health, but they were also experiencing everyday survival issues and struggles. Sensitive providers needed to deliver a culturally relevant health service in a geographically convenient area. Women aged 40 and older were eligible for this service. Breast cancer is higher among women over 50; therefore researchers focused on this group. The intended target audience was Hispanic MSFW and Caucasian or Hispanic rural women, but it also included women from diverse ethnic backgrounds.

Goal: To prevent premature death and disability from breast cancer through early detection, screening, and culturally and linguistically relevant education.

Objectives: To increase education, mammograms, clinical breast examinations, and follow-up programs among medically underserved women in rural Hillsborough County.

TABLE 7-6

Teaching-Learning Formats

Teaching Format	Application to Health Education
Brainstorming session	Allows participants the freedom to generate ideas and discuss them in a group setting. Cultivates creativity. Fosters empowerment to allow members to identify the issue and find solutions.
Community-wide programs	Can reach large numbers of community members through a systematic plan. May include individual or group approaches with a defined intended audience.
Demonstration	Effective in learning perceptual motor skills. Aids in visual identification.
Group discussion	Members can learn from each other and receive support. Nurses can tailor teaching content to group needs. Ideal for groups combining patients and families. Nurses, health professionals, or lay members can lead the groups. Facilitator must be comfortable with group method and familiar with group characteristics.
Lecture	Varying group sizes can use formal oral presentations. Group members share expertise and experiences. Presenter must be comfortable and possess speaking ability. Requires organizational skills and ability to highlight key points in interesting and creative ways. A combination of lecture and media may enhance learning. Audience participation is linked to the presenter's speaking style and ability. Audience feedback is limited.
Personal discussion (i.e., individual and one-on-one)	Allows individual assessment and identification of cultural barriers, physical impairments, learning needs, literacy, and anxiety. Promotes the tailoring of health education plans. Ideal to capture "teachable moments." Does not allow sharing and support from others. High cost of staff time.
Role playing	Effective in influencing attitudes and opinions. Encourages problem-solving and critical thinking skills. Enhances learner participation. Some members may be hesitant to become involved.
Task force committee	Joins individuals with diverse backgrounds and expertise to achieve a goal. May represent many interests and perspectives.

Based on data from Babcock and Miller, 1994; Rankin and Stallings, 1995; Redman and Klug, 1996.

materials. The nurse must consider how to reach the intended audience and use supporting materials and media. The community nurse must consider the best way to reach the audience and what methods to use. *Channel* refers to how the nurse will reach communication sites (i.e., churches, clinics, nurses, or community-based organizations). *Format* refers to how the nurse will communicate the health message (e.g., individually or group discussion) (Table 7-6).

Materials and media are the program's tools, not the program itself (Table 7-7). Education is a human activity and should not focus on audiovisuals exclusively.

Questions to Ask
- What channels are best?
- What formats should be used?
- Are there existing resources?

TABLE 7-7

Materials and Media

Media	Considerations in Health Education Settings
Audiotapes	Do not require reading Portable and small Individuals can use them at home in a comfortable setting and can replay and use them at their own pace Economical Helpful for individuals with visual difficulties or low literacy skills
Bulletin boards	Inexpensive and easy to develop Direct attention to a specific message; uses few words
Exhibits and displays	Graphics offer appeal Placement in high-traffic areas (e.g., waiting rooms and exam rooms reach wide audiences)
Flip charts and chalkboards	Excellent format to enlarge teaching concepts or cue reader to salient points; may add graphics and diagrams Chalkboards are reusable; flip charts have replacement pads Inexpensive
Games and simulations	Involve patients in a fun manner; involve the entire family Highly effective with children
Graphics Drawings and visuals	Can convey important points in a salient and visual fashion Can aid understanding for low-literacy audiences Humorous messages may attract the attention of intended members Visual messages should be pretested to ensure acceptability and understanding (Michielutte et al., 1992)
Interactive videotapes (i.e., multimedia)	A variety of computer programs, interactive videodisks, and computer-assisted instructions are available and are undergoing testing Algorithms and branching decisions aid patients in decision making, problem solving, and fact acquisition (Campbell et al., 1994) Interactive patient education is becoming more common via kiosks in waiting rooms Nurses should assess computer comfort level Software development may be time intensive and costly
Models and real objects	Bring the teaching concept to the patient in a familiar way
Demonstrations	Helpful when conveying psychomotor skills; encourage patient involvement and tactile learning (e.g., penis model for condom placement or breast model to show breast self-exam) No reading needed Helpful in individual and group instruction Nurses can incorporate models and real objects into displays or fairs

Based on data from Babcock and Miller, 1994; Breckon et al., 1998; Doak et al., 1998; Meade, 1996; Rankin and Stallings, 1995.
Media are the tools of a health education program and encounter. They can inform, reinforce, and convey health messages. Education is a human activity and should not be reduced to the exclusive use of audiovisuals. Media should match the target audience. If developing new media, the nurse should field test the media with members of the intended group to ensure relevancy.

T A B L E **7-7—cont'd**

Materials and Media—cont'd

Media	Considerations in Health Education Settings
Overheads	Useful in small and large group settings Highlight key points and help patients focus ideas Use of color and advance organizers, large type, and key points are recommended; avoid busy and cluttered overheads Can be prepared in advance Inexpensive
Photographs, picture books, and slide series (i.e., Powerpoint slides) Photoessay and photo-voice	Help promote understanding by showing realistic images and real situations Help patients make connections to their life Photographs may appear alone or in combination with other photographs or slides or placed in an album Powerpoint slides are easily updated Helpful for patients with limited literacy skills; offers visual presentation of concepts Effective with an individual and with small groups (i.e., self-study or reflection) Easily updated (Paskett, 1996; Wang and Burris, 1997)
Printed materials (brochures, leaflets, or booklets)	Portable, widely available, and economical Useful in reinforcing health concepts and interactions Patients can set and adjust the pace and refer back to information later Can be effective with individuals, families, groups, or community-wide dissemination Materials written at simple levels can be effective and acceptable for both low-level and high-level readers (Doak et al., 1998; Meade et al., 1989) Personalized materials are highly effective (Skinner et al., 1994) and are a promising strategy for health education (Kreuter et al., 1999) Nurses should assess issues of readability, design, layout, cultural relevance, and appropriateness of content. (Guidry and Walker, 1999; Michielutte et al., 1999).
Programmed materials, self-help guides, slide and tape programs	May involve printed materials combined with visuals to allow self-pacing Helpful to learn facts Nurse should assess individual or group to determine whether independent learning style is preferred
Teaching cards	Portable, use few words, and offer visual interpretations
Flashcards	The nurse can create them economically and update them easily. Effective with individual, small group, or family instruction
Radio and newspapers	Reach large audiences within the community Effective in conveying general health information in a user-friendly manner Nurses can play an active role in disseminating health information (Meade, 1992)

Continued

TABLE 7-7—cont'd

Materials and Media—cont'd

Media	Considerations in Health Education Settings
Television and cable television	Reach large audiences within the community
	Can help enhance community members' general health and well-being
	Effective in influencing attitudes and behaviors
	Offer a familiar medium for viewers to learn about health topics
	Nurses can play key roles in reaching the community (Meade, 1992)
Videotapes	Combine audio and visual medium to convey realistic images (Meade, 1996).
	Videotapes should incorporate role modeling concepts (Gagliano, 1988)
	Expensive to produce and update; requires access to audiovisual equipment and viewing sites
	Videotapes may be costly to produce, purchase, and update.
	Tailoring of content to target audience enhances effectiveness (Rimer, 1999)
Online resources (i.e., Internet, simple dial-up services, and World Wide Web)	Electronic information sources can link individuals, families, and groups to health information, data bases, and bulletin board services (Bush, 1999)
	Common Internet providers are America On-Line and Prodigy
	World Wide Web is a software system that facilitates creating and sharing multimedia across the Internet (Andrews, 1999; Sikorski and Peters, 1997)
	Access World Wide Web sites for accuracy, credibility, and relevancy
	New technologies can help consumers find health information, advice, and support (Sharp, 1999)

Based on data from Babcock and Miller, 1994; Breckon et al., 1998; Doak et al., 1998; Meade, 1996; Rankin and Stallings, 1995.

Collaborative Actions to Take

- Identify messages and materials.
- Decide whether to use existing materials or produce new ones.
- Select channels and formats.

Stage III: Developing Materials and Pretesting

The nurse may develop several types of communication concepts in the first stages and can test them with the audience for feedback.

Questions to Ask

- How can the nurse present the message?
- How will the intended audience react to the message?
- Will the audience understand, accept, and use the message?
- What changes may improve the message?

Collaborative Actions to Take

- Develop relevant materials with the target audience.

- Pretest the message and materials and obtain audience feedback (e.g., interviews, questionnaires, focus groups, and readability testing). Pretesting helps ensure comprehension, acceptability, and personal relevance.

Stage IV: Implementation

At this stage, the nurse introduces the health education message and program to the target audience and reviews and revises necessary components.

Questions to Ask

- Is the message and program reaching the intended audience?
- Do any channels require alteration?
- What are the strengths of the health program?
- What changes would enhance effectiveness?

Collaborative Actions to Take

- Work with community organizations, businesses, and other health agencies to enhance effectiveness.
- Monitor and track progress.

Illustration: Selecting Channels and Methods

Nurses selected a combination of channels to communicate health information about breast cancer, screenings, and early detection methods (e.g., community-based clinics, missions, and social service agencies). Nurses conducted individual interactions at the mobile site.

Nurses collected a variety of health materials and media about breast cancer from national, state, and local sources and determined that many of the printed materials were not culturally or educationally relevant (e.g., high reading levels). Few Spanish language materials were available.

Illustration: Developing Materials

In 1994, through a grant from Avon, or the National Alliance of Breast Cancer Organizations (NABCO), Suncoast and Moffitt designed bilingual English and Spanish materials to educate and encourage women to practice self-breast exams and receive screening. A series of focus groups and pretesting measures ensured the materials were culturally and educationally relevant. Additionally, a grant from the Cancer Research Foundation of America, Inc. funded the development of a 14-minute Spanish videotape on breast

and cervical cancer. Women now view this tape in the mobile unit while waiting for their appointments.

Community agencies, missions, and clinics received printed service schedules. Although translators were sporadically present in the van, it became apparent that permanent bilingual staff was necessary. Ongoing dialogue with community members and clinics helped refine the screening process, the education component, and the follow-up services to ensure effectiveness, efficiency, appropriateness, and timely follow-up.

Illustration: Implementation

The mass media introduced the service at a press conference. Each year, several spokespersons helped kick off the program. An outreach worker distributed lists in the community that publicized the mobile unit's sites and operation dates. The outreach worker posted flyers at a variety of sites (e.g., beauty shops, laundromats, unemployment offices, and community centers).

Twice per month, the mobile unit traveled to Suncoast. There, the outreach worker or the mobile unit staff greeted the women and answered questions about procedure and follow-up. The health educator offered instruction on breast self-examination and encouraged women to watch the video on breast and cervical health. Staff consisted of the outreach worker, NP, mammography technician, and health educator.

■ Establish process evaluation measures (e.g., follow-up with users of the service, number of women who used the service, and expenditures).

Stage V: Assessing Effectiveness

The nurse analyzes the program and health message for effectiveness and tracks the mechanisms identified in Stage I. Both process and summative are helpful. Process evaluation examines the procedures

and tasks involved in the program or message such as monitoring media, identifying the intended audience's interim reactions, and addressing internal functioning (e.g., work schedules and expenditures). Outcome evaluation examines short-term or long-term results such as the number of sites covered, the number of women reached, inquiries about the program or service, and change in audience awareness, knowledge, attitude, behaviors, and mortality and morbidity figures.

Illustration: Assessing Efficiency

Process Evaluation: A number of newspaper, television, and radio advertisements publicized the free/low-cost mammography service and highlighted the importance of breast health. Also, several human-interest stories emerged, which communicated the screening services to a wider audience. Since 1993, an increase in the number of staff involved in the program and the number of funded projects that support the program enhanced the breadth and depth of the services. The on-site service logistics have made continual improvements, most notably in adding a dedicated outreach worker and part-time health educator to the program.

In the first few years of operation, a total of 200 women underwent screening, which is a modest number. Assessment revealed that many women failed to appear for breast screenings because they had a "fear of cancer" and were uncertain how to navigate the health care system. Typically, many women from the community did not seek preventative health care; they sought care only for acute illness. Assessment showed that peer outreach was necessary to ensure participation. Therefore a subsequent request to Avon-NABCO in 1997 aimed to link 350 women to screening by proposing an outreach component, which consisted of a bilingual lay worker who would provide customized recruitment, culturally and linguistically appropriate instruction, and follow-up care.

This program produced dramatic results, reaching 352 women for screening services and education. Within this group, there were 53 abnormal findings, or 15%, and follow-up detected cancer in one person. In 1998, the program implemented stronger outreach and education elements to reach 400 women. Peer outreach continued to be the program's key component. Fortunately, the outreach worker continued with the project in 1998, which allowed continuity. During 1998, the program exceeded its goal by linking 471 women to screening. In 1999, the most recent screening year, the program produced over 600 screenings. Sixty-four women, or 14%, had abnormal results and received follow-up until diagnosis and treatment was complete. Two women received cancer diagnoses and underwent treatment.

Women expressed gratitude for the sensitivity and personal attention given by the peer outreach worker and mobile unit staff. The program's goal is to provide screenings and education to 800 women per year and increase the number of community partners in the next millennium. Formal and informal feedback revealed that women responded well to the service and were especially satisfied with the Spanish language educational materials.

Outcome Evaluation: During the program's first six years, less than 200 women received screening per year. The number of women now screened approaches 800 per year. The number of community partners increased and includes a partnership with the CDCs Breast and Cervical Early Detection Program, the Hillsborough Health Department, the ACS, Avon-NABCO, the Cancer Research Foundation of America, and other migrant organizations. Regular health fairs and health events are scheduled and the program's leaders continually refine its mechanisms for follow-up care. The program ensures that participating women receive respectful and relevant care.

Questions to Ask

- Were objectives met? What was the impact (i.e., change in morbidity or mortality)?
- How well did each step work (i.e., process evaluation)?
- Did the changes result from the program or from other factors (i.e., outcome evaluation)?

Collaborative Actions to Take

- Conduct process and outcome evaluations.

Stage VI: Feedback to Refine Program

The nurse may prepare for a new development cycle using information gained from audience feedback, communication channels, and the program's intended effect. This phase helps to continually refine the health message and respond to the target audience's needs. This stage yields information that helps validate the programs' strengths and allows necessary modifications. Feedback is necessary to continually refine the message.

Illustration: Feedback

Reports describing process and outcome evaluation, and analysis provide a point of reference for continual improvements. Such reports apply knowledge and outline methods to enhance and improve the service's efficiency and effectiveness. Lifetime's mobile mammography van continues to provide service to women in rural Hillsborough County. Each year, the number of women receiving the service increases. The program persists under the auspices of the cancer center's Lifetime Cancer Screening Center and the Education Program and ongoing funding opportunities sustain the program.

The program has incorporated a network of outreach and educational components to reach rural MSFW and low-income elderly women in South and East Hillsborough County. The program will progress and build upon the knowledge, experience, and lessons garnered to reach even more underserved rural women and link them to culturally relevant services. The program's leaders aim to extend its reach into surrounding counties such as rural Pasco. Although the program provided desired links to screening services and formed successful community partnerships, it is important to develop and refine community empowerment strategies through outreach and education to sustain and widely disseminate the program.

The primary outcome of the education and outreach screening program ensured direct access and education for breast self-exams, mammogram screenings, and clinical breast exams; however, the next goal is to achieve a reproducible model for effective education and outreach through community partnership. Likely, the project will culminate in a series of approaches that other rural communities can apply to deliver breast cancer prevention and early detection messages. Aiming to reach the community rather than the individual produces health benefits for the entire community. Such a model will provide critical information about successful approaches that can combine with other resources for local, statewide, and national dissemination.

Questions to Ask

- What was learned?
- What can be improved?
- What worked well and what did not work well?
- Are the goals and objectives relevant?
- Has anything changed about the intended audience?
- Was the assessment complete?
- Did the audience perceive the problem?
- Are the methods and formats tailored to the intended audience?
- Were barriers overlooked?
- Overall, what lessons were learned and what modifications could strengthen the health education activity?

Collaborative Actions to Take

- Reassess and revise goals and objectives.
- Modify unsuccessful strategies or activities.
- Generate continual support from businesses, health care agencies, and other community groups for ongoing collaboration and partnerships.
- Summarize the health education program or message in an evaluation report.
- Provide justification for continuing or ending the program.

The reader should consider how to plan other health messages or programs using this model. The exercise in Fig. 7-2 will help the reader organize ideas systematically.

HEALTH EDUCATION RESOURCES

A variety of health education materials and resources are available from local, state, and national organizations and agencies. Such associations can provide helpful information about services, educational materials, and links to support groups or self-help groups. Often printed and electronic materials are available for free or for a nominal cost. Nurses can help individuals, families, and groups access materials, services, or equipment loan programs. Nurses who are knowledgeable about available resources can support community education programs and messages. Additionally, identifying gaps in services or resources may yield data to help nurses create the necessary services or materials.

The nurse can locate many health resources through a variety of search engines on the Internet. Andrews (1999) examines Internet and CD-Rom resources containing information on transcultural nursing and health subjects. University or college

FIGURE 7-2

Planning the health education message.

Planning Your Health Education Message

Instructions: Think about a target group that you are currently working with and planning to deliver/create a health education program or message. Complete the exercise by asking yourself the following questions:

Questions to Ask	Action Plan
• What is the overall intended message/goal? What are my reasons for planning this message? How do I know that it is needed or wanted by the target audience?	
• Who is the intended audience? (Write a brief statement describing the characteristics of the target group.)	
• What will be the benefits of this message to the target group?	
• What channels will I use to deliver the message? Provide a rationale.	
• Will I need to create materials? Are there available materials that are appropriate for my target group?	
• How will I know if my message gets across to the target audience? Did the target audience respond? How many people were reached? Who responded?	
• Was there change? What are the reasons the message was or was not effective? What can be modified to strengthen the message?	

---

libraries often provide information on beginning and advanced search strategies. The nurse can use the following sources for health education information. The book's website contains a summary of major organizations and resources at ⟨SIMON⟩ www.wbsaunders.com/SIMON/nies/.

Rankin and Stallings (1995) also provide the following comprehensive resource listing:

■ local and regional hospitals, clinics, libraries, health education centers, and businesses;

■ local and state governmental sources (e.g., health departments and social service agen-

cies); check the yellow pages or Internet for listings;

■ community-based organizations (i.e., advertised, nonadvertised, and those recommended by community leaders);

■ universities and colleges, community colleges, and academic nursing centers;

■ professional organizations (e.g., APHA, ANA, and National Black Nurses Association);

■ commercial organizations (e.g., pharmaceutical companies, medical supply companies, and patient and health education companies); written and audiovisual sources are often available;

- federal government sources (e.g., National Institutes of Health [NIH]; National Cancer Institute; National Heart, Lung, Blood Institute; PHS; CDC; National AIDS Clearinghouse; Office of Minority Health [OMH]; and Office on Smoking and Health);
- voluntary agencies and their local affiliates (e.g., American Heart Association, Amyotrophic Lateral Sclerosis Association, American Council for Drug Disorders, American Dairy Council, and American Lung Association);
- Directory of Information Resources onLINE (DIRLINE) is available on the National Library of Medicine's software package called Grateful MED; this data base offers a directory of organizations providing information services;
- World Wide Web Internet searches;
- Medline Plus Health Information (i.e., a service of the National Library of Medicine for patient and consumer information); Internet appliances such as Web TV ™.

Assessing the Relevancy of Health Materials

It is critical that nurses use materials that are appropriate for the intended target audience in community health education initiatives. The nurse should ask the following questions:

- Does the material match the intended audience?
- Are the materials appealing?
- Is the message clear and understandable?
- Will the intended audience relate to the content, the visuals, and the written style?

Literacy and Health

In her 1944 text, *The Public Health Nurse in the Community,* Rue stated that the community's illiteracy level is an important factor in health program planning. This factor remains a significant issue in planning health education programs and materials. Millions of Americans are unable to process and use information that is often vital to their survival. Approximately one of five Americans is faced with the challenges of low literacy skills. A U.S. Department of Education survey indicated that over half the population aged 16 and older have very basic reading skills and limited critical thinking

skills (Kirsch et al., 1993). The nurse may ask the following questions:

Will parents know what to do if their infant gets a fever?
Do parents know how to read a thermometer?
Does the patient know how to take four different types of medications?
Will the family understand how to get through the health care system?
Do community members understand food labels?
Are printed immunization schedules clear?
Can the patient understand warning messages if they are written in complex technical language?

Research indicates serious disparities between the reading levels of materials and most Americans' reading skills (Alexander, 2000; Baker et al., 1998; Gazmararian et al., 1999b; Glazer et al., 1996; Guidry and Fagan, 1997; Macario, 1998; Meade and Byrd, 1989; Meade, 1999; Meade et al., 1992; Meade et al., 1994; Mohrmann et al., 2000; Swanson et al., 1990; Weiss and Coyne, 1997; Wells et al., 1994; Williams et al., 1995; Williams et al., 1998a; Wilson, 1996). Additionally, materials often fail to incorporate the target audience's cultural beliefs, values, languages, and attitudes (Guidry and Walker, 1999; Wilson, 1996).

Weiss and colleagues (1992) reported significant links between health status and literacy even in adjusting for sociodemographic variables. The relational mechanisms between literacy and health are unclear; however, individuals with very low literacy skills are at an increased risk for poor health. Baker and colleagues (1997) studied two public hospitals with 2659 patients. Data showed that patients with an inadequate literacy level were more likely to have poor self-reported health status than patients with adequate literacy skills. Gazmararian and colleagues (1999a) studied 3260 elderly managed care enrollees and found they may not possess the literacy skills necessary to function adequately in the health care environment. In another study, Bennett (1998) revealed that a low literacy level was a better predictor than race or age at presentation for prostate cancer.

In 1999, the Report of the Council on Scientific Affairs of the AMA reported that patients with the most health care needs are often the least able to read and understand information to function successfully within the health care system. Patients with low literacy skills have many complex communication difficulties that may interact with other factors such as income and age and may ultimately impact their health outcomes. It was recommended that a broad policy agenda on health literacy be crafted to involve decision makers from the public and private sector. *Healthy People 2010 Objectives: Draft for Public Comments* states that health literacy is critical to help the public evaluate health information and make health decisions (USDHHS and PHS, 1998). Future research must focus on finding effective health education methods to improve communication and better delineate the causal pathway to poor literacy's effect on health. Also, health organizations (i.e., nursing and medical associations) need to partner with professional and consumer groups to find solutions to the health literacy problem (Ad Hoc Committee on Health Literacy for the Council on Scientific Affairs and AMA, 1999; Davis et al., 1998; Meade, 1999).

The Doaks, who brought the literacy issue to the forefront in public health, indicated that "the health community is a written culture. Unfortunately, many written instructions are over the heads of patients" (Doak et al., 1998). There is often a serious mismatch between the readability levels of health instructions and the reading skills of patients. Health care providers and nurses can control the literacy levels of their instructions and are responsible for reducing the mismatch. Techniques for accomplishing this are available and easy to apply (Doak et al., 1996). The Doaks' excellent book, *Teaching Patients with Low Literacy Skills* (1995), offers practical suggestions for preparing and testing materials.

Nurses can assume important roles in the creation and dissemination of relevant health materials and media. Within Stage I of the "Framework for Developing Health Communications" model, the nurse should use assessment skills to determine the reading level of the intended target audience. For example, the nurse should ask patients a series of simple questions to assess their reading skills (e.g., whether they read, whether they enjoy reading, what they like to read, and how often they read). Skilled readers like to read and enjoy a variety of materials. The nurse should determine how they get their health information and if the information is from written sources. The nurse should ask patients to read a paragraph from a health material aloud. Skilled readers enjoy reading, are fluent readers, understand content, interpret the meaning of words, and look up unfamiliar words. Limited readers read slowly, miss the intended meaning, take words literally, tire quickly from reading, and skip over uncommon words. Also, the nurse should ask the patients a few questions about the information they read. They should be able to answer questions about the material's content (Doak et al., 1996; Doak et al., 1998). The nurse should remember that reading skills are not necessarily equated with years of schooling. In fact, studies have often indicated a three to four grade level difference in reading skills compared with education level (Meade and Byrd, 1989; Meade et al., 1994; Streiff, 1986; Williams et al., 1998b).

The nurse may couple such informal assessment techniques with more formal, easily administered assessment methods to create a reading profile for patients. Davis and colleagues (1998) provided a helpful review of literacy assessments, discussed their implementation in a variety of settings, and offered suggestions nurses must consider before applying such tools. Tools used to estimate reading level in health care settings include the Wide-Range Achievement Test, Level III (Jastak and Wilkinson, 1993) and the Rapid Estimate of Adult Literacy in Medicine (REALM) by Davis and colleagues (1993) (Fig. 7-3). In developing health programs and materials for community groups, the nurse should apply informal or formal assessment techniques with a sample of potential intended members to ensure a match between health communications and readers.

Helpful Tips for Effective Teaching

- Assess reading skills using informal and formal methods.
- Determine what *patients* know and want to know.
- Stick with the essentials. Limit the number of concepts or key points. The focus may need to be on critical survival skills.
- Set realistic goals and objectives. Take cues from *patients* about what they want to learn and how to help them learn.
- Use clear and concise language. Avoid technical terms if possible. For example, substitute the word *problem* for *complication.* Use the term *stick to* instead of the word *compliant,* or use the word *chance* instead of *possibility.* However, do not needlessly simplify if the intended meaning is lost. Although the words *insulin* and *infection* may be polysyllabic words, diabetic patients are usually familiar with them. See Example 1.
- Consider developing a glossary or vocabulary list for common words on the health topic. For example, in teaching a family about dental health, create a list of common words about the topic (e.g., toothbrush, flossing, cavity, decay, checkups, and X-rays).

FIGURE 7-3

The Rapid Estimate of Adult Literacy in Medicine (REALM) is a screening instrument to assess an adult patient's ability to read common medical words and lay terms for body parts and illnesses. It is designed to assist medical professionals in estimating a patient's literacy level to use the appropriate level of patient education materials or oral instructions. The test takes two to three minutes to administer and score (Reprinted with permission of Dr. Terry Davis, Louisiana State University. From Davis TC et al: Rapid estimate of adult literacy in medicine: a shortened screening instrument, *Fam Med* 25:56-57, 1993).

Rapid Estimate of Adult Literacy in Medicine (Realm)©

Terry Davis, PhD • Michael Crouch, MD • Sandy Long, PhD

Patient's name/
Subject #_____

Reading Level _____ Grade Completed_____

Date of Birth_____

Date_____ Clinic_____ Examiner_____

List 1	List 2	List 3
fat	fatigue	allergic
flu	pelvic	menstrual
pill	jaundice	testicle
dose	infection	colitis
eye	exercise	emergency
stress	behavior	medication
smear	prescription	occupation
nerves	notify	sexually
germs	gallbladder	alcoholism
meals	calories	irritation
disease	depression	constipation
cancer	miscarriage	gonorrhea
caffeine	pregnancy	inflammatory
attack	arthritis	diabetes
kidney	nutrition	hepatitis
hormones	menopause	antibiotics
herpes	appendix	diagnosis
seizure	abnormal	potassium
bowel	syphilis	anemia
asthma	hemorrhoids	obesity
rectal	nausea	osteoporosis
incest	directed	impetigo

Score
List 1_____
List 2_____
List 3_____
Raw Score_____

Directions:

1. Give the patient a laminated copy of the Realm and score answers on an unlaminated copy that is attached to a clipboard. Hold the clipboard at an angle so that the patient is not distracted by your scoring procedure. Say:
"I want to hear you read as many words as you can from this list. Begin with the first word on List 1 and read aloud. When you come to a word you cannot read, do the best you can or say 'blank' and go on to the next word."

2. If the patient takes more than five seconds on a word, say "blank" and point to the next word, if necessary, to move the patient along. If the patient begins to miss every word, have him/her pronounce only known words.

3. Count as an error any word not attempted or mispronounced. Score by marking a plus (+) after each correct word, a check (√) after each mispronounced word, and a minus (−) after words not attempted. Count as correct any self-corrected words.

4. Count the number of correct words for each list and record the numbers in the "Score" box. Total the numbers and match the total score with its grade equivalent in the table below.

Grade Equivalent	
Raw Score	**Grade Range**
0 to 18	**3rd Grade and Below** Will not be able to read most low literacy materials; will need repeated oral instructions, materials composed primarily of illustrations, or audiotapes or videotapes.
19 to 44	**4th to 6th Grade** Will need low literacy materials; may not be able to read prescription labels.
45 to 60	**7th to 8th Grade** Will struggle with most patient education materials; will not be offended by low literacy materials.
61 to 66	**High School** Will be able to read most patient education materials.

EXAMPLE 1

Prostate Cancer and Treatment Options

Original text (harder to grasp)

The doctor has recently communicated to you that you have localized prostate cancer, commonly labeled Stage I. In addition to managing the anxieties associated with a life-threatening illness, patients must carefully consider the available treatment modalities and account for the potential effect each one may have on QOL. Patients must seriously evaluate the benefits and side effects of each treatment modality and determine the most efficacious one for their lifestyle.

Revised text (easier to grasp)

Your doctor has told you that you have early-stage prostate cancer. Deciding on a treatment is difficult, but it is important. Besides dealing with fears that go along with a cancer diagnosis, the patient must explore treatment options.

- Get to know the benefits and side effects of each treatment.
- Think about how each treatment will affect your life.
- Ask questions.
- Choose the best treatment for you.

- Space your teaching out over time if possible. Incorporate health education activities into other activities. For example, ask patients about smoking habits at each prenatal visit. Relate teaching to their everyday concerns.
- Personalize health messages. Use the active voice. For example, instead of saying, "It is important that patients read labels if they want to cut down on fat intake," say "Learn to read food labels. This can help you cut down on fat intake." See Example 2.
- Incorporate methods of illustration, demonstration, and real life examples. Connect the health message to everyday events and real life situations.
- Give and get. Review information often. Ask the patient questions before, during, and after teaching.
- Summarize often. Provide the patient with feedback. Obtain feedback from the patient.
- Be creative. Use your imagination to convey

EXAMPLE 2

Testicular Self-exam

Version A (use of passive voice; more complex words; more difficult to grasp)

Performing TSE can increase the likelihood that abnormal growths can be located early. Current recommendations state that men should perform this procedure regularly every month after a warm bath or shower. This procedure is not difficult to perform and usually involves several minutes.

Version B (use of active voice; simpler words; easier to grasp)

You can increase your chances of finding growths or lumps early by doing a simple exam called TSE. Do TSE once a month after a warm bath or shower. It is easy and takes only a few minutes.

difficult concepts (e.g., use picture cards, drawings, real objects, and flip charts).
- Use appropriate resources and materials to enhance teaching and convey ideas (e.g., videotapes, computer-based interactive programs, and bulletin boards).
- Put patients at ease. Focus on inclusion and trust before delivering content.
- Praise patients, but do not patronize them.
- Be encouraging throughout the educational steps.
- Allow time for patients and family members to think and ask questions.
- Remember that understanding requires time and practice. Ongoing feedback helps refocus the teaching encounter.
- Conduct learner verification (i.e., process to verify suitability of information) to ensure understanding.
- Evaluate the teaching plan and continually infuse new information.

Assessing Materials: Become a Wise Consumer and User

Materials are collected, stored, and disseminated within community sites. In many instances, nurses distribute pamphlets, but patients either do not read them, or review them superficially. "People of this country have had so much pamphlet materials passed out to them free that some have lost respect for free

FIGURE 7-4

Assessment guide to review health materials (Adapted from University of Kentucky: *Assessment guide to review health materials*, Patient Education Materials Workshop, 1980). *Continued*

Directions:
Assess your printed material using the following tool. Use the rating scale of 1 to 4 for each item in a major category: 1 = poor, 2 = fair, 3 = good, 4 = very good, and N/A = not applicable. For each category, give it an overall category rating of (+) effective, (−) not effective, or (X) unsure.

Name of brochure: _____

Author: _____

Intended target audience: _____

Cost/availability/producer: _____

Category/criteria	Rating 1 to 4	Overall rating (+)(−)(x)	Comments
Format/layout			
Organizational style	____		_____
White/black space	____		_____
Margins	____		_____
Grouping of elements	____		_____
Use of headers/advance organizers	____	_____	_____
Type			
Size	____		_____
Style	____		_____
Spacing	____	_____	_____
Verbal content			
Clarity	____		_____
Difficulty	____		_____
Quantity	____		_____
Relevancy to target group (i.e., age, gender, and ethnicity)	____		_____
Use of active voice	____		_____
Readability level	____ grade level ____		_____
Accuracy	____		_____
Currency	____	_____	_____

literature. Health educators may have contributed to this delinquency by passing out health literature carelessly and indiscriminately. The nurse who expects the pamphlet to take the place of the health teacher is employing weak measures in the health education program" (Rue, 1944, p. 215). It is important that nurses evaluate health materials before they disseminate them to individuals, families, or the general public. Health materials are intended to strengthen previous teaching and should be an adjunct to health instruction.

Fig. 7-4 provides an assessment guide for reviewing health materials. The nurse can use this guide in critiquing printed materials; however, the nurse can make slight modifications in assessing other types of health resources (e.g., videotapes and interactive modules). This tool allows the nurse to review health materials systematically for appropriateness within the intended target audience. The material assessment should focus on the following criteria: format-layout, type, verbal content, visual content, and aesthetic quality.

Format-layout

- Is the information organized clearly? Does it make sense?
- Do headers or advance organizers cue the reader? Headers help the reader visualize what is next.

F I G U R E 7-4—cont'd

For legend see previous page.

Category/criteria	Rating 1 to 4	Overall rating (+)(−)(x)	Comments
Visual content			
Tone/mood	____		_____
Clarity	____		_____
Cueing	____		_____
Relevancy to target group (i.e., age, gender, and ethnicity)	____		_____
Currency	____		_____
Accuracy	____		_____
Detail	____	____	_____
Aesthetic quality/appeal			
Attractiveness	____		_____
Color	____		_____
Quality of production space for notes, glossary, or personalized instructions	____	____	_____

Comments:

_____

_____

_____

Overall, based on your scoring of 1 to 4 and an evaluation of its effectiveness with the target audience, how would you rate this educational tool? Circle one.

1 = poor: probably won't work with my target group. I would probably never use it.

2 = fair: has a low likelihood of success with my target group. I would use it rarely and only in combination with other sources.

3 = good: has a good likelihood of being suitable and relevant for about half of my target group. I would use it sometimes.

4 = very good: has a high likelihood of being suitable and relevant for most of my target group. I would most definitely use it.

■ Is there a 50% to 50% allocation of white and black space? This provides breathing space.

■ Is the information easy to read and uncluttered?

Type

■ Is the type or font a readable size? Consider the age of your intended group and whether visual difficulties are likely.

Verbal content

■ Is the information current, accurate, and relevant to the intended group?

■ Are difficult terms defined?

■ Does the text reflect the ethnic diversity of the intended audience?

■ What is the reading level?

Visual content

■ Are the graphics accurate, current, and relevant to the intended group?

■ Does cueing help the reader connect the printed words and pictures?

■ Will the reader understand the intended meanings of the pictures?

■ Are the pictures on the cover reflective of the material inside?

FIGURE 7-5

SMOG formula for estimating readability grade level of printed text (Adapted from McLaughlin HG: SMOG-grading: a new readability formula, *J Reading* 12:204-206, 1969. Used with permission). For more detailed information about the application of SMOG formulas, refer to USDHHS (1992); for information on other readability formulas, refer to Redman (1996).

SMOG Readability Formula

Directions:

- Count off 10 consecutive sentences near the beginning, in the middle, and near the end of the text (total of 30 sentences).

- Circle all polysyllabic words (those containing three or more syllables). This includes repetitions of words. Total the number of polysyllabic words.

- Estimate the square root of the total number of polysyllabic words counted. This is done by finding the nearest perfect square and taking its square root.

- Add a constant of three to the square root. This number gives the SMOG number, grade, or the reading grade level that a person must have reached to understand the text being evaluated.

Tips:

Count hyphenated words as one word.

Count a sentence as a string of words with a period (.), an exclamation point (!), or a question mark (?).

Count proper nouns.

Count numbers that are written out or, if in numeric form, pronounce them to assess whether they are polysyllabic.

- Do the pictures reflect the target audience's ethnic diversity?

Aesthetic quality and appeal

- Is the material appealing?
- Are there helpful special features (e.g., glossary, space for notes, and useful telephone numbers)?

Assessment of Reading Level

Part of the written material's assessment is reading level. Many formulas are available to estimate the printed text's readability and grade level including the SMOG readability formula (Fig. 7-5). Readability formulas are objective, quantitative tools that measure sentence and word variables. However, they do not consider factors related to understanding such as motivation, experience, or need for information (Meade and Smith, 1991). These formulas do estimate reading ease and provide guidelines for assessing and

rewriting health information. The Flesch-Kincaid Formula (Flesch, 1948) is another broad estimate of reading and is programmed into most computer software programs' grammar editing tools.

Learner Verification

The best way to identify material suitability is to deliver the materials to the intended audience and obtain feedback about acceptability, understanding, and usefulness. **Learner verification** engages intended members in dialogue and helps uncover unsuitable aspects of the material (i.e., content, visuals, or format) (Doak et al., 1995). If the nurse discovers a need for new educational materials or media, he or she may incorporate Freirian principles to produce empowering products. The Freire approach supports learner participation in the development process, ensures the learner is the active subject of the educational experience, and allows learners to define content and outcomes (Rudd and Comings,

1994; Wallerstein, 1992). Freire's approach focuses on people's experiences and ideas and creates themes to address them.

For example, the author used a series of learner verification processes to develop a breast and cervical cancer educational videotape for Hispanic migrant and seasonal farmworker women. In the preproduction phase, a series of six focus groups was conducted with members of the intended target audience. Focus groups revealed that women thought bumps and bruises caused cancer, that health was important for family, and that basic information was needed about how the body functions. The design and delivery of cancer messages integrated these emergent themes using a photonovella format. Later, more learner verification measures with the intended audience were conducted during the production phase. This verified the understanding of words and pictures, the acceptability of music and narrator, and the usability of the message (Meade et al., 1999). The study found that collecting information in the intended audience's own words helped to examine issues from their own perspective (Facione, 1999; Salazar, 1996). Farmworker women are a medically underserved population. The nurse can build effective community-based educational programs by providing them with cancer information that reduces educational barriers and addresses underlying knowledge, attitudes, and beliefs. In summary, effective health messages can be achieved by obtaining "rich" information directly from subjects and closely involving them in various aspects of the development process.

Although these strategies are especially helpful with low literacy individuals, people at all literacy levels prefer and better understand simply written, concise materials and are more motivated by materials that are relevant to their learning needs (Doak et al., 1998; Foltz and Sullivan, 1999).

CASE STUDY

APPLICATION OF THE NURSING PROCESS

The following case study and teaching plan provide an example of selected teaching approaches and learning needs for the individual, family, and community.

Emma Jackson, aged 29, received ongoing health care at her neighborhood's community-based clinic. She visited the NP and the nurse confirmed that Mrs. Jackson was two months pregnant. She was married and had a four-year-old child. Emma told the nurse she smoked and wanted to quit, but she was unable to quit during her last pregnancy. She told the nurse, "I smoke when I get stressed. I have so many things on my mind." Her husband was also a smoker. The nurse referred Mrs. Jackson to a community nursing student named Irene Green for counseling, education, and follow-up.

Assessment

Irene recognized that smoking during pregnancy is detrimental for the unborn infant, unhealthy for Mrs. Jackson, and harmful for the four-year-old child who breathes the second-hand smoke (Castles et al., 1999; Cnattingius et al., 1999; DiFranza and Lew, 1995; MacLeod and MacLain, 1992; Tuthill et al., 1999). Irene also knew that smokers often experience stages of readiness in their attempts to quit and relapse is often part of the process (Prochaska and DiClemente, 1983). She noted that family and community support systems are important.

Irene assessed Mrs. Jackson on an individual level, which follows:

- Smoking history, smoking patterns, and previous attempts to quit
- Support systems (e.g., family, friends, and peers)
- Perceived barriers to quitting
- Perceived benefits to quitting
- Perceived priority in addressing this health issue vs. other everyday stresses
- Perceived effect of smoking behavior on family communication patterns
- Confidence in ability to quit

Assessment of other groups includes families, neighborhoods, churches, community organizations, and environmental messages that promote smoking cessation.

Diagnosis

Individual

- Ineffective individual coping related to inadequate resources and support networks evidenced by unsuccessful management of stressors
- Decisional conflict related to previous unsuccessful attempts (lack of confidence in ability to quit smoking and stay quit)
- Altered health maintenance (tobacco use) in response to personal stressors, unawareness of available resources, and insufficient support systems
- Health seeking behavior (desire to quit smoking) for individual and family

Family

- Potential for altered family processes related to lack of agreement about household smoking patterns

Community

- Inadequate organized smoking cessation programs and initiatives for populations at risk related to lack of economic resources and community-building coalitions

Planning, Goals, and Interventions

Individual

Short-Term Goals
- Mrs. Jackson will recognize that continued smoking is unhealthy for herself, her unborn infant, and her young child.
- Mrs. Jackson will become aware of ways to enhance her confidence during smoking cessation.
- Mrs. Jackson will identify situations and stressors that influence her smoking patterns.
- Mrs. Jackson will learn two strategies to cope with stressful situations and apply those strategies.

Long-Term Goal
- Mrs. Jackson will quit smoking.

Planning and interventions encourage expression, offer positive reinforcement, help the patient use adaptive coping mechanisms, provide cultur-

ally and educationally relevant materials and media, and offer appropriate smoking cessation strategies. The nurse may apply the National Cancer Institute's "4 A's" approach to smoking cessation counseling (Ask, Advise, Assist, and Arrange). Irene offered empowerment strategies to help Mrs. Jackson cope with her smoking cessation attempts and identified daily hassles and stressors. Irene gave tailored smoking cessation messages and culturally and educationally appropriate materials (Mullen, 1999). The nurse initiates a follow-up plan that is acceptable to both the nurse and patient.

Family
Short-Term Goals
- Mr. and Mrs. Jackson will acknowledge the benefits of a smoke-free environment.
- Mr. Jackson will recognize the need to quit smoking.
- The couple will recognize the need to support each other in smoking cessation.
- Mr. and Mrs. Jackson will identify and discuss specific supportive actions during the smoking cessation phases. The couple will enlist the support of another person or network.

Long-Term Goal
- Mr. and Mrs. Jackson will quit smoking and become a smoke-free family.

Planning and interventions recognize the need for strong support systems within families. Irene provided education and counseling to promote family self-care and recognized that she must address and incorporate Mr. Jackson's support or lack thereof into the care plan. Irene made links to community resources (e.g., health classes, support groups, and networking with people who quit or are attempting to quit) to build Mrs. Jackson's support-system and self-confidence. Irene provided audiotapes and videotapes that contained relaxation methods.

Community
Short-Term Goals
- A coalition of community members will develop and implement policies to support a smoke-free environment.

Continued

- A consortium of health care agencies and community-based organizations will recognize the need to develop partnerships in creating smoking cessation strategies for the community.

Long-Term Goals
- The community will support and endorse a smoke-free environment and publicize these efforts through billboards and other media.
- Community agencies and organizations will integrate smoking cessation programs and messages into their existing health-related activities.
- Cigarette advertising will cease.

Planning and interventions implemented on an aggregate level identify key community leaders, agencies, legislators, and lay members who are committed to supporting smoking cessation initiatives at a sociopolitical level (e.g., producing counter billboard advertising and creating smoking cessation initiatives at various community channels). Program initiatives assist community members in defining issues and solutions to the effects of smoking on individuals, families, and community groups. Developing coalitions and partnerships among community-based organizations, health care groups, governmental agencies, and intended audience members through dialogue and increased awareness is essential.

Evaluation

- Evaluation is systematic and continuous and focuses on the individual, family, and community.

Individual

- An evaluation of Mrs. Jackson's smoking habits occurs within the health system and the community (clinics and WIC). These groups address both process (decrease in number of cigarettes smoked) and outcome (quit or not quit) endpoints. Mrs. Jackson experienced an increase in her coping skills and support system, which was evident in her personalized care plan.
- Irene tailored smoking cessation messages to Mrs. Jackson.
- Irene provided Mrs. Jackson with follow-up (e.g., telephone, letter, and personal visit).

Family

- Care plans include support pattern development with family or significant other in smoking cessation initiatives.
- Irene assessed family health patterns and screened for other at-risk behaviors.
- Irene identified and addressed family support and communication patterns in the care plan.

Community

- Irene introduced smoking cessation programs and smoking prevention initiatives to at least two channels of dissemination (e.g., churches, schools, work sites, and community-based organizations).
- Smoking cessation messages are infused throughout the community through radio, television, and billboards.
- Community task forces and coalitions demonstrate a collaborative partnership among lay members, community leaders, organizers, and legislators to address smoking-related health issues.

SUMMARY

Teaching is a significant component of community health nursing and it impacts virtually every nursing activity. The goal of health education is to facilitate a process that allows individuals, families, and groups to make well-informed decisions about health practices. An understanding of learning and the theoretical frameworks that explain behaviors and health actions is inherent in community health education. No single theory explains human behavior; the nurse must apply multiple theories and approaches.

Nurses must be knowledgeable about sociopolitical, cultural, environmental, and ecological forces affecting community health to ensure the success of health education strategies. Health education, which is relevant for a target group, is based on individual variables and social, structural, political, cultural, and economic factors within the larger community context. Nurses develop relevant teaching interventions by assessing the target audience and their characteristics thoroughly and by using an organized and systematic approach to delivering health messages and programs. Implementing social action strategies such as advocating health-promoting lifestyles, creating an environment for problem-posing dialogue, and providing links to health resources supports the philosophy of critical consciousness. Nurses can facilitate the principle of social justice by mastering health information delivery and committing themselves to creating empowerment strategies that equip individuals, families, and communities with knowledge and navigation skills for healthy lifestyles and environments.

Nurses can use a variety of methods, materials, and media to support health education activities including electronic and web-based information. The nurse should review and evaluate these resources for their appropriateness within the intended target group. Embracing the notion that health education is an ongoing interactive process influenced by many internal and external factors is key to meeting the needs of individuals, families, and communities. Nurses can make important contributions to the prevention of disease and the promotion of personal and community health with knowledge, spirit, and commitment to empowerment strategies.

LEARNING ACTIVITIES

1. In groups of two to four students, describe how theoretical frameworks help explain health behavior. Identify the strengths and limitations of models that focus on individual health determinants vs. models that encompass sociopolitical factors.
2. Identify a specific group in the community. Describe the group's characteristics and identify the methods for obtaining this information.
3. Select an aggregate (e.g., students, elderly people, pregnant women, homeless people, or MSFW). Describe how to apply Freire's empowerment education model to address health issues (e.g., identify with community members, develop

generative themes, and prioritize members' perspectives).
4. Select a health education brochure or health website and apply the assessment criteria presented to evaluate its appropriateness for the intended audience. Evaluate the relative strengths of the printed material or website and potential areas for improvement.
5. Review electronic or printed media in the community (e.g., Internet, television, radio, or newspaper) to identify health issues of concern (e.g., hospital or clinic closings or restaurant smoking bans). Discuss sociopolitical issues that impact the health issue. Outline specific activities and roles that the community nurse can perform to provide education regarding the health issue.

REFERENCES

Ad Hoc Committee on Health Literacy for the Council on Scientific Affairs, American Medical Association: Health literacy: report of the Council on Scientific Affairs, *JAMA* 281:552-557, 1999.

Airhihenbuwa CO: Health promotion and the discourse on culture: implications for empowerment, *Health Educ Q* 21:345-353, 1994.

Alexander DE: Readability of published dental educational materials, *J Am Dent Assoc* 131:937-42, 2000.

American Cancer Society: *Cancer facts and figures: 1999,* Atlanta, 1999, The Author.

American Hospital Association: *A patient's bill of rights in hospitals,* Chicago, 1972, The Author.

American Management Association: *Fifth annual multicultural forum: gaining the competitive edge,* New York, 1993, The Author.

American Nurses Association: *The professional nurse and health education,* Kansas City, Mo, 1975, The Author.

Andrews MM: How to search for information on transcultural nursing and health subjects: Internet and CD-ROM resources, *J Transcult Nurs* 10:69-74, 1999.

Babcock DE, Miller MA: *Client education: theory and practice,* St. Louis, 1994, Mosby.

Baker DW et al: Health literacy and the risk of hospital admission, *J Gen Intern Med* 13:791-81, 1998.

Baker DW et al: The relationship of patient reading ability to self-reported health and use of health services, *Am J Public Health* 87:1027-30, 1997.

Baldwin JH et al: MOM empowerment, too! (ME2): a program for young mothers involved in substance abuse, *Pub Health Nurs* 16:376-83, 1999.

Bandura A: Self-efficacy: toward a unifying theory of behavioral change, *Psychol Rev* 84:191-215, 1977a.

Bandura A: *Social learning theory,* Englewood Cliffs, NJ, 1977b, Prentice-Hall.

Becker MH, editor: *The health belief model and personal health behavior,* Thorofare, NJ, 1974, Charles B. Slack.

Becker MH et al: The health belief model and prediction of dietary compliance: a field experiment, *J Health Soc Behav* 18:348-366, 1977.

Bennett CL et al: Relationship between literacy, race, and stage of presentation among low-income patients with prostate cancer, *J Clin Oncol* 16:3101-3104, 1998.

Bernstein E et al: Empowerment forum: a dialogue between guest editorial board members, *Health Educ Q* 21:281-294, 1994.

Bigge ML: *Learning theories for teachers,* ed 5, Reading, Mass, 1997, Addison-Wesley Educational Publishers.

Boyle JS: Transcultural nursing: where do we go from here? *J Transcult Nurs* 11:10-11, 2000.

Braithwaite RL, Bianchi C, Taylor SE: Ethnographic approach to community organization and health empowerment, *Health Educ Q* 21:407-416, 1994.

Breckon DJ et al: *Community health education: settings, roles, and skills for the 21st century,* ed 4, Gaithersburg, Md, 1998, Aspen Publishers.

Bush NE et al: Web site design and development issues: the Washington State breast and cervical health program web site demonstration project, *Oncol Nurs Forum* 26:857-65, 1999.

Campbell MK et al: Improving dietary behavior: the effectiveness of tailored messages in primary care settings, *Am J Public Health* 84:783-787, 1994.

Castles A et al: Effects of smoking during pregnancy: five meta-analyses, *Am J Prev Med* 16:208-215, 1999.

Clark MJ: The health education process. In Clark MJ, editor: *Nursing in the community: dimensions of community health nursing,* ed 3, Stamford, Conn, 1998, Appleton & Lange.

Cnattingius S et al: The influence of gestational age and smoking habits on the risk of subsequent preterm deliveries, *N Engl J Med* 23:943-948, 1999.

Davis L et al: AAN expert panel report on culturally competent health care, *Nurs Outlook* 40:277-283, 1992.

Davis TC et al: Practical assessment of adult literacy in health care, *Health Educ Behav* 25:613-24, 1998.

Davis TC et al: Rapid estimate of adult literacy in medicine: a shortened screening instrument, *Fam Med* 25:56-57, 1993.

DiFranza JR, Lew RA: Effect of maternal cigarette smoking on pregnancy complications and sudden infant death syndrome, *J Fam Pract* 40:385-394, 1995.

Doak LG et al: Improving comprehension for cancer patients with low literacy skills: strategies for clinicians, *CA Cancer J Clin* 48:151-162, 1998.

Doak LG, Doak CC, Meade CD: Strategies to develop effective cancer education materials, *Oncol Nurs Forum* 23:1305-1312, 1996.

Doak CC, Doak LG, Root JH: *Teaching patients with low literacy skills,* Philadelphia, 1995, JB Lippincott.

Duryea EJ: Decision making and health education, *J Sch Health* 53:29, 1983.

Eisen A: Survey of neighborhood-based, comprehensive community empowerment initiatives, *Health Educ Q* 21:235-252, 1994.

Facione NC: Breast access screening in relation to access to health services, *Oncol Nurs Forum* 26:689-696, 1999.

Flesch RR: A new readability yardstick, *J Appl Psychol* 32:221-223, 1948.

Foltz AT, Sullivan JM: Limited literacy revisited: implications for patient education, *Cancer Prac* 7:145-150, 1999.

Frank-Stromborg M, Wassner LJ, Chilton B: A study of rural Latino women seeking cancer-detection examinations, *J Cancer Educ* 13:231-241, 1998.

Freire P: *Education for critical consciousness,* New York, 1973, Seabury Press.

Freire P: *Pedagogy of the oppressed,* New York, 1970, Herder and Herder (Translated from original manuscript, 1968).

Fugate Woods N: Cancer research: future agendas for women's health, *Semin Oncol Nurs* 11:143-147, 1995.

Gagliano ME: A literature review on the efficacy of video in patient education, *J Med Educ* 63:785-792, 1988.

Gardner MS: *Public health nursing,* ed 3, New York, 1936, MacMillan.

Gazmararian JA et al: Health literacy among medicare enrollees in a managed care organziation, *JAMA* 281:545-551, 1999a.

Gazmararian JA, Parker RM, Baker DW: Reading skills and family planning knowledge and practices in a low-income managed care population, *Obstet Gynecol* 93:239-44, 1999b.

Gillis AJ: Determinants of a health-promoting lifestyle: an integrative review, *J Adv Nurs* 18:345-353, 1993.

Glanz K, Lewis FM, Rimer BK, editors: *Health behavior and health education: theory, research and practice,* ed 2, San Francisco, 1990, Jossey-Bass.

Glanz K, Lewis FM, Rimer BK, editors: *Health behavior and health education: theory, research and practice,* ed 2, San Francisco, 1997, Jossey-Bass.

Glazer HR, Kirk LM, Bosler FE: Patient education pamphlets about prevention, detection, and treatment of breast cancer for low literacy women, *Patient Educ Couns* 27:185-89, 1996.

Goodman RM et al: Identifying and defining the dimensions of community capacity to provide a basis for measurement, *Health Educ Behav* 25:358-78, 1998.

Green L et al: *Health education planning: a diagnostic approach,* Mountain View, Calif, 1980, Mayfield.

Green L: Introduction to behavior change and maintenance: theory and measurement. In Schumaker S, Schron EB, Ockene JK, editors: *The handbook of health behavior change,* New York, 1998, Springer.

Green LW, Kreuter MW: *Health promotion planning: an educational and ecological approach,* ed 3, Mountain View, Calif, 1999, Mayfield.

Guidry JJ, Fagan P: The readability levels of cancer-prevention materials targeting African Americans, *J Cancer Educ* 12:108-113, 1997.

Guidry JJ, Walker VD: Assessing cultural sensitivity in printed cancer materials, *Cancer Prac* 7:291-296, 1999.

Hochbaum GM: *Public participation in medical screening programs: a sociopsychological study,* US Public Health Service Pub No 572, Washington, DC, 1958, US Government Printing Office.

Israel BA et al: Health education and community empowerment: conceptualizing and measuring perceptions of individual, organization, and community control, *Health Educ Q* 32:149-170, 1994.

Israel BA et al: Review of community-based research: assessing partnership approaches to improve public health, *Annu Rev Public Health* 19:173-202, 1998.

Janz NK, Becker MH: The health belief model: a decade later, *Health Educ Q* 11:1-47, 1984.

Jastak S, Wilkinson GS: *The wide-range achievement test III: revised administration manual,* Wilmington, Del, 1993, Jastak Associates.

Jezewski MA: Culture brokering as a model for advocacy, *Nurs Health Care* 14:78-85, 1993.

Joint Commission on Accreditation of Healthcare Organizations: *1996 accreditation manual for hospitals,* vol 1, Oak Brook, Ill, 1995, The Author.

Keck CW: Community health: our common challenge, *Fam Community Health* 172:1-9, 1994.

Kegeles SS et al: Survey of beliefs about cancer detection and papanicolaou tests, *Public Health Rep* 80:815-823, 1965.

Kendall J: Fighting back: promoting emancipatory nursing actions, *Adv Nurs Sci* 15:1-15, 1992.

Kirsch I et al: *Adult literacy in America: a first look at the findings of the National Literacy Survey,* Washington, DC, 1993, National Center for Education Statistics, US Department of Education.

Kleinman A: Concepts and a model for the comparison of medical systems as cultural systems, *Soc Sci Med* 12:85-93, 1978.

Knowles MS: *The making of an adult educator: an autobiographical journey,* San Francisco, 1989, Jossey-Bass.

Knowles MS: *The modern practice of adult education: from pedagogy to andragogy,* Chicago, 1980, Association Press/Follett.

Kreuter MW, Strecher VJ, Glassman B: One size does not fit all: the case for tailoring print materials, *Ann Behav Med* 21:276-83, 1999.

Kuehnert PL: The interactive and organizational model of community as client: a model for public health nursing practice, *Public Health Nurs* 12:9-17, 1995.

Labonte R: Health promotion and empowerment: reflections on professional practice, *Health Educ Q* 21:253-268, 1994.

Lewin K: *The conceptual representation and the measurement of psychological forces,* Durham, NC, 1938, Duke University Press.

Lipson JG: Cross-cultural nursing: the cultural perspective, *J Transcult Nurs* 10:6, 1999.

Lugo NR: Empowerment education: a case study of the resource sisters/companeras program, *Health Educ Q* 23:281-89, 1996.

Macario E et al: Factors influencing nutrition education for patients with low literacy skills, *J Am Diet Assoc* 98:559-64, 1998.

MacLeod C, MacLain K: The effects of smoking in pregnancy: a review of effects of approaches to behavioral change, *Midwifery* 8:19-30, 1992.

Maslow AH: *Motivation and personality,* ed 2, New York, 1970, Harper and Row.

McFarland J, Fehir J: De madres a madres: a community, primary health care program based on empowerment, *Health Educ Q* 21:381-394, 1994.

McLaughlin HG: SMOG-grading: a new readability formula, *J Reading* 12:204-206, 1969.

Meade CD: Approaching the media with confidence, *Public Health Nurs* 9:209-214, 1992.

Meade CD: Improving understanding of the informed consent process and document, *Semin Oncol Nurs* 15:124-137, 1999.

Meade CD: Producing videotapes for cancer education: methods and examples, *Oncol Nurs Forum* 23: 837-846, 1996.

Meade CD, Byrd JC: Patient literacy and the readability of smoking education literature, *Am J Public Health* 79:204-206, 1989.

Meade CD, Byrd JC, Lee M: Improving patient comprehension of literature on smoking, *Am J Public Health* 79:1411-1412, 1989.

Meade CD, Calvo A, Rivera M: *Creating an educational tool to reach rural and migrant seasonal farmworker women with breast and cervical cancer messages: platiquemos acerca de su salud!* Paper presentation at American Public Health Association's 127th Annual Meeting, Public Health Education and Promotion section, Chicago, Ill, November 1999.

Meade CD, Diekmann J, Thornhill D: Readability of American Cancer Society patient education literature, *Oncol Nurs Forum* 19:51-55, 1992.

Meade CD, McKinney WP, Barnas G: Educating patients with limited literacy skills: the effectiveness of printed and videotaped materials about colon cancer, *Am J Public Health* 84:119-121, 1994.

Meade CD, Smith CF: Readability formulas: cautions and criteria, *Patient Educ Couns* 17:153-158, 1991.

Meleis AI: Culturally competent care, *J Transcult Nurs* 10:12, 1999.

Michielutte R, Alciati MH, El Arculli R: Cancer control research and literacy, *J Health Care Poor Underserved* 10:281-297, 1999.

Michielutte R et al: The use of illustrations and narrative text style to improve readability of a health education brochure, *J Cancer Educ* 7:251-260, 1992.

Milio N: *Promoting health through public policy,* Philadelphia, 1981, FA Davis.

Minkler M, Wallerstein N: Improving health through community organization and community building. In Glanz K, Lewis K, Rimer BK, editors: *Health behavior and education: theory, research, and practice,* ed 2, San Francisco, 1997, Jossey-Bass.

Mohrmann CC et al: An analysis of printed breast cancer information for African American women, *J Cancer Educ* 15:23-7, 2000.

Mullen PD: Maternal smoking during pregnancy and evidenced-based intervention to promote cessation, *Prim Care* 26: 577-89, 1999.

Nichols A: (Director, University of Wisconsin-House of Peace Community Nursing Center) Personal communication, January, 2000.

Nightingale F: *Notes on nursing,* New York, 1859, Appleton-Century Crofts.

Padilla GV, Bulcavage LM: Theories used in patient/health education, *Semin Oncol Nurs* 7:87-96, 1991.

Paskett ED et al: Use of a photoessay to teach low-income African American women about mammography, *J Cancer Educ* 11:216-220, 1996.

Pavlov IP: *Experimental psychology, and other essays,* New York, 1957, Philosophical Library.

Pender NJ: *Health promotion in nursing practice,* ed 3, Stamford, Calif, 1996, Appleton & Lange.

Piaget J: *Adaptation and intelligence: organic selection and phenocopy,* Chicago, 1980, University of Chicago.

Prochaska JO, DiClemente CC: Stages and processes of self-change of smoking: toward an integrative model of change, *J Consult Clin Psychol* 51:390-395, 1983.

Rankin SH, Stallings KD: *Patient education: issues, principles, practices,* ed 3, Philadelphia, 1995, Lippincott-Williams and Wilkins.

Redman BK, Klug B: *The practice of patient education,* ed 8, St. Louis, 1996, Mosby.

Rimer BK et al: The impact of tailored interventions on a community health center population, *Patient Educ Couns* 37:125-140, 1999.

Robertson A, Minkler M: New health promotion movement: a critical examination, *Health Educ Q* 21:295-312, 1994.

Rogers CR: *A Carl Rogers reader,* Boston, 1989, Houghton Mifflin.

Rosenstock I: Why people use health services, *Milbank Memorial Fund Q* 44:94-127, 1966.

Rosenstock IM, Strecher VJ, Becker MH: Social learning theory and the health belief model, *Health Educ Q* 15:175-183, 1988.

Rudd RE, Comings JP: Learner developed materials: an empowering product, *Health Ed Q* 21:313-327, 1994.

Rue CB: *The public health nurse in the community,* Philadelphia, 1944, WB Saunders.

Salazar MK: Hispanic women's beliefs about breast cancer and mammography, *Cancer Nurs* 19:437-446, 1996.

Shalala DE: Nursing and society: the unfinished agenda for the 21st century, *Nurs Health Care* 14:289-291, 1993.

Sharp JW: The internet: changing the way cancer survivors obtain information, *Cancer Pract* 7:266-269, 1999.

Sikorski R, Peters R: Oncology ASAP: where to find reliable cancer information on the internet, *JAMA* 277:1431-32, 1997.

Skinner BF: *About behaviorism,* New York, 1974, Knopf.

Skinner CS, Strecher VJ, Hospers H: Physician's recommendations for mammography: do tailored messages make a difference? *Am J Public Health* 84:43-49, 1994.

Spellbring AM: Nursing's role in health promotion, *Nurs Clin North Am* 26:805-813, 1991.

Steuart GW, Kark SO: *A practice of social medicine: a South African team's experiences in different African communities,* Edinburgh, 1962, Livingstone.

Strecher VJ et al: The role of self-efficacy in achieving health behavior change, *Health Educ Q* 13:73-92, 1986.

Strecher VJ, Rosenstock IM: The health belief model: improving health through community organization and community building. In Glanz K, Lewis K, Rimer BK, editors: *Health behavior and education: theory, research and practice,* ed 2, San Francisco, 1997, Jossey-Bass.

Streiff L: Can clients understand our instructions? *Image J Nurs Sch* 18: 24-52, 1986.

Strickland J, Squeoch MD, Chrisman NJ: Health promotion in cervical cancer prevention among the Yakama Indian women of the Wa'Shat Longhouse, *J Transcult Nurs* 10:190-96, 1999.

Swanson JM et al: Readability of commercial and generic contraceptive instructions, *Image J Nurs Sch* 22:96-100, 1990.

Swanson JM, Dibble SL, Chapman L: Effects of psycho-educational interventions on sexual health risks and psycho-social adaptation in young adults with genital herpes, *J Adv Nurs* 29:840-851, 1999.

Thorndike EL: *Educational psychology,* New York, 1969, Arno Press.

Travers KD: Reducing inequities through participatory research and community empowerment, *Health Educ Behav* 24:344-356, 1997.

Tuthill DP et al: Maternal cigarette smoking and pregnancy outcome, *Paediatr Perinat Epidemiol* 13:245-253, 1999.

University of Kentucky: *Assessment guide to review health materials,* Patient Education Materials Workshop, 1980.

US Department of Health and Human Services, Public Health Services: *Healthy people 2010: draft for public comments,* Pub No PHS 91-50212, Washington DC, 1998, PHS.

US Department of Health Human Services: *Making health communication programs work,* NIH Pub No 92-1493, Bethesda, Md, 1992, Office of Cancer Communications, National Cancer Institute.

Wallerstein N: Health and safety education for workers with low-literacy or limited English skills, *Am J Ind Med* 22:751-765, 1992.

Wallerstein N, Bernstein E: Empowerment education: Freire's ideas adapted to health education, *Health Educ Q* 15:379-394, 1988.

Wallerstein N, Bernstein E: Introduction to community empowerment, participatory education, and health, *Health Educ Q* 21:141-148, 1994.

Wang C, Burris MA: Empowerment through photo novella: portraits of participation, *Health Educ Q* 21:171-186, 1994.

Wang C, Burris MA: Photovoice: concept, methodology, and use for participatory needs assessment, *Health Educ Behav* 24:369-87, 1997.

Weiss BC, Coyne C: Communicating with patients who cannot read, *N Engl J Med* 337:272-274, 1997.

Weiss BD et al: Health status of illiterate adults: relationship between literacy and health status among persons with low literacy skills, *J Am Board Fam Pract* 5:257-264, 1992.

Wells JA et al: Literacy of women attending family planning clinics in Virginia and reading levels of brochures on HIV prevention, *Fam Plann Perspect* 26:113-131, 1994.

Wertheimer M: *Productive thinking,* New York, 1959, Harper.

Williams MV et al: Inadequate functional health literacy among patients at 2 public hospitals, *JAMA* 274:1677-1682, 1995.

Williams MV et al: Inadequate literacy is a barrier to asthma knowledge and self-care, *Chest* 114:1008-1015, 1998a.

Williams MV et al: Relationship of functional health literacy to patients' knowledge of their chronic disease: a study of patients with hypertension or diabetes, *Arch Intern Med* 158:166-72, 1998b.

Wilson FL: Patient education materials nurses use in community health, *West J Nurs Res* 18:195-205, 1996.

World Health Organization: *Health promotion and community action in developing countries,* Geneva, 1994, The Author.

Zimmerman MA et al: An HIV/AIDS prevention project for Mexican homosexual men: an empowerment approach, *Health Educ Behav* 24:177-190, 1997.

8

Case Management

Jean Cozad Lyon

OBJECTIVES

Upon completion of this chapter, the reader will be able to do the following:

1. Define case management.
2. Discuss the purpose of providing case management services.
3. Identify the origin and purpose of case management.
4. Discuss trends that influence the development of case management programs.
5. Incorporate case management concepts into clinical practice settings.
6. Identify educational preparation and skills recommended for case managers.

KEY TERMS

case management
client-centered case management
continuum of care
discharge planning
system-centered case management
utilization review

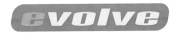

http://evolve.elsevier.com/Nies/

OVERVIEW OF NURSING CASE MANAGEMENT

Case management is a term that describes a wide variety of patient care coordination programs in acute hospital and community settings. The term **case management** applies to community health settings, which include public and mental health settings and population groups of all ages (Lyon, 1993).

From 1990 to 2000, case management evolved rapidly in response to changes in the health care environment and increased managed care programs. Client service use reflects a greater emphasis on health care costs; therefore third-party payers evaluate the appropriate use of health care resources such as diagnostical tests, laboratory tests, length of hospital visits, and duration of home health care services. MCOs may deny reimbursement to health care providers who exceed the expected costs. Health care providers must closely monitor their use of resources; therefore they introduced various forms of case management programs.

The development of case management models in acute hospital and community settings created confusion over what programs and services compose case management and how case management differs from other services like social services and **discharge planning.** A single definition of case management does not exist. The Case Management Society of America (1995) offered the following definition of case management:

> Case management is a collaborative process, which assesses, plans, implements, coordinates, monitors, and evaluates options and services to meet an individual's health needs through communication and available resources to promote quality cost-effective outcomes (p. 2).

According to the ANA, nursing case management is "a health care delivery process whose goals are to provide quality health care, decrease fragmentation, enhance the client's quality of life, and contain costs" (1992).

The case management process provides care to patients according to diagnosis, case type, or the individual's specific health needs and generally focuses on achieving patient outcomes within a specific period of time (Rice, 1996). Many labels describe case management. In addition to case management, other titles include case coordination, continuing care coordination, service integration, care management, service integration, continuity coordination, and ser-

BOX 8-1

Possible Case Management Functions

- Identifying the target population
- Determining screening and eligibility
- Arranging services
- Monitoring and follow-up
- Assessing
- Planning care
- Reassessing
- Assisting clients through a complex, fragmented health care system
- Care coordination and continuity

vice coordination. Multiple case management labels cause further confusion among health care professionals and heath care consumers.

Some hospitals, HMOs, and other insurance companies inaccurately use the term case management to describe "utilization management," "managed care," or the method of monitoring and controlling service use within a system or care episode to control cost (Lyon, 1993). Many of these providers have case management programs that transcend use control and monitor the patient following hospital discharge. Some of the programs provide continued services to high-risk clients for an indefinite time, regardless of the client's location (Box 8-1).

Case management programs aim to provide a service delivery approach to ensure the following: cost-effective care, alternatives to institutionalization, access to care, coordinated services, and patient's improved functional capacity (Lyon, 1993). These goals apply to community health and acute care settings.

ORIGINS OF CASE MANAGEMENT

Case management has a long history with the mentally ill, elderly patients, and the community setting (Steinberg and Carter, 1983). Public health, mental health, and long-term care settings have implemented and studied case management services and have reported them in the literature for many years (Mahn and Spross, 1996; Weil and Karls, 1985).

Public Health

Community service coordination, which was a fore-runner of case management, appeared in public health programs in the early 1900s. During this time, health care providers reported these community service and case management programs in the nursing literature. Programs focused on community education in sanitation, nutrition, and disease prevention became prevalent. Lillian Wald conducted many of these programs at the Henry Street Settlement House in New York City. The Metropolitan Life Insurance Company later expanded nursing services for individuals, families, and the community (Conger, 1999) to include disease prevention and health promotion.

The concept of **continuum of care** originated following World War II to describe the long-term services required for discharged psychiatric patients (Grau, 1984). Service coordination evolved into case management; this term first appeared in social welfare literature during the early 1970s.

Case Management in Mental Health

During the late 1960s and early 1970s, mental health care emphasized moving patients from mental health institutions to the community (Crosby, 1987; Pittman, 1989). The Community Mental Health Center Act of 1963 placed federal approbation on deinstitutionalization, which emphasized the importance of community mental health services. Mental health providers began to move patients from large state institutions to the community (Crosby, 1987).

Several problems resulted from the deinstitutionalization of mentally ill patients. In 1977, Congress acknowledged that many disabled people were deinstitutionalized without basic needs, proper follow-up, or health care monitoring. Congress further recognized that a systematic approach to service delivery could have prevented many state hospital readmissions. Case management in community mental health helped avoid client service fragmentation (Pittman, 1989).

Case Management and the Elderly

Specific elderly services recognized that age-generic programs do not adequately assist older people. Many older people have special, population-specific health care needs. Thus case management services frequently target the elderly population, specifically homebound individuals, or those with complex prob-

lems. However, not all older people who subscribe to multiple services require a case manager. Older adults may not need a case manager if they possess adequate functional status and can coordinate and access services for themselves, if they have family support, or if they have formal or informal caregivers who provide these functions for them. These individuals require information about options, available services, and follow-up assistance (Lyon et al., 1995).

PURPOSE OF CASE MANAGEMENT

Case management is client-centered and system-centered. **Client-centered case management** assists the client or patient through a complex, fragmented, and often confusing health care delivery system and achieves specific client-centered goals. **System-centered case management** recognizes that health care resources are finite. The upward spiral in health care costs causes third-party payers like Medicare, MCOs, and insurance companies to demand cost-effective health care. Client consumers insist on cost-effective, quality care. This demand forces health care providers to reevaluate the way they administer care, to emphasize quality improvement, and to focus on decreasing cost. This results in the need for the efficient use of goal-directed and time-limited resources (Rice, 1996).

Case management assists patients and families who need care coordination to access necessary resources in a time-efficient manner (Bower, 1992). For hospitalized patients, health care service coordination begins either upon the patient's admission or shortly thereafter and continues following the patient's discharge for an unspecified time. The patient's physical and psychosocial status and the plan's success will determine the length of the case manager's evaluation and intervention (Lyon, 1993; Lyon et al., 1995).

UTILIZATION REVIEW AND MANAGED CARE

Equity and cost-effectiveness require management and allocation of available resources in a hospital, community, city, state, or particular health care client population. System-centered case management rations and sets priorities for those in a larger group or population who could benefit from specific services.

Case management programs are often motivated by the need to evaluate, use, and allocate health care resources. Many case management programs evolved from **utilization review** departments. These departments showed that monitoring service use alone is insufficient for managing patient populations with diverse resource needs. Over time, the utilization review nurses assumed the additional case manager responsibilities.

TRENDS THAT INFLUENCE CASE MANAGEMENT

Numerous trends influenced case management programs. During the 1970s, hospitals billed Medicare, Medicaid, and other third-party payers for client services and received reimbursement. Health care costs skyrocketed and rapidly became the basis for discussion and concern throughout the health care industry and the country. In 1983, PL 98-21 of the Social Security Amendments introduced the prospective payment system (PPS) in the acute care setting. Under the PPS, health care providers receive a fixed amount of money based on the relative cost of resources they use to treat Medicare patients within each diagnosis-related group. Other third-party payers followed this example and negotiated reimbursement schedules through preferred provider programs or managed care contracts (US Department of Commerce, 1990).

Health care costs are escalating, the population is aging, and the elderly population is increasing. Many elderly suffer from chronic illness and require health care resources. These issues influenced the introduction of case management services to control costs and distribute health care resources.

CASE MANAGER EDUCATION PREPARATION

It is essential to determine what classification of health care provider is best qualified to provide case management services. Traditionally, case managers were social workers (SWs) who assumed the role of discharge planner. Client health care needs have become more complex, the need for ongoing patient assessment has emerged, and available resources have become more numerous and diverse; therefore nurses have become case managers. Several health care organizations exclusively employ SWs in case manager roles, others exclusively employ nurses in case management, and others use a combination of SWs and nurses, depending on the client population's needs. Combining the strength and knowledge of the nurse's clinical background with the SW's community service background is a combination that can efficiently move a client through the complex health care system (Lyon et al., 1995; Powell, 1996).

Nurse Case Managers

Although both nurses and SWs have proven themselves to be excellent case managers, this chapter focuses on the nurse case manager in discussing educational requirements. A nurse case manager's optimum education level is debatable. Basic nursing education for case managers required by employers can vary. Some may require a baccalaureate degree and others may not. In some settings, a master's degree may be required. Some programs are more interested in prior experience, continuing education, and case management certification than the entry-level nursing degree. Education and experience requirements may vary depending on the program's geographical location, specific client needs, and available staff.

Nurses with master's degrees and a focus in case management are readily available in urban settings. This gives facilities the opportunity to hire case managers who are academically prepared in theory and clinical experience. Rural areas that do not have master's level academic programs are at a great disadvantage in recruiting and hiring qualified nurses. To fill the case manager role, rural facilities promote nurses to case management positions, provide them with continuing education programs, and offer them necessary job-related experience. Although this is not the ideal solution, it is often the only option for smaller facilities and those in more remote parts of the United States.

Regardless of the educational requirements in the individual case management program, case managers need a minimum skill level to ensure success in the role. These skills include sound knowledge of reimbursement structures, knowledge of available resources within the institution, organization, or community, working knowledge of the identification and evaluation of quality outcomes, the ability to perform cost-benefit ratios, and an understanding of financial strategies. In addition to the required knowledge, the nurse case manager needs the following characteristics: flexibility, creativity, excellent communication skills, and the ability to work autonomously.

CASE MANAGER SERVICES

Although case management programs differ in structure and design, case managers provide some services regardless of the program's location. Case managers help clients and families who need care coordination across the health care continuum access necessary resources in a time-efficient manner (Bower, 1992). Examples of care coordination include assisting the client or family member with medical appointments, equipment acquisition, home meal delivery, home follow-up services (e.g., home health or public health nursing), appointment transportation, and medical insurance or Medicare form completion. The types of services differ depending on the location of the case management program, the population of clients, and the scope of case management services. Some case managers in managed care environments monitor whether the patient keeps medical appointments and follows the prescribed course of treatment.

The coordination of health care services for hospitalized patients begins at admission or shortly thereafter and continues after discharge for an unspecified time (Ethridge and Lamb, 1989; Lyon, 1991). Depending on setting, community case management services continue for varying lengths of time. Some programs continue service coordination indefinitely for populations like the high-risk elderly or the chronically ill. Other programs move patients' case management status from active to inactive when the patient no longer requires services. However, these clients become active again if their condition changes. Case management services continue in the home health setting until the client is discharged from the program.

CASE MANAGER ROLES AND CHARACTERISTICS

The individual case manager's role will vary depending on the specific program's services. The literature includes little information about the role or characteristics of nurse case managers and most studies and articles discuss patient outcomes and organizational program designs.

Conti's (1996) study of 59 nurse case managers reported that their most frequently used skills were business knowledge, efficiency and effectiveness skills integration, influential communication, and clinical knowledge. In a study of 413 case managers and staff nurses, Crabtree-Tonges (1998) found that nurse case managers believed the need for higher

levels of role autonomy and collaboration are essential. Novak (1998) evaluated the opinions of nurse case managers regarding their professional roles. She found that nurse case managers believed critical thinking and prioritizing are the highest rated personal attributes in their roles; the critical function of coordinating a multidisciplinary care plan was the second highest rated response.

Meisler and Midyette (1994) identified the following distinct roles of the nurse case manager: manager, clinician, consultant, educator, and researcher. The *manager* is responsible for evaluating and monitoring costs and resources. The *clinician* develops and manages the care plan for a patient or a population. The *consultant* works closely and collaboratively with a multidisciplinary team, patient, and family. The *educator* teaches the health care team and notifies the staff of any practice or program changes. The *researcher* performs continuing evaluation research and observation, and monitors and evaluates identified quality outcomes and costs.

Nurse case managers must be flexible. The health care environment experiences rapid change and new regulations and reimbursement schedules frequently emerge. The health care provider must respond to these changes rapidly to remain competitive. It is an ideal job for the self-directed nurse who enjoys being involved in a larger health care team within the organization and in the larger community.

CASE IDENTIFICATION

Identification of case management clients occurs in many ways and each program should determine the criteria for eligibility for case management services. These criteria depend on the services provided, the service's location, the population served, and whether the service is in an acute care or community setting. Some programs are diagnosis-based and use many community health care resources; for example, clients with chronic obstructive pulmonary disease (COPD) often require numerous hospitalizations. Programs may focus on a particular population (e.g., the elderly) and establish criteria to identify which clients to target for services (e.g., the high-risk elderly who are chronically ill or frail and would benefit from case management services).

All clients referred for case management must undergo screening to determine their appropriateness for inclusion in the program. Not all referred clients need the services of a nurse case manager. Often a nurse can arrange community services or instruct the client and family in the most appropriate follow-up per client need and program design. The screening instrument must be comprehensive enough to determine which clients meet the program's criteria and user friendly enough to allow the screener to evaluate the clients rapidly to determine their appropriateness for the program. The screener should refer clients to more suitable services within the community if they are not appropriate candidates for a particular case management program. For example, a nurse may refer an HIV-positive client to a case management program for high-risk clients in the community, but the program may not accept HIV and AIDS clients because the community already has a program for HIV-positive clients. Instead, the nurse should refer the client to a case management program that focuses exclusively on comprehensive service coordination for HIV and AIDS clients.

THE REFERRAL PROCESS

The nurse may perform program referrals in a variety of ways. In the acute care hospital setting, referrals are usually based on patient diagnosis or other criteria that trigger a nurse case manager referral (e.g., patient rehospitalization). Internal mechanisms alert the case manager of the patient's admission (e.g., a computerized list).

In community settings, referrals originate from a variety of sources such as a client's family, a primary care provider, or a hospital case manager. These referrals may be written or verbal. Staff in community agencies can also make service referrals; for example, the American Heart Association or ACS may receive calls from clients and families requesting information and assistance.

CASE MANAGEMENT MODELS

The literature has reported a variety of case management models. These models may be either hospital- or community-based and some provide client services across the health care continuum. Further, case management models are designed for a variety of populations.

Hospital-Based Case Management

The acute care setting uses the following essential models of case management: the New England model,

the discharge planner and arbitrator model, and the geriatric specialist model. In these models, the case manager provides patient services during hospitalization and performs short-term or limited intervention after discharge.

New England Model

The New England model of case management is a primary nursing care delivery system operated within the hospital (Bower, 1992; Zander, 1988; Zander, 1990). In this client-centered model, an RN provides primary nursing care to one patient group and case management to another patient group. The nurse may or may not provide primary nursing care to the case management group. In the case management role, the nurse is responsible for clinical nursing care and the financial outcome of each managed-care patient. The nurse measures the financial outcome through critical paths and aims to discharge each patient within the allotted number of hospital days under the PPS (Bower, 1992; Zander, 1988; Zander, 1990).

The New England model resembles a modified primary nursing model with additional managed-care responsibilities more closely than case management because the primary nurse provides direct patient care and financial managed-care responsibilities. An essential part of the nurse's responsibilities includes use of critical paths to determine the patient's progress and monitor consumed resources (a utilization review or managed-care function). The nurse performs a limited telephone follow-up after discharge and may make a single home visit. Using staff nurses for patient follow-up after discharge can create problems. Administration must find replacements for staff nurses in the acute-care setting when staff perform phone calls or home visits. They must also consider the education and experience level of the staff nurse acting in the community health nursing role.

Discharge Planner and Arbitrator Case Management Model

In this model, the RN patient care provider is the discharge planner and the manager of utilization review strategies and quality assurance activities. A multidisciplinary utilization review team also maximizes resource use and discharge planning services. The program's quality assurance component incorporates an evaluation process of patient outcomes that results from the community service discharge referrals from all discharge planning sources (Bair, Griswold, and Head, 1989).

Geriatric Clinical Nurse Specialist Model

The case managers in this model are master's-prepared geriatric clinical nurse specialists who augment the staff nurses' basic care. The case managers use a comprehensive discharge planning protocol for hospitalized elderly patients, which the staff nurses follow (Naylor, 1990; Neidlinger, Scroggins, and Kennedy, 1987). This protocol includes a comprehensive patient assessment and a comprehensive discharge plan for posthospital care. The protocol may include assessment of the patient's health status, orientation level, skill level, motivation level, sociodemographic data, and health status knowledge and perception levels. The discharge plan is based on patient assessment. Case managers often monitor patients on a short-term basis through telephone or home visits for at least two weeks following discharge.

Private Pay Case Management

Private pay case management is another type of service offered in many communities. In this program, a nurse case manager or SW offers case management services on a contract basis or in conjunction with an existing program. If the client does not meet the criteria for an existing case management program or if an existing program's services expire before the client is satisfied, the client or family must pay for the case manager's services. Families who need service coordination assistance often request this service. The length of time the case manager provides these services depends on the client's needs.

Case Management Models Across the Health Care Continuum

Some models provide patient discharge services from the acute hospital setting and continue with long-term case management services in the community setting after discharge. The Arizona model is one example of this case management model.

Arizona Model

In this case management model, nurse administrators, educators, researchers, and clinicians are case managers. They are responsible for patients during hospitalization and refer patients to appropriate community services following discharge (Ethridge, 1991; Ethridge and Johnson, 1996; Ethridge and Lamb, 1989). For several months or years, nurse case managers may work with chronically ill individuals who have frequent exacerbations or are entering terminal phases of their disease (Bower, 1992).

Community Case Management Models

Some case managers provide services exclusively in the community setting after discharge. Proponents argue that discharge planning and case management should be two separate and distinct functions with separate staff, procedures, and accountability. Supporters of this model believe case management's purpose is much broader than discharge planning and includes alternative planning to institutionalization, which ensures cost-effective care, access to comprehensive care, coordinating services, and improved client functional capacity (Simmons and White, 1988). The Denver model and the Indianapolis model are two exclusively community-based case management models.

Denver Case Management Model

In 1989, the Denver Regional Council of Governments evaluated counselor-facilitated hospital discharges in five metro area Colorado hospitals. The sample included 1040 people aged 75 or older and continued for eight weeks after discharge. The counselor intervention system resulted in fewer deaths, a 21% decrease in the number of discharged individuals in nursing homes, and an increase in those released into their homes rather than institutions. The research supported the trend toward case management services and services in the home for high-risk, high-cost cases in particular (Denver Regional Council of Governments, 1989).

Indianapolis Case Management Model

In 1985, a randomized control study stratified 1001 newly discharged patients by varying admission risk (low, medium, or high) and assigned them to intervention or control groups (Weinberger et al., 1988). Nurses in the outpatient setting closely monitored patients in the intervention, distributed appointment reminders, and rescheduled missed appointments. High-risk patients in the intervention group had higher outpatient costs ($131 per month compared with $107) and lower inpatient costs ($535 per month compared with $800). Shorter, less intensive hospital stays contributed to the high-risk intervention group's reduced inpatient costs. The Arizona model of case management produced similar results (Ethridge and Lamb, 1989).

RESEARCH IN CASE MANAGEMENT

Results of case management research is scarce in the literature; the documented studies describe the implemented programs and evaluate the program outcomes. Lyon et al conducted a randomized clinical control trial in a multidisciplinary case management program of HMO patients (Lyon et al., 1995). The study consisted of 156 adults who were aged 65 and older, lived at home with limited social support, and had multidimensional problems. The program provided comprehensive geriatric assessment and care coordination services to eligible adults enrolled in the HMO. Hospital discharge planners, outpatient clinic staff, home health nurses, and family members provided referrals for the program. After the case manager received the referral, he or she randomly assigned the client to either the control group for regular HMO services, or to one of two treatment groups. Group one received a detailed assessment and health care plan and group two received a detailed assessment and continuing case management services. Clients enrolled in group two, the case management group, had fewer HMO and nonHMO hospital admissions and shorter stays compared with group one, the control group. The differences in the number of admissions to long-term care facilities or mortality among the two treatment groups were insignificant. A detailed cost analysis showed that group two, the case management group, had a one year savings to the HMO of $187,504.

Case management programs in all settings require further study. The researcher or case manager must report the program's description, the case manager's role, the specific costs, and the quality outcome measures. The researcher or case manager must find and implement the most cost-effective programs for specific populations.

CASE STUDY

APPLICATION OF THE NURSING PROCESS

The following case study is an example of a comprehensive case management program. Case management programs and the served populations are diverse; this is only one example of case management implementation.

Judy, the case manager at an HIV early intervention program, received a call from Don, a white male aged 29. Don had just moved from a neighboring state where he recently discovered he was HIV-positive. A clinic administered his HIV test and he did not receive any health services. He found the HIV clinic's phone number in the phone book and did not have a local health care provider. He was a construction worker before he moved, but the company laid him off. He moved to Reno to find work because new building and growth abounded in the area. He moved into a local motel and paid rent for the following two weeks. He did not have health insurance, but he was eligible for continued health insurance coverage through the Consolidated Omnibus Budget Reconciliation Act (COBRA). Unfortunately, he could not afford to pay the COBRA premium because he was unemployed. He felt desperate, alone, isolated, and depressed and he needed help.

Judy performed an intake screening and assisted Don in receiving needed services. She scheduled appointments with the clinic's health care providers and met with him to identify the services he needed. Judy completed her assessment after Don attended the clinical appointment and met with her for case management.

Assessment

Don was HIV-positive, but he did not have any symptoms of AIDS. He took medication, ate well, maintained good physical condition and dentition, and owned a car. Although he had limited finances, he paid his rent for two weeks. He did not have health insurance and could not afford medications or laboratory tests. Judy developed the following plan:

Individual

Judy used Ryan White II grant funds to finance Don's services through the clinic. She applied for housing assistance and scheduled an appointment with the clinic's SW to discuss his financial situation and job prospects. The pharmacist provided his medications, which were funded by the clinic, explained the drugs in detail, and offered to answer questions. *Continued*

Family

Don was estranged from his family. His mother, who lived 2000 miles away, was aged 65, widowed, and retired. Don had not visited his two siblings in ten years and chose not to have family contact. Although Don had friends at his last job, he had not made friends in Reno. Prior to moving, he was in a relationship with a woman for two years. After the relationship ended, he did not know where she lived.

Community

Judy knew Don could access a solid network of community services. Don was new in the community and he did not have social support; therefore Judy identified that he needed to contact job placement services and attend an HIV support group.

Diagnosis

Judy developed the following nursing diagnoses for Don:

Individual

- Knowledge deficit related to HIV, including knowledge of the disease, medications, and available resources.
- Inadequate income from unemployment.

Family

- Lack of family and social support.
- Poor family communication patterns.

Community

- Adequate services through the HIV clinic.
- Coordination of services through case management.

Planning and Goals

Judy made the following plan, which is open for modification, and established goals with Don:

Individual

- Don will find employment within two months. If his employer does not provide health care

benefits, the clinic program will continue to provide them.
- If Don does not find work and cannot pay rent, local HIV funding will be used to provide housing assistance.
- The clinic will provide health care services, medications, laboratory tests, and other outpatient services.

Family

Don was not interested in communicating with his family. Judy respected his wishes and did not pursue the issue in the short term.

Community

Judy will collect information on available community resources to share with Don.

Intervention

Acting as his case manager, Judy connected Don with job opportunities, housing, and community support groups. Judy explained the available programs and allowed Don to choose his services.

Don had to attend his scheduled clinic appointments, take his medication, and contact his case manager regularly. The plan supplemented the services that Don could not afford. The plan focused on Don's individual needs in health care, employment, housing, and support groups.

Evaluation

Judy evaluated the results of Don's comprehensive case management plan on a continuing basis. If Don obtained employment in construction, he could support himself adequately and would require financial assistance primarily with his medications. If he did not find a job, or if his health status changed and he was unable to work in construction, then Judy would need to modify the plan. She would need to connect him with community support groups to establish friendships and gain social support.

LEARNING ACTIVITIES

1. Contact case management programs in the community and acute care setting.
2. Interview case management program directors. Ask them about their program's structure and process, the program's acceptance criteria, and their referral sources.
3. Ask the directors about their program's required education and experience levels for case managers.
4. Spend a day with a case manager and ask about their various roles and services.

REFERENCES

American Nurses Association: *Case management by nurses,* Washington, DC, 1992, The Association.

Bair NL, Griswold JT, Head JL: Clinical RN involvement in bedside-centered case management, *Nurs Economics* 7(3):150-154, 1989.

Bower KA: *Case management by nurses,* Washington, DC, 1992, American Nurses Publishing.

Case Management Society of America: *Standards of practice for case management,* Little Rock, Ark, 1995, The Author.

Conger MM: Nursing case management: a managed care organizational strategy. In *Managed care: practice strategies for nursing,* Thousand Oaks, Calif, 1999, Sage Publications.

Conti RM: Nurse case manager roles: implications for practice and education, *Nurs Adm Q* 21(1):67-80, 1996.

Crabtree-Tonges M: Job design for nurse case managers intended and unintended effects on satisfaction and wellbeing, *Nurs Case Management* 3:11-23, 1998.

Crosby RL: Community care of the chronically mentally ill, *J Psychosoc Nurs* 25(1):33-37, 1987.

Denver Regional Council of Governments: *DRCOG study may trigger new national policy,* Denver, 1989, The Author.

Ethridge PA: Nursing HMO: Carondelet St. Mary's experience, *Nurs Management* 22(7):22-27, 1991.

Ethridge PA, Johnson S: The influence of reimbursement on nurse case management practice: Carondelet's experience. In Cohen EL, editor: *Nurse case management in the 21st century,* St. Louis, 1996, Mosby.

Ethridge PA, Lamb GS: Professional nursing case management improves quality, access, and costs, *Nurs Management* 20(3):30-35, 1989.

Grau L: Case management and the nurse, *Geriatr Nurs* 5(8):372-375, 1984.

Lyon JC: *Descriptive study of models of discharge planning and case management in California,* doctoral dissertation, Ann Arbor, Mich, 1991, University of California, San Francisco, University Microfilms International.

Lyon JC: Models of nursing care delivery and case management: clarification of terms, *Nurs Economics* 11(3):163-169, 1993.

Lyon JC et al: *Case management for high risk elderly,* Paper presented at the 123rd annual meeting of the American Public Health Association, San Diego, 1995.

Mahn VA, Spross JA: Nursing case management as an advanced practice role. In Hamric AB, Spross JA, Hanson CM, editors: *Advanced nursing practice: an integrative approach,* Philadelphia, 1996, Saunders.

Meisler N, Midyette P: CNS to case manager: broadening the scope, *Nurs Management* 25(11):44-46, 1994.

Naylor MD: Comprehensive discharge planning for hospitalized elderly: a pilot study, *Nurs Res* 39(3):156-161, 1990.

Neidlinger SH, Scroggins K, Kennedy LM: Cost evaluation of discharge planning for hospitalized elderly, *Nurs Economics* 5(5):225-230, 1987.

Novak DA: Nurse case managers' opinions of their role, *Nurs Case Management* 3(6):231-237, 1998.

Pittman DC: Nursing case management: holistic care for the deinstitutionalized mentally ill, *J Psychosoc Nurs* 27(11):23-27, 1989.

Powell SK: *Nursing case management: a practical guide to success in managed care,* Philadelphia, 1996, Lippincott-Raven.

Rice R: Case management and leadership strategies for home health nurses. In *Home health nursing practice: concepts and application,* ed 2, St. Louis, 1996, Mosby.

Simmons WJ, White M: Case management and discharge planning: two different worlds. In Volland P, editor: *Discharge planning: an interdisciplinary approach to continuity of care,* Owings Mills, Md, 1988, National Health Publication.

Steinberg RM, Carter GW: *Case management and the elderly,* Lexington, Mass, 1983, Lexington Books, DC Health and Co.

US Department of Commerce/International Trade Administration: *Health and medical services: US industrial outlook,* US Document, Washington, DC, 1990, The Author.

Weil M, Karls J: *Case management in human service practice,* San Francisco, 1985, Jossey-Bass Publications.

Weinberger M et al: The cost-effectiveness of intensive post discharge care: a randomized trial, *Med Care* 26(11): 1092-1101, 1988.

Zander KS: Managed care and nursing case management. In Mayer GG, Madden MJ, Lawrenz E, editors: *Patient care delivery models,* Gaithersburg, Md, 1990, Aspen.

Zander KS: Nursing case management: strategic management of cost and quality outcomes, *J Nurs Admin* 18(5):23-30, 1988.

Factors that Influence the Health of the Community

9 The Health Care System

10 Economics of Health Care

11 Policy, Politics, Legislation, and Community Health Nursing

12 Cultural Diversity and Community Health Nursing

13 Environmental Health

The Health Care System

Anita W. Finkelman

OBJECTIVES

Upon completion of this chapter, the reader will be able to do the following:

1. Analyze landmark health care legislation and its influence on the delivery system.
2. Describe the organization of the public health care subsystem at the federal, state, and local levels.
3. Compare and contrast the scope of the private health care subsystem and the public health care subsystem.
4. Describe the roles of the members of the health care team.
5. Discuss the relationship of critical health care issues to the health care organization and health care providers.
6. Discuss future concerns for the health care delivery system.

KEY TERMS

accreditation
alternative therapies
client's rights
health care reform
managed care
managed care organizations (MCOs)
Medicaid
Medicare
outcomes measures
provider organizations
public health
quality care
redesigning
reengineering
reregulating
rightsizing and downsizing
telehealth

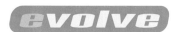

http://evolve.elsevier.com/Nies/

The health care system of the United States is dynamic, multifaceted, and not comparable with any other health care system in the world. It is regularly praised for its technological breakthroughs, frequently criticized for its high costs, and often difficult to access by those most in need. This chapter describes landmark health care legislation, the components of the health care system, critical health care organization and provider issues, the role of government in public health, and health care reform and presents a futuristic perspective.

MAJOR LEGISLATIVE ACTIONS AND THE HEALTH CARE SYSTEM

An examination of the major legislative actions that federal and state governments have taken and recognition of their influence on health and health care delivery are critical to understand the evolution of the health care system in the United States. Throughout the twentieth century, the United States Congress enacted bills that had a major influence on the private and public health care subsystems. Legislation pertaining to health increased in scope in each decade of the twentieth century, with the goal of improving the health of populations and coping with changing health care needs. During the last two decades, concerns about an increase in health care costs and the growth of managed care stimulated even more legislation.

Federal Legislation

The following discussion describes some of the landmark federal laws that have influenced health services and health care professionals. These are summarized in Table 9-1.

- Pure Food and Drugs Act of 1906: This Act established a program to supervise and control the manufacture, labeling, and sale of food. Subsequent legislation included meat and dairy products, pharmaceuticals, cosmetics, toys, and household products. Since 1927, the Food and Drug Administration (FDA) has administered elements of this Act.
- Children's Bureau Act of 1912: The Children's Bureau was founded to protect children from the unhealthy child labor practices of the time and to enact programs that had a positive effect on children's health. In 1921, the Sheppard-Towner Act extended children's health care programs by

TABLE 9-1

Critical Federal Legislation Related to Health Care

Date	Legislation
1906	Pure Food and Drugs Act
1912	Children's Bureau Act
1921	Shepard-Towner Act
1935	Social Security Act
1944	Public Health Act
1945	McCarren-Ferguson Act
1946	Hill-Burton Act
1953	Department of Health, Education, and Welfare as a cabinet-status agency; in 1979 divided into US Department of Education and USDHHS
1956	Health Amendments Act
1964	Nurse Training Act
1965	Social Security Act amendments: Title XVIII Medicare; Title XIX Medicaid
1970	Occupational Safety and Health Act
1972	Social Security Act amendments: Professional Standards Review Organization; further benefits under Medicare and Medicaid, including dialysis
1973	Health Maintenance Act
1974	National Health Planning and Resources Act
1981, 1987, 1989, 1990	Omnibus Budget Reconciliation Act
1982	Tax Equity and Fiscal Responsibility Act
1985	Consolidated Omnibus Budget Reconciliation Act
1988	Family Support Act
1990	Health Objectives Planning Act
1996	Health Insurance Portability and Accountability Act
1996	Welfare Act

providing funds for the health and welfare of infants.

- Social Security Act of 1935 and its amendments (1965, 1972): The Social Security Act and its subsequent amendments have had a far-reaching effect on health care for many groups. The Social Security Administration (SSA) provides welfare for high-risk mothers and children. Benefits were later expanded to include health care provisions for older adults and the handicapped. This major governmental action was the enactment of legislation for Medicare and Medicaid.

- **Medicare**, Title XVIII Social Security Amendment (1965): A federal program, administered by the Health Care Financing Administration (HCFA), that pays specified health care services for all people 65 years of age and older who are eligible to receive Social Security benefits. People with permanent disabilities and those with end-stage renal disease are also covered. The objective of Medicare is to protect older adults and the disabled against large medical outlays. The program is funded through a payroll tax of most working citizens. Private funds in the form of payroll taxes go to the federal government. Individuals or providers may submit payment requests for health care services and are paid according to Medicare regulations. See Chapter 10 for more information on Medicare.

- **Medicaid**, Title XIX Social Security Amendment (1965): A combined federal and state program. The program provides access to care for the poor and medically needy of all ages. Each state is allocated federal dollars on a matching basis (i.e., 50% of costs are paid with federal dollars). Each state has the responsibility and right to determine services to be provided and the dollar amount allocated to the program. Basic services (i.e., ambulatory and inpatient hospital care, physical therapy, laboratory, radiography, skilled nursing, and home health care) are required to be eligible for matching federal dollars. States may choose from a wide range of optional services including drugs, eyeglasses, intermediate care, inpatient psychiatric care, and dental care. Limits are placed on the amount and duration of service. Unlike Medicare, Medicaid provides long-term care services (e.g., nursing home and home health) and personal care services (e.g., chores and homemaking). In addition, Medicaid has eligibility criteria based on level of

TABLE 9-2

1999 Health and Human Services Poverty Guidelines

Size of Family Unit	48 Contiguous States and DC	Alaska	Hawaii
1	$8240	$10,320	$9490
2	$11,060	$13,840	$12,730
3	$13,880	$17,360	$15,970
4	$16,700	$20,880	$19,210
5	$19,520	$24,400	$22,450
6	$22,340	$27,920	$25,690
7	$25,160	$31,440	$28,930
8	$27,980	$34,960	$32,170
For each additional person, add:	$2820	$3520	$3240

From Annual update of the HHS poverty guidelines, *Federal Register* 64(52):13428-13430, March 18, 1999.

income. Table 9-2 provides the USDHHS poverty guidelines for 1999. Medicaid is also turning to managed care, but it is still unclear how successful this will be. The Medicaid population has complex needs and MCOs may not be able to provide optimum services to these beneficiaries. See Chapter 10 for more information on Medicaid.

- Public Health Act of 1944: The Public Health Act consolidated all existing public health legislation into one law. Many new pieces of legislation have become amendments in subsequent years. Examples of some of its provisions, either in the original law or in amendments, provided for or established the following:
  - Health services for migratory workers
  - Family planning services
  - Health research facilities
  - NIH
  - Nurse training acts
  - Traineeships for graduate students in public health
  - Home health services for people with Alzheimer's disease
  - Prevention and primary care services

- Rural health clinics
- Communicable disease control

■ McCarren-Ferguson Act of 1945: The McCarren-Ferguson Act has had a major influence on the insurance industry by giving states the exclusive right to regulate health insurance plans (Knight, 1998). No federal government agency is solely responsible for monitoring insurance. Some federal agencies are involved in insurance reimbursement; however, the structure of the benefit program for federal employees and military personnel, Medicare, and Medicaid, allows congress to pass laws that can override state laws if the laws meet certain criteria.

■ Hill-Burton Act of 1946: The Hill-Burton Act authorized federal assistance in the construction of hospitals and health centers with stipulations about services for the uninsured. As a result, hospitals with obligations to care for the uninsured were built in towns and cities across the United States. Through these measures, hospital care became more accessible, but by the late 1990s, the high cost of health care, combined with decreasing lengths of stay and increasing use of primary care, forced the closure of many of the hospitals built with Hill-Burton funds. Fig. 9-1

FIGURE 9-1

Decline in the U.S. hospital occupancy rate (From U.S. Census Bureau: *Statistical abstract of the United States,* Washington, DC, 1996, US Government Printing Office).

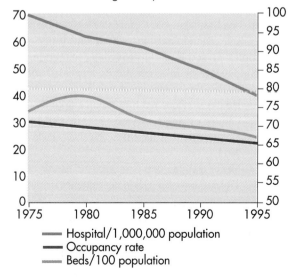

- Hospital/1,000,000 population
- Occupancy rate
- Beds/100 population

provides data demonstrating the decline in U.S. hospital occupancy rates.

■ Health Amendments Act of 1956: The Health Amendments Act, Title II, authorize funds to aid RNs in full-time study of administration, supervision, or teaching. In 1963, the Surgeon General's Consultant Group on Nursing noted that there were still too few nursing schools, nursing personnel were not put to good use, and there was limited nursing research. As a result, in 1964, the Nurse Training Act provided funds for loans and scholarships for full-time study for nurses and funds for construction of nursing schools.

■ Occupational Safety and Health Act of 1970: The Occupational Safety and Health Act focuses on the health needs and risks in the workplace and environment. It continues to provide critical programs important to the workplace and the community. See Chapter 27 for more information on the Occupational Safety and Health Act and OSHA.

■ Health Maintenance Organization Act of 1973: The HMO Act provides grants for HMO development. The Act requires that employers offer federally qualified HMOs as a health care coverage option to employees and established that states were responsible for the oversight of HMOs. Although initially it was not successful in stimulating HMO growth, this legislation has had a long-term effect on the growth of managed care.

■ National Health Planning and Resources Act of 1974: The National Health Planning and Resources Act assigned health planning responsibility to the states and local health systems agencies. In addition, it requires health care facilities to obtain prior approval from the state for expansion in the form of a CON.

■ Omnibus Budget Reconciliation Acts (1981, 1987, 1989, and 1990): The Omnibus Budget Reconciliation Acts were each enacted in response to the huge federal deficit. They have influenced funding for nursing homes, home health agencies, and hospitals and set up guidelines and regulations about several issues including a move from process to outcome evaluation, use of restraints, and prescription drugs for Medicaid recipients.

■ Tax Equity and Fiscal Responsibility Act of 1982: The Tax Equity and Fiscal Responsibility Act (TEFRA) was a major amendment to the Social Security Act of 1935, establishing the PPS for Medicare, the diagnostic-related group (DRG) system. This law changed health care radically by introducing a new reimbursement method. See Chapter 10 for more information on DRGs.

■ Consolidated Omnibus Budget Reconciliation Act of 1985: COBRA is a federal law that affects health care delivery and reimbursement. It requires all hospitals with emergency services that participate in Medicare to treat any client in their emergency services, whether or not that client is covered by Medicare or has the ability to pay. This legislation includes requirements for Medicaid services for prenatal and postnatal care to low-income women in two-parent families in which the primary spouse is unemployed. Another important requirement of COBRA focuses on the problem of the loss of insurance when a person loses his or her job. Employers who terminate an employee must now continue benefits for the employee and dependents for a specified period of time if the employee had health benefits before the termination. COBRA is an example of how a federal law can affect state health care practices. The federal government must determine who receives federal Medicare funds; therefore COBRA provides the opportunity for the federal government to legislate health care delivery at the state level.

■ Family Support Act of 1988: The Family Support Act expanded coverage for poor women and children and required states to extend Medicaid coverage for 12 months to families who have increased earnings but are no longer receiving cash assistance. This Act also required states to expand Aid to Families with Dependent Children (AFDC) coverage to two-parent families when the principal wage earner is unemployed.

■ Health Objectives Planning Act of 1990: The Health Objectives Planning Act was initiated in response to the 1979 report *Healthy People: The Surgeon General's Report on Health Promotion and Disease Prevention.* After that report, the federal government began to take a directive approach in identifying and monitoring national health care goals. *Healthy People 2000* and *Healthy People 2010* are also results of the Health Objectives Planning Act.

■ Health Insurance Portability and Accountability Act of 1996: The Health Insurance Portability and Accountability Act (HIPAA) addressed several insurance issues. Critical issues were the portability of coverage and preexisting condi-

tions. This law established that insurers cannot set limits on coverage of longer than 12 months. This is a complex law, but it is important for consumers with preexisting conditions.

■ Welfare Reform Act of 1996: The Welfare Reform Act placed restrictions on eligibility for AFDC, Medicaid, and other federally funded welfare programs. This law decreased the number of people on welfare and forced many individuals to take low-paying jobs, many of which do not offer health insurance. Between 1994 and March of 1999, welfare roles dropped 47% (DeParle, 1999). Concerns are raised that many individuals, particularly underserved women and children, subsequently lost Medicaid coverage.

The thrust of federal legislation has been on either prevention of illness through influencing the environment (e.g., Occupational Safety and Health Act of 1970) or provision of funding to support programs that influence health care (e.g., Social Security Act of 1935). Beginning with the Shepard-Towner Act of 1921 and continuing to the present, federal grants have increased the involvement of state and local governments in health care. The involvement of the federal government through fiscal allocations to state and local governments provided money for programs not previously available to state and local areas. Similar services became available in all states. Funds supporting these services were accompanied by regulations that applied to all recipients. Many state and local government programs were developed based on availability of federal funds. The involvement of the federal government through funding has served to standardize the public health policy in the United States (Pickett and Hanlon, 1990).

State Legislative Role

State governments are also directly involved in health care policy, legislation, and regulation. State governments particularly focus on financing and delivery of services and oversight of insurance. The latter has become important as managed care has grown. The states have major input in the following basic health care areas (Robert Wood Johnson Foundation, 1997):

■ Public health and safety: States are responsible for protecting public welfare through such areas as prevention and treatment of communicable diseases, monitoring of environmental health conditions, prevention of harm from violence, and prevention of workplace accidents.

- Provision of indigent care: Most state constitutions require that the state, either alone or with local governments, provide health care to those who cannot pay for it. This is usually provided by facilities run by state or local governments.
- Purchase care: Many states have been changing from the role of provider of health care to purchaser of care. States must purchase care, or contract for care, for state employees and for Medicaid beneficiaries.
- Regulation: States are responsible for licensing and credentialing facilities and professionals to ensure safety and quality. They are also responsible for regulation of insurers. States use CONs to control health care costs, particularly related to long-term care facilities and specialized technology. CONs require that the health care organization meet certain criteria to receive approval to build or expand physical facilities and to purchase expensive equipment (e.g., computed tomography [CT] and magnetic resonance imaging [MRI] equipment).
- Resource allocation: Traditionally states have not been responsible for financial support of medical and nursing education, which has been primarily through federal funding. However, states are more involved in identifying need (e.g., number of health care professionals that the state needs to graduate to meet state health care needs). Some states still assist in funding some public health care facilities.

Legislation Influencing Managed Care

Much of the recent legislation (i.e., usually state level) influencing **Managed Care Organizations** (MCOs) is in response to consumers' concerns about MCO's efforts to control costs. Considerable variability exists across states in MCO legislation and usually these acts are in response to consumer calls for reform (Levy, 1999). The following examples describe a growing number of legislative acts that provide more control over managed care:

- Provider protection initiatives (PPIs): The need for the removal of "gag rules" has been one area of concern for providers and clients. MCOs use gag rules to control what their providers discuss with clients about all treatment options. Additionally, many MCOs provide financial incentives to providers to control costs. These incentives are paid to providers based on their performance data (e.g., number of hospital admissions, length of stay, types of treatment, and types and number of prescriptions ordered).
- Any willing provider initiatives: Provider panels are the lists of providers that are approved by an MCO for reimbursement. These initiatives require that MCOs accept any provider on their provider panels who meets plan requirements and is willing to agree to the contract.
- Direct access legislation: Client freedom-of-choice legislation is rapidly growing as clients become more concerned about their lack of provider choice and want direct access to providers without obtaining prior approval.
- Mandated benefits requirement: This legislation mandates specific minimum health care benefits. Examples of these are the designation of specific basic services, emergency care without prior approval, coverage for experimental treatments, mental health parity, diabetes management, prostate screening, chiropractic treatment, and hospice services.
- Consumer rights: Consumers are demanding more rights than just provider choice. Examples include coverage for specific benefits, such as emergency services without prior approval; longer lengths of stay (e.g., obstetric and mastectomy); detailed disclosure of benefits and plan procedures; provider choice; and impartial mechanism for grievances (Mariner, 1996).

COMPONENTS OF THE HEALTH CARE SYSTEM

The current health care system consists of private and public health care subsystems (Fig. 9-2). The private health care subsystem includes personal care services from various sources, both nonprofit and profit, and numerous voluntary agencies. The major focus of the public health subsystem is prevention of disease and illness. These subsystems are not always mutually exclusive and their functions sometimes overlap.

With the rapid growth of technology and increased demands on the private and public health care subsystems, health care costs have become prohibitive. Cost-effectiveness and containment have become a critical driving force as health care delivery system changes are made and cost-effectiveness often conflicts with the provision of quality care.

U.S. health care system.

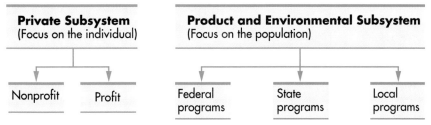

Community health nursing requires an understanding of the mission, organization, and role of the private and the public health care subsystems and the context within which they function. An organizational framework in which private and voluntary organizations and the government work collaboratively to prevent disease and promote health is essential. Public health and community health nurses are in a unique position to provide leadership and facilitate change in the health care system.

Private Health Care Subsystem

Most personal health care services are provided in the private sector. Services in the private subsystem include health promotion, prevention and early detection of disease, diagnosis and treatment of disease with a focus on cure, rehabilitative-restorative care, and custodial care. These services are provided in clinics, physicians' offices, hospitals, hospital ambulatory centers, skilled care facilities, and homes. Increasingly, these private sector services are available through MCOs.

Private health care services in the United States began with a simple model. Physicians provided care in their offices and made home visits. Clients were admitted to hospitals for general care if they experienced serious complications during the course of their illness. Currently, a variety of highly skilled health care professionals provide comprehensive, preventive, restorative, rehabilitative, and palliative care. A broad array of services is available, which are general to highly specialized with multidelivery configurations.

Personal care provided by physicians is delivered under the following five basic models:

1. The solo practice of a physician in an office continues to be present in some communities.
2. The single specialty group model consists of

physicians in the same specialty who pool expenses, income, and offices.
3. Multispecialty group practice provides for interaction across specialty areas.
4. The integrated health maintenance model has prepaid multispecialty physicians.
5. The community health center, developed through federal funds in the 1960s, addresses broader inputs into health such as education and housing.

Managed care has become the dominant paradigm in health care, affecting all aspects of health care delivery. Managed care involves capitated payments for care rather than fee-for-service. Health care providers, including physicians, hospitals, community clinics, and home care providers, are integrated in a system such as an HMO. See Chapter 10 for a more detailed discussion of managed care and reimbursement.

Voluntary Agencies
Voluntary or nonofficial agencies are a part of the private health care system of the United States and developed at the same time that the government was assuming responsibility for public health. In the United States during the 1700s and early 1800s, voluntary efforts to improve health were virtually nonexistent because early settlers from Western Europe were not accustomed to participating in organized charity. Immigration expanded to include slaves from Africa and people from Eastern Europe and their well-being received little attention.

Toward the end of the nineteenth century, new immigrants brought a heritage of social protest and reform. Wealthy business people, such as the Rockefellers, Carnegies, and Mellons, responded to the needs and set up foundations that provided health and welfare money for charitable endeavors. District nurses, such as Lillian Wald, established nursing practices in the large cities for the poor and destitute. Services did not just focus on illness but also on work conditions, health, communicable diseases, living conditions, and language skills.

Voluntary agencies can be classified into the following categories (Hanlon and Pickett, 1984):

1. Specific diseases, such as the American Diabetes Association, ACS, and Multiple Sclerosis Society
2. Organ or body structures, such as the National Kidney Foundation or the American Heart Association
3. Health and welfare of special groups, such as the National Council on Aging
4. Particular phases of health, such as the Planned Parenthood Federation of America

Philanthropical groups also support research and programs. Many professional organizations, such as the AMA and the ANA, have a significant role in advocacy and in providing professional expertise.

Voluntary organizations provide major sources of help in prevention of disease, promotion of health, treatment of illness, advocacy, consumer education, and research. For example, private and voluntary organizations currently support AIDS clients. In many cities, the Chicken Soup Brigade provides meals for AIDS clients who are unable to cook for themselves and AIDS support groups exist in most larger communities.

Overlap of services often occurs among the numerous private, voluntary, and public agencies. The private and public agencies provide a wide array of services, but sometimes duplication causes them not to be cost-effective. Without voluntary and official agencies, the array of services would be less than what is currently available.

The future is somewhat uncertain for voluntary agencies because major changes are occurring in health care. In 1995, the Pew Health Professions Commission projected that the emerging health care system would be an amalgam of different public and private forces that would work together to provide integrated, resource-conscious, population-based services (O'Neil and Pew Health Professions Commission, 1998). It was projected that the system would also be more innovative and diverse in how it responded to health needs and more concerned with disease prevention and promotion of health. Five years later the health care system continues to struggle, change, and then change again. The Pew Health Professions Commission's projection has not yet been fully realized.

Public Health Subsystem

The U.S. Constitution mandates that the federal government "promote the general welfare of its citizens." The public health subsystem is mandated by law to address the health of populations. Activities are covered by legal provisions at the local, state, and federal levels of government. At the federal level, Congress enacts laws and writes rules and regulations. The various departments of the executive branch implement and administer them. Interpretations of and amendments to the Constitution and Supreme Court decisions over time have changed and increased the role of the federal government in health activities.

Federal policies and practices have had an increasing influence on local and state governments in meeting health and social problems and many laws have been enacted to respond to changing health needs. Coordination of federal services under several agencies culminated in the establishment of the Department of Health Education and Welfare under President Eisenhower in 1953. In 1979, this department was separated into the Department of Education and the USDHHS. The USDHHS is currently the second largest department of the federal government; only the Department of Defense (DOD) is larger.

Public health refers to the efforts organized by society to protect, promote, and restore the people's health. The programs, services, and institutions involved emphasize the prevention of disease and address the health needs of the population as a whole. Public health activities typically respond to changing technology and social values, but the goals remain the same (i.e., to reduce the amount of disease, premature death, and disease-produced discomfort and disability).

The public health subsystem is concerned with the health of the population and a healthy environment. The scope of public health is broad and encompasses activities that promote good health. The public health subsystem is organized into multiple levels (i.e., federal, state, and local) to more effectively provide services to those who are unable to obtain health care without assistance and to establish laws, rules, and regulations to protect the public.

Federal Level Subsystem

Most health-related activities at the federal level are implemented and administered by the USDHHS. This department is directed by the Secretary of the USDHHS, numerous undersecretaries, and assistant secretaries. The Surgeon General is the principal deputy to the assistant secretary of the USDHHS. The USDHHS has five major agencies as described in Box 9-1.

Other federal agencies perform activities related to health. For example, the Department of Education is involved with health education and school health. The Department of Agriculture administers the inspection of meat and milk and provides funds for the supplemental nutrition program for WIC, the food stamp program, and the school-based nutrition program.

Scope of Health Services of the Federal Level Subsystem

The federal government targets the following major health areas: the general population, special populations, and international health. For the general population, federal activities include protection against hazards, maintenance of vital and health statistics, advancement of scientific knowledge through research, and provision of disaster relief. In recent years, public health efforts have been directed toward changing behaviors by fostering healthy eating habits, exercise, and prevention of tobacco, drug, and alcohol use. Other programs have provided nutritional food and food stamps to individuals and families to ensure adequate food intake.

Services for special populations include protection of workers against hazardous occupations and work conditions and health care for veterans, American-Indians, Alaskan natives, federal prisoners, and members of the armed services. In addition, the federal government provides special services for children, older adults, the mentally ill, and the vocationally handicapped.

In the international arena, the federal government works with other countries and international health

---

BOX **9-1**

Structure of the U.S. Department of Health and Human Services

The USDHHS is composed of several units that provide different services related to U.S. health care.

- The *Office of Human Development Services* is an umbrella agency responsible for programs for special needs of populations, such as congregate meals for older adults.
- The *HCFA* administers Medicare and Medicaid programs and carries out activities related to assurance of quality care.
- The *SSA* coordinates all activities related to implementing the Social Security law, including Supplemental Security Income for the Aged, Blind, and Disabled (SSI).
- The *Family Support Administration* carries out functions to strengthen the family unit.
- The *PHS* has multiple units. To facilitate coordination and provide more direct assistance to the states, the PHS has 10 regional offices. The regional offices carry out selected health programs, activities, and initiatives under the direction of the Assistant Secretary for Health.
  - The *CDC* conducts and supports programs directed to prevent and control infectious diseases; they assist states during epidemics. In addition, they provide services related to health promotion and education and professional development and training.
  - The *FDA* provides surveillance over the safety and efficacy of foods, pharmaceuticals, and other consumer goods.
  - The *HRSA* is concerned with the development of health services programs and facilities. The Division of Nursing is in this unit. A major focus of this agency is funding grants for nursing education and training. The Indian Health Service (IHS) is also in this unit, providing health services for Native-Americans and Alaskan Natives.
  - The *NIH* perform and support research programs. The focus of their efforts is to develop and extend the scientific knowledge base related to their respective areas. The National Institute for Nursing Research (NINR) is part of NIH and it focuses on nursing research.
  - The *Alcohol, Drug Abuse, and Mental Health Administration* awards grants related to problems with substance abuse and mental health.

organizations (e.g., the WHO and the Red Cross) to promote various health programs throughout the world.

State Level Subsystem

States are responsible for the health of their citizens and are the central authorities in the public health care system. The organization and activities of public health services among the states are widely varied. Most state agencies are directed by a health commissioner or secretary of health who is typically appointed by the governor. Each state also has a health officer, usually a physician with a degree and experience in public health. In some states, the health officer directs the health department. Many states have boards of health, which determine policies and priorities for allocation of funds. Staffing of the state agency varies among states; however, compared with other state programs, state health programs usually have a large staff.

Scope of Health Services of the State Level Subsystem

Each state is responsible for its own public health laws; therefore state policy is widely varied. Factors that affect the level of state services include per capita income, political factors related to division of power between state and local health departments (LHDs), and competition among officials, providers, and the business community.

As discussed in Chapter 1, the three core functions of public health are assessment, policy development, and assurance (IOM, 1988). Assessment activities include the collection of data pertaining to vital statistics, health facilities, and human resources; epidemiological activities, such as communicable disease control, health screening, and laboratory analyses; and participation in research projects. In the area of policy development, states formulate goals, develop health plans, and set standards for local health agencies. Assurance activities involve inspection in a variety of areas, licensing, health education, environmental safety, personal health services, and resource development.

Nurses represent the largest group of professionals providing health services. State legislatures determine licensure requirements and enact nurse practice acts. State boards of nursing are the administrative arm for implementation of these laws and regulations.

Local Health Department Subsystems

LHDs are generally responsible for the direct delivery of public health services and protection of the health of citizens. State and local governments (i.e., city and county) delegate the authority to conduct these activities. The organization of LHDs varies widely depending on community size, economics, partnerships with the private health care system, health care facilities, business support, health care needs, transportation, and the number of citizens requiring public health care. Some LHDs function as district offices of the state health department, others are responsible to local government and the state, and still others are autonomous, particularly those in large cities. LHDs may be a separate agency or a division within an agency, such as the USDHHS.

A health officer or administrator appointed by local government directs the LHDs. At least half of the states require that the health officer of a LHD have a medical degree. An interdisciplinary team carries out the activities of the department. Public health nurses and health inspectors represent the two largest groups of professional staff members. Other professional staff members include dentists, SWs, epidemiologists, nutritionists, and health educators.

Scope of Services of the Local Health Department Subsystem

LHDs are responsible for determining the health status and needs of their constituents. This involves identifying unmet needs and taking actions to meet these needs. Most services to groups and individuals are provided at the local level. These services fall into the following four major categories:

1. *Community health services* include control of communicable disease (i.e., surveillance and immunizations), maternal-child health programs, nutrition services, and education. Specific service activities are health promotion education directed toward changing behavior by eating healthy foods; increase of exercise; and decrease of tobacco, drug, and alcohol use. Other programs provide nutritional food and food stamps to individuals and families. Preventive screening for potential problems throughout the life span is a major activity of LHDs.

2. *Environmental health services* include food hygiene (e.g., inspection of food-producing and

food-processing plants and restaurants); protection from hazardous substances; control of waste, air, noise, and water pollution; and occupational health. The objective of these activities is to provide a safe environment.

3. *Personal health services* provide care to individuals and families in clinics, schools, and prisons. In many areas, home health care services are provided through the LHD.

4. *Mental health services* are provided through the LHDs in many communities. These services are supported by funds offered by local and regional mental health and mental retardation (MHMR) facilities and programs. See Chapter 22 for more information on community-based mental health care.

In the preceding description of the three government levels that provide public health services (i.e., local, state, and federal), distinctive and overlapping roles have been discussed. The federal government has been assuming a larger role in the protection of the population through regulation and funding. It finances specific programs (e.g., Medicare and categorical programs for mothers and infants) and provides direct care to special populations (e.g., veterans). States establish health codes, regulate the insurance industry, and license health care facilities and personnel. States also provide funds for services offered through Medicaid. Direct care activities funded by state health departments may include care in mental hospitals, state medical schools, and associated hospitals. LHDs are the primary agencies that provide direct services to communities, families, and individuals.

LHDs establish local health codes, fund public hospitals (i.e., city-county) and provide services to populations and individuals at risk. Programs and services for state health departments and LHDs vary across jurisdictions. The services provided reflect the values of the residents and officials, available resources, and perceived needs of their respective populations within their state and local area. Although the goals of the public health subsystem do not change, the programs and services provided change to meet the changing needs of the public.

Health Care Providers

Providers of health care are individuals, groups, and organizations that deliver or support health care

services. This section describes health care providers, including provider organizations, health care professionals, and nontraditional providers.

Provider Organizations

The following are examples of health care **provider organizations**:

- Hospital
- Clinic
- Physician practice
- Ambulatory care center
- Home health agency
- Long-term care facility
- Skilled nursing facility
- Rehabilitation center
- Hospice service
- Public health department
- School health clinic
- Birthing center
- Ambulatory surgical center
- Occupational health clinic
- Crisis clinic
- Any other type of organization that provides health care to the community

Health care provider organizations are undergoing tremendous changes. This is particularly true of hospitals, which are merging, consolidating, and closing. As discussed previously, the Hill-Burton Act provided funds to increase hospital beds and accomplished this goal. However, currently there are too many beds. With the increasing shift to ambulatory and primary care, hospital stays have shortened and the clients who are admitted to the hospital are more acutely ill and require more intensive care. Consequently, decreased hospital stays cause more home care admissions or more discharges from long-term care facilities for short-term recovery and rehabilitation.

The terms that are used to describe these changes are reengineering, redesigning, and rightsizing and downsizing the workforce, and reregulating professional practice.

Reengineering

Reengineering is a management technique that was borrowed from industry and recently applied to the health care delivery system. Reengineering involves more than a few simple changes in an organization. It requires a reinvention or recreation of processes, work, and systems.

Reengineering has become common in health care because the consumer has demanded it. The consumer in the current managed care environment is not just the client, but also businesses who contract for employee health care, all levels of government, third-party payers, and MCOs. Another important factor is competition among all the providers as they seek managed care contracts to increase client volume.

To be successful, reengineering needs to include a cross-functional approach, emphasizing that people do not work in isolation. This has resulted in many organizations that are cross training staff to work in several roles or settings. It emphasizes efficiency, effectiveness, role redesign, and the knowledge of staff to provide the best care or product available (Beyers, 1999; Flarey and Smith, 1999; Hammer and Champy, 1993; Turner, 1999).

Redesigning, Rightsizing, and Downsizing
Redesigning, rightsizing, and downsizing the workforce are terms that typically cause nurses to become alert and concerned. Staffing levels in health care organizations have dropped during the 1990s and the effect that this has had on care is of great concern to consumers and health care professionals, particularly nurses and physicians. Managed care demands cost-effectiveness, which has placed health care organizations in the position of increasing their productivity. The most common method used to increase productivity is to cut staff members; however, the result is not always improved productivity. Staff members may then be overworked, quality suffers, and morale drops, all of which affect overall productivity. However, staff roles need to be carefully assessed and redesigned. More research needs to be done about the effects of staffing, delivery models, and use of unlicensed assistive personnel (UAP). Strategies that help make redesigning, rightsizing, and downsizing more successful are staff education, staff involvement in the process, communication at all staff levels, support and reward, and evaluation (Buerhaus and Staiger, 1997; Dumpe, Herman, and Young, 1998; Hall, 1997; Hoover, 1998).

A national survey of 7560 nurses was conducted in 1996, focusing on staffing and problems that nurses encountered. The results indicated that nurses were experiencing major problems in providing safe care and they were experiencing morale problems. Some of the concerns identified were decreased continuity of care, increased use of temporary staff and UAPs, increased work-related injuries and violence, increased number of clients assigned, and less time to provide care (Shindul-Rothschild, Berry, and Long-Middleton, 1996).

Nurses are speaking out about their concerns through their professional organizations and their state legislative process. California nurses initiated a major effort to affect staffing levels in their hospitals. In October of 1999, California passed a law requiring California hospitals to meet fixed nurse-to-client ratios. This landmark legislation was the first in the United States. This law is important because California is the state that has experienced the influence of managed care for the longest period of time and it is recognizing critical concerns about the effects of some managed care approaches (Purdon, 1999).

Reregulating
The Pew Report identifies **reregulating** professional practice as a critical issue. Currently, health care delivery is less and less limited by boundaries, particularly state boundaries. Large medical centers have satellite delivery centers that may cross state boundaries and in some cases international boundaries; staff members may be expected to move from one to another. Home health agencies may have clients in adjacent states. Telehealth has eliminated all boundaries as long as the equipment is available. Mobility and globalization will have effects on the health care organization and health care professionals (O'Neil and Pew Health Professions Commission, 1998). In 1998, the Pew Health Professions Commission identified critical health care professional competencies for the twenty-first century (Box 9-2).

Health Care Professionals
The health care team has been growing and changing over the last few years with new types of health care professionals added and other members of the

team taking on new responsibilities. The following is a brief review of the major types of professional and nonprofessional members of the health care team:

- Registered Nurse (RN): This appears to be a simple designation that should be familiar to the reader. However, different educational routes exist to obtain a license to practice nursing, including diploma, associate degree, and baccalaureate degree. In addition, many nurses now obtain masters degrees and doctorates. These advanced degrees provide them with the opportunity to do more independent practice, teach, and conduct research. RNs practice in all types of health settings.
- Nurse practitioner (NP): This is a nurse who has obtained education beyond a baccalaureate degree and has had special content related to primary care. A NP specializes in such areas as adult health, pediatrics, neonatology, gerontology, and psychiatric nursing. NPs may work in clinics, the community, a private practice, the home, the hospital, and long-term care facilities (i.e., any setting in which health care is provided).
- Nurse midwife (NM): This is a nurse who has completed an additional educational program focused on midwifery. NMs work in all types of settings in which women's health and obstetrical services are provided.
- Licensed practical nurse or licensed vocational nurse (LPN or LVN): LPNs and LVNs perform some specific nursing functions and play a critical role in providing direct client care. They have high school degrees and additional training. They work in all types of settings, typically under the direct supervision of an RN or a physician.
- Physician (MD or DO): A physician has a medical degree and typically specializes in a specific area of practice (e.g., internal medicine, surgery, pediatrics, and gynecology). Currently, many physicians are specializing in primary practice or family practice because managed care has increased the need for physicians who will act as the primary care provider for clients. In this role, the physician acts as the "gatekeeper" for the client. Many insurance plans require that the client first see his or her primary care provider before seeing a specialist to receive reimbursement for the care. Some insurers are now allowing NPs and NMs to act as primary care providers.

BOX **9-2**

Health Care Professional Competencies for the Twenty-First Century

- Embrace a personal ethic of social responsibility and service.
- Exhibit ethical behavior in all professional activities.
- Provide evidence-based, clinically competent care.
- Incorporate the multiple determinants of health in clinical care.
- Apply knowledge of the new sciences.
- Demonstrate critical thinking, reflection, and problem-solving skills.
- Understand the role of primary care.
- Rigorously practice preventive health care.
- Integrate population-based care and services into practice.
- Improve access to health care for those with unmet health needs.
- Practice relationship-centered care with individuals and families.
- Provide culturally sensitive care to a diverse society.
- Partner with communities in health care decisions.
- Use communication and information technology effectively and appropriately.
- Work in interdisciplinary teams.
- Ensure care that balances individual, professional, system, and societal needs.
- Practice leadership.
- Take responsibility for quality of care and health outcomes at all levels.
- Contribute to continuous improvement of the health care system.
- Advocate for public policy that promotes and protects the health of the public.
- Continue to learn and help others learn.

From O'Neil E, Pew Health Professions Commission: *Recreating health professional practice for a new century.* San Francisco, 1998, Pew Health Professions Commission.

- Physician assistant (PA): The PA is a "physician extender" who provides medical services under the supervision of a licensed physician. The role was developed in the 1960s in response to a shortage of primary care physicians in certain areas. PAs generally work in primary care.

- Registered dietitian (RD): This health care professional assesses the client's nutritional status and needs. RDs work in hospitals, long-term care facilities, clinics, community health, and homes. An RD has knowledge about nutrition and food and in a community setting would recommend healthy diets and provide nutrition counseling and education.
- Social Worker (SW): SWs assist clients and their families with problems related to reimbursement, access to care, housing, care in the home, transportation, and social problems. They have been used as discharge planners, particularly in acute care facilities or hospitals, often as case managers; however, they work in all types of settings.
- Occupational therapist (OT): OTs assist clients with impaired functions to reach the clients' maximum level of physical and psychosocial independence. They work in all types of settings.
- Speech-language pathologist: Speech-language pathologists assist clients who need rehabilitative services related to speech and hearing. They work in all types of settings.
- Physical therapist (PT): PTs focus on assisting clients who are experiencing musculoskeletal problems. PTs typically work in rehabilitation and focus on maximizing physical functioning. They work in all types of settings.
- Pharmacist: Pharmacists are concerned with ensuring that clients receive the appropriate medication by preparing and dispensing medications. Pharmacists have become much more involved in client education about medications and in monitoring and evaluating the effects of medications. They work in all types of settings, including the local drug store, where they play a critical role in ensuring safe prescriptions and providing consumer education.
- Respiratory therapist (RT): RTs provide care to clients with respiratory illnesses. They use oxygen therapy, intermittent positive pressure respirators, artificial mechanical ventilators, and inhalation therapy. Most RTs work in hospitals and long-term care, but they are becoming more common in home health care.
- Chiropractor: Chiropractors are concerned with improving the function of the clients' nervous system with various treatment modalities (e.g., spinal manipulation, diet, exercise, and massage).

Interest in using chiropractors has been increasing as the consumer has become more interested in nontraditional medical interventions. Chiropractors are mostly community-based.

- Paramedical technologists: Paramedical technologists work in various medical technology areas (e.g., radiology, nuclear medicine, and other laboratories).
- Unlicensed Assistive Personnel (UAP): This member of the health care team has caused some controversy in last few years; however, the UAP is a critical member of the team. Aides and assistants have been in existence for a long time. Their responsibilities have changed over the years and they are currently providing more direct client care. They are supervised by RNs, who must ensure that they are able to provide safe care to the client. The amount of education and training of UAPs is highly variable and this has caused much concern about practice parameters and the effect on the quality of care.

Nontraditional Health Care Providers

Nontraditional health care providers deliver alternative or complementary therapies. Although they are among the oldest group of providers, they are now more accepted as members of the team. The consumer has also become more interested in this type of care and has demanded that it be available (Burcham, 1999; Korczyk and Witte, 1998).

Although many large medical centers are now developing programs and centers that offer complementary therapies, reimbursement for these services is still lagging. The NIH agreed to conduct research focused on a wide array of alternative therapies and their effects on health and disease. In 1998, the NIH established the National Center for Complementary and Alternative Therapies to meet the need. This represents a major change in the scientific and medical communities.

Alternative therapies, provided by a variety of health care providers, include massage therapy, herbal therapy, healing touch, energetic healing, acupuncture, and acupressure. Ethnic healers, such as curanderos, and folk healers are also found in some communities. Training and licensure requirements vary, but will probably become more standard as their care becomes more accepted in established medical practice. Many nurses have incorporated alternative therapies in their practice and are seeking continuing education on this topic.

CRITICAL ISSUES IN HEALTH CARE DELIVERY

Managed Care

Managed care refers to any method of health care delivery designed to reduce unnecessary use of services, increase cost containment or effectiveness, and ensure high quality care. Managed care is currently the most dominant force in health care delivery. It affects health care organizations, health care providers, and reimbursement. It has a direct influence on what care is provided and by whom, where, when, and whether it is to be provided.

Managed care is complex and many MCO models exist, such as HMOs, preferred provider organizations (PPOs), integrated delivery systems (IDSs), and physician hospital organizations (PHOs). Each of these models has different characteristics and often clients can choose their health policy from several different models. For example, an employer may offer employees the option of choosing an HMO plan or a PPO plan. See Chapter 10 for additional information on managed care and reimbursement.

Quality Care

Quality care has been a concern of consumers and providers for many years. **Quality care** is a difficult concept to define and more difficult to measure. In 1996, President Clinton established the Advisory Commission on Consumer Protection and Quality in the Health Care Industry and its final report was published in 1999 (Advisory Commission on Consumer Protection and Quality in the Health Care Industry, 1999). As identified in this report, "the purpose of the health care system must be to continuously reduce the impact and burden of illness, injury, and disability and to improve the health and functioning of the people of the United States." The report strongly supports public-private partnerships, strong leadership with clearly defined goals for improvement, an increase in consumer strength and rights, a focus on vulnerable populations, promotion of accountability, reduction in errors and an increase in health care safety, fostering of evidence-based practice, adaptation of organizations for change, an increase in health care workforce involvement, and investment in information systems. Box 9-3 provides additional information found in the report.

BOX **9-3**

The President's Advisory Commission on Consumer Protection and Quality in the Health Care Industry: Recommendations

The purpose of the health care system must be to continuously reduce the influence and burden of illness, injury, and disability and to improve the health and functioning of the people of the United States.

Initial Set of National Aims:
- Reducing the underlying causes of illness, injury, and disability
- Expanding research on new treatments and evidence on effectiveness
- Ensuring the appropriate use of health care services
- Reducing health care errors
- Addressing oversupply and undersupply of health care resources
- Increasing patients' participation in their care

Measurable objectives need to be specified for each of these aims.

Advancing Quality Measurement and Reporting: A core set of quality measures should be identified for standardized reporting by each sector of the health care industry. There should be a stable and predictable mechanism for reporting. Steps should be taken to ensure that comparative information on health care quality is valid, reliable, comprehensible, and widely available in the public domain.

From The President's Advisory Commission on Consumer Protection and Quality in the Health Care Industry: *Quality first: better health care for all Americans*, Washington, DC, 1999, US Government Printing Office.

Continued

BOX **9-3—cont'd**

**The President's Advisory Commission on Consumer Protection and Quality
in the Health Care Industry: Recommendations—cont'd**

Creating Public-Private Partnerships: An Advisory Council for Health Care Quality should be created in the public sector to provide ongoing national leadership in promoting and guiding continuous improvement of health care quality. The Council would track and report on the progress of achieving the national aims for improvement, undertake related quality measurement and reporting, and implement the Consumer Bill of Rights and Responsibilities. A Forum for Health Care Quality Measurement and Reporting should be created in the private sector to improve the effectiveness and efficiency of health care quality measurement and reporting. Widespread public availability of comparative information on quality care needs to be provided.

Encouraging Action by Group Purchasers: Group purchasers, to the extent feasible, should provide their individual members with a choice of plans. State and federal governments should create further opportunities for small employers to participate in large purchasing pools that, to the extent feasible, make a commitment to individual choice of plans. All public and private group purchasers should use quality as a factor in selecting the plans they will offer to their individual members, employees, or beneficiaries. Group purchasers should implement strategies to stimulate ongoing improvements in health care quality.

Strengthening the Hand of Consumers: Widespread and ongoing consumer education should be developed to deliver accurate and reliable information and encourage consumers to consider information on quality when choosing health plans, providers, and treatments. Some consumers will require assistance in making these choices. Further research should be conducted addressing the use of consumer information.

Focusing on Vulnerable Populations: Additional investment should be provided for developing, evaluating, and supporting effective health care delivery models designed to meet the specific needs of vulnerable populations.

Promoting Accountability: The Consumer Bill of Rights and Responsibility should be included in private and public sector contractual and oversight requirements.

Reducing Errors and Increasing Safety in Health Care: Interested parties should work together to develop a health care error-reporting system to identify errors and prevent their recurrence.

Fostering Evidence-Based Practice and Innovation: Federal funding for health care research, including basic, clinical, prevention, and health services research, should be increased and the necessary research infrastructure supported. Collaborative arrangements between researchers and private and public sectors should be developed. Research should target those areas where the greatest improvements in health and functional status of population can occur and where gaps in knowledge exist.

Adapting Organizations for Change: Health care organizations should provide strong leadership to confront quality challenges and pursue aims for improvement. They should commit to reducing errors and increasing safety. Organizations need to develop long-term relationships with all stakeholders.

Engaging the Health Care Workforce: The training of physicians, nurses, and other health care workers must change to meet the demands of a changing health care industry. Minimum standards for education, training, and supervision of unlicensed paraprofessionals should be established. Steps should be taken to improve the diversity and the cultural competence of the health care workforce. Health care workers must be encouraged to identify and report clinical errors and instances of improper or dangerous care. Action must be taken to reduce the unacceptably high rate of injury in the health care workforce. Efforts must be taken to address the serious morale problems that exist among health care workers in many sectors of the industry. Further research should be conducted into how changes in the roles and responsibilities of health care workers are affecting quality.

Investing in Information Systems: Purchasers of health care services should insist that providers and plans be able to produce quantitative evidence of quality as a means of encouraging investment in information systems.

From The President's Advisory Commission on Consumer Protection and Quality in the Health Care Industry: *Quality first: better health care for all Americans,* Washington, DC, 1999, US Government Printing Office.

Accreditation is one means to assess the quality of services and care of the organization. Specific minimum standards must be met by an organization to obtain accreditation. Many groups provide accreditation for health care providers and managed care MCOs. The JCAHO accredits hospitals, home care agencies, long-term care facilities, ambulatory care centers, and MCOs. The National Committee on Quality Assurance (NCQA) accredits MCOs and uses the Health Plan Employer Data Information Set (HEDIS) to collect data about plans and consumer satisfaction. Medicare also uses HEDIS. The American Healthcare Commission (URAC) also accredits MCOs (Diamond, 1998; O'Malley, 1997; Snowden, 1998).

Purchasers of care are concerned about the accreditation status of MCOs when they negotiate MCO contracts. Insurers and MCOs are concerned about the accreditation status of health care provider organizations, as are nursing schools that use clinical sites for educational purposes. Health care providers should also be concerned about the accreditation status of their employers. The Consumer Assessment of Health Plans (CAHPS) is a new survey and reporting tool sponsored by the Agency for Health Care Policy and Research (AHCPR), Harvard Medical School, the Research Triangle Institute, and RAND. CAHPS collects data and reports on consumer experience with specific aspects of their health plans. This type of survey provides data that help purchasers of plans compare and contrast plans (AHCPR et al., 1998).

Currently, quality care monitoring focuses on improvement. With the improvement approach, **outcomes measures** have moved to the forefront. Accrediting organizations require outcomes data and use them to assess overall performance. Practitioners use outcomes to identify the treatment goals with the client. Report cards are used to compare and contrast health care organizations and health care plans. These report cards are available to the consumer, providers, and insurers. Quality data are no longer hidden and will continue to be available as new methods are developed to assess improvement based on outcomes (Hibbard et al., 1997).

Fraud and Abuse

Health care fraud is widespread. The billions of dollars spent on health care and struggles for control between providers, consumers, and MCOs have provided an arena that lends itself to fraud and abuse (Kassirer, 1995). The Government Accounting Office estimates that 10% of the total health care expenditures, or about $100 billion, is lost to fraud and abuse. In 1994, a U.S. congressional committee concluded that an effective antifraud program is crucial to stopping fraud throughout the health care system (US House of Representatives, 1994).

Major health care fraud and abuse incidents have influenced the most vulnerable of the population (i.e., the mentally ill and older adults). In the 1980s and 1990s, a major psychiatric scandal occurred, involving large sums of money and abuse of clients (Meier, 1997; Mohr, 1996, 1997). This scandal involved many patient abuses, including inappropriate admissions, administration of medications and treatment that were not required, unsafe physical restraint for long periods of time, verbal abuse, and denial of patient rights. Hospitals falsified documentation to receive higher levels of reimbursement and discharged patients as soon as their insurance ran out with limited or no discharge planning. All of these examples indicate what can happen when a health care organization confronts the dilemma of care vs. the bottom line and chooses the bottom line.

Other major incidents concerning fraud include a case involving Columbia/HCA, in which federal investigations found widespread fraud, overcharges, and substandard care (Eichenwald, 1997). Medicare also found similar problems in its program; consequently, the federal government initiated Operation Restore Trust to combat further Medicare fraud in home care and long-term care organizations (Pear, 1997).

Many nurses have been directly influenced by fraud and abuse by participating in it, by trying to fight it, and by their apathy. Nurses need to assert their role as advocates and know how to cope with unethical behavior in health care organizations (Camunas, 1998; Meier, 1997; Mohr, 1996, 1997).

Information Technology

The development of information technology over the last decade has been phenomenal. Clinical staff members use computers in all health care settings. **Telehealth** is growing, which means that clients can receive care via technology, such as computer, video, or interactive television. The Internet has opened doors for consumers and providers and health information has exploded. Although information availability has been enhanced to millions of people, which resulted in an explosion of knowledge regarding health and health issues, the quality of this information is sometimes questionable. Providers must address the source and content of Internet information (Brody, 1999).

Consumerism, Advocacy, and Client Rights

The growth of managed care has increased the strength of consumerism. Over the past decade, the Baby Boom generation has been subsidizing the health care system and paying more in premiums than it has taken out in claims. However, growing concern exists that as this generation ages, it will demand more care than previous generations (Gosfield, 1997; Kleinke, 1998). Consumers are now critical of the health care system and demanding changes as they encounter problems. MCOs and providers are recognizing the importance of the consumer voice and the need for explanations. *Client-* or *customer-centered health care* is a term that has become commonly used in health care and more effort has been made to provide the consumer with information.

Client rights are now an important health care issue that individual states and the federal government have been addressing through legislation. In the fall of 1999, the House and Senate passed bills that focused on client rights in the managed care environment (Pear, 1999a). These bills are different and ultimately a combined bill will have to be passed. There is no doubt that this will be a critical issue in the future. Client rights issues that are vitally important are information disclosure, physician and provider choice, direct access to specialists, reimbursement for emergency care, and reimbursement denial.

Coordination and Access to Health Care

The social justice foundation of public health is yet to be realized because many inequalities in access to health care still exist. The United States has more than 43 million uninsured individuals (Pear, 1999b). Characteristics of uninsured people reflect a wide range of incomes, races, and occupations, although children, minorities, the poor, and those with less education are overrepresented.

Health care providers often function in isolation from one another and provide fragmented services. Although multiple services are available for the wellness-serious illness continuum, coordination is lacking. Services range from office-clinic, home care, adult day care, acute care institutions, and specialized institutions to skilled nursing facilities. The services provided by one agency or one provider do not help the individual transit, or move, across boundary lines and receive services offered by others. In addition, the services tend to be geographically separated and each agency has different criteria for access. The focus of services has not kept pace with the changing needs of individuals and populations. Millions of Americans lack access to health care services and inadequate financial resources are a deterrent to available health services.

The current health care system is pluralistic and competitive and it provides fragmented and uncoordinated care. Private care agencies and institutions are in competition with one another for clients, health professionals, and resources. Even with recent reforms, two hospitals in the same geographical area may be competing for the same clients. Hospital home care programs are in direct competition with private home care agencies. Hospitals diversify services to become economically viable; therefore they compete with HMOs for the ambulatory market. Public health services can be viewed as indirectly competing for resources (Rice, 1990; Schulz and Johnson, 1990). This fragmentation and duplication must be overcome to provide coordinated, collaborative, and accessible service to all citizens.

The health care system in the United States is complex, with social policies that favor pluralism, free choice, and free enterprise. The private sector personal care subsystem provides the majority of care to individuals. The private sector includes nonprofit agencies, for-profit agencies, and voluntary organizations. The public health subsystem provides limited personal care services for socially-marginalized populations, but for the most part subsidizes the private sector through Medicare and Medicaid reimbursement to provide these services.

Health Care Reform: The Clinton Health Reform Initiative

The United States appeared to be ready for **health care reform** when the Clinton administration took office (Skocpol, 1994). By 1990, support for reform had reached a 40-year high in the polls and the election of Bill Clinton in 1992 brought the health care debate onto the national agenda. Believing reform of the health care system to be part of his election mandate, the new president assembled an ambitious plan to produce legislation for national reform of the health care system. The process was initially supported by diverse sectors of the system. As the shape of the Clinton proposals began to emerge, some participants began to distance themselves and ultimately opposed the reform approach. This was true in the case of many major power constituents (i.e., businesses, physicians, and insurance companies). The insurance sector was probably the most vocal making its objections known.

The approach used by the administration was inclusive, with strong support for public health. The bill eventually proposed in Congress included a version of the core functions outlined in the 1988 IOM study *The Future of Public Health.* Public health's inclusion in the reform agenda fostered a renewed interest in prevention and health promotion. The focus was to improve health status and contain costs. After defeat of the reform bills in 1994, the consensus emerged that despite the American public's recognition of the need for reform, little recognition existed that such reform would have specific consequences for individual Americans in terms of cost and choice (Starr, 1993).

FUTURE OF PUBLIC HEALTH AND THE HEALTH CARE SYSTEM

The debate continues as the new century begins.

What health care services should be provided?
Who should have access to health care services?
Who should pay for health care services?
How should health care be delivered?

Changes in the health care system are necessary to meet the changing needs of populations. The private care subsystem needs to set limits on the care provided, setting criteria for use of technology and determining which conditions will be treated, which interventions are effective, and who should receive the care (Banta, 1990). Managed care has pressured the private care subsystem into focusing more on health promotion and prevention; however, the success of this pressure is unclear.

At the beginning of the twenty-first century it is difficult to speculate on the role of community health in the new century. However, the community health focus on health promotion, disease prevention, and the population-based approach to health care are finding a new audience. The concept of upstream thinking is also coming to the forefront with new listeners. Local, state, and national political leaders must begin to grapple with the health of the population and the need to reduce the levels of health care expenditures in a voluntary environment.

Futurists rarely identify the public health subsystem as a component of the health care system. Perhaps the historic involvement of the public health subsystem with the poor and disenfranchised is a major influence in inattention to their problems. The assumptions underlying the ecological model demand that attention be paid to the poor and underserved, but the political aspects of health care frequently demand a focus in another direction. Furthermore, focus on environmental influences on population is critical for the future health of any nation.

Predicting future trends in human values is more difficult than predicting scientific discoveries or the patterns of disease. However, Koop (1989) stated that the ultimate test of the public health subsystem is whether it effectively serves the people by *their* measurements, not those of the public health profession. A significant shift has occurred in thinking about the future of the health care system since the beginning of the 1990s. Consumer rights and further efforts to control or limit managed care will be critical issues to be resolved in the future. How these decisions will affect public health is unclear.

SUMMARY

The health care system is complex and changes quickly. Federal, state, and local legislation and policies affect the system and understanding the legislation and its effect on the health care delivery system is critical for any nurse. In addition, the development of managed care has demonstrated how important it is for health care providers to understand the reimbursement system and to learn how to advocate for their clients.

The many different types of health care organizations and health care providers also affect the health care system. Interdisciplinary care will be necessary for success in the system and to ensure that the client receives cost-effective, quality care. There are many concerns about health care such as cost, access, the number of uninsured, quality, and health care fraud and abuse. Resolving these concerns will not be an easy task, but it must be done. Understanding the system helps as health care providers learn to function in the rapidly changing system.

LEARNING ACTIVITIES

1. Describe the organization of the state and local health departments.
2. Visit the LHD and learn what services are provided. How do these services relate to *Healthy People 2010* objectives?
3. Identify regional and state health services.
4. Visit a voluntary agency. Determine the services they offer and how the agency collaborates with the local public health agency. Does the agency have a website? If so, visit it and find out what information is available for consumers and professionals.
5. Discuss how critical health care issues (e.g., managed care, quality care, fraud, and abuse) affect health care organizations in the community.
6. Site examples of health care consumerism in the local community.
7. Give a personal reaction to health care fraud and abuse. How should the principles found in the *Code for Nurses* apply in practice?

REFERENCES

Advisory Commission on Consumer Protection and Quality in the Health Care Industry: *Quality first: better health care for all Americans,* Washington, DC, 1999, US Government Printing Office.

Agency for Health Care Policy and Research, Harvard Medical School, Research Triangle Institute, RAND: *Consumer assessment of health plans,* Washington, DC, 1998, AHCPR.

Annual update of the HHS poverty guidelines, *Federal Register* 64(52):13428-13430, March 18, 1999.

Banta H: What is health care? In Kovner A, editor: *Health care delivery in the United States,* ed 4, New York, 1990, Springer.

Beyers M: Re-engineering patient care in a multi-institutional system. In Smith S, Flarey D, editors: *Process-centered health care organization,* Gaithersburg, Md, 1999, Aspen.

Brody J: The health hazards of point-and-click medicine, *New York Times,* August 3, 1999.

Buerhaus P, Staiger D: Future of the nurse labor market according to health executives in high-managed care areas of the United States, *Image J Nurs Sch* 29(4):313, 1997.

Burcham M: Credentialing alternative medicine: a challenge for managed care organizations, *Managed Care Q* 7(2):39, 1999.

Camunas C: Ethical dilemmas of nurse executives, *J Nurs Admin* 24(7-8):45, 1998.

DeParle J: States struggle to use windfall born of shifts in welfare law, *New York Times,* August 29, 1999.

Diamond F: NCQA adds performance to accreditation reviews, *Managed Care* 8(5), 1998, The Author, www.managedcaremag.com.

Dumpe M, Herman J, Young S: Forecasting the nursing workforce in a dynamic health care market, *Nurs Econ* 16(4):170, 1998.

Eichenwald K: Hospital chain cheated U.S. on expenses, documents show, *New York Times,* August 22, 1997.

Flarey D, Smith S: Re-engineering: the journey to a process-centered organization. In Smith S, Flarey D, editors: *Process-centered health care organization,* Gaithersburg, Md, 1999, Aspen.

Gosfield A: Who is holding whom accountable for quality? *Health Affairs* 16(3):39, 1997.

Hall L: Staff mix models: complementary or substitution roles for nurses, *Aspen's Advisor for Nurse Executives* 21(2):31, 1997.

Hammer M, Champy J: *Re-engineering the corporation: a manifesto for business revolution,* New York, 1993, Harper Business.

Hanlon G, Pickett J: *Public health administration and practice,* ed 8, St. Louis, 1984, Mosby.

Hibbard J et al: Will quality report cards help consumers? *Health Affairs* 16(3):281, 1997.

Hoover K: Nursing work redesign in response to managed care, *J Nurs Admin* 28(11):9, 1998.

Institute of Medicine: *The National Academy of Science: the future of public health,* Washington, DC, 1988, National Academy Press.

Kassirer J: Managed care and the morality of the marketplace, *N Engl J Med* 333(1):50, 1995.

Kleinke J: *Bleeding edge: the business of health care in the new century,* Gaithersburg, Md, 1998, Aspen.

Knight W: *Managed care: what it is and how it works,* Gaithersburg, Md, 1998, Aspen.

Koop CE: An agenda for public health, *J Public Health Policy* 10:7, 1989.

Korczyk S, Witte H: *The complete idiot's guide to managed health care,* New York, 1998, Alpha Books.

Levy D, editor: *1999 state by state guide to managed care law,* Gaithersburg, Md, 1999, Aspen.

Mariner W: State regulation of managed care and the Employer Retirement Income Security Act, *N Engl J Med* 335(26):1986, 1996.

Meier B: For-profit care's human cost: Tenet Health Care to settle some old accounts, *New York Times,* August 8, 1997.

Mohr W: Dirty hands: the underside of marketplace health care, *Adv Nurs Sci* 19(1):28, 1996.

Mohr W: Outcomes of corporate greed, *Image* 29(1):39, 1997.

O'Malley C: Quality measurement for health systems: accreditation and report cards, *Am J Health Syst Pharm* 54(7):1528, 1997.

O'Neil E, Pew Health Professions Commission: *Recreating health professional practice for a new century,* San Francisco, 1998, Pew Health Professions Commission.

Pear R: House passes bill to expand rights on medical care, *New York Times,* October 8, 1999a.

Pear R: Insurers ask government to extend health plans, *New York Times,* May 23, 1999b.

Pear R: Investigators say a Medicare option is rife with fraud: violations in home care, *New York Times,* July 27, 1997.

Pickett G, Hanlon JJ: Public health administration and practice, ed 9, St. Louis, 1990, Mosby.

Purdon T: California to set level of staffing for nursing care, *New York Times,* October 12, 1999.

Rice DP: The medical care system: past trends and future projections. In Lee PR, Estes CL, editors: *The nation's health,* ed 3, Boston, Mass, 1990, Jones and Bartlett.

Robert Wood Johnson Foundation: *State health care reform: looking back toward the future,* Princeton, NJ, 1997, The Author.

Schulz R, Johnson AC: *Management of hospitals and health services,* ed 3, St. Louis, 1990, Mosby.

Shindul-Rothschild J, Berry D, Long-Middleton E: Where have all the nurses gone? final results of our patient care survey, *Am J Nurs* 96(11):25, 1996.

Skocpol T: From social security to health security? *J Health Polit Policy Law* 19:239, 1994.

Snowden F: National benchmarking is on the way, *Inside Case Management* 5(9):2, 1998.

Starr P: The framework of health care reform, *N Engl J Med* 329:1666, 1993.

The President's Advisory Commission on Consumer Protection and Quality in the Health Care Industry: *Quality first: better health care for all Americans,* Washington, DC, 1999, US Government Printing Office.

Turner S: *The nurse's guide to managed care,* Gaithersburg, Md, 1999, Aspen.

US Census Bureau: *Statistical abstract of the United States,* Washington, DC, 1996, US Government Printing Office.

US House of Representatives: *Deceit that sickens America: health care fraud and its innocent victims.* Hearings before the Subcommittee on Crime and Criminal Justice of the Committee on the Judiciary House of Representatives, One Hundred and Third Congress, Second Session, Washington, DC, 1994, US Government Printing Office.

10

Economics of Health Care

Carrie Morgan

Carrie Morgan

OBJECTIVES

Upon completion of this chapter, the reader will be able to do the following:

1. Discuss factors that influence the cost of health care.
2. Identify terms used in the financing of health care.
3. Discuss public financing of health care.
4. Discuss private financing of health care.
5. Discuss health insurance plans.
6. Describe trends in health care financing.
7. Describe the effects of economics on health care access.
8. Identify the future of health care economics.

KEY TERMS

See the list provided in Box 10-1 for terms pertaining to consumers, terms pertaining to providers, and terms pertaining to third party payers.

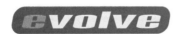

http://evolve.elsevier.com/Nies/

Economics affects all aspects of health care, yet nurses have traditionally avoided the arena of health care economics, preferring to focus on the actual, direct care of the client. So strong is the feeling of social justice that some nurses express a reluctance to be informed of the individual client's health care financing source for fear that this knowledge will influence their care. Community health nurses who deal with the medically underserved have had more experience in this area. However, even these nurses may have only rudimentary knowledge. Health care costs have risen rapidly; therefore nursing can no longer ignore the intricacies of health care financing.

This chapter focuses on the economics of health care. It specifically discusses factors that influence health care costs, terminology of health care financing, and future trends of health care economics. This chapter also addresses the future of health care financing. Box 10-1 presents terms and definitions that are important to the discussion of these topics.

BOX **10-1**

Terminology Used in Health Care Financing

The financing of health care has given rise to new terminology. Nurses, as providers of care and consumers of services, need to be knowledgeable about these terms to increase their understanding of health care financing. These terms are in bold within the chapter.

Terms Pertaining to Consumers
Access: Ability to obtain health care services in a timely manner, at a reasonable cost, by a qualified practitioner, and at an accessible location.
Carve-out service: A service (i.e., mental health care) provided within a standard benefit package, but delivered exclusively by a designated provider or group.
Charges: The posted prices of provider services.
Coinsurance: Cost sharing required by a health plan whereby the individual is responsible for a set percentage of the charge for each service.
Copayment: Cost sharing required by the health plan whereby the individual must pay a fixed dollar amount for each service.
Deductible: Cost sharing whereby the individual pays a specified amount before the health plan pays for covered services.
Fee schedule: List of predetermined payment rates for medical services.
Flexible spending account (FSA): A mechanism by which an employee may pay for uncovered health care expenses through payroll deductions.
Gatekeeper: Person in a MCO who decides whether a patient will be referred for specialty care. Doctors, nurses, NPs, and PAs function as gatekeepers.
Health care provider: An individual or institution that provides medical services (e.g., physicians, hospitals, or laboratories).
Health plan: A health insurance plan that pays a predetermined amount for covered services.
Indemnity plan: A health plan that pays covered services on a fee-for-service basis.
HMO: A managed care plan that acts as an insurer and sometimes a provider for a fixed prepaid premium. HMOs usually employ physicians.
Managed care plan: A health plan that uses financial incentives to encourage enrollees to use selected providers who have contracted with the plan.
Medicaid: Joint federal- and state-funded programs that provide health care services for low-income people.
Medicare: A health insurance program for people over 65 years of age, those who are disabled, and sufferers of end-stage renal disease.

Continued

BOX 10-1—cont'd

Terminology Used in Health Care Financing—cont'd

Medicare+Choice: Medicare recipients may choose to enroll in a coordinated care plan, private fee-for-service, or medical savings account plan created by the Balanced Budget Act of 1997.

Medigap insurance: Privately purchased individual or group health insurance plan designed to supplement Medicare coverage.

Out-of-pocket expenses: Payment made by the individual for medical services.

Point of service (POS): A managed care plan that combines prepaid and fee-for-service plans. Enrollees may choose to use the services of an uncontracted provider by paying an increased copayment.

Portability: An individual changing jobs is guaranteed coverage with the new employer without a waiting period or having to meet additional deductible requirements.

PPO: A health plan that contracts with providers to furnish services to the enrollees of the plan. Usually no insurance copayment is required.

Premium: Amount paid periodically to purchase health insurance benefits.

Primary care provider: A generalist physician, typically family physicians, internists, gynecologists, and pediatricians, who provides comprehensive medical services.

Terms Pertaining to Providers

Ambulatory care: Medical services provided on an outpatient basis in a hospital or clinic setting.

Capitation: Payment mechanism that pays health care providers a fixed amount per enrollee to cover a defined set of services over a specified time period regardless of actual services provided.

Care management: Process used to improve quality of care by analyzing variations in and outcomes for current practice in the care of specific health conditions.

Cost containment: Reduction of inefficiencies in the consumption, allocation, or production of health care services.

Customary charge: Physician payment based on a median charge for a given service within a 12-month period.

DRG: A system of payment classification for inpatient hospital services based on the principal diagnosis, procedure, age and gender of the patient, and complications.

Effectiveness: Net health benefit provided by a medical service or technology for a typical patient in community practice.

Fully capitated: A stipulated dollar amount established to cover the cost of all health care services delivered for a person.

Maximum allowable costs: Specified cost level established by the health plan.

Outcome: The consequences of a medical intervention on a patient.

Physician's current procedural terminology (CPT) codes: A list of codes for medical services and procedures performed by physicians and other health care providers that has become the health care industry's standard for reporting physician procedures and services.

Practice guidelines: An explicit statement of what is known and believed about the benefits, risks, and costs of particular courses of medical action intended to assist decisions made by practitioners, patients, and others about appropriate health care for specific and clinical conditions.

Utilization review: A formal prospective, concurrent, or retrospective assessment of the medical necessity, efficiency, and appropriateness of health care services.

Terms Pertaining to Third-Party Payers

Actuarial classification: Classification of enrollees that is determined by use of the mathematics of insurance, including probabilities to ensure adequacy of the premium to provide future payment.

BOX **10-1—cont'd**

Terminology Used in Health Care Financing—cont'd

Administrative costs: Costs that the insurer incurs for utilization review, marketing, medical underwriting, agents' commissions, premium collection, claims processing, insurer profit, quality assurance activities, medical libraries, and risk management.

Adverse selection: Larger proportion of people with poorer health status enroll in specific plans or options. Plans that enroll a subpopulation with lower-than-average costs are favorably selected.

Capital cost: Depreciation, interest, leases and rentals, taxes, and insurance on tangible assets.

Carrier: An organization that contracts with the HCFA to administer claims processing and make Medicare payments to health care providers.

Cost contract: Arrangement between a managed health care plan and the HCFA for reimbursement of the costs of services provided.

Cost shifting: The cost of uncompensated care is passed on to the insured, resulting in higher costs for those with insurance coverage.

Mandate: A state or federal statute or regulation that requires coverage for certain health services.

Risk assessment: Statistical method used to estimate claims costs of enrollees.

FACTORS INFLUENCING HEALTH CARE COSTS

Historical Perspectives

Until the 1930s, the predominant method of health care financing in the United States was private payment. Physicians charged a fee for the services they rendered and the patient paid these **out-of-pocket expenses**. The following types of hospitals existed:

1. Public hospitals, which received public funds and served the health care needs of the entire population regardless of ability to pay
2. Private hospitals, which cared mainly for those whose ability to pay was greater than the general population.
3. For-profit hospitals, which were limited in number, received funds from investors and cared for those who could definitely pay. Most hospitals and **health care providers** donated a portion of their services to charity.

This system worked well as long as the number of those who could pay outnumbered those who could not. The Great Depression of the 1930s changed this. With 25% of the population out of work, the number of those capable of financing the health care system was greatly reduced. Hospitals and physicians went bankrupt because they were no longer able to collect fees.

In 1929, Texas schoolteachers negotiated a pre-paid health provision contract with Baylor Hospital. The teachers paid a sum of money each month, which guaranteed them health care at that hospital. The idea was successful and other hospitals began to form such plans.

The concept of paying a small fee for guaranteed health care became popular. Employers regarded health insurance as a means of supplementing their worker's benefits without granting a wage increase. Workers enjoyed freedom from fear that illness would impoverish them. Health care providers envisioned guaranteed payment for their services (Higgins, 1997).

Use of Health Care

According to economic principles, use is influenced by the availability of financial funding for a product, demand for the product, and the existence of a desirable product. By viewing health care as a product, the individual begins to gain insight into the problem. Emphasis placed on illness care with little or no provisions for health promotion, together with providers who receive a fee only when a service is rendered, has resulted in an incentive for use and an expectation of the most elaborate and costly care. When they are insulated from rising health care costs, health care consumers demand complex and technologically advanced services whenever illness strikes.

These demands represent the major driving force in rising health care costs (Weinick and Drilea, 1996).

Attempts to decelerate the escalation of health care costs by reducing use have been only minimally successful. Insurance plans have begun to limit coverage for certain services and people. Restrictions on use of health care, such as establishment of a "gate-keeper" that requires preauthorization, limited coverage for preexisting illnesses, and exclusion of those participants whose use was deemed exorbitant, have been instituted. These attempts have sparked resentment and resistance by the general public. Protests and legal torts involving denied services have begun to increase.

Health Behaviors

Until recently, little to no incentive has existed to prevent illness or promote health. Curative measures have traditionally been the focus of health care. Soaring costs and an improved knowledge of health have heightened the public's awareness of their obligation to assume responsibility for their health by amending many unhealthy behaviors. As a result, more people are demanding preventive health care from the provider and their health care contractors. Public financing of health care has increased funding for such preventive care as screening tests, periodic examinations, and immunizations.

Lifestyle

A healthy lifestyle does not ensure everlasting good health. However, the leading causes of death and illness can be positively affected by changes in lifestyle. Recent studies have found that a low-fat diet, exercise, and stress reduction will curtail the influence of CVD, the leading cause of death. Smoking cessation reduces the incidence of lung cancer. Seat belt use reduces the severity of injuries incurred during moving vehicle accidents. Effective treatment of illness must be coupled with a change in lifestyle. In the near future, access to expensive and unique medical treatment will probably be influenced less by the patient's ability to pay and more by the person's commitment to compulsory lifestyle changes.

Old movies dramatize the change in lifestyle that has taken place in the last 30 years. The current "smoke-free" environment appears shocking contrasted to the nonchalant attitude toward smoking that was pervasive at that time. The advent of the HBM and Pender's HPM has given rise to numerous studies into methods of achieving lifestyle changes. The total effects of these changes are just now being seen. Meanwhile, the health care system must continue to contend with the results of years of unhealthy lifestyles.

Societal Beliefs

With the advent of such wonders as penicillin, society began to believe that the eradication of disease was just a few years away. More resources were dedicated to this illusive search. Armed with the belief that disease would soon be eliminated, societal interest in preventive care was limited. The general belief was that more money available for health care meant better health care and the greater likelihood that illness would be cured.

Health care professionals were also slow to embrace preventive care. Most efforts were directed toward curing illness. With what seemed to be an unending source of financing, illness prevention seemed counterproductive.

As health care costs accelerated at an alarming rate and technological advances did not keep up with the increase in illnesses, the health of society had to become a collaborative effort between society itself and the health care industry. Insurance would pay for needed care; therefore the lack of concern for health has been replaced with the concept of preservation of health. Although people still expect the health care industry to cure them when they are ill, increased interest in preventive care has developed.

Technological Advances

Modern society has come to expect miraculous technological advances. In response to this demand, technological advances have become too numerous to mention. Available technological advances can save the lives of people who would otherwise die. These advances, although remarkable, are expensive and result in 20% of the population consuming 80% of the health care resources (Vermont Medical Roundtable, 1999). As the health care dollar shrinks, these advances raise ethical questions involving health care access and rationing.

The availability of these technological advances also contributes to health care use. In countries such as Canada and Germany, the latest technology, such as

MRI, is available only in large hospitals. In contrast, most community hospitals in the United States provide a wide variety of tertiary services, including the most current technological advances.

Availability restriction on technology has resulted in significantly reduced cost of health care; however, the delays, inconvenience, and lack of care that plague these countries would not be tolerated by the American public (Vermont Medical Roundtable, 1999).

PUBLIC FINANCING OF HEALTH CARE

As the popularity and benefits of employer-provided insurance plans were recognized, it became evident that the health care of some segments of society were being neglected. The 1960s, with a pervasive interest for social justice in the public and political arenas, presented the ideal opportunity for governmental participation in health care financing. In 1965, the federal government enacted the first movement toward universal health care coverage. Titles XVIII and XIX of the Social Security Act created Medicare and Medicaid, respectively.

Medicare

Medicare was intended to provide health care to the growing population of those 65 years of age or older. Medicare Part A coverage is an entitlement program, or provided free of charge, to older individuals and those people who are disabled or suffer from end-stage renal disease. Services covered by Medicare Part A include services delivered in a hospital.

For those eligible for Medicare part A, Medicare Part B may be purchased for a monthly fee. Covered services under Part B include outpatient services, home health services, therapies, and physician services. Participation in Medicare part B is not compulsory. Currently, reimbursement for covered services under Medicare part B is provided on a fee-for-service basis, but that is being changed to a **capitation** method of reimbursement.

Medicaid

Medicaid provides universal health care coverage for the indigent and children. A joint state and federal venture, eligibility to this program is dependent on the size and income of the family. The created purpose of this program is support for the health care needs of the medically indigent. Priority participation is given to children, pregnant women, and the disabled.

The federal government sets baseline eligibility requirements. State governments who wish to provide care to more of its citizens through this program can lower the eligibility requirements. For example, the federal government may set 110% of poverty as an eligibility requirement, but Kentucky may set the requirement as 100% of poverty. This means that a family living in Kentucky can have an income slightly above the federal standard and still qualify for Medicaid. The federal government **mandates** covered services, but again state governments may provide more services. Currently, Medicaid payments are based on a fee-for-service system, but this is rapidly changing as states experiment with various methods of prospective payment.

Effect of Medicare and Medicaid on Health Care Economics

The enactment of Medicare and Medicaid created an unprecedented demand for services. By the end of the first five years, Medicare costs had more than doubled the original estimates (Vermont Medical Roundtable, 1999). The cost-based reimbursement used by these programs established a new source of funding that dramatically influenced hospital use. By 1975, the average length of stay for Medicare patients was twice that of their younger insured counterparts (Turner, 1999). Medicare reimbursement rates generally became the standard for all insurance **carriers.**

Government funding of health care has admirably provided more people with access to high quality care who otherwise could not afford it, but the cost of this care amounts to $350 billion dollars per year. Approximately 47% of the total cost of health care in the United States is paid by the government, but Medicare and Medicaid recipients represent less than 20% of the total population (Vermont Medical Roundtable, 1999).

PRIVATE FINANCING OF HEALTH CARE

A limited amount of the nation's estimated $1 trillion health care bill is paid by private funding whose services are usually capricious and research- or disease-oriented. Eligibility for services through these associations is generally limited to the specific disease or population of interest, as with the American Heart Association. Few direct services are rendered and these are awarded on individual case consideration. Associated health care needs such as transportation may be addressed. Informational and research activities constitute the majority of services provided by these types of organizations.

Exceptions do exist. National organizations such as the Shriners operate health care institutions designed to provide specialty care for a specific population group. These services and all costs related to this care, including transportation, are provided to the eligible person free of charge. The only requirement for this care is sponsorship by a member of the supporting organization.

HEALTH INSURANCE PLANS

Historical Perspective

During the 1930s, in an effort to provide care and avoid bankruptcy, health care providers began to establish health insurance plans. One of the most recognizable of these plans is Blue Cross and Blue Shield. Those enrolled in the plan, called *enrollees,* paid a monthly fee for a guarantee of health care. Providers delivered services to the enrollees and collected payment from the health insurance plan. The insurance plan paid fees plus their **administrative costs** from money collected from the enrollees.

During World War II when prices and wages were frozen, industries began to offer health insurance as a fringe benefit. Workers' union groups began to negotiate for these benefits. In 1953, as a further incentive to obtain health care coverage, money spent on health insurance was declared tax exempt. With more available financial resources, the health care industry grew. Reimbursement based on operational costs represented a strong incentive for expansion (Higgins, 1997).

Types of Health Care Plans

Blue Cross and Blue Shield was an example of an **indemnity plan.** This plan paid all of the costs of covered services provided to the enrollee. The enrollee had free choice of the provider and services. Although indemnity plans are still available, the monthly cost of enrollment has increased to exorbitant amounts, making these plans cost-prohibitive. Mechanisms of cost sharing were introduced to lower the cost. These cost-sharing methods include **copayment, deductible** amounts, and **coinsurance.** Indemnity plans preserve the enrollee's right of choice and allow the person to manage his or her own health care.

As health care costs escalated, variations in health care insurance plans were developed. Industries, the major providers of insurance coverage, began to look for a more economical means of providing health care to their employees. Large industrial giants, such as Kaiser Permanente, decided to assemble their own health care program. They built hospitals, hired physicians, and provided health care services to their employees. In an effort to market this concept, Dr. Paul Elwood coined the phrase **"Health Maintenance Organization"** (Higgins, 1997). Although comprehensive in the care provided, this type of program lacks freedom of choice. More preventive care is covered, but the care is restricted to the services rendered by the HMO. Health care providers are encouraged to reduce costs by providing only the most necessary services. Despite participants dissatisfied with the lack of choice and other health care provider complaints about the lack of competition, by the end of the 1980s, HMOs represented approximately 25% of the health care plans (Higgins, 1997).

In an effort to compete with the HMO, physicians and hospitals organized the Independent Practice Model (IPM). The IPM was a separate entity that provided services to enrollees of one insurance company. This model evolved into the **PPO.** These types of plans negotiated with care providers for services at a specific rate in exchange for a guaranteed increase in consumers. A negotiated reimbursement rate allows the cost of the plan to be somewhat controlled. Plan enrollees are offered cost incentives for choosing health care from within the plan's network. Providers are encouraged to be cost-conscious in the services provided as they receive a specific amount regardless of the rendered services.

Health insurance purchasing cooperatives are large multistate networks or alliances that establish purchasing pools responsible for negotiating health insurance arrangements for employers, employees, and state Medicaid recipients. These alliances use the sheer volume of health consumers that they represent as leverage to negotiate contracts for health care coverage. Provider membership into the alliance is voluntary but exclusive. If the provider is located in an area in which the alliance is the predominant insurance plan, the provider is financially forced to join and accept the negotiated reimbursement.

Currently, insurance providers may offer the enrollee or consumer a wide variety of choices. Employers may specify the amount of money that will be contributed toward health care. The consumers may then customize their health care coverage, depending on their needs and willingness to pay. By picking the types of services they want covered and the provider of these services, the consumer has some control over his or her health care. The consumer assumes financial responsibility for the cost of any plan over the employer's contributing amount.

Reimbursement Mechanisms of Insurance Plans

The customary method of reimbursement has been a fee for the service rendered, or retrospective reimbursement. Calculation of the fee was based on the cost of providing the service. Included in this "umbrella" of costs were such things as salaries, supplies, equipment, building depreciation, utilities, and taxes. Cost-based reimbursement encouraged inflated prices and fraud. Physicians were encouraged to overtreat and the participant was encouraged to overuse the health care system. Soon, health care was costing Americans more than any other industrialized country. The health care system needed to be reformed, but there was no clear consensus on how this was to be accomplished (Higgins, 1997).

Prospective reimbursement, a concept derived from the HMO method of payment, seemed to be an effective financial alternative to cost-based reimbursement. Prospective reimbursement meant that care, no matter what the provider's cost, would be paid according to a predetermined amount. The government introduced this method of reimbursement for Medicare in 1983 and an immediate savings was noted. For determination of the prospective amount, Medicare depended on the **DRG** to calculate the reimbursement amount according to the client's primary and secondary diagnoses, age, gender, and complications. This amount was deemed sufficient for health care ascertained to be adequate for treatment (Higgins, 1997). If the provider, who was limited to hospitals at first, could provide the treatment below this amount, a profit was made. If the services required were delivered above this amount, then the provider took a loss. Hospitals developed **cost shifting,** another means of supplementing the loss of

Medicare funding. By 1983, Medicare paid $0.87 for each hospital dollar and the insurance provider paid $1.27 (Higgins, 1997).

To further reduce costs, hospitals looked at their largest expense, nursing care. Reductions in the number and the types of nurses followed. Staffing patterns changed from a staff of all RNs to just a few RNs supplemented with more LPNs, LVNs, or UAPs. Lengths of stay were shortened, giving an impetus for more outpatient services.

Other health care plans followed the government's lead. More sophisticated methods of calculating the relative cost of health care were developed. **Actuarial classifications** ensured that adequate **premiums** were charged for the projected health care needs of those enrolled. Managed care groups began to emerge and negotiated with health care providers to render care for a specified amount based on community ratings modified by group-specific demographics (Turner, 1999). Prospective reimbursement created incentives to undertreat and underuse the system. Soon, the public clamored for guarantees that the quality of care provided was being monitored as closely as the cost of care (Higgins, 1997).

Covered Services

Insurance plans have always designated the types of services for which the plan would be financially responsible as covered services. Usually these included such things as hospitalization at the rate of a semiprivate room, x-ray examinations and laboratory tests performed during the hospitalization, medications, and nursing care. As provision of insurance became incorporated into the employee fringe benefit package, the scope of covered services began to increase to such things as physician's office visits, medication, and dental costs. Unions began to negotiate for these expanded covered medical services in lieu of additional wages.

When health care costs increased, the price of enrollment into the insurance plans increased. Industries began to balk at paying these higher premium rates. Workers also became disgruntled when their employers passed these increased rates onto them. To curtail the escalating price, insurance companies began to limit the covered services and dictate the conditions under which these services would be covered. Many methods of treatment were required to be delivered outside the hospital, or in **ambulatory care** centers. As the patient was held financially responsible for "uncovered" services, substantial pressure was placed on health care providers to comply with these requirements. Providers began to modify the delivery of health care to accommodate for these changes.

Conflicts arise between providers, patients, and the insurance plans when services the consumer and provider believe are necessary, are denied insurance coverage. In some instances, the state governments have passed legislation mandating insurance coverage for certain services (Vermont Medical Round-table, 1999).

National Health Insurance

National health insurance is not a new concept. European countries began a social model of health insurance in the early 1900s. In 1916, President Theodore Roosevelt advocated enactment of a form of national medical coverage. President Franklin Roosevelt wanted national health insurance to be part of the Social Security Act of 1935 (Higgins, 1997). During the administration of President Lyndon Johnson, a modified form of national health insurance was instituted.

During the 1992 presidential campaign, Bill Clinton promised to reform America's health care system, ensure universal coverage, and reduce medical care costs without damaging the economy. According to Robert Shapiro (1993), basic health care coverage for all individuals could be achieved over several years. The necessary changes required by the current health care system are as follows:

- Consumers will have to bear more of the costs for their own choices and accept treatment from nonphysician providers.
- Health care businesses will have to become more efficient.
- Physicians will have to practice in HMO-type organizations.
- Politicians will have to resist appeals to add benefits to the basic coverage.

Unfortunately, most Americans want a guarantee that all of the medical services that they and their families need, now and in the future, will be available no matter what the medical condition, age of the patient, job status, or ability to pay. The current system is a $900 billion-per-year business and the price tag for this type of universal coverage would be astronomical (Shapiro, 1993).

ACCESS TO HEALTH CARE

Access to health care is a complex situation that is defined by the circumstances of the individual. The primary concern is inadequate access to health care, which leads to unnecessary illness (Gostin, 1994). As stated previously, most Americans want to feel that the best possible health care will be available at any time regardless of their age, sex, race, or ability to pay. Anything that obstructs this pursuit can be considered a barrier to the access of health care.

About 50% of Americans surveyed worry that they would be unable to finance a long illness (Himmilstein and Woodhandler, 1994). Delay in seeking health care or not following through with the recommended health care is most often associated with an inability to pay. Lack of insurance coverage, preexisting conditions, unapproved care, or nonparticipating physicians represent the most frequent factors attributed to difficulty in obtaining care (Weinick and Drilea, 1996). Within the past year, financial barriers have inhibited an estimated 40 million adults from obtaining needed medical care (Budetti and Shikles, 1999). About 300,000 people are refused care each year at hospital emergency rooms because they are uninsured or inadequately insured (Himmilstein and Woodhandler, 1994).

Other impediments to health care access are physical barriers, including structural inaccessibility, lack of appropriate equipment, or inability to communicate. North Carolina State University developed a universal design for health care providers, which would render their services handicap accessible. Some of these features include chairs for people who cannot sit, wheelchair scales, adjustable-height examination equipment, communication amplifiers, and the use of interpreter services. Inequality in the distribution of health care services represents another type of physical barrier. Transportation difficulty, conflict with work hours, and failure to provide services exemplify these types of physical barriers.

Even those with insurance coverage may be unable to locate "participating" health care providers (Weinick, Zuvekas, and Drilea, 1996). Rural areas and inner cities have been recognized as medically underserved for many years. Government incentives for increasing medical services in these areas have not solved the problem. Lack of transportation, either public or private, contributes to health care deprivation. Even when adequate transportation is available, the "office hours" tend to be the same as typical "work hours." Opportunities to seek health care during these work times, especially preventive health care, is often discouraged and sometimes forbidden.

Sociological barriers to health care access exist among the poor and ethnic Americans. When researching health care among the poor, Helen Burstin (1992) found that the major sociological risk factor for substandard care was lack of insurance. Poor outpatient diagnosis and treatment, increased use of emergency rooms for primary care, and reluctance to hospitalize were possible explanations. Ethnic Americans, although insured, are at risk for deprivation of services as guidelines and standards for determining the medical necessity of services are based on data derived from healthy European-American males. Application of restrictions derived from these data results in inadequate and unreliable health care for the poor and for ethnic Americans (Randall, 1994). Provision of ethnically sensitive health care is almost nonexistent.

Universal Coverage

The United States uses more of the gross national product (GNP) for health care than any other industrialized county, but it ranks only seventh in the world with regard to the health of the population. Even though about $2700 is spent on health care per year per person, not everyone in the United States receives health care (Himmilstein and Woodhandler, 1994). Currently, one in seven people in the United States is without basic health care (Shapiro, 1993).

Medicare and the expanded eligibility of Medicaid have brought about national health insurance coverage for older adults, the disabled, and those living below the poverty level. With these advances toward universal coverage, a new genre of uninsured has emerged (i.e., the working poor). According to the Commonwealth Fund 1999 National Survey of Workers' Health Insurance, 32% of workers with annual incomes less than $32,000 were uninsured. About 42% of workers with incomes below $20,000 and 20% with incomes between $20,000 and $30,000 responded that their employer did not offer a health care plan. Of this group, 25% were reported to be in fair or poor health and 37% admitted to going without needed medical care because they lacked resources.

The current dilemma is how to provide affordable health care at a level acceptable to the American public. Other countries provide their citizens with universal health care, but the consequences of this, such as waiting several months for nonemergent treatment, are probably not acceptable to most Americans. No successful solution to the problem of escalating health care costs exists.

COST CONTAINMENT

Costs have to be controlled to meet the public's demand for unlimited health care. This is known as **cost containment**. Numerous attempts have been made over the years, but none have been more than marginally successful.

Historical Perspectives of Cost Containment

By the late 1970s, the government realized its mistake. The political compromise necessary for passage of Medicare and Medicaid had resulted in a health care explosion. Hospitals were reimbursed at cost plus 2%, physicians received reimbursement for inflated fees, and private insurance companies were paid to process Medicare and Medicaid claims. All of this led to an unprecedented increase in use and escalation of health care costs (Higgins, 1997).

The first attempts at institution of cost containment were directed at curtailing unnecessary proliferation of medical technology. Health care providers were required to demonstrate a community necessity or a CON for additional services. This information was then presented to a CON board, who made the decision of need. If deemed necessary, the project progressed. These boards were soon rendered impotent by political pressures.

To further reduce use, hospitalization records were reviewed for the appropriateness of care provided. Peer standard review organizations (PSRO) were made up of physicians whose purpose was to prevent unnecessary stays in the hospital by reviewing the hospital records and counseling the attending physician about the unwarranted services.

Both of these efforts proved ineffective. In 1970, medical care represented 7% of the GNP. By 1990, 14% of the GNP was devoted to medical care (Shapiro, 1993). The only effective means of controlling costs were rate regulation or price control, which limited flexibility to account for the patient's condition acuity adjustment. Prospective payment based on DRGs was the effective compromise.

The cost reduction, as a result of prospective payment, gave rise to the managed care revolution. Price competition became the new health care dynamic. Health care plans began to negotiate for the best value for their premiums. Health care providers were forced to be cost efficient. By 1995, 70% of U.S. workers were enrolled in some type of managed health care. In the early 1990s, health care spending increases dropped to the lowest level in 30 years and many credit the managed care phenomenon for this reduction (Shapiro, 1993).

Current Trends in Cost Containment

The managed care form of health care financing changes economic incentives, which forces health care providers to rethink medical management decisions. Costs of the service rendered rather than enhancement of revenue through service provision must be considered. These economic incentives can be divided into the following broad categories: capitated reimbursement, access limitation, and rationing.

Capitated Reimbursement

The increasing visibility of HMOs and their associated success with the use of reimbursement to influence provider practice gave rise to various arrangements that link health care financing to service delivery or managed care. MCOs create partnerships with health care providers using financial incentives to prevent overuse. Statistical norms, practice parameters, and population data determine the capitated payment. Health care providers must provide appropriate medical care while being cognizant of medical costs. As a reward for conservative medical practices, health care providers may receive a specified amount of money or a percentage of the agreed reimbursement if services are delivered below the limit set by the third party payer (Vermont Medical Roundtable, 1999). Providers whose services exceed this limit are excluded from the network.

Cost Containment through Access Limitation

All third-party payers, or insurance plans, control access to health care through designation of covered services. **Managed care plans** designate the type of covered services and specify the conditions under which the service is covered. Some services may only be accessed upon approval or referral from physicians who are used as a **gatekeeper.** The enrollee must consult his or her **primary care provider** before seeking specialty services. Without this referral, the enrollee is financially responsible for the service.

Even with the referral, choices may be limited to the providers who have contracted with the managed care plan.

Managed care plans may require that less costly health care modalities or medications be used. More technologically advanced and expensive treatment modalities may be accessed under the most stringent conditions. Preauthorization requirements determine the medical necessity of the service. The process is so complex that the client may not be aware that the service is not covered until the reimbursement for the service is denied.

Cost Containment through Rationing

Rationing of health care is particularly distasteful to the public. Dr. David Eddy eloquently stated that health care deals with "the ultimate issues of human existence: life versus death, peace versus suffering and discomfort, function versus dysfunction" (Vermont Medical Roundtable, 1999). Every developing nation has various mechanisms in place that ensures inability to pay does not prevent receipt of health care.

Rationing is best described as determining the most appropriate use of health care or directing the health care where it can do the most good. The following case dramatizes the problem:

> A middle-age woman was diagnosed with ovarian cancer. After conventional and high-dose chemotherapy failed, her physician recommended an autologous bone marrow transplant, which was considered experimental at the time. The procedure was approved and performed. Medical costs exceeded $200,000, but the patient died two months later.

Health care is not an exact science; too many variables exist. What appears to be the best course of action for one is not the best course of action for another. Therefore making these decisions accurately is difficult and the ramifications of a mistake are great. Health care providers and third-party payers, including the federal government, are currently investigating the **outcomes** of health care practices to determine what methods, if any, can be instituted to improve the accuracy of these choices.

CARING FOR THE UNINSURED

More than 43 million Americans are uninsured. People under 65 years of age who were uninsured were 38% more likely to lack a usual source of health care and more than twice as likely to experience difficulty or delay in receiving needed medical care. Lack of insurance is the major factor associated with lack of access to medical care (Weinick, Zuvekas, and Drilea, 1996). Uninsured adults are more than three times as likely to go without needed medical care than those insured. By 2007, up to 54 million people or more may be uninsured.

Historical Perspective

Before the 1930s, most Americans were uninsured. Most health care providers considered it their duty to donate time and services to charity. Hospitals and clinics maintained charity wards. Society believed that those who could, and those who could not, should help themselves. The enactment of governmental entitlement programs changed this belief. Quickly the feeling was that those who could not help themselves should get government assistance (Higgins, 1997).

Societal Perceptions

Social justice, or equal medical care for all, is a concept that the American public thinks they embrace. Most people state that health care should be one of those necessities available to all without cost. However, when asked if they would agree to finance this unlimited health care through higher taxes, the answer is a resounding no (Himmilstein and Woodhandler, 1994). Managed care has curtailed escalating health care costs by diminishing and limiting use. The public perceives this limitation as diminished quality of care although no clear body of evidence exists to support this concern (Vermont Medical Roundtable, 1999). Considering the needs of the individuals and the community, health care is currently distributed through the fairest and just means available.

Ethical Dilemmas

Economics and technological advances have presented health care providers with the ethical dilemma of allocation of health care. An ethical act is one that leads to the greatest benefit for the most people and increases the self-esteem of the person performing the act. Changes and shifts in the population have added a strain on the nation's limited health care resources (Klainberg et al., 1998).

Concern over possible changes in the basic goal of equal health care for all has prompted the creation of the *Consumer Bill of Rights and Responsibilities* of

health care. Created by the President's Advisory Commission (1997), the goals of this document are as follows:

- To strengthen consumer confidence by ensuring that the health care system is fair and responsive to consumer needs
- To reaffirm the importance of a strong relationship between patients and their health care providers
- To reaffirm the consumer's role in safeguarding his or her health

TRENDS IN HEALTH FINANCING

The public's demand for affordable health care has created a new environment for health care financing. Competition among health care providers and third-party payers has led to new and innovative health care. Increased competition has required insurance plans to be sensitive to the needs of the employee organizations and its enrollees. Individualized plans of covered services can be created. Health care providers are advertising to ensure that the consumer selects an insurance plan in which their services are included.

Cost Sharing

Aware of the amount that the employer is willing to contribute for basic coverage, a third-party payer may propose several options, giving the employee freedom to choose services desired. Employees willing to pay may be able to increase the covered services not provided by the basic plan. Cost sharing may also require the consumer to pay a portion of the bill for covered services in return for lower premiums. This can result in increased consumer control of health care.

Health Care Alliances

The creation of powerful regional or statewide insurance purchasing pools or health alliances is seen as one means of reform for the health care industry. The alliance would define basic benefits that all insurers would have to offer to everyone at the same price despite their health status. These alliances would be chartered to not regulate insurance prices. Health alliances would collect premiums and help consumers choose among competing insurers and plans. The consumer's choice would be based on published simple standard information about benefits and outcomes of the different available plans. Plans would have to compete by offering better outcomes or less cost. Insurers would have to contract with providers that find ways of delivering cost-efficient care (Shapiro, 1993).

Self-Insurance

Some organizations have used health care information collected by insurance plans to self-insure their employees. This has enabled organizations to reduce the administrative cost of insurance, which has been estimated to represent 12.5% of the cost of insurance (Himmilstein and Woodhandler, 1994). Unlike the large industrial HMOs, self-insured status organizations administer their own health care plan but purchase health care services from an established insurance plan.

Flexible Spending Accounts

Another source of funding for uncovered services is the **flexible spending account** (FSA). The employee determines how much he or she will have to spend for uncovered services and has this much deducted from his or her paycheck. When these services are incurred, the employee can secure payment for these services from this account. The employee continues to pay into the account until the estimated amount is reached. If the employee overestimates the cost, the remaining amount is forfeited. If the cost of the services exceeds the estimate, only the amount estimated will be paid.

SUMMARY

Health care economics is influencing health care practice at all levels. Nurses must become aware of the economics of health care to practice in this new era. Patient outcomes are quickly being seen as a measurement for health care financing. As the health care system evolves toward health promotion and disease prevention, nursing will play a pivotal role. Community health nurses, whose domain of practice has encompassed these areas, will be in the forefront of this change.

This chapter has presented the basics of health care economics. An understanding of these elements is essential for the practice of nursing. This is an ever-changing field with new innovations and changes coming every day. To be effective, the nurse must be attentive to these developments.

LEARNING ACTIVITIES

1. Create a health care system including services, eligible recipients, funding resources, and qualifying requirements for these services.
2. Evaluate a family's health care coverage. Investigate the type of coverage and the ability of this coverage type to meet the needs of the family. Is there another type of insurance coverage that would meet more of the family's needs and what prohibits their ability to obtain this coverage?
3. Investigate health care reform from the point of view of the consumer, health care provider, and third-party payer. How would a change in the current health care system affect each of these concerns?
4. Interview representatives from health care provider groups, insurance plans, and consumer groups regarding their suggestions for health care reform.

REFERENCES

Budetti J, Shikles J: Can't afford to get sick: a reality for millions of working Americans. In *1999 national survey of workers' health insurance,* Washington DC, 1999, The Commonwealth Fund.

Burstin H: Socioeconomic status and risk of substandard medical care, *JAMA* 2383:268, 1992.

Gostin L: Securing health or just health care? the effects of the health care system on the health of America, 39 St. Louis, 1994.

Higgins W: How did we get this way? *Health Care Economics* 11:35, 1997.

Himmilstein D, Woodhandler S: *Paying for health care: the National Health Program book,* Monroe, Maine, 1994, Common Courage Press.

Klainberg M et al: *Community health nursing: an alliance for health,* New York, 1998, McGraw-Hill.

President's Advisory Commission on Consumer Quality in the Health Care Industry: *Consumer bill of rights and responsibilities,* Washington, DC, 1997, US Government Printing Office.

Randall V: Racist health care: reforming an unjust health care system to meet the needs of African-Americans, *Health Matrix* 127, 1994.

Shapiro R: Health care reform and the laws of economics, *Policy Briefing,* July 16, 1993.

Turner SO: *The nurse's guide to managed care,* Gaithersburg, Md, 1999, Aspen.

Vermont Medical Roundtable: *Can we have it all? balancing access, quality and cost in health care,* Montpelier, Vt, 1999, Vermont Business Roundtable: Healthcare Task Force.

Weinick R, Drilea S: Usual sources of health care and barriers to care, AHCPR Pub. No. 98-R024, *Statistical Bulletin,* 1996.

Weinick R, Zuvekas S, Drilea S: Access to health care in America, AHCPR Pub. No. 98-001, *Sources and Barriers,* 1996.

Policy, Politics, Legislation, and Community Health Nursing

Cecilia M. Tiller and Melanie McEwen

OBJECTIVES

Upon completion of this chapter, the reader will be able to do the following:

1. Describe the philosophical and historical foundations of government.
2. Identify the legislative process involved in establishing state or federal health policy.
3. Identify the social and political processes that influence health policy development.
4. Discuss current health policy issues, including restructuring of the health care system, patient safety, quality, accountability, and effective use of nurses.
5. Discuss nurses' roles in political activities.

KEY TERMS

Achieving Access for All Americans
administrative law
Clara Barton
coalition
Florence Nightingale
government
health policy
Hill-Burton Act
interstate nursing practice
institutional policies
judicial law
Lavinia Dock
Lillian Wald
lobby
Margaret Sanger
nursing policy
organizational policies
policy
policy analysis
political action committee (PAC)
politics
public accountability
public health law
public policies
Sojourner Truth
statutory law

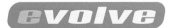

http://evolve.elsevier.com/Nies/

The health care delivery system, including nursing practice, is profoundly influenced by policies set by government and private entities. Nurses must understand the system of health policy development and implementation to effectively interpret and influence policies that affect nursing practice and the health of individuals, families, groups, and communities.

The more an individual knows about the political process, the more he or she tends to become involved. Individual nurses may become politically active on a local, state, or national level or they may work collectively within groups such as the ANA or their state nurses association (SNA) to lobby for health causes. All nurses should be encouraged to become change agents, develop active political roles, and mentor younger nurses into the political arena. With united efforts, nurses can influence political figures to make changes to the health care system that are beneficial to all.

INTRODUCTION TO HEALTH POLICY AND THE POLITICAL PROCESS

Politics and legislation are processes through which health policies are instituted. Policy, politics, and legislation are the forces that determine the direction of health programs at every level of government. These programs are critical to the health and well-being of the nation and of every individual. This chapter addresses the interrelationships of these processes and outlines the importance of nurses' continual efforts to maintain and improve the health of individuals, groups, and communities.

Definitions

Policy denotes a course of action to be followed by a government or institution to obtain a desired end (Bonick, 2000). Policy reflects values and encompasses the choices that a society, segment of society, or organization makes regarding goals and priorities and the criteria used to allocate resources (Leavitt and Mason, 1998). Furthermore, policy involves the application of reason and evidence to problem solving in public and private settings (Helms, Anderson, and Hanson, 1996).

Politics, in contrast, is defined as the art of influencing others to accept a specific course of action (Bonick, 2000). It is a process by which an individual exerts control over situations and events (Leavitt and

Mason, 1998). In general, politics constitutes a means and policy is the end or outcome (Helms, Anderson, and Hanson, 1996). All policies are shaped by politics and reflect social values, beliefs, and attitudes (Leavitt and Mason, 1998).

Public policies are authoritative decisions made in the legislative, executive, or judicial branch of government intended to direct or influence the actions, behaviors, or decisions of others (Shi and Singh, 1998). Public policies are intended to serve the interests of the public as a whole. **Health policy** refers to public policies that pertain to or influence the pursuit of health, or a course of action to obtain a desired health outcome for an individual, family, group, community, or society (Bonick, 2000; Shi and Singh, 1998). **Nursing policy** can be viewed independently as its own policy sector or as a subset within the larger health policy arena.

Public health law consists of legislation, regulations, and court decisions enacted by governments at the federal, state, and local levels to protect the public's health (Brooke, 2000). According to Hanlon and Pickett (1984), public health law exists by the authority of the U.S. Constitution to promote the general welfare of society.

Institutional policies govern work sites and identify the institution's goals, operation, and treatment of employees. **Organizational policies** are rules that govern organizations and their positions on issues with which the organization is concerned (Leavitt and Mason, 1998).

HISTORICAL FOUNDATIONS OF HEALTH LEGISLATION AND POLICY

In the United States, the government has been involved in efforts to improve or maintain the health of citizens since the late 1700s. As a result, over the past two centuries, federal, state, and local initiatives, laws, and organizations have fostered significant improvements in the health and life expectancy of Americans. However, the strength and focus of health policy efforts from the federal level were largely imparted during the latter part of the twentieth century.

One of the earliest pieces of comprehensive health care legislation was the Hill-Burton Hospital Construction Act, which was passed during the Truman administration in 1946 (Shi and Singh, 1998). The **Hill-Burton Act** provided grants to states for the construction of new hospitals, targeting low-income and rural areas (Dowling, 1999). Two decades later, President Johnson's terms in office marked a time of dramatic growth in federal health policy, highlighted by the passage of Medicare and Medicaid in 1965. This landmark legislation strengthened the government's role in the health care system and dramatically shaped its rapid growth.

During the 1970s, the Nixon administration tried to shift emphasis in health policy issues to state and local agencies by combining local initiatives with policy input and national standards. In Nixon's presidential term, two important pieces of health legislation were passed. The HMO Act was passed in 1973 and required employers to offer an HMO alternative to conventional health insurance. The National Health Planning and Resources Development Act of 1974 required states to obtain a CON for new hospital construction and modernization projects, including technology, to procure federal funding (Shi and Singh, 1998). During this period, many of the federal responsibilities for a uniform, cooperative national public health system were removed and individual states were expected to assume those responsibilities.

The federal government's involvement in public health services revived when Ronald Reagan took office in 1980. In response to the alarming inflation of health care costs under Reagan, new Medicare cost-control approaches for hospitals and physicians (e.g., DRGs) were created (Shi and Singh, 1998; Sultz and Young, 1999).

In the early 1990s, the public was anxious for reform and President Clinton's administration worked diligently to set up a national health policy. This attempt to bring about national health insurance was the first since Truman's initiatives to provide nationally sponsored health coverage for all Americans in the late 1940s. However, like Truman's, Clinton's policy initiative was not successful.

As a result, health care insurance costs and coverage have worsened. A 1997 report indicated that the number of people under 65 years of age who have private insurance dropped from 75% in 1989 to 71% in 1995, a 5.3% change. Children are more likely to be uninsured than adults. Children's coverage dropped from 73% to 66%, a 9.6% reduction, during that period (Smith, 1997). The lack of coordinated government influence, coupled with the decline in insurance coverage, has increased the emphasis on managed care. Reductions in federal payments for health care have resulted in even more Americans being unable to obtain care.

The publication of *Healthy People 2000* in 1990 led to a resurgence of interest by the federal government in the welfare of Americans. However, fiscal resources for public health interventions continued to decline and only marginal progress was made in meeting the goals. In early 2000, *Healthy People 2010* marked the beginning of the new millennium and an enhanced focus on population-based health promotion strategies. Many *Healthy People 2010* objectives directly or indirectly involve health policy. Virtually all of the areas have multiple policy-related objectives and Table 11-1 lists only a few of them. New objectives for the new century are to see a reduction in health disparities among groups and witness even greater improvements in the health of all Americans.

NURSES WHO MADE A DIFFERENCE

The significance of nurses' involvement in influencing health policy is not new. Many nurses in the past and present have been instrumental in working with legislation and politics. A few exemplary nurse heroines who illustrate this point follow:

- **Florence Nightingale** was the first nurse to exert political pressure on a government (Hall-Long, 1995). She transformed military health and knew the value of data in influencing policy. Even after she became ill, policymakers consulted her. She was a leader who knew how to use the support of followers, colleagues, and policymakers.
- **Sojourner Truth** became an ardent and eloquent advocate for abolishing slavery and supporting women's rights. Her words helped transform the racist and sexist policies that limited the health and well-being of African-Americans and women. She fought for human rights and lobbied for federal funds to train nurses and physicians (Leavitt and Mason, 1998).
- **Clara Barton** was responsible for organizing relief efforts during the U.S. Civil War. In 1882, she successfully persuaded Congress to ratify the Treaty of Geneva, which allowed the Red Cross to perform humanitarian efforts in times of peace. This organization has had a lasting influence on national and international policies (Hall-Long, 1995; Kalisch and Kalisch, 1995).
- **Lavinia Dock** was a prolific writer and political activist. She waged a campaign for legislation to allow nurses to control the nursing profession instead of physicians. In 1893, with

TABLE 11-1

Selected *Healthy People 2010 Objectives* Related to Public Policy

Objective	Baseline	Goal
6-8: Eliminate disparities in employment rates between working-age adults with and without disabilities.	52%	82%
7-4: Increase the proportion of the nation's elementary, middle or junior, and senior high schools that have a nurse-to-student ratio of at least 1:750.	34%	50%
8-5: Increase the proportion of people served by a community water system who receive a supply of drinking water that meets the regulations of the Safe Drinking Water Act.	73%	95%
8-23: Reduce the proportion of occupied housing units that are substandard.	6.2%	3%
13-8: Increase the proportion of substance abuse treatment facilities that offer HIV and AIDS education, counseling, and support.	58%	70%
14-23: Maintain vaccination coverage levels for children in licensed day care facilities and children in kindergarten through first grade.	93% to 97%	95%
15-10: Increase the number of states and the District of Columbia with statewide emergency department surveillance systems that collect data on external cause of injury.	12 states	50 states and DC
15-22: Increase the number of states and the District of Columbia that have adopted a graduated driver licensing model law.	23 states	50 states and DC
15-24: Increase the number of states and the District of Columbia with laws requiring bicycle helmets for bicycle riders.	11 states	50 states and DC
16-20: Ensure appropriate newborn bloodspot screening, follow-up testing, and referral services.	NA	NA
21-9: Increase the proportion of the population served by community water systems with optimally fluoridated water.	11 states	50 states
25-13: Increase the proportion of STD programs that routinely offer hepatitis B vaccination to all STD clients.	5%	90%
26-24: Extend legal requirements for maximum blood alcohol concentration levels of 0.08% for motor vehicle drivers 21 years of age and older.	16 states	50 states and DC
26-26: Extend administrative license revocation laws or programs of equal effectiveness for people who drive under the influence of intoxicants.	41 states	50 states and DC
27-11: Increase smoke-free and tobacco-free environments in schools, including all school facilities, property, vehicles, and school events.	37%	100%
27-13: Establish laws on smoke-free indoor air that prohibit smoking or limit it to separately ventilated areas in public places and work sites.	13% work sites 3% restaurants 16% public transportation	51%
27-21: Increase the average federal and state tax on tobacco products.	$0.63 cigarettes $0.27 smokeless tobacco	$2.00
28-11: Increase the proportion of newborns who are screened for hearing loss by one month of age, have audiologist evaluation by three months of age, and are enrolled in appropriate intervention services by six months of age.	NA	NA

From U.S. Department of Health and Human Services: *Healthy people 2010,* Conference edition, Washington, DC, 2000, The Author.

the assistance of Isabel Hampton Robb and Mary Adelaide Nutting, she founded the politically active organization, the American Society of Superintendents of Training School for Nurses, which later became the National League for Nursing (NLN) (Kalisch and Kalisch, 1995). She was also active in the suffrage movement, advocating that nurses support the woman's right to vote (Lewinson, 1998).

■ **Lillian Wald's** political activism and vision were shaped by feminist values. Working in the early 1900s, she recognized the connections between health and social conditions. She was a driving force behind the federal government's development of the Children's Bureau in 1912. Wald appeared frequently at the White House to participate in the development of national and international policy (Leavitt and Mason, 1998).

■ **Margaret Sanger** was a nurse-activist who transformed the nation's attitudes and approaches to family planning. Her actions and political voice spoke out for women and the need for birth control. Despite legal opposition and frequently intense criticism, in 1916 she opened the first birth control clinic in the United States in Brooklyn. She continued her crusade for many decades, giving lectures and organizing meetings. In 1928, she founded the National Committee on Federal Legislation for Birth Control, which was a forerunner of Planned Parenthood (Kalisch and Kalisch, 1995; Leavitt and Mason, 1998).

STRUCTURE OF THE GOVERNMENT OF THE UNITED STATES

Government is broadly defined as the exercise of political authority, direction, and restraint over the actions of inhabitants of communities, societies, or states. Government is crucial to human interdependence and the concomitant necessity for cooperative action. Among its purposes are regulation of conditions beyond individual control and provision of individual protection through a population-wide focus. These tasks are accomplished through passage and enforcement of laws, regulations, and policies. Requirements of childhood immunizations for school attendance, vector control, and sewage treatment are examples of government activities and policies to protect the health of the population.

The delineation of the government's responsibility for health in the United States evolved from statements of policy that express the values of the founders of the country. These statements have been issued in a series of historic documents. The earliest was the Mayflower Compact, through which the Pilgrims committed themselves to making "just and equal laws" for the general good. The Declaration of Independence later established the doctrine of inalienable rights, life, liberty, and the pursuit of happiness. The U.S. Constitution, the foundation of national democracy and the supreme law of the land, established the responsibilities of the federal government, including the responsibility to promote the general welfare. The following year, the first 10 amendments to the Constitution, known as the Bill of Rights, ensured the sovereignty of the states in all areas not constitutionally reserved for the federal government. The Bill of Rights also emphasizes specific individual freedoms.

States retain powers not delegated to the federal government; therefore much of public health law is under state jurisdiction and, as a result, varies considerably among states. In the United States, legislative activities of the three levels of government (federal, state, and local) may vary greatly in their expectations, actions, and results. The state legislatures, for the most part, are directly involved in health care, yet the federal government influences health policy, directly and indirectly, through financing of health care for many groups (e.g., Medicare), regulation activities (e.g., approval of drugs), and setting of standards (e.g., air quality).

Intermediary policies have developed to provide more specific guidance to government in its daily operations. Some of these policies have been explicitly declared and some have been implied through programs or other activities. An *implicit policy* basic to public health is that the right to health of the majority must be preserved over individual freedoms. For example, a corporation may not dump hazardous waste into a river that is a source of drinking water for a community; the welfare of the people must prevail over short-term corporate profits. Another example is local or regional efforts to prevent the sale of tobacco or alcohol to minors. Again, this is a policy that implicitly serves to protect health.

Balance of Powers

As described previously, the three basic levels of government in the United States are federal, state, and

TABLE **11-2**

Comparison of Statutory Law, Administrative Law, and Judicial Law

Type of Law	Source	Characteristics	Activities	Examples
Statutory law	Legislative branch	Prohibits or declares as lawful certain behaviors or actions	Sets state and federal laws (i.e., statutes) and local laws (i.e., ordinances)	Social Security Act; state nurse practice acts; city ordinance against smoking in public places
Administrative law	Administrative branch	Consists of orders, rules, and regulations set by administrative bodies (e.g., regulatory agencies [state boards], government agencies [CDC, HCFA, local health department])	Defines policies and procedures; sets rules and guidelines	Conditions of participation in Medicare; notifiable communicable diseases; pediatric immunization schedule
Judicial or common law	Court decisions	Based on case precedents	Interprets laws and statutes	Malpractice cases; product liability rulings; informed consent cases; supervisory liability

Adapted from Brooke PS: Legal context for community health nursing practice. In Smith CM, Maurer FA, editors: *Community health nursing: theory and practice,* ed 2, Philadelphia, 2000, W.B. Saunders; Leavitt JK, Mason DJ: *Policy and politics in nursing and health care,* Philadelphia, 1998, W.B. Saunders.

local. Each level has a legislative, executive, and judicial branch and each may be the source of health law and health policy (Brooke, 2000). The three branches of government enact different types of law. The legislative branch enacts **statutory law**, the administrative branches set **administrative law**, and court decisions determine **judicial law**, or common law (Brooke, 2000). Table 11-2 compares these three basic types of law.

Decisions affecting the public's health are made not only at every level of government, but also in each branch. The separation of powers is as important to health as it is to the economic or military status of the country. Box 11-1 describes checks and balances for immunization requirements.

The legislative branch (i.e., Congress at the federal level and the legislature, general assembly, or general court at the state level) enacts the statutory laws that are the basis for governance. The executive branch administers and enforces the laws, which are broad in scope, through regulatory agencies. These agencies, in turn, define more specific implementation of the statutes through rules and regulations (i.e.,

BOX **11-1**

Checks and Balances on Immunization Requirements

Immunization requirements for school attendance are an example of the checks and balances among the three branches of government. To protect the public welfare, most state legislatures have passed laws mandating that all primary school children be immunized against certain communicable diseases. The appropriate executive agency, usually the state health department, develops the regulations through which the law is implemented and enforced. The legislative branch has no further power over the administration of the law except to change it when necessary through amendment or repeal. The few parents who object to their children being immunized have recourse through the judicial system to have the law waived in their case.

regulatory or administrative law). The judiciary body provides protection against oppressive governance and against professional malpractice, fraud, and abuse. Its function, through the courts, is to determine the constitutionality of laws, interpret them, and decide on their legitimacy when they are challenged. The courts also have jurisdiction over specific infractions of laws and regulations.

OVERVIEW OF HEALTH POLICY

As mentioned previously, *public policy* refers to decisions made by legislative, executive, or judicial branches of one of the three levels of government (i.e., local, state, or federal). These decisions are intended to direct or influence actions, behaviors, or decisions of others. When public policy addresses health issues, it is *health policy.* Health policies influence health care through monitoring, production, provision, and financing of health care services. Virtually everyone, from providers (e.g., physicians, nurses, pharmacists, and dentists) to consumers are affected by health policies. Likewise, health policy influences organizations, such as insurers, medical schools, HMOs, nursing homes, producers of medical equipment and technologies, and employers.

Health policies are developed, regulated, and enforced at all of the three levels of government. Furthermore, policies vary with the population, location, and level of government (Shi and Sing, 1998). In addition to the public policy-making sector, health policies can also be made through the private sector. For example, an insurance company or employer will determine such matters as what illnesses will be covered by the insurance program, what drugs will be included in a formulary, and how much to charge for coverage.

Policies can be used as regulatory tools to prescribe and control the behavior of a specific group. An example is the federally funded peer review organizations (PROs), which develop and enforce standards for care received under Medicare programs. Health policies may also be used as allocative tools in that they direct provision or delivery of income, services, or goods. Examples of allocative support include subsidies for providers to deliver care to older adults, the poor, or veterans; construction of facilities through the Hill-Burton program; development of personnel (e.g., primary care physicians or NPs) by financing education; creation of HMOs; and production and dissemination of knowledge (e.g., through the numerous research programs of the NIH).

PUBLIC POLICY: BLUEPRINT FOR GOVERNANCE

Policy is directed by values. It articulates the guiding principles of collective endeavors, establishes direction, and sets goals. It influences and, in turn, is influenced by politics. Through the political process, policy directives may become realized or obstructed at any step along the way.

Policy Formulation: The Ideal

In ideal circumstances, authorized authoritative bodies (e.g., state health departments, OSHA, HCFA, and a fiscal oversight subcommittee) rationally determine actions to create, amend, implement, or rescind health care policy. These groups would decide what is right or best and then develop the political strategies to affect the desired outcomes. The question of whether a particular policy is advocated or adopted would depend on the degree that a group or the society as a whole may benefit without harm or detriment to subgroups. Of all the seemingly limitless factors that may influence policy formation, group need and group demand should be the strongest determinants. The premises supporting the goals of health policy should be equitable distribution of services and the ensurance that the appropriate care is given to the right people, at the right time, and at a reasonable cost.

Policy Formulation: The Real World

In the "real world," policy for health care exemplifies both conflict and social change theories. Health policy is the product of continuous interactive processes in which interested professionals, citizens, institutions, industries, and other groups compete with one another for the attention of various branches of government. The most obvious and prominent among these is the legislative branch, although policy is also made through executive orders, regulatory mechanisms, and court decisions as described previously. Health policy may also issue from the recommendations of fact-finding commissions established by the legislative or executive branch.

Health policy is rarely created through discrete, momentous determinations in relation to single problems or issues. It often evolves slowly and incrementally as an accumulation of many small decisions. It also changes slowly because changes in the social beliefs and values that underlie established policy develop within the context of actual service delivery. Once a direct health care service is offered, especially an official tax-funded service, it is often difficult to discontinue it. Existing programs create tradition by establishing vested interest and a sense of entitlement on the part of the public. This tradition also exerts political influence in a natural effort for self-preservation.

Steps in Policy Formulation

The tangible formulation of public policy begins with the most critical step, which is defining the problem and placing it on the agenda. The next step is the commitment of resources, most often, through the passage of legislation. A regulatory schedule for the implementation of the law into program is formulated. Then an evaluation process is designed that satisfies regulatory and legislative remedies should they be needed.

Policy Analysis

Analysis of health policy is an objective process that identifies the sources and consequences of policy decisions in the context of the factors that influence them. Health **policy analysis** determines those who benefit and those who experience a loss as the result of a policy (Fig. 11-1). These considerations are

FIGURE **11-1**

Policy analysis model (Redrawn from Spradley B: *Community health nursing,* ed 2, Boston, 1985, Little, Brown).

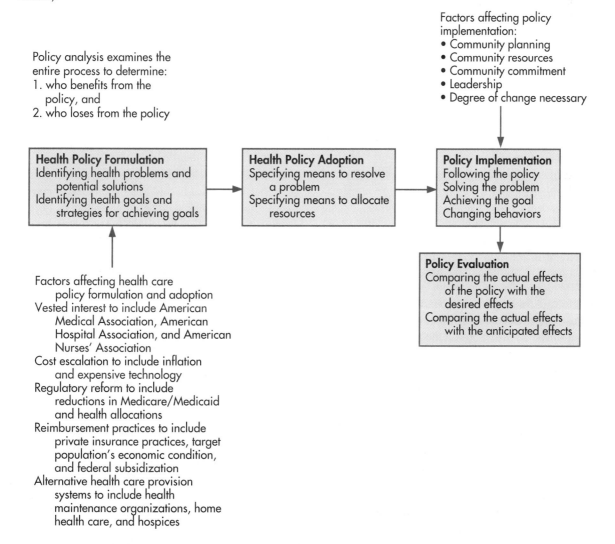

**Policy Analysis: Immunization
Recommendations vs. Vaccine Costs**

In February 2000 the CDC's Advisory Committee on Immunization Practices (ACIP) met to debate a recommendation on the addition of Prevenar, a vaccine to enhance immunity against pneumococcal bacteria, which causes most cases of meningitis, pneumonia, blood poisoning, and ear infections, to the routine pediatric immunization schedule. The major concern against the policy was the cost—$232 for the four-dose series. If added, Prevenar would cost as much as all other childhood vaccinations combined.

Currently the federal government pays for half of all childhood immunizations in the United States. As manufacturers have targeted less-severe illnesses, policy makers have been forced to debate whether the cure is worth the cost. Because the FDA is only concerned with whether a vaccine is safe and effective, the ACIP must determine whether a vaccine is worth the price.

From Vaccine's price drives a debate about its use, *Wall Street Journal*, Feb. 16, 2000.

critical to ensure health policies that are fair to all those affected.

President Clinton's attempt to reform health care in the mid1990s reflected ethical and practical considerations for a national health policy. The fundamental principle was access to health care for all Americans. Those benefiting would be the American public, as consumers of health care and payers for health care, through tax-supported insurance programs. The opposition consisted of those envisioning major financial losses from the proposed changes. Among these, the insurance industry was a dominant antagonist, with some provider groups joining the opposition forces. The public was confused by the complexity of the issues and wary of change. This effort to make an overdue change in health care policy eventually failed.

Recently policy analysis has begun to place even more attention on economic issues in health care. For example, proposed changes in Medicare to add coverage for prescription medications was stalled by concerns over the massive increase in costs. Box 11-2

presents another example in which the addition of a vaccine to the recommended childhood immunization schedule was modified over cost concerns.

GOVERNMENT AUTHORITY FOR THE PROTECTION OF THE PUBLIC'S HEALTH

The authority for the protection of the public's health is largely vested with the states and most state constitutions specifically delineate this responsibility. Municipal subdivisions of states, such as counties, cities, or towns, usually have the power of local control of the services conferred by the state legislature (Fig. 11-2).

The responsibility of local, state, and federal governments for health services under varying conditions sometimes complicates attempts to determine the locus of political decision making. The supremacy of the state prevails in most situations; therefore the state is a critical arena for political action. An example is the state's authority to license health professionals, such as nurses and physicians, and health care institutions, such as hospitals, nursing homes, and day care centers.

Each state establishes policies or standards for goods or services that influence the health of its citizens. However, several factors may affect that authority. For example, the standards for pasteurization of milk sold within a state are determined by that state, but if the milk is sold in another state, it comes under the interstate commerce jurisdiction of the federal government. This could mean that a higher standard must be met, which negates the state standard. Alternatively, when public health authority is delegated to political subdivisions within the state, they too may impose a standard that is higher, and never lower, than that of the state.

The federal government also has a strong influence on health services. Constitutionally, this authority is derived from the federal role in regulation of interstate commerce (e.g., meat inspection) and through broad interpretation of the general welfare clause (e.g., Medicare). States vary considerably in resources allocated to provide health programs; therefore significant de facto authority derives from the promise of revenues or threats to remove funding (e.g., funds for interstate highway repair are often tied to air quality). Federal funds fully or partially fund many of the programs discussed in this and other chapters.

FIGURE **11-2**

Mandate of powers (Redrawn from Bagwell M, Clements S: *A political handbook for health professionals,* Boston, 1985, Little, Brown).

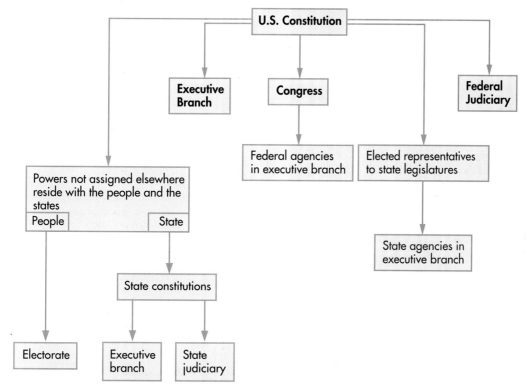

Compliance by states to federal program standards is voluntary, but the advantage of the revenue, which is withheld from the states if they do not comply, is seldom ignored. Programs such as control of STDs and the statistical reporting system are standardized across the country in response to the indirect but marked effect of federal funding.

THE LEGISLATIVE PROCESS

How a Bill Becomes a Law

The procedure through which legislation must pass to eventually become law is similar for all U.S. legislative bodies. Once a concept has been drafted into legislative language, it becomes a bill, is given a number, and moves through a series of steps depicted in Fig. 11-3. The bill's passage is sometimes smooth, but more often than not the bill is extensively altered through amendments or even killed at various stages.

In Congress and in the 49 states that have a two-house legislature, a bill must succeed through the two legislative bodies, the House of Representatives, and the Senate. Nebraska, which has a single house legislature, is the exception. A bill that has moved successfully through the legislative process has one final hurdle, which is the chief executive's approval. The approval may be a clear endorsement, in which case the governor or president signs it. If the executive neither signs nor vetoes it, the bill may become law by default. An explicit veto conclusively kills the bill, which then can be revived only by a substantial vote of the legislature to override the veto. This is another example of the checks and balances of the government process (Smith, 1997).

Issues that find their way into the legislative arena are commonly controversial and proponents and opponents quickly align themselves. Defeating a bill is much easier than getting one passed; therefore the opposition always has the advantage. Health legislation, which usually requires preventive action (e.g.,

F I G U R E **11-3**

How a bill becomes a law at the federal level.

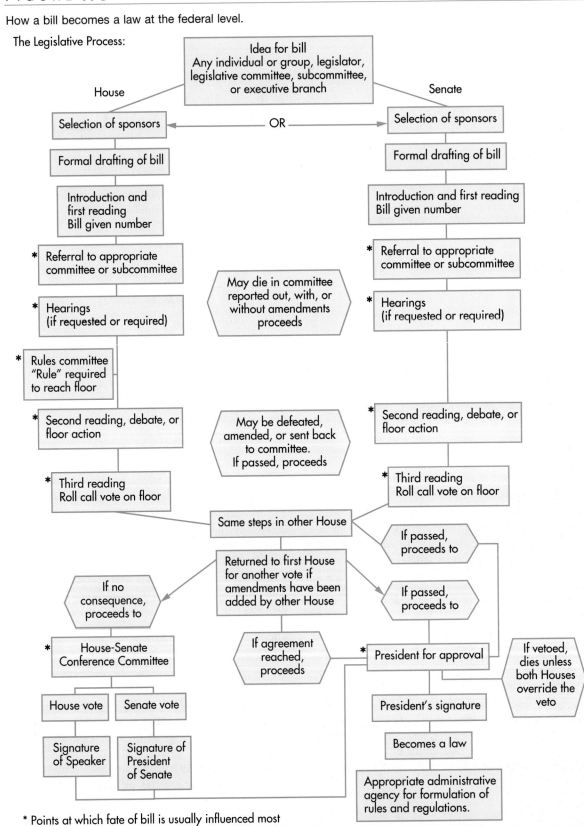

* Points at which fate of bill is usually influenced most

toxic waste management) or creates a new service (e.g., nursing center organizations for Medicare recipients), is at a disadvantage from several other standpoints.

Few elected officials are knowledgeable about the health care field. Although health is readily recognized as a national resource, it is not easily quantified into the economic terms that make the issue easy to grasp. Other disadvantages are the backgrounds, biases, and ambitions of each legislator. The decision to run for public office is often made in keeping with personal goals that are likely to differ from health values for the public good.

Despite these obstacles, good health laws can be passed when concerned nurses and other health care workers understand the legislative process and use it effectively. For nurses, this is yet another mode of intervention on behalf of clients. Legislation passed to reduce abuse for all children is as important as physical and emotional care of the abused child.

HEALTH POLICY AND THE PRIVATE SECTOR

As described previously, the government has a profound role in setting and implementing health policy, but nurses must recognize that health policy is also made in the private sector. The private sector includes professional organizations (e.g., AMA and AHA), nonprofit health care organizations (e.g., Red Cross and ACS) and for-profit corporations that deliver, insure, or fund health care services outside direct government control. Health insurance companies and MCOs in particular are increasingly setting policies that influence a large number of individuals (Pulcini et al., 2000).

In the private sector, health policy evolves differently than in the public sector. One difference is that private health policy is largely influenced by theories of economics and business management as opposed to the social and political theories that predominate in the public sector. In the private sector, economics are central, whereas in the public sector, economic considerations are one of many factors. In the private sector, decisions can be swift and are often proactive; whereas in the public sector, decision making is more deliberate and tends to be reactive. Private sector change is dictated by consumer needs, economics, and market trends, whereas voting shifts and electoral realignments often delineate the need to change policy in the public sector. The private sector

is managed by stockholders and boards of directors who are generally less accessible to the public than elected officials (Pulcini et al., 2000).

Nursing's Involvement in Private Health Policy

Nursing should incorporate private health policy into its policy agenda. Nurses can influence private health care organizations from internal and external positions. From an internal perspective, nurses can hold important management positions in MCOs. This would allow direct involvement in policy setting. Nurses can also support and use nursing research that demonstrates positive clinical and economic outcomes. This would serve to validate the importance of nursing within the health system (Pulcini et al., 2000).

External strategies that nurses can use to influence private health policy include participation in discussions regarding quality and managed care (Pulcini et al., 2000). Nurses should monitor the quality ratings of MCOs and suggest changes in providers accordingly. Nurses can also build entrepreneurial practices to provide lower-cost services for underserved groups and can encourage clients to call and write their managed care plan organization to request that nursing services be reimbursable. Nurses should work cooperatively with other health professions to influence MCOs to improve quality of care.

CURRENT HEALTH POLICY ISSUES

Health policy is continually evolving and changing and new issues are constantly emerging; therefore nurses must be aware of current health policy issues. Among the most pressing issues facing health policy makers at the beginning of the twenty-first century are restructuring of the health care industry, protection of safety and quality, accountability, and effective use of nurses (Keepnews and Marullo, 1996).

Restructuring of the Health Care Industry

Few nurses will argue that reform is needed in the health system in the United States. In virtually every practice arena, nurses see the inequalities and inadequacies that diminish the nation's level of wellness. In the market-driven system that dominated through much of the twentieth century, and in the managed care system that is currently developing, control of health decisions has moved from physician providers to MCOs and often the patient seems to be a helpless bystander. Identification of problems is an important initial step, but development of direction for their correction is essential follow-up.

In the 1990s, *Nursing's Agenda for Health Care Reform* was developed through collaborative efforts of the ANA and the NLN. Once completed, more than 75 nursing associations added their endorsements (de Vries and Vanderbilt, 1994). The agenda was a powerful tool to promote understanding of nursing and its special contributions to health care.

Armed with the plan set forth in the *Agenda,* nurses were active participants in Clinton's efforts at health care reform. Soon after his inauguration, Clinton appointed a task force that included nursing association representatives and eventually designed a universal plan. Reducing barriers to practice for advanced NPs and redesigning personnel systems for use by nurses in a reformed system were two issues critical to nursing (ANA, 1993).

The insurance industry and some provider groups opposed the unprecedented effort to redesign the health care system. The complexity of the plan and the issues involved confused the public. Despite general acknowledgment of the problems with the health care system, many were wary of the proposed changes. By the fall of 1994, efforts to support the plan waned and it eventually died. Litman (1997) summarized the following reasons for the failure of Clinton's plan:

■ Opposition forces were strong and well organized, whereas those in favor were disorganized and frequently at odds over the best way to attain reform.
■ Ideological differences arose between the President and Congress.
■ A lack of consensus existed between the majority party and the numerous House and Senate committees.
■ The plan was too complex and bureaucratic.
■ The plan's objectives were not easily understood and therefore were easily distorted.
■ Although the administration consulted numerous individuals, groups, and organizations, it deliberated and made decisions in secret. This precluded prenegotiated arrangements with potential allies.
■ The administration took too long to introduce its plan, which allowed opponents to gather momentum.

■ The plan's core reform was directed at a politically weak constituency and opposed by well-financed special interest groups.
■ An improved economy and moderation in health insurance premium costs lessened the sense of urgency.

After the failed attempt at comprehensive reform, more intermediate reform steps have been proposed and taken. For example, in early 2000, President Clinton delivered a proposal that called for Medicare to pay a portion of prescription drugs for older adults. Box 11-3 outlines this proposal.

A lack of a national policy causes the inequalities and inadequacies in health care to continue. Nurses must continue to work to chart a course for a healthy nation. In January 2000, the ANA proposed *Achieving Access for All Americans*, a "universal Medicare program" to address the fragmented health care system. The proposal recommends restructuring Medicare into a seamless, universal program of health care for all Americans. A universal system may provide substantial health care savings by reducing

---

BOX **11-3**

Medicare Coverage of Prescription Drugs

Seniors spend about 21% of their income on health care, with prescription drugs being the second highest expense after insurance premiums. Many older adults do not fill prescriptions that they desperately need because they lack finances. Citing statistics that approximately 35% of seniors have no insurance coverage for medications, in February 2000, President Clinton proposed that Medicare pay for seniors' prescription drugs. The proposal calls for subsidization of the costs of prescription drugs for Medicare's 39 million older adult and disabled beneficiaries. To participate in the plan, Medicare recipients would pay a monthly premium that would start at $26 and rise to $51 within a few years. Under the plan, Medicare would pay for about half of an individual's prescriptions—up to $5000 a year. The plan would cost approximately $160 billion over 10 years.

From Shapiro JP: Medicare's drug woes: a costly but crucial plan, *U.S. News and World Report,* Feb 21, 2000.

administrative costs and limiting duplicative paper-work (ANA, 2000a). Box 11-4 summarizes the changes proposed to implement the program. More information is available at the ANA website, which can be accessed through the WebLinks section of the book's SIMON website.

Protection of Safety and Quality

The emphasis on cost containment that has been pervasive in health care for the past 15 years has lead to questions about safety and quality of health care. Many people are concerned that the fundamental principle of protecting patient safety is being compromised in the drive to cuts costs (Keepnews and Marullo, 1996). Currently, mechanisms to ensure patient safety and quality of care have proved inadequate to address many issues. A need also exists to establish understandable, objective measures by

---

BOX **11-4**

Steps in Implementing the ANA's *Achieving Access for All Americans*

1. Merge Medicare Parts A and B to reduce administrative costs and provide a basis for a unified system of health care financing.
2. Raise the Medicare payroll tax to 5% (2.5% each from employers and employees).
3. Shift current employer-employee insurance premiums into a national trust fund.
4. Phase-in a system of financing based on a combination of payroll taxes and general fund revenues.
5. Institute and employ competitive bidding and competitively set rates.
6. Integrate physician and facility payment for inpatient cases using a DRG or high-cost medical staff's approach.
7. Expand current graduate medical education to include payment for graduate nursing education with particular emphasis on advance practice nursing to meet primary care needs.

From American Nurses Association: *ANA proposes universal Medicare program as solution to fragmented health care system,* American Nurses Association Press Release, Jan 13, 2000b, The Author, www.nursingworld.org/rnrealnews.

---

which to measure quality in nursing and health care.

In a December 1999 report on patient safety, the IOM responded to a national study estimating that medical errors kill between 44,000 and 98,000 people each year by describing a fragmented health care system that is prone to errors and detrimental to safe patient care. Most errors result from flaws in the health care system and although errors are more easily detected in hospitals, they affect all health care settings, including outpatient clinics, pharmacies, nursing homes, and home care. The report listed the following recommendations for addressing safety issues:

- Congress should create a center for patient safety within the Agency for Health Care Research and Quality. This center would set national goals for patient safety and develop knowledge and understanding of errors in health care by developing a research agenda, evaluation methods for identification and prevention of errors, and funds for dissemination and communication activities to improve patient safety.
- State governments should establish a mandatory reporting system to provide for the collection of standardized information about adverse events in the health system that result in death or serious harm.
- Congress should pass legislation to extend peer review protection to data related to patient safety and quality improvements.
- Regulators and accreditors should focus greater attention on patient safety and set specific performance standards and expectations for health care organizations.
- Performance standards and expectations for health professionals should focus greater attention on patient safety.
- The FDA should increase attention to the safe use of drugs in the premarketing and postmarketing processes.
- Health care organizations and affiliated professionals should continually improve patient safety programs with defined executive responsibility.
- Health care organizations should implement proven medication safety practices.

Safety and quality issues in health care are numerous and diverse. They include practice patterns of health care providers, use and misuse of technology, appropriate use of medications, and several related issues influencing various groups

BOX 11-5

Safety Issues and Health Policy: Anthrax Vaccine

In March 1998, the DOD implemented the Anthrax Vaccine Immunization Program (AVIP) to immunize all active duty personnel against anthrax, a bacterial disease that can be used as a biological weapon in spore form. This program was the result of contentions by the DOD that mass vaccination is the safest way to protect U.S. military forces against a potential threat that is 99% fatal to unprotected individuals. The DOD cited several sources supporting conclusions that the anthrax vaccine is safe and effective.

Responding to increasing questions and concerns voiced by military personnel, in February 2000, a subcommittee comprised of representatives from the National Security Council, Department of Veterans Affairs, and the House Committee on Government Reform issued recommendations repealing the program. The subcommittee reported that the AVIP is a "well-intentioned but overwrought response to the threat of anthrax as a biological weapon." They determined that the program was:

1. Unrealistic (vaccinating 2.4 million active duty and reserve members with six injections)
2. Based on dated medical technology (a 1950s-era vaccine)
3. Questionably effective (vaccine was developed to protect against cutaneous infection of anthrax and has not been tested against aerosolized spores)
4. Potentially unsafe (adverse events are twice as high for women as men)
5. Vulnerable to supply shortages and price increases (only one manufacturer)

Despite the subcommittee's testimony and detailed report, the DOD persisted with the program, declaring it safe and effective. By March 2000, more than 320,000 military personnel had received the vaccine. As a result of concerns about safety, servicemen and women have refused to take the inoculations and have quit, been discharged, and been threatened with court martial.

From Subcommittee on National Security, Department of Veterans Affairs and International Relations, House Committee on Government Reform: *Unproven force protection: summary report,* 2000, The Author, www.house.gov/reform/ns/1; www.cnn.com/2000/health.

throughout the United States. Box 11-5 describes an issue that has been recently debated dealing with patient safety.

Accountability

Public accountability in health care refers to the public's right to know and the provider's duty to disclose information on the health care system. Public accountability encourages the open reporting and sharing of data across institutions and organizations (Malone and Keepnews, 1998). Consumers and purchasers should have information on outcomes and costs of health care to make informed choices on where and from whom to seek health care services.

MCOs are increasingly called upon to take accountability measures so that enrollees can make informed decisions. HEDIS and other health plan report cards have been designed to provide assessment data and improve the quality of care (Shi and Singh, 1998).

As part of its efforts to enhance public accountability, the ANA has advocated public disclosure by health care institutions regarding staffing levels and patient outcome data. The ANA sponsored the Patient Safety Act (PSA) of 1999 for this purpose. If implemented, the PSA would require Medicare providers to publicly disclose the following information (ANA, 1999c):

- Staffing regarding the number of RNs providing direct care
- Number of unlicensed personnel used to provide direct patient care
- Average number of patients per RN
- Patient mortality rate
- Incidence of adverse patient care incidents
- Methods used for determination and adjustment of staffing levels

BOX 11-6

RN Staffing Levels and Patient Outcomes

Two recent studies examined the relationship be-tween RN staffing levels and patient outcomes. One large-scale study conducted in hospitals in California, Massachusetts and New York exam-ined length of stay and patient outcomes based on RN staffing levels. The study found that shorter lengths of stay were strongly related to higher RN staffing per acuity-adjusted day and that patient morbidity indicators for preventable conditions (e.g., pressure ulcers, pneumonia, postoperative infections, and urinary tract infections) were also tied to staffing levels. A second study found that a higher proportion of RNs was directly related to a lower incidences of negative outcomes, including medication errors, pressure ulcers, and com-plaints by patients and families.

From American Nurses Association: *Nursing-sensitive quality indicators for acute care settings,* 1999, The Author, www.ana.org/readroom/fssafe99.htm.

The PSA would also make available the follow-ing performance indicators to promote improved consumer information and choice (ANA, 1999c):

- Data regarding complaints filed with the state, HCFA, or a provider accrediting agency
- Compliance with conditions of Medicare participation
- Data regarding investigations and findings result-ing from complaints

The bill is currently pending in Congress.

The importance of staffing levels of RNs and other personnel is particularly important in providing the optimum level of health care and improving patient outcome. Box 11-6 illustrates this principle.

Effective Use of Nurses

In addition to the influence on financing and delivery of health care, health policy also directly influences nursing practice. Efforts to cut the use of nurses and replace nursing staff with lower-paid unskilled substi-tutes have been of particular concern to the nursing profession.

In response to this issue, significant health policy was enacted in California in October 1999. The California A.B. 394 Staffing Bill (AB 394) requires California's Department of Health Services to adopt regulations that establish minimum, specific, and numerical licensed nurse-to-patient ratios by licensed nurse classification and hospital units for general acute care hospitals, psychiatric hospitals, and special hospitals. AB 394 requires nurse staffing to be determined based on illness severity, need for special-ized equipment and technology, complexity of clinical judgment needed for care, and the ability for self-care. The measure prohibits hospitals from assigning an unlicensed person to perform the following nursing functions:

- Medication administration
- Venipuncture
- Intravenous therapy
- Parenteral or tube feedings
- Invasive procedures (e.g., inserting nasogastric tubes or catheters, tracheal suctioning)
- Assessment of patient condition
- Patient education

AB 394 also requires a RN assigned to a unit or clinical area to receive orientation in the area (ANA, 1999a).

Nursing policies include other issues such as prescriptive authority for NPs, third-party reimburse-ment for service, and work site safety (e.g., safe needles). Box 11-7 describes another recent policy issue influencing nursing practice, that of **interstate nursing practice**.

NURSES' ROLES IN POLITICAL ACTIVITIES

A recent research study looked at facilitators and hindrances for political involvement among nurses. Factors identified that facilitated political involve-ment included being raised in a family that was politically active, positive role models (e.g., a politi-cally involved nurse-mentor or national figure) who exemplified the importance of involvement in social issues, and education. Hindrances to political action included lack of resources (e.g., financial burdens of membership dues), the slow nature of the political process, time constraints, perceived lack of support from society and peers, gender issues, administrative structure, negative experiences, frustration, burnout, and apathy (Winter and Lockhart, 1997).

BOX **11-7**

Interstate Nursing Practice

The National Council of State Boards of Nursing (NCSBN), the ANA, specialty organizations, and state legislatures have examined the concept of interstate nursing practice, or multistate licensure, for several years. Multistate licensure is a system in which one license allows a nurse to practice in multiple states and has resulted from three major influences, which are the rapid growth of tele-health and telemedicine; the expansion of multistate health care systems; and the increased mobility of RNs.

For multistate licensure, an interstate contract or agreement between two or more states has been advocated as a mechanism to promote interstate nursing practice. These interstate contracts establish relationships among states for jurisdiction, discipline, and information sharing. Each participating state's nurse practice act does not change and each state continues to have authority in determining licensure requirements and disciplinary actions on nurses' licenses.

The NCSBN approved the implementation of multistate licensure for RNs at the Delegate Assembly in August 1997 and adopted the outcome of implementation of a Mutual Recognition Master Plan. Utah was the first state to adopt the NCSBN's plan and enacted legislation that became effective January 1, 2000. Several other states have expressed interest in adopting interstate licensure.

From Glazer G: Legislative and policy issues related to interstate practice, *Online J Issues Nurs* May 4, 1999; Lasseter F: Legislative activity on the interstate compact for the mutual recognition model on nursing regulation, *AORN J* 69:647, 1999.

More effort needs to be given to educate nurses about the importance of being informed on health policy issues and to encourage them to become politically active. Exposure to positive role models is particularly important. Nurses also need to overcome the factors that may impede political involvement. This section describes several ways that nurses can become involved in the political process.

Nurses as Change Agents

Although nurses have historically been recognized as a necessary resource during wars and other emergencies, since the 1950s all levels of government have begun to consider nurses as indispensable in ordinary times. The public now recognizes nurses as necessary and valued national resources. In their advocacy role, nurses are seen as professionals whose knowledge, skills, and concern are used to promote society's well-being.

Nurses have a unique status in caring for patients, they are interpreters of the health care system to the public, and their professional activities are influenced by government-funded programs; therefore public health nurses must know how to participate in the political process. To do this effectively, they need a sound knowledge of community, state, and national government organization and function and a clear understanding of how these bodies interact collectively to influence policy. Nurses must know how to influence the creation of health care legislation and how to contribute to the election and appointment of key officials. Policy is fundamental to governance; therefore nurses need to know about the formulation of public policy and the acts of government and its agencies. To assist in these activities, Table 11-3 presents sources for legislation information and Table 11-4 gives sources for information on electoral issues.

Nurses as Lobbyists

To **lobby** is to try to influence legislators; it is an art of persuasion. A lobbyist is, by definition, a person who represents special interests (Loquist, 1999). Influencing lawmakers to pass effective health legislation requires the participation of individual nurses and nursing organizations. The initial step in this process involves a telephone call to make an appointment with an elected official. Although exceptions exist, most officials are interested in meeting only with their own constituents (i.e., those registered to vote in their political jurisdiction) because the power of generating votes is the primary determinant of political influence.

The goal of the first contact with the official is to establish that the nurse is a concerned constituent and a credible source of information on health issues. The image of nurses as caring and helping people is a definite advantage at this point. In communities in which nurses have already established strong political credentials, their colleagues will be more readily

TABLE 11-3

Sources for Legislative Information

Government Level	Information Available	Location
Federal	Background of members of Congress Committee assignments Terms of service	Congressional Directory Government documents section of selected public or university libraries
	Congressional news Vote tabulations	Congressional Quarterly Weekly Report Government documents section of selected public or university libraries
	Bills in process or legislated (bill number needed)	U.S. representative or senator (may have local office)
	Health and nursing issues in U.S. Congress ANA-PAC (The American Nurse)	ANA 600 Maryland Ave, SW Suite 100 Washington, DC 20024 (202) 554-4444
	Public health issues in U.S. Congress (The Nation's Health)	APHA 1015 15th St NW Washington, DC 20005 (202) 789-5600
State	Bills in process or legislated (bill number needed)	State representative or senator (may have local office)
	Health and nursing issues in state legislature, State PACs for nursing	SNA (for location, see April directory issue of the *American Journal of Nursing*)

TABLE 11-4

Sources for Electoral Information

Government Level	Information Available	Location
State	State government operations Political subdivisions Legislative information telephone number State election laws and procedures Campaign finance reports	Secretary of state (state capitol) Office of Lieutenant Governor (state capitol)
County or municipal	Similar to state as appropriate to local government Political jurisdictions for each household address	County clerk (county courthouse) City clerk (city hall)
General	Government information Political jurisdictions for each household address Names of current office holders in local jurisdictions	League of Women Voters 1730 M Street, NW Washington, DC 20036 (202) 429-1965 Telephone directory (major cities)

BOX 11-8

Lobbying Activities of the ANA: Medicare Balanced Budget Act Revisions

In October 1999, the ANA issued a statement to address refinements to the Medicare provisions included in the Balanced Budget Act of 1997 (BBA 97). In this statement the ANA reported that the BBA 97 made cuts that were severe and negatively influenced quality of health care and a reduced access to health care for vulnerable people. The following were the major areas of concern voiced in this statement:

- Home health care: The interim payment system (IPS) implemented by the BBA 97 caused severe problems for home health providers and their patients. Among the influences of the IPS were 550,000 fewer Medicare beneficiaries receiving home health services in 1998 than 1996, closing of nearly 25% of all home health agencies in the United States, and a 29% reduction in home health agency reimbursement since 1996.
- Skilled nursing facilities: The implementation of a PPS for skilled nursing facilities has resulted in greater reductions in payments than originally intended. The intended reduction was 6%, but a 15% reduction in payments occurred, causing substantial financial difficulties.
- Acute care: The BBA resulted in decreased quality of care and access to care by cutting payments some 33% more than anticipated to acute care institutions.

The ANA concluded that the legislators must "take immediate action to reduce the harm by the BBA 97." Among the recommendations were to eliminate a 15% cut in home health care funding scheduled for October 1, 2000; increase IPS per visit reimbursement for home health care; provide relief for hospitals serving the uninsured by carving out Medicare managed care payments; and pass legislation that would limit payment losses created by the move to outpatient PPS.

From American Nurses Association: *Written testimony of the ANA before the U.S. House of Representatives Committee on Ways and Means Subcommittee on Health,* October 1, 1999, The Author, www.ana.org/gov/federal/legis/testimon/1999/medbn101.htm.

accepted. An individual who establishes a reputation as a reliable and accurate resource as a lobbyist has substantial influence.

Legislators rely heavily on lobbyists for education on issues and they usually want to hear from opposing sides before taking a position. The official must trust lobbyists to give accurate, though predictably biased, information. If a lobbyist does not have the information requested, he or she should obtain it and give it to the official quickly.

Each official represents a constituency with varied needs and interests and each vote must be weighed within this context. The positions taken by legislators will not always be to an individual's liking and evaluation of their performance should be based on their overall voting patterns, not on their votes on isolated issues. The ANA and the APHA regularly tally and publish the records of each federal legislator on all issues related to the organization's priorities. This information can be helpful in evaluating elected officials. Internet addresses for these two organizations can be found through the SIMON website.

Professional Associations and Lobbying

Collective action by nursing and health care organizations (e.g., ANA and APHA) is critical to their goals. These associations monitor legislative activity related to health issues and link the process to their membership. This continual surveillance of the legislative environment is critical because even seemingly minor amendments can have profound effects on health services.

Thorough monitoring requires the participation of people who are knowledgeable about nursing, health care, and the political intricacies of the legislative process. The ANA and the APHA have full-time staff lobbyists who work with Congress. Many of their state constituent associations also work with state legislatures. However, regardless of the effectiveness of association lobbyists in promoting the interests of nurses and society, they always need grassroots cooperation to truly influence decisions. In the final analysis, a sufficiently high number of communications, via letters and telephone calls, from individual constituents have the greatest influence.

Lobbying is an ongoing activity for health policy issues influencing nursing and health care delivery. Box 11-8 presents an example of a recent effort by the ANA to influence the House of Representatives Committee on Ways and Means, Subcommittee on Health, to address problems related to the Medicare Beneficiary Access to Care Act.

Nurses and Political Action Committees

Political action committees (PACs) have been important sources of collective political influence since the 1970s. These nonpartisan entities promote the election of candidates believed to be sympathetic to their interests. PACs are established by professional associations and business and labor groups under federal and state laws that stipulate how they may contribute financially to campaigns. The advantage of a PAC is that small donations from many members, when added together, make an impressive addition to a campaign fund in the name of an organization. This gains the attention of the candidate and earns good will for the group.

Valid concern exists about the correlation of major PAC contributions and the legislator's votes on special interest legislation. However, as long as PACs are a reality of political life, nurses need to recognize their power and support those that are committed to electing candidates sympathetic to health care issues.

Most national associations of health care providers have PACs. Among the strongest are those representing hospitals, nursing homes, home health agencies, pharmaceutical interests, and insurance companies. A PAC that makes major political contributions is the American Medical Political Action Committee (AMPAC), sponsored by the AMA. State medical associations also have strong PACs. This means that organized medicine has a powerful influence on national and state elections and on health care legislation at both levels.

The ANA and many other nursing organizations have PACs. According to the information posted on their website, the ANA-PAC works "to ensure that nurses have the best representation possible in the United States Congress." Among other achievements, in 1998 the ANA-PAC helped procure funding increases for the Nurse Education Act and the National Institute of Nursing Research. Box 11-9 gives additional information on the ANA-PAC.

Nurses and Coalitions

When two or more groups join to maximize resources, increasing their influence and improving their chances of success in achieving a common goal, it is called a **coalition**. Coalitions of health care providers often work together on issues such as family violence and fluoridation of water supplies. An outstanding example of such cooperative action has been the establishment of rehabilitation programs for health profession-

---

BOX 11-9

American Nurses Association-Political Action Committee

- In 1998, the ANA-PAC raised more than $1 million from nurses across the United States (average contribution is $42 per year).
- The ANA-PAC is a bipartisan PAC and works directly with both parties to recruit and support candidates.
- The ANA-PAC endorses candidates for public office based on the following:
  - Potential for winning the election
  - Support for ANA's legislative agenda
  - Sponsorship of key nursing bills at the federal, state, or local level
  - Support of issues and programs
  - Active solicitation of nursing input into the development of policy and position statements and congressional races in which the ANA or the SNA have a specific interest.
- Financial support of a candidate is based on the following:
  - Their party's leadership position
  - Congressional committee assignments
  - Demonstrated support for ANA's legislative agenda
  - Evaluation of opposition
  - Political viability of the race
  - Nonincumbent with a strong chance of winning
  - Nurse candidate (SNA membership)
- Female or minority candidate

From American Nurses Association: *American Nurses Association Political Action Committee: PAC FAQ,* 2000, The Author, www.ana.org/gova/federal/anapac/gpacfaq.htm.

als whose practice has been impaired by substance abuse or mental health problems.

Nursing and consumer groups often form coalitions to advance their shared interests in health promotion. In September 1999, the ANA joined 16 other organizations (e.g., American College of NPs, American Red Cross, Department of Veteran's Affairs, and Sigma Theta Tau) to form a coalition called Nurses for a Healthier Tomorrow. Responding to concerns about a potentially dangerous shortage of nurses, this coalition hopes to raise funds for a national advertising campaign designed to recruit new nurses and encourage existing ones to remain in the profession. The coalition hopes to attract major health insurers, managed care companies, pharmaceutical firms, health care providers, nursing schools, and hospitals to support the campaign. The campaign focuses on the message that nurses are essential to the health care team and that they save health care dollars. The campaign shows that an increased demand exists for nurses, including employment opportunities outside the hospital and an increased demand for nurses in specialty areas (ANA, 1999b).

Nurses in Public Office

A profession derives its status from a contract with society to provide essential services under conditions of altruism and trust. Nurses are demonstrating this professionalism by serving the healthy and sick and by serving future generations through their influence in promoting wellness through public policy development. Although a few nurses are directly involved in health policy development, more are needed. Nurses and the public should be constantly attuned to opportunities to promote the appointment or election of nurses to policymaking positions.

Many women have become spokespeople for nursing and have a strong voice in politics. During the 1998 election cycle nurses were very visible. The ANA endorsed 252 candidates for the 106th Congress with an 88% success rate. Three nurses (Lois Capps, RN [D-CA]; Carolyn McCarthy, LPN [D-NY]; and Eddie Bernice Johnson, RN [D-TX]) were reelected to the U.S. House of Representatives (ANA, 1999d). In February 2000, a total of 97 nurses were serving as state legislators in 38 different states.

Nurse-legislators play a crucial role in interpreting health issues and influencing appropriate legislation. Nurses serve in county and city governments and on special governing bodies, such as school boards. Nurses also influence health policy through politically appointed positions. These appointments are based on individual qualifications for the position but may involve political connections.

Other women who have been active in the federal government are Carolyne Davis, who served as the administrator of the HCFA, and Shirley Chater, who was Commissioner of the Social Service Administration. Virginia Trotter Betts, who served as the President of the ANA, was also the Senior Advisor on Nursing and Policy to the Secretary of the USDHHS

in Washington, DC. Likewise, Dr. Beverly Malone resigned as President of the ANA in 1999 to assume the position of Deputy Assistant Secretary of the USDHHS. In this capacity, she advises the assistant secretary for the USDHHS, Dr. David Satcher, in program and political matters, policy and program development, and setting of legislative priorities.

Finally, nurses head 2 of the 10 regional offices of the USDHHS. Pat Monoya, MA, RN, is director for Region VI headquartered in Dallas and Pat Ford-Roegner, MS, RN, oversees Region IV headquartered in Atlanta.

In the future, more nurses need to run for public office at all three levels of government. Whether serving as political appointees or career bureaucrats, nurses have much to offer. Young and beginning nurses should take the challenge as many of these nurses have and advance the nursing practice and the nation's health.

Nurses and Health Policy Development

As nurses' role in changing health care policy increases, more nurses are needed who are equipped for this challenge. A strong cadre of nursing leaders who have the vision for change is essential to promoting nursing's policy agenda. National fellowships and internships are available for nurses who are interested in taking leadership roles (Sharp, 1999).

The Robert Wood Johnson (RWJ) Health Policy Fellowship is a one-year career development program for midcareer health professionals. The goal of this program is to help nurses gain an understanding of the health policy process and contribute to the formulation of new policies and programs. RWJ Health Policy fellows are selected from academic faculties from diverse disciplines, including medicine, dentistry, nursing, public health, health services administration, economics, and social services. After an extensive orientation on the legislative and executive branches of government, the fellows work with a member of Congress or on a congressional health committee (Sharp, 1999).

The President's Commission on White House Fellowships offers 20 fellowships each year to nurses early in their careers; the average age is 33. The White House fellows participate in an education program that involves working with government officials, scholars, journalists, and private-sector leaders to explore U.S. policy in action. Nurses who have been White House fellows may work at the HCFA and the

Health Policy Fellowships

RWJ Health Policy Fellowships:
Marion Ein Lewin
2101 Constitution Ave, NW
Washington, DC 20418
(202) 334-1505

Commission on White House Fellowships:
712 Jackson Place, NW
Washington, DC 20503
(202) 395-4522

The website of each program can be accessed through the book's website at SIMON www.wbsaunders.com/SIMON/nies/.

Office of Science and Technology Policy, among others (Sharp, 1999). These fellowship programs are competitive, but strong leaders are desperately needed. For more information on both programs, contact sources are provided in Box 11-10.

Nurses and Campaigning

Helping someone win an election is a sure way of gaining influence. All candidates are grateful for campaign assistance and usually remember those who have helped. Although campaign contributions are commonly thought of as financial, they can also take the form of participation in campaign activities.

Nurses are frequently unable to contribute much money; therefore they can provide these invaluable services. For the novice, veteran campaigners are eager to help him or her learn the necessary skills. Initially, a volunteer can address or stuff envelopes for mailings. The volunteer can also invite friends and neighbors for a social gathering to meet the candidate, thereby providing an opportunity to discuss issues of concern with constituents.

Telephone banks help a candidate identify supporters, opponents, and the critical undecided voter. These latter voters can make a difference on election day and are courted by all candidates. The telephone interviews are highly structured and easily handled by inexperienced campaign workers. Direct contact with potential voters may occur later in the form of house-to-house block walks or poll work on election day. The confidence that this requires comes with

experience and a strong commitment to the candidate and the cause.

Hosting a social function to allow nurse colleagues to meet the candidate is a welcome contribution to the campaign. Nurses are substantial in number and their voting record is humanistic; therefore they are valued as a political force.

Government employees may be restricted by policies that limit or disallow political activism. Nurses employed at any level of government should be aware of such prohibitions.

Nurses and Voting Strength

With more than 2.5 million members, nurses make up the largest profession in health care; one in 44 women voters is an RN (Hadley, 1996). Therefore if every RN would vote, the power to make an influence on health policy would be tremendous. If the nursing profession is to meet the challenges of the twenty-first century and work as a profession to positively influence the health of populations, political action is necessary and an understanding of the factors that motivate or impede political action is needed (Winter and Lockhart, 1997).

Nurses' interest in affecting health policies and legislation has expanded in recent years as they realize the influence on their practice and profession. As a body of more than 2.5 million, they can wield enormous power. This power of numbers is never more apparent than in the legislative process. A legislator carefully weighs the number of constituents supporting or opposing a bill before deciding how to vote. A sizable block of constituents on one side of an issue can significantly affect that vote. Representing the district is important to a legislator for ethical reasons and for political pragmatism.

INTERNET AND POLITICAL PROCESS

A 30-day window of opportunity is typical for public input into the development of regulations. Written comments about a political issue are made part of the public record. To facilitate correspondence, websites have been set up to promote contacting agencies, governmental organizations, and political figures. Nurses need to be aware of some of the important websites. Furthermore, many legislators may have their own web page so that the nurse could easily access his or her office. Numerous websites related to health policy issues may be accessed through the WebLinks section of this book's website at [SIMON] www.wbsaunders.com/SIMON/nies/.

The Internet can provide almost unlimited access to information. However, access to information does not ensure the quality or credibility of the information. The user is responsible for evaluation of the information and separation of quality information from misinformation.

SUMMARY

Historically, nurses have been able to make significant differences in the QOL experienced by the members of the communities in which they serve. By understanding how government works, how bills become law, and how legislators make decisions, nurses can influence policy decisions through individual efforts such as letter writing, participation in political campaigns, and selection of candidates who support policies conducive to improving the health and welfare of all citizens. When organized in lobbying groups, coalitions, and PACs, or when holding office, nurses can be a powerful force that brings about change in the delivery and quality of the health care of aggregates.

LEARNING ACTIVITIES

1. Develop an "insight" bulletin board, with each class member contributing cartoons, anecdotes, and clippings about issues affecting public health or nursing.
2. Develop expertise on a current public health or nursing issue, including an understanding of the causes, effect on the public, and possible solutions. Influence its resolution through any of the following activities:
   a. Write a succinct letter to the editor of a local newspaper.
   b. Write a position paper and submit it to the "opinion page" of a local newspaper.
   c. Write to elected or appointed officials whose jurisdiction may be influential on the issue.
   d. Meet with an elected or appointed official to discuss the issue in groups of two or three.
   e. Call in to a radio talk show about the issue.
   f. Volunteer to speak on the issue to appropriate consumer or professional groups.

3. With a group of two or three, meet with an elected official for a 15-minute appointment to ask about the official's concerns and priorities. If the official is not familiar with health issues, do not preach; instead, begin an educational process.
4. Invite an elected official who is sympathetic to nurses to speak to the local chapter of the National Nursing Students Association to discuss the political process and health policy.
5. Invite an elected official to spend a day with a public health nurse or nursing student in appropriate activities. Take black-and-white pictures for press use.
6. Invite a medical reporter from the press, radio, or television to observe public health nursing activities that would appeal to the public.
7. Participate in a group organized around a public health issue (e.g., disposable diapers, toxic waste, and fluoride).
8. Serve as a volunteer in a campaign for a candidate who is supportive or potentially supportive of public health or nursing issues.
9. Serve as a volunteer for a political party.

REFERENCES

American Nurses Association: ANA advises on health care reform, *Capital Update* 11(8):1, 1993.

American Nurses Association: *Written testimony of the ANA before the U.S. House of Representatives Committee on Ways and Means Subcommittee on Health,* October 1, 1999, The Author, www.ana.org/gov/federal/legis/testimon/1999/medbn101.htm

American Nurses Association: *State government relations: California A.B. 394 Staffing Bill,* October 10, 1999a, The Author, www.nursingworld.org/rnrealnews.

American Nurses Association: *ANA joins coalition formed to promote nursing* (Press Release), Sept 28, 1999b, The Author, www.nursingworld.org/rnrealnews.

American Nurses Association: *Patient Safety Act,* 1999c, The Author, www.ana.org/gova/federal/legis/106/gpsaintr.htm.

American Nurses Association: *Nurse state legislators,* 1999d, The Author, www.nursingworld.org/rnrealnews.

American Nurses Association: *American Nurses Association Political Action Committee:* PAC FAQ, 2000, The Author, www.ana.org/gova/federal/anapac/gpacfaq.htm.

American Nurses Association: *Achieving access for all Americans: a proposal from the American Nurses Association for Health Coverage 2000,* Jan 13, 2000a, The Author, www.ana.org/readroom/rwjpaper.htm.

American Nurses Association: *ANA proposes universal Medicare program as solution to fragmented health care system,* American Nurses Association Press Release, Jan 13, 2000b, The Author, www.nursingworld.org/rnrealnews.

American Nurses Association: *Nursing-sensitive quality indicators for acute care settings,* 1999, The Author, www.ana.org/readroom/fssafe99.html.

Bagwell M, Clements S: *A political handbook for health professionals,* Boston, 1985, Little, Brown.

Bonick J: Policy, politics and the law. In Stanhope M, Lancaster J, editors: *Community and public health nursing,* ed 5, St. Louis, 2000, Mosby.

Brooke PS: Legal context for community health nursing practice. In Smith CM, Maurer FA, editors: *Community health nursing: theory and practice,* ed 2, Philadelphia, 2000, W.B. Saunders.

de Vries C, Vanderbilt M: Nurses gain ground during reform debate, *Am Nurse* 26(10):2, 1994.

Dowling WL: Hospitals and health systems. In Williams SJ, Torrens PR, editors: *Introduction to health services,* ed 5, Albany, NY, 1999, Delmar.

Glazer G: Legislative and policy issues related to interstate practice, *Online J Issues Nurs,* May 4, 1999.

Hadley EH: Nursing in the political and economic marketplace: challenges for the 21st century, *Nurs Outlook* 44(1):6, 1996.

Hall-Long BA: Nursing's past, present, and future political experiences, *Nurs Health Care Perspect* 16:24, 1995.

Hanlon GE, Pickett JJ: *Public health: administration and practice,* ed 8, St. Louis, 1984, Mosby.

Helms LB, Anderson MA, Hanson K: 'Doin' politics: linking policy and politics in nursing, *Nurs Admin Q* 20:32, 1996.

Institute of Medicine: *To err is human: building a safer health system,* Washington, DC, 1999, The Author.

Kalisch PA, Kalisch BJ: *The advance of American nursing,* ed 3, Philadelphia, 1995, J.B. Lippincott.

Keepnews D, Marullo G: Policy imperatives for nursing in an era of health care restructuring, *Nurs Admin Q* 20:19, 1996.

Lasseter F: Legislative activity on the interstate compact for the mutual recognition model on nursing regulation, *AORN J* 69:647, 1999.

Leavitt JK, Mason DJ: Policy and politics: a framework for action. In Mason DJ, Leavitt JK: *Policy and politics in nursing and health care,* Philadelphia, 1998, W.B. Saunders.

Lewinson, SB: In Mason DJ, Leavitt JK: *Policy and politics in nursing and health care,* Philadelphia, 1998, W.B. Saunders.

Litman T: *Health, politics and policy,* ed 3, Albany, NY, 1997, Delmar.

Loquist RS: Regulation: parallel and powerful. In Milstead JA, editor: *Health policy and politics: a nurse's guide,* Gaithersburg, Md, 1999, Aspen.

Malone BL, Keepnews, D: Ensuring the future of nurses in clinical practice: issues and strategies for staff nurses and advanced practice nurses. In Mason DJ, Leavitt JK, editors: *Policy and politics in nursing and health care,* Philadelphia, 1998, W.B. Saunders.

Pulcini J et al: Health policy and the private sector: new vistas for nursing, *Nurs Health Care Perspect* 21:22, 2000.

Shapiro JP: Medicare's drug woes: a costly but crucial plan, *U.S. News and World Report,* Feb 21, 2000.

Sharp N: Wanted: nurse leaders to craft health policy, *Nurse Pract* 24(10):85, 1999.

Shi L, Singh DA: *Delivering health care in America: a systems approach,* Gaithersburg, Md, 1998, Aspen.

Smith BM: Trends in health care coverage and financing and their implications for policy, *N Engl J Med* 337(14):1000, 1997.

Spradley B: *Community health nursing,* ed 2, Boston, 1985, Little, Brown.

Subcommittee on National Security, Department of Veterans Affairs and International Relations, House Committee on Government Reform: *Unproven force protection: summary report,* 2000, The Author, www.house.gov/reform/ns/1; www.cnn.com/2000/health.

Sultz HA, Young KM: *Health care USA: understanding its organization and delivery,* ed 2, Gaithersburg, Md, 1999, Aspen.

US Department of Health and Human Services: *Healthy people 2010,* Conference edition, Washington, DC, 2000, The Author.

Vaccine's price drives a debate about its use, *Wall Street Journal* Feb 16, 2000.

Winter MK, Lockhart JS: From motivation to action: understanding nurses' political involvement, *Nurs Health Care Perspect* 18(5):244, 1997.

Cultural Diversity and Community Health Nursing

Margaret M. Andrews

OBJECTIVES

Upon completion of this chapter, the reader will be able to do the following:

1. Critically analyze racial and cultural diversity in the United States.
2. Analyze the influence of sociocultural, political, economic, and religious factors that influence the health of culturally diverse individuals, groups, and communities.
3. Identify the cultural aspects of nursing care for culturally diverse individuals, groups, and communities.
4. Apply the principles of transcultural nursing to community health nursing practice.

KEY TERMS

biomedical
cultural code
cultural imposition
cultural negotiation
cultural stereotyping
culture
culture-bound syndrome
culture shock
culture specific
culture universal
culturological assessment
dominant value orientation
epidemiological paradox
ethnocentrism
family-community HPM
magicoreligious
naturalistic
norms
poverty rate
socioeconomic status (SES)
spirituality
subculture
transcultural nursing
value
yin-yang theory

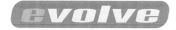

http://evolve.elsevier.com/Nies/

TRANSCULTURAL PERSPECTIVES ON COMMUNITY HEALTH NURSING

The nurse's knowledge of culture and cultural concepts can serve to improve the health of the community. Culturally competent community health nursing requires that the nurse understand the lifestyle, value system, and health and illness behaviors of diverse individuals, families, groups, and communities. The nurse should also understand the culture of institutions that influence the health and well-being of communities. Nurses who have knowledge of and an ability to work with diverse cultures are able to devise effective interventions to reduce risks in a manner that is culturally congruent with community, group, and individual values.

In the United States, metaphors such as *melting pot, mosaic,* and *salad bowl* describe the cultural diversity that characterizes the population. Although there is a tendency to identify the federally defined racial and ethnic minority* groups when referring to the cultural aspects of community health nursing, *all* individuals, families, groups, communities, and institutions, including nurses and the nursing profession, have cultural characteristics that influence community health. When planning and implementing health care, community health nurses need to balance cultural diversity with the universal human experience and common needs of all people.

POPULATION TRENDS

The population of the United States is becoming increasingly diverse. In recent years, individuals from the federally defined minority groups have grown faster than the population as a whole. In 1970, minority groups* accounted for 16% of the population. By 1999, this share increased to 27%. Assuming that current trends continue, the U.S. Census Bureau (1999a) projects that by the middle of the twenty-first century, minorities will account for 51.1% of the total population. For the first time in U.S. history, minorities will make up a majority of the total population. If

current demographic trends continue, the United States will have the following population composition by the year 2080: Hispanic, 23.4%; black, 14.7%; and Asian and Pacific Islander, 12% (US Census Bureau, 1999a). At the same time, the Native-American and Alaska Native population is projected to remain at 0.9% or perhaps decrease slightly in intermarriage. Table 12-1 summarizes the current population composition by race, number, percentage, and percentage of change from 1990 to 2000.

Although the nursing profession has representatives from diverse groups, minorities are continually underrepresented. Approximately 11%, or 216,000, of the nation's 2.12 million RNs come from racial and ethnic minority backgrounds. Estimates for each minority group are as follows: 91,000 black; 35,800 Hispanic; 79,000 Asian and Pacific Islander; and 10,500 Native-American and Alaska Natives (USDHHS/Division of Nursing, 1996). Each minority group is distributed differently around the country. Black nurses are more likely found in the South, Hispanics in the West or South (i.e., especially states bordering Mexico), and Asian and Pacific Islanders in the West or Northeast. Native-American and Alaska Native nurses are predominantly in states with reservations.

The United States has grown and achieved its success largely through immigration. Since 1972, more than 10 million legal immigrants have come to United States. The number of immigrants and refugees in the United States is projected to continue to increase. People from other countries will probably continue to seek treatment in U.S. hospitals, particularly for cardiovascular, neurological, and cancer care, and U.S. nurses will continue to have the opportunity to travel abroad to work in a variety of health care settings in the international marketplace. In the course of a nursing career, it is possible to encounter foreign visitors, international university faculty members, international high school and university students, family members of foreign diplomats, immigrants, refugees, members of more than 130 different ethnic groups, and Native-Americans from more than 550 federally recognized tribes. A serious conceptual problem exists within nursing in that, without formal preparation, nurses are expected to know, understand, and meet the health needs of culturally diverse individuals, groups, and communities.

Members of some cultural groups, most notably blacks and Hispanics, demand culturally relevant health care that incorporates their specific beliefs and

*The term *minority* is used here because the U.S. Census Bureau has reported its data according to the following federally defined minority groups: blacks (African, Haitian, or Dominican Republic descent); Hispanics (Mexican, Cuban, Puerto Rican, and others); Asians (Japanese, Chinese, Filipino, Korean, Vietnamese, Hawaiian, Guamian, Samoan, or Asian Indian descent); and American Indians and Alaska Natives (550 federally recognized nations). Because the term connotes inferiority and marginalization, members of some groups object to its use.

TABLE 12-1

Composition of United States Population and Percentage of Change, 1990 to 2000

Population Group	Population 1990 (4/90)	% of Population	Population 2000 (1/00)	% of Population	% Change from 1990
Total	248,765,000	100	273,866,000	100	10
White (nonHispanic)	188,307,000	75.7	196,409,000	71.7	4.3
Black (nonHispanic)	29,299,000	11.8	33,278,000	12.2	13.6
Native-American, Eskimo, and Aleut	1,796,000	0.7	2,033,000	0.7	13.2
Asian and Pacific Islander	6,992,000	2.8	10,379,000	3.8	48.4
Hispanic (any race)	22,372,000	9.0	31,767,000	11.6	42.0

From US Census Bureau: *Population estimates program,* 1999a, Population Division, www.census.gov.

practices. An increasing expectation exists among members of certain cultural groups that health care providers will respect their "cultural health rights," an expectation that frequently conflicts with the unicultural, Western biomedical worldview taught in most U.S. educational programs that prepare nurses and other health care providers.

Given the multicultural composition of the United States and the projected increase in the number of individuals from diverse cultural backgrounds, concern for cultural beliefs and practices of people in community health nursing is becoming increasingly important. Nursing is inherently a transcultural phenomenon in that the context and process of helping people involves at least two people who usually have different cultural orientations or intracultural lifestyles.

CULTURAL PERSPECTIVES AND *HEALTHY PEOPLE 2010*

Healthy People 2010, the prevention agenda for the nation, identifies priority areas and objectives aimed at increasing the years of healthy life and reducing the health disparities for Americans. By developing a set of national health targets, which includes eliminating racial and ethnic disparities in health and holding forums for public response to those targets, U.S. health officials, together with state and local officials and members of the private sector, are setting goals to increase the quality and years of healthy

life for all Americans (Brooks, 1998; Lurie, 1999; USDHHS, 2000).

The *Healthy People 2010* objectives encompass the government's *Initiative to Eliminate Racial and Ethnic Disparities in Health* and focus on ways to close the gaps in health outcomes, particularly racial and ethnic disparities in diabetes, AIDS, heart disease, infant mortality rates, cancer screening and management, and immunizations. The objectives bring focus to disparities among racial and ethnic minorities, women, youths, older adults, people of low income and education, and people with disabilities (Brooks, 1998; USDHHS, 2000).

The aims of *Healthy People 2010* are the promotion of healthy behaviors, promotion of healthy and safe communities, improvement of systems for personal and public health, and prevention and reduction of diseases and disorders. The initiative is a tool for monitoring and tracking health status, health risks, and use of health services. Table 12-2 lists selected objectives from *Healthy People 2010* specific to cultural health issues.

Healthy People 2000: Research Overview and Cultural Issues

Improvement has been demonstrated for 56% of the *Healthy People 2000* objectives, and substantial progress has been made on 43% (Simpson, 1998). For example, more black, Hispanic, Chinese-American, and Vietnamese-American women are participating in

TABLE 12-2

Culture and *Healthy People 2010* Objectives

Objective	Baseline (1998)	Target
1-1: Increase the proportion of persons with health insurance.		
American-Indian or Alaska Native	79%	100%
Asian or Pacific Islander	83%	
Black	84%	
White	87%	
Hispanic	70%	
1-8 e-h: Increase nursing degrees awarded to underrepresented populations.		
e. American-Indian or Alaska Native	0.7%	1%
f. Asian or Pacific Islander	3.2%	4%
g. Black	6.9%	13%
h. Hispanic	3.4%	12%
3-1: Reduce the overall cancer death rate.	201.4 per 100,000	158.7 per 100,000
American-Indian or Alaska Native	131.8	
Asian or Pacific Islander	127.2	
Black	262.1	
White	202.2	
Hispanic	125.5	
5-3: Reduce the overall rate of diabetes that is clinically diagnosed.	40 per 1000	25 per 1000
American-Indian or Alaska Native	NA	
Asian or Pacific Islander	NA	
Black	74	
White	36	
Hispanic	61	
8-11: Eliminate elevated blood lead levels in children.	4.4% (one to five years of age)	0
American-Indian or Alaska Native	NA	
Asian or Pacific Islander	NA	
African-American	11.5%	
White	2.6%	
Hispanic	4%	
9-7: Reduce pregnancies among adolescent females (overall).	72 per 1000	42 per 1000
American-Indian or Alaska Native	NA	
Asian or Pacific Islander	NA	
Black	133	
White	61	
Hispanic	110	
12-1: Reduce coronary heart disease deaths (overall).	208 per 100,000	166 per 100,000
American-Indian or Alaska Native	134	
Asian or Pacific Islander	125	
Black	257	
White	214	
Hispanic	151	

From US Department of Health and Human Services: *Healthy people 2010,* Washington, DC, 2000, US Government Printing Office.

Continued

TABLE 12-2—cont'd

Culture and *Healthy People 2010* Objectives—cont'd

Objective	Baseline (1998)	Target
13-1: Reduce AIDS among adolescents and adults (overall).	19.5 new cases per 100,000	1 new case per 100,000
American-Indian or Alaska Native	9.4	
Asian or Pacific Islander	4.3	
Black	82.9	
White	8.5	
Hispanic	33	
15-3: Reduce firearm-related deaths (overall).	11 per 100,000	4.9 per 100,000
American-Indian or Alaska Native	11.4	
Asian or Pacific Islander	5	
Black	23.7	
White	10	
Hispanic	10.7	
16-1 h: Reduce deaths from SIDS.	0.77 per 1000	0.3 per 1000
American-Indian or Alaska Native	1.56	
Asian or Pacific Islander	0.51	
Black	1.46	
White	0.71	
Hispanic	0.47	
18-1: Reduce the suicide rate (overall).	10.8 per 100,000	6 per 100,000
American-Indian or Alaska Native	12.4	
Asian or Pacific Islander	7	
Black	6.5	
White	12.8	
Hispanic	6.4	
19-2: Reduce the proportion of adults who are obese (overall).	23%	15%
American-Indian or Alaska Native	NA	
Asian or Pacific Islander	NA	
Black	30%	
White	21%	
Hispanic	29%	
26-1: Reduce deaths caused by alcohol-related motor vehicle crashes.	6.1 per 100,000	4 per 100,000
American-Indian or Alaska Native	19.2	
Asian or Pacific Islander	2.4	
Black	6.4	
White	6	
Hispanic	NA	
27-1 a: Reduce cigarette smoking by adults (overall).	24%	12%
American-Indian or Alaska Native	34%	
Asian or Pacific Islander	16%	
Black	26%	
White	25%	
Hispanic	20%	

From US Department of Health and Human Services: *Healthy people 2010*, Washington, DC, 2000, US Government Printing Office.

mammography screening for breast cancer detection, largely as a result of partnerships between health care providers and ethnic community-based agencies (Lurie, 1999; USDHHS, 1997). Frank-Stromberg and colleagues (1998) report that they were able to improve rural Hispanic women's participation in breast and cervical cancer screening by collaborating with a Catholic community outreach program, a local university, a university nursing program, and a rural nurse-managed clinic. By addressing barriers to access such as language, transportation, cost, and child care, the outreach program addressed the cultural and economic needs of the women who participated. The use of female family NP students promoted culturally congruent care by eliminating the traditional cultural embarrassment associated with examination by a male health care provider.

Fox and colleagues (1998) report similar strategies in a program for "hard-to-reach" urban Hispanic women. Bird and colleagues (1998) report significant increases in mammograms and Papanicolaou (PAP) tests among Vietnamese-American women when trained community-based Vietnamese lay health workers were used. The neighborhood-based intervention includes small-group educational sessions, material distribution, and promotional events all in the Vietnamese language (Jenkins et al., 1999).

Research that focuses on the prevention and treatment of specific diseases among minority populations includes studies on the prevention of CVD in blacks (Ofili, Igho-Pemu, and Bransford, 1999), cancer prevention and control among Hispanics (Ramirez et al., 1995), influence of the social environment on Asian-American diabetics (Rankin, Galbraith, and Huang, 1997), and the use of Native-American medicine in the treatment of multiple illness (e.g., diabetes).

Recognizing that lifestyle change is a major avenue for reducing illness and promoting health throughout the life span, Duffy, Rossow, and Hernandez (1996) examined the health-promoting behaviors of employed Mexican-American women. More than one half of Mexican-American women are employed outside the home, with about one third in semiskilled, nonprofessional occupations. The results of the study indicate that age, education, self-efficacy, the influence of powerful significant others, and current health status affect Mexican-American women's health-promoting lifestyle behaviors. Employed, middle-age Mexican-American women who perceive that their lifestyle behaviors can influence their health were more likely to engage in regular exercise;

maintain appropriate weight, cholesterol level, and blood pressure; drink alcohol in moderation; and practice "heart-healthy" lifestyles.

Strickland, Squeoch, and Chrisman (1999) designed a culturally appropriate cervical cancer prevention program with Yakama Indian women residing in Eastern Washington. In this program, several teaching strategies were used including storytelling, talking circles, and use of role models. Conclusions after this three-year study included the need for the following:

1. Cervical cancer prevention goals to be holistic and focused on wellness.
2. Teaching methods that include religious considerations such as the use of circular symbols.
3. Interventions that include elders and are linked to the natural communication patterns.

As health care continues to shift toward community-based ambulatory care, the need to provide meaningful and satisfying services at home for people from diverse cultures becomes more urgent. Pacquiao, Archeval, and Shelley (1999) studied informants' experiences with home care by multidisciplinary health care providers. Study findings support the importance of culture as the context for defining and interpreting satisfaction with care. In contrast to hospital care, informants perceived home care as enhancing their ability to remain in their familiar, valued home environment and supportive of their restorative and health maintenance needs. All informants viewed their home as the optimum location for continuity of their lifestyles, family relationships, and cultural values.

HISTORIC PERSPECTIVES ON CULTURAL DIVERSITY

At no other time in the history of nursing have cultures been interacting and communicating with one another more frequently than today. However, nurses have been concerned with the cultural dimensions of care for many years. This section is a brief historic overview of the ways in which nurses have responded to the health care needs of those from various cultural backgrounds.

Although the nineteenth-century concept of culture was limited and focused on physiological differences, Florence Nightingale's provision of care to wounded soldiers during the Crimean War and her concern with the fate of the Australian aborigines made her the first nurse in modern history to consider cultural aspects of nursing care. Concern for the health care needs of culturally diverse groups is also reflected in early nineteenth-century U.S. history. In 1870, Linda Richards became the first nurse known to engage in international nursing when, under the auspices of the American Board of Missions, she established a school of nursing in Japan. In the early 1900s, Lillian Wald, Lavinia Dock, and other public health nurses provided nursing care for European immigrants, many of whom resided in low-income tenement houses in New York City.

In the 1960s and 1970s, many racial and ethnic groups, most notably blacks and Hispanics, became increasingly concerned with their civil rights and raised the consciousness of the U.S. public. Influenced by the social and political climate, U.S. nurses responded with growing professional awareness and increased sensitivity to attitudes, values, beliefs, and practices about health, illness, and caring among culturally diverse clients. The nursing profession responded to the sociocultural and historic events of this era with the development of a specialty called **transcultural nursing** (Andrews, 1992).

TRANSCULTURAL NURSING IN THE COMMUNITY

In 1959, Madeleine Leininger, a nurse-anthropologist, used the term *transcultural nursing* to define the philosophical and theoretical similarities between nursing and anthropology. In 1968, Leininger proposed her theory-generated model, and in 1970 she wrote the first book on transcultural nursing, *Nursing and Anthropology: Two Worlds to Blend* (Leininger, 1970). According to Leininger, transcultural nursing is "a formal area of study and practice focused on a comparative analysis of different cultures and subcultures in the world with respect to cultural care, health and illness beliefs, values, and practices with the goal of using this knowledge to provide culture-specific and culture-universal nursing care to people" (Leininger, 1978, p. 493). **Culture specific** refers to the "particularistic values, beliefs, and patterning of behavior that tend to be special, 'local,' or unique to a designated culture and which do not tend to be shared with members of other cultures" (Leininger, 1991, p. 491), whereas **culture universal** refers to the "commonalties of values, norms of behavior, and life patterns that are similarly held among cultures about human behavior and lifestyles and form the bases for formulating theories for developing

cross-cultural laws of human behavior" (Leininger, 1978, p. 491).

Although many nurse-scholars have developed theories of nursing, Leininger's theory of culture care diversity and universality is the only one that gives precedence to understanding the cultural dimensions of human care and caring. Leininger's theory is concerned with describing, explaining, and projecting nursing similarities and differences focused primarily on human care and caring in human cultures. Leininger used worldview, social structure, language, ethnohistory, environmental context, and the generic (i.e., folk) and professional systems to provide a comprehensive and holistic view of influences in cultural care and well-being. The following three models of nursing decisions and actions may be useful in providing culturally congruent and competent care (Andrews and Boyle, 1997, 1999; Leininger, 1978, 1991, 1995):

1. Culture care preservation and maintenance
2. Culture care accommodation and negotiation
3. Culture care repatterning and restructuring

Among the strengths of Leininger's theory is its flexibility for use with individuals, families, groups, communities, and institutions in diverse health systems. Leininger's sunrise model (Fig. 12-1) depicts the theory of cultural care diversity and universality and provides a visual representation of the key components of the theory and the interrelationships among its components.

Although this text does not review all the recognized nursing theories from a transcultural perspective, the reader should critically evaluate the cultural relevance of a theory before using it in community health nursing. The nurse should examine the underlying assumptions of theories from a transcultural perspective. For example, those theories emphasizing self-care fail to recognize that many cultures and subcultures value group interdependence, cooperation, and responsibility for others. When clients' cultural values and expressions of care differ from those of the nurse, the nurse must exercise caution to ensure that mutual goals have been established.

The term *cross-cultural nursing* is sometimes used synonymously with *transcultural nursing*. The terms *intercultural nursing* and *multicultural nursing* and the phrase *ethnic people of color* are also used. Since Leininger's early work, many nurses have contributed significantly to the advancement of nursing care of culturally diverse clients, groups, and

F I G U R E **12-1**

Leininger's sunrise model to depict the theory of cultural care diversity and universality (From Leiniger MM: *Culture, care, diversity, and universality: a theory of nursing,* Pub No 15-2402, New York, 1991, NLN).

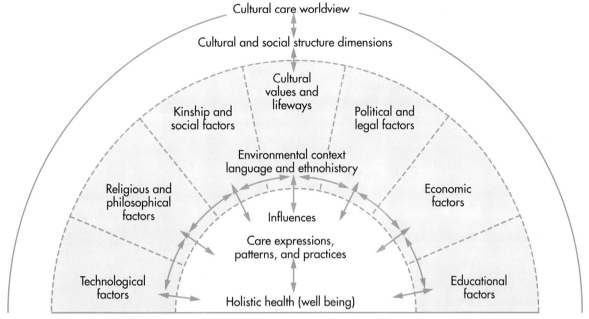

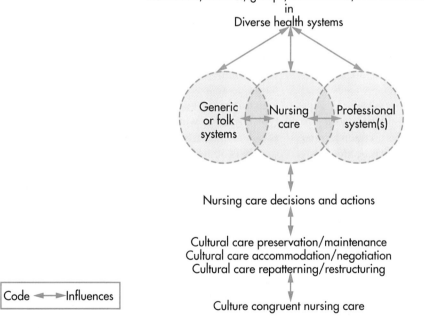

communities, and some of their contributions are mentioned in this chapter.

One of the major challenges that community health nurses face in working with clients from culturally diverse backgrounds is overcoming individual **ethnocentrism**, which is a person's tendency to view his or her own way of life as the most desirable, acceptable, or best and to act in a superior manner toward another culture. Nurses must also beware of **cultural imposition**, which is a person's tendency to impose his or her own beliefs, values, and patterns of behavior on individuals from another culture.

OVERVIEW OF CULTURE

In 1871, the English anthropologist Sir Edward Tylor was the first to define the term **culture.** According to Tylor (1871), *culture* refers to the complex whole, including knowledge, beliefs, art, morals, law, customs, and any other capabilities and habits acquired by virtue of the fact that one is a member of a particular society. Culture represents a person's way of perceiving, evaluating, and behaving within his or her world and it provides the blueprint for determining his or her values, beliefs, and practices. Culture has four basic characteristics.

1. It is learned from birth through the processes of language acquisition and socialization.
2. It is shared by all members of the same cultural group.
3. It is adapted to specific conditions related to environmental and technical factors and to the availability of natural resources.
4. It is dynamic.

Culture is an all-pervasive and universal phenomenon. However, the culture that develops in any given society is always specific and distinctive, encompassing all of the knowledge, beliefs, customs, and skills acquired by members of that society. Within cultures, groups of individuals share beliefs, values, and attitudes that are different from those of other groups within the same culture. Ethnicity, religion, education, occupation, age, sex, and individual preferences and variations bring differences. When such groups function within a large culture, they are termed *subcultural groups.*

The term **subculture** is used for fairly large aggregates of people who share characteristics that are not common to all members of the culture and enable them to be a distinguishable subgroup. Ethnicity, religion, occupation, health-related characteristics, age, sex, and geographical location are frequently used to identify subcultural groups. Examples of U.S. subcultures based on ethnicity (e.g., subcultures with common traits such as physical characteristics, language, or ancestry) include blacks, Hispanics, Native-Americans, and Chinese-Americans. Subcultures based on religion include members of the more than 1200 recognized religions such as Catholics, Jews, Mormons, Muslims, and Buddhists. Those based on

occupation include health care professionals (e.g., nurses and physicians), career military personnel, and farmers. Those based on health-related characteristics include the blind, hearing impaired, or mentally retarded. Subcultures based on age include adolescents and older adults, and those based on sex or sexual preference include women, men, lesbians, and gay men. Those based on geographical location include Appalachians, Southerners, and New Yorkers.

Culture and the Formation of Values

According to Leininger (1995), **value** refers to a desirable or undesirable state of affairs. Values are a universal feature of all cultures, although the types and expressions of values differ widely. **Norms** are the rules by which human behavior is governed and result from the cultural values held by the group. All societies have rules or norms that specify appropriate and inappropriate behavior. Individuals are rewarded or punished as they conform to or deviate from the established norms. Values and norms, along with the acceptable and unacceptable behaviors associated with them, are learned in childhood (Herberg, 1995).

Every society has a **dominant value orientation**, a basic value orientation that is shared by the majority of its members as a result of early common experiences. In the United States, the dominant value orientation is reflected in the dominant cultural group, which is made up of white, middle-class Protestants, typically those who came to the United States at least two generations ago from northern Europe. Many members of the dominant cultural group are of Anglo-Saxon descent; therefore they are sometimes referred to as White Anglo-Saxon Protestants (WASPs). In the United States, the dominant cultural group places emphasis on educational achievement, science, technology, individual expression, democracy, experimentation, and informality (Herberg, 1995).

Although an assumption is sometimes made that the term *white* refers to a homogeneous group of Americans, a rich diversity of ethnic variation exists among the many groups that constitute the dominant majority. Countries of origin include Eastern and Western Europe (e.g., Ireland, Poland, Italy, France, Sweden, and Russia), and Canada, Australia, New Zealand, and South Africa Origins can ultimately be traced to western Europe. Appalachians, the Amish, Cajuns, and other subgroups are also examples of whites who have cultural roots that are recognizably different from those of the dominant cultural group.

According to Kluckhohn and Strodtbeck (1961), several basic human problems exist for which all people must find a solution. They identified the following five common human problems related to values and norms:

1. What is the character of innate human nature (human nature orientation)?
2. What is the relationship of the human to nature (person-nature orientation)?
3. What is the temporal focus (i.e., time sense) of human life (time orientation)?
4. What is the mode of human activity (activity orientation)?
5. What is the mode of human relationships (social orientation)?

Human Nature Orientation

Innate human nature may be good, evil, or a combination of good and evil. Some consider human nature to be unalterable or able to be perfected only through great discipline and effort because they believe that life is a struggle to overcome a basically evil nature. For others, human nature is perceived as fundamentally good, unalterable, and difficult or impossible to corrupt.

According to Kohls (1984), the dominant U.S. cultural group chooses to believe the best about a person until that person proves otherwise. Concern in the United States for prison reform, social rehabilitation, and the plight of less fortunate people around the world is a reflective perception of the belief in the fundamental goodness of human nature, although human nature may also be viewed as a combination of good and evil.

Person-Nature Orientation

The following three perspectives examine the ways in which the person-nature relationship is perceived:

1. Destiny, in which people are subjugated to nature in a fatalistic, inevitable manner.
2. Harmony, in which people and nature exist together as a single entity.
3. Mastery, in which people are intended to overcome natural forces and put them to use for the benefit of humankind.

Most Americans consider humans and nature clearly separated, which is an incomprehensible perspective for many individuals of Asian heritage. The idea that a person can control his or her own destiny is alien to many individuals of culturally diverse backgrounds. Many cultures believe that people are driven and controlled by fate and can do very little, if anything, to influence it. Americans, by contrast, have an insatiable drive to subdue, dominate, and control their natural environment (Kohls, 1984).

For example, the reader should consider three individuals who have been diagnosed with hypertension, where each embraces one of the values orientations described. The person whose values orientation is destiny may say, "Why should I bother watching my diet, taking medication, and getting regular blood pressure checks? High blood pressure is part of my genetic destiny and there is nothing I can do to change the outcome. There is no need to waste money on prescription drugs and health checkups." The person whose values orientation embraces harmony may say, "If I follow the diet described and use medication to lower my blood pressure, I can restore the balance and harmony that were upset by this illness. The emotional stress I've been feeling indicates an inner lack of harmony that needs to be balanced." The person whose values orientation leads to belief in active mastery may say, "I will overcome this hypertension no matter what. By eating the right foods, working toward stress reduction, and conquering the disease with medication, I will take charge of the situation and influence the course of my disease."

Time Orientation

People can perceive time in the following three ways:

1. *The focus may be on the past, with traditions and ancestors playing an important role in the client's life.* For example, many Asians, Native-Americans, East Indians, and Africans hold particular beliefs about ancestors and tend to value long-standing traditions. In times of crisis, such as illness, individuals with a values orientation emphasizing the past may consult with ancestors or ask for their guidance or protection during the illness.
2. *The focus may be on the present, with little attention paid to the past or the future.* These individuals are concerned with the current situation and they perceive the future as vague or

unpredictable. Nurses may have difficulty encouraging these individuals to prepare for the future (e.g., participate in primary prevention measures).

3. *The focus may be on the future, with progress and change highly valued.* These individuals may express discontent with the past and present. In terms of health care, these individuals may inquire about the "latest treatment" and the most advanced equipment available for a particular problem.

The dominant U.S. cultural group is characterized by a belief in progress and a future orientation. This implies a strong task or goal orientation. This group has an optimistic faith in what the future will bring. Change is often equated with improvement and a rapid rate of change is usually normal.

Activity Orientation

This value orientation concerns activity. Philosophers have suggested the following three perspectives:

1. Being, in which a spontaneous expression of impulses and desires is largely nondevelopmental in nature.
2. Growing, in which the person is self-contained and has inner control, including the ability to self-actualize.
3. Doing, in which the person actively strives to achieve and accomplish something that is regarded highly.

The person often directs the doing toward achievement of an externally applied standard, such as a code of behavior from a religious or ethical perspective. The Ten Commandments, Pillars of Islam, Hippocratic oath, and Nightingale pledge are examples of externally applied standards.

The dominant cultural value is action oriented, with an emphasis on productivity and being busy. As a result of this action orientation, Americans have become proficient at problem solving and decision making. Even during leisure time and vacations, many Americans value activity.

Social Orientation

Variations in cultural values orientation are also related to the relationships that exist with others. Relationships may be categorized in the following three ways:

1. Lineal relationships: These exist by virtue of heredity and kinship ties. These relationships follow an ordered succession and have continuity through time.
2. Collateral relationships: The focus is primarily on group goals, and family orientation is important. For example, many Asian patients describe family honor and the importance of working together toward achievement of a group vs. a personal goal.
3. Individual relationships: These refer to personal autonomy and independence. These goals dominate and group goals become secondary.

The social orientation among the dominant U.S. cultural group is toward the importance of the individual and the equality of all people. Friendly, informal, outgoing, and extroverted members of the dominant cultural group tend to scorn rank and authority. For example, nursing students may call faculty members by their first names, patients may call nurses by their first names, and employees may fraternize with their employers.

Members of the dominant culture have a strong sense of individuality. However, family ties are relatively weak, as demonstrated by the high rate of separation and divorce in the United States. In many U.S. households, the family has been reduced to its smallest unit—the single-parent family.

When making health-related decisions, clients from culturally diverse backgrounds rely on relationships with others in various ways. If the cultural values orientation is lineal, the client may seek assistance from other members of the family and allow a relative (e.g., parent, grandparent, or elder brother) to make decisions about important health-related matters. If collateral relationships are valued, decisions about the client may be interrelated with the influence of illness on the entire family or group. For example, among the Amish, the entire community is affected by the illness of a member because the community pays for health care from a common fund. Members join together to meet the needs of the patient and family for the duration of the illness and the roles of many in the community are likely to be affected by the illness of a single member.

A values orientation that emphasizes the individual is predominant among the dominant cultural majority in the United States. Decision making about health and illness is often an individual matter, with the client being responsible, although members of the nuclear family may participate to varying degrees.

Culture and the Family

Despite the alarmingly high rate of divorce in the United States, the family remains the basic social unit. Although various ways exist to categorize families, the following are commonly recognized types of constellations in which people live together in society:

- Nuclear (i.e., husband, wife, and child or children)
- Nuclear dyad (i.e., husband and wife alone, either childless or with no children living at home)
- Single parent (i.e., either mother or father and at least one child)
- Blended (i.e., husband, wife, and children from previous relationships)
- Extended (i.e., nuclear plus other blood relatives)
- Communal (i.e., group of men and women with or without children)
- Cohabitation (i.e., unmarried man and woman sharing a household with or without children)
- Gay (i.e., same-gender couples with or without children)

In addition to structural differences in families cross-culturally, accompanying functional diversity may exist. For example, among extended families, kin residence sharing has long been recognized as a viable alternative to managing scarce resources, meeting child care needs, and caring for a handicapped and/or older family member. Sometimes the shared household is an adaptation for survival and protection. In general, families with a culturally diverse heritage include a large number of adults and a larger number of children.

More than half, or 55.3%, of all black children younger than three years of age are born into single-parent families. Among Puerto Ricans living in the United States, 44% of families are headed by single women. Among black families, grandmothers have the most active involvement with the grandchildren when they live with their single adult daughters. This is not the case in families with two parents or in single-parent families when the grandmother lives in a different household. Black infants are exposed to a variety of primary care providers and experience different patterns of social interaction compared with their counterparts in the dominant cultural group (Garcia Coll, 1990; NCHS, 1999).

In addition to a higher incidence of single heads of household, some cultural groups also have a higher incidence of teenage parents. Both blacks and Hispanics, especially Mexican-Americans and mainland Puerto Ricans, have higher percentages of births to mothers younger than 20 years of age (24% and 18%, respectively) than do whites (10%). Blacks also have a higher rate of adolescent pregnancy than whites, especially for births to unmarried teenagers. Adolescent pregnancies among whites have declined markedly in recent years as a result of such factors as sex education programs in schools, availability of contraceptives, and legalization of abortion (NCHS, 1999).

The family constellations associated with teen parenting are unique and provide a special socialization context for infants. For example, Hispanic teen mothers receive more child care help from grandmothers and peers than do white teen mothers. Among blacks and Puerto Ricans, the presence of the maternal grandmother ameliorates the negative consequences of adolescent childbirth on the infant. In addition, grandmothers are more responsive and less punitive in their interactions with the infant than their daughters. These data suggest the following two mechanisms by which three-generational households can have an influence on the infant's development: by influencing the mother's knowledge about development and providing other more responsive social interactions with infants (Garcia Coll, 1990).

Ethnic families are often characterized as being more conservative in terms of sex roles and parenting values and practices than white families. For example, traditional Japanese-American and Mexican-American families are family centered, enforce strict gender and age roles, and emphasize children's compliance with authority figures. Children of culturally diverse backgrounds are involved in different family interactions than children from the dominant U.S. cultural group.

Relationships that may seem apparent sometimes warrant further exploration when interacting with clients from culturally diverse backgrounds. For example, the dominant cultural group defines siblings as two people with the same mother, the same father, the same mother and father, or the same adoptive parents. In some Asian cultures, a sibling relationship is defined as involving infants who are breast-fed by the same woman. In other cultures, certain kinship patterns, such as maternal first cousins, are sibling relationships. In some African cultures, anyone from the same village or town may be called "brother" or "sister."

Certain subcultures, such as Roman Catholics, who may be further subdivided by ethnicity into those who are Italian, Polish, Spanish, Mexican, etc., recognize relationships such as "godmother" or "godfather;" in which an individual who is not the biological parent promises to assist with the moral and spiritual development of an infant and agrees to care for the child in the event of parental death. The godparent makes these promises during the religious ceremony of baptism.

When providing care for infants and children, the nurse must identify the primary provider of care because this individual may or may not be the biological parent. For example, among some Hispanic groups, female members of the nuclear or extended family (e.g., sisters or aunts) are sometimes the primary providers of care. In some black families, the grandmother may be the decision maker and primary caregiver of the children.

CULTURE AND SOCIOECONOMIC FACTORS

No single indicator can adequately capture all facets of economic status for entire populations, but measures such as median or average annual income, employment rate, poverty rate, and net worth are most often used. The economic status of most individuals, especially children, is better reflected by the pooled resources of family or household members than by their individual earnings or income. **Socioeconomic status** (SES) is a composite of the economic status of a family or unrelated individuals based on income, wealth, occupation, educational attainment, and power. It is a means of measuring inequalities based on economic differences and the manner in which families live as a result of their economic well-being. Most families with racially or ethnically diverse backgrounds have a lower SES than the population at large, with a few exceptions (e.g., Cuban-Americans and subgroups of Asian-Americans).

The average income of U.S. families increased significantly during the past 50 years. However, between the 1970s and the 1990s, the median family incomes of blacks and Hispanics were stagnant, whereas the median incomes of nonHispanic whites increased. The income of nonHispanic whites and Asian families was nearly twice that of black and Hispanic families. The ratio of black to nonHispanic white median family income is about the same today as it was in the 1970s, whereas the ratio of Hispanic to nonHispanic white income has fallen markedly during the same period (Council of Economic Advisors for the President's Initiative on Race, 1999).

The decline in the relative economic well-being of Hispanics is due, in part, to immigration of Hispanics with relatively low levels of education and income. The lack of relative progress by black families is a result of the large rise in single-parent families among blacks. Other factors contributing to differences in family income include differences in educational attainment, unemployment rates, and wage rates. The median family income of Asians is slightly higher than that of nonHispanic whites and is consistent with Asians' high levels of educational attainment and the higher percentage of Asian families with two or more wage earners (Council of Economic Advisers for the President's Initiative on Race, 1999).

Unemployment is consistently high among blacks, Hispanics, Native-Americans, and Alaska Natives. For example, most Native-American reservations report an unemployment rate of approximately 30% (IHS, 1997).

Poverty is another factor that dramatically influences health and well-being. The **poverty rate** refers to the proportion of the population who lack the economic resources needed to purchase a minimally acceptable standard of living. Despite their higher median income, Asian-Americans have a 50% higher poverty rate than nonHispanic whites. This reflects the economic and educational diversity of the Asian populations. Blacks, Hispanics, and Native-Americans have much higher rates of poverty than nonHispanic whites and Asians. Although it remains high, the black poverty rate has declined since the early 1990s and reached an all-time low in 1996. The poverty rate for Native-Americans is higher than that of any other group.

Although child poverty rates exceed overall individual poverty rates, differences between racial and ethnic groups in child poverty mirror those in overall poverty. Blacks, Hispanic, and Native-American children have higher poverty rates than nonHispanic white and Asian children (Council of Economic Advisers for the President's Initiative on Race, 1999).

Distribution of Resources

Status, power, and wealth in the United States are not distributed equally throughout society. Rather, a small percentage of the population enjoys most of the nation's resources, primarily through ownership of multibillion-dollar corporations, large pieces of real estate in prime locations, and similar assets. Using SES as an indicator of status, power, and wealth, the U.S. population has traditionally been divided into the following three social classes: upper, middle, and lower. SES may be calculated by considering a variety of factors, but it is customarily determined by examining factors such as total family income, occupation, and educational level. In a less formalized examination of SES, factors such as age, sex, material possessions, health status, family name, location of residence, family composition, amount of land owned, religion, race, and ethnicity may also be considered.

A disproportionate number of individuals from the racially and ethnically diverse subgroups are members of the lower socioeconomic class, whereas a larger percentage of members of the dominant cultural group (i.e., WASPs) belong to the upper and middle socioeconomic classes (Council of Economic Advisers for the President's Initiative on Race, 1999). The United States has socioeconomic stratification; therefore the idealization of America as the land of opportunity often applies more to members of the upper and middle classes than to those of the lower class. The outcome of social stratification is social inequality. For example, school systems, grocery stores, and recreational facilities vary significantly between the inner city, which has a high percentage of minority residents, and the suburbs, which are overwhelmingly WASP.

Blacks, Hispanics, and Native-Americans experience the most severe economic deprivation of all ethnic groups in the United States. In 1990, when husband-wife families were compared, blacks earned 84% and Hispanics earned 69% of the median income of whites. When both husband and wife worked, the gap narrowed to 85% for blacks and 74% for Hispanics. When age, education, experience, and other factors are equal to those of white men, the earnings of racial and ethnic minorities and whites become more similar, but the income ratios among the groups still favor whites (Council of Economic Advisers for the President's Initiative on Race, 1999; US Census Bureau, 1992).

Members of racial and ethnic minorities make up a disproportionately high percentage of people in poverty. Of the white population, 11% fall below the poverty level compared with 32% of the black population and 38% of the Hispanic population. Within the Hispanic population, 41% of Puerto Ricans suffer from poverty. One cause and effect of poverty is that people from racial and ethnic minorities tend to be more segregated than white families. For example, 70% of black households are located in low-income areas, whereas 66% of poor white families live in suburban or rural areas (US Census Bureau, 1999a). Table 12-3 summarizes the percentage of minority populations living below the poverty level.

For many years, health care settings have been the subject of study and concern regarding distribution of resources, with members of racial and ethnic minority groups clamoring with indignation at the inequalities. As the only industrialized Western nation in the world without a national health care delivery system, the United States provides the best health care

TABLE **12-3**

Percentage of Minority Populations Living Below Poverty Level: 1998

Race	Total (%)	Children Younger than 18 Years of Age (%)	Female Head of Household (%)
Total	12.7	18.3	29.9
Black	26.1	NA	40.8
Hispanic	25.6	NA	43.7
Asian and Pacific Islander	12.5	NA	NA
White nonHispanic	8.2	NA	20.7

From US Census Bureau: *Poverty 1998: poverty by selected characteristics,* 1999b, The Author, www.census.gov/hhes/poverty/poverty98/pv98est1.html.

to those with the highest SES and substantially inferior health care to those with low SES. In the United States, SES largely determines the quality of health care.

Education

One of the components considered in determining SES is educational level. Educational attainment is perhaps the single most important factor. For example, Native-Americans and Alaska Natives, who have a relatively poor health status, average 9.6 years of formal education, which is the lowest rate for any major U.S. ethnic group (IHS, 1997).

Research suggests that differences between white and Mexican-American home teaching strategies can be accounted for by differences in levels of formal schooling rather than by cultural differences or economic indices. Mothers who had received more years of formal education inquired and praised more often than did mothers with less education. In contrast, the lower the mother's level of formal education, the more often she used modeling as a teaching strategy. Compared with white mothers, Hispanic mothers inquired and praised less often and used modeling, visual cues, directives, and negative physical control more often. However, these differences disappeared entirely when the mother's or father's educational level was controlled statistically (Garcia Coll, 1990). These studies contribute to an understanding of the ways in which educational level attained by people from culturally diverse backgrounds affects the didactic aspects of the child-rearing environment.

The importance of other correlates of SES, such as home language and family size, has also been studied. In a study that examined the levels of performance on various abilities by children from Hispanic and white families of diverse socioeconomic levels, home language backgrounds, and family size, Hispanic and white children performed equally well when the socioeconomic factors were controlled. However, the combination of low SES and language minority status negatively affected the children's performance in areas such as verbal ability, quantitative ability, and short-term memory.

CULTURE AND NUTRITION

Long after assimilation into the U.S. culture has occurred, clients from various ethnic groups will continue to follow culturally-based dietary practices and eat ethnic foods. When a new group of immigrants arrives in the United States, neighborhood food markets and ethnic restaurants are often established soon after arrival. The ethnic restaurant is often a place for members of the cultural group to meet and mingle and customers from the dominant cultural group may be of secondary interest. Food is an integral part of cultural identity that extends beyond dietary preferences.

Nutrition Assessment of Culturally Diverse Groups

Among factors that must be considered in a nutrition assessment are the cultural definition of food, frequency and number of meals eaten away from home, form and content of ceremonial meals, amount and types of food eaten, and regularity of food consumption. Potential inaccuracies may occur; therefore the 24-hour dietary recalls or three-day food records traditionally used for assessment may be inadequate when dealing with clients from culturally diverse backgrounds. Standard dietary handbooks may fail to provide culture-specific diet information because nutritional content and exchange tables are usually based on Western diets. Another source of error may originate from the cultural patterns of eating. For example, among low-income urban black families, elaborate weekend meals are frequently eaten, whereas weekday dietary patterns are markedly more moderate.

Although community health nurses may assume that *food* is a culture-universal term, they may need to clarify its meaning with the client. For example, certain Latin-American groups do not consider greens, an important source of vitamins, to be food and fail to list intake of these vegetables on daily records. Among Vietnamese refugees, dietary intake of calcium may appear inadequate because low consumption rates of dairy products are common among members of this group. However, they commonly consume pork bones and shells, providing adequate quantities of calcium to meet daily requirements.

Food is only one part of eating. In some cultures, social contacts during meals are restricted to members of the immediate or extended family. For example, in some Middle Eastern cultures, men and women eat meals separately or women are permitted to eat with their husbands but not with other males. Among some Hispanic groups, the male breadwinner is served first, then the women and children eat. Etiquette during meals, use of hands, type of eating utensils (e.g., chopsticks or special flatware), and protocols governing the order in which food is consumed during a meal all vary cross-culturally.

Dietary Practices of Selected Cultural Groups

Cultural stereotyping is the tendency to view individuals of common cultural backgrounds similarly and according to a preconceived notion of how they behave. However, not all Chinese like rice, not all Italians like spaghetti, and not all Mexicans like tortillas. Nevertheless, aggregate dietary preferences among people from certain cultural groups can be described (e.g., characteristic ethnic dishes and methods of food preparation, including use of cooking oils); the reader is referred to nutrition texts on the topic for detailed information about culture-specific diets and the nutritional value of ethnic foods.

TABLE 12-4

Dietary Practices of Selected Religious Groups

Religion	Dietary Practice
Hinduism	All meats are prohibited.
Islam	Pork and intoxicating beverages are prohibited.
Judaism	Pork, predatory fowl, shellfish, other water creatures (fish with scales are permissible), and blood by ingestion (e.g., blood sausage and raw meat) are prohibited. Blood by transfusion is acceptable. Foods should be kosher (i.e., meaning "properly preserved"). All animals must be ritually slaughtered by a sochet (i.e., quickly with the least pain possible) to be kosher. Mixing dairy and meat dishes at the same meal is prohibited.
Mormonism (Church of Jesus Christ of Latter-Day Saints)	Alcohol, tobacco, and beverages containing caffeine (e.g., coffee, tea, colas, and selected carbonated soft drinks) are prohibited.
Seventh-Day Adventism	Pork, certain seafood (including shellfish), and fermented beverages are prohibited. A vegetarian diet is encouraged.

Religion and Diet

Cultural food preferences are often interrelated with religious dietary beliefs and practices. As indicated in Table 12-4, many religions have proscriptive dietary practices and some use food as symbols in celebrations and rituals. Knowing the client's religious practice as it relates to food makes it possible to suggest improvements or modifications that will not conflict with religious dietary laws.

Fasting and other religious observations may limit a person's food or liquid intake during specified times. For example, many Catholics fast and abstain from meat on Ash Wednesday and each Friday of Lent, Muslims refrain from eating during the daytime hours for the month of Ramadan but are permitted to eat after sunset, and Mormons refrain from ingesting all solid foods and liquids on the first Sunday of each month.

CULTURE AND RELIGION

According to the *Yearbook of American and Canadian Churches* (National Council of Churches, 1999), 354,194 congregations represent more than 1200 religious denominations in North America. In a Gallup poll conducted by the Princeton Religion Research Center (1996), 96% of the U.S. population said that they believe in God or a universal spirit, 90% pray, and 87% believe that God answers prayers. About 82% of respondents to a CNN/*Time* poll reported that they believed in the healing power of prayer and 79% indicated that spiritual faith can help people recover from illness, disease, or injury. About 63% believe that physicians should talk to patients about spiritual faith. People in the United States, with or without health problems, are consistent in their belief that religion plays an important role in their health and well-being

Although the nurse cannot be an expert on each of the estimated 1200 religions practiced in the United States, knowledge of health-related beliefs and practices and general information about religious observances are important in providing culturally competent nursing care. For example, the nurse should have a general understanding of the religious calendar, including designated holy days, when planning home visits or scheduling clinic visits for members of a specific religious group. The nurse should also know the customary days of religious worship observed by members of the religion. Although most Protestants worship on Sundays, the sacred day of worship may vary for other religious groups. For example, the Muslims' holy day of worship extends from sunset on Thursday to sunset on Friday, whereas for Jews and Seventh-Day Adventists, the holy day extends from sunset on Friday to sunset on Saturday. Roman Catholics may worship in the late afternoon or evening of Saturday or all day Sunday. Some religions may meet more than once weekly.

In addition to regularly scheduled weekly religious services, most major religions also recognize special days of observance or celebration that last from one day (e.g., Christmas, Easter, Rosh Hashanah, and Janamasthtmi) to one month (i.e., Ramadan). Some days of commemoration or observation are based on a lunar calendar and some have rotating dates; the nurse may consult official information sources such as religious leaders or religious calendars to verify exact dates. The nurse should also ask clients what religious practices they follow because individual activity within the religious organization may vary widely.

As an integral component of the individual's culture, religious beliefs may influence the client's explanation of the cause of illness, perception of its severity, and choice of healer. In times of crisis, such as serious illness and impending death, religion may be a source of consolation for the client and family and may influence the course of action believed to be appropriate.

Religion and Spirituality

Religious concerns evolve from and respond to the mysteries of life and death, good and evil, and pain and suffering. Nurses frequently encounter clients who find themselves searching for a spiritual meaning to help explain illness or disability. Some nurses find spiritual assessment difficult because the topic is abstract and personal, whereas others feel comfortable discussing spiritual matters. Comfort with personal spiritual beliefs is the foundation for effective assessment of spiritual needs in clients.

Although religions offer various interpretations to many of life's mysteries, most people seek a personal understanding and interpretation at some time in their lives. Ultimately, this personal search becomes a pursuit to discover a supreme being (e.g., Allah, God, Yahweh, or Jehovah) or some unifying truth that will render meaning, purpose, and integrity to existence.

An important distinction must be made between religion and spirituality. *Religion* refers to an orga-

nized system of beliefs concerning the cause, nature, and purpose of the universe, especially belief in or the worship of a god or gods. More than 1200 religions are practiced in the United States. **Spirituality** is born out of the individual's unique life experience and personal effort to find purpose and meaning in life. Box 12-1

BOX **12-1**

Methods of Assessing Spiritual Needs in Culturally Diverse Clients

Environment
- Does the client have religious objects in the environment?
- Does the client wear outer garments or undergarments that have religious significance?
- Are get-well greeting cards religious in nature or from a representative of the client's church?
- Does the client receive flowers or bulletins from a church or other religious institution?

Behavior
- Does the client appear to pray at certain times of the day or before meals?
- Does the client make special dietary requests (e.g., kosher diet; vegetarian diet; or diet free from caffeine, pork, shellfish, or other specific food items)?
- Does the client read religious magazines or books?

Verbalization
- Does the client mention a supreme being (e.g., God, Allah, Buddha, or Yahweh), prayer, faith, church, or religious topics?
- Does the client request a visit by a clergy member or other religious representative?
- Does the client express anxiety or fear about pain, suffering, or death?

Interpersonal Relationships
- Who visits the client? How does the client respond to visitors?
- Does a church representative visit?
- How does the client relate to nursing staff and roommates?
- Does the client prefer to interact with others or remain alone?

Data from Andrews MM, Boyle JS, editors: *Transcultural concepts in nursing care*, ed 3, Philadelphia, 1999, Lippincott, Williams & Wilkins.

provides suggested guidelines for assessing the spiritual needs of culturally diverse clients.

Religion may influence decisions regarding prolongation of life, euthanasia, autopsy, donation of a body for research, disposal of a body and body parts including fetus, and type of burial. The nurse should use discretion in asking clients and their families about these issues and gather data only when the clinical situation necessitates that the information be obtained. The nurse should encourage clients and families to discuss these issues with their religious representative when necessary. Before dealing with potentially sensitive issues, the nurse should establish rapport with the client and family by gaining their trust and confidence in less sensitive areas.

Childhood and Spirituality

Serious illness during childhood is especially difficult. Children have spiritual needs that vary according to the child's developmental level and the religious climate that exists in the family. Parental perceptions about the illness of their child may be partially influenced by religious beliefs. For example, some parents may believe that a transgression against a religious law is responsible for a congenital anomaly in their offspring. Other parents may delay seeking medical care because they believe that prayer should be tried first. Certain types of treatment (e.g., administration of blood or medications containing caffeine, pork, or other prohibited substances and selected procedures) may be perceived as cultural taboos, which are to be avoided by children and adults.

CULTURE AND AGING

Values held by the dominant U.S. culture, such as emphasis on independence, self-reliance, and productivity, influence aging members of society. Americans define people aged 65 years as "old" and limit their work. In some other cultures, people are first recognized as being unable to work and then identified as being old. In some cultures the wisdom, not the productivity, of the older adult is valued; the diminishment of one's activity level and reduction of physical stamina associated with growing old are accepted more readily without loss of status among culture members. Retirement is also culturally defined, with some older adults working as long as physical health continues and others continuing to be active but assuming less physically demanding jobs.

The main task of older adults in the dominant culture is to achieve a sense of integrity in accepting responsibility for their own lives and having a sense of accomplishment. Individuals who achieve integrity consider aging a positive experience, make adjustments in their personal space and social relationships, maintain a sense of usefulness, and begin closure and life review. Not all cultures value accepting responsibility for an individual's own life. For example, among Hispanics, Asians, Arabs, and other groups, older adults are often cared for by family members who welcome them into their homes when they are no longer able to live alone. The concept of placing an older family member in an institutional setting to be cared for by strangers is perceived as an uncaring, impersonal, and culturally unacceptable practice by many cultural groups.

Older adults may develop their own means of coping with illness through self-care, assistance from family members, and social group support systems. Some cultures have developed attitudes and specific behaviors for older adults that include humanistic care and identification of family members as care providers. Older adults may have special family responsibilities (e.g., the older Amish adults provide hospitality to visitors, and older Filipinos adults spend considerable time teaching the youth skills learned during a lifetime of experience).

Older adult immigrants who have made major lifestyle adjustments in the move from their homeland to the United States or from a rural to an urban area, or vice versa, may need information about health care alternatives, preventive programs, health care benefits, and screening programs for which they are eligible. These individuals may also be in various stages of **culture shock**, the state of disorientation or inability to respond to the behavior of a different cultural group because it holds sudden strangeness, unfamiliarity, and incompatibility to the newcomer's perceptions and expectations (Leininger, 1995).

CROSS-CULTURAL COMMUNICATION

Verbal and nonverbal communication are important in community health nursing and are influenced by the cultural background of the nurse and client. *Cross-cultural,* or *intercultural, communication* refers to the communication process occurring between a nurse and a client who have different cultural backgrounds as both attempt to understand the other's point of view from a cultural perspective.

Nurse-Client Relationship

From the introduction of the nurse to the client through termination of the relationship, communication is a continuous process for the community health nurse. First impressions are important in all human relationships; therefore cross-cultural considerations concerning introductions warrant a few brief remarks. To ensure a mutually respectful relationship, the nurse should introduce himself or herself and indicate how the client should refer to the nurse (i.e., by first name, last name, or title). Having done so, the nurse should ask the client to do the same. This enables the nurse to address the client in a manner that is culturally appropriate and could avoid embarrassment in the future. For example, some Asian and European cultures write the last name first; confusion can be avoided in an area of extreme sensitivity (i.e., the client's name).

Space, Distance, and Intimacy

The client's and nurse's own sense of spatial distance is significant because culturally appropriate distance zones vary widely. For example, nurses may back away from clients of Hispanic, East Indian, or Middle Eastern origin who invade personal space with regularity in an attempt to bring the nurse closer into the space that is comfortable to them. Although nurses are uncomfortable with clients' close physical proximity, clients are perplexed by the nurse's distancing behaviors and may perceive the community health nurse as aloof and unfriendly. Table 12-5 summarizes the four distance zones identified for the functional use of space that are embraced by the dominant cultural group, including most nurses.

Interactions between clients and nurses may also depend on the client's desired degree of intimacy, which may range from formal interactions to close personal relationships. For example, some Southeast Asian clients expect those in authority (e.g., nurses) to be authoritarian, directive, and detached.

In contrast, Appalachian clients traditionally have close family interaction patterns that often lead them to expect close personal relationships with health care providers. The Appalachian client may evaluate the nurse's effectiveness on the basis of interpersonal skills rather than professional competency. Appala-

TABLE 12-5

Functional Use of Space

Zone	Remarks
Intimate zone (0 to 1.5 feet)	Visual distortion occurs. Best for assessing breath and other body odors.
Personal distance (1.5 to 4 feet)	Perceived as an extension of the self, similar to a "bubble." Voice is moderate. Body odors are inapparent. Visual distortion does not occur. Much of the physical assessment will occur at this distance.
Social distance (4 to 12 feet)	Used for impersonal business transactions. Perceptual information is much less detailed. Much of the interview will occur at this distance.
Public distance (12 feet)	Interaction with others is impersonal. Speaker's voice must be projected. Subtle facial expressions are imperceptible.

Data from Hall E: Proxemics: the study of man's spatial relations. In Galdston I, editor: *Man's image in medicine and anthropology,* New York, 1963, International Universities Press.

chian clients are likely to be uncomfortable with the impersonal, bureaucratic orientation of most health care institutions. Likewise, clients of Arab, Latin-American, or Mediterranean origin often expect an even higher degree of intimacy and may attempt to involve the nurse in their family system by expecting participation in personal activities and social functions. These individuals may come to expect personal favors that extend beyond the scope of professional nursing practice and may believe it is their privilege to contact the nurse at home at any time of the day or night for care.

Overcoming Communication Barriers

Nurses tend to have stereotypical expectations of the client's behavior. In general, nurses expect behavior to consist of undemanding compliance, an attitude of respect for the health care provider, and cooperation with requested behavior throughout the examination.

Although clients may ask a few questions for clarification, slight deference to recognized authority figures (e.g., health care providers) is expected. However, individuals from culturally diverse backgrounds may have significantly different perceptions about the appropriate role of the individual and family when seeking health care. If nurses find themselves becoming annoyed that a client is asking too many questions, assuming a defensive posture, or otherwise feeling uncomfortable, they may pause for a moment to examine the source of the conflict from a cross-cultural perspective.

During illness, culturally acceptable "sick-role" behavior may range from aggressive, demanding behavior to silent passivity. Complaining, demanding behavior during illness is often rewarded with attention among Jewish and Italian-American patients, whereas Asian and Native-American patients are likely to be quiet and compliant during illness. Furthermore, during the interview, Asian clients may provide the nurse with the answers they think the nurse wants to hear, which is behavior consistent within their cultural value for harmonious relationships with others. The nurse should attempt to phrase questions or statements in a neutral manner that avoids foreshadowing an expected response. Appalachian clients may reject a community health nurse whom they perceive as prying or nosy because a cultural ethic of neutrality mandates that people mind their own business and avoid assertive or argumentative behavior.

Nonverbal Communication

Unless the nurse makes an effort to understand the client's nonverbal behavior, he or she may overlook important information such as that which is conveyed by facial expressions, silence, eye contact, touch, and other body language. Communication patterns vary widely cross-culturally, even for seemingly "innocent" behaviors such as smiling and handshaking. For example, among many Hispanic clients, smiling and handshaking are considered an integral part of sincere interaction and essential to establishing trust, whereas a Russian client may perceive the same behavior by the nurse as insolent and frivolous.

Gender issues also become significant. For example, among some groups of Middle Eastern origin, men and women do not shake hands or touch each other in any manner outside of the marital relationship. However, if the nurse and client are both female, a handshake is usually acceptable.

Wide cultural variation exists when interpreting silence. Some individuals find silence extremely uncomfortable and make every effort to fill conversational lags with words. In contrast, Native-Americans consider silence essential to understanding and respecting the other person. A pause after a question signifies that what the speaker has asked is important enough to be given thoughtful consideration. In traditional Chinese and Japanese cultures, silence may mean that the speaker wishes the listener to consider the content of what has been said before continuing. The English and Arabs may use silence out of respect for another person's privacy, whereas the French, Spanish, and Russians may interpret it as a sign of agreement. Asian cultures often use silence to demonstrate respect for elders.

Eye contact is among the most culturally variable nonverbal behaviors. Although most nurses have been taught to maintain eye contact while talking with clients, individuals from culturally diverse backgrounds may misconstrue this behavior. Asian, Native-American, Indochinese, Arab, and Appalachian clients may consider direct eye contact impolite or aggressive, and they may avert their own eyes during the conversation. Native-American clients often stare at the floor when the nurse is talking. This culturally appropriate behavior indicates that the listener is paying close attention to the speaker.

In some cultures, including Arab, Hispanic, and some black groups, modesty for women is interrelated with eye contact. For Muslim women, modesty is achieved in part by avoiding eye contact with men, except for their husband, and keeping the eyes downcast when encountering members of the opposite sex in public situations. In many cultures, the only women who smile and establish eye contact with men in public are prostitutes. Hassidic Jewish men also have culturally based norms concerning eye contact with women. The male may avoid direct eye contact and turn his head in the opposite direction when walking past or speaking to a woman. The preceding examples are intended to be illustrative and are not exhaustive; nor do they represent values, actions, and beliefs of all members of the cultural group described.

Language

When assessing nonEnglish-speaking clients, the nurse may encounter one of the two following situations: choosing an interpreter or communicating effectively when no interpreter is available. Interviewing a nonEnglish-speaking person requires a bilingual interpreter for full communication. Even the person from another culture or country who has a basic command of English may need an interpreter when faced with the anxiety-provoking situation of becoming ill, encountering a strange symptom, or discussing sensitive topics, such as birth control, gynecologic concerns, or urologic problems. The nurse may be tempted to ask a relative or friend of another client to interpret because this person is readily available and is anxious to help. However, this is disadvantageous because it violates confidentiality for the client who may not want personal information shared with another. Furthermore, the friend or relative, although fluent in ordinary language, is likely to be unfamiliar with medical terminology, clinical procedures, and medical ethics.

Whenever possible, the nurse should use a bilingual team member or trained medical interpreter. This person knows interpreting techniques, has a health care background, and understands patients' rights. The trained interpreter is also knowledgeable about cultural beliefs and health practices, can help bridge the cultural gap, and can provide advice concerning the cultural appropriateness of recommendations.

Although the nurse is in charge of the client-nurse interaction, the interpreter is an important member of the health care team. Whenever feasible, the nurse should ask the interpreter to meet the client before the visit to establish rapport and learn about the client's age, occupation, educational level, and attitude toward health care. This enables the interpreter to communicate on the client's level.

The nurse should allow more time for visits with culturally diverse clients who require an interpreter. With the third person repeating everything, it can take considerably longer than interviewing English-speaking clients. The nurse will need to focus on the major points and prioritize data.

Line-by-line and summarization are interpretation styles. Translation of line-by-line ensures accuracy, but it takes more time. The nurse and client should speak only a sentence or two and then allow the interpreter time to interpret. The nurse should use simple language, not medical jargon that the interpreter must simplify before translating it. Summary translation is faster and useful for teaching relatively simple health techniques with which the interpreter is already familiar. The nurse should be alert for nonverbal cues as the client talks because they can give valuable data. A good interpreter will also note

BOX 12-2

Overcoming Language Barriers: Use of an Interpreter

- Before locating an interpreter, the nurse should know what language the patient speaks at home because it may be different from the language spoken publicly (e.g., French is sometimes spoken by aristocratic or well-educated people from certain Asian or Middle Eastern cultures).
- The nurse should avoid interpreters from a rival tribe, state, region, or nation (e.g., a Palestinian who knows Hebrew may not be the best interpreter for a Jewish client).
- The nurse should be aware of the gender difference between the interpreter and client to avoid violation of cultural mores related to modesty.
- The nurse should be aware of the age difference between the interpreter and client.
- The nurse should be aware of socioeconomic differences between the interpreter and client.
- The nurse should ask the interpreter to translate as closely to verbatim as possible.
- An interpreter who is not a relative may seek compensation for services rendered.

nonverbal messages and communicate those to the community health nurse. Box 12-2 summarizes suggestions for the selection and use of an interpreter.

Although use of an interpreter is ideal, the nurse may find himself or herself in a situation with a nonEnglish-speaking client when no interpreter is available. Box 12-3 provides some suggestions for overcoming language barriers when an interpreter is not available.

Touch

Touching the client is a necessary component of a comprehensive assessment. Although benefits exist in establishing rapport with clients through touch, including the promotion of healing through therapeutic touch, physical contact with clients conveys various meanings cross-culturally. In many cultures (e.g., Arab and Hispanic), male health care providers may

BOX **12-3**

Overcoming Language Barriers When an Interpreter is not Available

- The nurse should be polite and formal.
- The nurse should greet the client using his or her last or complete name. The nurse should gesture to himself or herself and say his or her name. The nurse should offer a handshake or nod and smile.
- The nurse should proceed in an unhurried manner. The nurse should pay attention to efforts by the client or family to communicate.
- The nurse should speak in a low, moderate voice. The nurse should remember that he or she may have a tendency to raise the volume and pitch of his or her voice when the listener appears not to understand and the listener may perceive that the nurse is shouting or angry.
- The nurse should use words that he or she may know in the patient's language. This indicates that the nurse is aware of and respects the patient's culture.
- The nurse should use simple words, such as "pain" instead of "discomfort." The nurse should avoid medical jargon, idioms, and slang. He or she should avoid using contractions such as "don't," "can't," and "won't." The nurse should use nouns repeatedly instead of pronouns. For example, the nurse should say "Does Juan take medicine?" instead of "He has been taking his medicine, hasn't he?"
- The nurse should pantomime words and simple actions while verbalizing them.
- The nurse should give instructions in the proper sequence. For example, he or she should say, "First, wash the bottle. Second, rinse the bottle," instead of "Before you rinse the bottle, sterilize it."
- The nurse should discuss one topic at a time. He or she should avoid use of conjunctions. For example, the nurse should say, "Are you cold [while pantomiming]?" and "Are you in pain?" instead of, "Are you cold and in pain?"
- The nurse should determine if the client understands by having the client repeat instructions, demonstrate the procedure, or act out the meaning.
- The nurse should write out several short sentences in English and determine the client's ability to read them.
- The nurse should try a third language. Many Indo-Chinese speak French. Europeans often know three or four languages. The nurse should try Latin words or phrases.
- The nurse should ask who among the client's family and friends could serve as an interpreter.
- The nurse should obtain phrase books from a library or bookstore, make or purchase flash cards, contact hospitals for a list of interpreters, and use both formal and informal networking to locate a suitable interpreter.

be prohibited from touching or examining all or certain parts of the female body. During pregnancy, the client may prefer female health care providers and may refuse to be examined by a man. The nurse should be aware that the client's significant other may also exert pressure on health care providers by enforcing these culturally meaningful norms in the health care setting.

Touching children may also have variable meanings cross-culturally. For example, Hispanic clients may believe in mal ojo (i.e., "evil eye") in which an individual becomes ill as a result of excessive admiration by another. Many Asians believe that personal strength resides in the head and that touching

the head is considered disrespectful. The nurse should approach palpation of the fontanelle of an infant of Southeast Asian descent with sensitivity. The nurse may need to rely on alternative sources of information (e.g., assessing for clinical manifestations of increased intracranial pressure or signs of premature fontanelle closure). Although it is the least desirable option, the nurse may need to omit this part of the assessment.

Gender

Violating norms related to appropriate male-female relationships among various cultures may jeopardize the therapeutic nurse-client relationship. Among Arab-Americans, a man is never alone with a woman, except his wife, and is usually accompanied by one or more other men when interacting with women. This behavior is culturally significant and failure to adhere to the **cultural code** (i.e., set of rules or norms of behavior used by a cultural group to guide their behavior and interpret situations) is viewed as a serious transgression, often one in which the lone male will be accused of sexual impropriety. The best way to ensure that cultural variables have been considered is to ask the client about culturally relevant aspects of male-female relationships, preferably at the beginning of the interaction before an opportunity arises to violate culturally based practices.

HEALTH-RELATED BELIEFS AND PRACTICES

One of the major aspects of a comprehensive cultural assessment concerns the collection of data related to culturally-based beliefs and practices about health and illness. Before determining whether cultural practices are helpful, harmful, or neutral, the nurse must first understand the logic of the belief system underlying the practice and then be sure to grasp fully the nature and meaning of the practice from the client's cultural perspective.

Health and Culture

The first step in understanding the health care needs of clients is to understand personal culturally-based values, beliefs, attitudes, and practices. Sometimes this requires considerable introspection and may necessitate that the nurse confront his or her own biases, preconceptions, and prejudices about specific racial, ethnic, religious, sexual, or socioeconomic groups. The next step is to identify the meaning of health to the client, remembering that concepts are derived in part from the way in which members of their cultural group define *health*.

Considerable research has been conducted on the various definitions of *health* that may be held by various groups. For example, Jamaicans define *health* as having a good appetite, feeling strong and energetic, performing activities of daily living without difficulty, and being sexually active and fertile. For traditional Italian women, *health* means the ability to interact socially and perform routine tasks such as

cooking, cleaning, and caring for oneself and others. On the other hand, some individuals of Hispanic origin believe that coughing, sweating, and diarrhea are a normal part of living rather than symptoms of ill health, because the frequency of these problems in the clients' country of origin is high. Individuals may define themselves or others in their group as healthy even though the nurse identifies symptoms of disease.

Cross-Cultural Perspectives on Causes of Illness

For clients, symptom labeling and diagnosis depend on the degree of difference between the individual's behaviors and those the group define as normal. Other issues that the nurse should consider include the client's beliefs about the causation of illness, level of stigma attached to a particular set of symptoms, prevalence of the disease, and meaning of the illness to the individual and family.

Throughout history, humankind has attempted to understand the cause of illness and disease. Theories of causation have been formulated on the basis of religious beliefs, social circumstances, philosophical perspectives, and level of knowledge. Disease causation may be viewed from the following three major perspectives: biomedical (i.e., sometimes used synonymously with the term *scientific*), naturalistic (i.e., sometimes used synonymously with the term *holistic*), and magicoreligious.

Biomedical Perspective

The **biomedical** (i.e., scientific) theory of illness causation is based on the following:

1. All events in life have a cause and effect.
2. The human body functions more or less mechanically (i.e., the functioning of the human body is analogous to the functioning of an automobile).
3. All life can be reduced or divided into smaller parts (e.g., the human person can be reduced into body, mind, and spirit).
4. All of reality can be observed and measured (e.g., with intelligence tests and psychometric measures of behavior).

Among the biomedical explanations for disease is the germ theory, which posits that microscopic organisms such as bacteria and viruses are responsible for specific disease conditions. Most educational programs for nurses and other health care providers embrace the biomedical or scientific theories that explain the causes of physical and psychological illnesses.

Naturalistic Perspective

Another way in which clients may explain the cause of illness is from the **naturalistic** (i.e., holistic) perspective. This viewpoint is found most frequently among Native-Americans, Asians, and others who believe that human life is only one aspect of nature and a part of the general order of the cosmos. Individuals from these groups believe that the forces of nature must be kept in natural balance or harmony to maintain health and well-being.

Many Asians believe in the **yin-yang theory** in which health is believed to exist when all aspects of the person are in perfect balance. Rooted in the ancient Chinese philosophy of Tao, the yin-yang theory states that all organisms and objects in the universe consist of yin or yang energy forces. The origin of the energy forces is within the autonomic nervous system, where balance between the opposing forces is maintained during health. *Yin* energy represents the female and negative forces (e.g., emptiness, darkness, and cold), whereas *yang* forces are male and positive, emitting warmth and fullness. Foods are classified as hot and cold in this theory and are transformed into yin and yang energy when metabolized by the body. Yin foods are cold, and yang foods are hot. Cold foods are eaten when one has a hot illness, and hot foods are eaten when one has a cold illness. The yin-yang theory is the basis for Eastern or Chinese medicine and is commonly embraced by Asian-Americans.

The naturalistic perspective posits that the laws of nature create imbalances, chaos, and disease. Individuals embracing the naturalistic view use metaphors such as the healing power of nature and they may call the earth "Mother." For example, from the perspective of the Chinese, illness is not seen as an intruding agent, but rather as a part of life's rhythmic course and an outward sign of the disharmony that exists within.

Many Hispanic, Arab, black, and Asian groups embrace a hot-cold theory of health and illness, an explanatory model with its origin in the ancient Greek humoral theory. Blood, phlegm, black bile, and yellow bile, the four humors of the body, regulate basic bodily functions and are described in terms of temperature, dryness, and moisture. The treatment of disease consists of adding or subtracting cold, heat, dryness, or wetness to restore the balance of the humors.

Beverages, foods, herbs, medicines, and diseases are classified as hot or cold according to their perceived effects on the body, not on their physical characteristics. Illnesses believed to be caused by cold entering the body include earache, chest cramps, paralysis, gastrointestinal discomfort, rheumatism, and TB. Illnesses believed to be caused by overheating include abscessed teeth, sore throats, rashes, and kidney disorders.

According to the hot-cold theory, the individual as a whole, rather than a specific ailment, is significant. Those who embrace the hot-cold theory maintain that health consists of a positive state of total well-being, including physical, psychological, spiritual, and social aspects of the person. Paradoxically, the language used to describe this artificial dissection of the body into parts is a reflection of the biomedical-scientific perspective, not a naturalistic or holistic one.

Magicoreligious Perspective

Another way in which people explain the causation of illness is from a **magicoreligious** perspective. The basic premise of this explanatory model is that the world is seen as an arena in which supernatural forces dominate. The fate of the world and those in it depend on the action of supernatural forces for good or evil. Examples of magical causes of illness include the belief in voodoo or witchcraft among some blacks and others from circum-Caribbean countries. Faith healing is based on religious beliefs and is most prevalent among selected Christian religions, including Christian Scientists. Various healing rituals may be found in many religions, such as Roman Catholicism, Mormonism (i.e., Church of Jesus Christ of Latter-Day Saints), and others (Hanson and Andrews, 1999).

A combination of worldviews is possible and many clients are likely to offer more than one explanation for the cause of their illness. As a profession, nursing largely embraces the biomedical-scientific worldview, but some aspects of holism have begun to gain popularity. These include a wide variety of techniques for management of chronic pain (e.g., hypnosis, therapeutic touch, and biofeedback). Many nurses hold a belief in spiritual power and readily credit supernatural forces with various unexplained phenomena related to clients' health and illness states.

Folk Healers

All cultures have their own recognized symptoms of ill health, acceptable sick-role behavior, and treatments. In addition to seeking help from the nurse as a biomedical-scientific health care provider, clients from many groups may also seek help from folk or religious healers.

Numerous types of folk healers exist, each with a unique scope of practice. Hispanic clients may turn to a curandero (male folk healer) or curandera (female folk healer), spiritualist, yerbo (herbalist), or sabador (healer who manipulates muscles and bones). In a study of the use of folk healing and healers by Latinos in New England, Zapata and Shippee-Rice (1999) found that none of the study participants relied exclusively on folk healers, but they combined folk and biomedicine. The main reason cited by informants for seeking care from folk healers relates to their perception that biomedical practitioners (e.g., physicians and nurses) fail to provide holistic care and use medicines that are not natural.

Some black clients may mention having received assistance from a hougan (voodoo priest or priestess), spiritualist, or "old lady" (an older woman who has successfully raised a family and specializes in child care and folk remedies). Likewise, Native-American clients may seek assistance from a shaman or a medicine man or woman. Clients of Asian descent may mention that they have visited herbalists, acupuncturists, or bone setters.

Each culture has its own healers, most of whom speak the native tongue of the client, make house calls, and cost significantly less than healers practicing in the biomedical-scientific health care system. In addition to folk healers, many cultures have lay midwives (e.g., parteras for Hispanic women) or other health care providers who meet the needs of pregnant women.

In some religions, spiritual healers may be found among the ranks of the ordained or official religious hierarchy ranks and are called priest, bishop, elder, deacon, rabbi, brother, or sister. Other religions have a separate category of healer (e.g., Christian Science "nurses" [not licensed by states] or practitioners) (Hanson and Andrews, 1999).

A comprehensive discussion of the variety of healing beliefs and practices used by the numerous cultural groups is beyond the scope of this chapter. However, the nurse should be aware of alternative practices and folk healers that are used by the groups for which they care. The nurse should also be aware that most indigenous healing practices are innocuous, regardless of whether they are effective.

Cultural Expressions of Illness

A wide cultural variation exists in the manner in which certain symptoms and disease conditions are perceived, diagnosed, labeled, and treated. The disease that is grounds for social ostracism in one culture may be reason for increased status in another. For example, epilepsy is contagious and untreatable among Ugandans; a cause for family shame among Greeks; a reflection of a physical imbalance among Mexican-Americans; and a sign of having gained favor by enduring a trial by God among the Hutterites.

Bodily symptoms are also perceived and reported in a variety of ways. For example, individuals of Mediterranean descent tend to report common physical symptoms more often than people of northern European or Asian heritage. The Chinese do not have a translation for the English word "sadness," yet all people experience the feeling of sadness at some time in their life. To express emotion, Chinese clients sometimes somaticize their symptoms. For example, a client may complain of cardiac symptoms because the center of emotion in the Chinese culture is the heart. If the client has experienced a loss through death or divorce and is grieving, he or she may describe the loss in terms of a pain in the heart. Although some biomedical-scientific clinicians may refer to this as a psychosomatic illness, others will recognize it as a culturally acceptable somatic expression of emotional disharmony.

Cultural Expression of Pain

To illustrate the manner in which symptom expression may reflect the client's cultural background, pain, an extensively studied symptom, is used. Pain is a universally recognized phenomenon and an important aspect of assessment for clients of various ages. Pain is a private, subjective experience that is greatly influenced by cultural heritage. Expectations, manifestations, and pain management are all embedded in a cultural context. The definition of *pain,* like that of health or illness, is culturally determined.

The term *pain* is derived from the Greek word for penalty, which helps explain the long association between pain and punishment in Judeo-Christian thought. The meaning of painful stimuli for individuals, the way people define their situation, and the influence of personal experience combine to determine the experience of pain.

Much cross-cultural research has been conducted on pain (Ludwig-Beymer, 1999; Zborowski, 1969). Pain has been found to be a highly personal experience that depends on cultural learning, the meaning of the situation, and other factors unique to the individual. Health care professionals have identified silent suffering as the most valued response to pain. The majority of nurses have been socialized to believe that in virtually any situation, self-control is better than open displays of strong feelings.

Studies of nurses' attitudes toward pain reveal that the ethnic background of patients is relevant to the nurses' assessment of physical and psychological pain. Nurses view Jewish and Spanish patients as suffering the most and Anglo-Saxon Germanic patients as suffering the least. In addition, nurses who infer relatively greater patient pain tended to report their own experiences as more painful. In general, nurses with an eastern or southern European or African background tend to infer greater suffering than do nurses of northern European background. Years of experience, current position, and area of clinical practice are unrelated to inferences of suffering (Ludwig-Beymer, 1999).

In addition to expecting variations in pain perception and tolerance, a nurse should expect variations in the expression of pain. Individuals turn to their social environments for validation and comparison. A first important comparison group is the family, which transmits cultural norms to its children.

Culture-Bound Syndromes

Clients may have a condition that is culturally defined, known as a **culture-bound syndrome**. Some of these conditions have no equal from a biomedical or scientific perspective, but others, such as anorexia nervosa and bulimia, are examples of health problems found primarily among members of the dominant U.S. cultural group. Table 12-6 presents selected examples from among more than 150 culture-bound syndromes that have been documented by medical anthropologists.

Pica, the ingestion of nonfood substances such as starch, clay, and dirt, is another example of a culture-bound health condition. Although pica has been observed in various cultural groups for centuries, the cause remains unknown. Boyle and Mackey (1999) studied pica in black women and recommended strategies for the clinical management of pica during pregnancy.

MANAGEMENT OF HEALTH PROBLEMS: A CULTURAL PERSPECTIVE

After a symptom is identified, the first effort at treatment is often self-care. In the United States, an estimated 70% to 90% of all illness episodes are treated first, or exclusively, through self-care, often with significant success. The availability of over-the-counter medications, a relatively high literacy level, and influence of the mass media in communicating health-related information to the general population have contributed to the high percentage of self-treatment. Home treatments are attractive because they are accessible compared with the inconvenience associated with traveling to a physician, NP, and pharmacist, particularly for clients from rural or sparsely populated areas. Furthermore, home treatment may mobilize the client's social support network and provide the sick individual with a caring environment in which to convalesce.

However, the nurse should be aware that not all home remedies are inexpensive. For example, urban black populations in the Southeast sometimes use medicinal potions that cost much more than an equivalent treatment with a biomedical intervention.

Various nontraditional interventions are gaining the recognition of health care professionals in the biomedical-scientific health care system. Acupuncture, acupressure, therapeutic touch, massage, biofeedback, relaxation techniques, meditation, hypnosis, distraction, imagery, and herbal remedies are interventions that clients may use alone or in combination with other treatments.

Cultural Negotiation

Cultural negotiation refers to the process in which messages, instructions, and belief systems are manipulated, linked, or processed between the professional and lay models of health problems and preferred treatment. In each act, the nurse gives attention to eliciting the client's views regarding a health-related experience (e.g., pregnancy, complications of pregnancy, or illness of an infant).

Katon and Kleinman (1981) describe negotiation as a bilateral arrangement in which two principal parties attempt to work out a solution. The goal of negotiation is to reduce conflict in a way that promotes cooperation. Cultural negotiation is used

TABLE 12-6

Selected Culture-Bound Syndromes

Group	Disorder	Remarks
Whites	Anorexia nervosa	Excessive preoccupation with thinness, self-imposed starvation
	Bulimia	Gross overeating, then vomiting or fasting
Blacks	Blackout	Collapse, dizziness, or inability to move
	Low blood	Not enough blood or weakness of the blood that is often treated with diet
	High blood	Blood that is too rich in certain components from ingesting too much red meat or rich foods
	Thin blood	In women, children, and the elderly; renders the individual more susceptible to illness in general
	Diseases of hex, witchcraft, or conjuring	Sense of being doomed by a spell, part of voodoo beliefs
Chinese or Southeast Asians	Koro	Intense anxiety that that penis is retracting into the body
Greeks	Hysteria	Bizarre complaints and behavior because the uterus leaves the pelvis and goes to another part of the body
Hispanics	Empacho	Food forms into a ball and clings to the stomach or intestines, causing pain and cramping
	Fatigue	Asthma-like symptoms
	Mal ojo ("evil eye")	Fitful sleep, crying, and diarrhea in children caused by a stranger's attention; sudden onset
	Pasmo	Paralysis-like symptoms of face or limbs; prevented or relieved by massage
	Susto	Anxiety, trembling, and phobias from sudden fright
Native-Americans	Ghost	Terror, hallucinations, and sense of danger
Japanese	Wagamama	Apathetic childish behavior with emotional outbursts

when conceptual differences exist between the client and the nurse, a situation that may occur for one or more of the following reasons:

- The nurse and client may be using the same words but have different meanings.
- The nurse and client may apply the term to the same phenomenon but have different notions of its causation.

- The nurse and client may have different memories or emotions associated with the term and its use.

In cultural negotiation, the nurse provides scientific information while acknowledging that the client may hold different views. If the client's perspective indicates that behaviors would be helpful, positive, adaptive, or neutral in effect, the nurse should include these in the plan of care. However, if the client's perspective would result in behaviors that may be harmful, negative, or nonadaptive, the nurse should attempt to shift the client's perspective to that of the practitioner (Herberg, 1995; Spector, 2000).

Pregnancy and childbirth are social, cultural, and physiological experiences; therefore an approach to culturally sensitive nursing care of childbearing women and their families must focus on the interaction between cultural meaning and biological functions. Childbirth is a time of transition and social celebration that is of central importance in any society; it signals realignment of existing cultural roles and responsibilities, psychological and biological states, and social relationships. Child rearing is also a period during which culturally-bound values, attitudes, beliefs, and practices permeate virtually all aspects of life for the parents and child (Andrews and Boyle, 1999). Careful assessment and attention to culturally based practices are particularly important during these occasions.

MANAGEMENT OF HEALTH PROBLEMS IN CULTURALLY DIVERSE POPULATIONS

The factors responsible for the health disparity between minority and white populations are complex and defy simplistic solutions. Health status is influenced by the interaction of physiological, cultural, psychological, and societal factors that are poorly understood for the general population and even less so for minorities. Despite the shared characteristic of economic disadvantage among minorities, common approaches for improving health are not possible. Rather, solving problems among minorities necessitates activities, programs, and data collection that are tailored to meet the unique health care needs of many different subgroups. Solutions to health care problems among culturally diverse populations include the following:

- Providing health information and education
- Delivering and financing health services
- Developing health professionals from minority groups
- Enhancing cooperative efforts with the nonfederal sector
- Improving methods of data development
- Promoting a research agenda on minority health issues

Providing Health Information and Education

According to the ACS (1999), minority populations are less knowledgeable or aware of some specific health problems than whites. This is demonstrated by the following:

- Blacks and Hispanics receive less information about cancer and heart disease than nonminority groups.
- Blacks tend to underestimate the prevalence of cancer, give less credence to the warning signs, obtain fewer screening tests, and are diagnosed at later stages of cancer than whites.
- Hispanic women receive less information about breast cancer than white women. Hispanic women are less aware that family history is a risk factor for breast cancer and only 25% of Hispanic women have heard of breast self-examination.
- Many professionals and lay people, both minority and white, do not know that heart disease is as common in black men as in white men and that black women die from coronary heart disease at a higher rate than white women.
- Hypertensive Japanese women and younger men (i.e., aged 18 to 49) are less aware of their hypertension than nonminority subgroups.
- Among Mexican-Americans, cultural attitudes regarding obesity and diet are often barriers to achieving weight control.

Programs to increase public awareness about health problems have been well received in several areas. For example, the Healthy Mothers and Healthy Babies Coalition, which provides an education program in both English and Spanish, has contributed to increased awareness of measures to improve the health status of mothers and infants. In addition, increased knowledge among blacks of hypertension as a serious health problem is one of the accomplishments of the National High Blood Pressure Education program. The success of these efforts indicates that carefully planned programs have a beneficial effect, but efforts must continue and expand to reach even more of the target population and focus on additional health problems.

Planning Health Information Campaigns

Sensitivity to cultural factors is often lacking in the health care of minorities. Key concepts for the nurse to consider in designing a health information campaign include meeting the language and cultural needs of each identified minority group, using minority-specific community resources to tailor educational approaches, and developing materials and methods of presentation that are commensurate with the educational level of the target population. Furthermore, the powerful influences of cultural factors over a lifetime in shaping people's attitudes, values, beliefs, and practices concerning health require health information programs to be sustained over a long period. The following are examples of ways in which the nurse can interweave these concepts into health promotion efforts:

- The nurse should involve local community leaders who are members of the targeted cultural group to promote acceptance and reinforcement of the central themes of health promotion messages.
- Health messages are more readily accepted if they do not conflict with existing cultural beliefs and practices. Where appropriate, messages should acknowledge existing cultural beliefs.
- The nurse should involve families, churches, employers, and community organizations as a support system to facilitate and sustain behavior change to a more healthful lifestyle. For example, although hypertension control in blacks depends on appropriate treatment (e.g., medication), blood pressure can be improved and maintained by family and community support of activities such as proper diet and exercise.
- Language barriers, cultural differences, and lack of adequate information on access to care complicate prenatal care for Hispanic and Asian women who have recently arrived in the United States. By using lay volunteers to organize community support networks, programs have been developed to disseminate culturally appropriate health information.

Health Education

Although printed materials and other audiovisual aids contribute to the educational process, client education is inherently interpersonal. The success of educational efforts is often determined by the credibility of the source and is highly dependent on the skill and sensitivity of the nurse in communicating information in a culturally appropriate manner. Education programs are particularly critical and necessary for several health problems with the greatest influence on minority health, such as hypertension, obesity, and diabetes. For example, if diabetics could improve

their self-management skills through education, an estimated 70% of complications (e.g., ketoacidosis, blindness, and amputations) could be avoided, saving human misery and health care dollars.

Delivering and Financing Health Services

Innovative models for delivering and financing health services for minority populations are needed. According to community health experts, models should increase flexibility of health care delivery, facilitate access to services by minority populations, and improve efficiency of service and payment systems. One of the most commonly used indicators of adequacy of health services for a population is distribution of health care providers; however, this is an inadequate measurement. The following facts exemplify the problems associated with health services for minorities:

- The disparities in death rates between minorities and whites remain despite overall increases in health care access and use.
- Language problems hinder refugees and immigrants when they seek health care.
- Blacks with cancer postpone seeking diagnosis of their symptoms longer than whites and delay initiation of treatment once diagnosed.
- A smaller proportion of black women than white women, or 63% vs. 76%, begin prenatal care in the first trimester of pregnancy.

Models of Health Promotion

In most health models, SES is assumed to affect health status through environmental or behavioral factors. These models posit that poor families may not have the economic, social, or community resources needed to remain in good health. For example, poverty is thought to affect children's well-being by influencing health and nutrition, the home environment, caregiver interactions with children, caregiver mental health, and neighborhood conditions. The deficits associated with poverty may lead to inadequate diets, which results in poor growth and delayed development. Likewise, poor housing results in increased risk for exposure that leads to other environmental hazards; overcrowding results in increased risk for infectious diseases such as TB, meningitis, influenza, and related conditions; and community violence threatens the safety and well-being of children. The combined effects of these stressors is thought to provide the foundation for a cycle of hopelessness and depression among family members, who in turn engage in risky health behaviors (e.g., smoking, substance abuse, poor dietary habits resulting in obesity, high cholesterol levels, and other risk factors) and unfavorable family interactions (Mendoza and Fuentes-Afflick, 1999).

In studying the health of Latino children, Mendoza and Fuentes-Afflick (1999) noted that although the majority of Latino children live in poverty, unlike other children in the lower socioeconomic group, they enjoy relatively good health. This has been called an **epidemiological paradox**. In an effort to explain this paradox, Mendoza and Fuentes-Afflick proposed an alternative model of risk factors for adverse health outcomes called the **family-community HPM**.

The family-community HPM emphasizes the family-community complex compared with the three classic factors (i.e., genetics, environment, and high-risk behaviors) used in traditional HPMs. It also offers a new conceptual approach to understanding the unexpectedly low rates of adverse health outcomes among some culturally diverse groups with high levels of poverty.

The family-community HPM stresses the capacity of the family to support the optimum health behaviors of its family members and the ability of the family's community to support it in this endeavor. The assumption is that if the family promotes beneficial health behaviors among its members, these behaviors will become integrated into the culture. Healthy lifestyle behaviors become an integral component of the family identity, traditions, and history. The model also distinguishes between physical and mental disorders (Mendoza and Fuentes-Afflick, 1999).

Continuity of Care

Continuity of care is associated with improved health outcomes and is presumably greater when a client is able to establish an ongoing relationship with a care provider. Many of the leading causes of death among minorities (e.g., cancer, CVD, and diabetes) are chronic rather than acute problems; therefore they require extended treatment regimens. Consider the following:

- A higher percentage of blacks and Hispanics than whites report that they have no usual source of health care (29% and 19%, respectively vs. 13%) (NCHS, 1999).

- Refugees are eligible for special refugee medical assistance during their first 18 months in the United States. However, after this period, refugees who cannot afford private health insurance and are ineligible for Medicaid or state medical assistance may become medically indigent.
- Many Native-Americans and Alaska Natives live in areas where the availability of health care providers is half the national average.

Financing Problems

As mentioned previously, problems associated with financing health care tend to be more common in minority groups. The following are statistics reported by the NCHS (1999):

- Economic inequalities cause members of minority groups to rely on Medicaid and charity for their health care needs.
- Older minority people are less likely than whites to supplement Medicare with additional private insurance.
- Proportionately, three times as many Native-Americans, blacks, Hispanics, and certain Asian and Pacific Islander groups as whites live in poverty.
- Proportionately twice as many blacks and three times as many Hispanics as whites have no medical insurance (18% and 26%, respectively vs. 9%).
- Of those who had no insurance, 35% had not seen a physician during the past 12 months, compared with 22% of those who had insurance.

To better manage health problems and reduce the disparity in health indicators, these issues of financing must be addressed. Failure to do so will result in continued inequity in access to services and poor health among minority groups.

Developing Health Professionals from Minority Groups

The need to increase the number of health professionals from minority groups has been recognized for decades. With few exceptions, minorities are underrepresented as students and practitioners of the health professions. Although the number of minority nursing students has been steadily increasing, there still are proportionately more white nursing students (Rosella, Regan-Kubinski, and Albrecht, 1994; USDHHS/DON, 1996).

Differences in the availability of health personnel resources in minority communities are apparent regardless of the minority group being considered. Communities located in urban-metropolitan areas have significantly more professional resources. Among the factors that contribute to the imbalances in minority representation in health professions are the size of a minority population, number of cultural subgroups, and demographic features (Rosella et al., 1994; Satcher, 1998).

Efforts to encourage more students from minority groups are ongoing. The OMH (1996) has recommended a review of programs having an influence on the actual or potential availability of health professionals to minority communities in an effort to improve the number of practitioners. Grants, scholarships, and low-cost loans are readily available in many areas. Minority and nonminority health professional organizations, academic institutions, state governments, health departments, and other organizations from the public and private sectors should work together to develop strategies to improve the availability and accessibility of health care professionals to minority communities.

Enhancing Cooperative Efforts with the Nonfederal Sector

Activities to improve minority health should involve participation of organizations at all levels (i.e., community, municipal, state, and national). Community involvement in developing health promotion activities can contribute to their success by providing credibility and visibility to the activities and facilitating their acceptance. Changes in health behavior frequently depend on personal initiative and are most likely to be triggered by efforts from locally based sources.

However, not all minority communities have the ability to identify their own health problems and initiate activities to address them. Support from the state and federal governments and private sector assistance is needed to assist with identifying and solving health-related problems afflicting the minority community. Assistance may be provided to minority communities in the following ways:

1. The use of technical assistance to identify high-risk groups
2. Assistance with planning, implementing, and evaluating programs to address identified needs

3. Specialized community services (e.g., federally funded projects for infants and frail older adults)
4. Programs supported by businesses and industries (e.g., health promotion programs organized by unions)

The private sector can also serve as an effective channel for programs targeted to minority health projects. National organizations concerned with minorities, such as the National Urban League and the Coalition of Hispanic Mental Health and Human Services Organizations, include health-related issues in their national agendas and are actively seeking effective ways to improve the health of minorities. Organizations such as these have a powerful potential for affecting change among their constituencies because they have strong community-level grassroots support.

Improving Methods of Data Development

The OMH (1996) recommended that existing sources of health data be improved by including racial and ethnic identifiers in data bases and oversampling selected minorities in national surveys. Analyses such as cross-comparisons from different data sets and specialized studies should be encouraged because they can contribute to understanding the health status and needs of minority populations. Unfortunately, many studies conducted in the past have failed to include data categories for culturally diverse groups and subgroups.

Promoting a Research Agenda on Minority Health Issues

The OMH (1996) recommended that a research agenda be developed to investigate factors affecting minority health. The influences include risk factor prevalence, health education interventions, preventive services interventions, treatment services, and sociocultural factors and health outcomes.

For further information on current research related to culture and community health nursing, the reader should search library data bases for reports of completed studies (Andrews, 1999). Electronic bulletin boards also may be valuable when searching for research in progress and for communicating with researchers studying a particular phenomenon of interest. Box 12-4 contains

BOX 12-4

Selected Research on Culture and Community Health Nursing

To assist older adults who want to remain in their homes, the Baltimore City Commission on Aging and Retirement Education (CARE) studied 288 (66% response rate) MOW recipients to evaluate their medical and social needs. The MOW nutritional assistance program was combined with a comprehensive assessment of the seniors, which included physical assessment, mental health assessment, housing assessment, transportation assessment, client interests, legal issues, and use of other agencies and community resources.

The majority of the sample were black (51%), Protestant (39%), and women (77%), but some were Hispanics, Asian and Pacific Islanders, and white men from various religions in the study. One-third were aged 80 and older, 39% were aged 71 to 80, 27% were aged 61 to 70, and only 1% (one informant) was under 60 years of age. Monthly incomes ranged from $450 to $900.

Study findings revealed that the majority of seniors reported independent functioning in their activities of daily living. About 17% required assistance with bathing, shopping, and light housework. About 30% indicated that they needed transportation to medical appointments. Although the majority were cognitively intact, 40% reported being depressed and 12% were interested in counseling services. About 50% indicated that they needed information about living wills, will preparation, or burial plans. About 50% expressed interest in obtaining assistance with finances to determine eligibility for social services. When asked to describe their greatest need to improve their home or apartment, 31% requested smoke detectors and 28% needed home repairs. Other areas of concern to the seniors included trash and an unclean environment and control of rodents and insects.

These findings can help community health nurses better meet the needs of low-income homebound older adults from diverse cultures as they endeavor to remain in their homes or apartments vs. becoming institutionalized. Study results suggest that the Baltimore MOW Assessment Project is an example of one intervention that assisted older adults through a comprehensive assessment of their needs and through effective referrals to local area health and social services agencies.

Lubaczewski J, Pezzoli SA: Alternatives to institutionalization: identifying and addressing the needs of urban homebound elderly, *J Multicultural Nurs Health* 4:49, 1998.

Breast cancer is the leading cause of death among black women in the United States. According to the ACS, black women have a higher risk that the disease will be more advanced when it is diagnosed. The purpose of this study was to describe the barriers for low-income black women for breast screening and education. Using a semistructured questionnaire, researchers interviewed 83 black women ranging from 51 to 91 years of age who had no history of cancer. Of the women interviewed, 41 (44%) had less than a high school education, 33 (40%) had a high school diploma or equivalent, and 10 (12%) had some college. The subjects were volunteers residing in a Midwestern metropolitan area.

Findings indicated that most subjects believed that prevention of breast cancer was an important reason for mammography screening. Recommendations for the procedure by the subject's health care provider and previously having a mammogram increased the likelihood that the subject would repeat the procedure. Reasons cited by subjects for not having a mammogram include cost, lack of transportation, illness, and fear of pain.

Community health nurses often are in a position to recommend preventive measures such as mammography and breast self-examination to black clients and women over 40 in general. Improving access by offering assistance with transportation or bringing mobile mammography units to neighborhoods may substantially increase participation among those women at highest risk. Another strategy that has been used successfully is involvement of local churches, mosques, temples, and other religious organizations in promoting regular mammography screening for at-risk populations.

Lambert S, Newton M, deMeneses M: Barriers to mammography in older, low-income African American women, *J Multicult Nurs Health* 4:16, 1998.

summaries of selected research on topics of relevance to community health nurses in providing culturally competent care. The website for this book SiMON www.wbsaunders.com/SIMON/nies provides links to other websites related to cultural issues.

ROLE OF THE COMMUNITY HEALTH NURSE IN IMPROVING HEALTH FOR CULTURALLY DIVERSE PEOPLE

This chapter provides data detailing the health care problems of culturally diverse individuals, families, groups, and communities. Given the complexity of the problems and the wide variation in incidence and distribution of these problems within specific subgroups, no simple method exists for providing culturally sensitive community health nursing care to all clients. However, the following strategies may assist the community health nurse when working with culturally diverse clients:

- Conduct a "culturological" assessment.
- Conduct a cultural self-assessment.
- Seek knowledge about local cultures.
- Recognize political issues of culturally diverse groups.
- Provide culturally competent care.
- Recognize culturally-based health problems.

Culturological Assessment

All nursing care is based on a systematic, comprehensive assessment of the client; therefore the community health nurse must gather cultural data on clients from racially and ethnically diverse backgrounds. A **culturological assessment** refers to a systematic appraisal or examination of individuals, groups, and communities regarding their cultural beliefs, values, and practices to determine explicit nursing needs and intervention practices within the cultural context of the people being evaluated (Leininger, 1995). The term *culturological* is a descriptive reference to culture phenomena in their broadest sense.

Culturological assessments are as vital as physical and psychological assessments. Culturological assessments tend to be broad and comprehensive because they deal with cultural values, belief systems, and ways of living now and in the recent past. In conducting a culturological assessment, the community health nurse should be involved in determining

and appraising the traits, characteristics, or smallest units of cultural behavior as a guide to nursing care. The following section summarizes major data categories pertaining to the culture of clients and offers suggested questions that the nurse may ask to elicit needed information.

Brief History of Ethnic and Racial Origins of the Cultural Group with which the Client Identifies

- With what ethnic group or groups does the client report affiliation (e.g., Hispanic, Polish, Navajo, or a combination)? To what degree does the client identify with the cultural group (e.g., "we" concept of solidarity or a fringe member)?
- What is the client's reported racial affiliation (e.g., black, Native-American, or Asian)?
- Where was the client born?
- Where has the client lived (i.e., country and city) and when (i.e., during what years)? If the client has recently relocated to the United States, knowledge of prevalent diseases in the country of origin may be helpful.

Values Orientation

- What are the client's attitudes, values, and beliefs about birth, death, health, illness, and health care providers?
- Does culture influence the manner in which the client relates to body image change resulting from illness or surgery (e.g., importance of appearance, beauty, strength, and roles in cultural group)?
- How does the client view work, leisure, and education?
- How does the client perceive change?
- How does the client value privacy, courtesy, touch, and relationships with individuals of different ages, of different social class, or caste, and of the opposite sex?
- How does the client view biomedical-scientific health care (e.g., suspiciously, fearfully, or acceptingly)? How does the client relate to people in a different cultural group (e.g., withdrawal, verbal or nonverbal expression, or negative or positive attitude)?

Cultural Sanctions and Restrictions

- How does the client's cultural group regard expression of emotion and feelings, spirituality, and religious beliefs? How are dying, death, and grieving expressed in a culturally appropriate manner?

■ How is modesty expressed by men and women in the client's cultural group? Does the client's cultural group have culturally defined expectations about male-female relationships, including the nurse-client relationship?

■ Does the client have restrictions related to sexuality, exposure of body parts, or certain types of surgery (e.g., amputation, vasectomy, or hysterectomy)?

■ Does the client have restrictions against discussion of dead relatives or fears related to the unknown?

Communication

■ What language does the client speak at home? What other language does the client speak or read? In what language would the client prefer to communicate with you?

■ What is the written and spoken English fluency level of the client? Remember that the stress of illness may cause clients to use a more familiar language and temporarily forget some English.

■ Does the client need an interpreter? If so, is a relative or friend available whom the client would like to have interpret? Is anyone available with whom the client would prefer not to interpret (e.g., member of the opposite sex, a person younger or older than the client, or a member of a rival tribe or nation)?

■ What are the rules (i.e., linguistics) and modes (i.e., style) of communication?

■ Is it necessary to vary the technique of communication during the interview and examination to accommodate the client's cultural background (e.g., tempo of conversation, eye contact, sensitivity to topical taboos, norms of confidentiality, and style of explanation)?

■ How does the client's nonverbal communication compare with that of individuals from other cultural backgrounds? How does it affect the client's relationship with the nurse and with other members of the health care team?

■ How does the client feel about health care providers who are not of the same cultural background (e.g., black, middle-class nurse, or Hispanic of a different social class)? Does the client prefer to receive care from a nurse of the same cultural background, sex, or age?

■ What are the overall cultural characteristics of the client's language and communication processes?

■ With which language or dialect is the client most comfortable?

Health-Related Beliefs and Practices

■ To what cause or causes does the client attribute illness and disease (e.g., divine wrath, imbalance in hot-cold or yin-yang, punishment for moral transgressions, hex, or soul loss)?

■ What does the client believe promotes health (e.g., eating certain foods, wearing amulets to bring good luck, exercise, prayer, ancestors, saints, or intermediate deities)?

■ What is the client's religious affiliation (e.g., Judaism, Islam, Pentecostalism, West African voodooism, Seventh-Day Adventism, Catholicism, or Mormonism)?

■ Does the client rely on cultural healers (e.g., curandero, shaman, spiritualist, priest, minister, or monk)? Who determines when the client is sick and when the client is healthy? Who determines the type of healer and treatment that should be sought?

■ In what types of cultural healing practices does the client engage (e.g., herbal remedies, potions, massage, wearing talismans or charms to discourage evil spirits, healing rituals, incantations, or prayers)?

■ How does the client perceive biomedical-scientific health care providers? How do the client and family perceive nurses? What are the expectations of nurses and nursing care?

■ What comprises appropriate "sick-role" behavior? Who determines what symptoms constitute disease and illness? Who decides when the client is no longer sick? Who cares for the client at home?

■ How does the client's cultural group view mental disorders? Do they show differences in acceptable behaviors for physical vs. psychological illnesses?

Nutrition

■ What nutritional factors are influenced by the clients cultural background?

■ What are the meanings of *food* and *eating* to the client? With whom does the client usually eat? What types of foods does the client usually eat? What does the client define as food? What does the client believe comprises a "healthy" vs. an "unhealthy" diet?

■ How does the client prepare foods at home (e.g., type of food preparation; cooking oils used;

length of time foods, especially vegetables, are cooked; amount and type of seasoning added to various foods during preparation)?

■ Do religious beliefs and practices influence the client's diet (e.g., amount, type, preparation, or delineation of acceptable food combinations such as kosher diets)? Does the client abstain from certain foods at regular intervals, on specific dates determined by the religious calendar, or at other times?

■ If the client's religion mandates or encourages fasting, what does the term *fast* mean to the client (e.g., refraining from certain types or quantities of foods, eating only during certain times of the day)? For what period of time is the client expected to fast?

■ During fasting, does the client refrain from liquids or beverages? Does the religion allow exemption from fasting during illness, and if so, is the client believed to have an exemption?

Socioeconomic Considerations

■ Who constitutes the client's social network (i.e., family, peers, and healers)? How do they influence the client's health or illness status?

■ How do members of the client's social support network define *caring* (e.g., being continuously present, doing things for the client, or looking after the client's family)? What are the roles of various family members during health and illness?

■ How does the client's family participate in the client's nursing care (e.g., bathing, feeding, touching, and being present)?

■ Does the cultural family structure influence the client's response to health or illness (e.g., beliefs, strengths, weaknesses, and social class)? Does a key family member have a role that is significant in health-related decisions (e.g., grandmother in many black families or eldest adult son in Asian families)?

■ Who is the principal wage earner in the client's family? What is the total annual income? This is a potentially sensitive question that should be asked only if necessary. Does the family have more than one wage earner? Does the family have other sources of financial support (e.g., extended family or investments)?

■ What influence does economic status have on lifestyle, place of residence, living conditions, ability to obtain health care, and discharge planning?

Organizations Providing Cultural Support

■ What influence do ethnic and cultural organizations have on the client's receiving health care (e.g., Organization of Migrant Workers, National Association for the Advancement of Colored People, Black Political Caucus, churches, schools, Urban League, and community-based health care programs and clinics)?

Educational Background

■ What is the client's highest educational level obtained? Does the client's educational background affect the client's knowledge level concerning the health care delivery system, how to obtain the care needed, teaching and learning skills, and written material that is distributed in the health care setting (e.g., insurance forms, educational literature, information about diagnostical procedures and laboratory tests, and admissions forms)?

■ Can the client read and write English, or does he or she prefer another language? If English is the client's second language, are materials available in the client's primary language?

■ What learning style is most comfortable or familiar? Does the client prefer to learn through written materials, oral explanation, or demonstration?

Religious Affiliation

■ How does the client's religious affiliation influence health and illness (e.g., death, chronic illness, body image alteration, and cause and effect of illness)?

■ What is the role of the client's religious beliefs and practices during health and illness?

■ Does the client believe in healing rituals or practices that can promote well-being or hasten recovery from illness? If so, who performs these?

■ What is the role of significant religious representatives during health and illness? Does the client have recognized religious healers (e.g., Islamic imams, Christian Scientist practitioners or nurses, Catholic priests, Mormon elders, and Buddhist monks)?

Cultural Aspects of Disease Incidence

■ Does the client have specific genetic or acquired conditions that are more prevalent in a specific cultural group (e.g., hypertension, sickle cell anemia, Tay-Sachs disease, or lactose intolerance)?

■ Are any socioenvironmental diseases more prevalent among the client's specific cultural group (e.g., lead poisoning, alcoholism, AIDS, drug abuse, or ear infections)?

■ Do diseases exist against which the client has an increased resistance (e.g., skin cancer in darkly pigmented individuals)?

Biocultural Variations

■ Does the client have distinctive physical features that are characteristic of a particular racial group (e.g., skin color or hair texture)? Does the client have variations in anatomy that are characteristic of a particular racial or ethnic group (e.g., body structure, height, weight, facial shape and structure [nose, eye shape, and facial contour], or upper and lower extremity shape)?

■ How do anatomical and racial variations affect the assessment?

Developmental Considerations

■ Does the client have distinct growth and development characteristics that vary with his or her cultural background (e.g., bone density, psychomotor patterns of development, or fat folds)?

■ What factors are significant in assessing children from the newborn period through adolescence (e.g., expected growth on standard grid, culturally acceptable age for toilet training, introduction of various types of foods, sex differences, discipline, and socialization to adult roles)?

■ What is the cultural perception of aging (e.g., is youthfulness or the wisdom of old age more highly valued)?

■ How are older people handled culturally (e.g., cared for in the home of adult children or placed in institutions for care)? What are culturally acceptable roles for older adults?

■ Does the older adult expect family members to provide care, including nurturance and other humanistic aspects of care?

■ Is the older adult isolated from culturally relevant supportive people or enmeshed in a caring network of relatives and friends?

■ Has a culturally appropriate network replaced family members in performing some caring functions for older adults?

Cultural Self-Assessment

Community health nurses can engage in a cultural self-assessment. Through identification of health-related attitudes, values, beliefs, and practices that are part of the personal cultural meaning brought to the nurse-client interaction, the nurse can better understand the cultural aspects of health care from the perspective of the client, family, group, or community. Everyone has ethnocentric tendencies that must be brought to a level of conscious awareness so that efforts can be made to temper ethnocentrism and view reality from the perspective of the client.

Knowledge about Local Cultures

Community health nurses can learn about the cultural diversity characteristics of the subgroup or subgroups that are most prevalent within their communities. The nurse cannot know about all health-related beliefs and practices of the diverse groups served; therefore he or she can study selected ones. The nurse can accomplish this cultural study by a review of nursing, anthropology, sociology, and related literature on culturally diverse groups; in-services held at community health agencies, educational institutions in the community, or organizations serving minority groups; enrollment in courses on transcultural or cross-cultural nursing and medical anthropology; and interviews with key members of the subgroups of interest, such as clergy members, nurses, physicians, and others, to obtain information about the influence of culture on health-related beliefs and practices.

Recognition of Political Issues of Culturally Diverse Groups

Awareness of the political aspects of health care for culturally diverse groups and communities can enable community health nurses to have increased involvement in influencing legislation and funding priorities aimed at improving health care for specific populations. Recognized for their leadership role in community health matters involving culturally diverse groups, community health nurses may be invited by political leaders to participate in political decision making affecting the health of a targeted subgroup. Community health nurses should also be active politically, both individually and collectively, to influence legislation affecting culturally diverse individuals, groups, and communities, and they should offer to serve on key community committees, boards, and advisory councils that impact the health of culturally diverse groups.

Provide Culturally Competent Care

When caring for individuals and families from culturally diverse backgrounds, the community health nurse can assess, diagnose, implement, and evaluate nursing care in a manner that is culturally congruent, competent, relevant, and appropriate. To provide this culturally appropriate nursing care, the nurse must be aware of the cultural similarities and differences between the nurse and the client to create a relationship of mutual respect. A guideline for gathering cultural data has been presented and the nurse may use this guideline or a similar one for identifying significant areas in which the nurse and client differ. Knowledge about biocultural variations in health and illness is particularly important when conducting cultural assessments (Andrews, 1992).

Recognition of Culturally Based Health Practices

As discussed previously, the community health nurse should attempt to understand the nature and meaning of culturally based health practices of clients, groups, and communities. Once the practices are understood, the nurse can make a determination regarding their appropriateness in a particular context. Generally, the nurse should decide whether a cultural practice is useful, neutral, or harmful to the client, group, or community. The nurse should encourage or "tolerate" helpful and neutral practices, whereas he or she should discourage harmful practices.

The classification of some cultural healing practices is not so easily determined. For example, many Southeast Asians practice *coining,* which is the rubbing of a coin over body surfaces to expel "bad winds" that are believed to cause illness. Coining leaves abrasions on the skin; therefore community health nurses are sometimes faced with an ethical dilemma when coining is practiced on young children because this practice may be construed by some members of the dominant cultural group as child abuse. This practice is not useful, so the nurse must make the decision whether it is neutral or harmful. An argument for the practice being neutral is based on the facts that the abrasions usually heal quickly, no harm is done to the child as a result of the practice, and the practice is meaningful to parents who have much confidence in the healing powers associated with coining.

The argument can also be made that the practice is harmful. The red marks and skin abrasions caused by the coining places the child at increased risk for skin infection. Given that the child may require antibiotics or other medication for a respiratory disorder, encouragement of coining may prevent the child from receiving needed medical intervention and delay treatment.

As a solution, the community health nurse may suggest that parents combine traditional treatment with Western biomedicine (i.e., they can use coining in conjunction with a biomedical intervention). Therefore the healing will occur in a manner that has involved the use of both folk and professional health care systems.

RESOURCES FOR MINORITY HEALTH

Community health nurses will find federal resources for improving the health care of the federally defined minority populations through the USDHHS and PHS. Within the PHS, the OMH and the IHS relate to health promotion, disease prevention, service delivery, and research on minority groups.

U.S. Department of Health and Human Services

Office of Minority Health

The OMH is the unit of the USDHHS that coordinates federal efforts to improve the health status of racial and ethnic minority populations (i.e., blacks, Hispanics, Native-Americans and Alaska Natives, and Asians and Pacific Islanders). Located within the office of the PHS, the OMH is directed by the deputy assistant secretary for minority health.

The OMH was established by the Disadvantaged Minority Health Improvement Act of 1990 (PL 101-527), which was signed by President Bush on November 6, 1990. Under the directives of the Act, the OMH has the following responsibilities:

- Establish short- and long-range goals and objectives relating to disease prevention, health promotion, service delivery, and research on the health of minority people.
- Promote increased participation of disadvantaged people, including minorities, in health service and health promotion programs.
- Create a national minority health resource center.
- Support research, demonstrations, and evaluations of new and innovative models that increase

understanding of disease risk factors and support better information dissemination, education, prevention, and service delivery to minority communities.

■ Promote minority health-related activities in the corporate and voluntary sectors.

■ Develop minority-focused health information and health promotion materials and teaching programs.

■ Assist providers of primary care and preventive services in obtaining assistance of bilingual health professionals when appropriate.

Initiatives for Improved Minority Health Care

As the focal point for minority health efforts, the OMH plays a key role in major initiatives launched by the USDHHS secretary and the PHS. Table 12-7 lists some of the initiatives.

Indian Health Service

The IHS is also a component of the PHS. The IHS is responsible for providing federal health services to Native-Americans and Alaska Natives. Federal Indian health services are based on the laws that Congress has passed pursuant to its authority to regulate commerce with the Indian Nations as specified in the Constitution and other documents.

The primary responsibility of the IHS is to elevate the health status of Native-Americans and Alaska Natives to the highest level possible. The mission is to ensure quality, availability, and accessibility of a comprehensive high-quality health care delivery system, providing maximum involvement of Native-Americans and Alaska Natives in defining their health needs, setting health priorities for their local areas, and managing and controlling their health programs. The IHS also acts as the principal federal health

TABLE 12-7

Federally Sponsored Initiatives to Improve the Health of Minority Groups

Initiative	Description
Program Direction 9: Improving the Health of Minority and Low-Income People	A broad multiyear plan sponsored by the USDHHS encompassing nine program directions for health and social services. The two-part strategy, in which all divisions of the USDHHS participate, involves improving access to health care for minority and low-income persons and reducing the risks of chronic and preventable diseases and conditions that disproportionately affect minority and low-income people through expanded biomedical, behavioral, and health services research, prevention, and early detection and treatment.
Grant programs	The grant programs of the OMH have been developed to help communities deal with specific problems, such as the high death rates among minority males and the continuing high prevalence of numerous acute and chronic conditions. The grants also have a larger goal—to empower communities both large and small to help themselves and overcome the myriad social and health problems facing communities.
Minority Community Health Coalition Demonstration Grant Program	The OMH provides grants to community coalitions for risk-reduction projects that target health problem areas in minority populations. These demonstration grants have provided coalitions with up to two years of funding to initiate community-designed programs that would address disease risk factors affecting minority populations.
Minority HIV Education and Prevention Grant Program	The OMH provides grants to minority community-based and national organizations for risk-reduction projects that target HIV infection and the diseases that often precede or accompany it: STDs, cervical cancer, and TB. These education and prevention grants provide minority organizations with up to three years of funding to develop new approaches to prevent and reduce HIV transmission among minority populations.
Minority Male Grant Program	The Minority Male Grant Program was initiated to address the multiple health and human service problems that disproportionately affect minority males. Two components make up the program. Coalition development projects address the specific needs of the defined high-risk minority male populations in each community. Coalition demonstration grants will go beyond the initial steps of sharing information and developing coalitions to the actual implementation of educational, support, and service programs for high-risk minority males.

advocate for Native-Americans by ensuring that they have knowledge of and access to all federal, state, and local health programs to which they are entitled as American citizens. The IHS also works with these programs so Native-Americans will be cognizant of their entitlements.

The IHS carried out its responsibilities through development and operation of a health services delivery system designed to provide a broad-spectrum program of preventive, curative, rehabilitative, and environmental services. This system integrates health services delivered directly through IHS facilities and staff with those purchased by IHS through contractual arrangements. Tribes are also actively involved in program implementation.

The 1975 Indian Self-Determination Act (PL 93-638) as amended builds on IHS policy by giving tribes the option of staffing and managing IHS programs in their communities and provides funding for improvement of tribal capability to contract under the act. The 1976 Indian Health Care Improvement Act (PL 94-437) as amended was intended to elevate the health care status of Native-Americans and Alaska Natives to a level equal to that of the general population through a program of authorized higher resource levels in the IHS budget. Appropriated resources were used to expand health services, build and renovate medical facilities, and step up the construction of safe drinking water and sanitary disposal facilities. It also establishes programs designed to increase the number of Native-American health professionals for Native-American needs and to improve health care access for Native-Americans living in urban areas.

The operation of the IHS health care delivery system is managed through local administrative units called *service units.* A service unit is the basic health organization for a geographical area served by the IHS program, just as a county or city health department is the basic health organization in a state health department. These are defined areas usually centered around a single federal reservation in the continental United States or a population concentration in Alaska. The IHS serves approximately 50% of the total Native-American and Alaska Native population in the United States, primarily those residing on reservations.

CASE STUDY

APPLICATION OF THE NURSING PROCESS

Community health nurse Maria Gonzales visited the home of five-year-old Nguyen Van Nghi, who was discharged from the hospital on the previous day. The pediatrician had diagnosed the child with pneumonia and "suspected failure to thrive" because the child's growth fell below the third percentile on a standard growth chart for height and weight and he performed poorly on a screening test used to identify developmental delays for a five-year-old child.

Residing in the home were the child's parents, four siblings, grandmother, aunt, uncle, and three cousins. Although the child's father and uncle spoke some English, other members of the household communicated in a language unfamiliar to Maria, which "sounded like Chinese." When Maria approached the child, he did not look at her or speak to her, even when she called him Nguyen (pronounced "we'en").

During her initial assessment, Maria observed multiple tender, ecchymotic areas with petechiae between the ribs on the front and back of the body, resembling strap marks. Suspecting child abuse, Maria told the family that she would return later in the day with an interpreter. She located an interpreter who spoke Mandarin Chinese and briefed him about her concerns with child abuse. When Maria and the interpreter returned to the client's home, she instructed the interpreter to ask the parents for an explanation of the bruises. The interpreter told Maria that the family was Vietnamese and could not understand his Chinese dialect. Both the interpreter and the child's father knew a little French and awkwardly managed to communicate.

The interpreter advised the nurse that, in the Vietnamese culture, the person's family name is given first, followed by the middle name and then the first name. Only a few different family names exist among the Vietnamese; therefore it is common practice to call people by their given first name. At this point, Maria also learned that the child was actually four-years-old, because the Vietnamese consider a newborn to be one-year-old at birth.

The interpreter explained that a Vietnamese healer performed *cao gio,* or coining, to exude the "bad wind" from Nghi. *Cao gio* is performed by applying a special menthol oil to the painful or symptomatic part of the body and then rubbing a coin over the area with firm, downward strokes. When Nghi's condition seemed to worsen after his hospital discharge, his grandmother convinced his parents that Western biomedicine had failed and that their son required the stronger power of folk healing.

Assessment

Although a systematic and comprehensive cultural assessment is necessary, the community health nurse must set priorities and focus on selected cultural data categories because they seem most relevant for the Nguyen family at present. After the nurse and family resolve the immediate concerns of a worsening case of pneumonia and potential child abuse, the nurse can complete the remaining data categories of the cultural assessment. To guide the data collection in an orderly manner, the community health nurse may find it useful to follow Leininger's cultural and social structure dimensions (see Fig. 12-1).

Technological Factors
- Use of prescription medicines and adherence by family to a recommended medical regimen for the child's pneumonia
- Use of x-ray examinations for identifying healed fractures in children who may be habitually abused by caregivers

Religious and Philosophical Factors
- Culturally based health-related values, beliefs, and practices pertaining to children
- Yin-yang beliefs and practices concerning health and illness, foods, seasons, and organs of the body

Kinship and Social Factors
- Family configuration, degree of assimilation, and acculturation; extended family roles and responsibilities
- Sex-role–related behavior of parents, siblings, grandmother, aunt, uncle, and cousins
- Children expected to respect and obey adults and others in authority

Cultural Values and Ways of Life
- Cross-cultural communication and use of primary language
- English as a secondary language
- Normal regression in language skills and stress
- Culturally based child-rearing practices, including expected parent-child relationships and cultural definitions of abuse and neglect
- Cultural value for respecting authority figures, including health care providers
- Patterns of parenting: mothering, fathering, and substitute or surrogate parents
- Identification of primary provider of care and decision maker for health-related matters affecting the child because this may or may not be the biological parent

Political and Legal Factors
- Cultural fear of authority, which sometimes includes health care providers, resulting from abuse of power by officials during the Vietnam War
- U.S. laws governing child abuse and neglect
- U.S. immigration laws

Economic Factors
- Financial situation of family
- Employment and income of breadwinners in family
- Health insurance
- Cost for cultural healer and folk remedies vs. professional Western biomedical practitioners and medical-surgical interventions
- Access to transportation for health care purposes
- Family's ability to afford utility bills, insurance premiums, food, rent and mortgage payments, and other household expenses

Continued

Educational Factors
- Parents and other family members
- Correct placement of children in educational settings given cultural conceptualization of age, normal height and weight for children of Asian descent, language, and other sociocultural considerations

Generic or Folk Health Systems
- Role of cultural healers and relationship with families
- Appropriateness of cultural healers as members of the health care team
- Folk healing practices in care of children
- Yin-yang beliefs in causation and cure of diseases in children
- Cultural practice of *cao gio*
- Interrelationship with Western biomedical practices

Professional Health Systems
- Biocultural variations in normal growth and development
- Use of appropriate growth and development instruments for Asian-American children
- After correction of the erroneous age reported by the hospital, reassessment of growth and development based on norms for Asian children
- Reevaluation of the pediatrician's diagnosis of failure to thrive

Nursing Care
- Role of the community health care nurse in serving ethnic populations
- Overcoming of potential barriers to providing culture-congruent and culturally competent nursing care, such as ethnocentrism, cultural imposition, cultural stereotyping, and cross-cultural miscommunication
- Role of the community health nurse in reporting cases of suspected child abuse
- Determination of the difference between harmless cultural healing practices, such as coining, and child abuse
- Home health care for Vietnamese-American child with clinical manifestations of respiratory disease
- Health education for the child, parents, and other family members

Application of Leininger's Theory of Culture Care Diversity and Universality: Nursing Care Decisions and Actions

To provide culturally congruent or culturally competent nursing care for individuals, families, groups, communities, and institutions, the community health nurse must review and evaluate all data gathered in the cultural assessment. When making nursing care decisions or actions, nurses will find the following three options available: cultural care preservation and maintenance, cultural care accommodation and negotiation, or cultural care repatterning and restructuring (Leininger, 1991, 1995).

In the case study, Maria learned in her assessment that the cultural healing practice called *cao gio* was responsible for red marks on the torso of a minor child. She must first determine whether this cultural healing practice is helpful, neutral, or harmful to the child. If the practice is believed to be helpful, Maria may choose cultural care preservation and maintenance (i.e., encourage the family to continue using *cao gio*). If it is neutral, she also is likely to choose cultural care preservation and maintenance. If she determines that the practice is harmful (e.g., has concern that the abrasions will become infected or that the practice is preventing the child from receiving biomedical care that will cure the pneumonia), she will choose either cultural care accommodation and negotiation or cultural care repatterning and restructuring. Examples of accommodation or negotiation might include involving the cultural healer as a member of the health care team and suggesting to the family that both *cao gio* and Western biomedical treatments be used to cure the child. Examples of repatterning or restructuring might include asking the family to stop *cao gio* and reporting the case to authorities representing a child protective services agency.

Gaining skills necessary to address this Vietnamese-American child's health needs requires ability in cultural, or culturological, assessment. If the community health nurse determines that the agency's assessment instrument is inadequate in cultural data categories, it will be necessary to adopt or adapt published cultural assessment guides (e.g., Andrews and Boyle, 1999; Leininger, 1995).

SUMMARY

To provide community health nursing for individuals, groups, and communities representing the hundreds of different cultures and subcultures found in the United States, the nurse should include cultural considerations in nursing care. Guidelines for gathering data from clients of culturally diverse backgrounds have been suggested in this chapter and are interwoven throughout the text. Knowledge about culture-specific and culture-universal nursing care is foundational and is an integral component of community health nursing.

LEARNING ACTIVITIES

1. Examine the vital statistics of a community and compare differences in morbidity and mortality rates for whites and racial and ethnic subgroups. What data are available according to racial and ethnic heritage? What data are missing?
2. Visit an inner-city grocery store and compare quality, prices, customer services, and variety of products with those of a suburban grocery store.
3. Select a client from a racially or ethnically diverse background and conduct a cultural assessment.
4. Interview someone from a different racial or ethnic background to determine beliefs about illness causation, use of the lay and professional health care delivery systems, and culturally based treatments.
5. Dine at an ethnic restaurant. While dining, notice the type of cultural heritage in restaurant decor and information about the culture available from the menu, placemats, or elsewhere in the restaurant. Ask the owner or manager about the history of the restaurant.
6. Attend religious services at a church, temple, synagogue, or place of worship for an unfamiliar religion.
7. Interview an official representative (e.g., priest, elder, monk, or bishop) from an unfamiliar religion. Ask about health-related beliefs and practices, healing rituals, support network for the sick, and dietary practices.
8. Watch prime-time television and note the racial and ethnic diversity that is present during the commercials. During the program, note the role played by racially and ethnically diverse characters. Are they heroes or heroines or the "bad guys"? What are their occupations, SES, religions, and lifestyles?
9. Skim a popular magazine for references to racially and ethnically diverse subgroups. What is being written? Is the nature of the article favorable or unfavorable?

REFERENCES

American Cancer Society: *Cancer facts and figures—1997: racial and ethnic patterns,* December 29, 1999, The Author, www.cancer.org/statistics.

Andrews MM: Cultural perspectives on nursing in the 21st century, *J Prof Nurs* 8:7, 1992.

Andrews MM: How to search for information on transcultural nursing and health subjects: internet and CD-ROM resources, *J Transcult Nurs* 10:69, 1999.

Andrews MM, Boyle JS: Competence in transcultural nursing care, *Am J Nurs* 97:16AA, 1997.

Andrews MM, Boyle JS, editors: *Transcultural concepts in nursing care,* ed 3, Philadelphia, 1999, Lippincott, Williams & Wilkins.

Bird JA et al: Opening pathways to cancer screening for Vietnamese-American women: lay health workers hold a key, *Prev Med* 27:821, 1998.

Boyle JS, Mackey MC: Pica: sorting it out, *J Transcult Nurs* 10:65, 1999.

Brooks J: *Healthy people 2010 and beyond: closing the gap,* Washington, DC, 1998, OMH.

Council of Economic Advisers for the President's Initiative on Race: *Changing America: indicators of social and economic well-being by race and Hispanic origin,* Washington, DC, 1999, US Government Printing Office.

Duffy ME, Rossow R, Hernandez M: Correlates of health-promotion activities in employed Mexican American women, *Nurs Res* 45:18, 1996.

Fox SA et al: A trial to increase mammography utilization among Los Angeles Hispanic women, *J Health Care Poor Underserved* 9:309, 1998.

Frank-Stromberg M et al: A study of rural Latino women seeking cancer-detection examination, *J Cancer Educ* 13:231, 1998.

Garcia Coll CT: Developmental outcome of minority infants: a process-oriented look into our beginnings, *Child Dev* 61:270, 1990.

Hall E: Proxemics: the study of man's spatial relations. In Galdston I, editor: *Man's image in medicine and anthropology,* New York, 1963, International Universities Press.

Hanson PA, Andrews MM: Religion, culture and nursing. In Andrews MM, Boyle JS, editors: *Transcultural concepts in nursing care,* ed 3, Philadelphia, 1999, Lippincott, Williams & Wilkins.

Herberg P: Theoretical foundations of transcultural nursing. In Andrews MM, Boyle JS, editors: *Transcultural concepts in nursing care,* Philadelphia, 1995, J.B. Lippincott.

Indian Health Service: *Trends in Indian health,* Washington, DC, 1997, US Government Printing Office.

Jenkins CNH et al: Effect of a media-led education campaign on breast and cervical cancer screening among Vietnamese-American women, *Prev Med* 28: 395, 1999.

Katon W, Kleinman A: Doctor-patient negotiation and other social science strategies in patient care. In Eisenberg L, Kleinman A, editors: *The relevance of social science for medicine,* Boston, 1981, D. Reidel.

Kluckhohn F, Strodtbeck F: *Variations in value orientations,* Evanston, Ill, 1961, Row, Peterson.

Kohls LR: *Survival kit for overseas living,* Yarmouth, Me, 1984, Intercultural Press.

Lambert S, Newton M, deMeneses M: Barriers to mammography in older, low-income African American women, *J Multicult Nurs Health* 4:16, 1998.

Leininger MM: *Culture, care, diversity, and universality: a theory of nursing,* Pub No 15-2402, New York, 1991, NLN.

Leininger MM: *Nursing and anthropology: two worlds to blend,* New York, 1970, Wiley.

Leininger MM: *Transcultural nursing: concepts, theories, and practice,* New York, 1978, Wiley.

Leininger MM: *Transcultural nursing: concepts, theories, research and practice,* Columbus, 1995, McGraw Hill and Enden Press.

Lubaczewski J, Pezzoli SA: Alternatives to institutionalization: identifying and addressing the needs of urban homebound elderly, *J Multicult Nurs Health* 4:49, 1998.

Ludwig-Beymer PA: Transcultural aspects of pain. In Andrews M, Boyle JS, editors: *Transcultural concepts in nursing care,* ed 3, Philadelphia, 1999, Lippincott, Williams & Wilkins.

Lurie N: *Statement of Nicole Lurie, M.D., M.S. P.H., Principle Deputy Assistant Secretary for Health,* September 15, 1999, US Public Health Services for the Senate Committee on Health, US Senate, www.waisgate.hhs.gov.

Mendoza FS, Fuentes-Afflick E: Latino children's health and the family-community health promotion model, *West J Med* 170(2):85, 1999.

National Center for Health Statistics: *Health, United States: 1999,* Hyattsville, Md, 1999, US PHS.

National Council of Churches: *Yearbook of American and Canadian churches,* New York, 1999, National Council of the Churches of Christ in the United States of America.

Office of Minority Health, Public Health Service, US Department of Health and Human Services: *Empowerment zones and enterprise communities, closing the gap,* Washington, DC, July/August, 1996, OMH.

Ofili E, Igho-Pemu P, Bransford T: The prevention of cardiovascular disease in blacks, *Curr Opin Cardiol* 14:169, 1999.

Pacquiao DF, Archeval L, Shelley EE: Transcultural nursing study of emic and etic care in the home, *J Transcult Nurs* 10:112, 1999.

Princeton Religion Research Center: *Religion in America,* Princeton, NJ, 1996, The Gallop Poll.

Ramirez AG et al: The emerging Hispanic population: a foundation for cancer prevention and control, *J Natl Cancer Inst Monogr* 18:1, 1995.

Rankin SH, Galbraith ME, Huang P: Quality of life and social environment as reported by Chinese immigrants with non–insulin-dependent diabetes mellitus, *The Diabetes Educator* 23:171, 1997.

Rosella J, Regan-Kubinski M, Albrecht S: The need for multicultural diversity among health professionals, *Nurs Health Care* 15:242, 1994.

Satcher D: *U.S. to fight racial health disparities,* 1998, The Author, www.afamnet.com.

Simpson CE: *Healthy People 2010: what can we do to shape the objectives? closing the gap,* Washington, DC, Aug/Sept. 1998, OMH.

Spector R: *Cultural diversity in health and illness,* Norwalk, Conn, 2000, Appleton-Lange.

Strickland CJ, Squeoch MD, Chrisman, NJ: Health promotion in cervical cancer prevention among the Yakima Indian women of the Wa'Shat longhouse, *J Transcult Nurs* 10:190, 1999.

Tylor EB: *Primitive culture,* London, 1871, Murray.

US Census Bureau: *Population estimates program, population division,* Washington, DC, 1999a, US Government Printing Office.

US Census Bureau: *Poverty 1998: poverty by selected characteristics,* 1999b, The Author, www.census.gov/hhes/poverty/poverty98/pv98est1.html.

US Census Bureau: *Statistical abstract of the United States, 1992,* ed 108, Washington, DC, 1992, US Government Printing Office.

US Department of Health and Human Services: *Healthy people 2010,* Washington, DC, 2000, US Government Printing Office.

US Department of Health and Human Services, Office of Disease Prevention and Health Promotion: *Developing objectives for Healthy People 2010,* Washington, DC, 1997, US Government Printing Office.

US Department of Health and Human Services, Public Health Service, Bureau of Health Professions, Division of Nursing: *Fact sheet: selected facts about minority registered nurses,* Washington, DC, 1996, US Government Printing Office.

Zapata J, Shippee-Rice R: The use of folk healing and healers by six Latinos living in New England: a preliminary study, *J Transcult Nurs* 10:136, 1999.

Zborowski M: *People in pain,* San Francisco, 1969, Jossey-Bass.

Environmental Health

Patricia E. Stevens and Joanne M. Hall

Upon completion of this chapter, the reader will be able to do the following:

1. Describe the broad areas of environmental health about which community health nurses must be informed and name environmental hazards in each area.

2. Recognize potential social, cultural, economic, and political factors affecting environmental health.

3. Apply the basic concepts of critical theory to environmental health nursing problems.

4. Identify aggregates at risk for particular environmental health problems.

5. Distinguish between environmental health approaches that focus on altering individual behaviors and those that aim to change health-damaging environments.

6. Formulate critical questions about environmental conditions that limit the survival and well-being of communities.

7. Understand the skills needed to facilitate community participation and partnership in identifying and solving environmental health problems.

8. Propose collective strategies in which community health nurses can participate to address the environmental health concerns of specific aggregates.

aggregate
atmospheric quality
community
environment
environmental racism
food quality
health
living patterns
participatory action research
sick building
waste control
water quality

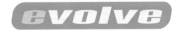

http://evolve.elsevier.com/Nies/

Environmental health is of ever-increasing importance to community health nursing practice. Accumulated evidence shows that the environmental changes of the past few decades have profoundly influenced the status of public health. The safety, beauty, and life-sustaining capacity of the physical environment are unquestionably of global consequence. The ecological approach of the 1960s and 1970s tended to focus on clean water, clean air, and protected natural resources in specific locales. By the end of the twentieth century, it was acutely apparent that the world was fraught with urgent environmental difficulties including extinction of many species, diminishment of tropical rain forests, proliferation of toxic waste dumps, effects of acid rain, progressive destruction of the ozone layer, shortage of landfill sites, consequences of global warming, development of deadly chemical and ballistic weapons, adulteration of food by pesticides and herbicides, oceanic contamination through toxic dumping and petroleum spills, overcrowding of urban areas, traffic congestion of thoroughfares, and evergrowing industrial hazards that pose health risks to workers.

This chapter will explore the health of communities in relation to the environment. Critical theory is useful in examining environmental health (Stevens and Hall, 1992). It offers a framework for discussion and a basis for described community health nursing practices. Applying critical theory is a way of thinking upstream (Chapter 3). Critical theory is an approach that raises questions about oppressive situations, involves community members in the definition and solution of problems, and facilitates interventions that liberate people from the health-damaging effects of environments. By applying the nursing process in a critical fashion, nurses can be dynamically involved in the design of interventions that alter the precursors of poor health.

Throughout this chapter, case examples illustrate how environmental health problems affect the everyday lives of aggregates. The term **aggregate** refers to a group that shares a common aspect such as age, gender, race, economic status, cultural perspective, chronic illness, and area of residence. Aggregates may be a **community** in which the members know and interact with each other such as a barrio neighborhood or a labor union. Aggregates may also be "theoretically defined" categories of individuals who may or may not interact regularly with others in the defined group, such as "all crack cocaine users,"

TABLE 13-1

Concept	Definition
Aggregate	An aggregate is a group of people who share some common aspect such as age, economic status, cultural background, gender, race, area of residence, and chronic illness.
Community	Community is an aggregate in which the members know and interact with each other and have a collective identity such as a barrio neighborhood or a labor union.
Environment	Environment is the accumulation of physical, social, cultural, economic, and political conditions that influence the lives of communities.
Health	Health of communities depends on the integrity of the physical environment, the humaneness of the social relations within it, the availability of resources necessary to sustain life and to manage illness, the equitable distribution of health risks, attainable employment and education, cultural preservation and tolerance of diversity among subgroups, access to historic heritage, and a sense of empowerment and hope.

"women with physical disabilities," or "all men over the age of 65."

This chapter uses two other terms throughout. **Environment** is the accumulation of physical, social, cultural, economic, and political conditions that influence the lives of communities. The community's **health** depends on the integrity of the physical environment, the humaneness of the social relations in the environment, the availability of resources necessary to sustain life and manage illness, the equitable distribution of health risks, attainable employment and education, cultural preservation and tolerance of diversity among subgroups, access to historical heritage, and a sense of empowerment and hope (Table 13-1).

A CRITICAL THEORY APPROACH TO ENVIRONMENTAL HEALTH

Questioning what appears to be "given" in the environment and challenging "the way things have always been done" are the core dynamics of critical thinking. For example, public buildings, schools, work places, and mass transportation systems are environmental structures that are vital to people's everyday functioning. Ordinarily, society takes them for granted. However, the experiences of physically challenged people bring into question what society takes for granted about the environment.

Can disabled people board local buses?

Are public facilities wheelchair-accessible?

Can sight- or hearing-impaired children attend public schools and receive an equitable education?

Will a company deny employment to disabled people because it lacks entrance ramps, wheelchair-accessible rest room facilities, and elevators?

Critical theory suggests that community health nurses must be critical of environmental obstructions that affect the safety and well-being of particular aggregates or deprive them of access to necessary resources for the pursuit of health. In identifying environmental sources of health problems, nurses must be involved with the affected communities. Rather than impose assessments of the problem, nurses should share their ideas and dialogue with community members. For example, nurses should listen to what the community believes is problematic, help raise consciousness about environmental dangers, and help bring about change (Stevens and Hall, 1992).

Again, the experiences of disabled people provide examples of how to critically approach environmental health. Often subconsciously, able-bodied people infantilize physically challenged individuals and assume they are passive, powerless, and victimized by their physical incapacity. Community health nurses frequently approach members of this aggregate to assist them in coping with their disabilities by arranging home environments to facilitate their daily activities. This may be an appropriate goal, but many disabled people identify broader problems such as architectural and discriminatory constraints in the environment that have systematically barred them from employment, education, housing, and health care. From their perspective, these may be the most essential health problems. Many disabled people "eschew the telethon's 'politics of pity' and abhor the 'poster child' image, demanding instead to be regarded as self-determining adults, capable of militant political action" (Anspach, 1979, p. 766).

If nurses become involved in open, respectful dialogue with this aggregate, they can learn how the disabled perceive themselves, their health, and their environmental influences. From a critical standpoint,

helping communities become more aware of the environmental effects on health and helping them make needed changes in their environment are legitimate nursing actions. The ultimate goal of the critical practice of community health nursing is liberating people from health-damaging environmental conditions.

Since the 1980s, people with disabilities and their advocates have achieved changes in environmental conditions, including federal legislation mandating accessibility of public facilities and services, changes in municipal building codes and state employment regulations, and increased enforcement of laws regarding nondiscrimination in hiring, educational opportunities, and health services. Collective actions were instrumental in accomplishing these environmental changes. Some of the strategies included strategic organization, litigation, public hearing testimony, letter-writing campaigns, legislative lobbying, and mass demonstrations.

A critical perspective can help nurses plan and implement aggregate-level interventions because it emphasizes collective strategies for change. Acting collectively can empower nurses to impact environmental health just as collective action empowered disability rights activists to achieve their objectives. In assessing environmental health problems, planning and implementing interventions, and evaluating the effectiveness of community-based actions, the community health nurse should be aware of physical surroundings and the effects of cultural realities, social relations, economic circumstances, and political conditions on communities. Several sources that discuss critical theory and its application to community health nursing are available in the literature (Allen, 1986; Butterfield, 1990; Hall, Stevens, and Meleis, 1994; Stevens, 1989; Stevens and Hall, 1992; Thompson, 1987; Watts, 1990).

AREAS OF ENVIRONMENTAL HEALTH

Although many conceptual schemes are possible, this chapter divides the vast field of environmental health (Alexander and Fairbridge, 1999; Kemp, 1998; Moore, 1999) into the following subcategories: living patterns, work risks, atmospheric quality, water quality, housing, food quality, waste control, radiation risks, and violence risks (Table 13-2). The brief discussions of these areas are only introductions to environmental health and focus on basic problems and strategies rather than statistical detail. The following sections define these nine areas of environmental

TABLE 13-2

Areas of Environmental Health

Area	Definition
Living patterns	Living patterns are the relationships among people, communities, and their surrounding environments that depend on habits, interpersonal ties, cultural values, and customs.
Work risks	Work risks include the quality of the employment environment and the potential for injury or illness posed by working conditions.
Atmospheric quality	Atmospheric quality refers to the protectiveness of the atmospheric layers, the risks of severe weather, and the purity of the air for breathing purposes.
Water quality	Water quality refers to the availability and volume of the water supply and the mineral content levels, pollution by toxic chemicals, and the presence of pathogenic microorganisms. Water quality consists of the balance between water contaminants and existing capabilities to purify water for human use and plant and wildlife sustenance.
Housing	Housing is an environmental health concern and refers to the availability, safety, structural strength, cleanliness, and location of shelter, including public facilities and family dwellings.
Food quality	Food quality refers to the availability, relative costs, variety and safety of foods and the health of animal and plant food sources.
Waste control	Waste control is the management of waste materials resulting from industrial and municipal processes, human consumption, and efforts to minimize waste production.
Radiation risks	Radiation risks are health dangers posed by the various forms of ionizing radiation relative to barriers preventing exposure of humans and other life forms.
Violence risks	The environmental risks of violence include the potential for victimization through the violence of particular individuals and the general level of aggression in psychosocial climates.

health, provide examples of problems relevant to each category, and present vignettes that illustrate community health nursing responses to environmental health concerns. Table 13-3 lists some of the environmental health problems included in this chapter.

Living Patterns

Living patterns are the relationships among people, communities, and their surrounding environments that depend on habits, interpersonal ties, cultural values, and customs. Drunk driving, second-hand smoke, urban crowding, noise exposure, unabated traffic, and the stress of increased mechanization could pose environmental health problems because people live within sociocultural patterns that limit their ability to escape these realities (Aday, 1993; Harper and Lambert, 1994; Kozol, 1991; Lunberg, 1998; Sidel, 1992).

Living patterns do not reflect an individual's lifestyle choices (e.g., eating a diet rich in saturated fats, leading a sedentary lifestyle, or becoming emotionally involved with a substance abuser). Rather, living patterns reflect population exposure to environmental conditions affected by mass culture, social policy, ethnic customs, and technology (Eckersley, 1992; Lawrence, 1999).

For example, community responses to a toxic chemical spill are mediated by many cultural, psychological, social, and economic conditions in the affected residential areas (Vyner, 1988a). Exposure to toxic substances in the environment is an increasingly common event. The situation becomes a toxicological disaster when an entire community suffers exposure (Havenaar and van den Brink, 1997). The technological hazard represented by a toxicological disaster can be more difficult for communities to cope with than natural disasters. The human failure symbolized by technological hazards can evoke anger, hopelessness, and helplessness that manifests in heightened community stress and deepening personal depression (Vyner, 1988b).

Difficulties in alerting state and federal officials

TABLE 13-3

Examples of Environmental Health Problems

Area	Problems
Living patterns	Drunk driving
	Second-hand smoke
	Noise exposure
	Urban crowding
	Technological hazards
Work risks	Occupational toxic poisoning
	Machine-operating hazards
	Sexual harassment
	Repetitive motion injuries
	Carcinogenic work sites
Atmospheric quality	Gaseous pollutants
	Greenhouse effect
	Destruction of the ozone layer
	Aerial spraying of herbicides and pesticides
	Acid rain
Water quality	Contamination of drinking supply by human waste
	Oil spills in the world's waterways
	Pesticide or herbicide infiltration of groundwater
	Aquifer contamination by industrial pollutants
	Heavy metal poisoning of fish
Housing	Homelessness
	Rodent and insect infestation
	Poisoning from lead-based paint
	Sick building syndrome
	Unsafe neighborhoods
Food quality	Malnutrition
	Bacterial food poisoning
	Food adulteration
	Disrupted food chains by ecosystem destruction
	Carcinogenic chemical food additives
Waste control	Use of nonbiodegradable plastics
	Poorly designed solid waste dumps
	Inadequate sewage systems
	Transport and storage of hazardous waste
	Illegal industrial dumping
Radiation risks	Nuclear facility emissions
	Radioactive hazardous wastes
	Radon gas seepage in homes and schools
	Nuclear testing
	Excessive exposure to x-rays
Violence risks	Proliferation of handguns
	Increasing incidence of hate crimes
	Pervasive images of violence in the media
	High rates of homicide among young black males
	Violent acts against women and children

In an urban Chinese community, the economic after-shocks of a major earthquake caused the closure of many businesses. Some of these family businesses moved to parts of the city less characterized by the use of Chinese languages. These moves caused many elderly, nonEnglish-speaking family members to experience depression, which is characterized by loss of appetite.

The community health nurses in the area began visiting these elders and brought interpreters with them. In their assessments, the nurses focused on psychiatric symptoms and suggested ventilation of emotions. They encouraged many elderly Chinese to attend a local senior center staffed and attended mostly by European-Americans. In some cases, they recommended psychiatric evaluations. In almost every instance, the elderly Chinese resisted these interventions.

The nurses failed to establish an alliance with the very strong Chinese family organizations before imposing their solutions. They also neglected to investigate Chinese cultural patterns before attempting to assist them with the life pattern ramifications of the earthquake. Generally, Chinese people do not readily talk about feelings with outsiders and they do not conceptualize distress in psychiatric terms. They interpret the presence of fatigue and disturbances in eating and sleeping patterns as physical illness. They expect health care personnel to recognize and help them with these physical symptoms. The suggestion that socializing in clubs populated by English speakers would cure their illness seemed quite incredulous to the families.

---

about environmental health dangers and difficulties in obtaining compensation for environmental toxin-causing disease and death often result in resident revictimization (Smets, 1988; Soble and Brennan, 1988). Tightly knit social structures in the affected community and a lack of low-cost housing in other neighborhoods may hinder residents from leaving an area that poses potentially severe health risks from exposure to hazards. Residents may be unwilling to disrupt family ties and cultural roots to start over elsewhere or they may be unable to afford a move. These residents may live with uncertainty and conflict. Long-term community-wide effects of division, animosity, distrust, cynicism, and despair can abound in these situations.

Another living pattern problem is the marginalization of unwanted sites (e.g., waste incinerators, sewage treatment plants, landfills, refineries, and prisons) in urban environments that are already strewn with obsolete and abandoned derelict sites (e.g., deserted factories, warehouses, railways, mines, and vacant garbage-strewn lots). People of all age groups, races, and genders who live near such environmental hazards are in danger of becoming victims of violent death from falls, fires, homicides, poisonings, suicides (Greenberg and Schneider, 1994), and malignant and nonmalignant disease. The environmental movement of the 1960s and 1970s succeeded in building political power capable of

passing monumental environmental reforms; however, it failed to address charges that poor and minority communities are dumping grounds for environmental hazards (Northridge and Shepard, 1997).

Discriminatory land use ensures that poor people and people of color live in close proximity to industrial contamination. This is called **environmental racism** (Alston, 1990; Bryant and Mohai, 1992). Bullard (1993) concluded, "Whether by conscious design or institutional neglect, communities of color in urban ghettos, in rural 'poverty pockets,' or on economically impoverished Native-American reservations face some of the worst environmental devastation in the nation" (p. 17). Many communities lack sufficient resources to engage in the expensive litigation that becomes inevitable when urban development and technological advances jeopardize the health and well-being of families in affected areas (Peña and Gallegos, 1993).

In the 1990s, the central issues of equity and justice emerged in environmental health policy. In 1994, President Clinton signed Executive Order 12898, which required all federal agencies to develop comprehensive strategies for achieving environmental justice. Both the US Environmental Protection Agency (EPA) and the NIH responded with increased staffing and research funds to meet the needs of environmentally degraded communities (Northridge and Shepard, 1997).

Sanitation workers in an urban area experienced an increasing incidence of puncture injuries while transporting hazardous wastes from the public medical center, which caused several hepatitis cases. When the story became public, members of the city health commission contacted community health nurses and instructed them to politically support the interests of the city and the medical center "at all costs." Subsequently, the sanitation workers' union contacted the community health nursing office and requested information about procedures for safely packaging medical wastes. They also requested that a nurse speak to their membership about immediate measures for preventing further injuries on the job.

The nurses met to resolve the conflict. Most agreed that the union membership had pressing needs for education and support. Despite the city's demand for loyalty, they decided to "choose sides" with the workers and respond to their requests. They collectively drafted a letter to the city health commission and arranged a meeting with the commissioners to discuss their plan to assist the sanitation workers. The health commission held a press conference, which depicted the nurses' actions as mediational efforts that benefited the union and the city. Eventually, the nurses and the commission developed a new medical waste disposal plan and injured workers received reasonable compensation through an out-of-court settlement.

Work Risks

Work risks include poor employment environments and potential injury or illness within working conditions. Environmental health problems posed by work risks include sexual harassment, occupational toxic poisoning, machine-operation hazards, electrical hazards, repetitive motion injuries, and carcinogenic particulate inhalants (e.g., asbestos), dust pollutants (e.g., coal dust), and heavy metal poisoning (Cralley, Cralley, and Cooper, 1990; Davies, 1998; Gaillard, 1993; Grondona, 1993; Smith, 1990; Steenland, 1993; Sumrall and Taylor, 1992). Prevention of work-related health problems requires integrated action to improve job content and the working environment (Kogi, 1993).

Annually, more than 20 million injuries and 400,000 new cases of disease in the United States are work related (Levy and Wegman, 1995). Across the nation, approximately 7000 traumatic occupational fatalities occur each year. Mining, construction, and agriculture are the three industries with the highest rates of traumatic deaths to workers (Veazie et al, 1994). These statistics do not reflect unreported health problems. For example, a clerical worker leaves the office every day with back strain and a headache. After five years on the job, the employee develops carpal tunnel syndrome. A midwestern farmer suffers the loss of his hand when it is caught in his new hay-baler. He is unaware that several other farmers in the state suffered similar injury using the same model of hay-baler. An operating room nurse who has a miscarriage remembers that many of her coworkers have also been unable to carry their babies to term. A dry cleaner often leaves work feeling light headed and dizzy from inhaling solvents at the shop; one day she has a car accident on her way home (Brender and Suarez, 1990; Connon, Freund, and Ehlers, 1993; Dumont, 1989; McAbee, Gallucci, and Checkoway, 1993).

Atmospheric Quality

Atmospheric quality refers to the amount of protection in the atmospheric layers, the risks of severe weather, and the purity of the air. Environmental dangers related to atmospheric quality include chlorofluorocarbon destruction of the ozone layer and loss of carbon dioxide-consuming resources such as forests, tornadoes, electrical storms, smog, gaseous pollutants (e.g., carbon monoxide), excessive hydrocarbon levels, aerial herbicide spraying, and acid rain (Elsom, 1992; Foster, 1994; Wijnen and vander Zee, 1998).

The amount of protection in the atmospheric layers is diminishing (Last, 1993). Chlorofluorocarbons, which are in widespread use for refrigeration, air conditioning, and aerosol propellants, remain in the atmosphere. These molecules cause depletion of the atmosphere's ozone layer. The resulting "holes" in the ozone layer allow excess ultraviolet radiation to penetrate, which cause harmful effects on living organisms. Another problematic atmospheric condition is increasing atmospheric carbon dioxide. This carbon dioxide allows sunlight to pass through the

A sudden increase occurred in the number of emergency calls from residents of a particular urban neighborhood to a medical hotline. These calls often involved elderly women who collapsed in their homes. In one case, an asthmatic child developed severe dyspnea. A community health nurse commented that these problems may be psychosocial.

The emergency calls continued and two other community health nurses noted that respiratory difficulties were often implicated. These nurses decided to visit the neighborhood and investigate. It neared rush hour and within minutes the traffic on the nearby freeway slowed to a crawl, apparently from road construction. Through their direct observations and critical assessment, these nurses determined that heavy car exhaust fumes seemed to stagnate around several residential buildings in the area. The nurses notified an environmental protection agency and the city transportation department and recommended further investigation and resolution of the problem.

One week later, the nurses returned to the neighborhood and determined that the traffic moved more efficiently, although road construction continued. Within several weeks, the number of emergency medical calls decreased.

earth's atmosphere, but it absorbs and traps part of the heat reemitted by the earth. Thus the earth's surface temperature is increasing (i.e., the "greenhouse effect"), causing irreversible global climate changes, a rise in the sea level, and other potentially catastrophic ecological consequences (Jepma and Munasinghe, 1998; Tchounwou, 1999). Scientists predict that by the year 2010, regional climate changes of 10 degrees centigrade will occur around the world and a 49 centimeter mean global sea-level rise will cause coastal wetland loss worth $46 billion U.S. dollars (Raymo et al., 1998).

Burning fossil fuels such as coal and oil releases carbon dioxide into the atmosphere, which stimulates the greenhouse effect. In addition, there is a disruption in the key processes that break down atmospheric carbon dioxide. The ongoing devegetation of the earth's surface, especially cutting the tropical rain forests, not only releases the carbon stored in the biomass, but it also eliminates sources of photosynthesis (i.e., the process by which plants absorb carbon and release oxygen) (Barnes et al., 1998; Bergstrom and Kirchmann, 1998). The rate at which the world's forests are being cut is nearly inconceivable. According to the United Nations Food and Agriculture Organization's (FAO) biannual review, State of the World's Forests 1999, a forested area of approximately 42,460 square miles is lost throughout the world each year from over-harvesting industrial wood and fuel wood, overgrazing, poor harvesting practices, air pollution, insect pests and diseases, and fire (State of the World's Forests, 1999). This massive worldwide deforestation is destroying countless species of animals and plants (Wilson, Myers, and Ehrenfeld, 1991). Overgrazing, over cultivation, and soil erosion is spreading desertlike conditions and yielded an 18% loss of all arable land on the globe during the final quarter of the twentieth century (Myers, 1993).

Severe weather conditions, another aspect of atmospheric quality that affects the public's health, can have dramatic results in the form of injury and loss of life, destruction of plants and wildlife, and property damage. Climatic changes associated with global warming are increasing the frequency and severity of the earth's weather extremes (Mungall and McLaren, 1990).

Hazardous atmospheric pollutants cause lung cancer, chronic respiratory disease, and death (National Toxic Inhalation Study Group, 1998) and exterminate animal and plant species (Rose, 1990). For instance, an estimated 50,000 lakes in the United States and Canada are "dead" (i.e., fish and plant life destroyed by acid rain) (Perdue and Gjessing, 1989). In addition to ruining aquatic ecosystems, acid rain affects terrestrial ecosystems by increasing soil acidity, reducing nutrient availability, mobilizing toxic metals, leaching soil chemicals, and altering species composition (Foster, 1994).

Water Quality

Water quality refers to the water supply's availability, volume, and mineral content levels, toxic chemical pollution, and pathogenic microorganism levels.

In a midwestern farm community, there is growing concern about agricultural pesticide and herbicide seepage into groundwater. Families obtain water from their own wells rather than a central municipal source. The families recognized the long-range carcinogenic effects of the chemicals involved. Although family farmers decreased their use of these chemicals, the large-scale agribusiness companies continued to use excessive amounts of these chemicals, sacrificing environmental integrity for larger crop yields.

County community health nurses lobbied local officials to begin a comprehensive program to monitor groundwater pollutants and enforce standards for herbicide and pesticide use; however, the powerful agribusiness companies pressured these officials to stand

back. Together, some county farmers and nurses organized grassroots information and support groups among rural families. The families and nurses, in coalition with environmental activist groups in the state, established several participatory action research projects. These projects included collecting and testing samples from each family well, forming a local umbrella organization called "Water Watch" to coordinate actions and communications, coordinating a research project with a federal health agency to track the health problems of local residents who consumed these water sources on a long-term basis, and disseminating an emergency plan for drinking water distribution if wells have toxic levels of pesticides, herbicides, or other pollutants.

Water quality consists of the balance between water contaminants and the existing capabilities to purify water for human use and plant and wildlife sustenance. Water quality problems include experiencing droughts, dosing reservoirs with copper sulfate to reduce algae, contaminating the drinking supply with human wastes, contaminating pesticide aquifers, poisoning fish in the Great Lakes with mercury, leaching lead from water pipes, spilling oil in the world's waters, spreading water-borne bacteria, and causing toxicity with excessive chlorination (Schuurmann and Markert, 1998).

Advances in water treatment technologies in industrialized countries such as the United States have controlled many water-related diseases such as cholera, typhoid, dysentery, and hepatitis A (McKeown, 1991). However, disease outbreaks resulting from contamination by untreated groundwater and inadequate chlorination are increasing in both urban and rural areas (Gelberg et al., 1999; Myers, 1993). Poverty is accompanied by poor-quality water supplies associated with water-borne disease. Accelerated soil erosion caused by construction, agriculture, and deforestation leads to high sediment levels in drinking water supplies. This necessitates higher levels of water treatment to remove heavy metals and chemicals. Heavy metal and toxic chemical pollution may originate in the water treatment process or in the drinking water distribution system (Krieps, 1989).

Some of the most serious problems are found in drinking water sources (Blumenthal and Ruttenber,

1995; Foster, 1994). Microcontaminants escape landfills, effluent lagoons, and petroleum storage facilities and enter water supplies. Residential, commercial, and industrial outputs increase the pollutant load of surface water, such as rivers and lakes. Pesticides, herbicides, and carcinogenic industrial waste infiltrate an increasing amount of groundwater, the underground source of half the U.S. population's drinking water (Sutherland, 1998). This is particularly tragic because groundwater is uniquely susceptible to long-term contamination. Unlike river or lake water, once groundwater becomes contaminated, it is impossible to cleanse.

Housing

Housing is an environmental health concern and it refers to the availability, safety, structural strength, cleanliness, and location of shelter, including public facilities and individual or family dwellings. Environmental health problems related to housing include homelessness; fire hazards; lack of access for disabled people; illnesses caused by overcrowding, dampness, and rodent or insect infestation; lead-based paint poisoning; psychological effects of architectural design (e.g., low-cost, high-rise housing projects); injuries sustained from collapsed building structures; and exposure deaths from inadequate indoor heating.

A housing's structure and its immediate surroundings can affect health (e.g., population density of the neighborhood, proximity to industry, safety of

In a large northeastern city, an economic recession led to massive unemployment, rising housing costs, and drastically reduced housing subsidies. Simultaneously, funding was cut for several public health and mental health facilities. The result left approximately 4000 people "houseless." Over a dozen people died from exposure to the elements during the winter. The local shelters housed a total of 500 people each night, although none of these shelters accepted women.

Community health nurses met with local church groups who started a shelter for women. This coalition acquired a building in an area where many shelterless people congregated. They began to offer accommodations for 75 women. After three months, the city took over the women's shelter because the churches

experienced difficulties filling the beds and maintaining the project's financial solvency. The city changed the shelter to a dwelling for 50 men and 25 women because women did not use it sufficiently.

In their evaluation, the nurses consulted with several shelterless women and workers from a popular soup kitchen. The answer was relatively simple. The women did not feel safe going to the shelter because the area had a high-crime reputation and lacked street lighting. Eventually, a new coalition formed, composed of community health nurses, several women who were or had been shelterless, a representative from the police force, and the church groups. A new women's shelter opened in a safer, well-lit neighborhood close to public transit lines.

adjacent buildings, level of security, and noise and pollution from nearby traffic) (Kay, 1991b; Mielke et al., 1999).

Poor housing conditions can spread infectious disease (Jackson and McSwane, 1992; Kerner, Dusenbury, and Mandelblatt, 1993) and it is becoming more apparent that poor housing conditions may also contribute to cardiovascular and respiratory disorders, cancers, allergies, and mental illnesses (Lemus et al., 1998; Mariethoz et al., 1999). The term **sick building** describes a phenomenon in which public structures and homes cause occupants to experience toxic syndromes from poor ventilation and building operations, hazardous building materials, furniture and carpeting substances, and cleaning agents (Brooks, 1991).

Commercial buildings with offices near underground parking garages may cause workers to suffer carbon monoxide intoxication. Formaldehyde, asbestos, and volatile organic compounds, which are common components of thermal insulation, cement, flooring, furnishings, and household consumer products have carcinogenic properties. Much controversy surrounds the economic hardship that industry, government, business, and multidwelling owners would face if they were forced to reduce concentrations of such toxic elements. Unlike most states, Massachusetts has a 22-year-old policy that requires lead paint abatement of children's homes and holds property owners liable for lead paint poisoning. This environmental management effort has been successful and

has significantly reduced the state's childhood lead poisoning rate (Sargent et al., 1999). The development and enforcement of laws that mandate toxic abatement will ensure a safer future and represent aggregate level responses to environmental problems.

Traditionally, U.S. economic development has produced optimal wealth with the assumption that the environmental health consequences would be minor (Young, 1990). This notion of sustainable development has proven inadequate. The country suffers major ecological threats to human health via cumulative hazardous episodes and must depend on pollution control technologies (Jain et al., 1997).

Food Quality

Food quality refers to availability and relative cost of food, variety and safety of food, and the health of animal and plant food sources. Food quality problems include malnutrition, bacterial food poisoning, carcinogenic chemical additives (e.g., nitrites, alar, and cyclamate), improper or fraudulent meat inspection or food labeling, viral epidemics among livestock (e.g., cholera), food products from diseased animal sources, and disruption of vital natural food chains by ecosystem destruction.

Foods may be contaminated by foodborne viruses and bacteria (Powell and Atwell, 1999). Foods may also be affected by toxic chemicals passing through the food chain, potentially resulting in reproductive and mutagenic effects in humans (Foster, 1994;

A southern town with a population of 10,000 has a large population of African-American farm workers and a smaller, but significant, number of Euro-American residents who work as textile workers. Located well off the interstate arteries, the town experienced very high food costs from shipping difficulties. Many families tapered their diets and ate mostly bread, rice, beans, and eggs. Health assessments of school-aged children and toddlers indicated deficiencies of vitamins contained in fresh fruits and vegetables.

Local physicians, county health nurses, and the Parent-Teacher Association joined forces to improve the nutritional situation. The most popular proposed solution involved a community garden project. The groups leased land from the county, and the project began. Conflict arose when African-American community leaders realized that the mostly Euro-American textile workers formed their own garden project and competed with the original garden project for the town's support. Racial tensions intensified.

The nurses and parents originally involved in planning the project met to avert a crisis. They decided to focus on reaching church leaders and women in both African- and Euro-American sectors of the town in the hope of supporting a dialogue and a just solution to the problem. Parents and church leaders spread the word in their respective communities. A community meeting was held at a convenient time for women in the town and at a neutral place that was acceptable for both African-Americans and Euro-Americans.

Although tensions were strong enough to prevent the formation of a joint garden, the solution reached in the meeting caused each group to feel successful and like it was able to save face. On a per-capita basis, town funds were allocated to two gardening projects. The groups agreed that they would share vegetable and fruit yields equitably depending on the yield from each site. In addition, the cooperative plan increased the total garden space allotted by 50% and began a gardening "tool library" so neither group had to purchase new tools.

Guillen, Sopelana, and Partearroyo, 1997). For instance, farmers spray dioxin-containing weed killers on range land. Beef cattle graze on the land and the herbicide accumulates in their fatty tissue. The contaminated meat is sold in markets along the West Coast. Dioxin accumulates in human mothers' milk in the western United States and increasing numbers of children experience birth defects in these states.

A plethora of agrichemicals such as pesticides and fertilizers, materials from mechanical handling devices, detergents, and organic packaging materials can poison food and may induce immune suppression (Foster, 1994; Whalen, Loganathan, and Kannan, 1999). Unsuitable handling, storage, processing, and transport techniques can damage and contaminate foodstuffs (Covello and Merkhofer, 1993). Adulterating food to increase its volume or weight or to improve its color or flavor is also problematic because adulterants are usually less nutritious and often harmful. Residues from the overuse of antibiotics in animal husbandry remain in meat and milk products, causing consumers to develop resistance to a wide range of antibiotics, thus rendering these antibiotics ineffective in treating human infections (Krieps, 1989; Neu, 1992).

A relatively new and potentially dangerous threat to food quality involves scientific gene mutations through "gene splicing." This method produces livestock that grows faster and fattens easier, thereby generating an earlier slaughter and greater yields at a lower cost (Teitelman, 1989). This controversial genetic engineering is producing new animal species. The unregulated introduction of these genetically mutated species onto range land and into farm herds threatens the survival of food-producing animal species and has unknown consequences for human nutrition.

Waste Control

Waste control is the management of waste materials resulting from industrial and municipal processes, human consumption, and efforts to minimize waste production. Environmental health problems related to waste control include nonbiodegradable plastics, expensive and inefficient recycling programs, unlicensed waste dumps, inadequate sewage systems (i.e., ill prepared for actual population demand), unsafe dumping of industrial toxic wastes, exportation of hazardous radioactive medical wastes to Third World countries, cover-ups of illicit dumping, and nonenforcement of environmental protection legislation.

In a city on the Mississippi River, an outbreak of shigellosis was traced to a group of high school students who had been swimming in a particular area of the river. The local meat-packing plant was releasing waste material, including human and animal feces, directly into the river.

After intervening to contain the shigella outbreak, the local community health nurses began to assess the situation. Their research indicated that the meat packing facility was in violation of waste control laws for some time. City officials imposed fines, which the company paid, but the dumping continued. A sign at the riverside prohibited swimming.

Frustrated by their attempts to negotiate with the city and the plant, the nurses wrote a letter to the state capital newspaper, which had a large state readership, and the local newspaper. In the letter, they voiced concern about the community's health and the river's ecological integrity. Both papers published their informative letter as a commentary, which prompted responses from two local environmental groups, several activist groups located downriver, and a national organization concerned with clean water. These groups provided legal support and brought a collective suit against the meat-packing company. Subsequently, the company improved its waste treatment process to avoid paying a large award in the civil suit.

American consumers' increasing trash production and the improper treatment, storage, transport, and disposal of waste are a mounting concern (DeLong, 1993; Haun, 1991; Reinhardt and Gordon, 1991; Rom, 1992). Multiple problems exist. The increasing use of petroleum-based plastics in products (e.g., disposable diapers) creates grave ecological problems. Routinely, commercial and institutional wastes are dumped with household waste in the same municipal incinerator, landfill, or sewer system. These commercial enterprises are generally exempt from the strict waste regulation applied to industry, although they often generate the same hazardous materials. Small businesses such as dry cleaners, photography laboratories, pesticide formulators, construction sites, and car repair shops use and discard a variety of substances that can cause serious public health problems.

Solid waste landfills present a problem because methane gas, a byproduct of decomposing organic wastes, accumulates in the ground. Without proper venting, this volatile gas can move through soil and cause fires and explosions in nearby areas. Waste incineration is not the best solution because it causes particulate air pollution and it is ineffective in the combustion of many hazardous wastes.

The United States produces between 250 and 400 million metric tons of toxic waste per year, about one ton per person per year. No viable solution to this mounting waste exists (Hamilton, 1993). Consequently, the United States has an estimated 32,000 to 50,000 uncontrolled waste disposal sites (Keller, 1992). Improper design, operation, or waste site location causes hazardous substances to spread through air, soil, and water to poison humans, animals, and plant life. Alarmingly, only a small percentage of hazardous wastes actually reach the designated waste sites. The EPA estimates that 90% of hazardous waste is improperly disposed in open pits, surface impounds, vacant land, farmlands, and bodies of water (Anderson, 1987).

In 1980, Congress passed the Environmental Response Compensation and Liability Act, which established a revolving fund called the Superfund, to clean up several hundred of the worst abandoned chemical waste disposal sites. However, funds are insufficient and improvements have been minor (Keller, 1992; Kilburn, 1999). One of the most notorious sites is the Love Canal in Niagara Falls, New York. For 40 years prior to the 1960s, more than 80 different types of chemicals including benzene, dioxin, dichlorethylene, and chloroform were dumped in an abandoned canal. Afterwards, the covered area became the site for a school and several hundred homes. In the winters of 1976 and 1977, heavy snowfall and rain caused toxic wastes to reach the surface. Subsequently, the inhabitants experienced elevated miscarriage rates, blood and liver abnormalities, birth defects, and chromosome damage.

Radiation Risks

Radiation risks are health dangers posed by various forms of ionizing radiation relative to barriers that prevent human exposure and other life form exposure. Radiation risks include nuclear power emissions, radioactive hazardous wastes, medical and dental

During wartime, federal standards related to radioactive environmental contamination and the public's "right to know" are suspended for military projects. In the middle of the Persian Gulf War, information "leaked" about a military installation in the southwestern desert near Deserttown. The installation planned test explosions of several new nuclear bombs, which they called nuclear "devices."

Local townspeople expressed concern, but the military did not confirm or deny these plans. The possible dates for the tests were also unknown. Residents began to panic and several families moved. Others built makeshift shelters and began stockpiling food. There was an increase in psychiatric hospitalization rates. The town reached a crisis when a spate of three related adolescent suicides occurred in two months. The entire community appeared disorganized, helpless, and hopeless.

Town officials organized town meetings. Public health nurses offered community education about the health effects of ionizing radiation and answered questions, but this did not raise resident morale. The nurses decided to contact other communities that faced similar threats to determine how they dealt with them.

When these communities received word about Deserttown, they organized a letter-writing campaign and a support demonstration. They converged on Deserttown for a weekend rally and celebration of solidarity. The youth of Deserttown extended this demonstration by performing weekly vigils at the military site. One year later, the community was more united and less depressed and the adolescent suicide rate decreased significantly. The nuclear threat remained.

---

radiographs, radon gas leaks in homes, and wartime nuclear weapon dangers.

Nuclear industries are barraged with environmental problems (Blumenthal and Ruttenber, 1995). People and animals living near nuclear facilities such as power plants, waste storage sites, uranium-processing plants, nuclear weapons factories, and nuclear test sites have manifested increased rates of cancer, stroke, diabetes, cardiovascular and renal disease, immune system damage, premature aging, infertility, miscarriage, and birth defects (Elsom, 1992; International Physicians for the Prevention of Nuclear War, 1991; Keller, 1992; Marino, 1994). In addition, there is the ever-present risk of nuclear accidents that release large amounts of radioactivity into surrounding areas (Gould, 1990). It is unknown what will happen to nuclear facilities after exceeding their three- or four-decade life span. At the end of the life span, these facilities will be saturated with radioactivity from everyday operation and will require some form of decommission and decontamination.

Nuclear wastes remain dangerously radioactive for thousands of years; a safe way to dispose of them does not exist. Interim collection centers currently stockpile much of the waste. There is a quandary not only about how, where, and when to dispose of newly-generated nuclear wastes, but also how to manage improperly disposed radioactive materials.

Countless drums of radioactive wastes dumped at sea or buried in the earth are leaking (Council on Scientific Affairs, 1989; Keller, 1992).

Millions of Americans are exposed to dangerous levels of radiation in their homes, schools, and work places (Platt, 1993; Sandman and Weinstein, 1993). The EPA determined that radon contamination is the second leading cause of lung cancer mortality in the United States, with an estimated 5000 to 20,000 deaths each year (USEPA, 1992). Radon is a radioactive radium decay product that occurs naturally in certain kinds of phosphate- and uranium-containing rock such as granite and black shale. Radon may be present in building materials, drinking water, and soil. Radon gas diffuses into dwellings, mostly through soil, and is prevalent where uranium-bearing land is common. Radon seeps through basement walls, pipes, and cracks in the foundation and is trapped in buildings with inadequate ventilation.

Cumulative exposure to excessive or ill-performed radiographs can also cause radiation damage in the body (McAbee, Gallucci, and Checkoway, 1993; Miller, 1990; Mole, 1990). People who work with medical sources of radiation, such as radium or radioactive iodine, are at increased risk for developing cancers and producing children with birth defects. Older x-ray machines may emit excessive levels of radioactivity; all such equipment should undergo regular testing for leakage.

Violence Risks

Environmental violence risks include potential victimization through the violence of particular groups and the general level of aggression in psychosocial climates. Violence-fostered environmental health problems can arise from conditions such as extreme poverty, widespread unemployment, handgun proliferation, pervasive violent media images, lacking child abuse services, insufficient police follow-up for women's reports of sexual molestation, and increasingly common hate crimes.

The environment's social, political, and economic characteristics influence the potential for violent crimes, including verbal abuse, harassment, battery, sexual assault, abduction, and murder (Greenberg and Schneider, 1994; Hall, Stevens, and Meleis, 1994; Rosenberg and Fenley, 1991; Ruback and Weiner, 1994). The phenomenon of urban youth gangs exemplifies how poverty and powerlessness foster aggressiveness and territorial defensiveness in young males. Specifically, chronic deterioration of urban centers and the systematic withdrawal of services and resources are connected with violent behavior (Earls, Cairns, and Mercy, 1993).

Social stigmatization of racial, ethnic, and religious minorities and lesbians and gay men can take the form of violent hate crimes against these groups (Stevens and Morgan, 1999). For example, official talk of registering, placing under surveillance, and possibly interning "suspicious" Arab-Americans during the Persian Gulf War was accompanied by an increase in malicious innuendoes, threats, and violent crimes against Arab-Americans throughout the United States (Hall and Stevens, 1992). Also, women and children become frequent targets of violence because they hold relative little political power (Stevens and Hall, 1990).

It is debatable whether films, television, recorded music, and sexually explicit materials foster the commission of violent crimes. Regardless of whether they do or not, it is reasonable to conclude that if media images portray violence against certain groups (e.g., women, children, and minorities), individuals with violent impulses will be likely to target these vulnerable groups. Key factors in the incidence and severity of violent aggression are the availability and regulation of ballistic weapons. Handguns, rifles, and automatic weapons are easily obtained in the United States. Although multiple mass killings in schools and work places at the end of the twentieth century horrified and transfixed the public in front of their television sets, gun control legislation remained elusive. Meanwhile, communities face very difficult questions about how to curtail the violence in their environments. Increasing dependence on the police force, the penal system, and censorship tactics may produce a situation of diminishing returns; forceful repression may provoke an increase in social aggression.

EFFECTS OF ENVIRONMENTAL HAZARDS

Environmental effects on the public's health are complex and usually interconnected (DeRosa, Stevens, and Johnson, 1993; Jaga and Brosius, 1999; Lawrence, 1999). Nurses must understand the multidimensional nature of citizens' health disorders. For example, nuclear power plant emissions may contaminate water and air supplies, affecting water quality, atmospheric quality, and radiation risk. Overcrowded housing may exacerbate problems in managing human wastes, which may taint foodstuffs and contribute to the spread of communicable disease.

Oppressive environments may affect health directly. In one case, an American company dumped dangerous waste material in Mexico rather than pay for proper disposal (Schrieberg, 1991). Poor children who lived nearby and scavenged for food in the dump picked up and played with the shiny, brightly colored radioactive medical waste. The severe burns they suffered and the wine-colored spots on their skin were very direct effects of the illegally dumped toxic waste (Center for Investigative Reporting, 1990). Effects may also be indirect, such as global warming (Foster, 1994). Over decades, farming regions will warm up, dry out, and become less productive. The sea level will eventually rise from the melting polar ice caps. The resulting coastal inundation and permanent flooding will threaten large areas of low-lying agricultural land and food supplies in many regions of the world. Rising global temperatures will enhance the quantity and distribution of parasites, insects, and other disease vectors, thus increasing the prevalence of a variety of infectious diseases.

Effects of environmental hazards may be general or specific. For example, the ramifications of massive unemployment, drought, and extensive smog cover affect the public generally, whereas the particular housing needs of elderly people who use walkers or canes, the occupational risks of electrical line repair workers, and the mentally incapacitating effects of

At a prestigious private university, a survey revealed that over 30% of the female students experienced "date rape." The university appealed to the school's student health service to respond to this growing problem. The university asked the nurses at the health service to organize classes for female students about self-defense and "what to do if raped."

One nurse voiced opposition, pointing out that rape is a violent act perpetrated by men and not a health matter that only concerns women. She suggested that male students receive education about the bodily rights of others and classes about "how not to rape women." This caused a deep polarization among the nurses and other health workers at the student health service. Many believed the self-defense classes were useful even if they did not address the core problem. Others believed that ignoring the male responsibility for rape encouraged or condoned a "climate of violence."

The self-defense classes were not well attended. One year later, the rates of date rape and other sexual assaults involving university students increased. In reevaluating their intervention, the nurses decided to mingle with the student body and visit places that students frequent. They informally interviewed groups of students about what they thought caused the high incidence of date rape. The consensus was that the campus fraternity culture encouraged heavy drinking and sexual aggressiveness on the part of male students. With these new data, the nurses approached university officials and suggested several student services and policy changes.

Together, the nurses and university staff developed new interventions. First, the university invited an alcohol-problems researcher to institute an alcohol self-awareness research project and a bartender-education program on campus. Second, the university required fraternity leaders to participate in four weekend seminars about sexual assault and interpersonal violence. Third, the university gave incentives to fraternities based on how many members attended the seminars and extended commendations and prizes for collective projects that demonstrated effectiveness in decreasing the number of date rapes and other violent campus crimes. Last, the university adopted a new policy in which it pledged to vigorously pursue criminal and civil actions in all cases of sexual assault involving students.

---

lead poisoning in children affect the public more specifically.

Environmental health effects can also be immediate, long term, or transgenerational. Burns, gunshot wounds, hurricane damage, and outbreaks of gastrointestinal distress among cafeteria customers are examples of immediate effects from health-damaging environments. Examples of long-term health effects include gradual occupational hearing loss, "black lung" in coal miners, and increased rates of cancer among migrant farm workers who ingested the pesticide DDT from aerial spray in the 1980s (Jaga and Brosius, 1999; Werner and Olson, 1993). Transgenerational effects occur with female factory workers exposed to radiation at plutonium-processing plants. The radiation caused chromosomal anomalies, which resulted in birth defects in their children. Another transgenerational effect occurs in the repetition of domestic violence in successive family generations.

Some negative environmental health effects are reversible. For example, the lungs of nonsmokers who inhale second-hand smoke from their smoking family members and coworkers can heal and restore healthy function if the smoke is eliminated. However, radiation damage to human cells and silicosis damage to lung capacity are irreversible. Heavy metal exposure represents many environmental hazards that cause cumulative effects. Lead slowly collects in the long bones and the lead can rerelease into the body. This release may cause acute poisoning and may cause additional damage over time (Needleman et al., 1992).

EFFORTS TO CONTROL ENVIRONMENTAL HEALTH PROBLEMS

The 1970s were the decade of environmental concern. Cynicism toward institutions grew during the Vietnam era and legislative activism for environmental preservation exploded (Burger, 1989). Table 13-4 outlines the essential statutes. During the 1970s, Congress created new agencies to regulate environmental conditions on a national level, including the EPA, OSHA, and the Nuclear Regulation Commission (NRC). The EPA has enormous responsibilities for protecting the

TABLE 13-4

Landmark Federal Environmental Legislation

Year	Legislation
1970	Clean Air Act
1970	Poison Prevention Packaging Act
1970	Occupational Health and Safety Act
1970	Hazardous Materials Transportation Control
1970	National Environmental Policy Act
1971	Lead-Based Paint Poisoning Prevention Act
1972	Federal Water Pollution Control Act Amendments
1972	Noise Control Act
1976	Resource Conservation and Recovery Act
1976	Toxic Substances Control Act
1977	Clean Water Act
1980	Low Level Radiation Waste Policy Act
1980	Comprehensive Environmental Response, Compensation, and Liability Act (i.e., Superfund)

environment and minimizing environmental risks to human health. Among its roles are health surveillance and monitoring; setting standards for air and water quality; evaluating environmental risks; acquiring information; screening new chemicals; performing basic research and training; maintaining the data base; and establishing, evaluating, and enforcing regulatory efforts.

The legislative activism of the 1970s was responsible for unprecedented movement toward a comprehensive national environmental policy. For example, stricter automobile fuel and emissions standards created improvements in air quality, which caused lead levels in urban air to decrease 87% from 1977 levels (Bingham and Meader, 1990). The momentum to control environmental corruption in the United States slowed in the 1980s and 1990s with several policy reversals and the defunding of regulatory mechanisms. For instance, the Reagan administration's deregulation of industry seriously weakened the

Occupational Health and Safety Act and other statutes. In the 1990s, Congress staged unprecedented attacks on environmental legislation, threatening to rollback two and a half decades of progress towards environmental protection. Big business and industry strongly opposed environmental protection efforts in the 1990s and launched publicity campaigns against efforts such as stricter air-quality standards, regulated logging in old-world forests, and bans on marine dumping. These groups claimed that environmentalists were a threat to local jobs and profits.

Dumont (1989, p. 1077) offered the following critique:

> Truly alarming assessments of the dangers inherent in current levels of soil, air, and water pollution are reduced to the level of cliché, mere ambient noise. We have become accustomed to revelations about clusters of birth defects and cancer in communities near landfills, chemical spills in the major rivers of the world, contamination of wells and aquifers with industrial waste, and bursts of toxic gases from 'human errors' at factories. It is only when catastrophes of such tremendous magnitude occur like Bhopal or Chernobyl that North Americans take note of the tortured biosphere.

Political dynamics, social values, and powerful industry and business interests influence the attention paid to environmental problems and the economic commitment to their solution (Reich, 1988). For example, the widespread agricultural use of neurotoxic organophosphate pesticides continues even though they cause lasting central nervous system damage (Jaga and Brosius, 1999). Advocates for farm workers claim the EPA should ban pesticide use registered in the highest toxicity category. Instead, the EPA requires that employers provide general pesticide safety information to all farm workers. The EPA also suggests regular blood tests to monitor toxin levels in those who apply the pesticides. Monitoring is required only for commercial applicators (i.e., companies that apply chemicals, not farm workers who apply pesticides in their job). The EPA has limited the scope of its monitoring requirement because large agribusiness corporations have begun to apply pressure.

Legislators and other policy makers have often made pesticide-use decisions based on economic impact, (i.e., how it will affect crop yield).

Regulators have thus ignored the costs: To farm-workers from pesticide poisoning, disability, loss of income, and increased risk of chronic health effects; To society from pesticide pollution and contamination of the air, water, soil, and food; To wildlife from the killing of fish, birds, bees, and other species; and To the planet generally from the widespread environmental and ecological damage that continues unchecked because of the failure to develop safer, healthier, and more sustainable methods of growing crops

(Moses, 1993, p. 171).

Weaknesses in legislation and regulatory structures in regard to other environmental health problems also exist (Walker, 1990). For instance, federal mandates for recycling do not exist, although local communities have made great strides in this area. Comprehensive groundwater legislation, similar to adopted measures to preserve marine and surface waters, also does not exist (Bingham and Meader, 1990). In general, environmental laws have often been too detailed or inflexible, causing problems in the articulation of federal and local regulatory efforts. Much to the chagrin of states and municipalities, the federal EPA tends to set priorities for the reduction of environmental problems, but does not allocate the resources necessary to accomplish these goals.

In general, most of the U.S. environmental health efforts have aimed for short-term goals rather than anticipating future needs and problems. In this regard, U.S. industries are underinvested in development of renewable resource technologies for the sake of transient profits (Jain et al., 1997). However, counter efforts are underway to conserve the habitat of endangered species and contain the ecological disturbance of suburban sprawl (Dupuis and Vandergeest, 1996).

A crucial need also exists in the development of human resources in the area of environmental health (Walker, 1990). Nursing careers in environmental health science (Neufer, 1994; Neufer and Narkunas, 1994; Salazar and Primomo, 1994) would be an excellent move toward integrating health and environmental theory and practice at the community level.

The scientific research and ongoing systematic surveillance necessary to fully inform environmental health policy are costly and time consuming, yet absolutely necessary to assure public health (Thacker et al., 1996). Government, industry, and big business have hesitated to adequately support these efforts.

This is in part because determination of damages caused by past hazardous practices would cause a vast liability. Effectively enforced environmental legislation may thwart some technological advances and economic growth. Communities suffer the health consequences and laws often excuse industry, business, and government from environmental clean-up because high costs would incur.

GLOBAL ENVIRONMENTAL HEALTH

Nurses must work with the public to promote more stringent and actively enforced environmental legislation, regulation, and greater social control over corporations, domestic and foreign governments, and other entities that contribute to health-damaging environments. In the new millennium, actions must include not only national, but also worldwide environmental policies. Ozone depletion, global warming, fossil fuel burning, marine dumping, active land mine abandonment in war-torn areas, mass relocation of refugees across national borders, and destruction of tropical rain forests are among key global environmental health concerns.

In an era of globalization of many sorts, nursing must support global actions for biodiversity, including pushing back the deserts, replanting the forests, stabilizing climate, and seeking alternative development pathways that do not destroy plant and animal species (Swanson, 1997). The development of state-of-the-art methods for removing pollutants from the biosphere, managing ecosystems, handling hazardous waste treatment, and preserving oceans depends on the integration of scientific knowledge, complex sociopolitical processes, and values. In times of excessive abuse of the global biosphere and exploitation of the world's ecosystems, environmental integrity over the long term will require international assistance, ameliorative actions, and an environmentally-educated global public.

Environmental concerns for clean air, clean water, and freedom from noxious chemicals must become global nursing concerns. Furthermore, human-caused disasters, such as bombings, biological warfare, hostage taking, disappearances, and mass killings can no longer be tolerated (Hall and Stevens, 1992). To bring home this fact, the public need only consider the mass killings perpetrated by angry workers and school-aged children that occurred in post offices, businesses, and schools in the 1990s. These incidents made tremendous changes in the public's notion of safety in everyday settings.

Community health nurses can be catalysts to neighborhood efforts to produce collective security from gun violence and healing after such events. Nurses should also be aware of anniversaries of violent events to remind communities to use these days to foster restoration instead of retraumatization. Posttrauma counseling should extend beyond the initial shock; this requires planning and redirection of resources in anticipation of the aftermath of such disasters in the social environment.

The changing physical, interpersonal, and cross-cultural aspects of the global environment greatly complicates nursing decision making. For example, major cities in the United States are home to sizable enclaves of immigrants and refugees. The larger the enclave, the easier it is to maintain original language and religious patterns. Nurses must be knowledgeable about transgenerational cultural expectations in these communities and potential family conflicts that may occur when children become acculturated to mainstream American values more quickly than parents (Lee, 1997). State laws that enforce English as the official language in schools, workplaces, and other public spaces exemplify how additional obstacles to health and well-being can result from fear-based public reactions towards people from other parts of the globe.

Immigrants and refugees obviously face special problems in terms of culture and language. However, international relocation also poses environmental obstacles. Adjustments to technology, diet, and climate can make the transition even more difficult to bear. In one instance, a woman from a Middle Eastern country was relocated to California and felt a seismic tremor, which was a frequent experience for acclimated Californians. However, this woman lacked extended family support and was unfamiliar with earthquakes. She began to have pains in her heart. A trip to the emergency room did not yield medical confirmation of disease and did not ease her distress. Within a month of her arrival, she was convinced she could not stay in the United States. For the majority of refugees who relocate to the United States, returning to their country is not an option.

In relation to the postmodern world, community health nursing must expand its theory and practice to incorporate the reality that individual and com-

munity health ultimately depends on global environmental integrity. Countless organizations work to preserve and protect the environment and could benefit from the active involvement and support of nurses. Box 13-1 lists several of these organizations. In the new millennium, nursing must broaden its borders to include a global perspective in all its business. Global sustainability will be achieved through commitment to strong ethical principles and social justice and with initiatives for environmental responsibility in daily personal activity. Not only are personal environmental responsibility and grassroots inventiveness needed, cooperation among multina-

---

BOX 13-1

Environmental Organizations

American Farmland Trust
Animal Preservation League
Citizens for a Better Environment
Clean Water Action
Earth Regeneration Society
Forests Forever
Greenpeace
International Rivers Network
National Environmental Law Center
National Toxics Campaign
Natural Resources Defense Council
Ocean Alliance
Pesticide Action Network
Radioactive Wastes Campaign
Rainforest Action Network
Sierra Club
Toxics Coordinating Project
Trust for Public Land
U.S. Public Interest Research Group
Wilderness Society

Websites for these organizations can be accessed through the WebLinks section of the book's website at ⓢⓘⓜⓞⓝ www.wbsaunders.com/SIMON/nies/.

For further information, see the report by the Institute of Medicine Committee on Enhancing Environmental Health Content in Nursing Practice: *Nursing, health, and the environment*, Washington, DC, 1995, National Academy Press.

tionals and governments across the world is also required.

APPROACHING ENVIRONMENTAL HEALTH AT THE AGGREGATE LEVEL

In the United States, the ideas of personal independence and individual responsibility for success and failure have always been very important. However, these values can lead nurses to blame individual clients for their health problems and overlook glaring environmental hazards (Crawford, 1977; Stevens, 1989). By placing responsibility for the cause and cure of health problems exclusively on the individual, the belief is reinforced that all individuals are free to exert meaningful control over the quality and length of their lives (Hall, Stevens, and Meleis, 1994). Such a perspective absolves society, government, industry, and business from accountability for changing dangerous conditions under which people live and work. Existing research evidence suggests that changing individual behaviors does not lead to significant reductions in overall morbidity and mortality in the absence of basic social, economic, and political changes (Freudenberg, 1984-1985; Milio, 1986). Emphasizing only public health interventions that attempt to modify deleterious personal habits through exercise programs, weight-loss regimens, smoking-cessation classes, and stress-reduction tactics fails to engage the broader environmental origins of disease, injury, and ecological destruction.

Nursing is not alone in its focus on individual health-promoting interventions. With federal directives such as the 1979 Surgeon General's report on health promotion and disease prevention (USDHHS, 1979), most health agencies, health care institutions, and corporate workplaces have principally addressed the idea of "controllable risk" in the individual, with much less effort directed toward reducing risks in the environment. The government has also reduced its overall focus on environmental health. In the 1980s and 1990s, the effectiveness and power of agencies such as the EPA and the National Institute for Occupational Safety and Health declined; therefore they are less able to study environmental health risks and enforce regulatory policies.

By focusing on the individual, nurses may overlook other levels of intervention (Stevens and Hall, 1992). Interventions designed for individuals alone leave environments that "sicken" people unchallenged. Although environmental dangers posed by contaminated drinking water, carcinogenic food additives, the depleted ozone layer, and occupational hazards are often serious, the implication persists that little can alter the inevitability of technological and industrial growth around the world. Therefore individuals are compelled to simply accommodate environments that cause them illness and injury.

Recognition of the gravity and pervasiveness of environmental hazards can be overwhelming. Looking beyond the individual to recognize the environmental determinants of illness and wellness can be complicated and threatening. Intervening to improve the quality of air, water, housing, food, and waste disposal and reducing the risks of occupational injury, radiation, and violence requires basic social, economic, and political changes in the process. Bringing about changes in health-damaging environments must be an aggregate-level endeavor.

Community health nurses who base their practices on the principles of critical theory are better prepared to respond to these challenges (Stevens and Hall, 1992). In the vignettes, nurses focus their efforts on organizing groups of people. Nurses can facilitate community participation in identifying and solving environmental health problems and bring about changes that improve environments and eliminate hazards.

CRITICAL COMMUNITY HEALTH NURSING PRACTICE

Community health nurses must take action to approach environmental health critically (Stevens and Hall, 1992). The vignettes illustrate how nurses take sides. Nurses ask critical questions, become involved with the communities they serve, form coalitions, and become familiar with various collective strategies. In the interest of educating future practitioners about the critical practice of community health nursing in environmental health, the following sections discuss each of these interventions.

Taking a Stand; Choosing a Side

An old labor union folk song asks, "whose side are you on?" Although a nurse may acknowledge that there are multiple sides to health and environmental issues, nurses cannot ultimately avoid taking a stand. Nurses must make individual and collective decisions about which interests they want to serve with their specialized knowledge and skills. To say that all must be served is certainly an ideal; however, people often experience consequences of hazardous environments inequitably. Vulnerable groups are exposed to more health-damaging effects than less vulnerable groups. A growing body of research substantiates that communities with people of color and economically impoverished neighborhoods face greater environmental risks (Bullard, 1990; Goldman, 1991). Nurses have the potential to increase or decrease these inequities through the decisions they make about the positions they accept and the interventions they undertake.

Community health nurses have a mandate to assist vulnerable aggregates who are less able to protect themselves from pollution, inadequate housing, toxic poisoning, unsafe products, and other hazards. NonEnglish-speaking refugees, African-American children, poor women, and illiterate manual laborers are just some of the groups in the United States who hold little power to broker with industry, government, business, and other large institutions for environmental changes and compensations for harm from environmental hazards.

Environmental problems are clearly intertwined with social, political, and economic policies, resource barriers, and the interests of those in positions of control. Nurses need to connect the immediate and long-term health problems experienced by particular communities to this larger sphere of influence.

Asking Critical Questions

Community health nurses must consider the relationships between nonhealth and health policies. They should ask how policies concerning ecological preservation, energy, housing, immigration, civil rights, crime, nutrition, minimum wage, occupational safety, and defense may affect the well-being of people in the United States. Addressing critical questions such as who has access to resources in this country, and whose interests are served in the existing system, provides a way to include social, political, and economic factors in environmental nursing assessments. Box 13-2 pro-

BOX 13-2

Critical Questions about Environmental Health Problems

What is the problem?
Who is defining the problem?
In what terms is the problem described?
How are others in the situation viewing the problem?
What is the history of the problem?
How did things get the way they are?
What other situations does this problem directly affect?
Who does the problem impact?
Whose health is damaged because things are this way?
Who benefits from the way things are?
Whose interests do current solutions serve?
What are the economic inequities in the situation?
Who has political power in the situation?
Who knows about the problem?
Who needs to know or know more about the problem?
How effective are current programs, strategies, and policies?
What are the barriers to solving the problem?
What strategies may alleviate the problem?
How successful have these strategies been?
What existing groups might deal with this problem?
What resources are needed to solve the problem?
How accessible are the resources?
How can nurses evaluate potential solutions?

vides a sample set of questions that are useful in this endeavor. Nurses can ask these critical questions when approaching environmental health problems.

Dialogue resulting from critical questioning can frame the problem and assist in building collective strategies. Ideally, those directly affected by the problem should explore these questions collectively. However, even one individual involved in the situation can begin to explore a problem from this perspective and define an initial basis for action.

Facilitating Community Involvement

Approaching community health from a critical perspective requires working to improve health conditions and creating the context in which people can identify health-damaging problems in their environments. One important nursing goal is to help people learn from their own experiences and analyze the world with an intention to change it. It is essential that the affected people participate in the process of identifying and working to solve environmental problems.

To create this openness, nurses must abandon asymmetrical leadership positions and join in mutual exchanges with community members that consider each person's experience. The nurse's role changes from presenting solutions and directing lifestyle changes, to asking critical questions and helping groups reflect on the problematic environmental realities of their lives. A second nursing role is to provide support, information, and expertise to groups to assist them in meeting their goals for environmental change. In each of these roles, nurses use the concept of solidarity, in which the relationship with the community and its individual members is maintained and nurtured despite disagreements that may occur over what is the best course of action.

Rather than trying to compel people to behave in certain ways, nurses should assist aggregates in their collective search for effective change strategies. Actions dictated from those outside the situation are often culturally inappropriate and doomed to be ineffective. Lasting rapport with aggregates depends on honesty, fairness, and mutuality in interactions over extended periods.

Using critical questions, community health nurses can help community members look beyond immediate environmental problems and explore social, cultural, economic, and political circumstances. Nurses can share their knowledge about the scientific basis for health problems, their insights about the historical origins of particular environmental hazards, their technical skills, and their expertise in communicating and organizing. Nursing expertise is not used to dominate a group, but rather to develop a mutual plan of action to deal with the problems a group has collectively identified. By addressing people's everyday concerns and targeting the problems they identify, nurses situate their efforts in community struggles.

Forming Coalitions

Another very important nursing task that arises from approaching environmental health from a critical perspective involves forming coalitions to produce social change. By initiating dialogue and building a strong base of collective support, nurses can demand structural changes that eliminate hazards and improve public health. In dealing with health-damaging environments, nurses can approach existing community organizations and family and friendship networks to help mobilize aggregate members who have not previously socialized or acted together. Nurses can then expose hazards, assess needs, plan actions, report abuses, and secure appropriate resources, personnel, funding, and legislative changes.

The environmental justice movement (Bullard, 1993) is an excellent example of coalition-building wherein people of color have organized grassroots groups to address lead contamination, pesticide use, water and air pollution, Native self-government, nuclear testing, and workplace safety. These groups focus on the disproportionate environmental challenges they face. Drawing insights from the civil rights movement and the environmental movement, environmental justice groups have forged alliances with many conventional environmental and civil rights organizations to mount formal responses to environmental threats. The Mothers of East Los Angeles, one grassroots organization fighting for environmental justice, acquired the support of Greenpeace, Natural Resources Defense Council, Environmental Policy Institute, Citizens' Clearinghouse on Hazardous Waste, National Toxics Campaign, and Western Center on Law and Poverty to bring a lawsuit against state and federal agencies who granted a private corporation permission to build and operate a toxic waste incinerator in their urban neighborhood. The permission was granted although the incinerator corporation failed to prepare an environmental impact report. The mainstream environmental organization allies provided the Mothers of East Los Angeles with valuable technical advice, expert testimony, lobbying, research, and legal assistance. The grassroots group spearheaded efforts in which hundreds of East Los Angeles residents placed intense political pressure on the state and federal agencies by attending every public hearing about the incinerator project. In the ensuing State Supreme Court battle, the decision prevented construction of the proposed facility.

Nurses can be instrumental in these efforts by helping community groups make connections with larger, more powerful organizations. Nurses can organize forums whereby community groups meet with scientific experts who can help them gather evidence about health threats, with businesses managers whose actions impinge on the economic life of the community, with industry leaders whose companies create ecological hazards, and with legislators who can bring community concerns to law-making bodies. Using available institutional resources, skills, and knowledge, nurses can also explore what is happening elsewhere. Making connections with groups in other locales who are struggling for similar environmental changes can enhance collective strength and solidarity. Press releases, media events, interviews, television spots, speeches, newsletters, and leaflets are important means of calling attention to a situation and raising awareness among communities.

In working for various municipalities, agencies, and health care corporations, nurses may find some of the philosophies, policies, resources, and relations of these organizations to be constraining in their community work. Although nurses may not always agree with everything their employers stand for, communities perceive them to be representatives of the organizations for whom they work. These institutional connections may cause problems for nurses working with people who consider themselves abandoned by the system, disregarded in policy decisions, or denied access to resources. Nurses usually find that establishing alliances with disenfranchised communities is a complex and often long-term process of building trust. Nurses must advocate for the fiscal, logistical, ideological, and labor support necessary to make community alliances possible. In many cases, this requires nurses to struggle collectively for institutional changes to develop resources and make the environment safer. When mobilizing aggregates for improvement in environmental health, it is essential that a withdrawal of resources does not undermine the process; withdrawal will cause further alienation and mistrust on the part of vulnerable groups.

It may appear that what is being discussed here is an "us-them" approach that advocates an alignment with the vulnerable against outside "enemies." This is an unfortunate oversimplification. When nurses work to build coalitions for improving environmental conditions, each issue or problem requires appropriate strategic action based on its own merits. Allies in a current struggle may have been adversaries in a previous struggle. For example, although a bank refused to help farm families by granting farm loan extensions last month, it may still be an ally this month when a superhighway development project threatens its location and an adjacent poor neighborhood. An ally need not be in complete agreement with the core group's philosophy, political agenda, or moral beliefs. The federal government may be an adversary in regards to restrictive immigration policies, but it is an ally in enforcing the provisions of the Rehabilitation Act. Virtually no person or faction can be completely discounted as an ally or remain untouched by environmental health issues. It is a good idea to brainstorm about all the possible groups in a locale that may have a stake in the outcome of an issue. A good coalition-building strategy is to consider the future and contemplate how one struggle, or one set of allies, can extend its network and subsequently form new coalitions for emerging issues.

Using Collective Strategies

Nurses can use a variety of collective strategies in coalition with others to intervene at the aggregate level and facilitate liberating changes in a community's health. Nurses can organize people to change health-damaging environments through combinations of strategies including coalition building; consciousness-raising groups; educational forums in neighborhoods, workplaces, schools, churches, and social clubs; seminars for health care providers, city officials, teachers, and employers; community needs assessments; dissemination of clinical research and policy analyses; use of mass media; canvassing; litigation; legislative lobbying; testimony at public hearings; demonstrations; and participatory research. Stotts (1991) demonstrated several of these collective strategies in his community health nursing intervention aimed at limiting second-hand smoke in public buildings and work sites.

Although nurses have not traditionally used all of these collective strategies to intervene in community health matters, environmental hazards are multiplying geometrically, pushing nurses to expand their skill repertoire. If nurses have not learned these types of organizational skills, they can learn from experts in the community who have experience with conducting mass media campaigns, organizing demonstrations, canvassing neighborhoods, participating in class-action litigation, and testifying at public hearings. Nurses can also consult many available books about political action.

One collective strategy that is an effective aggregate-level community health nursing intervention is **participatory action research**. Participatory action research calls for nurses, community members, and other resource people to work together in identifying environmental health problems, designing the studies, collecting and analyzing the data, disseminating the results, and posing solutions to the problems (Greenfield and Zimmerman, 1993; Hildebrandt, 1994; Whyte, 1991). With the assistance of community health nurses, community members gather information on suspected environmental hazards, document their effects on health, educate their communities, persuade corporations to clean up, and lobby local, state, and federal governments for stricter regulations and improved enforcement. The goal of the research process is not merely the production of knowledge, but rather the generation of open discussion and debate that intensifies a community's consciousness of health-impairing environmental constraints. Box 13-3 presents an abstract of an article about popular epidemiology (Brown, 1987), which is a type of participatory action research related to environmental health.

In towns across the United States, concerned residents are conducting surveys to determine the severity of community health threats posed by water-polluting factories, nuclear power plants, herbicide-spraying planes, vehicle exhaust pollution, off-shore oil drilling, and excessive lumbering. The following effort, detailed by Freudenberg (1984-85), was very successful:

In response to unregulated toxic contamination in Pennsylvania during the early 1980s, a coalition of tenant associations, environmental groups, senior citizens, labor unions, and Vietnam veterans who had been exposed to Agent Orange organized in Philadelphia. The Delaware Valley Toxics Coalition, as it was called, elicited the help of scientists and epidemiologists to write environmental impact reports about chemical contamination, implemented massive community and workplace education, staged protest demonstrations at polluting companies, organized testimony at public hearings, and helped draft legislation. The coalition also used the media creatively to publicize their concerns. For example, one labor union member sprayed from an unmarked canister into the city council chamber

BOX 13-3

Participatory Action Research about Environmental Health

Abstract
The residents of Woburn, Massachusetts worked together with civic activists and professionals to collect data that confirmed the existence of a leukemia cluster. The group demonstrated that the cluster was traceable to industrial waste carcinogens that leached into the drinking water supply. These residents collectively took part in years of actions that led to successful civil suits against the corporations at fault. The actions of the Woburn citizenry offered a valuable example of lay communication of risk to scientific experts and government officials and demonstrated a concerted collective effort at investigating disease patterns and their likely causes. This case, which drew national attention during the 1980s, catalyzed similar efforts across the country and expanded knowledge on the effects of toxic wastes. The Woburn residents introduced evidence to show that the health effects of toxic wastes are not restricted to physical disease, but also include emotional problems.
Using this case study of popular epidemiology, which involved community-propelled investigation, the author provided a framework for participatory action research about environmental health.

Data from Brown P: Popular epidemiology: community response to toxic waste-induced disease, *Sci Technol Hum Value* 12:78-85, 1987.

during public testimony. When the city council members protested, the unionist replied, "This can contains only air, but every day we have to work with chemicals we know nothing about." As a result of the coalition's efforts, the city of Philadelphia enacted the nation's first Right-to-Know law. The statute stipulated that workers and community residents had the right to know the names and health effects of chemicals used, manufactured, stored, or released into the air.

In December 1990, the *San Francisco Examiner* reported an extensive lead exposure problem in the city of Oakland, California (Kay, 1990). This case study expands upon some of the reported facts of the situation to construct hypothetical nursing interventions.

Assessment

Oakland's community health nurses have long been involved with city residents and have been aware of high rates of lead poisoning in particular neighborhoods. In the wake of alarming newspaper articles about the dangerous incidence of lead exposure in the city, the nurses decided to make lead exposure a priority. The community health nurses and several nursing students assigned to their department divided assessment tasks and uncovered the following conditions.

In 1988, a California study of lead exposure reported that approximately 50,000 California children had enough lead in their serum to lower intelligence, alter behavior, create neurological dysfunction, damage kidneys, and depress growth (Kay, 1990). One fifth of inner-city Oakland children had toxic levels of lead in their blood. Although city, state, and federal authorities were aware of the ubiquitous danger of lead poisoning for decades, they failed to establish routine testing for children. They did not create programs to remove lead-based paint from existing structures and they did not eliminate lead emissions from industrial sources and overcrowded freeways.

An economically depressed neighborhood in Oakland, hypothetically called "Rosario," is situated near numerous railways, freeways, and industrial yards. High numbers of African-American, Latino, and Southeast Asian residents live in the older homes that line the streets of Rosario. The concentration of lead in the neighborhood's soil averages 1200 parts per million (Kay, 1991a). A soil lead concentration of 500, or 1000 parts per million, is sufficient to cause dangerously high blood levels of lead in children (Alliance to End Childhood Lead Poisoning, 1991). Lead levels are also significant in Rosario's drinking water because much of its plumbing consists of lead pipes that leach lead into standing water. Lead-based paint peels from most of the houses. Many heads of households who work in the nearby radiator shops, scrap metal yards, and battery-manufacturing plants carry lead dust home on their clothing and shoes. Isolated by language and economic circumstances, many Rosario residents do not know they are exposed to these environmental health hazards.

Children absorb 50% of the lead they eat, drink, or breathe, whereas adults absorb only 10% (Phoenix, 1993). Children come in contact with lead by playing in contaminated dirt and eating paint chips. Substandard nutrition also increases lead absorption. People inhale lead from car exhaust and industrial emissions and the lead contaminates the ground near busy freeways and factories. Unfortunately, lead remains in soil for thousands of years (Bailey et al., 1994).

Lucia, a 7-year-old girl who lives in Rosario, developed a lead level several times higher than necessary to cause intelligence impairment. Her hair fell out and she became emaciated, weak, and often tearful. She experienced constant nosebleeds and fell down frequently. She received painful and risky intravenous treatment with chelating agents over a period of one year and most of her symptoms receded. However, her mother said, "No one cleans up the area. People move in and out, but the poison remains here." In fact, local hospital spokespersons claim that 25% of the children they treat for lead poisoning become repoisoned after they return home (Kay, 1990).

Although the federal government requires lead tests to qualify for Medicaid funding, the state's Child Health Program, which provides health examinations for poor children, refused to add lead tests to their routine examinations. California officials claimed they provide testing when a physician recommends the test, but private physicians in the city generally assume that lead poisoning is an East Coast phenomenon. Therefore they often fail to recommend the blood test and are unlikely to recognize lead poisoning when it does occur.

Continued

Furthermore, the Child Health Program reaches only about one third of those who are eligible. The governor vetoed $160,000 in funding for a lead-testing program for high-risk children in Oakland.

Based on this assessment, the city's community health nurses devised the following list of unresolved problems:

- Lead-screening programs for children are not in place.
- Private physicians are not recommending lead tests for vulnerable children.
- Health care providers at local public hospitals and clinics may not recognize lead-poisoning symptoms.
- Children are being repoisoned after treatment.
- Industrial and vehicular emissions are poorly controlled.
- A comprehensive plan for removing lead-based paint from the city's older structures does not exist.
- Many Rosario residents work in lead-related industries.
- Poverty and malnutrition are widespread in Rosario.
- Residents are poorly informed about lead hazards in the environment.
- Multiracial, multicultural, and language characteristics of Rosario make organizing education efforts more complex.

Planning

Given their assessment, the community health nurses decided they needed to assist members of the Rosario community to affect environmental changes that reduce lead-poisoning risks. They realized they should involve members of the Rosario community at planning meetings and include African-American, Latino, and Southeast Asian community members. They contacted neighborhood leaders, church leaders, ethnic clubs, the local Parent-Teacher Association, a senior citizen organization in the neighborhood, the Black Women's Health Project, and a local Latina women's political organization. In their initial meetings, nurses learned about a budding multicultural grassroots effort by People United for a Better Oakland (PUEBLO) (Calpotura, 1991; Kay, 1990) that travels door to door educating Oakland residents about the dangers of lead.

Nurses and community members discussed how all parties viewed the problem, what resources were available to them, how they might align with PUEBLO, how they might generate more community involvement, who might serve as potential allies, what functions the community health nursing agency could perform, and what potential actions they might take. The nurses also asked questions about other circumstances affecting Rosario's residents. Community members expressed that they were still reeling from the damages caused by a major earthquake a few years before. They also reported that many of their neighbors were fearful about coming to the meetings or joining PUEBLO because they were undocumented workers and worried about deportation. In addition, the state highway commission pressed for the construction of another freeway close to Rosario; the community worried about this. After several meetings, members decided to establish a permanent Rosario Coalition and nurses played an important part.

The nurses discussed their competing priorities; the lead problem was only one of the issues they faced. They concluded they could advocate for Rosario's residents most efficiently by using their established ties with local physicians, nurses, and health care institutions. They allocated adequate funds and personnel to accomplish the coalition's goals and established a time frame for evaluating the Rosario project. The coalition encouraged nursing students and community health nursing faculty from the local university and college programs to participate in the interventions.

Intervention

The actions of the community health nurses in coalition with community members divide into interventions at the individual, family, and aggregate levels.

Individual

- Identify Rosario children who were diagnosed and treated for lead poisoning and plan follow-up nursing home visits to prevent repoisoning.
- Redesign the community health agency's child health assessment protocol, adding several observations designed to detect symptoms of lead poisoning and several questions that establish

whether there are specific risks for lead poisoning in the home.

- Coordinate with school nurses to ensure they incorporate similar changes in their health assessment protocols.
- Establish an agreement with the state's Child Health Program that ensures they will obtain lead levels on children if physicians, school nurses, or community health nurses recommend it.
- Prepare an educational pamphlet with members of the Rosario Coalition that details Rosario residents' lead-poisoning risks. With the coalition's endorsement, the nurses mail the pamphlet to individual physicians and nurses who provide services to children in Oakland.
- Prepare translations of the pamphlet in languages and reading levels appropriate for Rosario residents and mail it to individual households.
- Follow-up on pamphlet mailings with announcements about community health nurses' willingness to offer lead-poisoning education programs at churches, schools, hospitals, workplaces, medical association meetings, and nursing association meetings.

Family

- Initiate a family-to-family program in which a core group of Rosario community members attend educational meetings with the community health nurses. In these meetings, share information about the environmental origins of lead poisoning and its prevention, diagnosis, and treatment. These specially trained community members then take charge of the program, sharing their knowledge with extended family members and neighboring families.
- Coordinate with school nurses to establish a health education program in Rosario schools in which school-aged children learn about lead poisoning. Encourage these children to take their knowledge home and teach younger preschool-aged brothers and sisters about washing their hands and keeping their hands out of their mouths.
- Investigate how community health nurses might better assist Rosario families by helping them apply for and obtain nutritional resources such as food stamps, food bank supplements, and school lunch programs. With improved nutritional status, lead absorption may decrease.

- Facilitate the formation of a support group for families with children who have suffered lead poisoning damage. The community health nurses offer their offices for evening meeting space and provide information about health care, social services, and government disability assistance.

Community

- With the Rosario Coalition, form broader coalitions with PUEBLO, Oakland churches, local nurses association, several preschool and day care centers, and the Oakland School Board to design a comprehensive, nonduplicative, cost-effective lead-screening program that will test all children in Oakland on a regular basis.
- Lobby state legislatures, municipal officials, local medical associations, local hospitals, and city clinics regarding plan implementation.
- Contact researchers at a local university's environmental sciences program and request that they work with the coalition to conduct a house-to-house study of lead poisoning sources. The nurses and other members of the coalition cooperate with the researchers in teaching Rosario residents about questionnaires and data gathering that will involve soil, water, and paint samples. They also should offer to coordinate the services of bilingual research assistants from the Rosario community.
- Coordinate efforts at abatement, the process of removing the exposure source of the environmental hazard, by performing the following: obtain federal guidelines for lead abatement in private homes (US Department of Housing and Urban Development, 1990); determine municipal, state, and federal accountability for financing lead abatement in low-income owner-occupied households; explore strategies that compel multiple-dwelling owners to de-lead their properties to ensure tenant safety; and initiate fund-raising activities to cover Rosario residents' out-of-pocket expenses from the abatement process.
- Contact the occupational health nurses at local lead-based industries to ascertain policies related to heavy metals, enforcement of regulations regarding lead disposal, and number of cases of lead poisoning among workers.

Continued

- Contact state environmental groups for advice on local efforts and join in their fight for stricter regulation of lead emissions and toxic wastes.
- Contact local media (e.g., television, radio, and newspaper) about running a series of stories about local lead-poisoning risks. Nurses and other coalition members should supply information and contacts for interviews and photographs.

Evaluation

In regular meetings of the original Rosario Coalition, the nurses facilitated the evaluation of ongoing interventions. Among their many evaluation activities, the nurses tracked the number of lead-screening tests Rosario children received and the rates of lead poisoning and repoisoning to determine the effectiveness of their efforts in these areas. They documented participation levels at educational programs and family-to-family training sessions and interest in nutrition referrals and support groups, all of which appeared to be successful.

The community health nurses also kept close contact with the school nurses and occupational health nurses. At one point, the occupational health nurses reported they were too overburdened in their jobs to perform the necessary worker education concerning prevention of heavy metal poisoning. The community health nurses and coalition members offered to help. They organized an after-work educational program for foremen at local industries and another program for union shop stewards. They hoped both groups would disseminate the information at their workplaces. The community health nurses and coalition asked occupational health nurses to report on the educational sessions' success.

Although local officials supported their plan, the broader coalition's efforts at pushing for a comprehensive lead-screening program met a great deal of opposition from the state legislature. When repeated negotiations continued to fail, the coalition decided to align with environmental and civil rights groups who were suing the state of California for failure to provide federally mandated lead poisoning tests for low-income children. The coalition became plaintiffs in the class-action suit. The community health nurses from Rosario gave expert testimony in the case.

The court case proceeded and some members of the state legislature began to show more interest in a lead-screening program; another vote was scheduled. The Rosario Coalition participated in a Lead Poisoning Awareness Day at the state capitol the week before the vote. They were active in the demonstration and gave speeches about their local experiences. They visited the offices of individual legislators, informing them of Rosario's situation. Citing the tentative results from the environmental sciences' house-to-house research study and the community health nurses' screening and poisoning rate statistics proved very useful. This evidence strengthened the coalition members' arguments about the need for a comprehensive lead-screening program in the state. The coalition also shared these data with the national environmental groups they worked with. These groups used the data in testimony before federal legislators to secure federal funding for a new program to remove lead-based paint from existing structures.

Examples of Levels of Prevention

Primary Prevention
Educating the community regarding lead poisoning and lead hazards in the environment.

Secondary Prevention
Screening at-risk populations for exposure to lead and testing lead blood levels.

Tertiary Prevention
Follow-up treatment for people with lead poisoning and removing lead hazards from the community environment.

SUMMARY

This chapter provided a glimpse into the complex world of environmental health from a critical community health nursing perspective. The case study, vignettes, and examples illustrate that nurses must evaluate the broader picture in assessing the environmental health status of communities and the vulnerable aggregates within communities. In preventing, minimizing, and resolving environmental health problems, nurses must recognize patterns, detect subtle changes, identify underlying issues, and work collaboratively with a variety of individuals and groups. In the past, environmental threats to health were usually suspected only when other possible causes of illness were ruled out. Nurses can expect this pattern to change drastically in the new millennium as environmental health moves increasingly to the forefront of the public health agenda.

LEARNING ACTIVITIES

1. Identify a health-related problem associated with some aspect of the environment. It may be a problem in a nearby community, a problem publicized in the media, or a difficulty experienced by a family. Examine the problem using the sample series of critical questions listed in Box 13-2. Without sharing the results, present the problem to the group and ask them to discuss it by responding to the same questions. Were there differences or similarities in the initial results and the group's answers? On what points did everyone agree? Why? What questions caused the most disagreement? Why? Now repeat the entire activity by involving people other than nursing students in the group discussion. How did this discussion compare with the previous discussion and responses?

2. Attend meetings that hold environmental hazard discussions. If meetings or public forums are not available in the vicinity, write for information about the state's actions to fight environmental hazards. The reference librarians at colleges or public libraries can suggest ways of contacting sources and will supply addresses. Organizations that are likely to sponsor forums and provide information include those listed in Box 13-1, the EPA, the National Institute for Occupational Safety and Health, state and municipal agen-

cies for environmental protection and occupational health, environmental caucuses of political parties, the APHA, the local public health department, farmers' organizations, and labor unions.

3. This chapter describes how to use participatory research as an intervention in dealing with ecological hazards. In a group, brainstorm about possibilities for participatory action research projects in the area. Try to identify examples from a variety of environmental health areas. Be creative in planning. How might a nurse mobilize community support and participation in the research? What groups would be approachable? What critical questions might facilitate dialogue about the problem? What kinds of data could be collected and how could they be used? How could research results be publicized? What ramifications could the completed study have for community members, other communities in the state, and community health nurses in other locales?

4. Nurses may have to supplement their knowledge of collective strategies by reading books about political action and by learning from community members who are experienced in political organizing. Visit a college or public library to investigate books and journal articles outside the nursing literature. Compile a list of references related to one of these political strategies (e.g., grassroots organizing, legislative lobbying, community education, policy analysis, use of the media, coalition building, citizen surveys, public protest, letter-writing campaigns, or consciousness-raising groups). Exchange reference lists with peers to benefit from their efforts. Then choose one or two books of interest and read them.

REFERENCES

Aday LA: *At risk in America: the health and health care needs of vulnerable populations in the United States,* San Francisco, 1993, Jossey-Bass.

Alexander DE, Fairbridge RW: *Encyclopedia of environmental science,* Higham, Mass, 1999, Kluwer Academic Publishers.

Allen DG: Using philosophical and historical methodologies to understand the concept of health. In Chinn PL, editor: *Nursing research methodology issues and implementation,* Rockville, Md, 1986, Aspen.

Alliance to End Childhood Lead Poisoning: *Childhood lead poisoning prevention: a resource directory,* ed 2, Washington, DC, 1991, National Center for Education in Maternal and Child Health.

Alston D: *We speak for ourselves: social justice, race, and environment,* Washington, DC, 1990, Panos Institute.

Anderson RF: Solid waste and public health. In Greenberg MR, editor: *Public health and the environment: the United States experience,* New York, 1987, Guilford Press.

Anspach RR: From stigma to identity politics: political activism among the physically disabled and former mental patients, *Soc Sci Med* 13A:765-773, 1979.

Bailey AJ et al: Poisoned landscapes: the epidemiology of environmental lead exposure in Massachusetts children: 1990-1991, *Soc Sci Med* 39(6):757-766, 1994.

Barnes BV et al: *Forest ecology,* ed 4, New York, 1998, John Wiley and Sons.

Bergstrom L, Kirchmann H: *Carbon and nutrient dynamics in natural and agricultural tropical ecosystems,* New York, 1998, CAB International.

Bingham E, Meader WV: Governmental regulation of environmental hazards in the 1990s, *Annu Rev Public Health* 11:419-434, 1990.

Blumenthal DS, Ruttenber J, editors: *Introduction to environmental health,* ed 2, New York, 1995, Springer.

Brender JD, Suarez L: Paternal occupation and anencephaly, *Am J Epidemiol* 131:517-521, 1990.

Brooks BO: Indoor air pollution: an edifice complex, *Clin Toxicol* 29(3):315-374, 1991.

Brown P: Popular epidemiology: community response to toxic waste-induced disease, *Sci Technol Hum Value* 12:78-85, 1987.

Bryant B, Mohai P: *Race and the incidence of environmental hazards,* Boulder, Colo, 1992, Westview Press.

Bullard RD, editor: *Confronting environmental racism: voices from the grassroots,* Boston, 1993, South End Press.

Bullard RD: *Dumping in Dixie: race, class, and environmental quality,* Boulder, Colo, 1990, Westview Press.

Burger EJ: Human health: a surrogate for the environment: the evolution of environmental legislation and regulation during the 1970s, *Regul Toxicol Pharmacol* 9:196-206, 1989.

Butterfield PG: Thinking upstream: nurturing a conceptual understanding of the societal context of health behavior, *Adv Nurs Sci* 12:1-8, 1990.

Calpotura F: *PUEBLO (People United for a Better Oakland) and lead poisoning,* Speech presented at the National Conference on Preventing Childhood Lead Poisoning, Washington, DC, October 7, 1991.

Center for Investigative Reporting: *Global dumping grounds: the international trade in hazardous waste,* Washington DC, 1990, Seven Locks Press.

Connon CL, Freund E, Ehlers JK: The occupational health nurses in agricultural communities program: identifying and preventing agriculturally related illnesses and injuries, *Am Assoc Occup Health Nurs J* 41(9):422-428, 1993.

Council on Scientific Affairs: Low-level radioactive wastes, *JAMA* 262:669-674, 1989.

Covello VT, Merkhofer MW: *Risk assessment methods: approaches for assessing health and environmental risks,* New York, 1993, Plenum Press.

Cralley LV, Cralley LJ, Cooper WC, editors: *Health and safety beyond the work place,* New York, 1990, John Wiley and Sons.

Crawford R: You are dangerous to your health: the ideology and politics of victim blaming, *Int J Health Serv* 7:663-680, 1977.

Davies DB: *Phosphorus, agriculture and water quality,* Wallingford, UK, 1998, CABI Publishing.

DeLong JV: Public policy toward municipal solid waste, *Annu Rev Public Health* 14:137-157, 1993.

DeRosa CT, Stevens Y, Johnson BL: Cancer policy framework for public health: assessment of carcinogens in the environment, *Toxicol Ind Health* 9(4):559-575, 1993.

Dumont MP: Psychotoxicology: the return of the mad hatter, *Soc Sci Med* 29(9):1077-1082, 1989.

Dupuis M, Vandergeest P: *Creating the countryside: the politics of rural and environmental discourse,* Philadelphia, 1996, Temple University Press.

Earls F, Cairns RB, Mercy JA: The control of violence and the promotion of nonviolence in adolescents. In Millstein SG, Petersen AC, Nightingale EO, editors: *Promoting the health of adolescents: new directions for the twenty-first century,* New York, 1993, Oxford University Press.

Eckersley R: *Environmentalism and political theory: toward an ecocentric approach,* Albany, NY, 1992, State University of New York Press.

Elsom EM: *Atmospheric pollution: a global problem,* Oxford, UK, 1992, Basil Blackwell.

Foster HD: Health and the physical environment: the challenge of global change. In Hayes MV, Foster LT, Foster HD, editors: *The determinants of populations health: a critical assessment,* Victoria, BC, Canada, 1994, University of Victoria.

Freudenberg N: Training health educators for social change, *Int Q Comm Health Educ* 5:37-52, 1984-1985.

Gaillard AWK: Comparing the concepts of mental load and stress, *Ergonomics* 36(9):991-1005, 1993.

Gelberg KH et al: Nitrate levels in drinking water in rural New York State, *Environ Res* 80(1):34-40, 1999.

Goldman B: *The truth about where you live: an atlas for action on toxins and mortality,* New York, 1991, Random House.

Gould P: *Fire in the rain: the democratic consequences of Chernobyl,* Baltimore, 1990, The Johns Hopkins University Press.

Greenberg M, Schneider D: Violence in American cities: young black males is the answer, but what was the question? *Soc Sci Med* 39(2):179-187, 1994.

Greenfield TK, Zimmerman R, editors: *Experiences with community action projects: new research in the prevention of alcohol and other drug problems,* Center for Substance Abuse Prevention, Monograph 14, Rockville, Md, 1993, USDHHS.

Grondona C: Lead revisited: a case study on lead exposed painters, *Am Assoc Occup Health Nurs J* 41(1):33-38, 1993.

Guillen MD, Sopelana P, Partearroyo MA: Food as a source of polycyclic aromatic carcinogens, *Rev Environ Health* 12(3):133-146, 1997.

Hall JM, Stevens PE: A nursing view of the U.S.-Iraq war: psychosocial health consequences, *Nurs Outlook* 40: 113-120, 1992.

Hall JM, Stevens PE, Meleis AI: Marginalization: a guiding concept for valuing diversity in nursing knowledge development, *Adv Nurs Sci* 16(4):23-41, 1994.

Hamilton C: Coping with industrial exploitation. In Bullard RD, editor: *Confronting environmental racism: voices from the grassroots,* Boston, 1993, South End Press.

Harper AC, Lambert LJ: *The health of populations: an introduction,* ed 2, New York, 1994, Springer.

Haun JW: *Guide to the management of hazardous waste,* Golden, Colo, 1991, Fulcrum.

Havenaar JM, van den Brink W: Psychological factors affecting health after toxicological disasters, *Clin Psychol Rev* 17(4):359-374, 1997.

Hildebrandt E: A model for community involvement in health program development, *Soc Sci Med* 39(2):247-254, 1994.

Institute of Medicine Committee on Enhancing Environmental Health Content in Nursing Practice: *Nursing, health, and the environment,* Washington, DC, 1995, National Academy Press.

International Physicians for the Prevention of Nuclear War: *Radioactive heaven and earth: the health and environmental effects of nuclear weapons testing, in, on, and above the earth,* New York, 1991, Apex Press.

Jackson MP, McSwane DZ: Homelessness as a determinant of health, *Public Health Nurs* 9(3):185-192, 1992.

Jaga K, Brosius D: Pesticide exposure: human cancers on the horizon, *Rev Environ Health* 14(1):39-42, 1999.

Jain RK et al, editors: *Environmental technologies and trends: international and policy perspectives,* New York, 1997, Springer Verlag.

Jepma CJ, Munasinghe M: *Climate change policy: facts, issues and analyses,* Cambridge, UK, 1998, Cambridge University Press.

Kay J: Ethnic enclaves fight toxic waste, *San Francisco Examiner* April 9, 1991a:1,8.

Kay J: Minorities bear brunt of pollution: Latinos and blacks living in state's 'dirtiest' neighborhood, *San Francisco Examiner* April 7, 1991b:1,12.

Kay J: State's kids still exposed to lead, *San Francisco Examiner* December 9, 1990:1,16.

Keller EA: *Environmental geology,* New York, 1992, Macmillan.

Kemp DD: *The environmental dictionary,* London, 1998, Routledge.

Kerner JF, Dusenbury L, Mandelblatt JS: Poverty and cultural diversity: challenges for health promotion among the medically underserved, *Annu Rev Public Health* 14:355-377, 1993.

Kilburn KH: Neurotoxicity from airborne chemicals around a superfund site, *Environ Res* 81(2):92-99, 1999.

Kogi K: Practical approaches to the assessment of work-related risks, *Int Arch Occup Environ Health* 65:S11-S14, 1993.

Kozol J: *Savage inequalities: children in America's schools,* New York, 1991, Harper Collins.

Krieps R, editor: *Environment and health: a holistic approach,* Brookfield, Vt, 1989, Avebury.

Last JM: Global change: ozone depletion, greenhouse warming, and public health, *Annu Rev Public Health* 14:115-136, 1993.

Lawrence RJ: Urban health: an ecological perspective, *Rev Environ Health* 14(1):1-10, 1999.

Lee E, editor: *Working with Asian Americans: a guide for clinicians,* New York, 1997, Guilford Press.

Lemus R et al: Potential health risks from exposure to indoor formaldehyde, *Rev Environ Health* 13(1-2):91-98, 1998.

Levy BS, Wegman DH, editors: *Occupational health: recognizing and preventing work-related disease,* ed 3, Boston, 1995, Little, Brown and Co.

Lunberg A: *The environment and mental health: a guide for clinicians,* Mahwah, NJ, 1998, Lawrence Erlbaum.

Mariethoz E et al: Allergy and the environment: a meeting report, *Rev Environ Health* 14(2):63-78, 1999.

Marino G: The nuclides in town: does danger lurk in low-level radioactivity in sewage? *Sci News* 146(14):218-219, 1994.

McAbee RR, Gallucci BJ, Checkoway H: Adverse reproductive outcomes and occupational exposures among nurses: an investigation of multiple hazardous exposures, *Am Assoc Occup Health Nurs J* 41(3):110-119, 1993.

McKeown T: *The origins of human disease,* Oxford, UK, 1991, Basil Blackwell.

Mielke HW et al: The urban environment and children's health, *Environ Res* 81(2):117-129, 1999.

Milio N: *Promoting health through public policy,* Ottawa, Ontario, 1986, Canadian-Public-Health Association.

Miller R: Effects of prenatal exposure to ionizing radiation, *Health Phys* 59:57-61, 1990.

Mole R: Childhood cancer after prenatal exposure to diagnostic x-ray examinations in Britain, *Br J Cancer* 62:152-168, 1990.

Moore GS: *Living with the earth: concepts in environmental health science,* Boca Raton, Fla, 1999, Lewis Publications.

Moses M: Farmworkers and pesticides. In Bullard RD, editor: *Confronting environmental racism: voices from the grassroots,* Boston, 1993, South End Press.

Mungall C, McLaren DJ: *Planet under stress: the challenge of global change,* Toronto, Canada, 1990, Oxford University Press.

Myers N: *Gaia: an atlas of planet management,* New York, 1993, Doubleday.

National Toxic Inhalation Study Group: Environmental pulmonary edema: an update, *Rev Environ Health* 13(1-2):27-58, 1998.

Needleman HL et al: The long-term effects of exposure to low doses of lead in children: an 11-year follow-up report, *N Engl J Med* 322:83-88, 1992.

Neu HC: The crisis in antibiotic resistance, *Science* 257:1064-1072, 1992.

Neufer L: The role of the community health nurse in environmental health, *Pub Health Nurs* 11(3):155-162, 1994

Neufer L, Narkunas D: Hazardous substance releases at the community level: a practical approach to analyzing potential health threats, *Am Assoc Occup Health Nurs J* 42(7):329-335, 1994.

Northridge ME, Shepard PM: Environmental racism and public health, *Am J Public Health* 87(5):730-732, 1997.

Peña D, Gallegos J: Nature and Chicanos in southern Colorado. In Bullard RD, editor: *Confronting environmental racism: voices from the grassroots,* Boston, 1993, South End Press.

Perdue EM, Gjessing ET, editors: *Organic acids in aquatic ecosystems,* New York, 1989, John Wiley and Sons.

Phoenix J: Getting the lead out of the community. In Bullard RD, editor: *Confronting environmental racism: voices from the grassroots,* Boston, 1993, South End Press.

Platt JR: Radon: its impact on the community and the role of the nurse, *Am Assoc Occup Health Nurs J* 41(11):547-550, 1993.

Powell SC, Atwell R: The use of epidemiological data in the control of foodborne viruses, *Rev Environ Health* 14(1):31-38, 1999.

Raymo ME et al: Millennial-scale climate instability during the early Pleistocene epoch, *Nature* 392:699-702, 1998.

Reich MR: Social policy for pollution-related diseases, *Soc Sci Med* 27:1011-1018, 1988.

Reinhardt PA, Gordon JG: *Infectious and medical waste management,* Chelsea, Mich, 1991, Lewis Publishers.

Rom W, editor: *Environmental and occupational medicine,* ed 2, Boston, 1992, Little, Brown, and Co.

Rose J, editor: *Environmental health: the impact of pollutants,* New York, 1990, Gordon and Breach Science Publishers.

Rosenberg ML, Fenley MA, editors: *Violence in America: a public health approach,* New York, 1991, Oxford University Press.

Ruback RB, Weiner NA: *Interpersonal violent behaviors: social and cultural aspects,* New York, 1994, Springer.

Salazar MK, Primomo J: Taking the lead in environmental health: defining a model for practice, *Am Assoc Occup Health Nurs J* 42(7):317-324, 1994.

Sandman PM, Weinstein ND: Predictors of home radon testing and implications for testing promotion programs, *Health Educ Q* 20(4):471-487, 1993.

Sargent JD et al: The association between state housing policy and lead poisoning in children, *Am J Public Health* 89(11):1690-1695, 1999.

Schrieberg D: Death from a healing machine: radioactive waste goes on Mexican odyssey after sale of medical device, *San Francisco Examiner* June 23, 1991:1,12.

Schuurmann G, Markert B, editors: *Ecotoxicology, ecological fundamentals, chemical exposure, and biological effects,* New York, 1998, John Wiley and Sons.

Sidel R: *Women and children last: the plight of poor women in affluent America,* New York, 1992, Penguin.

Smets H: Major industrial risks and compensation of victims: the role of insurance, *Soc Sci Med* 27:1085-1095, 1988.

Smith BE: Black lung: the social production of disease. In Conrad P, Kern R, editors: *The sociology of health and illness: critical perspectives,* ed 3, New York, 1990, St. Martin's Press.

Soble SM, Brennan JH: A review of legal and policy issues in legislating compensation for victims of toxic substance pollution, *Soc Sci Med* 27:1061-1070, 1988.

State of the World's Forests 1999: *Environment news: state of the world's forests 1999,* 1999, The Author, http://ens.lycos.com/ens/mar99/1999L-03-04-02.html.

Steenland K: *Case studies in occupational epidemiology,* New York, 1993, Oxford University Press.

Stevens PE: A critical social reconceptualization of environment in nursing: implications for methodology, *Adv Nurs Sci* 11:56-68, 1989.

Stevens PE, Hall JM: Abusive health care interactions experienced by lesbians: a case of institutional violence in the treatment of women, *Response Victimization Women Children* 13:23-27, 1990.

Stevens PE, Hall JM: Applying critical theories to nursing in communities, *Public Health Nurs* 9:2-9, 1992.

Stevens PE, Morgan S: Health of lesbian, gay, bisexual, and transgender youth, *J Child Fam Nurs* 2(4):237-249, 1999.

Stotts RC: Application of the salmon model: a tale of two cities, *Public Health Nurs* 8:10-14, 1991.

Sumrall AC, Taylor D, editors: *Sexual harassment: women speak out,* Freedom, Calif, 1992, Crossing Press.

Sutherland WJ: *Conservation science and action,* Oxford, UK, 1998, Blackwell Science.

Swanson T: *Global action for biodiversity,* London, 1997, Earthscan Publications.

Tchounwou PB: Climate change and its potential impacts on the Gulf Coast region of the United States, *Rev Environ Health* 14(2):91-102, 1999.

Teitelman R: *Gene dreams: wall street, academia, and the rise of biotechnology,* New York, 1989, Basic Books.

Thacker SB et al: Surveillance in environmental public health: issues, systems, and sources, *Am J Public Health* 86(5):633-638, 1996.

Thompson JL: Critical scholarship: the critique of domination in nursing, *Adv Nurs Sci* 10:27-38, 1987.

US Department of Health and Human Services: *Healthy people: the surgeon general's report on health promotion and disease prevention,* Pub No (PHS) 75-55071, Washington, DC, 1979, US Government Printing Office.

US Department of Housing and Urban Development: *Comprehensive and workable plan for the abatement of lead-based paint in privately owned housing: a report to Congress,* Rockville, Md, 1990, The Author.

US Environmental Protection Agency: *Technical support document for the 1992 citizen's guide to radon,* EPA 400-R-92-011, Washington, DC, 1992, The Author.

Veazie MA et al: Epidemiologic research on the etiology of injuries at work, *Annu Rev Public Health* 15:203-221, 1994.

Vyner HM: *Invisible trauma: the psychosocial effects of invisible environmental contaminants,* Lexington, Mass, 1988a, Lexington Books.

Vyner HM: The psychological dimensions of health care for patients exposed to radiation and the other invisible environmental contaminants, *Soc Sci Med* 27:1097-1103, 1988b.

Walker B: Environmental health policies in the 1990s, *J Public Health Policy* 11:438-447, 1990.

Watts RJ: Democratization of health care: challenge for nursing, *Adv Nurs Sci* 12:37-46, 1990.

Werner MA, Olson DK: Identifying sources of disease in agriculture: a role for occupational health nurses, *Am Assoc Occup Health Nurs J* 41(10):481-490, 1993.

Whalen MM, Loganathan BG, Kannan K: Immunotoxicity of environmentally relevant concentrations of butyltins, *Environ Res* 81(2):108-116, 1999.

Whyte WF, editor: *Participatory action research,* Newbury Park, Calif, 1991, Sage.

Wijnen JH, vander Zee SC: Traffic-related air pollutants: exposure of road users and populations living near busy roads, *Rev Environ Health* 13(1-2):1-26, 1998.

Wilson EO, Myers N, Ehrenfeld D: Species diversity and extinction. In Bormann FH, Kellert SR, editors: *Ecology, economics, ethics,* New Haven, Conn, 1991, Yale University Press.

Young J: *Sustaining the earth,* Cambridge, Mass, 1990, Harvard University Press.

Populations in the Community

14 Child and Adolescent Health

15 Women's Health

16 Men's Health

17 Family Health

18 Senior Health

19 Populations Affected by Disabilities

20 Homeless Populations

21 Rural and Migrant Health

CHAPTER

14

Child and Adolescent Health

Mary Brecht Carpenter and Susan Rumsey Givens

OBJECTIVES

Upon completion of this chapter, the reader will be able to do the following:

1. Identify major indicators of child and adolescent health status.
2. Describe how socioeconomic circumstances influence child and adolescent health.
3. Discuss the individual and societal costs of poor child health status.
4. Discuss public programs and prevention strategies targeted to children's health.
5. Apply knowledge of child and adolescent health needs in planning appropriate, comprehensive care at the individual, family, and community levels.

KEY TERMS

adolescent pregnancy
child abuse and neglect
childhood immunization
Early and Periodic Screening, Diagnosis, and
    Treatment (EPSDT)
fetal alcohol syndrome (FAS)
Head Start
infant mortality
lead poisoning
low birth rate
Medicaid
preconception counseling
prenatal care
State Children's Health Insurance Program (SCHIP)
Women, Infants, and Children (WIC)

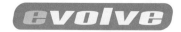

http://evolve.elsevier.com/Nies/

A nation's destiny lies with the health, education, and well-being of its children. Children are the nation's smallest and most vulnerable population. The United States has made tremendous progress over the last century toward improving children's lives. Improvements in public health measures, such as sanitation, infectious disease control, environmental regulation, health screening and education, and remarkable strides in medical care have all contributed to the good health status that most children enjoy. However, these improvements have not equally benefited children of all races and ethnic groups, children at all income levels, or children in all geographical areas of the country. For example, significant disparities persist in the health status of black and white children. Children living in suburban areas and most outer urban areas experience superior access to health care services compared with children living in rural areas and inner cities, especially if they are poor.

Although most of the nation's children are healthy and succeed in school, many are not enjoying optimal health, are failing academically, and are not reaching their full potential as contributing members of society. The mortality and morbidity rates for children in all age groups are unacceptably high.

■ In 1997, over 28,000 infants died before reaching their first birthday.
■ In that same year, over 291,000 babies were born with low birth weights (i.e., less than 5.5 pounds) and many suffered long-term debilitating respiratory, vision, or mental conditions.
■ An estimated three million children are victims of child abuse and neglect; most are under the age of four.
■ More than 900,000 adolescent girls become pregnant every year.
■ In children aged 12 to 17, 19% use alcohol and nearly 10% use an illegal drug other than alcohol.
■ Violence is the second leading cause of death among adolescents.

The health of a child has long-term implications. Today's youth develop health habits that will profoundly influence their potential for a healthy, productive future. The physical and emotional health of a child plays a pivotal role in his or her overall development and the well-being of the entire family. Children who go to school sick or hungry, who cannot see the chalkboard or hear the teacher, who abuse drugs or miss school frequently, who are troubled by abusive parents or disruptive living circumstances, or who fear for their safety at home or in school often do not perform on the level of their counterparts who are healthy, well-nourished, well cared for at home, and safe and secure in their world.

In 1998, 69.7 million children in the United States were under age 18 (Fig. 14-1). They formed 26% of the country's population, which was down from 36% at the end of the "baby boom" when the child population was at its peak. The demographic composition of the United States' child and adolescent population is changing. In 1998, the U.S. child population consisted of the following:

■ 65% nonHispanic whites,
■ 15% nonHispanic blacks,
■ 15% Hispanic,
■ 4% Asian and Pacific Islander, and
■ 1% American-Indian and Alaska Native (US Bureau of the Census, 1999).

Children are a dependent population and rely primarily on working adults, especially parents, to protect and promote their health and well-being. Community health nurses can learn more about this important population group and the positive and negative factors that influence their health. Nurses can use this information to help improve the chances that children will grow up to be healthy, contributing members of society.

FIGURE **14-1**

U.S. child population by race and Hispanic origin, 1998 (From US Bureau of the Census: *Current population reports,* Series P-25, No 311, Washington, DC, 1999, The Author).

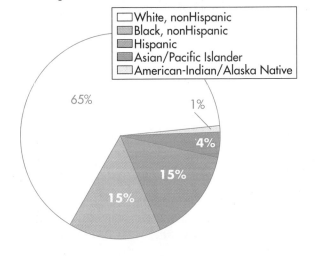

COMMUNITY HEALTH VISIT

- *Story by Leonard Kaku, RN, MSN*
- *Photography by George Draper*

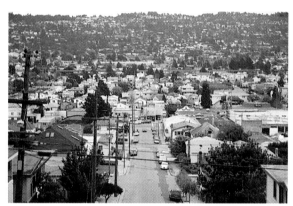

What is community health nursing? The American Nurses Association's definition says it is *a synthesis of nursing practice applied to promoting and preserving the health of populations.* It is, therefore, general, comprehensive, and continuous. The focus of care is directed to individuals, families, or groups (aggregates). Many community health nurses (CHNs) provide care to families in clinic settings.

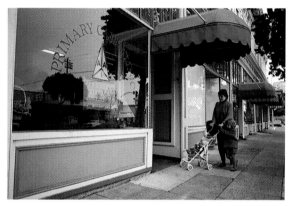

This clinic provides services through the Early Periodic Screening Diagnostic Treatment (EPSDT) Program, which was developed to provide health care for children in low-income families.

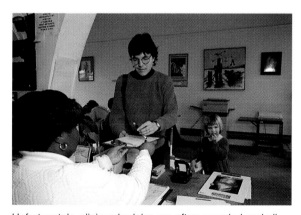

Unfortunately, clinic schedules are often crowded and clients may not be able to get appointments for several weeks.

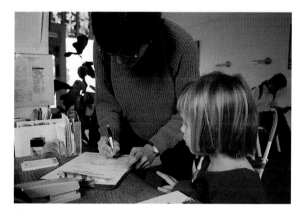

The nurse has an opportunity to observe the client and the family as they register and wait for their appointment. The parent registers the 5-year-old daughter for a school entry health physical. Medicaid insurance is verified for the physical exam.

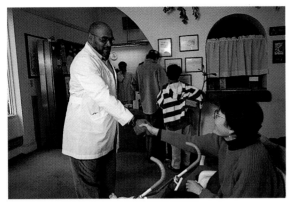

Introduction of the nurse to the client should include your name and role with the agency. It is important to address clients by their proper names and titles—Mr., Mrs., Ms.

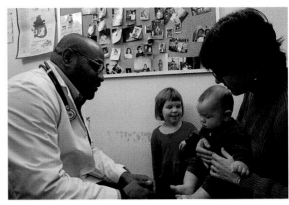

The nurse understands the importance of developing a comfortable atmosphere by beginning with social talk and general questions about the client and family.

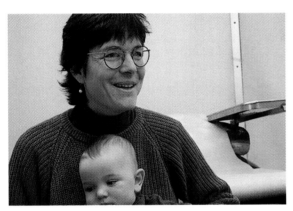

Trust can be established in a short period of time. The nurse can begin by explaining the steps in the clinic process so that the client knows what is expected. Always listen to the client attentively, and allow enough time for the client to reflect and respond to questions.

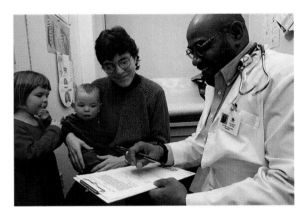

Asking an introductory question, such as "What brought you here today?", provides an open range of responses from the client. The parent's signature is required on a consent form in order for a physical examination and laboratory tests to be performed. The nurse explains the consent form to the parent.

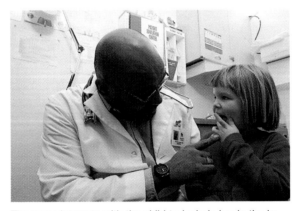

The nurse interacts with the child to include her in the interview process. This provides an opportunity for the nurse to develop a clearer picture of the relationship between the child and parent. It will promote a smoother transition through the examination process.

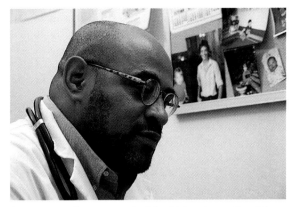

As you move from one part of the history to another, it is helpful to orient the client with brief transitional phrases such as, "Now I would like to ask you some questions about. . . "

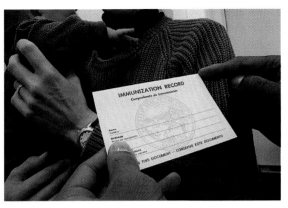

Reviewing immunization records is an important primary prevention role for the community health nurse. This is a teachable opportunity for the nurse to stress the importance of maintaining immunizations for the child. In California parents are provided with a yellow state immunization record for the child, which they should use for recording all immunizations and showing proof of immunizations when needed.

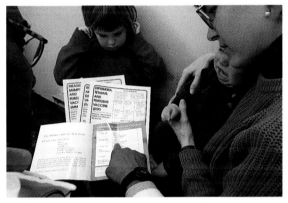

The child requires booster immunizations. The immunization consent forms are given to the parent for a signature. The nurse goes over the consent form with the parent and obtains a signature.

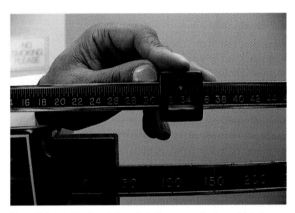

The clinic staff often take vital signs on clients, which include height and weight.

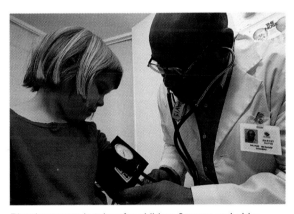

Blood pressure is taken for children 3 years and older.

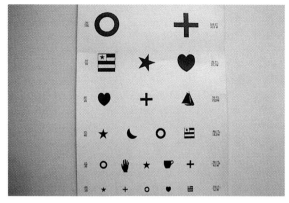

A vision screen is first attempted on a 4-year-old child. If the child is younger, a verbal report is taken from the parent.

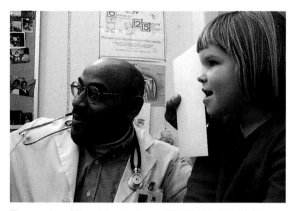

The results of the vision test are: OS: 20/40; OD: 20/50; and OU: 20/50.

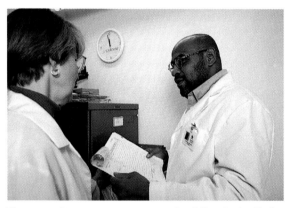

The nurse discusses any concerns about the client with the practitioner prior to the examination. The nurse reports the vision test results to the practitioner as well as any other concerns the nurse may have about the family.

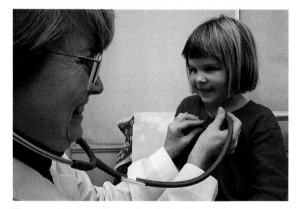

The practitioner performs the physical examination on the child with the help of the parent. The practitioner discusses the result of the vision test with the parent and the need for a follow-up appointment with an ophthalmologist. The child has not had a lead level done and requires booster immunizations. The practitioner orders laboratory tests, immunizations, and a referral to an ophthalmologist.

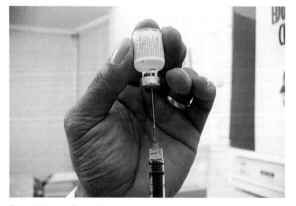

The clinic staff perform the laboratory work: Hct, UA, Pb level. The immunization consent forms have been signed by the parent. The nurse administers the immunizations and takes this opportunity to reinforce the importance of immunizations for both children.

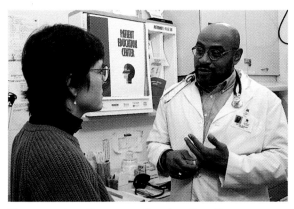

The nurse also offers suggestions to relieve the common side effects of immunizations.

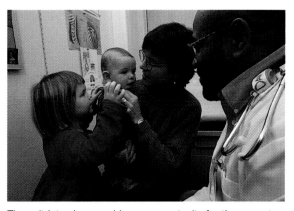

The exit interview provides an opportunity for the nurse to review any issues the parent has raised about the child. The nurse may ask, "Is there anything else I can assist you with?"

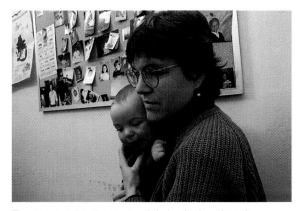

The parent asks about an ophthalmologist who takes Medicaid and about day care facilities in the area for the younger child. The parent also asks about family planning services in the community.

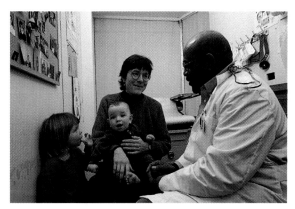

The family agrees to maintain immunizations on the children and to follow-up with appointments with an ophthalmologist and a family planning clinic. The nurse returns the immunization record to the parent documenting today's immunization as well as when the next immunizations are due. The nurse will call with a referral for an ophthalmologist, a family planning clinic, and a day care facility.

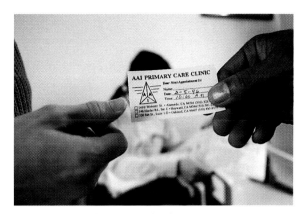

The nurse gives the parent a business card with the nurse's name and agency's address and phone number. The CHN advises the parent to call the nurse if there is anything else that the family may need.

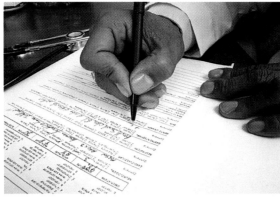

The nurse charts accurately, clearly, and concisely after the clinic visit.

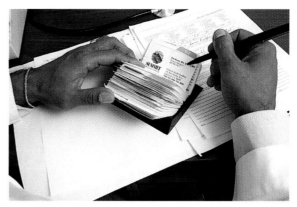

The nurse searches for resources for an ophthalmologist and a family planning clinic that accept Medicaid and a resource for day care providers. The nurse obtains phone numbers for a couple of ophthalmologists, a family planning clinic, and a day care consortium service.

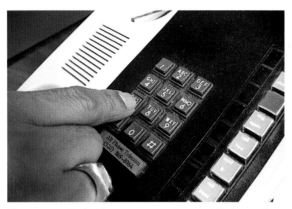

The nurse calls the day care consortium and finds out that there is a list of day care providers available.

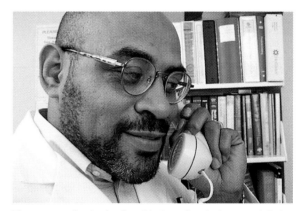

The nurse calls the family with the referrals for an ophthalmologist and a phone number to obtain a list of day care providers.

This chapter focuses on the health status of children and adolescents; the medical, socioeconomic, environmental, educational, safety, and public health factors that nurses must address to improve child and adolescent health; and the community health nursing implications. This chapter also discusses indicators of child and adolescent health status, the individual and societal costs of poor child health, public programs targeted to children's health, and strategies to improve child and adolescent health at the individual, family, and community levels.

ISSUES OF PREGNANCY AND INFANCY

Genetic endowment, maternal health, and intrauterine and neonatal environments strongly influence early child health status. The protection and promotion of early child health can help ensure a healthy future. However, neglecting early child health may cause the following:

- Children who suffer prenatally from the intrauterine effects of maternal smoking, alcohol use, and illicit drug use are more likely to be born with serious health conditions that require immediate attention. These conditions can lead to permanent damage such as mental retardation from fetal alcohol syndrome.
- A fetus exposed to maternal conditions such as hypertension, poor nutrition, anemia, and infectious disease is more likely to suffer from chronic conditions that affect health and well-being.
- Similarly, children exposed to unsafe environmental conditions such as lead-based paint are more likely to suffer from chronic conditions throughout childhood and, in some cases, through adolescence and adulthood.
- Children who do not receive preventive health care and do not obtain all necessary immunizations by their second birthday are more likely to suffer from preventable diseases or chronic conditions that could have been prevented or minimized and controlled.

The first year of life is the most hazardous until the age of 65. Therefore it is particularly important for pregnant women to receive **prenatal care** and adopt healthy lifestyle choices and for infants to receive primary health care to maintain health and prevent or minimize serious, long-lasting health problems.

Infant Mortality

Infant mortality, the death of an infant during the first year of life, is an important gauge of children's health status and pregnant women's health. It is an important marker because it is related to several factors including maternal health, medical care quality and access, socioeconomic conditions, and public health practices. Infant mortality reflects the health and welfare of an entire community or society. The incidence of infant mortality decreased over the past century because public health measures emerged (e.g., improved sanitation, a clean milk supply, immunizations against deadly childhood diseases, and improved availability of nutritious food and improved access to maternal health care).

The 1997 infant death rate of 7.2 deaths per 1000 live births (Martin et al., 1999) is the lowest recorded rate. However, the United States ranks poorly among industrialized nations. The nation's 1995 rate (the most recent year with final international data) of 7.6 was an abysmal twenty-fifth behind other nations including Finland, Japan, France, and Canada (Table 14-1). This reflects the differences in women's health before and during pregnancy; access to prenatal care; access to infant health care; nutritional status; and other health, social, and economic factors.

In the United States, about two thirds of infant deaths occur during the first month of life (the neonatal period). These deaths are attributable to infant health problems or problems with the pregnancy itself such as preterm birth or birth defects. The other one third of infant deaths occur in the remaining 11 months (the postneonatal period) and are attributable to social or environmental factors such as medical care access and accidents (Box 14-1).

The three leading causes of infant death in the United States are congenital anomalies, disorders relating to short gestation and unspecified low birth weight, and sudden infant death syndrome (SIDS) (Hoyert, Kochanek, and Murphy, 1999). These three conditions account for nearly half of all infant deaths. Although the overall infant mortality rate has declined steadily since the 1960s, African-American infants continue to die at twice the rate of white infants (Fig. 14-2). Higher rates of low birth weight infants among African-American women account for this disparity.

TABLE 14-1

Infant Mortality Rates: Ranking of the Developed Countries: 1995

Rank	Country	Infant Mortality Rate*	Rank	Country	Infant Mortality Rate*
1	Finland	3.93	15	Belgium	6.05
2	Singapore	4.01	16	Italy	6.12
3	Norway	4.13	17	Canada	6.14
4	Sweden	4.13	18	England and Wales	6.14
5	Japan	4.26	19	Scotland	6.24
6	Hong Kong	4.57	20	Ireland	6.37
7	France	4.86	21	New Zealand	6.68
8	Switzerland	5.05	22	Israel	6.86
9	Denmark	5.07	23	Northern Ireland	7.08
10	Germany	5.30	24	Portugal	7.51
11	Austria	5.42	25	United States	7.59
12	Netherlands	5.46	26	Czech Republic	7.70
13	Spain	5.49	27	Greece	8.15
14	Australia	5.66	28	Cuba	9.40

From National Center for Health Statistics: *Health, United States: 1999*, Hyattsville, Md, 1999, USDHHS.
*Number of infant deaths per 1000 live births.

BOX 14-1

Sources of Vital Statistics Data for Children

Information concerning an infant's birth, including the mother's total prenatal care visits, the mother's name and father's name, and the infant's weight and birth date appear on a baby's birth certificate. Information concerning an infant's death, such as the cause(s), date, and other details appear on the death certificate. In each state, the state vital statistics office in the state health department stores these certificates. This agency collects and regularly reports the aggregated data and forwards it to the NCHS. The NCHS collects, analyses, and publishes numerous reports on the health and well-being of the nation's infants. These data sources are very important in tracking the health of infants and the health of other population groups; they help determine necessary interventions from various perspectives (e.g., clinical, public health, public policy, and environmental).

Infant mortality rates are lowest for Asian and Pacific Islander mothers (5.0 per 1000 live births), followed by white mothers (6.0), American-Indian mothers (8.7), and African-American mothers (13.7). Infant mortality rates vary considerably among Hispanic subgroups (Puerto Rican rate of 7.9 and Cuban rate of 5.5). Identifying and remedying the causes of higher infant mortality rates among certain population subgroups remains a vexing societal problem.

FIGURE 14-2

U.S. infant mortality rates by race, 1960-1997 (From Hoyert DL, Kochanek KD, Murphy SL: Deaths: final data for 1997, *Natl Vital Stat Rep* 47[19], 1999).

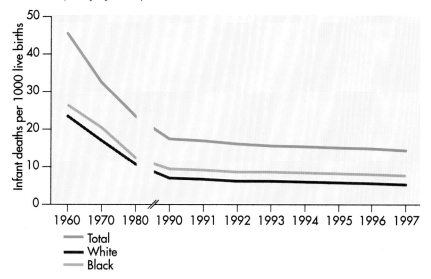

Low Birth Weight and Prematurity

Infants born too soon (before 37 weeks' gestation) and too small (less than 5.5 pounds) have a far greater risk of death and physical and mental disabilities such as blindness, deafness, learning disabilities, and mental retardation than infants born at term with normal weight. The leading predictor of infant mortality is **low birth weight**. Although low birth weight affects only a small proportion of infants (7.6% in 1997), these infants account for nearly 65% of all infant deaths (MacDorman and Atkinson, 1999).

The percentage of infants born with low birth weight has increased. Over 291,000 low-birth-weight babies were born in 1997 (Ventura et al., 1999). African-American infants are affected disproportionately and are twice as likely to be born with low birth weight than white infants (Martin et al., 1999).

Low-birth-weight infants raised in disadvantaged households have a higher risk of experiencing long-term disabilities. Risk factors associated with low birth weight include the following:

- minority status,
- lack of prenatal care,
- low SES, and
- unhealthy maternal habits (e.g., poor nutrition, alcohol and drug use, and cigarette smoking).

The development of advanced life-support technologies for small infants has significantly improved the survival rate of low-birth-weight babies. Although technology can save many of these infants, preventing the occurrence of low birth weight is a high priority for clinical and public health research and public policy. Public health interventions to reduce these risks among target population groups are important strategies to improve the health of these vulnerable children and their families.

Prenatal Care

Obtaining early and regular prenatal care greatly enhances a woman's chance of delivering a healthy, full-term baby. In addition to the important public health measures that improved the health of women and children early in the twentieth century, recent medical, public health, and public policy developments increased the availability of quality prenatal care. For example, the Medicaid program expanded to cover more low-income pregnant women and infants in the 1980s. The proportion of women receiving prenatal care early in pregnancy (i.e., in the first trimester) has risen over the past decade. However, 17% of women in the United States do not receive prenatal care beginning in the first trimester, which is the care standard that health care professionals recognize (Martin et al., 1999).

Women who do not receive prenatal care or those who receive late prenatal care deliver babies with an infant mortality rate nearly 50% higher than mothers who receive first trimester care (MacDorman and Atkinson, 1999). Examples of population groups who do not receive early prenatal care include the following:

- poor women who are under age 20 and unmarried;
- African-American, Hispanic, or Native-American women;
- women who live in isolated rural areas or medically underserved urban areas; or
- women who completed less than 12 years of education.

Timely and comprehensive prenatal care increases the identification and treatment possibilities for specific causes of infant morbidity and mortality such as maternal anemia, diabetes, hypertension, urinary tract infections, STDs, and poor nutrition. Comprehensive prenatal care is particularly important for low-income women. It can help them obtain other services such as the WIC program, food stamps, housing, child care, job training, substance abuse treatment, and domestic violence counseling.

Health education and counseling during prenatal visits can provide women with the information they need to make lifestyle changes to help ensure a healthy pregnancy. Ideally, such counseling should begin before a woman becomes pregnant, This is known as **preconception counseling** (Box 14-2).

Prenatal Substance Use

Tobacco, alcohol, and illicit drug use are social factors that affect health. During pregnancy, substance use profoundly affects the fetus' neurological and physical development. The use of these substances in any combination worsens infant health and development outcomes.

Smoking

Smoking is far more common than alcohol and illicit drug use during pregnancy. The percentage of women who smoke during pregnancy ranges from 1% for Chinese mothers to 21% for American-Indian mothers. The infant mortality rate for infants of smoking mothers is 60% higher than infants of nonsmoking mothers (MacDorman and Atkinson, 1999). The elimination of tobacco use among pregnant women would significantly reduce the percentage of low-birth-weight infants, preterm delivery, intrauterine growth retardation, and infant mortality.

BOX **14-2**

Preconception Counseling

Preconception counseling is a prevention strategy that helps women identify potential risks to a fetus before pregnancy. Tiny developing fetal organ systems are highly vulnerable to the effects of maternal nutrition, drugs, alcohol, tobacco, chronic maternal diseases, environmental toxins, and other exposures. Preconception assessment encourages health and lifestyle modifications that can lead to healthier babies. Many pregnancies are unintended and the fetus can suffer damage before a woman knows she is pregnant; therefore all women capable of childbearing should have a source of regular medical care and adapt healthy lifestyles. This includes consuming 0.4 μg of the B vitamin folic acid every day, even before conception, to decrease the likelihood of delivering a child with NTDs (CDC and PHS, 1992).

Tobacco use passes nicotine, hydrogen cyanide, and carbon monoxide into the fetal blood supply, which restricts fetal access to oxygen (Wilcox, 1993). Maternal cigarette smoking and secondhand smoke exposure are closely linked to SIDS (Schoendorf and Kiely, 1992) and childhood asthma (Cunningham, Dockery, and Speizer, 1994). Many local health departments, hospitals, MCOs, and clinics offer smoking cessation programs for pregnant women.

Alcohol and Illegal Drug Use

Although the effect of low alcohol consumption during pregnancy is uncertain, high consumption during pregnancy can lead to spontaneous abortion, low birth weight, and a cluster of congenital defects including the nervous system dysfunction called **fetal alcohol syndrome** (FAS). FAS has become increasingly common and has surpassed Down syndrome as the leading cause of mental retardation in the United States (Streissguth et al., 1991).

According to the National Pregnancy Health Survey, 5% of women who delivered in 1992 used illegal drugs during pregnancy. Illegal drug use was higher among single, unemployed women with less than a college education (Leshner, 1994).

The prenatal transmission of STDs, especially HIV, is among the most serious potential consequences of drug abuse during pregnancy. Heterosexual HIV transmission is increasing most rapidly among women. The following women are at the highest risk of contracting HIV:

■ women whose sex partners have high-risk behaviors (e.g., IV drug use and failure to use condoms),
■ adolescent women,
■ women with multiple sex partners, and
■ women with other STDs.

CHILDHOOD HEALTH ISSUES

At all ages, appropriate and timely medical care plays an important role in children's health status. However, other factors including parental influences, nutrition, environmental hazards, community safety, and the overall quality of home life exert stronger influences over a child's well-being. Childhood is generally a healthy time of life, as evidenced by the improvement in many indicators of child health status over the past century. For example, the incidence of childhood disease has decreased because the majority of children receive a full complement of immunizations during infancy and toddlerhood.

The causes of childhood death vary with age, but accidental injury is the leading cause of death for all children over the age of one. Parents and the community have important responsibilities in promoting healthy lifestyles, creating safe environments, and ensuring access to medical care. They must take steps to protect children from the leading threats to children's health (i.e., accidental injury and exposure to environmental toxins, abuse, and violence).

Accidental Injuries

After the first year of life, accidental injury (e.g., motor vehicle accidents, drowning, burning, and suffocation) is the leading cause of death in children. Motor vehicle accidents are the greatest danger to their life and health. Many injuries occur because adults fail to secure children in car seats and the most important step that a parent can take to ensure a child's safety in a motor vehicle is to correctly secure them into car seats for each and every ride.

Head injury from cycling and other sports is another leading cause of child death and disability. Although studies have shown that helmets reduce the risk of head injuries in biking accidents by 85%,

BOX 14-3

Toy-Related Injuries Among Children and Teenagers: United States, 1996

Although most toys are safe, children are at risk from toy-related injuries and death. During 1996, a total of 13 toy-related deaths and an estimated 117,000 nonfatal injuries among children requiring emergency department care were reported. Of those injuries, 65% occurred in males and 56% involved children from birth to age four. Most toy-related injuries (45%) were lacerations, but injuries also included abrasions or contusions (21%), ingestion or lodging of a foreign body (12%), fractures or dislocations (7%), and miscellaneous injuries (15%). Approximately two thirds of injuries occurred above the neck and involved the face, head, mouth, and eye.

Strategies recommended to prevent toy-related injuries include the following: use only age-appropriate toys; children should be directly supervised when playing with balloons, which result in 7 to 10 deaths each year, or in activities when potentially dangerous household objects are required; parents should ensure that toys are used in a safe and proper environment; and parents should be particularly cautious when children use projectile toys (e.g., dart guns).

The Child Safety Protection Act (PL 103-267, 1994) was designed to reduce toy-related choking and requires manufacturers to place choking hazard warning labels on balloons, marbles, small balls, and games with small parts intended for use only by children aged three and above. The Act also requires manufactures, importers, distributors, and retailers to report choking incidents involving such products to the Consumer Product Safety Commission.

From Centers for Disease Control and Prevention, US Public Health Service: Toy-related injuries among children and teenagers: United States, 1996, *Mor Mortal Wkly Rep* 46(50):1185-1189, 1997.

fewer than 5% of child riders wear helmets (American Academy of Pediatrics, 1995). Many children who survive serious motor vehicle and bicycle accidents suffer severe, permanent neurological damage. Box 14-3 discusses how toys can be another threat to small children.

Lead Poisoning

Lead poisoning is a preventable cause of childhood death, mental retardation, cognitive and behavioral problems, decreased growth, and neurological disabilities. Although the average blood lead level dropped over 80% since the late 1970s, nearly one million U.S. children have blood lead levels high enough to cause long-term health damage.

The great reduction of lead levels in both children and adults is among the greatest public health stories of the last half of the twentieth century. Over the past three decades, lead has been removed from the manufacture of gasoline, household paint, food and drink cans, and plumbing systems. Public health, legislative, and commercial measures tremendously reduced the problem of lead poisoning in the United States.

Lead is an invisible threat. The neurotoxic properties of lead have been apparent for at least a century, but the nature and extent of subtle long-term effects are newly realized. Unlike the obvious signs of measles or polio, it is difficult to recognize low-level lead poisoning in children. Lead poisoning affects virtually every system in the body and rarely yields distinctive symptoms.

Before 1950, lead-based paint was quite common, but the 1972 Lead Paint Poisoning Prevention Act limited the manufacture of lead-based paint. However, an estimated 42 million housing units in the United States still contain lead-based paint. Most of these units are located in poor, inner-city neighborhoods. Contamination can result from contact with paint dust or chips (e.g., raising and lowering windows) and from exposure to contaminated soil. Despite dramatic declines in blood lead levels for most U.S. populations, levels remain high among children in low-income families who live in older housing with lead-based paint. More than one fifth of nonHispanic black children living in older homes have elevated lead levels. To continue to help reduce the menace of lead poisoning, the CDC recommended blood lead screening for children who receive public assistance or for infants and toddlers who reside in, or frequently visit, pre1950s housing (CDC and PHS, 1997).

Immunization

Childhood immunization is a benchmark of child health. Maintaining appropriate immunization protects all members of the community, especially immuno-compromised individuals and pregnant wo-men who are particularly vulnerable to certain infectious diseases. Adequate immunization protects children against several diseases that killed or disabled many children in the past.

U.S. immunization levels have improved over the past decade. The federal USDHHS, state and local health departments, and health care providers administered the national Childhood Immunization Initiative of 1993 and the Vaccines for Prevention Program of 1994, which contributed to this improvement. In 1998, the United States achieved some of the highest rates of childhood immunization ever reported (i.e., 79% of children between 19 and 35 months of age received full immunization). The full range of childhood immunizations include vaccinations against the following:

- diphtheria,
- tetanus,
- pertussis,
- polio,
- measles,
- mumps,
- rubella,
- hepatitis B,
- Haemophilus influenzae type B (Hib), and
- varicella.

However, an estimated one million children are not fully immunized by age two and need one or more vaccinations to meet CDC guidelines (CDC and PHS, 1999). Typically, these children do not have a primary care provider, their families cannot pay for the immunizations and do not have access to free or reduced cost vaccinations, and their parents choose not to immunize their children.

Child Abuse and Neglect

Child abuse and neglect rates are other indicators of children's physical and emotional health status. In 1997, child protection agencies in 45 states received reports alleging the maltreatment of nearly three million children. Approximately half of the reports were from community professionals, which illustrates the important role nurses play in protecting children's safety.

An estimated 1000 children die each year from abuse and neglect. Most often the perpetrators of abuse and neglect are parents (USDHHS, 1999). Approximately one quarter of all reported cases involve children younger than four years. The two dominant characteristics of abusive parents are a history of substance abuse and abuse from their own parents. A very disturbing trend is the growing population of young children being raised by drug-abusing parents who are ill equipped to cope with the physical and psychological demands of caring for young children. Community organizations must become involved in preventing child abuse and creating a climate that supports families and provides alternatives to abusive behavior. Tragically, such services are in short supply in most communities.

ADOLESCENT HEALTH ISSUES

Adolescence is a time of generally good health. It is a period when adolescents form lifelong health habits including dietary and exercise habits and emotional health skills such as problem solving and coping strategies. Typically, adolescents do not use health services unless they have an underlying chronic condition or an acute illness. They rarely use preventive health services.

In their struggle to gain independence and with their sense of immortality, many adolescents engage in risk-taking behaviors that threaten their health, including alcohol and drug abuse, early and unprotected sexual activity, unsafe driving, and participation in delinquent and violent activities. The leading cause of death for those aged 15 to 24 years is unintentional injury, but the second and third leading causes of death for older children and young adults are homicide and suicide (Hoyert, Kochanek, and Murphy, 1999). Injury and violence are the leading threats to adolescent life and health. These "new morbidities" that adolescents face at the beginning of the twenty-first century are very different from those that threatened the health of this age group only a generation or two ago. The community health nurse can help parents and communities understand the nonmedical, public health nature of these morbidities and assist in developing community-wide strategies to effectively deal with them.

Violence

For too many of the nation's youth, violence is a way of life, a way of coping with challenging and difficult situations, and a significant public health problem. Nearly 13 children in America die each day from gunfire (Children's Defense Fund, 2000). Although violence is most predominant in inner cities, adolescents in suburbs and rural areas are increasingly faced with violence and its direct and indirect impact on the entire community.

African-American youths are at the greatest risk for homicides, suicides, and firearm accidents. Since 1978, homicide has been the leading cause of death among African-American males aged 15 to 24 years (Kochanek and Hudson, 1995).

Violence among youth is a multifaceted problem. It disproportionately affects minorities, but social factors such as unemployment and poverty strongly influence this excess (Durant et al., 1994). Factors such as gang exposure; violence in the home, in the media, and in the community; gun ownership; and child abuse, violence, or severe corporal punishment may socialize youth to viewing violence as an expected and unavoidable part of life.

Handguns are readily accessible to America's youth. Federal law prohibits anyone under age 21 from purchasing a handgun from a licensed dealer, but it does not prohibit anyone under age 21 from purchasing a handgun from a nonlicensed dealer. No one under age 18 is permitted to purchase or possess a handgun, but only 10 states prohibit the sale of handguns to individuals under age 21 (Children's Defense Fund, 2000).

Teen violence does not have simple remedies. Solutions require community and neighborhood efforts to help young people diffuse anger and frustrations before they escalate; help parents, religious organizations, and schools assist their youth in managing anger and resolving conflicts; and work with children and teenagers to assure them that they are loved, appreciated, and accepted for who they are and that help is available.

Adolescent Pregnancy and Childbearing

Adolescent childbearing is not a new phenomenon at all. What is new, at least since the 1930s, is the increase in out-of-wedlock birthrates. Years ago, the teenage birth rates were high, but teenagers were usually married before conception or by the time the infant was a young child. The proportion of premarital first births for women aged 15 to 19 years increased from 28% in the early 1930s to 89% in the early 1990s (Bachu, 1999).

Despite trends toward a lower teenage birth rate, **adolescent pregnancy** is a persistent and troubling problem. In the United States, over 880,000 girls and women under age 20 become pregnant each year (Ventura, Matthews, and Curtin, 1998). The great majority of teen pregnancies are unintended and over one third end in abortions (Henshaw, 1999).

Among white, Hispanic, and black teens, Hispanics have the highest birth rate. Although birth rates for African-American teens remain high compared with white teens, the African-American rate is falling faster than other races (Fig. 14-3) (Ventura, Matthews, And Curtin, 1998).

One of the many risk-taking adolescent behaviors is sexual intercourse among unmarried teenagers. Adolescent sexual activity is often unprotected and can result in pregnancy and STDs. Among high school students, the percentage of females who report having had sexual intercourse increases from 34% of ninth graders, to 62% of seniors. For males, the percentage increases from 42% of ninth graders, to 60% of seniors (CDC and PHS, 1997).

Several factors predispose a child to engage in sexual activity in the early teen years. These include a history of sexual abuse, poverty, early pubertal development, cultural and family patterns, lack of parental guidance, difficulties in school, and lack of school and career goals (Alan Guttmacher Institute, 1994; Carter et al., 1994; Jaskiewicz and McAnarney, 1994).

Sexually active teens report increased contraception use, which corresponds with a lower teen pregnancy rate. Contraception use at first intercourse has risen to 78% mostly because teens have increased their condom use (Moore, 1998). Increased condom use may be linked to the threat of AIDS infection. Sexually active teens who do not use contraceptives have a 90% chance of becoming pregnant within a year (Harlap, Kost, and Forrest, 1991).

Consequences of Early Childbearing and Parenting

The consequences of early childbearing are significant. Teen childbearing poses serious health risks to the infant, including death, prematurity, low birth weight, abuse, and neglect. Research studies disagree on the causes of poor pregnancy outcomes among teenagers, but most agree on the importance of socioeconomic factors associated with young age, such as lacking education, low income, and inadequate prenatal care rather than biological factors (Goldenberg and Klerman, 1995).

Adolescent childbearing and parenting often have long-term, negative consequences for both child and mother, including the following:

■ Children born to teenage parents are more likely to have poor health, school problems, low intelligence quotient test scores, and emotional problems; they often become teen parents themselves (Lewit, 1992).

FIGURE 14-3

U.S. adolescent birth rates by age, race, and Hispanic origin, 1997 (From Ventura SJ et al: Births: final data for 1997, *Natl Vital Stat Rep* 47[18], 1999).

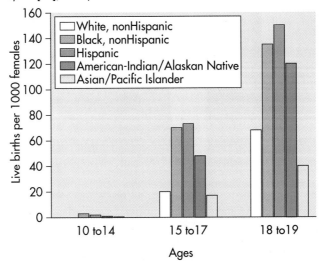

- Compared with those who begin parenting after age 20, adolescent parents are less likely to finish high school and less likely to gain employment.
- Teenage parents are more likely to have low incomes, face marital disruptions, and depend on welfare.

Adolescent Pregnancy Prevention Programs

The causes and effects of teen pregnancy are complex and the solutions are multifaceted. Primary prevention models are most successful when tailored to the community's individual needs. Components of such programs can include the following:

- abstinence promotion,
- education about contraception and its availability,
- sexual education,
- character development,
- problem solving skill development,
- strategies for ensuring teenagers' school success, and
- job training.

Such efforts benefit from partnerships between parents, adolescents, and agencies for health, education, religion, social service, and government. Nurses working within such organizations can play leadership roles in developing community programs for adolescent pregnancy prevention.

Sexually Transmitted Diseases

Every year, three million teenagers (i.e., about one in four sexually experienced teens) acquire an STD (Alan Guttmacher Institute, 1994). The most common STD among adolescents is chlamydia; gonorrhea is the second most common (CDC and PHS, 1998).

Although most STDs are treatable with antibiotics, they can have long-term health consequences. For women, untreated STDs can lead to pelvic inflammatory disease, ectopic pregnancy, cervical cancer, and infertility. Young men infected with STDs do not suffer the same health consequences as women because male symptoms typically appear earlier than female symptoms; men can obtain early treatment.

Not only is a woman's health affected, especially if the infections go untreated, but infants born to women with STDs are at risk of infection and can suffer long-term consequences. One of the most tragic is the perinatal transmission of HIV, which accounts for the majority of pediatric AIDS cases. Fortunately, the number of new pediatric AIDS cases from perinatal transmission declined significantly during the last decade from the increased use of zidovudine treatment during pregnancy. The American College of Obstetricians and Gynecologists now recommends routine HIV counseling and voluntary testing for all pregnant women.

Substance Abuse

Alcohol is the drug adolescents use and abuse most often. One in five adolescents aged 12 to 17 years are current drinkers (Substance Abuse and Mental Health Services Administration [SAMHSA], 1999). Teenage alcohol use is strongly associated with a number of health risks including early and unprotected sex, tobacco use, violence, and traffic fatalities.

Likewise, tobacco use is a prevalent and dangerous problem among adolescents. Smoking can lead to lung disease and cancer. Each day, approximately 3000 teenagers become smokers and an estimated one in five adolescents are cigarette smokers (CDC and PHS, 1996). Teenagers without college plans are more likely to smoke than teens with college plans; twelfth grade students are the most likely to smoke; and black teens are less likely to smoke than white teens (University of Michigan Institute for Social Research, 1998).

Nearly all initial tobacco use occurs before high school graduation (Elders et al., 1994). The Surgeon General's report to the nation (Elders et al., 1994) concluded the following:

- Most adolescent smokers are addicted to nicotine and report they want to quit but are unable to stop.
- Adolescents who have lower levels of school achievement, fewer skills to resist pervasive influences to use tobacco, lower self-images, and those who have friends who use tobacco are more likely to use tobacco than their peers.
- Cigarette advertising appears to increase young people's risk of smoking by affecting their perceptions of the image, pervasiveness, and function of smoking.

Illicit drug use is also too common among high school students. A national survey in 1998 found that nearly 10% of adolescents aged 12 to 17 used illicit drugs, specifically alcohol, marijuana, and cocaine. Fortunately, this rate was a significant decrease from the previous year's rate of 11.4%. The majority of adolescents reported that marijuana was easy to obtain. Of the adolescents surveyed, 14% reported that someone selling drugs approached them in the month before the survey (SAMHSA, 1999).

Adolescents perceive a low level of risk for illicit drugs in relation to the drug. Just under one third of adolescents believe marijuana use is risky and over one half believe cocaine use is risky (SAMHSA, 1999).

FACTORS AFFECTING CHILD AND ADOLESCENT HEALTH

Like all age groups, social, nonmedical factors largely determine children's health. Children are dependent on their families or caregivers for health and well-being; therefore the following factors significantly impact children's physical and mental health and overall well-being:

- parents' or caregivers' education, income, and stability;
- security and safety of the home;
- nutritional and environmental issues; and
- health care use.

Poverty

Poverty is the greatest threat to child health. Child poverty in the United States is higher than most other industrialized countries including Canada and most western European countries. Over 13 million of the nation's children, or nearly one in five, live below the poverty threshold (i.e., $16,660 for a family of four in 1998). One in every three black and Hispanic children is poor (Center on Budget and Policy Priorities [CBPP], 1999).

High economic growth in the late 1990s caused a significant reduction in overall poverty by 1998. However, children are disproportionately affected; children under age six are the poorest age group (Fig. 14-4). Those most at risk for poverty live in female-headed households, because over 55% of these children under age six live in poverty. For African-American children the rate is 60%; among Hispanic children the rate is 67%.

During the late 1990s, the Census Bureau reported that the gap between rich and poor families was at its widest recorded point (CBPP, 1999). By 1999, the wealthiest 2.7 million Americans (i.e., the top 1%) had as much money to spend as the poorest 100 million Americans did. That ratio has more than doubled in the past 20 years (CBPP, 1999).

Poverty alone does not always place a child at risk; children in higher income groups can also suffer similar health and related problems. However, poor children face the following health and socioeconomic risks that can compound the burdensome influence of poverty (Center for the Future of Children, 1997):

- Children in poverty have less access to nutritious food, shelter, and health care.
- Poor children are often deprived of advantages such as good schools, libraries, and other community resources.
- Deaths from unintended injuries, child abuse, homicide, SIDS, and infectious diseases including AIDS are more common among poor children.
- Many poor children live in substandard housing, have stressful home lives, may live surrounded by drugs and crime, and lack positive and nurturing adult role models.
- Poor children may feel hopeless about the future.
- Poor children often suffer from low birth weight, asthma, dental decay, elevated blood lead levels, learning disabilities, and teenage premarital childbearing.
- The extreme living conditions of poor children who are homeless or migrants usually compound their health problems.

FIGURE **14-4**

Percent of people in poverty by age group, 1998 (From US Census Bureau: *Current population survey,* Washington, DC, March 1999, The Author).

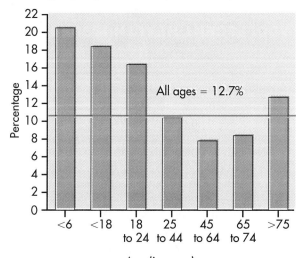

These social and economic burdens can be overwhelming to parents or caregivers and may cause them to neglect other matters such as providing a nutritious breakfast before school, taking a child for a well-child appointment, or getting his or her immunizations completed on schedule. They can create a sense of despair and hopelessness among parents and children, which greatly hinders healthy behavior. These factors clearly increase a child's physical and emotional health risks.

Single Parenting

Children in households headed by a single parent (usually the mother) are far more likely to live in poverty and 59% of these poor children live in homes headed by a single mother (Dalakar and Niafeh, 1998). Children living in single-parent households tend to score lower on many health indicators than those living in two-parent homes. These children are more likely to be exposed to drugs and alcohol before birth and do not have a regular source of health care (Klerman, 1991).

Parents' Educational Status

Children's health is also tied closely to their parent's education level. Low birth weight and infant mortality are more common in the children of less educated mothers. Women with higher education are more likely to obtain prenatal care, delay childbearing until after adolescence, and breast feed their babies. Women with less than 12 years of education are almost 10 times more likely to smoke during pregnancy than mothers with 16 years of education (NCHS, 1998; Ross, 1998).

Health Care Use

Children in low-income families are less likely to have a regular source of health care than children from more privileged families (NCHS, 1998). Children grow and develop rapidly between infancy and adolescence; therefore they are extremely vulnerable to the effects of illness and environmental factors that influence physical and emotional health. Preventive health and dental care offers children and parents a chance to periodically meet with a doctor or NP to address the following:

- discuss the child's growth and development,
- learn about good nutrition,

- receive immunizations and vision and hearing screening,
- learn about potential environmental threats to the child's health,
- begin prompt treatment for a condition if it is discovered during the exam, and
- ask other questions or obtain a referral if necessary.

Access to a regular health care source can facilitate prompt attention to *acute* medical problems, which can help prevent chronic, disabling conditions. For example, untreated ear infections can lead to hearing loss, which can lead to learning disabilities, school problems, and school dropout. Resulting low self-esteem can increase the likelihood for depression, behavior problems, early sexual activity, STDs, and unplanned pregnancy. Comprehensive, regular health care helps all children achieve their potential (Box 14-4).

BOX 14-4

The Medical Home

The American Academy of Pediatrics has long endorsed the concept of a "medical home." This ideal suggests that each child should have "accessible, continuous, comprehensive, family-centered, coordinated, and compassionate" health care (Dickens et al., 1992). A medical home has the following characteristics:

- the provision of preventive care,
- the assurance of ambulatory and inpatient care 24-hours-a-day,
- strategies and mechanisms to ensure continuity of care from infancy through adolescence, and
- appropriate use of subspecialty consultation and referrals.

Experts recommend that a health care provider should consistently examine children eight times during their first year, three times during their second year, and once a year until age six. This allows children and parents to build trusting relationships with their health care providers and enables providers to monitor growth and development.

Health Insurance Coverage

Children and pregnant women who have health care insurance are much more likely to obtain needed health care services (Newacheck et al., 1998). Although most children are insured through their parents' workplace, an increasing number of children are losing this coverage. The cost of health insurance has risen over the years and an increasing number of employers are no longer offering coverage for employees or their dependents. This is a more prevalent problem in small businesses and in businesses with mostly low wage earners. Between 1987 and 1995, the percentage of children with employment-based coverage fell from 67% to 59% (Employee Benefit Research Institute [EBRI], 1996).

Medicaid, the federal-state health coverage program for low-income families and individuals, covers a significant proportion of poor and near-poor children. However, Medicaid does not cover all these children. Over 14%, or nearly 11 million children, lack health insurance (EBRI, 1996). The **State Children's Health Insurance Program** (SCHIP), a publicly-subsidized health insurance program for children, formed in 1997 to help close the gap between higher-income and lower-income families whose children need insurance.

Children lack insurance or other health care coverage like Medicaid for many reasons. Some of these include the following:

- It is too expensive.
- Medicaid has a welfare stigma and parents do not want to be associated with it.
- Medicaid application forms and processes are complex, burdensome, and can intrude upon a family's privacy.
- Parents may not consider the importance of health insurance.
- Parents may not know their child is eligible for programs such as Medicaid or SCHIP.
- Applications and other information may not be available in the family's language.

Although insurance gives a child financial access to health care, some children may not obtain the health care they need. Numerous health care or family barriers can stand in the way, which may include the following:

- lack of transportation,
- misunderstanding or denial of the child's health problem,
- clinic hours that conflict with work or school schedules,
- overcrowded clinics with long delays in securing an appointment,
- long delays in the waiting room; often parents have more than one child in tow,
- competing family or personal priorities that reduce the importance of obtaining care,
- some doctors' unwillingness to see Medicaid or low-income patients, and
- parents' concerns that care providers are either unresponsive to their medical needs or interpersonally disrespectful.

To successfully meet the health needs of children and adolescents, especially those with known risk factors, the community health nurse must be cognizant of health care access issues, family and neighborhood influences, and other social concerns in a child's life. The nurse must be prepared to help the family solve problems, be their health care system advocate, and address the child's health needs.

STRATEGIES TO IMPROVE CHILD AND ADOLESCENT HEALTH

One of the most important ways to ensure the success and well-being of future generations is for each child to start life healthy and maintain their physical and emotional health status throughout childhood and adolescence. Since the beginning of the twentieth century, the nation has made remarkable progress in many areas of child and adolescent health, but the results are mixed. Fortunately, scientific, medical, environmental, parenting, and other knowledge can lessen or eliminate many of the problems. It is a matter of making these concerns a priority and taking the necessary steps to elicit change.

Healthy People 2010 and Child and Adolescent Health

Many professions establish goals and set measurable objectives. Educators use these techniques to organize their teaching materials, measure their students' progress, and evaluate the effectiveness of their teaching strategies and plans. Health care professionals use them for similar purposes in patient care. The individual community health nurse uses them in working with a family to ensure the nurse and family are organized and guided by common purposes. Goals and objectives help the nurse and family evaluate progress and make necessary midcourse corrections.

These strategies are also important at the macro level and the programmatic level, where multiple players must collaborate to address complicated statewide or national problems. In 1979, the Surgeon General of the United States embarked on an ambitious task of convening hundreds of public health experts, health care researchers, health professional organizations, and others to develop the first health goals and objectives for the nation. At each of the intervening decades, these groups have developed a new set of goals and objectives to help bring clear focus to the health concerns of the nation and to set measurable and attainable goals for different age groups and issues across the country.

Healthy People 2010 set broad national health goals for the first decade of the twenty-first century. This initiative, like its predecessors, helps define the nation's health agenda and guide policy development. *Healthy People 2010* addresses many challenges facing the country and will help the public and private sectors understand the nation's leading health problems, develop strategic plans for addressing them, and collaborate to reach common goals. Table 14-2 lists selected objectives from *Healthy People 2010* related to child and adolescent health.

Since the inception of the *Healthy People* initiative in 1979, child and adolescent health has improved. For instance, there has been a 50% improvement in infant mortality, a 40% improvement in child mortality, and a 26% improvement in adolescent and young adult mortality (Association of State and Territorial Health Officials [ASTHO], 1999).

Health Promotion and Disease Prevention

Health promotion and disease prevention is more significant and cost effective for children than for any other age group. Primary health care and early intervention for children and families can help prevent costly problems, suffering, and lost human potential. The following examples illustrate this need:

- Prenatal care, which can cost a few thousand dollars per pregnancy, can save hundreds of thousands of dollars by preventing conditions, such as low birth weight, that can require

expensive outpatient care, rehospitalization, special education, and special supplemental income for disabled children. A classic study by the IOM found that every dollar spent on prenatal care for high-risk women can save more than three dollars in medical care costs during the first year of an infant's life (IOM, 1985).

- Preventing pregnancy among school-aged mothers can reduce the dropout rate, welfare dependency, low birth weight, and infant mortality. Another classic cost-effectiveness study estimated that the public costs incurred in one year for families with adolescent parents total $16.65 billion in welfare payments, Medicaid, and food stamps (Burt and Levy, 1987).

Health promotion and disease prevention strategies for improving child and adolescent health come in many forms and originate in research institutions, public agencies, private businesses, and community-based organizations. They can include the following:

- clinical interventions;
- public health efforts that identify trends and develop population-based, community-wide, or individual strategies to affect these trends;
- philanthropic endeavors that fund initiatives at the community, state, and regional level for the purpose of testing a strategy or establishing an initiative; and
- public policy initiatives that create or improve public programs or provide incentives for nongovernmental entities to address identified problems.

PUBLIC HEALTH PROGRAMS TARGETED TO CHILDREN AND ADOLESCENTS

A number of public programs address the health needs of children and many help medically underserved or poor individuals specifically. In addition, local and state public health and social service agencies aim to protect the health of an entire community or state through programs such as water fluoridation, sanitation, and infectious disease control. Furthermore, broad-based strategies such as lead-based paint elimination, mandatory child safety seats in automobiles, bicycle helmet laws, lead-free gasoline, comprehensive school health clinics, and drug and violence prevention programs serve to improve the health of children through community-wide approaches.

TABLE 14-2

Selected *Healthy People 2010* Objectives: Child and Adolescent Health

Objective	Baseline (1998)	%Target
1-4b: Increase the proportion of children and youth aged 17 years and under who have a specific source of ongoing care	93%	96%
8-11: Eliminate elevated blood lead levels in children	4.5% of children aged one to five years	0
9-7: Reduce pregnancies among adolescent females	72 per 1000 females aged 15 to 17 years	46 per 1000 females aged 15 to 17 years
9-8a: Increase the proportion of adolescent females who have never engaged in sexual intercourse before age 15 years	81%	88%
13-17: Reduce new cases of perinatally acquired HIV infection	NA	NA
14-4: Reduce bacterial meningitis in young children	13.0 per 100,000	8.6 per 100,000
14-22a: Achieve and maintain effective vaccination coverage levels for universally recommended vaccines among young children (i.e., four doses of DtaP vaccine)	84%	90%
15-20: Increase use of child restraints	92%	100%
15-39: Reduce weapon carrying by adolescents on school property	8.5%	6%
16-1a: Reduce fetal and infant deaths during perinatal period (i.e., 28 weeks of gestation to seven days or more after birth)	7.5 per 1000	4.5 per 1000
16-15: Reduce the occurrence of spina bifida and other NTDs	6 per 10,000 live births	3 per 10,000 live births
18-2: Reduce the rate of suicide attempts by adolescents	2.6% per year	1% per year
19-3a: Reduce the proportion of children aged 6 to 11 years who are overweight or obese	11%	5%
21-1b: Reduce the proportion of children with dental caries experienced either in their primary or permanent teeth	52%	42%
22-11: Increase the proportion of children and adolescents who view television two or fewer hours per day	60%	75%
24-2a: Reduce hospitalizations for asthma in children under age five years	60.9 per 10,000	25 per 10,000
26-10: Reduce past-month use of illicit substances by adolescents aged 12 to 17	77%	89%
27-2a: Reduce tobacco use by adolescents in grades 9 to 12	43%	21%
28-12: Reduce otitis media in children and adolescents	344.7 visits per 1000	294 visits per 1000

From US Department of Health and Human Services: *Healthy people 2010: conference edition,* Washington, DC, 2000, USDHHS.

Health Care Coverage Programs

Medicaid

The ability to pay for health care greatly influences whether a parent takes a child to see a doctor or NP. This is especially true for preventive care. Access to health care services has significantly improved since the introduction of Medicaid and the **Early and Periodic Screening, Diagnosis, and Treatment** (EPSDT) program in the mid1960s. State and federal governments jointly finance Medicaid and Medicaid pays for health care services delivered to eligible individuals (i.e., primarily those receiving welfare payments). In the late 1980s, Congress and states passed legislation that expanded Medicaid eligibility for pregnant women, infants, and children in higher income groups in an effort to improve the nation's infant mortality rate and children's health status.

Over the years, Medicaid has become a primary payer for prenatal care and deliveries. Across the states, Medicaid now pays for 38% of all births (National Governors' Association, 1999). By 1997, Medicaid covered close to 23% of all children under age 18. Contrary to popular belief, all poor people do not have Medicaid coverage. Only 61% of poor children under age 18 have Medicaid coverage (EBRI, 1998).

Through the EPSDT program, a child covered by Medicaid can receive a range of health and health-related services beginning in infancy. The program's services far exceed those usually covered by private insurance, including the following:

- health, developmental, and nutritional screening;
- physical examinations;
- immunizations;
- vision and hearing screening;
- certain laboratory tests; and
- dental services.

Not all Medicaid-eligible children are enrolled in the program. The families, the Medicaid application and enrollment process, or the health care system present many barriers. These barriers are similar to those discussed earlier concerning insurance coverage.

State Children's Health Insurance Program

Again, Medicaid does not cover all poor children, nor does it cover children in the "gap group," (i.e., children whose family income is above Medicaid limits but do not receive health insurance through their parents' employment). This population group is often called the working poor. Over 14% of all children, or nearly 11 million, are uninsured and nearly all are in working poor families (EBRI, 1998).

How to insure the uninsured has been a perplexing public policy issue for years. However, in August 1997, Congress passed SCHIP into law with the support of the President, the states, countless organizations, advocacy groups, individuals, and others in an effort to solve this problem for children in working poor families. This program is the single largest public investment in children's health since the creation of the Medicaid program. Between federal fiscal years 1998 and 2003, SCHIP will allocate $24 billion in federal funds to states that choose to expand their Medicaid programs, establish a new insurance program for this group of children, or design a combination program using both approaches.

Direct Health Care Delivery Programs

Although Medicaid and SCHIP finance health care for their enrollees like private insurance, several other public programs deliver health care services directly to underserved populations. Most underserved aggregates live in inner cities or rural areas with few health care providers and facilities. Some have Medicaid, SCHIP, or insurance coverage, but many are uninsured.

Maternal and Child Health Block Grant

The Maternal and Child Health (MCH) Block Grant program has its roots in a number of smaller, categorical grant programs consolidated in 1981. The MCH Block Grants Program provides funds to the states for maternal and child health care. The MCH Block Grant program (also called Title V, because it is the fifth section, or title, of the Social Security Act) allocates federal funds to the states and the states must contribute their own funds.

In most states, these resources are combined with local funding to help ensure the delivery of basic health care to pregnant women and children and help deliver additional services to children with special health care needs. Title V agencies in state health departments also monitor the health status of mothers and children throughout their respective states and work with other state agencies to develop programs to improve the health of this population.

Community and Migrant Health Centers Programs

The Community and Migrant Health Centers Programs began in 1965 and were two of the early programs of the U.S. Office of Economic Opportunity. Through a network of approximately 550 centers that operate more than 2000 clinics, these health centers provide comprehensive primary health care to more than six million low-income people. Children under age 15 compose 2.1 million of this low-income group. Health centers are located in medically underserved areas, which are mostly rural and inner-city areas. Health centers often obtain funds from sources including local governments, foundations, corporations, and clients.

National Health Service Corps

The National Health Service Corps (NHSC) is another federal program that helps children receive primary health care services. The NHSC sends physicians, nurses, and other health care providers to underserved areas of the country. The program assists students with medical, nursing, and other training through scholarships and loan repayment plans if they agree to provide a certain number of service years in a rural or urban underserved area.

Although the NHSC funds were substantially reduced in the 1980s, Congress increased its funding in the early 1990s. This increase was in response to the continued lack of health care providers, especially obstetrical providers, in certain parts of the country.

School-Based and School-Linked Health Services

Adolescents are the least likely aggregate to use health care services, especially preventive services. Their adolescent health care needs are different from their childhood needs and they are often uncomfortable seeing a pediatrician or their childhood provider. Furthermore, they can discuss sensitive topics such as puberty, contraception, and peer relationships with their parents. They may not want their parents to know they have a health problem; therefore they may not want to see the family's health care provider out of concern for privacy and confidentiality. This can cause their health care needs to go unmet.

The school-based health movement began in the 1970s in a St. Paul, Minnesota high school. Since then, school-based health clinics have grown in both numbers and in the variety of available services. In the 1997 to 1998 school year, nearly 1200 school-based health centers operated across the country and most were located in the midAtlantic and New England states (Lear et al., 1999). Although centers are more common in high schools, they are spreading to elementary and middle schools. More conservative areas of the country are somewhat reluctant to allow adolescent health care at or near schools.

State dollars, mostly from general funds and the MCH Block Grant, are the primary sources of funding for school-based health care. An increasing number of health centers participate in the Medicaid and SCHIP programs and some provide services within a managed care network (Lear et al., 1999).

Women, Infants, and Children Program

Although it is not a health program exclusively, **Women, Infants, and Children** (WIC) provides highly nutritious foods and nutrition education to more than seven million low-income pregnant and breast-feeding mothers, their infants, and their children under age five each month (Food and Nutrition Service and US Department of Agriculture, 1999). To be eligible, women and children must meet income guidelines established by each state and a health professional must determine they are at "nutritional risk." Women and children who participate in Medicaid, the Food Stamp program, or the Temporary Assistance for Needy Families program are automatically income eligible for WIC.

Women participating in the program are encouraged to obtain prenatal care if they are pregnant. They also are encouraged to maintain healthy diets and obtain preventive health care for themselves and their children, including childhood immunizations. WIC participants receive checks or vouchers to purchase specific, nutritious foods. Most grocery stores and supermarkets participate in WIC and carry the foods designated by the program.

Established in 1972, WIC is one of the most successful, popular, and cost-effective public health programs. The benefits of WIC are tremendous. The rate of low birth weight births among infants born to women on WIC is 25% lower than for infants born to similarly-situated women not on WIC. Medicaid costs are lower for pregnant women on WIC (Food and Nutrition Service and US Department of Agriculture, 1999).

Although the level of WIC funding does not allow it to serve all eligible individuals, its reach has grown dramatically since it began over two decades ago. In 1998, about 81% of eligible women, infants, and children participated in WIC. Federal funding for WIC was $3.94 billion in fiscal year 1999.

Head Start

Formed in 1965, **Head Start** is a comprehensive, federally-funded early childhood program for low-income children aged three to five years. In 1994, Congress created Early Head Start, which serves children from birth to age three. Together, these programs are comprehensive child-development programs that aim to increase the school readiness of young children in low-income families. They provide educational opportunities and medical, dental, mental health, nutritional, and social services. They strongly emphasize parental involvement on a voluntary or paid-staff basis.

The Head Start Bureau in the USDHHS administers Head Start and Early Head Start. The Bureau awards grants to local public agencies, private non-profit organizations, Native-American groups, and school systems. The grantee organizations provide a range of services in the following areas:

- education and early childhood development;
- medical, dental, and mental health;
- nutrition; and
- parental involvement.

Head Start has served nearly 18 million children since its inception in 1965. Although it is a successful program, it does not reach all eligible children. Congress has steadily increased the funding level in an attempt to reach the goal of full enrollment for both Head Start and Early Head Start. Their fiscal year 1999 funding level was $4.66 billion (Administration on Children and Families, 1999).

SHARING RESPONSIBILITY FOR IMPROVING CHILD AND ADOLESCENT HEALTH

Most children in the United States are born healthy and remain healthy throughout childhood. However, the protective factors operating in the lives of healthy children and the interventions they receive are not available to all children. Although public sector programs have attempted to provide a "safety net" for children, these interventions cannot address all the children's needs. For example, the health care system may provide emergency care to a nine-year-old child injured by gunfire in a drive-by shooting, but it cannot address the community conditions that perpetuate violence.

Child health is affected by many factors; therefore the responsibility for improving children's health rests with the entire community. This responsibility begins with parents and includes health care professionals, community groups, businesses, and the public sector. When a child gets older, he or she can be responsible for practicing healthy behaviors and obtaining proper health care on his or her own.

Parents' Role

Even before conception, a mother is responsible for ensuring the health of her fetus. Before and during pregnancy, she should develop healthy behaviors including proper nutrition and avoidance of tobacco, alcohol, drugs, and other behaviors that could harm her developing baby. This is particularly important in the early stages of gestation when fetal organ systems are developing. It is also important for the mother to receive prenatal care early in pregnancy.

Starting with breast feeding, parents must give their children nutritious food and ensure that they are immunized, receive needed health care services, and acquire healthful lifestyles. It is important that parents model healthy behaviors for their children.

Another important task for parents is to ensure their children have a safe environment at home, in the neighborhood, and at school. They must protect their children from injury, violence, abuse, and neglect. Parents must learn how to nurture, guide, and protect their children effectively through the developmental stages of childhood.

Community's Role

Families need support from their community and society to fulfill their roles and responsibilities. This is particularly true for families who live in poverty and for parents who are isolated and disenfranchised. Ensuring access to health care is an important community role, but communities are responsible for promoting well-being, which goes far beyond the provision of traditional medical care.

Communities should work to create safe neighborhoods and support the development of community-based, comprehensive health, education, and social service programs. Also, communities can promote community health education campaigns concerning prenatal care, smoking, nutrition, teenage pregnancy, drug and violence prevention, and other health topics. Communities and community organizations can sponsor health fairs, immunization drives, car safety seat checks, bicycle safety helmet campaigns, crime prevention and reduction programs, and other projects that help families develop healthy lifestyles and gain access to needed health services.

Communities are well situated to facilitate the integration of health, education, and social services; to eliminate fragmentation and duplication of services; and to better organize more comprehensive and streamlined systems of care. Although many health and social service programs exist, they are usually poorly coordinated with each other and there is little collaboration among the professional disciplines. Through public awareness campaigns, communities can facilitate the integration and coordination of services. For example, these initiatives can alert parents about the importance of immunizations, a safer environment, prenatal care, and other services and can inform families about how and where to obtain these services.

The media is part of the community at large and should be involved in promoting child health. The media significantly influences children's lives, their perceptions of the world, and their self-image. From developing informational campaigns about prenatal care and immunizations, to discouraging violence and explicit sex in advertising and popular television programs, the media can have a profound effect on improving children's health and well-being.

Employer's Role

Business and industry have an enormous stake in the health of the nation's children. A strong, productive workforce is ensured only when the health, social, and educational needs of the next generation of workers are met. Furthermore, health risks cost employers in lost productivity and increased health care costs.

The private sector can play a role in improving the health of individual children or the community in general. An employer can make health care more accessible to families with children by offering affordable health insurance that covers employees and dependents. The provision of insurance plans that offer full pregnancy and well-child health care benefits is essential to employee health promotion.

Maintaining a work place that allows flexible leave for prenatal and pediatric health care and allows time off to care for newborn and sick children can also contribute to child health improvements. In 1993, the Family and Medical Leave Act mandated that employers with 50 or more employees must allow a total of 12 work weeks of unpaid leave during any 12-month period for the birth or adoption of a child or for the care of a sick family member.

In addition, employers can sponsor education opportunities for employees about healthy diets, healthy pregnancies, substance abuse, and stress management. Also, businesses can offer on-site child care and can work with community leaders and public officials to initiate community-wide health promotion

projects targeted to children. Finally, employers can be catalysts for linking health, education, and social services for children.

Government's Role

In the United States, government's role in promoting or ensuring children's health is more limited than many other countries. Other countries often have defined policies on children's health; the United States does not. Not only do such policies indicate that children are a priority of the citizenry, they also help shape the operation of programs and their funding.

As discussed earlier, U.S. state and federal governments have several public health programs that provide assistance to children, especially to those at risk from poverty or other disadvantages. Although these programs are not a substitute for a family's or caregiver's care and concern, they are important in protecting and promoting health and delivering services to those who would otherwise go without. Although many programs with significant funding exist, many children with health problems do not receive the services they need.

Managers and front-line workers (e.g., community health nurses, social workers, physicians, and caseworkers) in effective community programs should be encouraged to collaborate and thereby assist children with problems that adversely impact their health. "One-stop shopping" (i.e., user-friendly, accessible services for children and families) is an important concept for public programs to embrace to ensure that children easily receive needed services, especially preventive health and social services, before a problem becomes a crisis. Outreach efforts should be an integral part of health initiatives to provide children in need with the services they require. Community health nurses are often an essential part of these outreach efforts.

Community Health Nurse's Role

Public health nurses have always played pivotal roles in improving the health status of pregnant women and children. Within the community, the community health nurse is often most aware of children's health status, any barriers that prevent children from receiving necessary care, and other factors that may adversely affect their health. Armed with this information and knowledge about available health resources in the community, the community health nurse is an advocate for improved individual and community responses to children's needs, a participant in publicly funded programs, a promoter of social interventions that enhance the living situations of high-risk families, and a partner with other professionals to improve service collaboration and coordination.

One important role of the community health nurse is to help link local health and social services with the school system. Children must be healthy to learn; however, children often come to school with vision, hearing, and other health problems that appropriate education, screening, and treatment could have prevented or alleviated. When children pass the preschool years, sometimes the school health nurse is their only connection to the health care system. School health nurses can be an important source of primary health care and health information for students and their families.

Community health nurses can alert the health professional community, business leaders, religious groups, and voluntary organizations to children's needs and the strategies that can improve their health. Community health nurses, both individually and in groups, can influence the planning and implementation of necessary changes in the health care system to ensure improved children's health and to achieve the national health goals for the year 2010. Also, they can promote commitment within their own institutions for comprehensive, one-stop, user-friendly health services.

LEGAL AND ETHICAL ISSUES IN CHILD AND ADOLESCENT HEALTH

Every day, community health nurses are involved in making decisions. In each encounter with a patient, the nurse's decisions or the family's choices have the potential to impact the health and well-being of the family or the community at large for better or for worse.

People often assume that health care professionals, particularly nurses, are by nature attuned to the ethical implications of their decisions. In addition, the community trusts that nurses are aware of the legal ramifications of their actions and decisions, of their client's decisions, and of the health care and legal systems' decisions. In reality, the ever-changing pressures of serving the community's health care needs leave little time to reflect on the ethical and moral implications of a given situation. In some cases,

it may seem easier to avoid tough decisions. An ethical approach to decision making allows the community health nurse to evaluate a patient's needs or a population's needs more honestly and completely and take appropriate action. Understanding the legal environment will help the nurse make informed decisions and assist clients with their decision-making processes more effectively.

Ethical Issues

The complex nature of public health and health care delivery environments often sets the stage for conflicts of interest and values. Meanwhile, nurses and other health professionals must work within the system to improve child and adolescent health in a country of great differences. Such differences exist between races and cultures and great dichotomies, such as the affluence of some and the poverty of many others. The scope of ethical and legal dilemmas is broad, but the issues that community health nurses often see include the following:

- Allocation decisions: Given limited time and resources, what level of care should a nurse offer a child and his or her family?
- Patient autonomy: In each specific case, who should make health care decisions for a young patient, especially when opposing opinions arise? The patient? The parents or guardians? The nurse or other health care professional? At what age does a child become mature enough to participate in such decision making? What laws does any given state have that affect adolescent patient autonomy? What should the community health nurse do if he or she believes the patient's or parent's decisions are not in the best interest of the patient?
- Privacy and confidentiality: Is an intervention appropriate if the community health nurse identifies gross noncompliance, neglect, or abuse? Is it appropriate if the nurse must break confidentiality? When and how should the nurse take action?
- "Gaming the system": When the health care system's rules appear to impede the nurse's ability to serve the patient's best interest, is it acceptable to circumvent the system? If so, what are the moral and legal costs?
- Cultural competence: The United States will continue to experience huge demographic changes and increased diversity; nurses will face different

cultural definitions of what is and what is not acceptable or ethical. How should the community health nurse respond to a patient or population group that does not share the same cultural outlook on health? What is the nurse's legal justification, if any, for responding in a certain way?

These issues invariably involve value judgments and challenge a nurse's bounds of professional and personal duty. They also require the community health nurse to stay abreast of legislative changes at the local, state, and national levels and participate in professional activities that can help him or her stay current in these important matters.

Affecting Outcomes

Nurses will always address sensitive issues that require careful consideration and an effective plan of action. By recognizing the ethical implications of the care and advice they give or the actions they take, nurses can embrace their duty to promote the health and well-being of individual patients and the community more completely, protect their patients from harm, and strive for health care fairness and justice for all patients.

Recognizing the value of engaging in a shared dialogue with colleagues regarding ethical decision-making issues and understanding the possible legal implications of their decisions are equally important. The choices can be complex; therefore receiving the guidance of an ethics board or gaining a second opinion can be critical to making the right choices. On a broader scale, a community health nurse's ethical perspective can enhance any discussion about individual patient care and overall community health and it could impact the direction of the country's public health policy.

CASE STUDY

APPLICATION OF THE NURSING PROCESS

By applying the principles of the nursing process to the individual, family, and community, the community health nurse can provide services to children and adolescents more systematically and effectively. Most communities offer a range of preventive services and other important programs that children need. The community health nurse must thoroughly understand the needs of the individual child and family and must be aware of available community resources to help meet the child's health needs.

Maria Martinez, a community health nurse working for the county health department, received a call from the high school nurse informing her that a 16-year-old high school student named Tara Parkhurst would come in that afternoon for a pregnancy test. Tara had already missed three menstrual periods and was afraid to talk about it with her family. She had a long discussion with the school nurse and asked her boyfriend to take her to the health department clinic after school for the pregnancy test.

Assessment

Tara's pregnancy test was positive and she was an estimated three months pregnant. She was upset and would not speak with Maria at the health department. Maria arranged to make a home visit the next afternoon.

The school nurse told Maria that Tara wanted to keep her baby and Tara's family struggled financially. Tara and her siblings participated in the free and reduced lunch program at school. Knowing that she needed to address a number of issues at the first home visit, Maria prepared by developing a list of possible assessment areas that covered individual, family, and community concerns. Her list included the following:

Individual
- Medical risk factors
- Emotional well-being
- Cultural beliefs and attitudes toward pregnancy and medical care

- Barriers to communication with providers such as language, hearing, or sight
- Understanding and acceptance of pregnancy
- Health-promoting and risk-taking behaviors
- Understanding the importance of obtaining preventive care services
- Health insurance status
- Access to transportation

Family

- Adequacy of housing structure
- Safety of neighborhood
- Ability of family members to provide emotional support
- Ability of family to provide financial support

Community

- Availability of affordable and local prenatal and pediatric care
- Health and social services coordination
- Availability of culturally sensitive health care
- Emotional guidance and counseling
- Educational opportunities for pregnant and parenting teenagers
- Job training
- Nutrition services such as WIC and food stamps
- Pregnancy and parenting education
- Child care availability

Assessment Data

Individual

- The client was already in the early second trimester of pregnancy and did not receive prenatal care. She engaged in risk-taking behaviors (i.e., smoking, alcohol use, and poor eating habits).
- During the interview, Tara seemed quiet and reserved. She said she was excited to have a baby, but she feared labor and delivery. Her boyfriend wanted her to keep the baby.
- She said she did not think about prenatal care much, but would probably visit a health clinic sometime before her delivery. Her family did not have health insurance and she said they could not afford prenatal care.
- She wanted to keep the baby and remain in

school, yet she did not have a realistic understanding of parental responsibilities.

Family

- When Tara told her parents she was pregnant, they expressed disappointment. Her mother voiced a willingness to provide emotional support, but her seemingly emotionally-distant father expressed anger.
- Both parents expressed concern about how the family would manage financially.
- After a brief review of the family's financial situation, it appeared that Tara was eligible for either Medicaid or SCHIP.

Community

- Maria determined that prenatal services were available, but only during school hours. Although the only clinic that accepted Medicaid patients was on the other side of town, a nearby obstetrical practice with a certified NM on staff accepted patients with SCHIP coverage. However, their primary clientele was middle class, married women.
- Applying for Medicaid or SCHIP coverage and the WIC program required her to go to the welfare office and apply during school hours. However, the hospital outpatient department could make a preliminary Medicaid or SCHIP eligibility determination, which might be more convenient.
- Although Medicaid and SCHIP would pay for some prenatal classes, those nearby were geared to older, married couples.
- Tara's school encouraged her to remain in regular classes until her delivery date and participate in home study for a limited time thereafter.
- No parenting classes geared towards adolescents were available.
- Child care was not available at the high school, which made returning to school more difficult for Tara.
- Although the community has a lay home visitor program that matches mentors with pregnant and parenting teens and provides health information and encouragement, the project does not serve Tara's neighborhood. *Continued*

Diagnosis

Individual

- Altered health maintenance related to the lack of prenatal care and the effect of poor nutrition, smoking, and alcohol use on fetal development.
- Altered parenting potential related to unrealistic expectations about parenting responsibilities.
- Knowledge deficit of infant and child safety issues such as the use of child safety seats, prevention of lead poisoning, advantages of breast feeding, and use of preventive health care including immunization.

Family

- Altered family processes related to anger and disappointment over daughter's pregnancy.
- Altered financial status resulting from the addition of another dependent to the family.

Community

- Lack of coordinated, culturally sensitive, accessible prenatal and parenting services for adolescents.
- The existing Resource Mother (i.e., home visiting) program is a community strength, but the project must expand to reach all at-risk adolescents.

Planning

To ensure the action plan is complete, realistic, and successfully implemented, Maria must thoroughly identify the factors affecting Tara's health and well-being. In addition, Tara, her family, and Maria must set mutual goals.

Individual

Long-Term Goal

- Pregnancy outcome will be healthy for mother and infant.

Short-Term Goals

- Tara will obtain prenatal care.
- Tara will understand the reasons to change nutrition and substance use habits.

- Tara and the nurse will plan actions to change poor health habits.

Long-Term Goal

- Tara will demonstrate successful parenting behaviors.

Short-Term Goal

- Tara will enroll in parenting class. If classes are not available, she will use reading materials, films, videotapes, or visits with experienced parents.
- Tara will breast feed her baby.
- Tara will speak with the community health educator to determine methods to protect the health and safety of her newborn.

Long-Term Goal

- Tara will complete high school.

Short-Term Goal

- Tara will remain in school throughout her pregnancy and will use the home study program until she returns to school after her baby is born.

Family

Long-Term Goal

- The family's ability to handle crises will improve with their ability to discuss problems and engage in mutual problem solving.

Short-Term Goal

- Tara's parents will display supportive behaviors such as accompanying her to prenatal care appointments, helping her engage in healthy behaviors, and helping her arrange child care to remain in school.

Community

Long-Term Goal

- Accessible, comprehensive, culturally sensitive prenatal and other health care services will form, including home visiting and parenting classes targeted to adolescents.

Short-Term Goals

- The health department clinic will extend evening hours to accommodate students and working families.
- A child care facility will open in or near the high school.

Intervention

The nurse, family, and individual must address their immediate, mutual goals to help Tara achieve a healthy birth outcome and begin successful parenting. In addition, the nurse must be an advocate for community-wide change to ensure that the community is meeting individuals' needs.

To achieve aggregate-level goals, the community health nurse must communicate individuals' needs to program managers, community leaders, policymakers, and others in decision-making roles. For example, the health department director may not be aware that prenatal services are not readily available to high-risk groups of women such as adolescents. By bringing this information and possible solutions to the director's attention, clinics can expand their hours to benefit both pregnant teenagers and pregnant working women.

Likewise, it is in the best interest of the pregnant teenager, her child, her family, and the community for her to remain in school and obtain her high school diploma. The community health nurse is in an ideal role to stimulate dialogue about the consequences of dropping out of high school and facilitate action in policies such as child care for parenting teenagers to help them remain in school.

Evaluation

Evaluation strategies must involve both process and outcome measures on the individual, family, and community levels. For example, evaluating a strategy for an individual might entail considering processes (e.g., the number of prenatal appointments kept by the pregnant woman) or outcomes (e.g., whether the infant was born at full term). Evaluating a strategy at the community level requires assessing whether programs were established (e.g., an evening prenatal clinic) and whether the programs' establishment led to improved outcomes (e.g., a reduced rate of preterm births or a reduced dropout rate by adolescent mothers).

Levels of Prevention

Prevention is more important for children than any other aggregate. In particular, primary prevention strategies such as early prenatal care, good nutrition, and healthy behaviors among pregnant women help ensure that a child is born healthy and has a healthy start in life.

Primary

Primary prevention depends largely on the child's age. For the youngest children, strategies include preconception counseling and the practice of healthy behaviors by mothers before pregnancy and by parents and their children. Primary prevention also includes the prevention of unwanted pregnancy, which is especially important for adolescents.

Secondary

Once pregnant, the woman must receive early and adequate prenatal care, practice healthy behaviors, obtain necessary social and supportive services, and prepare herself for becoming a parent. Although the woman and her family are responsible for many of these practices, it is incumbent on the community to ensure that adequate preventive health services such as prenatal care, nutrition and dietary counseling, pregnancy and parent education, and social services are available. The community health nurse can alert community leaders to the individual and societal consequences of women not receiving prenatal care or of teenagers not completing high school because child care responsibilities are overwhelming. This information can help planners design programs and policies that are in the best interest of individuals and society.

Tertiary

Tertiary prevention involves the rehabilitation of individuals and aggregates to maximize potential functioning. In the case of adolescent pregnancy, the community health nurse is in an ideal position to initiate programs and services that prevent future unwanted pregnancy among teenagers and help the parenting teenager provide the best possible care to the child. These programs could include the establishment of parenting classes and support services to help adolescents complete their education; coordination of health and social services for the mother and her child, including family planning services; and the establishment of well-child care, immunizations, and nutrition services.

SUMMARY

Child and adolescent health status remains an important indicator of the nation's health. Child and adolescent health problems are a reflection of rapidly changing social conditions, not isolated events. Despite generally improving trends in health for most children, community health nurses must address discrepancies that exist between racial and ethnic groups. Poverty is the basis for many continuing health problems among children in this country and nurses must recognize and treat it as such.

The best way to ensure the success and well-being of future generations is for each child to begin life healthy and maintain that health status throughout childhood. Any health problem (e.g., hunger, poor vision or hearing, increased lead blood levels, asthma, anemia, dental caries, illicit drug use, or teen pregnancy) can interfere with school attendance, academic success, normal growth and development, learning ability, and life success.

The prevention of health problems is most significant and cost effective for children. Each dollar spent on the prevention of physical and emotional problems in children is a sound investment. Primary health care and early intervention for children and families can help prevent costly problems, suffering, and lost human potential.

Community health nurses can use their experience and "inside knowledge" of child health barriers to educate others. Rather than limiting their approach to caring for the individual and family only, community health nurses can maximize their roles to collaborate and forge necessary alliances to solve children's health problems. Nurses are authority figures in the least-expected places. Working on health care's front line is a powerful and very real position to members of Congress, state legislators, mayors, and others. By creatively using this kind of power, community health nurses can contribute greatly to improving the health and well-being of all children.

LEARNING ACTIVITIES

1. Examine infant mortality statistics in the community and compare the rates with state and national averages. Is infant mortality higher for any particular racial or ethnic group within the community?

2. Determine how a pregnant teenager without finances or available transportation would obtain prenatal care.

3. Accompany a pregnant woman to a local department of social services and observe as she tries to establish Medicaid eligibility for herself and her unborn child.

4. Develop strategies to inform parents whose children are uninsured about the availability of SCHIP.

5. Spend a day with a school health nurse and analyze what could help prevent the health problems and issues he or she encountered throughout the day.

6. Survey businesses in the community to determine whether they offer maternity health insurance benefits, paid or unpaid maternity or paternity leave for new parents, and leave for prenatal care appointments. Use this information to develop a strategy to encourage family-friendly policies and practices in the business community.

7. If the community has a lay home visitor program, meet with a home visitor and, if possible, accompany him or her during home visits.

8. Communicate with those in policy-making positions by writing letters or holding meetings about children's needs.

9. Identify the public health and advocacy organizations in the community that are working to address children's health needs and identify their strategies for promoting child health within the community.

REFERENCES

Administration on Children and Families: *Head start research and statistics: 1999 head start fact sheet,* November 22, 1999, The Author, www2.acf.dhhs.gov/programs/hsb/about/99_hsfs.htm.

Alan Guttmacher Institute: *Sex and America's teenagers,* New York, 1994, Alan Guttmacher Institute.

American Academy of Pediatrics, Committee on Injury and Poisoning Prevention: bicycle helmets, *Pediatrics* 95: 609-610, 1995.

Association of State and Territorial Health Officials: Healthy people initiative to launch nation's health goals for the new century, *ASTHO Report* 7(2), 1999.

Bachu A: *Trends in premarital childbearing: 1930 to 1994,* Washington, DC, 1999, US Census Bureau.

Burt MR, Levy F: Estimates of public costs of teenage childbearing: a review of recent studies and estimates on 1985 public costs. In Hofferth SJ, Hayes CD, editors: *Risking the future: adolescent sexuality, pregnancy, and childbearing,* vol 2, Washington, DC, 1987, National Academy Press.

Carter DM et al: When children have children: the teen pregnancy predicament, *Am J Prev Med* 10:108-113, 1994.

Center for the Future of Children: *Children and poverty,* vol 7(2), Los Altos, Calif, Summer/Fall, 1997, The David and Lucille Packard Foundation.

Center on Budget and Policy Priorities: *Low unemployment, rising wages fuel poverty decline: concerns remain amidst the good news,* Washington, DC, 1999, The Author.

Centers for Disease Control and Prevention, US Public Health Service: *National immunization survey: July 1997 to June 1998,* Atlanta, 1999, USDHHS, National Immunization Program.

Centers for Disease Control and Prevention, US Public Health Service: Recommendations for the use of folic acid to reduce the number of cases of spina bifida and other neural tube defects, *Mor Mortal Wkly Rep* RR-14, 1992.

Centers for Disease Control and Prevention, US Public Health Service: *Screening young children for lead poisoning: guidance for state and local public health officials,* Atlanta, 1997, USDHHS.

Centers for Disease Control and Prevention, US Public Health Service: *STD surveillance: 1997,* Atlanta, 1998, USDHHS.

Centers for Disease Control and Prevention, US Public Health Service: The great American smokeout: November 21, 1996, *Mor Mortal Wkly Rep* 45(44):961, 1996.

Centers for Disease Control and Prevention, US Public Health Service: Toy-related injuries among children and teenagers: United States, 1996, *Mor Mortal Wkly Rep* 46(50):1185-1189, 1997.

Children's Defense Fund: *Yearbook 2000: the state of America's children,* Washington, DC, 2000, The Author.

Cunningham J, Dockery D, Speizer F: Maternal smoking during pregnancy as a predictor of lung function in children, *Am J Epidemiol* 139:1139-1152, 1994.

Dalaker J, Niafeh M: *US Bureau of the Census: current population reports, series P60-201, poverty in the United States: 1997,* Washington, DC, 1998, US Government Printing Office.

Dickens MD et al: The medical home: ad hoc task force on definition of the medical home, *Pediatrics* 90(5):774, 1992.

Durant RH et al: Factors associated with the use of violence among urban black adolescents, *Am J Public Health* 84:612-617, 1994.

Elders JM et al: The report of the Surgeon General: preventing tobacco use among young people, *Am J Public Health* 84:543-547, 1994.

Employee Benefit Research Institute: Health insurance and characteristics of the uninsured, *EBRI Issue Brief* No 170, 1996.

Employee Benefit Research Institute: Sources of health insurance and characteristics of the ininsured: analysis of the March 1998 current population survey, *EBRI Issue Brief* No 204, 1998.

Food and Nutrition Service, United States Department of Agriculture: *Women, infants, and children: frequently asked questions,* December 1, 1999, The Author, www.fns.usda.gov/wic/menu/faq/faq.html.

Goldenberg RL, Klerman LV: Adolescent pregnancy: another look, *N Engl J Med* 332:1161-1162, 1995.

Harlap S, Kost K, Forrest JD: *Preventing pregnancy, protecting health: a new look at birth control choices in the United States,* New York, 1991, Alan Guttmacher Institute.

Henshaw SK: *U.S. teenage pregnancy statistics with comparative statistics for women aged 20-24,* New York, 1999, Alan Guttmacher Institute.

Hoyert DL, Kochanek KD, Murphy SL: Deaths: final data for 1997, *Natl Vital Stat Rep* 47(19), 1999.

Institute of Medicine: *Preventing low birthweight,* Washington DC, 1985, National Academy Press.

Jaskiewicz JA, McAnarney ER: Pregnancy during adolescence, *Pediatr Rev* 15:32-38, 1994.

Klerman LV: *Alive and well? a research and policy review of health programs for poor young children,* New York, 1991, National Center for Children in Poverty.

Kochanek KD, Hudson BL: Advance report of final mortality statistics: 1992, *Monthly Vital Stat Rep* 43(6, Suppl.), 1995.

Lear JG et al: The growth of school-based health centers and the role of state policies: results of a national survey, *Arch Pediatr and Adolesc Med* 153(11):1177-1180, 1999.

Leshner AI: *National pregnancy and health survey,* Washington, DC, 1994, USDHHS, PHS, NIH, National Institute on Drug Abuse.

Lewit E: Teenage childbearing. In *The future of children: U.S. health care for children,* Los Altos, Calif, 1992, The Center for the Future of Children, The David and Lucile Packard Foundation.

MacDorman MF, Atkinson JO: Infant mortality statistics from the 1997 period linked birth/infant death data set, *Natl Vital Stat Rep* 47(23), 1999.

Martin J et al: Births and deaths: preliminary data for 1998, *Natl Vital Stat Rep* 47(25):99-1120, 1999.

Moore KA: *A statistical portrait of adolescent sex, contraception and childbearing,* Washington, DC, 1998, National Campaign to Prevent Teenage Pregnancy.

National Center for Health Statistics: *Health, United States: 1998 with socioeconomic status and health chartbook,* Hyattsville, Md, 1998, The Author.

National Center For Health Statistics: *Health, United States: 1999,* Hyattsville, Md, 1999, USDHHS.

National Governors' Association: *MCH update,* Washington, DC, 1999, The Author.

Newacheck PW et al: Health insurance and access to primary care for children, *N Engl J Med* 338:513-9, 1998.

Ross Products Division, Abbott Laboratories: *Ross mothers survey: 1997,* Columbus, OH, 1998, Abbott Laboratories.

Schoendorf KC, Kiely JL: Relationship of sudden infant death syndrome to maternal smoking during and after pregnancy, *Pediatrics* 90:905-908, 1992.

Streissguth AP et al: Fetal alcohol syndrome in adolescents and adults, *JAMA* 265:1961-1967, 1991.

Substance Abuse and Mental Health Services Administration, Office of Applied Studies: *Summary of findings from the 1998 national household survey on drug abuse,* Rockville, Md, 1999, USDHHS.

University of Michigan Institute for Social Research: *Monitoring the future study: 1975-1998,* Rockville, Md, 1998, National Institute on Drug Abuse, NIH.

US Bureau of the Census: *Current population reports: population projections of the United States by age, sex, race, and Hispanic origin: 1995-2050,* Series P-25, No 1130, Washington, DC, 1999, US Government Printing Office.

US Bureau of the Census: *Current population reports,* Series P-25, No 311, Washington, DC, 1999, The Author.

US Census Bureau: *Current population survey,* Washington, DC, March 1999, The Author.

US Department of Health and Human Services, Children's Bureau: *Child maltreatment 1997 reports from the states to the national child and abuse data system,* Washington, DC, 1999, US Government Printing Office.

US Department of Health and Human Services: *Healthy People 2010: conference edition,* Washington, DC, 2000, USDHHS.

Ventura SJ et al: Births: final data for 1997, *Natl Vital Stat Rep* 47(18), 1999.

Ventura SJ, Matthews TJ, Curtin SC: Teenage births in the United States: state trends, 1991-96: an update, *Month Vital Stat Rep* 46(11) (suppl 2), 1999.

Wilcox A: Birthweight and perinatal mortality: the effect of maternal smoking, *Am J Epidemiol* 137:1098-1104, 1993.

15

Women's Health

Roma D. Williams

OBJECTIVES

Upon completion of this chapter, the reader will be able to do the following:

1. Discuss the major indicators of women's health.
2. Examine prominent health problems among women of all age groups (i.e., from adolescence to old age).
3. Identify barriers to adequate health care for women.
4. Discuss issues related to reproductive health.
5. Discuss the influence of public policy on women's health.
6. Discuss issues and needs for increased research efforts focused on women's health.
7. Apply the nursing process to women's health concerns across all levels of prevention.

KEY TERMS

Civil Rights Act
domestic violence
ectopic pregnancy
Family and Medical Leave Act (FMLA)
family planning
hypertension
life expectancy
maternal mortality
multiple family configurations
osteoporosis
pelvic inflammatory disease (PID)
sexual harassment

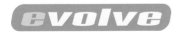

http://evolve.elsevier.com/Nies/

To achieve "health for all" in the twenty-first century, health care services must be affordable and available to all. Although adequate health care for women is a key to realizing this goal, a significant number of women and their families face tremendous barriers in gaining access to health care. Additionally, knowledge deficits related to health promotion and disease prevention activities prevent women from all educational and socioeconomic levels from assuming responsibility for their own health and well-being.

Beginning in the 1970s, the women's movement called for the reform of systems affecting women's health. Women were encouraged to become involved as consumers of health services and as establishers of health policy. More women entered health professions they previously underrepresented and those in traditionally female-dominated professions such as nursing and teaching became more assertive in their demands to gain recognition for their contributions to society.

In her *Preamble to a New Paradigm for Women's Health,* Choi (1985) declared that collaboration and an interdisciplinary approach are necessary to meet the health care needs of women. She further stated that "essential to the development of health care for women are the concepts of health promotion, disease and accident prevention, education for self-care and responsibility, health risk identification and coordination for illness care when needed" (p. 14). To realize this paradigm, community health nurses must work with other health care professionals to formulate upstream strategies that modify the factors affecting women's health. Many *Healthy People 2010* goals address health problems pertaining to women and include specific objectives and strategies to improve the health of this aggregate. Table 15-1 presents a small selection of these objectives.

This chapter examines the health of women from adolescence to old age. It explores the major

TABLE 15-1

Selected *Healthy People 2010* Objectives and Women's Health

Objective	Baseline	Target
3-3: Reduce breast cancer death rate.	27.7 deaths per 100,000	22.2 deaths per 100,000
3-4: Reduce death rate from cervical cancer.	3 deaths per 100,000	2 deaths per 100,000
3-11b: Increase the proportion of women 18 years of age and older who have received a PAP test within the preceding three years.	79%	90%
3-13: Increase the proportion of women 40 years of age and older who have received a mammogram within the preceding two years.	68%	70%
16-4: Reduce maternal deaths.	8.4 deaths per 100,000 live births	3.3 deaths per 100,000 live births
16-5a: Reduce maternal complications during labor and delivery.	32.1 per 100 deliveries	20 per 100 deliveries
16-6a: Increase the proportion of pregnant women who receive early and adequate prenatal care beginning in the first trimester.	83%	90%
16-15: Reduce the occurrence of NTDs.	6 cases per 10,000 live births	3 cases per 10,000 live births
25-1: Reduce the proportion of females 15 to 24 years of age with chlamydia infections.	12.2%	3%
25-6: Reduce the proportion of females who have required treatment for PID.	8%	5%

From US Department of Health and Human Services: *Healthy people 2010,* Conference Edition, Washington, DC, 2000a, The Author.

indicators of health, including specific health problems and the socioeconomic, sociocultural, and health policy issues surrounding women's health. This chapter also discusses identification of current and future research aimed at improving the health of women. An understanding of these points will enable community health nurses to appropriately apply expertise in a community setting to help improve women's health.

MAJOR INDICATORS OF HEALTH

In the United States, data collected on major causes of death indicate the health status of aggregates. These data are typically presented in terms of gender, age, or ethnicity and can help interpret the levels of health in different groups. The primary indicators of health this chapter covers are life expectancy, mortality (i.e., death) rate, and morbidity (i.e., acute and chronic illness) rate.

Many factors that lead to death and illness among women are preventable or avoidable. If certain conditions receive early detection and treatment, a significant positive influence on longevity and the QOL could ensue. Recognition of patterns demonstrated in these indicators can address problems preventatively. This section presents an overview of these major indicators of health among women.

Life Expectancy

Except in a few countries including Bangladesh, Bhutan, and Nepal, women typically experience greater longevity than their male counterparts (Paolisso and Leslie, 1995). For example, females born in the 1970s in the United States had an average life expectancy of 74.7 years, or 7.6 years longer than males born the same year. During the past two decades, this discrepancy has remained as males born in 1992 have a life expectancy of 72.3 years compared with 79 years for females (US Census Bureau, 1995).

However, **life expectancy** differs among aggregates based on variables other than gender. For example, racial background influences life span. Although black females born in 1992 gained an additional 6.5 years of life expectancy, which was up from the projected 69.4 years for those born in 1970, it falls behind the 79.7 years of life expectancy of white females born in 1992 (US Census Bureau, 1995).

Mortality Rate

Table 15-2 lists the five major causes of death among American women in 1995. The largest percentage of overall deaths is caused by CVD. Although the number of deaths decreased dramatically from 424.2 per 100,000 in 1950 to 186 per 100,000 in 1991, CVD continues to be the number one killer of women (AHA, 1999). Nevertheless, disparities continue related to prevention and management of heart disease in women (Bush, 1996; Schulman et al., 1999). Since 1984, a combination of all CVDs cause more deaths among females (505,930, or 52.7%) than among males (453,297, or 47.3%) (AHA, 1999). Some investigators believe the problem exists because women display different symptoms of heart disease and manage them differently. For example, women with heart disease may not respond positively to exercise

TABLE **15-2**

Five Leading Causes of Death among Women for All Races and Age Groups in 1995

Age Group (yr)	Cause of Death (in Rank Order)
15 to 24	Unintentional injury or accidents Homicide Suicide Malignant neoplasm Heart disease
25 to 44	Malignant neoplasm Unintentional injury or accidents HIV infection Heart disease Suicide
45 to 64	Malignant neoplasm Heart disease Cerebrovascular disease COPD Diabetes mellitus
65 to 74	Heart disease Malignant neoplasm Cerebrovascular disease COPD Influenza and pneumonia

Adapted from US Census Bureau: *Statistical abstract of the United States: 1995,* ed 115, Washington, DC, 1995, US Government Printing Office.

tests; therefore they are not treated the same way as men (e.g., with cardiac catheterization or heart surgery) (Mark et al., 1994).

Maternal Mortality Rate

Women are uniquely at risk during pregnancy and childbirth and they experience additional dangers associated with legal and spontaneous abortions. *The National Hospital Discharge Survey: Annual Summary, 1996* (Graves and Kozak, 1998) reported that 536,000 American women were hospitalized at least once during pregnancy, childbirth, or the puerperium from a complication.

Since the 1950s, **maternal mortality** rates have continued to decline in the United States. This decline is largely attributed to the use of blood transfusions, antimicrobial drugs, and the maintenance of fluid and electrolyte balance during serious complications of pregnancy and birth. The development of obstetric training programs and obstetric anesthesia programs is also important (Cunningham et al., 1997).

However, racial discrepancy persists in maternal mortality rates as in life expectancy. Table 15-3 illustrates how nonwhite women have a significantly higher incidence of death during pregnancy than whites (Cunningham et al., 1997). The gap in maternal mortality rates between black and white women has widened over the past several decades. Early in the twentieth century, black women were two times more likely to die of pregnancy-related complications than white women. Currently, black women are three times more likely to die as white women (CDC, 1999). Major risk factors for maternal death include lack of antepartal care and family planning services, inadequate health education, and poor nutrition. An additional risk factor, regardless of race, is advancing age. According to Cunningham (1997),

intrinsic maternal factors such as increasing frequency of hypertension and a greater likelihood of uterine hemorrhage explains this increase in the mortality rate. As more women postpone childbearing without appropriate prenatal care, the number of maternal deaths may increase.

In decreasing order of occurrence, the leading cause of maternal death is pulmonary embolism (17%) followed by pregnancy-induced hypertension, ectopic pregnancy, hemorrhage, stroke, and anesthesia (Cunningham et al., 1997). Death associated with legal surgical abortion is rare in the United States. Complications that result in death from legal abortion relate to the woman's age, the type of procedure, the fetus' gestational age, and general health problems at the time of the abortion (Cates and Ellertson, 1998).

Since 1988, a medical method of abortion using mifepristone (i.e., RU-486), an antiprogestin medication, together with prostaglandins has been used in European countries and China. Although this method is as effective as surgical abortion, public pressure in the United States caused a delay in the testing, licensing, and manufacturing of RU-486 until the mid1990s when it became available for clinical trials. In September 2000, the FDA approved the use of RU-486, yet news reports suggest that physicians may be reluctant to provide this method of abortion for fear of being targeted as an "abortion doctor."

In time, as clinicians gain experience with this medical method of abortion, protocols may be adapted for women to use it at home. Additional research is needed to examine the acceptability of the newer medical methods of abortion among American women, the relationship between the medical method of abortion and a woman's cultural beliefs, and her decision-making process to choose between a medical method or surgical abortion.

Abortion is a controversial issue for providers and for the women in their care. An upstream intervention would certainly be the best strategy; however, until that time, nurses must continue to keep abreast of all available pregnancy termination options to provide the best counsel (Cates and Ellertson, 1998; Donaldson, Briggs, and McMaster, 1995).

TABLE 15-3

Maternal Mortality Rate per 100,000 Live Births

Year	Total	Whites	Blacks	Other Nonwhite
1985	7.8	5.2	20.4	18.1
1987	6.9	5.1	14.2	12.20
1992	7.8	5.0	20.8	18.2
1995	7.1	4.20	22.1	18.5

According to the CDC, **ectopic pregnancy** is the leading cause of maternal death in the first trimester, accounting for 13% of maternal deaths. Since the 1980s, the incidence of ectopic pregnancy has increased fourfold to 11.3 per 1000 pregnancies among women 15 to 44 years of age (CDC, 1999). Racial discrepancy is evident and yields a rate of 14.7 per 1000 among nonwhites compared with 10.3 per 1000 among whites. This disparity continues to increase throughout the reproductive years of nonwhite women (Cunningham et al., 1997) possibly because, even though STDs are more frequent among nonwhite women, these patients have less access to health care.

The most significant risk for ectopic pregnancy is previous pelvic inflammatory disease (PID) or salpingitis; therefore women at risk for acquiring STDs must learn to protect themselves from these diseases. Prevention interventions are critical in reducing a woman's risk for an ectopic pregnancy because early diagnosis and treatment greatly reduce the mortality rate. An important task of health care providers is to assist women and men to reduce personal health risk-taking behaviors related to sexuality (Guest, 1998a).

Cancer

Cancer death rates among women increased from 136 per 100,000 women in 1960 to 141.9 per 100,000 women in 1990 (ACS, 1995). The ACS estimated that 272,000 deaths occurred among women as a result of cancer in 1999 (ACS, 1999). In 1987, lung cancer surpassed breast cancer as the leading cause of cancer deaths in women. Every year, breast cancer claims the lives of some 43,300 women, but an estimated 68,000 women will die from lung cancer in 1999. Colorectal cancer, the third most frequent cause of cancer deaths in women, claims the lives of 27,800 men and 28,800 women annually. The good news is that healthy lifestyle changes and early detection and intervention have contributed to the decrease in mortality rates from some cancers. For example, since the 1970s, colorectal cancer is down 29% for women and 7% for men (ACS, 1999).

Five-year survival rates vary according to the type of cancer and stage at diagnosis. For instance, the five-year survival rate for all patients with lung cancer is only 14%. For localized breast cancer it is 97%, but only 22% when diagnosed with distant metastases. Of cancers related to the reproductive tract, ovarian cancer has the lowest survival rate for all stages, which is 50% (ACS, 1999). When diagnosed at an early stage, five-year survival rate for women with colon cancer is 93% and for those with rectal cancer is 87%.

Early diagnosis and prompt treatment are major factors in surviving many types of cancer. In addition, certain health choices may reduce an individual's risk of cancer. All women need to avoid health-deteriorating practices and replace them with health-promoting behaviors that foster a health-protecting lifestyle. If providers and patients applied everything known about cancer prevention, approximately two thirds of cancer cases would not occur. For example, women could reduce their risk for cancer by never smoking or by quitting if they already use tobacco products. Eating a nutritious diet can decrease a woman's risk of both heart disease and cancer. Also, physical activity helps protect against heart disease and some cancers by achieving or maintaining a healthy body weight. Obesity has been associated with an increased risk for cancers such as colon and rectum, endometrium, and breast (i.e., among postmenopausal women) (ACS, 1999).

Community health nurses play a major role in providing cancer control services that should be culturally sensitive and appropriate to the targeted aggregate. Community health nurses must encourage all females (i.e., from childhood to old age) to avoid tobacco in any form, maintain healthy weight, stay physically active, and eat a low-fat, high-fiber diet filled with needed nutrients and calories (McElmurry and Tashiro, 1997; Woods and Mitchell, 1997; Young and King, 1997). The nurse should also recommend limiting alcohol and the consumption of salt-cured, smoked, and nitrite-cured foods (ACS, 1999).

For women, cancer is not just another chronic disease. It evokes more fear than heart disease, which is the number one killer. In addition, cancer's relevance for women changes across the lifespan. To read more about women and cancer, refer to Williams (1997).

Cardiovascular Disease

Each day more than 2600 Americans die from CVD. About one in five Americans has one or more forms of CVD (e.g., high blood pressure, coronary artery disease, stroke, and rheumatic heart disease). One in ten women under age 60 has some form of CVD; the ratio increases to one in three after age 65 (AHA, 1999). Black women are more likely to die from CVDs than white women. In 1996, the CVD death rate among white females was 145.7 per 100,000 compared with 165.2 per 100,000 for black females.

Correspondingly, the coronary heart disease death rates for white females is 58.9 per 100,000 in contrast to 80 per 100,000 for black females (36%

higher for blacks). Stroke, although 19% higher for males than for females, is more deadly for women than for men. Black women are more likely to die from stroke than white women (39.2 per 100,000 and 22.9 per 100,000, respectively, or 71% higher) (AHA, 1999).

Currently the health care industry is placing an increased emphasis on the cardiovascular health of women, and more research studies focus on women. Health care providers are learning about heart disease in women and recognize that women need different interventions than men to protect themselves from this deadly disease. Interventions must be culturally appropriate and nurse scientists have conducted interdisciplinary intervention studies designed to identify culturally appropriate behavioral risk-reduction strategies and chronic indicators and high-risk factors for young black women (i.e., 25 to 45 years of age) with coronary heart disease. These intervention studies are needed to test culturally appropriate models for their usefulness as educational tools that enhance and promote adherence (Giger and Strickland, 1995; Olson and Labat, 1995).

Further declines in CVD rates for women can only occur if individuals become more aware of risk factors and accept responsibility for managing their own health and well-being (Kuehn, McMahon, and Creekmore, 1999). Concerned and motivated providers must encourage women to practice heart-healthy behaviors.

Diabetes

Diabetes mellitus is another disease that causes the premature death of many women (American Diabetes Association, 1998). Diabetes ranks fourth as the cause of death among Native-American, black, Filipino, and Hawaiian women (CDC Diabetes Surveillance Report, 1998). The incidence of noninsulin-dependent diabetes (NIDDM) increases with age and is slightly higher for women than men (i.e., except among those aged 65 to 74 years). The highest prevalence of NIDDM is found among the Pima Indians (35%), which is significantly higher than among the entire Native-American population (17%). Blacks have a prevalence rate of 5%, which is twice that of the general population (2.5%) (Seltzer and Pearse, 1995).

Prevalence among blacks is higher than among whites at all ages for both men and women. In the United States, diabetes ranks as the seventh leading cause of death in black women (AHA, 1994).

In addition to being a serious illness in itself, diabetes is a risk factor for the development of coronary artery disease. Furthermore, it dramatically influences the severity and course of the CVD. When diabetic patients suffer heart attacks, their overall in-hospital mortality rate is much higher than for nondiabetic patients. The prognosis for diabetic women after a myocardial infarction (MI) is particularly grave; the overall in-hospital mortality rate is 37% for women, compared with 19% for men. According to Nesto and colleagues (1994), the aggregate at highest risk of death is obese, diabetic women. An upstream approach to this problem includes helping women maintain a desirable weight throughout life in an effort to avoid nutrition-related causes of death, such as diabetes and CVD.

Morbidity Rate

Hospitalizations

The 1996 National Hospital Discharge Survey reported that more women than men are hospitalized each year in the United States. However, the average length of hospitalization for males (5.8 days) exceeds that for females (4.9 days) until after age 65. Cerebrovascular disease resulted in the longest average hospital stays (6.7 days), which occurred most frequently among women aged 65 or older. Fractures accounted for an average of 5.9 days, malignant neoplasms for an average 7 days, and diseases of the heart for an average 5.2 days (Graves and Kozak, 1998).

The PPS for hospitalization resulted in an increased demand for skilled nursing services in the home. After hospitalization for several of these conditions, community health nurses may provide ongoing nursing care in the home by referral. Nurses practicing in home environments must be prepared to deliver high-tech and high-touch services. Chapter 30 discusses home health care in detail.

Chronic Conditions and Limitations

Women are more likely than men to be disabled from chronic conditions. Arthritis and rheumatism, hypertension, and impairment of the back or spine decrease women's activity level more often than they affect their male counterparts. In fact, almost twice as many women (24.6%) as men (12.4%) are limited in activity from arthritis and rheumatism. Women are more likely than men to have difficulty performing activities such as walking, bathing or showering, preparing meals, and doing housework (US Census Bureau, 1995).

Functional limitations may require home health care that community health nurses supervise and deliver. Nurses plan and implement interventions based on functional assessments. The care plan facilitates optimal resumption of the individual's independence in personal care activities.

Surgery

Hysterectomy is the second most frequently performed major surgical procedure among women of reproductive age; approximately 600,000 hysterectomies are performed each year (CDC, 1997). Hysterectomy rates for black women are slightly higher than those for white women (61.7 and 56.5 per 10,000 women, respectively).

The most common reason for hysterectomy is uterine fibroids or leiomyoma, which contributes to more than one third of all such surgeries, but considerably more for blacks (61%) than for whites (29%) (CDC, 1997). White women are more often diagnosed with endometriosis and uterine prolapse, which are the second and third most common reasons for hysterectomy. The mean age at hysterectomy is 40.9 years (Ravnikar and Chen, 1994).

In a recent study, focus groups and individual interviews helped obtain data from a sample of southern urban women who had a hysterectomy for benign conditions. Findings revealed that biophysical, psychosocial, and spiritual domains were important in their decision to have a hysterectomy. Most of the 38 women who participated described the hysterectomy experience as positive. However, many participants expressed a need for information about women's gynecological health for themselves and their male partners.

Black women expressed a need for change in the black community about women undergoing hysterectomy. Women reported that many spouses, brothers, uncles, and other black male friends were not supportive of their decision and a few women revealed that they had not told a new partner about the surgery (Williams and Clark, 2000).

New procedures and options have become available to women over the past few years such as myomectomy, or removing only the tumors with repair of the uterus, or the use of gonadotropin releasing hormone (GNRH) to shrink the tumors that decrease the need for hysterectomy; women may not know about these alternatives. Community health nurses function as advocates for women and can provide health education programs related to alternatives to hysterectomy, indications for hysterectomy and oophorectomy (i.e., removal of ovaries), and information regarding the type of surgical approach and the purpose of a second opinion. Second opinions and higher levels of education tend to decrease the rate of hysterectomies (Finkel and Finkel, 1990; Meilahan et al., 1989).

Birth by cesarean delivery is the most prevalent surgical procedure experienced by women in the United States and accounts for one out of every four births. Several factors contribute to the high rates of cesarean delivery, including physicians' fear of malpractice suits and progress in technology that facilitates fetal monitoring. The practice of vaginal birth after cesarean (VBAC) may decrease the high cesarean birth rate in the United States because almost half occur among women who had prior cesareans. As part of the childbirth curriculum, childbirth educators offer information related to the cesarean birth experience. Some hospitals or groups, such as Cesareans Support, Education, and Concern, hold classes in preparation for a repeat cesarean birth or for couples desiring VBAC (Olds, London, and Ladewig, 1996).

Mental Health

The most frequently occurring interruption in women's mental health relates to depression. Well-controlled epidemiological studies consistently demonstrate that women experience depression at two to three times the rate of men (Schmidt et al., 1997). Symptoms of depression range from depressed mood to apathy, anxiety, irritability, and thoughts of death and suicide (Evans et al., 1999; Szewczyk and Chennault, 1997). Women tend to be vulnerable to feelings of hopelessness and lowered self-esteem. Women with lower income and educational levels are at greater risk for depression than women with higher educational levels or economic status. Those lacking adequate financial or emotional support often express a sense of frustration and futility.

Nurses practicing in community health settings should be aware of depression's signs and symptoms

BOX 15-1

Signs and Symptoms of Depression

Mood disturbance and emotional distress
Sad, blue, and gloomy feelings
Feelings of helplessness, hopelessness, inadequacy, and worthlessness
Loss of interest in work, friends, family, and sex
Sleep pattern disturbances
Loss of appetite or voracious appetite
Feelings of heaviness in head or chest
Tendency to cry easily and sigh often
Complaints of headaches, backaches, and constipation
Difficulty in concentrating and making decisions
Flat to hectic gaiety
Everything drooping (i.e., mouth, eyes, posture, and body language)

and identify referral sources for professional help within the community. A woman experiencing depression may display some signs and symptoms listed in Box 15-1 (Smith, 1986).

SOCIAL FACTORS AFFECTING WOMEN'S HEALTH

Health Care Access

Approximately 44 million U.S. citizens lacked health insurance in 1998 (USDHHS, 2000b).Owing to the nature of their employment, women frequently lack health insurance but may not eligible for Medicaid benefits because their income is too high. Young adults (i.e., those between ages 16 and 24 years) make up approximately 50% of individuals without health insurance. Lacking economic means for meeting the costs of health care, these women are not likely to seek health care delivery until they or a family member is in acute distress. Others may rely on home remedies, over-the-counter drugs, lay midwives, or other folk healers for health care. Older adults, usually covered by Medicare may also delay seeking health care. Older women on fixed incomes may have difficulty meeting copayments required by Medicare and paying for prescription medications. Many senior citizens have paid hospitalization insurance premiums for policies that fail to meet the gap.

TABLE 15-4

Percentages of Degrees Received by Women

Degree	1970	1980	1988	1996
Medicine (MD)	8.4	23.4	33.3	40.9
Dentistry (DDS or DMD)	0.9	13.3	26.7	35.8
Law (LLB or JD)	5.4	30.2	40.8	43.4
Theology (BD, MDiv, or MHL)	2.3	13.8	19.3	23.3

From US Department of Education: *Digest of education statistics*, Pub No 99-036, 1998, Washington, DC, The Author.

Education and Work

In the workplace, women predominate as librarians, teachers, social workers, and nurses, which accounts for 65% of working women in 1990 (Pollard and Tordella, 1993). However, in the 1980s, more women began to enter professions traditionally held by men (e.g., lawyers, physicians, and dentists) and by 1990, more than half (57%) of young professionals were women. According to Pollard and Tordella, this is a revolutionary development and the likely trend of the future.

Statistics are also rising academically. In 1970, 55.4% of all women aged 25 or older were high school graduates compared with 75.9% in 1988 and 89.5% in 1998. Of this same age group 29.5% had completed college in 1988, which was more than three times the 1970 rate of 8.2%. In 1996, women earned 55.9% of all masters' degrees and 39.8% of all doctorates, which accounted for a 10% increase from 1980. An increasing number of women earned degrees in traditionally male-dominated professions. Table 15-4 reflects recent changes occurring in percentages of women receiving degrees in medicine, dentistry, law, and theology (US Department of Education, 1998).

Employment and Wages

In the early 1990s, nearly two of every three women of working age (aged 18 to 64 years) were employed (i.e., compared to four of every five men). More than half (57%) the married women with young children (younger than six years) were working

TABLE 15-5

Median Annual Earnings by Type of Household:
1969, 1979, 1989, and 1999 (in 1999 dollars)

Household Type	1969	1979	1989*	1999
Married couple with children	41,453	47,793	50,613	56,827
Female householder with children	16,327	18,468	17,651	26,164
Male householder with children	33,749	36,619	34,646	41,830

From US Census Bureau: *Money income in the United States, 1999,*
1999, The Author, www.census.gov/hhes/income/income99/
99tablea.html.

outside the home. In 1950, only 12% of women were combining these roles (Chadwick and Heaton, 1992).

Several questions concern women's health and well-being related to employment issues. A review of female-dominated vs. male-dominated jobs discloses inequalities in wage and salary scales; despite the diminishing gap between women's and men's incomes, there is still much room for improvement. Average annual earnings for both black and white women are lower than for their male counterparts. Recent data indicate that women earn only $0.73 for every $1.00 earned by men (US Census Bureau, 1999). Table 15-5 depicts median annual income by marital status of women and men.

Women and their children are the poorest aggregate in the United States. This phenomenon is labeled "the feminization of poverty." The nurse working with impoverished families should be aware of social services, child care programs, emergency services, and other resources for families in need. The community health nurse often needs to act as case manager and advocate for families with social service agencies and other public entities.

Working Women and Home Life

Added to inequalities outside the home are inequalities within the home. A working woman is less likely to have a spouse or partner help with the home and children. Even when a spouse or partner is present, the burdens of housework and child care usually fall more heavily on women regardless of ethnicity.

Mothers generally spend more time than fathers preparing meals and training and disciplining their children. These multiple-role demands and conflicting expectations contribute to stress (Bonam-Crawford and Orlick, 1994).

However, changes are occurring as younger and older men now report spending more time in family activities compared with middle-aged men. Blacks and Hispanics tend to spend a little more time working at family tasks than white men. Increasingly, books and articles encourage wives and husbands to make their needs known. As a result, many couples emphasize increased communication between partners. Marriage enrichment programs, often offered through churches and synagogues, teach couples how to communicate more effectively with each other. Such efforts should foster equality between partners.

Family Configuration and Marital Relationship Status

Women are members of **multiple family configurations** (e.g., nuclear families, extended family units, single-parent units, families of group marriages, blended family units, adoptive family units, nonlegal heterosexual unions, lesbian family units, and others). This diversity causes changing women's roles within families. Whether or not they function in a traditional role, most do whatever is necessary to maintain the integrity of their families. Early assessment of the strengths of family units by the community health nurse provides a data base for positive nursing interventions established on upstream strategies to enhance each family's level of health and well-being.

Many women are delaying marriage and an increasing number are not marrying. Overall marriage rates may have remained stable because the increasing number of remarriages balance the declining rate of first marriages. When a relationship ends in divorce or separation, more women than men have the responsibility of providing for themselves and their children. According to the U.S. Census Bureau (1994), single-parent households now represent 3 of every 10 family groups. Single mothers are most often the head of a single-parent family (6:1). Table 15-6 lists characteristics of black and white female-headed households. Percentages of single-parent households with children include 63% of black family groups, 35% of Hispanics, and 25% of whites. However, even in the face of changing lifestyles, divorce, and increased mobility, which leads to long-distance

TABLE 15-6

Characteristics of Black and White Female-Headed Households

Characteristic	Black	White
Never married	43%	18%
Married and spouse absent	20%	17%
Widowed	13%	22%
Divorced	23%	43%
Number of children per female-headed household	1.28	0.99

Adapted from US Census Bureau: *Statistical abstract of the United States: 1995,* ed 115, Washington, DC, 1995, US Government Printing Office.

relationships, most Americans report they remain connected to their extended families through parents, grandparents, siblings, aunts, and uncles.

One contemporary family configuration involves single women with one or more adopted children. Single-parent adoptions are legal; therefore an increasing number of single women are becoming adoptive parents. An often-ignored family structure is one headed by a lesbian parent. Lesbians who become parents have needs similar to those of all mothers. Many cities have lesbian-gay parent groups that provide support, anticipatory guidance, and strategies for coping in society. However, lesbian women often neglect their own health. This self-neglect may be traced to hostile and rejecting attitudes of health care providers (Andrews, 1997). However, the parents or guardians must remain healthy to ensure the child's well-being. A delay in health-seeking services may have devastating consequences.

HEALTH ISSUES FOR WOMEN

Health Promotion Strategies for Women

A woman's ability to carry out her important roles can affect her entire family; therefore women should receive services that promote health and detect disease at an early stage. Early detection and improved treatments for disease allow women to return to work or remain working throughout the course of an illness. Although work is essential to the economic and social well-being of many women's families, the

workplace itself creates physical and social stress. As more women enter the workforce and face many of the same risks and stressors as men, it is not surprising that their formerly favorable mortality and morbidity rates have been declining.

Many women seek information that will allow them to be in control of their own health. Since the early 1970s, women have met in self-help groups to develop a better understanding of their own health needs. Some of the health behaviors that women learn in self-help groups are the importance of nutrition, breast self-examination (BSE), pregnancy testing, and contraceptive awareness; recognition of the early signs of vaginal infections and STDs; and awareness of the variations in female anatomy and physiology.

Women desire to become more knowledgeable about their own health; therefore many books for consumers are available in bookstores, public libraries, and among the holdings of traditional women's groups such as sororities, federated women's clubs, and others. An excellent resource for women is the *FDA Consumer,* the official magazine of the FDA. The *FDA Consumer* reports on FDA studies that cover a variety of women's health issues such as mammography standards, menopause, cures for chlamydia, eating disorders, infertility, cosmetic safety, silicone breast implants, and osteoporosis (USDHHS, 1999).

Pender's (1996) Health Promotion Model (HPM) synthesizes the literature on health promotion and wellness. She indicates that "health promoting behaviors are directed toward sustaining or increasing the level of well-being, self-actualization and fulfillment of a given individual or group." The community health nurse can use this model in teaching health behaviors that lead to general health promotion among women. However, because many models were developed for the middle class, they may not be useful to community health nurses working with low-income families. Health promotion for low-income, underserved women may differ from that for their middle-class counterparts.

Williams and Lethbridge (1995) studied health promotion in low-income rural women. The ethnographic study of 49 black and white low-income women was aimed at eliciting views about the meaning of health and health promotion and gathering information on health maintenance behaviors, barriers, and facilitators.

The women identified health as the ability to do for themselves and their family. Findings revealed that they considered health promotion to be actions such as taking blood pressure medicine and watching what they ate. Many did not think strenuous exercise was good for most women and their exercise was in the form of walking, gardening, and taking care of children and grandchildren. These women did not distinguish between health promotion and health maintenance, which are concepts that may be more meaningful to health care providers than their clientele. Rural and other underserved women must be self-sufficient and have access to a culturally relevant, accessible, and appropriate health care delivery system that fits within the context of their lives.

When it comes to an awareness of their own bodies, knowledge deficits prevail among women regardless of socioeconomic or educational level. Regardless of whether a group is comprised of college-educated professional women or blue-collar working women, many of the questions are the same. For example, a woman may ask if she will menstruate after hysterectomy, when she should perform a BSE, or what she can do to prevent recurrent episodes of vaginitis. Nurses can play an instrumental role in helping women develop a greater sense of self-awareness. Furthermore, community health nurses can remove the mystery surrounding the woman's body and encourage clients to ask previously unmentionable questions.

Acute Illness

Females report a greater incidence of acute conditions than males. This section describes several of the most common.

Urinary Tract Infection

Approximately 5% of primary care visits by women are prompted by symptoms suggestive of bacteriuria (Seltzer and Pearse, 1995). By age 30, approximately 50% of women have at least one urinary tract infection (UTI) (Medimmune, 1999). The prevalence of infection directly correlates with age, increasing from about 3.5% to 10% between puberty and age 70

(Seltzer and Pearse, 1995). Often women experience their first UTI during pregnancy or soon after delivery (Clark, 1995). Trigonitis, or *honeymoon cystitis,* frequently occurs with a change in sexual activity from infrequent or no activity to more vigorous and frequent intercourse.

Diseases of the Reproductive Tract

Acute illnesses specific to the reproductive tract include conditions such as vulvovaginitis, PID, and toxic shock syndrome (TSS).

Vulvovaginitis

Vulvovaginitis may start in girls before puberty and is more common than in reproductive aged women. The labia of young girls lack fat and the vaginal mucosa is thin and friable. Vaginitis continues to be a frequent and often acute painful problem that thousands of women seek relief for annually. Women often report an increase in vaginal discharge, itching, burning, dysuria, and dyspareunia. The physical examination may reveal vaginal and/or vulvar edema and erythema and a discharge that varies in color, odor, and consistency (Mou, 1995). The reader is referred to a women's health text to learn more about the etiology of these conditions, their treatment, and comfort measures.

Pelvic Inflammatory Disease

Pelvic inflammatory disease (PID) starts with cervicitis and progresses to endometritis and eventual involvement of the fallopian tubes. Combinations of *N gonorrhea, C. trachomatis,* anaerobic bacteria, and a variety of other microbial agents can cause PID (Cates, 1998). More than one million episodes occur every year and one in seven American women of reproductive age report having received treatment for PID. Often women with PID have atypical or no symptoms. If symptomatic, a woman experiences pain and tenderness that involves the lower abdomen, cervix, and uterus, often with fever and chills.

The diagnosis of PID is often based on imprecise clinical findings. Diagnosis is critical because even mild to moderate forms of the disease have serious reproductive sequelae, including ectopic pregnancy and infertility. The causative organism is usually unknown at the time of initial therapy and treatment includes antimicrobial coverage against the broadest possible range of pathogens. Hospitalization and inpatient care are recommended with acute PID when the woman is severely ill and unable to receive outpatient care, is pregnant, is unable to follow or tolerate an outpatient regimen, or has failed to respond to outpatient therapy. All patients with PID must return for evaluation after initiation of therapy, usually in two to three days and again four days after completion of therapy. In addition, the woman's sex partner(s) needs evaluation and treatment. The woman and her partner or partners are advised to avoid sexual activity until they are cured. As with other STDs, counseling for women diagnosed with PID must include individualized behavioral messages aimed at risk reduction.

Toxic Shock Syndrome

TSS is caused by toxins released by some strains of *Staphylococcus aureus*. It is associated with tampon use during menses and carries nonmenstrual risk for women who use vaginal family planning methods (Stewart, 1998). The incidence of TSS has declined over the years owing to product changes and media warnings about tampon use (Farley, 1994). Although rare, TSS is a serious disorder to women's health, and providers must make women aware of this acute illness' potential, encourage them to report symptoms early, and exercise caution when using tampons and vaginal family planning methods (Creehan, 1995; Stewart F, 1998). Although TSS occurs most often in women of reproductive age who are menstruating, it has occurred in children and men (Creehan, 1995).

Chronic Illness

Included among chronic diseases that may affect a woman during her life span are arteriosclerotic heart disease (ASHD), hypertension, diabetes, arthritis, osteoporosis, and cancer.

Arteriosclerotic Heart Disease

According to clinical evidence, ASHD may have its beginnings in the second and third decades of a woman's life. Changing lifestyles are altering these statistics, but some risk factors such as race or family history of ASHD are nonmodifiable. As discussed earlier, black women are more vulnerable to ASHD than white women and experience congestive heart failure and angina pectoris after MI more frequently (AHA, 1999). Among the modifiable risk factors are the following:

- elevated serum lipid levels;
- a diet high in calories, total fats, cholesterol, refined carbohydrates, and sodium;

- hypertension;
- obesity;
- glucose intolerance;
- cigarette smoking;
- personality type;
- sedentary lifestyle; and
- stress.

Women should reduce their risk for ASHD by controlling as many of these factors as possible.

Hypertension

Hypertension, defined as blood pressure of 140/90 mm Hg or greater, significantly increases the risk of serious injury or death from coronary heart disease. Essential hypertension is the most common type of chronic hypertensive disorder in women of childbearing age, accounting for 85% of such cases. It is also responsible for approximately one third of all hypertension cases during pregnancy. Hypertension is more common in women than in men and affects more blacks than whites. Additional factors associated with primary hypertension are age (>35 years), family history of hypertension, obesity, cigarette smoking, and diabetes mellitus (AHA, 1999). Hypertension usually starts with an asymptomatic phase; therefore every woman should be screened on an average of every two years beginning in her teenage years. Diagnosis is crucial to prevent or modify possible complications of this disease.

Diabetes

According to the American Diabetes Association (2000), 15.7 million people (5.9% of the population) have diabetes in the United States. Furthermore, although an estimated 10.3 million have been diagnosed, some 5.4 million people are not aware they have the disease. In previous years, community health nurses have worked to educate women to assume responsibility in their management of diabetes mellitus. More recently, community health nurses have been actively involved in education and screening programs for groups at high risk. Included in these groups are individuals who have a family history of diabetes, those who are obese, and older adults.

According to Cunningham and colleagues (1997), pregnancy is potentially diabetogenic. Pregnancy may aggravate the condition and clinical diabetes may appear in some women only during pregnancy. Consequently, considerable attention has been given to screening for diabetes in pregnancy. Controversy surrounds the most effective method of screening for diabetes, but regardless of the selected method, the nurse is involved in explaining the purpose of the screening and how to prepare for the tests. In most public health settings, the nurse is responsible for explaining the results.

Arthritis

Arthritis afflicts an estimated 50 million people in the United States; therefore arthritis is a major health concern for women. The incidence of osteoarthritis is slightly higher in women than in men, but rheumatoid arthritis (RA) afflicts three times as many women as men (Arthritis Foundation, 1999; Verbrugge, 1995). Symptoms of RA, an autoimmune disease, include swelling, stiffness, and pain in joints and increasing evidence shows that ethnic minorities are at a disadvantage for arthritis-related disabilities (Jordan, 1999). The cause of arthritis is not known; however, recurring multiple factors in the development of arthritis include diet, environment, and stress. Smoking and female gender may also contribute to RA development (Karlson et al., 1999). Nursing interventions focus on prevention of joint deformity and lifestyle modification if necessary.

Osteoporosis

Osteoporosis is a major disorder affecting women. Estimates of its occurrence range from 25% to 50%. Although men may experience osteoporosis, it is more often associated with women. The National Osteoporosis Foundation estimates that between four million and six million nonHispanic white women in the United States have osteoporosis, and an additional 13 million to 17 million have osteopenia (Looker et al., 1997). Half of all nonHispanic white women in the United States will sustain an osteoporosis-related fracture during their lifetime. The most serious complication of osteoporosis is hip fracture. Some 280,000 Americans experience hip fractures each year; approximately 24% die within a year from complications from the injury (USDHHS, 2000b).

Postmenopausal white women are at highest risk for osteoporosis. In women, loss of bone begins at an earlier age and proceeds twice as rapidly as in men. The recent guidelines issued by the National Osteoporosis Foundation in the United States recommend bone mineral density (BMD) tests for selected postmenopausal women and the use of hormone replacement therapy (HRT) as a first-line pharmacological option for prevention and treatment of osteoporosis. Osteoporosis has no cure; therefore prevention is especially important early in life. Prevention involves an awareness of dietary practices such as maintaining a correct balance of calcium, vitamin D, and protein throughout life in addition to regular weight-bearing and muscle-strengthening exercises (National Osteoporosis Foundations, 1998).

Nurses in ambulatory health practices should encourage women to become more knowledgeable of the strategies to prevent osteoporosis. The nurse must discuss the risks and benefits associated with HRT and alternatives to HRT with the woman to facilitate her decision making. For women diagnosed with osteoporosis, nurses can assist in various aspects of management (e.g., education regarding prescribed medication, follow-up care, avoidance of complications, and dietary modifications as needed).

Breast Cancer

The incidence of breast cancer has been increasing since the 1950s. Presently, one of every eight women will acquire breast cancer sometime in her life. Risk factors include aging, personal or family history of breast cancer, early age at menarche, late age at menopause, never having children, or having a first child after age 30 (ACS, 1999). Female gender and aging are the most significant risk factors for breast cancer.

In the battle against breast cancer, women must understand and practice early detection methods. The practice of monthly BSE should begin in high school and continue throughout a woman's life. Nurses in any setting with an aggregate of women should possess the skills for teaching BSE. Most chapters of the ACS regularly offer classes. A breast examination by the woman's health care professional should be performed in addition to her annual pelvic examination and PAP smear. The ACS recommends that women aged 40 and older have an annual mammogram, an annual clinical breast examination, and perform monthly BSE (ACS, 1999). Mammography, which is low-dose radiography, is not usually indicated for asymptomatic women younger than age 30 years. The ACS recommendations are for asymptomatic women without a personal or family history of breast cancer.

When a palpable lump or an abnormality is found on mammography, health care providers use specific algorithms to evaluate the lump and determine a course of action (Love et al., 1996). All nurses must be familiar with resources that may assist women in the diagnostical process (Facione,

---

BOX **15-2**

Resource Materials for Breast Cancer

ACS Breast Cancer Resource Materials:
Breast Cancer: Nowhere to Hide (pamphlet)
Three Ways to Take Special Care of Your Breasts
  (card, fifth grade reading level, English on one
  side and Spanish on the other)*
Breast Health (poster)
BSE—Special Touch (video, instructor's guide,
  and flip chart)
How to Do BSE (pamphlet)
A Woman's Guide to Mammography (pamphlet)
For copies call (800) ACS-2345.

National Cancer Institute Breast Cancer
  Resources:
A Mammogram Once A Year . . . For a Lifetime
  (video)
*Smart Advice for Women 40 and Over: Have a
  Mammogram* (pamphlet)
Guidelines for Screening Mammography
  (pamphlet)
*A Mammogram Could Save Your Life**
*Take Care of Your Breasts**
For copies call (800) 4-CANCER or contact the
  NCI at (301) 496-8680.

USDHHS and HCFA:
*Get a Mammogram: A Picture That Can Save Your
  Life* (pamphlet)
Medicare Covers Mammograms (pamphlet)
For copies and more information call (800)
  4-CANCER (breast cancer and mammograms);
  (800) 638-6833 (Medicare coverage).

---

*Specifically designed for low-literacy audiences; some
resources are available in Spanish and English.
Additional information about these resources can be
found by accessing the websites of these organizations
through the WebLinks section on the book's website at
SIMON www.wbsaunders.com/SIMON/nies/.

1999) (Box 15-2). Breast health centers are excellent resources for women and many centers accept self-referrals.

Lung Cancer

Although breast cancer is the most common cancer among women (i.e., excluding skin cancer), cancer of the lung and bronchus is responsible for more cancer deaths. Currently, the United States has the highest death rate among women with lung cancer in the world (Landis et al., 1998). Of the 171,600 new lung cancer cases projected for 1999, 45.2% (77,600) will be among women (ACS, 1999). However, this disease has been largely missed or ignored as a woman's health issue. Although medical treatment may be similar for men and women, the symptom distress, QOL, and demands of illness experienced by women may be different than men because the competing household, child care, and other role-related demands take a toll on many women (Sarna and McCorkle, 1996). Women with advanced lung cancer report more psychological symptoms than men (Hopwood and Stephens, 1995). Data from female survivors of cancer indicate that women had significantly greater negative ratings on physical, psychological, and social components of QOL, but higher ratings of spiritual well-being (Ferrell, Hassey-Dow, and Grant, 1995).

Lung cancer is often a fatal illness because it is difficult to obtain early detection and effective treatment for advanced disease. Lung cancer at diagnosis is most commonly at an advanced stage. Women appear to have a survival advantage, but whether this has to do with the consequences of a shorter smoking history or hormonal, genetic, or other differences is unclear (Palomares et al., 1996). Many symptom management, QOL, and women's health issues in general have not been adequately researched in women diagnosed with lung cancer.

The primary factor in preventing lung cancer is for individuals to never start smoking or at least quit smoking. Nurses must work with other health care providers to reverse the morbidity and mortality rates related to this disease. The Agency for Healthcare Research and Quality (AHRQ), formerly the AHCPR, has developed a useful guideline for health care professionals to assist women and their families in smoking cessation efforts. The AHRQ has summaries of more than 400 guidelines on a wide variety of topics, which can be found on their website. It can be accessed through the book's SIMON website at www.wbsaunders.com/SIMON/nies/.

Gynecological Cancers

About 20% of all malignant diseases in women occur in the genital tract. Carcinoma of the cervix is the most common and accounts for 21% of all new genital tract malignancies. The cervix is accessible to cytologic study; therefore the mortality rate related to cervical cancer has decreased. Risk factors for cervical cancer include coitus at an early age, multiple sexual partners, history of sexually transmitted infections with certain types of human papillomavirus (HPV), cigarette smoking, and low SES (ACS, 1999).

The incidence of invasive cervical cancer has declined dramatically as a result of regular PAP tests that allow for identification of a precancerous condition (i.e., cervical carcinoma in situ). However, an estimated 4800 women will die from the disease in 1999 (ACS, 1999).

In recent years, a debate has arisen regarding how often a woman should have a PAP smear. Major authorities now recommend that women who are or have been sexually active or who have reached age 18 receive an annual PAP test, which is inexpensive, causes no known harm, and has the capacity for a high degree of sensitivity. After three or more annual examinations with normal findings, the test may be performed less frequently at the discretion of the woman and her clinician (ACS, 1999).

A new self-collected tissue sample that detects HPV may become an effective alternative to the PAP smear (Wright, 2000). This new test is especially important for use with populations at risk for HPV infection and for poor regions of the world (Box 15-3).

The incidence of carcinoma of the endometrium has increased significantly during the past three decades, being commonly found in women during their sixth and seventh decades of life (i.e., 80% of women with this condition are postmenopausal). Factors related to its occurrence are obesity, low parity, diabetes mellitus, and conditions in which high circulating estrogen levels are not countered by adequate progesterone levels. The most common sign of endometrial cancer, occurring in 90% of women, is abnormal vaginal bleeding. Postmenopausal women experiencing vaginal bleeding should seek immediate gynecologic evaluation (Seltzer and Pearse, 1995). In addition to an annual pelvic examination by a health professional, women should have an endometrial biopsy at menopause and high-risk women should be identified and encouraged to seek ongoing monitoring (ACS, 1999).

Cancer of the ovary causes more deaths than any other pelvic malignancy. In the United States, ovarian cancer's annual incidence usually ranges between 5 and 15 cases per 100,000 women. Approximately 1:70 will acquire ovarian cancer, a rate increasing fairly rapidly after age 40 years. Risk factors include increasing age, nulliparity, a history of breast cancer, and a family history of breast and ovarian cancer (ACS, 1999). Early-stage detection of ovarian cancer is difficult; therefore it has usually reached an advanced stage once discovered. The health professional should be alert to ovarian enlargement with suspicion that ovarian malignancy may be present. This is especially true in postmenopausal women (Seltzer and Pearse, 1995).

The most common sign a woman experiences is abdominal enlargement. She may complain that her skirts and slacks are getting tighter in the waist. This is a silent cancer; therefore any woman older than age 40 who experiences vague digestive complaints that persist and are not explained by another cause must have a thorough evaluation for ovarian cancer. According to the ACS (1999), transvaginal ultrasound and a blood test for tumor marker CA 125 may assist in the diagnosis of ovarian cancer; however, these are not recommended for routine screening of all women.

Mental Disorders and Stress

Various circumstances and conditions influence the mental health of women. Women face stressful decisions about career and family and many express anxiety in these decisions. A woman may feel pressured to make decisions regarding childbearing before she has fulfilled her career goals. Deciding to focus on a career may mean decreased authority and the suffering of stress in the workplace. Women combining motherhood and a career have additional decisions such as working during pregnancy and choice of child care. More women are occupying middle-management positions known for creating stress-related illness associated with high demands and little or no power.

A woman's emotional state is influenced by ovarian function from the onset of menstruation to the cessation of menstrual periods. Depressive symptoms have been associated with menarche, premenstrual dysphoric disorder or premenstrual syndrome, the postpartum period, and the perimenopause (Stotland, 1995). Depression is more prevalent among women than among men. Some attribute this difference to women's role socialization rather than to biological differences, whereas others emphasize the interactive

B O X **15-3**

Nurse Researchers Use Innovative Strategy to Increase Breast and Cervical Cancer Screening among Asian-American Women

The lack of breast and cervical cancer screening is more common among underserved women and women of color. To address the problem among Asian-American women, nurse researchers at the University of Alabama at Birmingham (UAB) School of Nursing are developing a program based on the community health advisor model. The project is funded through the Alabama State Department of Health CDC's Breast and Cervical Cancer Early Detection program and is outlined here.

Cancer Prevention Study Targets Asian-American Women:

Birmingham, Alabama: "While most cases of breast and cervical cancer can be treated effectively if detected early, nearly 60 percent of Asian-American women have never had a breast or cervical exam," said Youngshook Han, Ph.D., instructor with the School of Nursing at UAB. Han and colleagues are addressing an alarming statistic through a new study to improve cancer-screening practices among Asian-American women in Alabama.

Although Asian-American women are a small percentage of the population, "there is evidence of late stage cancer diagnosis and poor survival among Asian women. In America, the breast cancer risk rate in Asian-American women is seven times higher than it is in their home countries. We need to focus on intervention efforts for this population," said Han.

Researchers are developing culturally appropriate materials to overcome education barriers among Asian-American women. "Language is the biggest barrier to educating Asian-American women about cancer screenings," said Han. "There are also cost and attitude barriers. Mammograms are not free, and some Asian-American women do not feel comfortable being examined by male doctors."

The study will enroll 200 low-income Asian-American women from Birmingham, Huntsville, and Mobile, Alabama, where the majority of Asian-American women live in the state. "We are working with local churches and community organizations to identify women for the study," said Han. "Women must be at least 18 years old and able to read and write to participate."

A group of Asian-American women will become community volunteers and lay health advisors and work with the women to educate them about cancer, prevention, and early detection and to encourage them to have regular breast and cervical cancer screenings. "These women will be community leaders, well-respected by Asian-American women in the community as advisors and helpers," said Han.

After the one-year study, the intervention program will remain in place to provide ongoing cancer education and intervention support for Asian-American women in the community. "The success of this community-based intervention strategy will establish a lasting partnership and grassroots network between UAB and Asian-American communities," said Han.

For more information, contact Youngshook Han, Ph.D., at UAB (205) 934-6607 (Han, Williams, and Harrison, 1999).

biopsychosocial dynamics involved in the phenomenon of depression in women (Jones-Warren, 1995). According to Bhatia and Bhatia (1999), the higher prevalence of depression in women is most likely from a combination of gender-related differences in cognitive styles, certain biological factors, and a higher incidence of psychosocial and economic stressors. Community health nurses are in a good position to assess women's moods in diverse aggregates (see Box 15-1).

Reproductive Health

Community health nurses provide a variety of services in the area of women's reproductive health from menarche through the postmenopausal phase. Nurses, in collaboration with other health care professionals, have identified a persisting group of preventable and correctable problems related to maternal-child health. *Healthy People 2010* (USDHHS, 2000b) includes numerous recommendations for improving maternal

TABLE **15-7**

Healthy People 2010 Objectives and Family Planning

Objective	Baseline	Target
9-1: Increase the proportion of pregnancies that are intended.	51%	70%
9-7: Reduce pregnancies among adolescent females.	72 pregnancies per 1000 females 15 to 17 years of age	46 pregnancies per 1000 females 15 to 17 years of age
9-11: Increase the proportion of young adults who have received formal instruction before turning 18 years of age on reproductive health issues.	64%	90%
9-12: Reduce the proportion of married couples whose ability to conceive or maintain a pregnancy is impaired.	13%	10%

From US Department of Health and Human Services: *Healthy people 2010*, Conference Edition, Washington, DC, 2000a, The Author.

and infant health by activities such as reduction of cigarette smoking, reduction of alcohol and other drug use, better nutrition, better socioeconomic opportunities including education, and a decrease in environmental hazards.

For the *Healthy People 2000* initiative, family planning objectives witnessed progress. For example, the number of unintended pregnancies decreased from 56% to 49% between 1988 and 1995, yet the objective to reduce the rate of adolescent pregnancy still remains distant. With *Healthy People 2010* family planning objectives, the focus is on the positive that "all pregnancies should be intended." Table 15-7 shows examples of *Healthy People 2010* objectives related to family planning.

Nutrition

One of the most important factors related to a woman's reproductive health focuses on her total life nutritional experience from inception through infancy, childhood, and adolescence. Pregnancy may provide a motivational factor for developing an awareness of proper nutrition. During the nutritional assessment of a prenatal client, the community health nurse can take the opportunity to determine dietary habits and initiate a referral to the Special Supplemental Food Program for WIC when necessary. WIC provides food vouchers for pregnant or breast-feeding women, infants, and children who are at nutritional risk.

Good nutrition must consider factors other than kinds and amounts of foods. Other elements to consider include age, lifestyle, economic status, and culture. For example, when counseling a pregnant adolescent, the nurse can include the primary person responsible for meal preparation. However, the nurse should not ignore the adolescent in the planning of her diet, but should ask her to identify foods that she likes from those recommended. The nurse needs to make the adolescent aware of the influence of her nutrition on fetal growth and development. This information must be balanced with the young woman's individual needs.

Family Planning

The community health nurse has many opportunities to provide counseling in the area of **family planning**. Although the phrase "family planning" has come to imply planned limitation of pregnancies, another important aspect of family planning concerns couples attempting to increase their chances of conception.

Infertility occurs in a surprising number of otherwise healthy adults. Approximately 10% to 15% of couples in the United States are unintentionally childless (Stewart, 1998). On the other hand, slightly less than half of all pregnancies occurring in the United States are unintended (Seltzer and Pearse, 1995).

Community health nurses are in a strategic position to provide support and guidance for women in the area of fertility control. Numerous factors contribute to the decision of whether to use family planning methods and what methods to use. When counseling women on this matter, the nurse should use a holistic approach. The nurse must consider factors such as age, sexual activity, cost, health care access, and the woman's and her partner's values and beliefs. After a discussion with the nurse about benefits and risks, indications and contraindications, and advantages and disadvantages of the various contraception methods, the client selects a method that she believes is safe, effective, and comfortable.

> Health care professionals often neglect to mention natural family planning as a method of contraception. Although many consider this approach to be synonymous with the rhythm method, proponents of natural family planning are describing this method as natural reproductive technology, a term that is broader in scope and encompasses the health of a woman's reproductive system. Such knowledge allows feelings of empowerment and a sense of control over fertility. Women experience self-knowledge and thereby gain autonomy in relation to fertility. Family and community health care professionals need to have up-to-date information concerning natural family planning.

Women who decide that their families are large enough and do not wish to be concerned with temporary methods of fertility control may select voluntary surgical contraception (VSC) or contraceptive sterilization by tubal ligation. Vasectomy as a VSC continues to be a simpler, safer, and less expensive procedure than tubal ligation. The VSC is one of the most effective, safest, and cost-effective methods of family planning, and developed and developing countries use it widely (Stewart and Carignan, 1998). The client's decision must be based on clear, complete information for sterilization more than any other phase of family planning. The reversibility of sterilization procedures is not dependable; if a woman has doubts about her future childbearing, the nurse should encourage her to use other methods of fertility control.

Promoting responsible family planning is a goal of the International Council of Nurses (ICN). The ICN believes that family planning is basic to the health of the family and necessary to form a strong society. Furthermore, the ICN posits that all couples and individuals have the basic right to decide the number and spacing of their children and to have adequate knowledge to make these critical decisions (ICN, 1993). Major benefits of family planning services and counseling worldwide include preven-

tion of unwanted pregnancies and reduction in the high incidence of abortions. Worldwide, 300 million couples do not want more children but are not using effective methods of family planning.

Nurses worldwide have a major role to play if the health of women and their families is to improve. Besides being knowledgeable about family planning methods and services, all nurses must work for universally accessible maternal and child health care and seek to protect the rights of couples and individuals to receive good information about family planning. In addition, nurses must be involved in shaping policy that affects every woman's reproductive health. Research in the area of family planning will hopefully provide several safe options designed to meet the individual needs of all women.

STDs and HIV

STDs are commonly found among U.S. women. Community health nurses and other health providers, including physicians, NPs, nurse midwives, and social workers, must be prepared to provide age-appropriate STD prevention, education, and counseling.

STDs

Genital chlamydial infection is now the most commonly reported infectious disease in the United States (two to four million cases annually). Furthermore, more than 600,000 cases of gonorrhea are reported every year, making it the second most commonly reported communicable disease in the United States. The actual numbers are estimated to be about double owing to underreporting. A woman may acquire chlamydial infection simultaneously with gonorrhea; therefore she should be treated presumptively with a regimen effective against both organisms. Complications resulting from STDs include tubal occlusion, leading to infertility and ectopic pregnancy, pregnancy loss and neonatal injury caused by transmission of organism to fetus, genital cancers, and epidemiological synergy with HIV transmission (Cates, 1998).

Other commonly occurring STDs are HPV, herpes, trichomoniasis, and syphilis. Chapter 25 contains detailed information on these diseases, their incidence, symptoms, and treatment.

HIV and AIDS

HIV has become a woman's health problem in the United States after primarily affecting men for almost two decades. HIV infection is rising more rapidly among American women (15 to 44 years of age) than any other group. Worldwide, AIDS is a leading cause of death among young women (Joint United Nations Programme on HIV and AIDS, 1996). In the United States, AIDS is the third leading cause of death among women of reproductive age. However, many providers are unfamiliar with the symptoms of HIV infection as it infects women (Guest, 1998b).

Similar to other population groups with AIDS in the United States, the majority of women with AIDS are from racial and ethnic minority groups, with blacks comprising 49%, Latinas comprising 14%, and whites comprising 33% (USDHHS, 2000a). Women at highest risk for becoming HIV seropositive include the following:

- intravenous drug users who share needles or syringes,
- prostitutes,
- those who have sex with infected partners, and
- participants in unprotected sex.

> Bozzette and colleagues (1998) compared demographic variables of men vs. women living with HIV and AIDS in the United States in 1996. Women comprised 26% of 231,400 reported patients analyzed. HIV-infected women were more likely to be black than HIV-infected men (54% vs. 27%, P <0.001) and were more likely unemployed (76% vs. 59%). About 30% of the women had annual household incomes less than $5000 per year (vs. 17% of the men, P <0.001). The majority of both groups were without medical insurance, including 85% of the women and 63% of the men (P <0.001). The women were younger on average than the men and 44% of women were under age 35 vs. 31% of the men (P <0.001).

Recent employment of highly active antiretroviral therapy (HAART) in HIV-positive pregnant women has contributed to a rapid decline in the rate of perinatal transmission of HIV (Guest, 1998b; HIV Clinical Management, 1999). The nurse must counsel and recommend voluntary HIV testing for all pregnant women.

Other Issues in Women's Health

Unintentional Injury or Accidents
Although unintentional injury affects women less commonly than men, several areas of concern still exist for women. For example, older women are at increased risk for accidents such as falls. Falls account for the majority of serious unintentional injuries and lead to 40% of all deaths from injury in people older than 75 years of age. Factors that may be responsible for this major cause of injury among older adults are associated with an unsteady gait, reduced vision, or a hazardous environment. Older women experience an increasing number of falls; therefore the nurse must identify the preventable factors. Nurses, whether working with older adults in the home or in institutional settings, must be knowledgeable of hazards that may be corrected to decrease the incidence of falls.

Abuse in women is often explained as accidental injury. Approximately 6% of visits made by women to emergency rooms are for injuries that result from physical battering by their husbands, former husbands, boyfriends, or lovers. **Domestic violence** includes physical, sexual, and psychological attacks and economic coercion (Warshaw, Ganley, and Salber, 1995). Violent behavior toward women is epidemic with estimates of two to six million women from all socioeconomic levels abused annually (Elliot and Johnson, 1995). All women should be questioned directly about abuse. However, according to Blair (1999) barriers can interfere with such screening, including frustration when patients fail to leave the abusive situation after intensive intervention or counseling. Also, many nurses are past or current victims of abuse; assessing abuse with patients can evoke painful emotions that the nurse may not be ready to confront.

Nurses employed in community health settings need to know how to make assessments, provide support, and make referrals to agencies dealing with domestic violence. In addition, nurses and other health care professionals must know the laws in their state related to reporting known or suspected domestic violence (Fishwick, 1998).

Disability
More women than men have disabilities resulting from acute conditions, but women experience fewer disabilities resulting from chronic conditions because they report their symptoms earlier and receive necessary treatment. A disability may reduce the individual's activity; women report proportionately more days of restricted activity than men. Women average 16.1 days of disability per year compared with 12.7 days for men (US Census Bureau, 1990).

A frequently encountered disabling condition is dysmenorrhea, which is most often associated with ovulatory cycles and is one of the most common concerns of women. Dysmenorrhea affects approximately 50% to 80% of the female population between ages 15 and 24 years, but continues to plague women throughout the reproductive years (Nelson, 1998; Seltzer and Pearse, 1995). At least 10% to 20% of women with dysmenorrhea are incapacitated for one to three days each month; therefore dysmenorrhea is the greatest single cause of absenteeism from school and work among young women. Dysmenorrhea causes the loss of approximately 140 million working hours annually; therefore the economic influence of this condition is significant.

Disabling conditions limit the physical functional abilities of many women, but the health care delivery system has often overlooked the unique needs of this aggregate. In planning care for disabled women, community health nurses should focus attention on enabling women to strengthen their capabilities. In addition, nurses should be sensitive to barriers in the clinical setting that affect the access of disabled women to health care services. Chapter 19 discusses the needs of disabled people in greater detail.

End-of-Life Issues

The community gathered.
Preacher Thomas spoke of Meredith Jennings, Her parentage, The important dates of her life,
And said:
Unheralded, but day by day, As faithful as you'll find . . .
Unselfish in her ev'ry way, She was the steadfast kind.
Elton Fowler rose to state:
Unmoved, she always took her place. And doing all she could,
She filled, with grace, allotted space . . . Gave far more than she should.
Nellie Barker's face turned red. She had a word to say:
Freedom came to her at last.
Don't speak as if she's dead!
Departed yes, but she's not passed . . .
Our Meredith has fled!

From Sullivan E, Sullivan H: The departure. In Sullivan E, Sullivan H, editors: *Voices of a mother and daughter*, Norman, Okla, 1997, Hooper.

Meredith represents many active, female community members who have fled. They flee disease and suffering, but not before confronting many issues surrounding the end of life. Often women serve as caregivers when others face the end of life. At the end of life, many issues involve difficult decisions. Community health nurses must provide care, comfort, and support during this life stage (Ferrell, Virani, and Grant, 1998). Nurses must educate communities, families, and patients about advance directives as mandated in the Patient Self-Determination Act (Task Force on End of Life Decisions, American Nursing Association, 1991). However, the laws cannot legislate increased communication between patients and health care professionals as evidenced by the limited number of individuals with advance directives.

According to Stanley (2000), appropriate and effective communication about sequelae to a life-threatening illness and treatment is left undone because it provokes sheer discomfort. Transitioning patients from curative to palliative care occurs all too often in the final days of illness (Ferrell, 1996).

Women are "caregivers and communicators" in families and often face responsibilities related to end-of-life issues. Nurses involved in this process can make a critical difference in outcomes. As Stanley (2000) states, the nurse functions as "existential messenger" across the illness continuum. In this role, the nurse is comfortable and effective in working with patents and their families in making difficult, heart-wrenching decisions at the end of life. To make these decisions in isolation increases the anguish. According to Quill (1995), "there is a world of difference between facing an uncertain future alone and facing it with a committed partner." The community health nurse, in partnership with the patient and family, can help make this journey smoother.

MAJOR LEGISLATION AFFECTING WOMEN'S HEALTH SERVICES

Several legislative acts have a direct or indirect influence on the health of women. Many changes have been made in the past two decades that have the potential for improving the health and welfare of all women.

Public Health Service Act

The PHS Act, passed in 1982, provides biomedical and health services research, information dissemination, resource development, technical assistance, and service delivery. In the area of women's health, the PHS Act supports activities related to general health issues, reproductive health, social and behavioral issues, and mental health. Aggregates of women targeted by the PHS include those disabled by specific diseases, victims of sexual abuse and domestic violence, recent immigrants, and occupational groups.

The Family Planning Assistance Program, which is one component of the PHS Act, helps millions of women obtain family planning services each year. The need for subsidized family planning remains significant and federal funds should be made generously available to meet documented needs. With regard to the particular relationship of family planning and low birth weight, both young teenage status and poverty are major risk factors for delivering infants with low birth weight. The program is an important part of public effort to prevent low birth weight.

Civil Rights Act

Title VII of the **Civil Rights Act** of 1964 prohibits discrimination based on sex, race, color, religion, or national origin in determining employment eligibility or termination, wages, and fringe benefits. The Act was amended to prohibit discrimination against pregnant women or conditions involving childbirth or pregnancy. This landmark legislation makes it unlawful for employers to refuse to hire, employ, or promote a woman because she is pregnant. In addition, employee benefit plans that continue health insurance, income maintenance during disability or illness, or any other income support program for disabled workers must include disabilities resulting from pregnancy, childbirth, and other related conditions. If employers allow disabled employers to assume lighter or medically restricted assignments, the same considerations must extend to the pregnant woman (Craven, Greenberger, and Kolker, 1993).

The amendment does not require employers to pay health insurance benefits for abortions or abortion-related care unless the mother's life is endangered or she has medical complications after an abortion. Employers are prohibited from firing or refusing to hire a woman because she had an abortion.

Sexual harassment is a violation of the Civil Rights Act. Sexual harassment is "conduct of a sexual nature . . . unwelcome by the target . . . severe or pervasive enough to create an intimidating work environment" (Women Employed Institute, 1994). Female and male workers may face unwelcome sexual advances or requests for sexual favors or other verbal or physical conduct of a sexual nature. Awareness of sexual harassment in the workplace has increased dramatically over the past decade, but it has not been eliminated.

Social Security Act

The Social Security Act provides monthly retirement and disability benefits to workers and survivor benefits to families of workers covered by Social Security. Full retirement benefits are available to workers after 10 years of covered employment.

The Social Security Act permits a divorced person to receive benefits based on a former spouse's earning record when that spouse retires, becomes disabled, or dies if the marriage lasted at least 10 years. Since January 1985, a woman who has been divorced for at least two years can receive spousal benefits at age 62 if her former husband is eligible for benefits regardless of whether he is actually receiving them.

Medicare and Medicaid also resulted from the Social Security Act. Medicare is the insurance plan that covers the majority of the health care expenses of older adults, including payments for hospital care, physicians, home health care, and other services and supplies after copayments and deductibles. Medicaid covers health care for indigent and eligible children and includes family planning, obstetric care, and preventive cancer screening for women such as mammography and PAP smears. Chapters 9 and 10 describe Medicare and Medicaid in detail.

Occupational Safety and Health Act

The Occupational Safety and Health Act, enacted in 1970, helps ensure safe and healthful working conditions for workers throughout the United States. Although there is an increasing emphasis in the study of the health of women workers, gaps in knowledge exist. For example, little is known about women who work in cottage industries, as domestic workers, as prostitutes, in agriculture, and in the garment industry. In addition, the work of some women is classified as "women's work" and includes such things as housework, child care, caregiver of the sick, and farming (Misner, Beauchamp-Hewitt, and Fox-Levin, 1995). These women experience physical demands and

TABLE 15-8

Hazardous Occupations in which Women are Employed

Occupation	Health Hazard
Clerical workers	Organic solvents in stencil machines, correction fluids, rubber cement, and ozone from copying machines
Textile and apparel workers	Cotton dust, skin irritants, and chemicals
Hairdressers and beauticians	Hair, nail, and skin beauty preparations
Launderers and dry cleaners	Heat, heavy lifting, and chemicals
Electronics workers	Solvents and acids
Hospital and other health care workers	Infectious diseases, heavy lifting, radiation, skin disorders, and anesthetic gases
Laboratory workers	Biological agents; flammable explosive, toxic, or carcinogenic substances; exposure to radiation; and bites from and allergic reactions to research animals

hazards, yet government economic reports have not recognized these individuals as workers. Investigations of factors that influence the health of these women workers are needed. Table 15-8 lists specific positions in which a large number of women are employed and the potential for health hazards.

Community health nurses, occupational health nurses, and NPs need to be cognizant of environmental hazards wherever they find women at work. In taking health histories, the nurse should collect data regarding the client's occupational environment to assess the potential risk to emotional, general, and reproductive health. In addition, nurses must work individually and as an aggregate with their legislatures to maintain strong worker health and safety programs to protect the health of all women.

Family and Medical Leave Act

Enacted in 1993, the **Family and Medical Leave Act** (FMLA) allows an employee a minimum provision of 12 weeks unpaid leave each year for family and medical reasons such as personal illness; an ill child, parent, or spouse; or the birth or adoption of a child. This act guarantees the employee the same or equivalent job with the same pay and benefits upon the employee's return to work. In addition, health benefits must continue throughout the leave. Approximately 20% of the U.S. workforce needed some form of FMLA-covered leave after the law was enacted (Gilinson, 1999).

The FMLA is particularly important to female workers because they are more likely to use leave to care for seriously ill family members, whereas male workers more often use leave for personal illness (Gilinson, 1999). According to the Women's Legal Defense Fund, every employee who must be away from work for family and medical reasons loses income. However, the loss is most severe for those without job-protected leave. Annual earnings for female workers without job-protected leave reduced by 29.1% in the first year after giving birth, whereas those with leave lost only 18.2%. The FMLA is an important step toward equitable leave policies, but more change is needed. The ANA has been instrumental in securing passage of the FMLA and is currently advocating in Congress for paid FMLA.

HEALTH AND SOCIAL SERVICES TO PROMOTE THE HEALTH OF WOMEN

Medicaid is a health insurance program for the poor, exclusive of age eligibility. Medicaid is funded jointly by the federal government and each state but is administered by individual states. Many of the pregnant women who are eligible for Medicaid are at high risk for poor pregnancy outcome, including low birth weight. Ideally, a maternity care provider should examine women with high maternal risk immediately after conception. However, too often these women seek prenatal care late in the pregnancy or arrive at the emergency department without receiving prenatal care when delivery is imminent. Consider the clinical example on page 371.

This case is not unusual. Barriers limit access to prenatal care among those most in need. Medicaid allows some access to care. Greater public awareness of facilities and maternity care providers who accept Medicaid is necessary. Recent changes in payment plans that allow billing for care at higher rates have increased the number of providers who accept Medicaid patients.

Anita Rogers, a 16-year-old unemployed single woman, arrived at the Family Services Health Center seeking initial prenatal care at 36 weeks gestation. She stated that for a few days she noted some brown discharge from her vagina. She told the NP she knew she should have begun prenatal care earlier, but when she called several physicians' offices, the receptionist told her she should bring $1000 for her first visit. She said that neither she nor her parents had that much money. Her father was unemployed and her mother worked at a cafe as a waitress. She also had difficulty with transportation. Anita was sent to the hospital immediately for an ultrasound examination. The sonogram revealed triplets, but two of them died in utero. Anita was hospitalized and began to hemorrhage. She delivered a three-pound infant.

Women's Health Services

Since the mid1970s, women have sought health services beyond the conventional mode of care delivery. Many self-help groups have emerged and new approaches to women's health services have been accepted. Women have demanded a participatory role and have become more assertive; therefore health care facilities, including physicians' offices, are more responsive to women's perceptions of their health needs. A complete revolution in maternity care has occurred with the emergence of freestanding and hospital-based birth centers and family- and sibling-attended births. The health care needs of women go beyond their reproductive status and include their primary health care needs. The health care needs of women must be addressed more effectively and should include services for the following (Star et al., 1995):

1. Eating disorders
2. All forms of abuse
3. Disease prevention, including smoking cessation
4. Health promotion focusing on nutrition, exercise, and stress management

The National Women's Health Network has been a strong advocate for women's concerns and has provided testimony before congressional hearings dealing with women's issues. This organization is concerned with women's rights, environmental safety, reproductive rights, warnings regarding the effects of alcohol and drugs on the developing fetus, and safety in relation to medical devices. For example, the network was instrumental in the worldwide recall of the Dalkon Shield intrauterine device.

Another concern of the National Women's Health Network is drug safety, especially concerning drugs that may have teratogenic or carcinogenic effects. For example, the network has attempted to identify women who may have been exposed to diethylstilbestrol in utero.

Women's health consumers are requesting more emphasis in the area of well-women's health care (i.e., health care aimed at well-being, health promotion, and disease prevention). Several nurses throughout the United States have established collaborative practices with other health professionals to meet this demand for nonconventional services.

Other Community Voluntary Services

Networking has been one of the major movements during the last two decades. Networking is a system of interconnected or cooperating individuals. It is the means by which women seek to advance their careers, improve their lifestyles, and increase their income while helping other women become successful. Networks in business, professional support, politics and labor, arts, sports, and health have been established throughout the United States. These multiple networks have enabled women to develop new identities and become empowered to achieve mutual goals.

Many private voluntary organizations spend money, time, and energy in attempting to increase health awareness among its members and provide direct services to the public. Most urban areas have crisis hotline services in which women volunteer to provide counseling to battered women, battering parents, rape victims, those considering suicide, and those with multiple needs. A clinical example follows on page 372.

One of the most effective, low-cost, voluntary efforts to assist abused women involves shelters and safe houses scattered throughout the United States. Between two and six million American women are abused annually and abuse occurs in approximately 31% of all familial relationships (Tjaden and Thoenees, 1998). Many women needing shelter are

Helena Rowland arrived by taxi with her two-year-old child at the Truth Safe House for Women. Her left eye was bloodshot and her face was bruised and swollen. She was obviously pregnant. She stated that "my old man got mad and started beating on me. When he left, I found a friend who gave me some money to come to this place. I just don't know what gets into him, but every time I get pregnant he becomes even more abusive than usual. See my stomach? He kicked me right here," she said, pointing to the left side of her abdomen. After the intake worker received some preliminary information, Ms. Rowland was shown through the shelter and assigned a place for her and her child to sleep. She was greeted by the other six women and their children, who ranged in age from two weeks to 12 years. The women were working together to prepare the evening meal and invited Ms. Rowland to join them. During dinner they informed her that the nurse who talked with them and assisted them with personal and children's health concerns would come shortly to help her with her needs.

often denied emergency housing. One of the goals of *Healthy People 2010* relates to this problem.

Women's organizations have a long history of voluntary involvement with the community. An increasing number have added activities to their agenda to improve pregnancy outcomes, prevent teen pregnancy, and support older women's rights. Organizations such as the Older Women's League, United Methodist Women, other religious denomination women's groups, Urban League, sororities, Junior League, YWCA, National Association of Colored Women's Clubs, and many others have made women's health a major item on their agenda.

LEVELS OF PREVENTION AND WOMEN'S HEALTH

Primary Prevention

The author became involved in primary prevention with other community health nursing faculty as members of an ACS committee called Stop Cancer Among Minorities (SCAM). The SCAM committee members represented several ethnic groups from churches, schools, and health care agencies. The committee assessed the needs of a community that revealed a lack of knowledge of health promotion practices necessary to decrease the risk of cancer.

The committee planned a health fair to promote cancer awareness in the community. It was sponsored by the state chapter of the ACS and a local community health center. Nursing students and undergraduate faculty members from the local nursing college joined the committee to plan and implement the program.

Nursing students offered nutritious snacks (i.e., low in fat and high in fiber and complex carbohy-drates) and discussed the relationship of diet to cancer risk reduction. They also taught BSE and TSE. Other students shared the risks of smoking and the benefits of quitting. Seven booths located at the fair were associated with the seven danger signals of cancer.

Secondary Prevention

The focus of secondary prevention is on early diagnosis or health maintenance for people with chronic disorders. Women's health care NPs, family NPs, midwives from the community, the university baccalaureate nursing program, and the clinic's medical staff joined together to perform breast and pelvic examinations for each woman. PAP smears were also performed and sent for cytologic study to the state health department. The health center's director of nursing services carried out follow-up on PAP smear results.

Junior year nursing students became involved in a community study for a group of nuns in a local convent, who were a population at risk for breast cancer. The students prepared by becoming certified by the ACS as instructors in BSE. The ACS provided the students with current knowledge of breast cancer, its treatments, and early detection methods. The ACS also provided helpful films, pamphlets, and models for demonstration. Through the student's assessment, planning, and intervention, a group of women received skills for the early detection of a life-threatening disease.

Tertiary Prevention

Tertiary prevention consists of rehabilitation when sequelae of a condition have occurred. For example, Sandra Smith, a 55-year-old Native-American, had diabetes mellitus for the past three years. She attended

Jane Beaumont is a 20-year-old white woman who visited the clinic on the advice of her boyfriend. She appeared confused and frightened. She stated that her boyfriend had "clap" and that he told her to get treatment. She expressed little anger and stated that she knew he had sex with other women. During the interview, the nurse gathered information regarding the behavioral aspects of sexuality, physical symptoms, the client's knowledge of sexual health, and the client's emotional responses to the problem. During the examination, the nurse took chlamydia and gonorrhea cultures from appropriate sites. Then the nurse drew blood for serological diagnosis of syphilis. The patient was diagnosed with gonorrhea. The client also consented to HIV testing after the nurse discussed risk factors with her.

After the examination and the initiation of treatment according to protocol, the nurse answered questions and stressed the importance of follow-up and future protection against STDs. Ms. Beaumont asked why all this was necessary because she "felt okay." The nurse explained that 50% to 80% of all women have no complaints or symptoms and feel "okay" even though the disease is present. The nurse asked her to return in one week for the HIV test results. At that time, the nurse will evaluate whether the client understands her role in the prevention of STDs, including HIV.

Diana Cook came to the family planning clinic reporting that she missed two periods and "felt" pregnant. Ms. Cook was 33 years old and had two children aged 9 and 12 years. Her pregnancy test was positive and her pelvic examination was consistent with a six- to eight-week pregnancy. Ms. Cook did not plan the pregnancy and she needed counseling regarding her options. The nurse realized this was a crisis in Ms. Cook's life and that she needed support in whatever decision she made.

---

an urban clinic for monitoring her diabetes. After the physician examined her, he suggested that she have her annual pelvic examination. She was overdue for this and agreed to be seen by the women's health care NP. Ms. Smith described symptoms of a yeast infection (e.g., increase in vaginal discharge and itching) to the nurse. Her examination and a wet mount confirmed the diagnosis of *Candida albicans* infection, a common problem among diabetic women. The woman learned about the nature, predisposing factors, and treatment of the infection.

ROLES OF THE COMMUNITY HEALTH NURSE

Direct Care

The community health nurse provides direct care in a variety of settings. Often this is considered the "hands-on" nursing care given to a client in the home or a clinic. Direct care occurs in clinics many times every day. The first clinical example at the top of this page is representative of situations that arise numerous times every day.

Educator

The nurse encounters many opportunities for teaching. However, if the client is too anxious, the nurse will be unable to integrate new information. The present goal of the nurse is to develop trust so the young woman will return later for follow-up. See the second clinical example on this page.

Counselor

The counseling role of the nurse occurs in almost every interaction in the area of women's health. Before beginning counseling in the area of reproductive health, it is essential for effective intervention that the nurse become aware of his or her value system, including how biases and beliefs about human sexual behavior affect the counseling role. The third clinical example on this page is a representative scenario.

RESEARCH IN WOMEN'S HEALTH

Women have long been the major users of the health care system. However, until recently little research involving women provided information enabling prediction, explanation, or description of phenomena affecting health. In many cases, medical treatment for women is based on research with exclusively male subjects. This is also true in conditions that cause more deaths in women. Fortunately, increased effort includes women in studies related to cardiovascular health and lung and colon cancer. This emphasis came after a federal mandate that research must include women and minorities. If women are not included, a rationale must be given for their exclusion.

In a recent initiative, community health nursing faculty members interested in the health of women and their children received funding to offer a comprehensive breast cancer control program. They offered the program to the female parents or guardians of children enrolled in the Children's Rehabilitation Services (CRS) of Alabama. CRS is a state program that provides family-centered, community-based assistance to prevent, correct, or reduce physical disabilities of children.

Previous research has documented a decline in the personal health of parents of children with special health care needs. These caregivers, mostly mothers, often disregard personal symptoms of disease and avoid regular health checkups and important cancer detection practices in which delay may be catastrophic. In addition to providing breast health education, clinical breast examinations, and referral for mammography, the group is collecting data to compile a family profile and assess participants' breast cancer detection practices. This project allowed the nursing school, in cooperation with the CRS staff, to assist women in their pursuit of health promotion, provide clinical instruction to nursing students, and conduct needed research in the area of women's health (Williams and Turner-Henson, 1996).

The NIH established the Office of Research on Women's Health in 1990. Through a special task force, NIH recommendations are made for the research agenda for women's health for the next two decades. In addition, nurse researchers are encouraged to test interventions and question rituals in nursing by conducting ritual-busting research. The following are some of the areas for exploration and research among women:

- Health promotion
- Barriers to care
- Disease prevention
- Health education at various literacy levels
- Wellness across the life cycle
- Differences among women experiencing menopausal symptoms
- Dysmenorrhea
- Safe and effective contraception
- Promotion of breast feeding
- Infertility
- Coping with chronic illness such as systemic lupus erythematosus or arthritis
- Discomforts of pregnancy, including morning sickness
- Strengths of single female heads of households
- Adolescent sexuality
- Multiple-role adaptation
- Menstrual cycle variations
- Control of obesity
- Substance abuse and its effect on pregnancy
- HIV infection and pregnancy
- Influence of diet on osteoporosis
- Effect of socialization on role
- Domestic violence

More recently, research on the financing and delivery of health services for women has been supported. This research will address the changing health care environment; the unmet need for primary and preventive health services; the historic lack of research on women's health; and the importance of social, cultural, legal, economic, and behavioral factors influencing women's health care (Hinshaw, 2000).

With the increased emphasis on community health, community health nurses can make significant contributions toward the improvement of women's health through scholarly research either as principal investigators or through data gathering. Furthermore, they can become consumers of research and develop nursing interventions based on sound research and recommendations.

APPLICATION OF THE NURSING PROCESS

John Lawrence, an educator at the state women's correctional center, contacted Donna Williams, a women's health care NP and faculty member at the College of Nursing, and expressed concern for the health of an inmate, Lela Marvin. According to Mr. Lawrence, Lela, a 19-year-old pregnant primigravida, was being seen at the state-supported hospital for antepartal care; however, she was not permitted to attend perinatal education classes. He stated that other pregnant women in the facility could benefit from perinatal education. In fact, approximately 6.1% of female state prison inmates are pregnant when admitted to prison and could benefit from perinatal education (Snell, 1994).

Lawrence's call was followed by a call from Herman Martin, another RN who also expressed concern for the other women's needs for information regarding their personal hygiene. Although an RN, Mr. Martin was not knowledgeable of women's health because his primary clinical focus was emergency and trauma care. He indicated that many of the women were overweight, cared little about themselves, and lacked a general knowledge of how to maintain their health.

Assessment

After gaining clearance by the prison officials, Ms. Williams made an assessment of health care information needs and started offering classes for the inmates. The immediate need was for perinatal education for women in the last weeks of pregnancy. Lela said she wanted to learn about labor because she had heard only horror stories from other women. Donna noted that three other women were close to term and they also seemed eager to learn. Donna knew that students' readiness to learn was key to the course's success. Success of this course would be crucial to future course offerings.

The traditional perinatal education course was designed to promote healthy birth outcomes and an emotionally satisfying birth experience. These goals are also important to pregnant women in a correctional facility; however, perinatal education should be modified to meet this group's special needs. For example, information on newborn care is

not appropriate because the infant is usually placed with the mother's family or in foster care.

Assessment of nonpregnant women provided opportunities for other health education classes. The next spring and each spring thereafter, junior nursing students under the guidance of Ms. Williams were assigned to develop and carry out a one-hour weekly health education and awareness session at the correctional facility. Although each student expressed some initial anxiety toward the experience, each evaluated it as being worthwhile.

Diagnosis

After assessment, the community health nurse developed community and aggregate diagnoses, which served as the basis for the care plan.

Individual
- Inadequate preparation for childbirth related to lack of resources in prison (Lela)
- Lack of family support related to separation secondary to incarceration (Lela)
- Potential for feelings of loss related to separation from infant after birth (Lela)

Family
Lela's family visits are rare; therefore she looked for others to provide support during her pregnancy. Lela told Ms. Williams that her cellmate, Julieanna, offered to be her labor support person.

- Lack of knowledge of her role as a labor support person (Julieanna)

Community
- Knowledge deficit of adequate health-seeking behaviors of women in the correctional facility (i.e., pregnant and nonpregnant women)
- Lack of programs to promote health and prevent diseases among women prisoners

Planning

After validating the nursing diagnosis with the individual, family, or community, the plan of care is
Continued

developed. Examples of long- and short-term goals follow.

Individual

Long-Term Goal
- Individual family members will have a positive birth experience (Lela).

Short-Term Goal
- Family member or friends will help Lela use relaxation techniques to cope with discomforts of labor.

Family

Long-Term Goal
- The family members will be strengthened through their newly acquired knowledge and skills.

Short-Term Goal
- The family members will demonstrate increased ability to perform role as labor support people.

Community

Long-Term Goal
- The health and well-being of incarcerated women (i.e., pregnant and nonpregnant) will improve.

Short-Term Goal
- Health education programs will be instituted to individuals, families, and aggregates in the correctional facility.

Intervention

The community health nurse works with the individual, family, or community to achieve mutually established goals. Intervention is aimed at empowering individuals and groups to take responsibility for themselves and form links with others to accomplish goals.

Individual
Providing a perinatal education program for Lela is Ms. Williams first priority. In addition, counseling related to feelings of loss after birth may

be appropriate. Referral to a counselor may be necessary and Ms. Williams must become familiar with available resources.

Family
Teaching the family the roles and responsibilities of a labor support person is an important intervention. In the correctional facility, interventions must ensure that Lela has a labor support person to practice her relaxation techniques and be available for the birth. The nurse must negotiate with prison officials to make it possible for Lela to have a labor support person. If a family member is unavailable, then Ms. Williams may call on a childbirth educator in the community to assist during this time.

Community
Specific interventions with a group of pregnant women in the correctional facility are based on the specific needs of the group. The community health nurse must identify prison officials who are supportive of health education programs and request input as to which women should be targeted for such programs. Then the nurse meets with targeted women to assess level of knowledge and skills regarding women's health. For example, the nurse should survey what the woman perceives as learning needs (e.g., well-women's care, women's anatomy and physiology, self-care in health promotion, health protection, and disease prevention). Then the nurse tailors an intervention that is compatible with the community. Ms. Williams asked each nursing student to select a topic based on the survey and develop a teaching plan for presentation to female prisoners (i.e., pregnant and nonpregnant) at least once during the spring semester.

Evaluation

The community health nurse compares the actual and predicted outcomes to determine the efficacy of the plan of care and make revisions.

Individual
For example, Lela learned necessary relaxation techniques that were useful to her in labor and assisted in making the birth experience positive. Follow-up of Lela's psychosocial concerns in postpartum was also important.

Family

Evaluation of this nontraditional family would include their level of satisfaction with their role in the birth experience. Evaluation would also include learning how this interaction between family members (i.e., Lela and Julieanna) prepared them for other situations.

Community

The aggregate evaluation focuses on the community. For example, in health education programs designed for pregnant and nonpregnant women in the correctional facility, it is important to do the following:

- maintain attendance records;
- seek feedback from women, referring nurse-educator, and prison officials regarding changes in self-care behavior regarding health;
- obtain student response to learning experience; and
- make changes in health education programs based on evaluation.

SUMMARY

Women's health care has multiple facets. Many areas for community health nursing intervention exist. Nurses are advocates and activists for women's health through their involvement in health policymaking as a profession. Along with other multidisciplinary and consumer groups, professional nurses are in the forefront of making changes in the health care delivery system that will promote an overall quality- and research-based health plan for women. Women are at the center of the health of the United States; therefore if better models are developed for improving the health of women, the health of the entire nation will benefit.

LEARNING ACTIVITIES

1. Identify examples from everyday life that support or encourage violence against women (e.g., magazines, books, and television advertisements). Share findings with classmates.
2. Survey lay magazine advertisements and estimate the percentage of total pages that use a woman's image, including aging, menopause, overweight and obesity, and sexuality to sell products. Share these with classmates.
3. Discuss the need for cancer screening based on ACS guidelines with female relatives.
4. Discuss the need for a heart-healthy nutritional plan based on AHA guidelines with female relatives.
5. Investigate community resources for sites that offer instruction in BSE, clinical examination, and mammography accredited by the American College of Radiology.
6. Identify resources for mammograms and PAP smears for low-income women.
7. Visit with a women's group in the community (e.g., business, church, sorority, and Parents Without Partners) to discuss members' health care needs and concerns. From these data, develop research questions.
8. Call a family planning clinic and determine the population served (i.e., eligibility), available services, and costs.
9. Use the telephone directory to identify resources providing health care and psychosocial services to men, women, and children with HIV and AIDS.
10. Query a women's health care NP or NM regarding the changes made in gynecological care in women with physical disabilities.
11. Review county or state health department statistics for leading causes of death among women of varying ethnic or racial groups.
12. Determine the percentage of women in the county who begin prenatal care during the first trimester.
13. Identify how women's health care needs are met when they are in the correctional system in the county or state.
14. Investigate community services that offer support at end of life.
15. Explore a website related to a women's health issue and evaluate the quality of Internet information.

REFERENCES

American Cancer Society: *Cancer facts and figures 1995,* Atlanta, 1995, The Author.

American Cancer Society: *Cancer facts and figures, 1999,* Atlanta, 1999, The Society.

American Diabetes Association: *Diabetes facts and figures,* April 2000, The Author, www.diabetes.org/ada/facts.asp.

American Diabetes Association: *Vital statistics,* Alexandria, Va, 1998, The Association.

American Heart Association: *Heart and stroke facts: statistical supplement,* Dallas, 1994, National Center.

American Heart Association: *Heart and stroke statistical update,* 1999, The Author, www.americanheart.org/statsitics/index.html.

Andrews S: Gynecologic and obstetric care of lesbian and bisexual women. In Varney H, editor: *Varney's midwifery,* ed 3, Sudbury, Mass, 1997, Jones and Bartlett.

Arthritis Foundation: *Rheumatoid arthritis fact sheet,* 1999, The Author, www.arthritis.org/resource/racampaign/facts.asp.

Bhatia SC, Bhatia SK: Depression in women: diagnostic and treatment considerations, *Am Fam Physician* 60(1):225, 1999.

Blair T: Domestic abuse: what is the ob/gyn nurse's role? *Ob Gyn Nurse Forum* 7(2):1, 1999.

Bonam-Crawford D, Orlick M: Helping patients with cancer achieve their work potential, *Clin Perspect Oncol Nurs* 1:3, 1994.

Bozzette SA et al: The care of HIV-infected adults in the United States, *N Engl J Med* 339(26):1897, 1998.

Bush TL: Evidence for primary and secondary prevention of coronary artery disease in women taking estrogen replacement therapy, *European Society of Cardiology* 17(suppl D):9, 1996.

Cates W: Reproductive tract infections. In Hatcher RA et al: *Contraceptive technology,* ed 17, New York, 1998, Ardent Media.

Cates W, Ellertson C: Abortion. In Hatcher RA et al: *Contraceptive technology,* ed 17, New York, 1998, Ardent Media.

Centers for Disease Control and Prevention: Achievements in public health, 1900-1999: healthier mothers and babies. *MMWR Morb Mortal Wkly Rep* 48(38):849, 1999.

Centers for Disease Control and Prevention: *Diabetes surveillance report, 1997,* Atlanta, 1998, USDHHS.

Centers for Disease Control and Prevention: Hysterectomy surveillance, United States, 1980-93, *Morb Mortal Wkly Rep* 46(SS-2), 1997, www.cdc.gov/nccdphp/drh/wh_hysterec.htm.

Chadwick BA, Heaton TB, editors: *Statistical handbook on the American family,* Phoenix, 1992, Oryx Press.

Choi M: Preamble to a new paradigm for women's health, *Image* 17:14, 1985.

Clark RA: Infections during the postpartum period, *J Obstet Gynecol Neonatal Nurs* 24:552, 1995.

Craven S, Greenberger MC, Kolker A: *Reproductive health: an essential part of health care.* A report by the National Women's Law Center, Washington, DC, 1993, National Women's Law Center.

Creehan PA: Toxic shock syndrome: an opportunity for nursing intervention, *J Obstet Gynecol Neonatal Nurs* 24:557, 1995.

Cunningham FG et al: *Williams' obstetrics,* ed 20, Norwalk, Conn, 1997, Appleton & Lange.

Donaldson K, Briggs J, McMaster D: RU 486: an alternative to surgical abortion, *J Obstet Gynecol Neonatal Nurs* 23:555, 1995.

Elliot B, Johnson M: Domestic violence in a primary care setting: patterns and prevalence, *Arch Fam Med* 4:113, 1995.

Evans DL et al: Depression in the medical setting: biopsychological interactions and treatment considerations, *J Clin Psychiatry* 60(suppl 4):40, 1999.

Facione NC: Breast cancer screening in relation to access to health services, *Oncol Nurs Forum* 26(4):689, 1999.

Farley D: Preventing TSS: tampon labeling allows women to compare absorbencies. In USDHHS: *FDA consumer special report: current issues in women's health,* ed 2, Rockville, Md, 1994, The Author.

Ferrell BR: Humanizing the experience of pain and illness. In Ferrell BR, editor: *Suffering,* Boston, 1996, Jones & Bartlett.

Ferrell BR, Hassey-Dow K, Grant M: Measurement of the quality of life in cancer survivors, *Qual Life Res* 4:523, 1995.

Ferrell BR, Virani R, Grant M: HOPE: Home Care Outreach for Palliative Care Education, *Cancer Pract* 6(2):79, 1998.

Finkel ML, Finkel DJ: The effect of a second opinion program on hysterectomy performance, *Medical Care* 28:776, 1990.

Fishwick NJ: Assessment of women for partner abuse, *J Obstet Gynecol Neonatal Nurs* 27(6):661, 1998.

Giger J, Strickland O: *Behavioral risk reduction strategies for chronic indicators and high risk factors for premenopausal African American women (25-45) with coronary heart disease,* Grant Number N95-019, Bethesda, Md, 1995, DOD, Uniformed Health Services, University of Health Sciences, Tri-Service Nursing Research.

Gilinson T: Know family, medical leave rights for yourself, your patients, *The American Nurse,* July/August 1999.

Graves EJ, Kozak LJ: National hospital discharge survey: annual summary, 1996, *Vital Health Stat* 13(140):24, 1998.

Guest F: Education and counseling. In Hatcher RA et al: *Contraceptive technology,* ed 17, New York, 1998a, Ardent Media.

Guest F: HIV/AIDS and reproductive health. In Hatcher RA et al: *Contraceptive technology,* ed 17, New York, 1998b, Ardent Media.

Han Y, Williams RD, Harrison RA: Breast self-examination among Korean American women: knowledge, attitudes and behaviors, *J Cultural Diversity* 6(4):115, 1999.

Hinshaw AS: Nursing knowledge for the 21st century: opportunities and challenges, *J Nurs Sch* 32(2):117-123, 2000.

HIV Clinical Management: The 1999 National Conference on Women and HIV/AIDS: navigating into the new millennium through collaboration, 1999, Medscape, www.HIV.medscape.com/Medscape/CNO/1999/NCWH/public/index-NCWH.html.

Hopwood P, Stephens RJ, Medical Research Council (MRC) Lung Cancer Working Party: Symptoms at presentation for treatment in patients with lung cancer: implications for the evaluation of palliative treatment, *Br J Cancer* 71:633, 1995.

International Council of Nurses: *Healthy families for healthy nations,* Geneva, 1993, The Author.

Joint United Nations Programme on HIV/AIDS: The HIV/AIDS situation in mid-1996: global and regional highlights, *UNAIDS Fact Sheet,* July 1, 1996.

Jones-Warren B: The experience of depression in African American women. In McElmurry BJ, Parker R, editors: *Annual review of women's health,* vol 11, New York, 1995, NLN.

Jordan JM: Effect of race and ethnicity on outcomes in arthritis and rheumatic conditions, *Curr Opin Rheumatol* 11(2):98, 1999.

Karlson EW et al: A retrospective cohort study of cigarette smoking and risk of rheumatoid arthritis in female health professionals, *Arthritis Rheum* 42(5):910, 1999.

Kuehn J, McMahon P, Creekmore S: Stopping a silent killer: preventing heart disease in women, *AWHONN Lifelines* 3(2):31, 1999.

Landis SH et al: Cancer statistics: 1998, *CA Cancer J Clin* 48:6, 1998.

Looker AC et al: Prevalence of low femoral bone density in older U.S. adults from NHANES III, *J Bone Miner Res,* 12(11):1761, 1997.

Love S et al: Practice guidelines for breast cancer, *Cancer J Sci Am* 2(3A):S7, 1996.

Mark DB et al: Use of medical resources and quality of life after acute myocardial infarction in Canada and the United States, *N Engl J Med* 331(17):1130, 1994.

McElmurry BJ, Tashiro J: Health promotion and preventive health issues: young adulthood to the perimenopausal years (15-45). In Allen KM, Phillips JM, editors: *Women's health across the life span: a comprehensive perspective,* Philadelphia, 1997, J.B. Lippincott.

Medimmune: *MedImmune announces novel structure of urinary tract infection vaccine raget; x-ray structure of firm c-fim h complex published in science,* 1999, The Author, biz.yahoo.com/prnnews/990813md-medimmu-1.html.

Meilahan EN et al: Characteristics of women with hysterectomy, *Maturitas* 11:319, 1989.

Misner ST, Beauchamp-Hewitt JB, Fox-Levin P: Occupational issues in women's health. In McElmurry BJ, Parker RS, editors: *Annual review of women's health,* vol 11, New York, 1995, NLN.

Mou SM: Gynecologic infections. In Seltzer VL, Pearse WH, editors: *Women's primary health care,* New York, 1995, McGraw-Hill.

National Osteoporosis Foundation: *Physician's guide to prevention and treatment of osteoporosis,* Washington, DC, 1998, The Foundation.

Nelson AL: Menstrual problems and common gynecologic concerns. In Hatcher RA et al, editor: *Contraceptive technology,* ed 17, New York, 1998, Ardent Media.

Nesto RW et al: Heart disease in diabetes. In Kahn CR, Weir GC, editors: *Joslin's diabetes mellitus,* ed 13, Philadelphia, 1994, Lea & Febiger.

Olds S, London M, Ladewig P: *Maternal-newborn nursing,* ed 5, Menlo Park, Calif, 1996, Addison-Wesley.

Olson A, Labat J: Women, diet, and heart disease. In McElmurry BJ, Parker RS, editors: *Annual review of women's health,* vol 11, New York, 1995, NLN.

Palomares MR et al: Gender influence on weight loss pattern and survival of nonsmall cell lung carcinoma patients, *Cancer* 78:2119, 1996.

Paolisso M, Leslie J: Meeting the changing health needs of women in developing countries, *Soc Sci Med* 40(1):55, 1995.

Pender NJ: *Health promotion in nursing practice,* ed 3, Stamford, Conn, 1996, Appleton & Lange.

Pollard K, Tordella S: Women making gains among professionals, *Population Today* 21:1, 1993.

Quill TE: Nonabandonment: a central obligation for physicians, *Ann Intern Med* 122:368, 1995.

Ravnikar VA, Chen E: Hysterectomies: where are the indications? *Obstet Gynecol Clin North Am* 21:405, 1994.

Sarna L, McCorkle R: Burden of care and lung cancer, *Cancer Practice* 4:245, 1996.

Schmidt LA et al: Treatment of depression by obstetrician-gynecologists: a survey study, *Obstet Gynecol* 90(2): 296, 1997.

Schulman KA et al: The effect of race and sex on physicians' recommendations for cardiac catheterization, *N Engl J Med* 340:618, 1999.

Seltzer VL, Pearse WH: *Women's primary health care: office practice and procedures,* New York, 1995, McGraw-Hill.

Smith LS: Psychologic concerns. In Griffith-Kenney J, editor: *Contemporary women's health: a nursing advocacy approach,* Menlo Park, Calif, 1986, Addison-Wesley.

Snell T: *Survey of state prison inmates, 1991: women in prison,* United States Department of Justice, Bureau of Justice Statistics, Washington, DC, 1994, US Government Printing Office.

Stanley KJ: Silence is not golden: conversations with the dying, *Clin J Oncol Nurs* 4(1)34, 2000.

Star WL, Lommel LL, Shannon MT: *Women's primary health care: protocols for practice,* Washington, DC, 1995, American Nurses Publishing.

Stewart F: Vaginal barriers. In Hatcher RA et al: *Contraceptive technology,* ed 17, New York, 1998, Ardent Media.

Stewart GK: Impaired fertility. In Hatcher RA et al: *Contraceptive technology,* ed 17, New York, 1998, Ardent Media.

Stewart GK, Carignan CS: Female and male sterilization. In Hatcher RA et al: *Contraceptive technology,* ed 17, New York, 1998, Ardent Media.

Stotland NL: Psychiatric and psychosocial issues in primary care of women. In Seltzer VL, Pearse WH, editors: *Women's primary health care: office practice and procedures,* New York, 1995, McGraw-Hill.

Sullivan E, Sullivan H: The departure. In Sullivan E, Sullivan H: Voices of a mother and daughter, Norman, Okla, 1997, Hooper.

Szewczyk M, Chennault SA: Women's health: depression and related disorders, *Prim Care* 24(1):83, 1997.

Task Force on End of Life Decisions, American Nursing Association: *Position statements: nursing and the Patient Self-Determination Acts,* 1991, The Author, www.nursingworld.org/readroom/position/ethics/etsdet.htm.

Tjaden P, Thoenees N: *Prevalence, incidence and consequences of violence against women: findings from the National Violence Against Women Survey,* Research in Brief, Washington, DC, 1998, Institute of Justice.

US Census Bureau: *Money income in the United States, 1999,* 1999, The Author, www.census.gov/hhes/income/income99/99tablea.html.

US Census Bureau: Single parents maintain 3 in 10 family groups involving children: Mother's Day statistics of the United States, Washington, DC, 1994, US Government Printing Office.

US Census Bureau: Statistical abstract of the United States: 1990, 110th ed. Washington, DC, US Government Printing Office, 1990.

US Census Bureau: *Statistical abstract of the United States: 1995,* ed 115, Washington, DC, 1995, US Government Printing Office.

US Department of Education: *Digest of education statistics,* Pub No 99-036, Washington DC, 1998, The Author.

US Department of Health and Human Services: *FDA consumer magazine,* Washington, DC, 1999, The Author.

US Department of Health and Human Services: *Healthy people 2010,* Conference Edition, Washington, DC, 2000a, US Government Printing Office.

US Department of Health and Human Services: *Healthy people 2010: national health promotion and disease prevention objectives—Public Health Service,* Washington, DC, 2000b, U.S. Government Printing Office.

Verbrugge LM: Women, men and osteoarthritis, *Arthritis Care Res* 8:212, 1995.

Warshaw C, Ganley AL, Salber PR: *Improving the health care response to domestic violence: a resource manual for health care providers,* San Francisco, 1995, Family Violence Prevention Fund.

Williams RD: Cancer. In Allen KM, Phillips JM, editors: *Women's health across the life span: a comprehensive perspective,* Philadelphia, 1997, J.B. Lippincott.

Williams RD, Clark A: A qualitative study of women's hysterectomy experience, *J Womens Health Gend Based Med* 9(suppl 2):S15, 2000.

Williams RD, Lethbridge DJ: Health promotion behaviors for women in third world areas of industrialized countries. In Kristjansdottir G, Sveinsdottir H, Thoroddsen A, editors: *Connecting conversations: nursing scholarship and practice: proceedings of 1995,* Reykjavik, Iceland City, 1997, University of Iceland, Department of Nursing.

Williams RD, Turner-Henson A: *Breast health protection of female family caregivers,* Book of Abstracts, Jamaica, West Indies, 1996, Sigma Theta Tau International, Eighth International Research Congress.

Women Employed Institute: *Sexual harassment: the problem that isn't going away,* Chicago, 1994, The Author.

Woods NF, Mitchell ES: Preventive health issues: the perimenopausal to mature years (45-64). In Allen KM, Phillips JM, editors: *Women's health across the life span: a comprehensive perspective,* Philadelphia, 1997, J.B. Lippincott.

Wright TC: Patient-collected tissue samples may offer effective option to Pap smear, *JAMA* 283:81, 2000.

Young DR, King AC: Preventive health issues: the mature years (64 and older). In Allen KM, Phillips JM, editors: *Women's health across the life span: a comprehensive perspective,* Philadelphia, 1997, J.B. Lippincott.

Men's Health

Carrie Morgan

Upon completion of this chapter, the reader will be able to do the following:

1. Identify the major indicators of men's health status.
2. Describe two explanations for men's health status.
3. Discuss factors that impede men's health.
4. Discuss factors that promote men's health.
5. Describe men's health needs.
6. Apply knowledge of men's health needs in planning gender-appropriate nursing care for men at the individual, family, and community levels.

KEY TERMS

acute condition
androgen
chronic condition
illness orientation
life expectancy
medical care
morbidity
mortality
prevention orientation
sex-role socialization

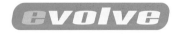

http://evolve.elsevier.com/Nies/

It is common knowledge that women live longer than men despite the fact that health care use is greater with women than men. Death rates for men are higher than for women in the major causes of death. Although the interest in health promotion and illness prevention has increased, men's health issues remain unaddressed. Women's health has become a specialty practice with courses and programs in women's health available in many colleges of nursing. A specialty in men's health has not been emphasized.

This chapter focuses on the health needs of men and the implications for community health nursing. Specific areas that are discussed include the current health status of men, theories that attempt to explain men's health, factors that impede men's health, factors that promote men's health, men's health needs, meeting men's health needs, and planning gender-appropriate care for men at the individual, family, and community levels.

MEN'S HEALTH STATUS

Traditional indicators of health include rates of longevity, mortality, and morbidity.

Longevity and Mortality in Men

Major gender differences in longevity and mortality rates reveal that men remain disadvantaged despite advances in technology. Although women are more likely to use health services and experience higher morbidity rates, mortality rates for men remain higher. Gender differentials are generally associated with behavioral factors, which place men at greater risk of death. These behavioral factors, together with men's reluctance to seek preventive and health services, have marked implications for community health nursing.

Longevity

Rates of longevity are increasing for both men and women. People can now expect to live more than 20 years longer than their forefathers and foremothers lived at the turn of the century. Infants born in the United States in 1996 can expect to live 76 years, whereas those born in 1900 lived an average of 47.3 years when the death rate was highest. Although **life expectancy** for both males and females has increased, the gender gap has also increased. This gender gap, which was 5.5 years in 1950, increased to 7.8 years in 1975. Males born in 1996 will live an

average of 73 years compared with females born in 1996, who will live an average of 79.1 years (McFalls, 1998).

STANDARDIZED TERMINOLOGY

In the fields of demography and sociology, the following terms are standardized:

- People of all ages: males and females
- Children younger than 18 years of age: boys and girls
- Adults 18 years of age or older: men and women
- Sex: the biological distinction between males and females
- Gender: The attitudes and behavior of men and women that are shaped by socialization and have a potential to be changed
- Role: The part one plays in society

Adapted from Skelton R: Man's role in society and its effect on health, *Nursing* 26:953, 1988; Verbrugge LM, Wingard DL: Sex differentials in health and mortality, *Women Health* 12:103, 1987.

Many health and vital statistics are not as complete as they could be. Educational attainment, as reported on the death certificate, has only been tabulated since 1989 (Kochanek and Hudson, 1995). Life expectancy is closely associated with SES throughout the world, including the United States. However, family income is more likely to be tabulated in morbidity, or illness reports, than in mortality rates. Reported by race and sex, mortality rates show that underserved populations in the United States, especially minorities, live significantly fewer years. Native-Americans live an average of four years less than white males and black males live approximately eight years less than white males. Hispanics have a life expectancy comparable with their white counterparts. The United States lags behind several other countries in mortality rates for males; in 1991 the United States was twenty-fifth in life expectancy for men and sixteenth in life expectancy for women (Table 16-1) (NCHS, 1996).

Mortality

Males in most industrialized countries have higher death rates than females (Waldron, 1995b). In the United States, males lead females in **mortality** rate in

TABLE 16-1

Life Expectancy at Birth According to Sex and Race, United States, 1900 to 1993

	All Races			White			Black		
Year	Both Sexes	Male	Female	Both Sexes	Male	Female	Both Sexes	Male	Female
1900	47.3	46.3	48.3	47.6	46.6	48.7	33.0	32.5	33.5
1960	69.7	66.6	73.1	70.6	67.4	74.1	63.2	60.7	65.9
1992	75.8	72.3	79.1	76.5	73.2	79.8	69.6	65.0	73.9

Data from National Center for Health Statistics: *Health, United States: 1994*, Hyattsville, Md, 1995, USPHS.

TABLE 16-2

Ratio of Age-Adjusted Death Rates for 12 Leading Causes of Death for the Total Population by Sex and Race: United States, 1992

Rank Order	Cause of Death (Ninth Revision, International Classification of Diseases, 1975)	Ratio	
		Male to Female	Black to White
—	All causes	1.72	1.61
1	Diseases of the heart	1.88	1.48
2	Malignant neoplasms	1.45	1.3
3	Cerebrovascular diseases	1.18	1.86
4	COPD and allied conditions	1.70	0.81
5	Accidents and adverse effects	2.63	1.27
—	Motor vehicle accidents	2.35	1.03
—	All other accidents and adverse effects	2.97	1.57
6	Pneumonia and influenza	1.69	1.44
7	Diabetes mellitus	1.14	2.41
8	HIV infection	6.97	3.69
9	Suicide	4.28	0.58
10	Homicide and legal intervention	3.98	6.46
11	Chronic liver disease and cirrhosis	2.42	1.48
12	Nephritis, nephrotic syndrome, and nephrosis	1.53	2.76

Data from Kochanek MA, Hudson BL: Advance report of final mortality statistics, 1992, *Mon Vital Stat Rep* 43(6 suppl):152, 1995.

each leading cause of death (Table 16-2). Men are about seven times as likely to die from AIDS as women. Men are more than four times as likely to die from suicide, four times as likely to die from homicide or legal intervention, and two to three times as likely to die from accidents or chronic liver disease or cirrhosis than women. They are nearly twice as likely as women to die of diseases of the heart, COPD, and pneumonia and influenza and lead in deaths resulting from cancer, kidney disease, cerebrovascular disease, and diabetes (Kochanek and Hudson, 1995).

Black men are always at the bottom of the longevity rates, being more than four times as likely to die from HIV infection than black women, nearly three times as likely to die from vehicle accidents, and over 1.6 times as likely to die from heart disease or cancer (NCHS, 1996). Black males die younger than white males because they are more vulnerable to 11 of the 15 leading causes of death (NCHS, 1998). The highest sex-to-mortality ratios shared by both white and black men were for HIV infection and homicide and legal intervention.

Morbidity

Despite the differences in mortality rates, men tend to perceive themselves to be in better health than women. In the National Health Interview Survey of 1993, which asked people to rate their health status, 40.3% of men rated their health as "excellent" compared with 35.0% of women; only 9.4% of men rated their health as "fair or poor" compared with 11.5% of women (Benson and Marano, 1994).

SOURCES OF DATA
NCHS: through the National Vital Statistics System, the NCHS collects data from each state, New York City, the District of Columbia, the U.S. Virgin Islands, Guam, and Puerto Rico on births, deaths, marriages, and divorces in the United States.
National Health Interview Survey: the National Health Interview Survey is a continuing nationwide sample survey in which data are collected by personal interviews about household members' illnesses, injuries, chronic conditions, disabilities, and use of health services.

Morbidity rates, or rates of illness, are difficult to obtain and have been available usually only in Western industrialized countries. For example, in the United States, reports of analyses of morbidity rates by gender lag several years behind analyses of mortality rates by gender. Gender differences in morbidity rates reflect the latest available reports. The following are common indicators of morbidity rate:

- incidence of acute illness,
- prevalence of chronic conditions, and
- use of medical care.

Although variations exist, women are more likely to be ill, whereas men are at greater risk for death.

Acute Illness
The incidence rate for acute infective and parasitic disease, digestive system conditions, and respiratory conditions is higher for women than for men (Benson and Marano, 1994). The only exception is for injuries, which were 12% greater for men in 1993. In addition, the severity of these injuries is reported to be greater in men than in women. When conditions associated with childbearing are excluded from the list of acute illnesses, the incidence rate for women remains 18% greater than men.

In the 1993 National Health Interview Survey, an **acute condition** was a type of illness or injury that usually lasted less than three months and either resulted in restricted activity (e.g., causing a person to limit daily activities for at least half a day) or caused the patient to receive medical care. In response to this survey, women slowed their activities and rested more often than men. The number of restricted-activity days associated with acute conditions per 100 people is 33% greater for women than for men; similarly, the number of bed days associated with acute conditions per 100 people is 38% greater for women than for men (Benson and Marano, 1994).

Chronic Conditions
A **chronic condition** is a condition that persists for at least three months or belongs to a group of conditions classified as chronic regardless of time of onset, such as TB, neoplasm, or arthritis (Benson and Marano, 1994). In general, women have higher morbidity rates than men. Table 16-3 illustrates major sex-to-morbidity ratios. Women are more likely than men to have a higher prevalence of chronic diseases that cause disability and limitation of activities but do not

TABLE 16-3

Morbidity Sex Ratios by Age, United States, 1993

Type of Condition	Male-Female Ratio per 1000 People		
	<45 Years	45 to 64 Years	>65 Years
Gout, including gouty arthritis	11.00	2.70	2.00
Absence of extremities (i.e., excludes tips of fingers or toes only)	5.50	7.10	7.40
Ischemic heart disease	2.27	2.45	1.63
Intervertebral disc disorders	1.50	1.40	0.94
Hypertension	1.08	0.94	0.85
Asthma	1.00	0.51	0.82
Hay fever or allergic rhinitis without asthma	0.88	0.87	0.79
Ulcer	0.79	0.62	0.84
Arthritis	0.76	0.65	0.74
Enteritis or colitis	0.68	0.42	0.62

Data from Benson V, Marano MA: *Current estimates from the National Health Interview Survey, 1993,* 1994, The Author, www.cdc.gov/nchs/data/10_190_1.pdf.

lead to death. However, men have higher morbidity and mortality rates for conditions that are the leading causes of death.

USE OF MEDICAL CARE

Medical care, the use of ambulatory care, hospital care, preventive care, or other health services, also illustrates the different gender patterns.

Use of Ambulatory Care

Men seek ambulatory care less often than women. According to the 1993 National Health Interview Survey, the physician's office is the primary setting for ambulatory care for both men and women. In this report, a physician contact is a consultation with a physician or another person working under the physician's supervision in person or via telephone for the purposes of examination, diagnosis, treatment, or advice (Benson and Marano, 1994). Women had 6.2 physician contacts outside a hospital (i.e., in a physician's office or via telephone) in 1993, whereas men had 4.3 contacts. Physicians see men more

frequently than women for conditions that correspond with their leading causes of death, such as ischemic heart disease. However, physicians see women more frequently than men for the chronic diseases that are more prevalent among them. Visit rates for boys and girls younger than age 18 are about the same (4.2 vs. 4.0).

Men were less likely than women to report seeing a physician within any previous year (72.8% vs. 84.1%) (Benson and Marano, 1994). Men were also more likely to report intervals of last contact with a physician between one and two years (11.1% vs. 8.3%), two and five years (11.2% vs. 5.5%), and five years or more (4.9% vs. 2.1%). These results indicate that the delay in seeking health care and the failure to use preventive health care resources cause men to be sicker when they do seek health care. They are sicker; therefore they require more intensive medical care.

Use of Hospital Care

The literature indicates that hospitalization rates also vary by sex. In 1993, rates of discharges from short-stay hospitals were lower for males (9.1%) than for females (12.3%) even when discharges for deliveries are excluded (9.7%) (Benson and Marano, 1994). However, males had a longer length of stay in the hospital than females (6.1 vs. 5.5 days). Boys up to age 15 are hospitalized more than girls, but females aged 15 to 44 are hospitalized more often than males in this age group (Verbrugge and Wingard, 1987). Discharge rates increase for both men and women after 45 years of age; however, rates for men increase more rapidly. After 65 years of age, men's discharge rates continue to be higher than women's rates.

Use of Preventive Care

Preventive examinations are necessary for early diagnosis of health problems. National health surveys indicate that women are more likely to receive physical examinations (NCHS, 1996). Women's examinations are also more likely to be recent than men's examinations. Young women aged 35 and under are more likely to have health insurance than young men; no difference exists after age 35 years (Salem, 1995).

Use of Other Health Services

Women are more likely to be admitted for psychiatric services to outpatient psychiatric settings, such as federally-funded, community mental health centers and more likely admitted for psychiatric services to private mental hospitals and psychiatric care units in nonfederal, general hospitals (NCHS, 1996). Women are also more likely to reside in nursing homes because they have longer life expectancy (NCHS, 1995). Men are more likely admitted for psychiatric services in state and county mental hospitals (NCHS, 1996).

THEORIES THAT EXPLAIN MEN'S HEALTH

As discussed previously, a gender gap exists in health. The data reviewed raise many questions for community health nurses to explore regarding sex differences in health and illness. Although men have shorter life expectancy and higher rates of mortality for all leading causes of death, women have higher rates of morbidity, including rates of acute illness and chronic disease and use of medical and preventive care services. Verbrugge and Wingard (1987) asked why "females are sicker, but males die sooner?" (p. 135). It is questionable whether health care providers

aggregate more male deaths and more female illnesses and injuries, or whether males and females respond to health problems differently. Several explanations exist for this paradox.

Nurses traditionally use developmental theories to explain individual behavior. Erickson's model was not gender specific (Erickson, 1963). Levinson focused somewhat on the male development (Levinson, 1978). There remains a need for literature detailing the factors and combinations of factors that influence gender differences in the health and illness of populations.

The following explanations proposed by Waldron (1995a, 1995b, 1995c, 1995d, 1995e) and Verbrugge and Wingard (1987) attempt to account for sex differences in this important area:

- biological factors, including genetics, effects of sex hormones, and physiological differences, which may be influenced by genetics, hormones, and environment;
- socialization;
- orientations toward illness and prevention; and
- reporting health behavior.

Biological Factors

Several biological factors influence sex differences in mortality and morbidity rates, including genetics, effects of sex hormones, and physiological differences, which may be influenced by genetics, hormones, and environmental factors (Waldron, 1995a, 1995b, 1995c, 1995d, 1995e). The embryo is unisexual until the seventh week of gestation. **Androgen**, a hormone from the Y-chromosome coupled with the maternal androgen source, results in the development of male gender. Male embryos outnumber female embryos 115 to 100. Higher rates of miscarriage and stillbirths in males reduce this gender difference to 105 to 100. More male births occur than female births, but higher male infant deaths during the first six months reduces this ratio (Legato, 1997). Sex ratios at birth appear to be lower for births to older fathers, black fathers, higher-order births (i.e., second, third, or fourth births), and births after induced ovulation.

Whether sex ratios at birth are influenced by sex ratios at conception or sex differentials in mortality rates before birth is unknown. Current evidence suggests that more than two out of three prenatal deaths occur before clinical recognition of the pregnancy. Sex differences in late fetal mortality rates, once favoring males in developed countries, have decreased since the early and midtwentieth century; currently, no differences exist from improved medical care and maternal health (Waldron, 1995c). These factors have decreased deaths resulting from difficult labor, injuries at birth, and maternal diseases and accidents. Although females have higher rates of late fetal mortality from congenital malformations, the male excess in late fetal mortality has disappeared.

However, the picture changes after birth. For example, in 1992, the neonatal (i.e., less than 28 days) mortality rate for males was higher than for females (5.8 vs. 4.9), as was postnatal (i.e., 28 days to 11 months) mortality rate (3.5 vs. 2.7) and infant (i.e., less than one year) mortality rate (9.4 vs. 7.6) (Kochanek and Hudson, 1995). Males' experience of higher mortality rates for perinatal conditions is attributed to biological disadvantages such as males' greater risk of premature birth, higher rates of respiratory distress syndrome, and infectious disease in infancy resulting from the influence of male hormones on the developing lungs, brain, and possibly the immune system of the male fetus (Waldron, 1995c). Sex chromosome-linked diseases such as hemophilia and certain types of muscular dystrophy are more common among males than females (Waldron, 1995c).

Biological advantages for females may also exist later in life because the mechanism produced by estrogen protects against heart disease, although studies must be interpreted cautiously (Waldron, 1995d). Some evidence supports the hypothesis that men's higher testosterone levels contribute to men's lower HDL levels. Body fat distribution may also contribute to sex differences in ischemic heart disease risk, specifically the tendency for men in Western countries to accumulate abdominal body fat vs. the tendency for women to accumulate fat on the buttocks and thighs (Waldron, 1995d). Men's higher levels of stored iron may also contribute to risk for ischemic heart disease.

Socialization

A second theory for explaining sex differences in health is socialization. Acquired risks may be different between males and females from differences in work, leisure, and lifestyle. **Sex-role socialization** may influence these differences.

More men than women are employed on a full-time basis in work environments outside the home. Usually, men's occupations are more hazardous than positions held by women. Injuries to male workers account for 60% of the reported occupational injuries and 94% of work-related fatalities (NCHS, 1998). Men's higher exposure to carcinogens at the work site is associated with high rates of mesothelioma and coal worker's pneumoconiosis (NCHS, 1995). In the United States, men score higher than women on measures of hostility and lack of trust of others, which may place them at higher risk of ischemic heart disease (Matthews et al., 1992). Although occupational hazards to women's health are being identified, evidence indicates that, unlike men, employment of U.S. women outside the home has a positive effect on their health (Waldron, 1995b).

Traits and characteristics of the traditional male gender role are combative and competitive, physically active, strong, coarse, and independent. Modern men must cope with the expectations of the traditional role coupled with the expectation that their relationships with women should include emotional intimacy, tenderness, and companionship (Harrison and Dignan, 1999).

FOUR DIMENSIONS OF STEREOTYPED MALE SEX-ROLE BEHAVIOR

No Sissy Stuff: the need to be different from women

The Big Wheel: the need to be superior to others

The Sturdy Oak: the need to be independent and self-reliant

Give 'Em Hell: the need to be more powerful than others, through violence if necessary

Adapted from David DS, Brannon R: The male sex role: our culture's blueprint of manhood, and what it's done for us lately. In David DS, Brannon R, editors: *The forty-nine percent majority: the male sex role*, Reading, Mass, 1976, Addison-Wesley.

Leisure, sports, and play activities also place men at high risk for injury. Greater risk-taking behavior by males is supported by boys' higher rates of accidents caused by riskier play (Rosen and Peterson, 1990), men's faster driving rates and higher rates of traffic violations and motor vehicle fatalities (Waldron, 1995a), men's greater use of illegal psychoactive substances, higher rates of alcohol consumption, and higher rates of cigarette smoking (NCHS, 1996). Men drive faster than women, but are less likely to wear seat belts. It is suggested that men are actively encouraged to drink and smoke as a validation of masculinity.

Men are more likely to be involved in violent crimes and violence is a typical precursor to homicide. Men are victims in four out of five homicides. Black males are involved in a homicide seven times more often than European-American males (NCHS, 1996).

Orientation Toward Illness and Prevention

Illness orientation, or the ability to note symptoms and take appropriate action, may also differ between the sexes. Most diseases, injuries, and deaths among men are preventable. Mechanic (1964) noted that boys in society are socialized to ignore symptoms. Symptom reporting may be more socially acceptable for girls (Waldron, 1995a). Women are more likely to cut down their activities when ill, seek health care, and report more details to health care providers (Waldron, 1995a). Surveys done by *Men's Health* reveal that nine million men have not seen a health care provider in five years. Men may be aware of being ill, but they make a conscious decision not to seek health care to avoid being labeled as "sick."

Prevention orientation, or the ability to take action to prevent disease or injury, may also vary between the sexes. Perhaps as a result of the women's movement of the 1970s, women's higher likelihood to seek preventive examinations may be a result of their need for routine reproductive health screening (i.e., the PAP test and breast examination). This examination includes some general screening, such as testing blood pressure and urine and blood for chronic problems. Men do not have routine reproductive health checkups that include screening, which would detect other health problems at an early stage. Uniformly recognized preventive screening programs for males have only recently been developed. With the advent of managed care, men who are eligible for coverage will have access to these routine health screenings. However, it is undetermined whether men will take advantage of these programs. Box 16-1 discusses matters related to men's reproductive health needs.

REPRODUCTIVE HEALTH AND RIGHT TO KNOW RESEARCH
Reproductive health hazard descriptions were analyzed on nearly 700 Material Safety Data Sheets (MSDS), important sources of information regarding health risks caused by exposure to toxic chemicals (e.g., lead or ethylene glycol ether-containing products). The descriptions were submitted by businesses in central Massachusetts to the Department of Environmental Protection under the provisions of the Massachusetts Right-to-Know Law. More than 60% of the MSDS failed to mention effects on the reproductive system, and among those that did, developmental risks rather than male reproductive effects were most often addressed. Those from larger firms (i.e., 100 or more employees) were more likely to mention reproductive effects than those from smaller firms (Paul and Kurtz, 1994).

MEN'S REPRODUCTIVE HEALTH SERVICES
Men's reproductive health services in family planning settings have existed but have been sorely underused by men (Swanson and Forrest, 1987). A national survey of 600 family planning clinics that were publicly funded with Title X money, conducted by The Urban Institute in 1993 (Schulte and Sonenstein, 1995), indicates that the trend continues. For example, of the 388 clinic managers who responded to the survey, only 13% reported that greater than 10% of their clients were men. Many services were available for men, including provision of condoms and contraceptive counseling, yet few men used them. Other services available to men in some clinics included testing, counseling, and treatment for STDs; HIV testing and counseling; vasectomy; infertility testing and counseling; and work and sports physicals.

Actual sex differences in preventive health behavior are variable and must be viewed with caution for the following reasons: little research has been completed and the efficacy of many behaviors is still in question (Waldron, 1995a). In addition, existing

BOX 16-1

Men's Reproductive Health Needs

Reproductive health needs are beginning to be recognized as important to men's health and to women's health. Usually the term *reproductive health* is applied to women of childbearing age. Used here, the term *reproductive health* applies to the health of reproductive organs, which develop in utero and with which a person is born, in both males and females, regardless of whether a person has sex or reproduces. Males may have reproductive health needs whether child or adult, straight or gay, or virgin or sexually experienced.

Many STDs are at epidemic proportions in the United States and are a major health hazard for many men and women. Sex differences exist in the incidence of STDs. AIDS in the United States is more likely to occur in males. For the 12-month period ending September 30, 1994, males 13 years of age and older accounted for 64.3 cases of AIDS per 100,000 population, whereas females of the same age accounted for only 12.6 cases of AIDS per 100,000 population (NCHS, 1996). Less well known perhaps, is that many STDs are considered intrinsically "sexist" because clinical evidence, more overt in men, is more likely to facilitate a correct diagnosis in men than in women. For example, in 1993, the rate of primary and secondary syphilis was higher for men (11.3 per 100,000 population) than for women (9.6 per 100,000 population) (CDC, 1994). The rate of gonorrhea was higher among men (185.1 per 100,000 population) than among women (147.2 per 100,000 population) because men are more likely to be treated for these STDs than women (CDC, 1994). These STDs are easier to detect in men because men are more likely to be symptomatic, laboratory tests are more reliable in men, efficiency of transmission is greater from male to female, and men are more likely to seek care for STDs that are symptomatic in men (CDC, 1994; Ehrhardt and Wasserheit, 1991; Temmerman, 1994; Wasserheit, 1994).

Testicular cancer is most likely to affect young men between ages 15 and 35 years and was estimated to account for 7100 new cases in 1995, up from an estimated 6100 in 1991 (ACS, 1991; Wingo, Tong, and Bolden, 1995). The incidence of testicular cancer has increased three to fourfold worldwide since the 1940s (Giwercman et al., 1993).

Cancer of the prostate is a leading cause of death from cancer in men and was estimated to account for 244,000 cases in 1995, up from an estimated 76,000 cases in 1984. The increase in the incidence of prostate cancer has been attributed to factors such as improved methods of detection and increased exposure to environmental carcinogens.

Incidence rates for all types of cancer increased between 1975 and 1979 and 1987 and 1991, but age-adjusted rates were higher among males (18.6%) than females (12.4%), which was largely from rising rates of prostate cancer among men (Devesa et al., 1995). Mortality rates for all cancers were less (3% among men and 6% among women) largely from rising rates of lung cancer mortality, whereas mortality rates for the majority of other types of cancer were stable or declining.

Many occupational and environmental agents associated with adverse sexual and reproductive outcomes in men have been identified, including pesticides, anesthetic gases in the operating room and dental office, inorganic lead from smelters, paint, printing materials, carbon disulfide from vulcanization of rubber, inorganic mercury manufacturing and dental work, and ionizing radiation from x-rays (Cohen, 1986; McDiarmid et al., 1991; Whorton, 1984). Nonchemical agents have also been identified as hazardous in men; for example, hyperthermia experienced by firefighters has been linked to male infertility (Agnew et al., 1991).

Many pharmacological agents, including prescription, over-the-counter, and recreational drugs, have been found to affect the reproductive outcomes or sexual functioning of men (Zilbergold, 1992). Examples include drugs from the following categories: antihypertensives, antipsychotics, antidepressants, hormones, sedatives, hypnotics, stimulants, chemotherapy agents used in cancer treatment, amphetamines, opiates, and alcohol, marijuana, cocaine, barbiturates, and lysergic acid diethylamide (LSD).

A focus on gay men's health has come about largely through the advent of the AIDS epidemic. For the role of the clinician in assessment, education, counseling, and providing support related to the reproductive health of the gay male client, see Swanson and Forrest (1984).

research shows decreasing gender differences for some health behaviors and increasing gender differences for others.

In the 1990 National Health Interview Survey of Health Promotion and Disease Prevention, women were more likely than men to report wearing seat belts, receiving blood pressure checks, having their blood cholesterol checked, and seeking help for an emotional or personal problem in the past year (Piani and Schoenborn, 1993). Men tended to spend more time in leisure activities than women, including playing sports regularly. The rapid growth of gymnasiums and health spas indicates a growing interest in maintaining physical fitness. Only 4.9% of men and 5.5% of women knew that exercise periods of 20 minutes per session three times per week are necessary to strengthen the heart and lungs.

OVERTRAINING AFFECTS MEN'S REPRODUCTIVE HEALTH STATUS

Overtraining physically, or strenuous exercise, has been recognized for its effect on the suppression of ovarian functioning in women. A study confirmed that overtraining in men also affects their reproductive functioning. Five endurance-trained men with normal spermatogenesis and hormone profiles engaged in overtraining, which doubled their average weekly mileage. After overtraining, basal testosterone levels decreased, basal cortisol levels increased, and sperm count decreased by 43%. Three months after overtraining, sperm count decreased by 52%, a significant decrease; the normal length of spermatogenesis is 72 ± two days. Although semen changes were also evident, such as the presence of immature sperm, semen reductions were within the normal range. Three months after resumption of normal training, testosterone and cortisol profiles returned to normal (Roberts et al., 1993).

Other studies suggest sex differences in other preventive health behaviors. Women are more likely to make dental visits (NCHS, 1995). In addition, women are more likely to attempt weight reduction (Piani and Schoenborn, 1993). Women consume more fruits, vegetables, and vitamin pills than men, contributing fiber and antioxidants such as vitamin C, which contributes to lower ischemic heart disease risk in women (Waldron, 1995d).

Females' illness and prevention orientations and their likelihood to seek routine medical and dental care in particular, contribute to higher morbidity rates. In addition, women are generally the caregivers of the family's health; they observe signs of illness, learn about sources of health care, set health care appointments and escort family members, and give direct care to ill family members. Although most women have more flexible schedules, their flexibility in scheduling time to see a physician balances out with men's flexibility from the little difference in the time it takes to perform their respective role obligations; men may work more hours, but women generally have more family demands (Waldron, 1995a).

Reporting of Health Behavior

Several differences in health behavior reporting may affect sex differentials (Verbrugge and Wingard, 1987). Women interviewers conduct most health surveys face to face or via telephone. Women may be better respondents than men, more likely to remember their health problems and actions, and more likely to talk with someone about aspects of their illness and health. A woman may respond more openly to another woman, whereas a man may be more inhibited. Women are usually solicited in health surveys to report the health behavior of men; therefore women are proxies and proxies have a tendency to underreport behavior (Montiero, 1976). Under these conditions, women may recall and report more health problems than men. Men may be less willing to talk, may not recall health problems, and may lack a health vocabulary. Men may not want to participate in the socialization of sickness and will make light of health problems.

Discussion of the Theories of Men's Health

Interpreting the Data

Verbrugge and Wingard (1987) cautioned that all four theories (i.e., biology, socialization, illness and prevention orientations, and health-reporting behavior) must be considered when interpreting data. When only diagnostic data from examinations or laboratory tests are considered (i.e., a highly medical perspective), sex differentials are most likely the result of inherited and acquired risks. However, when data have the potential to be affected by social factors such as sex differences in illness and prevention orientations and health-reporting behavior, these factors should not be ignored. The authors stated, "a sex differential in emphysema partly reflects risks men and women incur, but also whether they are aware of the condition or feel like reporting it" (Verbrugge and Wingard, 1987, p. 134). Health interview data such as those from the National Health Interview Survey and the National Survey of Health Promotion and Disease Prevention are the most common types available concerning a population's health. Verbrugge and Wingard (1987) cautioned that the social factors of sex differences in illness and prevention orientations and health-reporting behavior are critical in interpreting health interview data.

Many issues are raised for community health nurses, who are usually women and usually interact with female clients. The data obtained and interpreted by community health nurses may be influenced by one or more of these factors; therefore the nurse must consider the following questions:

- How does the health history reporting between male and female clients differ?
- How do data obtained by male nurses differ from those obtained by female nurses?
- What are the differences in data from health histories given by female "proxies" of absent members of the household or group and those given by the individual?
- What is the caregiving role of women in the family and how can men be supported in the caregiving role?
- How do these questions apply to men in the caregiving role (e.g., parent, partner, or other caregiving of a person with a chronic disease)?

In response to the question of why "females are sicker, but males die sooner," Verbrugge and Wingard (1987) provided several reasons. Conditions that affect morbidity rates (e.g., arthritis and gout) do not significantly affect mortality rates and conditions that affect mortality rates (e.g., heart disease) may not be as troublesome on a day-to-day basis. A difference exists in how the sexes respond to their health problems. Although mortality rates are in large part the outcome of inherited or acquired risks, sex differences in illness and prevention

orientations and the reporting of health behaviors suggest that social and psychological factors affect morbidity rates. Although males have higher prevalence and death rates for "killer" chronic diseases, injuries, and accidents, females have higher prevalence rates for a greater number of nonfatal chronic conditions. In addition, adult women report higher rates of morbidity from acute conditions than adult men. The authors stated that "females' greater willingness and ability to take care of themselves when ill, to seek preventive help, and to talk about health all boost their morbidity rate" (Verbrugge and Wingard, 1987, p. 136).

Sex-Linked Behavior

The largest sex differences in mortality rates occur for causes of death associated with sex-linked behavior and suggest that sex-linked behavior, which is more prevalent and encouraged in men, correlates with the following major categories of death (Harrison, 1984):

- Smoking: lung cancer, bronchitis, emphysema, and asthma
- Alcohol consumption: cirrhosis, accidents, and homicide
- Poor preventive health habits and stress: heart disease
- Lack of other emotional channels: cirrhosis, suicide, homicide, and accidents

Smoking, alcohol consumption, preventive health habits, and use of emotional channels are lifestyle factors that may be compounded by social and environmental conditions. These conditions include major physical and psychological public health concerns such as occupational hazards (e.g., carcinogens and stress), unemployment, and massive advertising campaigns that use sex and sex roles to sell alcohol and tobacco. Box 16-2 discusses the effect of unemployment on men's health. These lifestyle factors are compounded by men's lack of willingness to seek preventive care such as screening and to seek health care when a symptom arises. These concerns call for a major public health approach to men's health (Box 16-3).

To counter these types of factors, research is needed to determine gender-specific methods of education and practice aimed at health promotion, illness prevention, and political processes to create safer environments to enhance the well-being of males and females.

BOX 16-2

Unemployment and Men's Health

Although unemployment is not viewed as a major cause of injury, illness, or death, it has been recognized as a health risk (Hibbard and Pope, 1987; Lewis, 1988). Consequences of unemployment include a loss of personal and social identity, a life crisis and major change, loss of income or poverty, and higher rates of illness (e.g., CVD, hypertension, MI, cerebrovascular accidents, cirrhosis, and psychosis). Other increases noted are smoking, drinking, depression, aggression, and child abuse. For example, a study of employed people free of major depression reported that, on follow-up interview, those who had become unemployed had more than twice the risk of increased depressive symptoms and clinical depression than those who did not become unemployed (Dooley, Catalano, and Wilson, 1994).

Dooley, Catalano, and Wilson reported additional findings of initial and follow-up interviews with people who were initially employed and not violent. Those who were unemployed at reinterview had nearly six times the risk of violent behavior compared with those people who remained employed. Another study reported that the incidence of clinically significant alcohol abuse is greater among people who have lost their jobs than among people who have not. The current economic situation in a country may have marked implications for men's health. A U.S. study that investigated the relationship between states' public welfare spending and suicide rates from 1960 through 1990 reported that in 1990 states that spent less for public welfare had higher suicide rates (Zimmerman, 1995). The consequences of unemployment are felt not only at the individual level but also by the family and the community. Community health nurses may experience the deprivation associated with a community that experiences high rates of unemployment.

BOX 16-3

Images of Men and the Need for Marketing

Over a period of years, women have been reporting the harmful, sex-role–stereotyped images of women as passive, unintelligent, dependent sex objects in print, audio, and visual media (Bird, 1970; Steinem, 1983). Less has been written about the damaging sex-role–stereotyped images in the media's portrayal of men as aggressive, independent, powerful, and aloof (Allen and Whatley, 1986). Community health nurses are in a position to overcome the traditional medical and scientific approach to men's health as the presentation of "facts" only by marketing gender-appropriate health information directly to men. Recognizing the difference between the damaging sex-role–stereotyped images of men and the use of male culture as a way of communicating with men is important in marketing health concepts to men. For example, an early self-care book for men, *Man's Body: An Owner's Manual* (Diagram Group, 1976), uses language with which men can identify in their culture (i.e., "an owner's manual"). Another example of using this concept in marketing health information to men is an advertisement for seminars on fatherhood, "Come to Our Fatherhood Seminar . . . Because Babies Don't Come With an Owner's Manual."

Another example of marketing to men occurred within an HMO in Portland, Oregon (Plunkett, 1995). When traditional advertising of a series of 12 weeks of weight-reduction classes, "Freedom From Fat" targeting men, in the HMO's health education catalog failed to bring a response, an article about the class was placed in the business section of the daily newspaper. The response was immediate, and three classes of men signed up to take the series of classes, which were open to both members and nonmembers and required a fee. Many men may not read health education catalogs; more men may read the business section of the newspaper. The nurse must use a knowledge of men's culture in efforts to market programs and services to men.

FACTORS THAT IMPEDE MEN'S HEALTH

Many factors are barriers to men's health. Men's higher rates of mortality, greater risk taking, less use of the health care system, gaps in preventive health behavior, and differences in illness and health orientations and reporting health behavior all contribute to a diminished health status for men. Several other barriers have been proposed, including the patterns of medical care provided in the United States, access to care, and lack of health promotion.

Medical Care Patterns

DeHoff and Forrest (1984) stated, "the usual pattern of medical care in this country—'the system'—has contributed indirectly to men's health problems" (p. 5). During his lifetime, a man is likely to come into contact first with a pediatrician; then with a school nurse; next with a college, military, or company physician; and last with a family practitioner, internist, or geriatrician by the time he develops chronic disease later in life.

Many health professionals provide care for men with complex health needs in a wide variety of settings, yet DeHoff and Forrest pointed out that men do not have a specialist they could go to for care that "feels right" for them. Men were overlooked when new medical specialties were developed. No conscious effort was made to create a male-specific health care climate. Urologists, who may see men for genital abnormalities or diseases of the prostate, became the proxy "male health specialist." The medical specialty andrology, which originated in Europe to treat problems of fertility and sterility, is considered too narrow in focus to treat "the whole man." Without a primary care specialty that focuses specifically on men's needs, many needs such as sexual and reproductive problems and sex-role influences on health and lifestyle may not be attended to by anyone. In addition, these specialists and generalists have not received training that would enable them to focus on men's health needs specifically. In the current era of managed care, men will still be left without a gender-specific primary care provider with training focused specifically on their needs.

Access to Care

Mission Orientation

Public interest in men's health has focused on efforts necessary to maintain an effective workforce (DeHoff and Forrest, 1984). Men view health as a commodity

or resource that enables the body to work (Harrison and Dignan, 1999). Mission-oriented health care is a priority for large industries and organized sports. However, more general health care may be provided through insurance programs such as HMOs. Perhaps the most complete care is currently offered by the military; however, marked deficiencies exist in the lack of a focus on prevention and health promotion at the individual and aggregate levels and inattention to policy regarding environmental hazards.

Financial Considerations

Another barrier to health care for men is financial ability. A man may receive an annual physical examination if he belongs to an HMO or if he is an executive or an airline pilot, but many private insurance companies will reimburse more fully for a diagnosed condition (e.g., for pathology) and less fully for preventive care. A man is more likely insured for acute or chronic illness conditions than for health education, counseling, or other types of preventive health care. Women have annual gynecological examinations that include screening for other conditions and allow a woman to express other physical or psychological needs; however, men have lacked entrée to the health care system for a physical examination on a routine basis. Now, under managed care, health care professionals will be interested in whether gender differences in routine physical examinations for preventive reasons continue as they have in the past. However, socialization has a marked influence on behavior and current trends may prevail despite current behaviors, or attitudes, in health care delivery. Men must become advocates for programs to meet their own health care needs.

Time Factors

It is no longer true that men may not have access to the health care system as readily as women, because men have greater participation in the workforce and have schedules that usually correspond with clinicians' availability (Waldron, 1995b). Differences in role obligations balance out from family demands on women, although more men are employed. Men may still be reluctant to take time from work for a medical visit, fearing loss of income or the stigmatization of being "weak," "ill," or "less of a man."

Lack of Health Promotion

A concept of health that considers health as merely the absence of disease is limiting. Traditional mortality and morbidity rates, although reflective of the state of "health" of a population, fall short of desired health outcomes and tend to divorce the biological from the psychosocial (Choi, 1985). For example, the absence of overt pathology, even in the presence of behavioral risk factors such as smoking, alcohol consumption, obesity, and sedentary lifestyle, is enough to elicit a "clean bill of health." Men describe "healthy" as those with proportional body weight and height who do not excessively engage in behaviors detrimental to health. Physical recovery after impairment, illness, or injury is considered satisfactory. Although touted as the means to cost containment in managed care, prevention and health promotion are not always within the scope of the current system.

PRECURSORS OF DEATH
The following precursors of death are frequently unaddressed by the present health care system:

- Heart disease and stroke
- Hypercholesterolemia
- Hypertension
- Diabetes mellitus
- Obesity
- Type A personality
- Family history
- Lack of exercise
- Cigarette smoking
- Cancer
- Sunlight
- Radiation
- Occupational hazards
- Water pollution
- Air pollution
- Dietary patterns
- Cigarette smoking
- Alcohol
- Heredity
- Certain medical conditions

The disease focus of the present health care system persists. The ability to address the precursors of death is limited. Interventions by many disciplines are needed to prevent current health problems. Nursing's contribution to practice and research is instrumental in this process.

Coronary heart disease, cancer, and stroke are three conditions that account for two thirds of all deaths and the greatest use of resources. However, medical measures have not made a substantial influence on mortality rates. The increase in life expectancy has resulted in an increase in years of disability.

COMMUNITY HEALTH NURSING SERVICES FOR MEN
A male can be seen by a community health nurse in a well-baby clinic, by a school nurse, by an occupational health nurse, and by a community health nurse or home health nurse on a home visit for follow-up of a chronic disease. However, men are less likely to be seen by a community health nurse than women. Not only is MCH a major focus of many health departments, but neither a medical nor a nursing specialty within a health department routinely exists to specifically address men's health. Preventive reproductive health care (i.e., family planning, prenatal care, and cancer screening) and associated general screening are not routinely available for men. The hours of services offered by health departments do not usually provide ready access for men. The community health nurse's commitment to health for all requires an increased awareness of men's health issues in their social and cultural context and individual and group action that will improve men's physical, psychological, and social well-being.

Mortality rates for coronary heart disease declined approximately 40% between 1968 and 1987 (McKinlay, McKinlay, and Beaglehole, 1989). The causes of the decline are not clear and are associated with changes in risk behaviors. McKinlay, McKinlay, and Beaglehole (1989) cited evidence that the effects of pharmacological intervention, emergency response in the community, coronary care units, and coronary bypass surgery have been negligible with the exception of some benefits from beta-blocking agents in postMI patients (Goldman and Cook, 1984).

Age-adjusted mortality rates for all types of cancer increased slowly between 1950 and 1982 (McKinlay, McKinlay, and Beaglehole, 1989). Despite known environmental and personal risk factors for major cancers, funds and other resources have been allotted disproportionately into treatment and cure rather than into public health measures and primary prevention.

Mortality rates for stroke have been declining since the beginning of the twentieth century (McKinlay, McKinlay, and Beaglehole, 1989). Although the declines occurred well before antihypertensive therapy was available, McKinlay, McKinlay, and Beaglehole (1989) cited evidence for the contribution of medical treatment to only about 12% to 25% of the decline since 1970.

SOCIAL DEMOGRAPHY AND SOCIAL EPIDEMIOLOGY

Epidemiology is the method of research used to determine the nature and distribution of a health problem in a community. *Social demographers* and *social epidemiologists* study social and psychological factors that affect the distribution of health problems in a community. Factors associated with the occurrence of the problems can be identified and resources can be focused on prevention. Social epidemiologists have identified men as a population at risk for premature death. Concentrated efforts can improve men's health.

Financial resources are invested in traditional disease curative care rather than health promotion action. An inordinate amount of funds is poured into the health care system each year, with only minimum amounts allotted to public health promotion, as discussed in earlier chapters. In 1992, total health expenditures accounted for 13.6% of the gross domestic product, an increase from 5.9% in 1965 (NCHS, 1996). Of every dollar spent on health care in 1993, approximately $0.46 went to hospital care and physician services, which are in large part curative in focus, and less than $0.03 went to preventive government public health activities. The current health care system is limited in addressing the precursors of death. Therefore it is questionable whether medical care, or another medical specialty, is the answer to men's health needs when social, occupational, environmental, and "lifestyle" factors continue to place men at risk.

Milio (1983) asserted that healthy lifestyles are not a matter of free choice but rather a result of opportunities that are not always equally available to people. Although available, prevention and health pro-

motion are not uniformly applied at the aggregate and population levels. Health policies shape these opportunities for a healthy lifestyle for individuals and aggregates. Policies related to environmental and occupational changes beyond an individual's control are required to significantly impact the health of the population.

Community health nurses should be involved in political activities that develop health policies that will make a difference in men's health and in the population's health. Such activities are congruent with the philosophy of public health as "health for all" and a commitment to a social justice ethic of health care rather than a market justice ethic of health care. Examining men's health gives the community health nurse an opportunity to observe the market justice ethic of health care's influence on men's health in the United States from men's traditional roles in the family, the health of women, family, and community. The community health nurse can play a vital role in contributing to a social justice ethic of health care, particularly in relation to promoting men's health. Nurses must focus on health promotion and prevention at the aggregate and population levels rather than focus on treatment and cure.

MEN'S HEALTH CARE NEEDS

DeHoff and Forrest (1984) delineated men's health care needs that draw from the biological and the psychosocial causes of men's distinctive health situation. According to these authors, men need the following:

- Permission to have concerns about health and talk openly to others about them.
- Support for the consideration of sex-role and lifestyle influences on their physical and mental health.
- Attention from professionals regarding factors that may cause illness or influence a man's expression of illness, including occupational factors, leisure patterns, and interpersonal relationships.
- Information about how their bodies function, what is normal, what is abnormal, what action to take, and the contributions of proper nutrition and exercise.
- Self-care instruction, including testicular and genital self-examination.
- Physical examination and history taking that include sexual and reproductive health and illness across the life span.

- Treatment for problems of couples, including interpersonal problems, infertility, family planning, sexual concerns, and STDs.
- Help with fathering (i.e., being included as a parent in the care of children).
- Help with fathering as a single parent, in particular with a child of the opposite sex, in addressing the child's sexual development and concerns.
- Recognition that feelings of confusion and uncertainty in a time of rapid social change are normal and that they may mark the onset of healthy adaptation to change.
- Adjustment of the health care system to men's occupational constraints regarding time and location of health care sources.
- Financial ways to obtain these goals.

Additional health care needs of men are for primary prevention, and for secondary and tertiary prevention at the individual, family, and community levels, to address the precursors of death that influence males so greatly. Men are less likely to be consumers in the health care system than women; therefore alternative approaches must be developed that address their health needs. The most significant approaches in the future will be those that reach men in the community, schools, the workplace, and public settings. This calls for political processes that set policy, for health marketing techniques, and for advocacy.

Meeting men's health care needs can be viewed in a traditional public fashion. By viewing the problem from a primary, secondary, and tertiary intervention method, the nurse can look at the problem in a holistic manner. Factors that promote men's health are in the community, including interest groups in men and men's health, men's increasing interest in physical fitness and lifestyle, policy related to men's health, and health services for men.

GAINING SKILLS NECESSARY TO ADDRESS MEN'S HEALTH NEEDS

Assessment skills necessary to carry out screening activities with men to detect reproductive health needs may be lacking in nursing education. One community health nurse who worked in a rural health department felt unable to respond to male partners' requests for genital examinations when couples came to seek family planning services.

The community health nurse requested to work for specified periods of time with a urologist and in an STD clinic in a large urban area to gain the necessary skills. On return to the rural health department, she felt comfortable with male patients and taught the skills she had learned to nurse colleagues.

PRIMARY PREVENTIVE MEASURES

Health Education

Health care professionals, including the community health nurse, find that health education is the cornerstone of prevention. Although criticized by some as too narrow, health education can be a means of empowerment that assists individuals to make behavioral changes. Education about male health issues should begin early. At school, boys should learn the anatomical and physiological aspects of their bodies and the social aspects of taking responsibility for their health. Coeducational discussion classes that cover a variety of social and personal topics can be a venue to encourage boys to talk about their bodies and their feelings. This may lead to a less self-conscious attitude toward health seeking when boys reach adulthood.

Access to health education should follow males into the workplace. Many employers have experienced benefits such as lower health care costs when their employees receive health education programs coupled with health screening. Government incentives given to employers who provide such programs would provide further impetus. Men who are not in the workplace can access health education in other areas, such as shopping malls. Given the literacy level of some of the population, some health care professionals are concerned about this informal dispersion of health literature. Government benefits programs can be a medium for health education by including such in their benefit mailing. More control over the readability and the information included can be exerted over this material.

Interest Groups in Men and Men's Health

Unlike the consumer movement that occurred on behalf of women's health in the 1960s and early 1970s, a consumer movement has not taken place advocating men's health (Allen and Whatley, 1986). However, a viable men's consumer movement is forming. The National Organization for Changing Men is interested in redefining the male role, particularly those aspects of the male role that are detrimental to health and growth. The American Assembly for Men in Nursing sponsors annual meetings that address issues such as men's health, men's work environments, research on men's health, and networking and support among male nurses. Researchers are beginning to define and study men's health beyond men's occupational role (e.g., reproductive health) (Flaming and Morse, 1991; Smith and Babaian, 1992; Swanson, 1995).

Men's Increasing Interest in Physical Fitness and Lifestyle

Although CVDs are a major health hazard for men, research on the validity and usefulness of preventive and treatment modalities is an issue of considerable debate (Waldron, 1995d). Men's interest in altering behavior that places them at risk for cardiovascular and other major diseases is increasing. For example, men's smoking behavior has changed dramatically. Between 1965 and 1993, the age-adjusted percentage of men who smoked decreased from 51% to 27% (NCHS, 1996). As stated previously, more men report being physically active in leisure time sports in the past two weeks than women (36.6% vs. 22.6%) and men report exercising or playing sports more regularly than women (44% vs. 37.7%) (Piani and Schoenborn, 1993).

However, those health behaviors that have reported the greatest change in a positive direction have been those most influenced by legislative action (e.g., seat belt use, use of smoke detectors, and drunk driving) (Piani and Schoenborn, 1993).

Policy Related to Men's Health

Policies related to any group of people should include the opinions and perceptions of those directly affected. Policy related to men's health should include the male perception of health. Community health nurses can encourage and assist males to be advocates for policies regarding their health care. Male nurses can be extremely instrumental in this endeavor. Liaisons between male consumers and policy planners should be formed.

SECONDARY PREVENTIVE MEASURES

Health Services for Men

Fewer health care clinics are tailored to men's special needs than women's special needs. The "well-man clinics" set up in the 1980s were designed to identify lifestyle risk factors, not to provide screening clinics like the women's clinics. Once identified, a method or resolution was formulated. These clinics still exist with emphasis placed on CVDs (Sadler, 1979). Typically, male screening methods have been limited to detecting high blood cholesterol levels and cancers such as prostate cancer, skin cancer, and testicular lumps. This era of managed care may not encourage the concept of gender-specific care because men and women receive primary care from the same health services.

Screening Services for Men

The U.S. Preventive Services Task Force outlines the kinds of screening tests the population should have received. According to the Task Force, healthy men under age 50 should have the following:

Dental examination: yearly
Eye examination: every three to five years
Blood pressure check: every two years
Blood cholesterol check: every five years
Prostate examination: every year after age 50; blacks every year after age 40
Colorectal screening: every three to five years

Community health nurses should be familiar with these recommended screening test frequencies and take every opportunity to encourage men to have these screenings (Mayo Clinic Health Oasis, 1999).

TERTIARY PREVENTIVE MEASURES

Sex-Role and Lifestyle Rehabilitation

Traditional health services for males are available in both the private and governmental arenas. The emphasis of these services is on diagnosis and treatment. The traditional male role may change dramatically from treatment modalities. Rehabilitation services for males must include counseling on lifestyle, role changes, and job retraining. Men must be given permission to express their emotions such as fear and anxiety over the resultant change.

Goal setting and possible methods for achievement must be acceptable to the man. For example, after a heart attack a man may be told to stop smoking and begin an exercise program. To be successful, the male must be an active partner in the formation of the plan. He may be able to exercise by walking to the nearest automotive shop to talk with friends rather than spending time on a stationary bicycle at a local gym.

DOOR OPENERS: WAYS TO ADDRESS MEN ABOUT HEALTH CONCERNS

Strategies to address men about health concerns include the following:

- Ask a man to talk about the last time he had a physical examination, what was done, why it was done, where it was done, and what the recommendations were.
- Ask a man how he feels about his health insurance coverage and if he lacks health insurance; ask about the resources that have been used for medical care for him and his family.
- Ask a man about how he spends his leisure time, what he is doing to take care of himself, and what his usual physical activities are.
- Observe a man for signs of stress such as moist palms, nail biting, posture, and nervous movements. If signs of stress are present, ask about how he is coping with an identified health problem, family problem, or being unemployed.
- Observe a man for difficulty clearing airway (i.e., from smoking) and flushing of the face (i.e., from alcohol). Inquire as to habits of smoking and drinking and whether these habits have increased since the occurrence of the particular health or social problem.
- Involve men in decision making about health care to instill a sense of control over events.

New Concepts of Community Care

Specific services for men within health departments have been lacking in the United States, with the exception of STD clinics and selected family planning service models. Two male health visitors (i.e., British term for *public health nurses*) from the National Health Service (NHS) started an innovative public health nursing program directed at men in Glasgow, Scotland (Sadler, 1979). Health visitors Bill Deans and Bob Hoskins established a nurse-run Well-Man Clinic with the help of the NHS and the Scottish Council for Health Education. During home visits with mothers and infants, Deans and Hoskins observed that fathers excused themselves and went to the local pub when they arrived.

Noting characteristics of the male population in their community (e.g., overweight, heavy smoking, drinking, and high unemployment) Deans and Hoskins decided to modify their practice to their clients' needs. One afternoon per week, the clinic, which is based on a nursing model rather than a medical model, offers health screening, health education, and primary prevention to men. Marketing is important and men are referred from general practitioners' and specialists' practices and recruited through newspaper advertisements. Clients with clinical signs and symptoms are referred back to their physicians. Lifestyle counseling and education are offered in areas such as fat and fiber content in diet, smoking, alcohol use, and exercise.

Deans and Hoskins consider the clinic a way to extend the health visitor's role the NHS's efforts in health education with an aim to "nip potential diseases in the bud" (Sadler, 1979, p. 18). Deans and Hoskins are concerned that the NHS does not provide male services and are clear that "the unemployed chain-smoking husband needs as much care and health education from the health visitor as do his wife and baby" (Sadler, 1979, p. 18). The Well-Man Clinic and the Well-Woman Clinic models can now be found in several communities throughout Great Britain and have been expanded to serve inmates in prison (Fareed, 1994; Woodland and Hunt, 1994). For a description of the establishment and evaluation of a Well-Man Clinic and discussion of the clinic's ability to meet the health needs of men, see Brown and Lunt (1992).

Public health nurses working in the Benton County Health Department in Corvallis, Oregon, responded to the challenge of teen pregnancy in the 1970s by launching a community-wide effort that included developing a men's health clinic and marketing reproductive health services directly to teenage boys and men (Fig. 16-1). An early effort established an advisory committee that included people from churches, schools, and health care facilities. A public health nurse health educator launched an extensive education program in the high school, which focused on decision-making processes and services available in the community. Later efforts involved the establishment of a clinic for men. Teenage boys were members of a consumer advisory committee established by the nurses that recommended the wording and format for advertisements about the clinic that ran in the high school newspaper. The advisory committee also recommended a format for flyers that would be attractive to males. Specifically, they requested a card with information about the clinic and how to use condoms that would discretely fit into their wallets and be available to share with peers (Fig. 16-2).

FIGURE **16-1**

Men's health clinic brochure, Benton County Health Department, Corvallis, Oregon. Reprinted with permission.

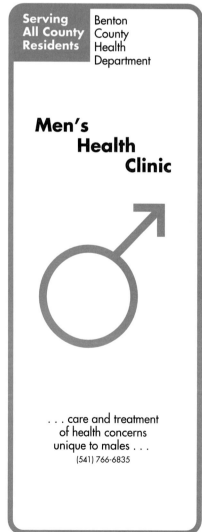

Serving All County Residents | Benton County Health Department

Men's Health Clinic

. . . care and treatment of health concerns unique to males . . .
(541) 766-6835

Services Available Include:
• Free condoms
• Information on birth control for men and their partners
• Vasectomy counseling and referral
• Full or partial payment of vasectomies for low income men
• Diagnosis and treatment of sexually-related diseases
• Medical treatment of genital and urinary problems
• Counseling and support for concerns related to sexuality
• Information for men involved in unplanned pregnancy
• Opportunity to share in female partner's clinic visit
• Books, pamphlets, and information on men's issues relating to sexuality

All Care and Counseling is Strictly Confidential
• Teenagers welcome. Parents' permission is not required
• Staffed by nurse practitioners and registered nurses
• No appointment necessary for condoms. Self-serve, free

Rev. 9/87

Benton County Health Department
530 NW 27th Street
Corvallis, Oregon 97330
(541) 766-6835

The nurses have expanded their focus to create inclusive service environments in which teenage girls and boys and adult men and women will feel accepted and comfortable. Particular attention is given to the clinic decor and advertising, reading materials, and posters to transmit a message that includes offering health care for males and females. Clinic staff will see males or females at any time; however, a room in which staff members see men has decor geared toward men (e.g., no gynecological stirrups on the examining table) and pamphlets available for men on topics such as testicular cancer and chewing tobacco. Integrated services exist in the areas of family planning, STDs, and HIV counseling and testing.

F I G U R E 16-2

Condom card, Benton County Health Department, Corvallis, Oregon. Reprinted with permission.

Condom Card
Produced by
Benton County
Health Department

Why use condoms (rubbers)
—Very effective in preventing pregnancy
—Protects against sexually transmitted diseases (VD), including **AIDS**
—Can be used with other birth control methods as added protection
—Inexpensive
—No exam needed
—No prescription needed; available at drugstores and Family Planning Clinics
—No health risks

REMEMBER
—Women can have supply for partner's use

—over—

Benton County Health Department
530 NW 27th Street
Corvallis, Oregon 97330
(541) 766-6835

Condom Card

HOW to use condoms (rubbers)
—Condoms must be put on penis **before** it gets close to vagina
—Keep condom rolled up until ready to use
—Roll gently onto hard penis
—Leave space at tip for semen; pinch tip of condom to expel air
—After ejaculation, promptly withdraw penis from vagina; hold condom at base of penis during withdrawal
—**Practice** putting a condom on before using for sexual intercourse
—Use only once. Condoms come in different varieties but only one size
—Condoms come lubricated or non-lubricated; if lubrication is needed, use contraceptive foam or KY jelly (not vaseline)
—Keep away from heat; do not keep in wallet for long periods of time; do not store in cars during hot weather

WHAT to do if a condom breaks or slips off
—Use contraceptive foam or jelly in vagina immediately
—Call Family Planning Clinic or physician for information on the Morning After Pill
—over—

C A S E   S T U D Y

APPLICATION OF THE NURSING PROCESS

Community health nurses are in an ideal position to address the health needs of men at the individual, family, and community levels. The community health nurse may promote self-care in male members of the family, facilitate men's health by addressing needed changes at the family level, buttress women's roles as caregivers of the family's health, and bring about change that influences policies that affect men at the community level.

Planning gender-appropriate care for males is outlined in the following case study, which is an application of the nursing process at the individual, family, and aggregate levels initiated in a home visit and applies the previous discussions about the levels of prevention, roles of the community health nurse, research, and men's health.

Application of the nursing process to aggregates is facilitated by the use of systems theory, in which the nurse identifies the system and sub-

systems involved. The nurse may use a deductive or an inductive approach. A deductive approach would involve carrying out a community assessment and identifying an area or areas, such as a program needed by the community. Planning, implementation, and evaluation of the program would be carried out at the family or group level. An inductive approach would involve entering the community system through a person or client via a referral about a problem or concern. Assessment of the individual would be followed by identification of those groups to which the client belongs, such as family and community, and assessment of those groups.

Beth Lockwood, a community health nursing student at a health department, received a referral from the high school nurse to visit the Connors family to assess Richard Connors' mental health status. Richard was a 16-year-old sophomore whose
Continued

academic work in school had declined rapidly after the premature death of his 46-year-old father. He died from a MI, which he suffered while cleaning the garage with Richard one evening after school. Richard and the neighbors failed to revive Mr. Connors and Richard carries feelings of guilt. Household members include Mrs. Connors, age 44, and Richard's sister Yvonne, age 12.

Assessment

The referral to assess the Connors family called for an inductive approach to assessment. Beth used a deductive approach later when her experience with the Connors family piqued her concern about the status of men's health in her community. Beth assessed Richard, his mother, and his sister as household members of the family. However, she could not stop with the immediate family; she had to continue to identify the other groups within the community to which each individual family member belonged. Viewing the community as a system and focusing on systems and subsystems helped Beth organize the data she collected during assessment. Knowing that "the whole is greater than the sum of its parts," Beth prepared for her visit by reviewing adolescent theories of development and family theory. Beyond individual assessment, she noted factors related to the development of sex-role–related behavior that may influence health. Examples of assessment areas include the following:

- family configuration, traditional or nontraditional
- sex-role–related behavior of parents, including work patterns in and out of the home, division of household labor, and decision-making patterns
- patterns of parenting: mothering, fathering, and substitute father figure(s)
- ability of male children to disclose feelings to family members and others
- degree of assertiveness in female children
- ability of family members to give emotional and physical support during crises and noncrises
- ability of family members to trade off role-related behavior during crises and noncrises
- risk-taking health behaviors
- processing stress and grief

- communal lifestyle patterns that place the individual or family at risk (e.g., lack of exercise, poor diet, smoking, and drinking)
- family history of death and illness
- health-care–taking patterns of family members
- preventive health behaviors
- leisure activities

Assessment of other groups includes neighborhood and other peer groups, school environments, sports, and church and civic activities.

Diagnosis

Through induction, the nurse makes a diagnosis for each individual and each system component, including family and the community. The following are examples of diagnoses.

Individual
- loss of interest or involvement in an activity related to conflicting stages of grief process secondary to premature death of father (Richard)
- expressed dissatisfaction with parenting role related to feelings of helplessness and hopelessness secondary to premature death of husband (Mrs. Connors)
- risk of interpersonal conflict resulting from prolonged, unrelieved family stress secondary to premature death of father (Yvonne)

Family
- decreased ability to communicate related to family stress secondary to premature death of father
- risk of family crisis related to disequilibrium

Community
- inadequate systematic programs for linking families in crisis to community resources
- inadequate systematic programs for populations at risk of premature death related to inadequate planning among community systems

Planning
Planning involves contracting and mutual goal setting and is an outcome of mutually derived assessment and diagnosis. A contract with the family alone is shortsighted and may provide little

community benefit over time. The following are examples of other aggregates with which a contract may be established:

- the school subsystem that does not provide ongoing counseling, but will meet periodically to evaluate pupil progression with family members;
- the school subsystem that provides physical education in football, basketball, and baseball (i.e., nonaerobic, nonlifetime sports), but offers extramural aerobic, lifetime sports such as swimming and track after school hours;
- the American Red Cross, which does not offer cardiovascular pulmonary resuscitation (CPR) courses on evenings or weekends, but offers to consider doing so for a defined minimum-size community.

Mutual goal setting requires collaboration regarding long- and short-term goals. Again, mutually defined needs and diagnoses are important to this process. Regardless of the diagnosis, each individual in the family and the subsystem must participate in developing a care plan. The following are examples of goals.

Individual

Long-Term Goal
- Individual family members will be able to trade off role-related behavior.

Short-Term Goal
- Individual family members will express feelings related to abandonment and loss.

Family

Long-Term Goal
- The family will exhibit an increased ability to handle crisis as evidenced by ability to discuss roles and interdependencies.

Short-Term Goal
- The family will identify specific ways to recognize and use support services.

Community

Long-Term Goal
- Systematic programs will be established for populations at risk of premature death from coro-

nary heart disease as evidenced by local planning bodies with ongoing program evaluation.

Short-Term Goals
- Dissemination is provided to individuals, families, groups, and planning bodies in the community about the incidence of coronary heart disease.
- Existing programs are identified that address coronary heart disease.
- Existing programs are coordinated to bridge gaps and avoid duplication of effort.

Intervention

The nurse, family, and other aggregates carry out interventions contracted during the planning phase to meet the mutually derived goals. Most importantly, the nurse empowers the family and community to develop the networks and linkages necessary to care for themselves.

Individual

Individual counseling regarding loss and grief may be beneficial to each family member, but options may need to be explored and referrals may need to be reevaluated for members of the rural family. Education regarding preventive measures that combat risk factors for heart disease include those aimed at individual family members and address areas such as diet, exercise, smoking, alcohol use, and stress management.

Family

Examples of interventions with the family include counseling, education, and referral aimed at family self-care promotion. For example, Beth's interventions with the Connors family were dependent on the family's ability to solve problems, investigate community resources, and create linkages between the family and resources. Periodic family conferences at school and more inclusive family therapy may enable the family to work through the death of Mr. Connors; this results in the development of new roles and the communication necessary to maintain family equilibrium. Education regarding preventive measures to combat risk factors for heart disease may need discussion at the family and individual levels (e.g., diet, exercise, smoking, alcohol use, and stress management).

Continued

Community

The nurse must also carry out interventions with other aggregates. These may involve activities such as educating, facilitating program expansion, or tailoring programs to meet community needs. Intervention at the aggregate level calls for group and community work. The nurse carries out interventions at this level in several ways (e.g., by communicating community statistics from a community analysis, relating anecdotes from families served, or linking family experience to program need by acting as an advocate and bringing family members to board meetings or hearings on community health issues).

Education regarding preventive measures to combat risk factors for heart disease also includes those interventions aimed at the community. A rationale for the development of lifetime aerobic sports is needed not only by Richard, but also by school districts. Exploration of options with the school nurse and review of the school district health education curriculum would be beneficial. A community assessment of heart disease awareness, including determination of the availability of resources such as emergency response and CPR courses, is an aggregate intervention. Taking the outcome of the assessment in the form of statistics and the anonymous anecdotal story of the Connors family to planning bodies in the community is also intervention at the aggregate level. Creative programs other communities used (e.g., teaching CPR within the school system) should be investigated and proposed.

Evaluation

Evaluation is multidimensional and ongoing. Using a systems approach to evaluation, the nurse evaluates each component of the system, from individual family member to family and community, in terms of goal achievement. Evaluation includes noting degrees of equilibrium established, degree of change, how the system handles change, whether the system is open or closed, and patterns of networking. Ongoing evaluation includes noting referrals and follow-up of the individual, the family, and other aggregates in resource use.

Individual

Use of resources such as support groups by the individual family member may be noted. These resources may include a teen support group, a women's support group, support groups for those experiencing the loss of a spouse or other family member, reentry programs for women at a local junior college or university, and parents without partners.

Family

Evaluation of the Connors family would include follow-up of their use of support services specifically for the family, such as counseling options for the family as a unit. Evaluation would also focus on the family's ability to handle crises in the future.

Community

Aggregate evaluation would focus on the community. For example, to what extent do school programs encourage sports options that promote lifetime aerobic activities and prevent premature death from heart disease? Are programs systematically planned in the community for populations that are at risk of premature death from heart disease?

Levels of Prevention

Society's expectations of men and women are in transition. Application of levels of prevention by the community health nurse must take into account men's health status, men's socialization, men's use of health care services, men's primary needs for prevention and health promotion, and the role of women as caregivers in family health.

Primary

Men are more likely to engage in risk-taking behavior than women and are less likely to engage in preventive behaviors; therefore primary prevention must be marketed specifically to men. Examples of primary prevention for the Connors family are applied at the following individual, family, and community levels:

- individual: assessment, teaching, and referral related to diet and exercise behaviors;
- family: assessment and teaching related to food selection and preparation at home and fast-food

restaurant food selection; teaching and role-modeling gender roles that allow male members of the family to use alternative expressions of emotion;
• community: provision of CPR courses for members of the community; consultation with schools regarding need for aerobic activities in physical education and sports programs.

The nurse must pull men from the family, workplace, or other aggregates into involvement with family planning, education, antepartum and postpartum care, parenting, dental prophylaxis, and accident prevention. In addition, assessment of need for immunizations and classes (e.g., retirement preparation) is considered action aimed at primary prevention.

Secondary

Men have higher mortality, morbidity, and health care use rates for many of the leading causes of death, but are second to women in overall use of health care services, including preventive physical examinations and screening; therefore early diagnosis and prompt intervention must also meet men's needs. Examples of secondary prevention regarding the Connors family include the following:

• individual: screening for risk factors related to CVD in the individual, such as how the individual handles stress;
• family: screening for risk factors related to CVD in the family, such as how the family processes stress;
• community: organizing screening programs for the community, such as health fairs.

The nurse must screen individuals and aggregates of men according to lifestyle risk factors, mortality

rates at different age levels, morbidity rates, and occupational health risks.

Tertiary

Activities that rehabilitate individuals and aggregates and restore them to their highest level of functioning are aimed at tertiary prevention. The nurse in the community is ideally situated to locate people in need of rehabilitation services. The nurse may provide evaluation and physical, mental, and social restoration services. Men in need of rehabilitation may have special needs because their disability influences themselves, their families, and ultimately their communities. Financial assistance and vocational counseling, training, and placement may be priorities for the well-being of the family. Socialization causes men to have difficulty admitting they need help. Community health nurses who teach men with chronic disease to rest at specified periods during the day or continue with medical regimens or speech or occupational therapy are providing tertiary prevention. Working with couples as a unit is also important because caregiving patterns may shift as a result of chronic disease and disability. Encouraging men to express their concerns about their health, families, and jobs and frustration with themselves is important. The following are examples of tertiary prevention with the Connors family:

• individual: assist individual family members in dealing with grief from the loss of the father and husband;
• family: assist family in dealing with grief and assuming alternate roles;
• community: assist the community in dealing with loss of a fully functioning family by providing grief support services that include males or target males and females.

LEARNING ACTIVITIES

1. Examine the vital statistics in the community and compare the sex-specific differences in mortality rates.
2. During a one-week period, determine the frequency of newspaper articles in the local major newspaper that identify the top 12 causes of death for men.
3. Survey the billboards in the community and determine the frequency of those that depict sex-linked behavior of men associated with risk-taking behavior.
4. Survey local businesses and industries in the community to determine what health promotion and prevention programs are available and used by men and women.
5. Select a family that has a man in the household

who is accessible. Select two "door openers" appropriate to initiate discussion of health concerns with this man. Devise a gender-appropriate nursing care plan that includes primary, secondary, and tertiary prevention for this man as an individual, for his family, and for his community.

6. Select a family that has a man in the household who is not readily accessible. Interview the female caregiver in the household and obtain information by proxy about the man's health. If possible, arrange to meet the man for lunch, at work, or after work and obtain information about his health. Compare the information obtained by proxy with that obtained from the client.

7. Review major nursing texts (e.g., medical-surgical); examine the tables of contents and the indexes for content on men's health vs. women's health.

RECOMMENDED READINGS

Adams KF Jr: Relation between gender, etiology, and survival in patients with symptomatic heart failure, *J Am Coll Cardiol* 28:1781-8, 1996.

Bozett FW, Forrester DA: A proposal for a men's health nurse practitioner, *Image J Nurs Sch* 21:158, 1989.

Brabant S, Forsyth C, Melancon C: Grieving men: thoughts, feelings, and behaviors following deaths of wives, *Hospice J* 8:33, 1992.

Brown I, Lunt F: Evaluating a "well man" clinic, *Health Visitor* 65:12, 1992.

Chalmers K: Working with men: an analysis of health visiting practice in families with young children, *Int J Nurs Stud* 29:3, 1992.

DiPasquale JA: The psychological effects of support groups on individuals infected by the AIDS virus, *Cancer Nurs* 13:278, 1990.

Flaming D, Morse J: Minimizing embarrassment: boys' experiences of pubertal changes, *Issues Compr Pediatr Nurs* 14:211, 1991.

Franciosa D, Shaw S: Breast cancer and benign breast disease in men, *Nurse Pract Forum* 5:56, 1994.

Go K: Recent advances in the treatment of male infertility, *Clin Issues Perinat Women's Health Nurs* 3:320, 1992.

Gregory DM, Peters N, Cameron CF: Elderly male spouses as caregivers: toward an understanding of their experience, *J Gerontol Nurs* 16:20, 1990.

Hahn W, Brooks J, Hartsouough D: Self-disclosure and coping styles in men with cardiovascular reactivity, *Res Nurs Health* 16:275, 1993.

Julian T, McKenry P, McKelvey M: Components of men's well-being at mid-life, *Issues Ment Health Nurs* 13:285, 1992.

Legato M: *Gender specific aspects of human biology for the practicing physician*, New York, 1997, Futura Publishing Company, Inc.

Lovejoy N et al: Potential predictors of information-seeking behavior by homosexual/bisexual (gay) men with a human immunodeficiency virus seropositive health status, *Cancer Nurs* 15:116, 1992.

MacIntyre R: Nursing loved ones with AIDS: knowledge development for ethical practice, *J Home Health Care Pract* 3:1, 1991.

Mackey V: Another look at the circumcision debate: opinions of nursing-home care-givers, *Nurse Pract* 17:63, 1992.

Mellick E, Buckwalter K, Stolley J: Suicide among elderly white men: development of a profile, *J Psychosocial Nurs Ment Health Serv* 30:29, 1992.

Smith D, Babaian R: The effects of treatment for cancer on male fertility and sexuality, *Cancer Nurs* 15:271, 1992.

Stoller EP: Males as helpers: the role of sons, relatives and friends, *Gerontologist* 30:228, 1990.

Underwood S: Cancer risk reduction and early detection behaviors among black men: focus on learned helplessness, *J Community Health Nurs* 9:21, 1992.

Wilson S, Morse JM: Living with a wife undergoing chemotherapy, *Image J Nurs Sch* 23:78, 1991.

Woodland A, Hunt C: Healthy convictions . . . well-man clinic for the inmates of Lindholme prison, *Nurs Times* 90:32, 1994.

REFERENCES

Agnew J et al: Reproductive hazards of fire fighting: I. non-chemical hazards, *Am J Ind Med* 19:433, 1991.

Allen DG, Whatley M: Nursing and men's health: some critical considerations, *Nurs Clin North Am* 21:3, 1986.

American Cancer Society: *Cancer facts and figures: 1991,* Atlanta, 1991, The Society.

Benson V, Marano MA: *Current estimates from the National Health Interview Survey, 1993,* 1994, The Author, www.cdc.gov/nchs/data/10_190_1.pdf.

Bird C: *Born female: the high cost of keeping women down,* New York, 1970, Pocket Books.

Brown I, Lunt F: Evaluating a "well man" clinic, *Health Visitor* 65:12, 1992.

Centers for Disease Control and Prevention: *Sexually transmitted disease surveillance, 1993,* Atlanta, 1994, USDHHS, PHS, CDC.

Choi MW: Preamble to a new paradigm for women's health care, *Image: J Nurs Sch* 17:14, 1985.

Cohen FL: Paternal contributions to birth defects, *Nurs Clin North Am* 21:49, 1986.

David DS, Brannon R: The male sex role: our culture's blueprint of manhood, and what it's done for us lately. In David DS, Brannon R, editors: *The forty-nine percent majority: the male sex role,* Reading, Mass, 1976, Addison-Wesley.

DeHoff JB, Forrest K: Men's health. In Swanson J, Forrest K, editors: *Men's reproductive health,* New York, 1984, Springer.

Devesa S et al: Recent cancer trends in the United States, *Cancer Inst* 87:175, 1995.

Diagram Group: *Man's body: an owner's manual,* New York, 1976, Paddington Press.

Dooley D, Catalano R, Wilson G: Depression and unemployment: panel findings from the epidemiologic catchment area study, *Am J Community Psychol* 22:745, 1994.

Ehrhardt AA, Wasserheit JN: Age, gender, and sexual risk behaviors for sexually transmitted diseases in the United States. In Wasserheit JN, Aral SO, Holmes KK, editors: *Research issues in human behavior and sexually transmitted diseases in the AIDS era,* Washington, DC, 1991, American Society for Microbiology.

Erikson E: *Childhood and society,* New York, 1963, WW Norton.

Fareed A: Equal rights for men, *Nursing Times* 90:26, 1994.

Flaming D, Morse JM: Minimizing embarrassment: boys' experiences of pubertal changes, *Issues Comprehensive Pediatric Nurs* 14:211, 1991.

Giwercman A et al: Evidence for increasing incidence of abnormalities of the human testis: a review, *Environ Health Perspect* 101(suppl 2):65, 1993.

Goldman L, Cook EF: The decline in ischemic heart disease mortality rates: an analysis of the comparative effects of medical interventions and changes in lifestyle, *Ann Intern Med* 101:825, 1984.

Harrison JB: Warning: the male sex role may be dangerous to your health. In Swanson J, Forrest K, editors: *Men's reproductive health,* New York, 1984, Springer.

Harrison T, Dignan K: *The state of man 1999: a special report,* New York, 1999, Churchill Livingstone.

Hibbard JF, Pope CR: Employment characteristics and health status among men and women, *Women Health* 12:85, 1987.

Kochanek MA, Hudson BL: Advance report of final mortality statistics, 1992, *Mon Vital Stat Rep* 43(6 suppl):152, 1995.

Legato M: *Gender-specific aspects of human biology for the practicing physician,* Armonk, NY, 1997, Futura.

Levinson D: *The seasons of a man's life,* New York, 1978, Alfred A. Knopf.

Lewis T: Unemployment and men's health, *Nursing* 26:969, 1988.

Matthews KA et al: Influence of age, sex, and family on type A and hostile attitudes and behaviors, *Health Psychol* 11:317, 1992.

Mayo Clinic Health Oasis: *Screening tests: interactive guide for men,* June 10, 1999, The Author, www. Mayohealth.Org/Mayo/9906/Htm/Screenings_Men. Htm.

McDiarmid MA et al: Reproductive hazards of fire fighting: II. chemical hazards, *Am J Ind Med* 19:447, 1991.

McFalls, JA: Population: a lively introduction, part II. mortality differences, *Popul Bull* 53(3):1-44, 1998.

McKinlay JB, McKinlay SM, Beaglehole R: A review of the evidence concerning the impact of medical measures on recent mortality and morbidity in the United States, *Int J Health Serv* 19:181, 1989.

Mechanic D: The influence of mothers on their children's health attitudes and behavior, *Pediatrics* 33:444, 1964.

Milio N: *Primary care and the public's health,* Lexington, Mass, 1983, Lexington Books.

Montiero L: *Monitoring health status and medical care,* Cambridge, Mass, 1976, Ballinger.

National Center for Health Statistics: *Health, United States, 1994,* Hyattsville, Md, 1995, USPHS.

National Center for Health Statistics: *Health, United States: 1995,* Hyattsville, Md, 1996, USPHS.

National Center for Health Statistics: *Health, United States, 1998,* Hyattsville, Md, 1998, USPHS.

Paul M, Kurtz S: Analysis of reproductive health hazard information on material safety data sheets for lead and the ethylene glycol ethers, *Am J Ind Med* 25:403, 1994.

Piani A, Schoenborn C: *Health promotion and disease prevention: United States, 1990.* Vital Health Stat 10, No. 185, 1993.

Plunkett A: Personal communication, October, 1995.

Roberts A et al: Overtraining affects male reproductive status, *Fertil Steril* 60:686, 1993.

Rosen BN, Peterson L: Gender differences in children's outdoor play injuries: a review and an integration, *Clin Psychol Rev* 10:187, 1990.

Sadler C: DIY male maintenance, *Nurs Mirror* 160:16, 1979.

Salem N: Health insurance coverage and receipt of preventive health services: United States, 1993, *Morb Mortal Wkly Rep* 44:219, 1995.

Schulte MM, Sonenstein RL: Men at family planning clinics: the new patients? *Fam Plann Perspect* 27:212, 1995.

Skelton R: Man's role in society and its effect on health, *Nursing* 26:953, 1988.

Smith DB, Babaian RJ: The effects of treatment for cancer on male fertility and sexuality, *Cancer Nurs* 15:271, 1992.

Steinem G: *Outrageous acts and everyday rebellions,* New York, 1983, Signet.

Swanson J: *Overview of men's health.* Invited paper presented at the continuing education program, "Including Men in Reproductive and Family Health," at the American Public Health Association's 123rd Annual Meeting, San Diego, Calif, October 28, 1995.

Swanson J, Forrest K, editors: *Men's reproductive health,* New York, 1984, Springer.

Swanson J, Forrest K: Men's reproductive health services in family planning settings: a pilot study, *Am J Public Health* 77:1462, 1987.

Temmerman M: Sexually transmitted diseases and reproductive health, *Sex Transm Dis* 24(suppl 2):S55, 1994.

Verbrugge LM, Wingard DL: Sex differentials in health and mortality, *Women Health* 12:103, 1987.

Waldron I: Changing gender roles and gender differences in health behavior. In Gochman DS, editor: *Handbook of health behavior research,* New York, 1995a, Plenum.

Waldron I: Contributions of biological and behavioral factors in changing sex differences in ischaemic heart disease mortality. In Lopez A, Caselli G, Valkonen T, editors: *Adult mortality in developed countries: from description to explanation,* New York, 1995d, Oxford University Press.

Waldron I: Contributions of changing gender differences in behavior and social roles to changing gender differences in mortality. In Sabo D, Gordon D, editors. *Men's health and illness: gender, power, and the body,* Thousand Oaks, Calif, 1995b, Sage.

Waldron I: Factors determining the sex ratio at birth. In United Nations, editors: *Sex differentials in infant and child mortality,* New York, 1995c, United Nations.

Waldron I: Sex differences in infant and early child mortality: major causes of death and possible biological causes. In United Nations, editors: *Sex differentials in infant and child mortality,* New York, 1995e, United Nations.

Wasserheit JN: Effect of changes in human ecology and behavior on patterns of sexually transmitted diseases, including human immunodeficiency virus infection, *Proc Nat Acad Sci US Am* 91:2430, 1994.

Whorton MD: Environmental and occupational reproductive hazards. In Swanson J, Forrest K, editors: *Men's reproductive health,* New York, 1984, Springer.

Wingo PA, Tong T, Bolden S: Cancer statistics, 1995, *Cancer J Clin* 45:8, 1995.

Woodland A, Hunt C: Healthy convictions . . . well-man clinic for the inmates of Lindholme prison, *Nursing Times* 90:32, 1994.

Zilbergold B: Appendix: the effects of drugs on male sexuality. In Zilbergold B, editor: *The new male sexuality,* New York, 1992, Bantam Books.

Zimmerman SL: Psychache in context: states' spending for public welfare and their suicide rates, *J Nerv Ment Dis* 183:425, 1995.

Family Health

Beverly Cook Siegrist

Upon completion of this chapter, the reader will be able to do the following:

1. State a definition of *family*.
2. Identify characteristics of the changing family that have implications for community health nursing practice.
3. Describe strategies for moving from intervention at the individual level to intervention at the family level.
4. Describe strategies for moving from intervention at the family level to intervention at the aggregate level.
5. Discuss the application of one conceptual framework to family studies.
6. Discuss a model of care for families.
7. Apply the steps of the nursing process to individuals within the family, the family as a whole, and the family's aggregate.

cohabitation
contracting
culture of poverty view
ecological framework
ecomap
expressive functioning
external structure
family
Family Health Assessment
family health tree
family interviewing
general systems theory
genogram
homosexual family
instrumental functioning
internal structure
network therapy
nuclear family

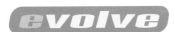

http://evolve.elsevier.com/Nies/

Rebecca Martin is a 72-year-old widow of 10 years who lives in a rural town in Tennessee. She resides in the home that she and her husband purchased before his death. Her primary source of income is Social Security benefits provided from her deceased husband and she also receives a small income from providing child care for infants at her church. Medicare benefits provide her only source of payment for health care. Her only child, a daughter from whom she has been estranged for many years, recently died. The daughter was a never-married, single mother of an 8-year-old medically fragile child with asthma. As the only surviving relative, Rebecca has become the custodial parent for her granddaughter.

Joe Hudson is a 74-year-old alcoholic who is being treated at an outpatient department in a large medical center. He lives in a hotel room in downtown Salt Lake City, Utah. He has one living relative, a 76-year-old brother. Mr. Hudson states, "I had a falling out with my brother 20 years ago. I never hear from him. I reckon he's still in Boston, if he's alive at all." Mr. Hudson frequently falls out of bed, dislodging the telephone that the desk clerk has placed precariously close to the bed, which signals the desk clerk that something is amiss. The clerk then goes to Mr. Hudson's room and puts him back in bed. Mr. Hudson's source of income is a check sent to him the first day of each month by a minister who lives in a town 75 miles away. The desk clerk cashes Mr. Hudson's check and assists him in paying his bill from the hotel, which provides congregate dining facilities.

Lai Chan is a refugee from Vietnam who moved with her family to San Francisco three months ago. Mrs. Chan is a single parent; Mr. Chan died in an automobile accident shortly after arriving in the United States. Mrs. Chan has two children, an 11-year-old son and a 5-year-old daughter. The family resides in a one-room efficiency apartment in the Tenderloin district in downtown San Francisco.

Jaime Gutierrez, a 72-year-old Mexican-American man, lives with his 36-year-old son, Roberto; his 34-year-old daughter-in-law, Patricia; and his three grandchildren who are 14, 13, and 12 years of age. Mr. Gutierrez was in good health until he fell from a tree while helping his son make roof repairs on the house in 1995. He suffered a concussion, right hemothorax, and fracture of vertebra T-11 and T-12. Confined to bed, he is receiving home health care. He requires intermittent catheterization but feels uncomfortable when the nurse suggests that his daughter-in-law is willing to carry out this procedure for him. Therefore Roberto quit work to provide this personal care to his father. Consequently, the family of six lives on Mr. Gutierrez's retirement income, which consists of $239 from Social Security and $244 from a pension plan per month. Roberto would like to increase his job skills while at home. He has finished the fourth grade and has failed the Graduate Equivalency Degree examination twice. Patricia would also like to return to school and pursue job training. Although agreeable to Patricia's interests, Roberto is hesitant to support active steps taken by Patricia to initiate her plan.

The four families described above depict broad contemporary definitions of *family* and are examples of families carried in caseloads by undergraduate community health nursing students. Assessments made by students during home, office, and hospital visits with these families triggered interventions that linked the families to resources provided by the community and, in turn, triggered questions about health needs of groups of families or larger aggregates living in the same communities.

Families have major health care needs that are not usually addressed by the health care system. Instead, the health care system most frequently addresses the individual. This holds true for nursing interventions within the health care system. The majority of nurses work in hospitals where interventions traditionally occur at the individual client level. However, nurses are on the forefront of a trend toward intervention at the family level.

UNDERSTANDING FAMILY NURSING

Family nursing is not a new concept and has been taught in schools of nursing since Nightingale's "district nursing" concept (Cook, 1913) and Lillian Wald's (1904) principles on how to nurse families in the home. The NLN has emphasized the importance of family nursing in standard curriculum guides for schools of nursing since 1917 (Beard, 1915; NLN, 1937). Early NLN publications directed nurses in "household science" and later required that 10 to15 hours of study should be directed toward understanding the "modern family," in which the nurse must consider the family as a unit (1937). Modern nurse theorists such as Newman, King, Orem, Roy, and others extensively discuss the family and its importance to individuals and society. Current discussion suggests that nursing defines *family* conceptually in the following ways: as the environment affecting individual clients; as small to large groups of interacting people; as a single unit of care with definable boundaries; or as a unit of care within a specific environment of a community or society (Whall, 1981). Family nursing care may be focused on the individual family member, within the context of the family, or the family unit. Regardless of the identified client, the nurse establishes a relationship with each family member within the unit and understands the influence of the unit on the individual and society (Box 17-1).

The family is composed of many subsystems and, in turn, is tied to many formal and informal systems outside the family. The family is imbedded in social systems that have an influence on health (e.g., education, employment, and housing). Many disciplines are interested in the study of families; interdisciplinary perspectives and strategies are necessary to understand the influence of the family on health and the influence of the broader social system on the family. Traditionally, nursing, and even community health nursing, has relied heavily if not solely on

---

BOX **17-1**

Nursing an Individual Client vs. Nursing a Family as Client

These authors discuss the similarities and differences between nursing an individual as client vs. nursing a family as client. Using the Betty Neuman systems model as a guide, they present factors that contribute to the decision to use one approach vs. the other. These factors include the following:

■ The perception of the client as to the need for nursing

■ The nature of the stressors as affecting only one member of the family or other family members

■ The risk of instability to the family as a whole posed by the health status of an individual member

■ The feasibility of the family-nurse collaboration (i.e., the availability of family members and the availability of nursing time to meet with family members)

■ The knowledge and skill of the nurse

Using a case study, the authors then make comparisons between an individual approach and a family approach by applying the nursing process to an individual client and to the family client.

Data from Ross MM, Helmer H: A comparative analysis of Neuman's model using the individual and family as the units of care, *Public Health Nurs* 5:30, 1988.

---

theoretical frameworks for intervention with families from disciplines of psychology or social psychology, which target individuals (Duvall, 1977; Erikson, 1963; Maslow, 1970). Dreher (1982) questioned the usefulness of these frameworks for the public health nurse "who is ministering to the health of socially and economically diverse populations. . . . Such psychological themes often draw our attention away from broader social issues that are the essence of public health nursing" (p. 505).

Intended for clinical rather than public health use, these models do not address why some social and economically advantaged populations are more likely to become self-actualized or why some populations experience greater mortality rates than other populations. Dreher (1982) stated that improvement must come about by addressing the socioeconomic conditions that make some families more dysfunctional than others and to alter the system itself that produces such inequities. Dreher cautioned that socioeconomic causes cannot be interpreted as psychological symptoms. Social and policy changes are necessary to alter the conditions under which families function. This chapter addresses how community health nurses work with families within communities to bring about healthy conditions for families at the family, social, and policy levels. This chapter focuses on the following five areas:

1. The changing family
2. Approaches to meeting the health needs of families
3. Family theory approach to meeting the health needs of families
4. Extending family health intervention to larger aggregates and social action
5. An example of the nursing process applied to a family

THE CHANGING FAMILY

Definition of Family

Many definitions of *family* exist. The nurse's definition of family is influenced by personal involvement with his or her own family and clinical experiences. Vaughan-Cole and colleagues (1998) suggest that traditional definitions of *family* are based on the following myths: the typical family as the nuclear family consisting of parents and children and the commonality of the extended family of several generations working toward a common family goal. The examples presented at the beginning of this chapter describe the variations found in today's families.

The term **family** as used in this chapter is defined as an aggregate made up of a body of units, the individuals that represent the whole, or the family. Definitions of *family* vary by discipline, the professional, and distinct groups of families. For example, psychologists may define *family* in terms of personal development and intrapersonal dynamics; the sociologist has used a classic definition of *family* in terms of a "social unit interacting with the larger society" (Johnson, 1984, p. 333). Other professionals have

classically defined *family* in terms of kinship, marriage, and descent (Farber, 1973).

> [A family is] a cluster of people, whose relationship is stipulated by law in terms of marriage and descent, and whose precise membership varies according to the circumstances (p. 2).

Other professionals have defined *family* in terms of household membership, as "a primary group of people living in a household in consistent proximity and intimate relationships" (Helvie, 1981, p. 64). According to Stuart (1991), the concept of family has the following five critical attributes:

1. The family is a system or unit.
2. Family members may or may not be related and may or may not live together.
3. The unit may or may not contain children.
4. Commitment and attachment exist among unit members and include future obligation.
5. The unit caregiving functions consist of protection, nourishment, and socialization of unit members.

Wright and Leahey (1994) stated that "the family is who they say they are" (p. 40). Most important, according to McGoldrick (1982), is the definition of *family* given by different family groups within the population. Patterson and colleagues (1999) define *family* as a "group of individuals (two or more) and the pattern of relationships between them" (p. 36).

The dominant American definition focuses on the intact nuclear family. Black families focus on a wide network of kin and community. The "nuclear" family does not exist for Italians. To them family means a strong, tightly knit three- or four-generational family, which includes godparents and old friends. The Chinese go beyond this and include in their definition of *family* all their ancestors and all their descendants (Patterson, 1999, p. 10).

The community health nurse interacts with communities made up of many types of families. When faced with great diversity in the community, the community health nurse must formulate a personal definition of *family* and be aware of the changing definition of *family* held by other disciplines, professionals, and family groups. The community health nurse who interacts with Mr. Hudson, the alcoholic who lives in a hotel, must have a broad conceptualization of the family. The surveillance activity of the hotel manager and the financial support of the minister could both be accounted for in Jordheim's

(1982) definition of *family* as a "relationship community of two or more persons" (p. 61) whether from the same or different kinship groups.

Characteristics of the Changing Family

The characteristics of the U.S. family continue to change. The typical family, the **nuclear family**, has traditionally been defined as "a small group consisting of parents and their non-adult children living in a single household" (Farber, 1973, p. 2). The stereotypical view of this family as father, mother, and nonadult children is eroding. For example, in 1970, 85% of children younger than 18 years of age were living with two parents (Saluter, 1994) and in 1998 this proportion declined to 59% (Casper and Bryson, 1999). Over the past 23 years, the percentage of black children living with both parents decreased from 58.5% in 1970, to 35.6% in 1993, with a slight increase in 1998 of 37.6% (US Census Bureau, 1999). About 76% of white children lived with both parents in 1998, whereas 64.3% of children of Hispanic origin lived with both parents.

Cohabitation, which is defined as "two unrelated adults of the opposite sex (one of whom is the householder) who share a housing unit with or without the presence of children under 15 years old," has also increased over time (Saluter, 1994, p. vii). Cohabiting unmarried people increased from 523,000 in 1970, to 4.2 million in 1998 (US Census Bureau, 1999). In 1998, about one third of the cohabiting-couple households included children. Cohen (1999) reported that differences in family income and education are significant in cohabiting families when compared with married couples, especially for white males. White cohabiting males tend to earn less income and have lower educational levels than their married counterparts.

Single parenting has also increased over time. In 1970, 12% of children lived with one parent (Saluter, 1994) and by 1998, 32% of children were found in single parent homes (with 23% of these homes headed by women) (US Census Bureau, 1999). The increase in the teenage birth rate among this group raises concern. During the years 1980 to 1998, the birth rate for unmarried women 15 to 17 years of age increased from 21 to 32 per 1000 in the United States. Of the children living with one parent, 38% live with a divorced parent and 19% live with a separated parent (US Census Bureau, 1997).

The proportion of children younger than 18 years of age who are living with their grandparents is also growing. In 1970, only 3% of children lived with their grandparents. By 1997, this figure rose to 6% of all children (i.e., four million children) and one parent was also present in 52% of these homes (US Census Bureau, 1997).

A **homosexual family** is made up of a cohabiting couple of the same sex who have a sexual relationship. The homosexual family may or may not have children. Estimates of the number of children who live in lesbian- or gay-parented families, including children conceived in heterosexual marriages, range from 6 to 14 million (Eliason, 1996; Singer, 1994). Between one and five million lesbian mothers and between one and three million gay fathers live in the United States (Patterson, 1992). These numbers are estimates because the U.S. Census Bureau does not count the number of lesbians and gay men. However, the 1990 census reported that in 3,187,772 "unmarried partners," 145,130 were counted as same-sex couples (Saluter, 1994). Studies have been conducted by Overlooked Opinions, a Chicago polling organization that has demographic data on gay and lesbian Americans (Singer, 1994). Despite societal attitudes, Kurdek (1994) found that 40% to 60% of gay men have stable, monogamous relationships and 45% to 80% live in long-term relationships.

Single parenting is associated with greater risk associated with lesser social, emotional, and financial resources, which affects the general well-being of children and families. About 45% of children in divorced families and 69% of children in never-married, single-parent families lived below or near poverty in 1997 (US Department of Commerce, 1997).

Families with an unmarried mother declined 1% to 44.6 births per 1000. This was the first decline in two decades and was evident primarily in the black population. During 1996, a 1% increase in births to unmarried white women occurred (Guyer and Martin, 1997).

APPROACHES TO MEETING THE HEALTH NEEDS OF FAMILIES

Community health nursing has long viewed the family as an important unit of health care, with an awareness that the individual can be best understood within the social context of the family. Observing and inquiring about family interaction enables the nurse in the community to assess the influence of family members on each other. However, direct intervention at the family rather than the individual client level is a new frontier for many nursing students, most of whom have experience in acute care settings before the community setting. A family model, largely a community health nursing or psychiatric-mental health intervention model, is now expanding into the areas of birthing and parent-child interventions, adult day care, chronic illness, and home care. However, nursing assessment and intervention must not stop with the immediate social context of the family, but must also consider the broader social context of the community and society. As Dunn (1961) stated, "the family stands in-between individual wellness and social wellness. You can't really have high-level wellness for either individuals or social groups unless you have well families."

Moving from Individual to Family

Community health and home care nurses have traditionally focused on the family as the unit of service. With the move to managed care throughout the United States, most of these nurses continue to focus their practice on individuals residing in the home. As a result of the current era of cost containment, constraints on the community health nurse and on nurses working within hospitals and in other settings will increase. For example, reimbursement, which is almost entirely calculated for services rendered to the individual, is a major constraint toward moving toward planning care for families as a unit. Various creative approaches to meeting the health needs of families are needed, reflecting interventions appropriate to the needs of the population as a whole.

Family Interviewing

Approaches to the care of families are needed and must be creative, flexible, and transferable from one setting to another. Community health nurses are generalists who bring previous preparation in communication concepts and interviewing to the family arena. Wright and Leahey (1994) proposed the realm of **family interviewing** rather than family therapy as an appropriate model. In this model, the community health nurse uses general systems and communication concepts to conceptualize health needs of families and a family assessment model to assess families' responses to "normative" events such as birth or retirement or to "paranormative" events such as chronic illness or divorce. Intervention is straightfor-

ward, as in asking a family to read a book about sex education of prepubescent teenagers, or dealt with through referral if the level of intervention is beyond the preparation of the nurse. For the purposes of this text, the model is extended to include intervention at the level of the larger aggregate. For example, the index of suspicion based on the health needs of a particular family would prompt the community health nurse to assess the need for similar information and the resources for intervention with other families in the community, schools, churches, or other institutions. Family interviewing requires thinking "interactionally" not only in terms of the family system, but also in terms of larger social systems.

Wright and Leahey (1999) identify the following critical components of the family interview: manners, therapeutic conservation, family genogram, and commendations. With experience, they believe that the family interview can be accomplished in 15 minutes.

Manners

Manners are common social behaviors that set the tone for the interview and begin the development of a therapeutic relationship. Wright and Leahey (1999) believe that erosion of these social skills prevents the family nurse from collecting essential data. Many nurses argue that too much formality establishes artificial barriers to communication; however, studies identify that the essentials of a therapeutic relationship begin with manners. The nurse introduces himself or herself by name and title, always addresses the family member by name (i.e., Mr., Mrs., or Ms., unless otherwise directed by patient), keeps appointments, explains the reason for the interview or visit, and brings a positive attitude (Leahey et al., 1995; Richardson, 1987).

Therapeutic Conversations

The second key element in the interview is the therapeutic conversation. This type of conservation is focused, planned, and engages the family. The nurse must listen and remember that even one sentence has the potential to heal or help a family member. The nurse encourages questions, engages the family in the interview and assessment process, and commends the family when strengths are identified.

Genogram and Ecomap

The genogram and ecomap constitute the third element and are described in detail later in this chapter. These tools provide essential information on family structure and are an efficient way to gather information such as family composition, background, and basic health status in a way that engages the family in the interview process.

Therapeutic Questions

Therapeutic questions are key questions that the nurse plans and asks the family to facilitate the interview. The questions are specific for the context or family situation, but have the following basic themes (Wright and Leahey, 1999): family expectations of the interview or home visit; challenges, concerns, and problems encountered by the family at the time of the interview; and sharing information (e.g., who will relate the family history or information).

Commending Family or Individual Strengths

The fifth element of the family interview is commending the family or individual strengths. The authors suggest identifying at least two strength areas and, during each family interview, sharing them with the family or individual. Sharing strengths reinforces immediate and long-term positive relationships between the nurse and family. Interviews that identify and build upon family strengths tend to progress toward more open and trusting relationships and often allow the family to reframe problems, thereby increasing problem solving and healing (Robinson, 1998; Wright and Leahey, 1999).

Issues in Family Interviewing

Creative family interviewing requires interviewing families in many types of settings. The prediction of decreased hospitalization supplemented by a wide variety of health care settings ranging from acute to ambulatory to community centers calls for flexible, transferable approaches. Clinical settings for family interviewing are reviewed by Wright and Leahey (1994) and include inpatient and outpatient ambulatory care and clinical settings in maternity, pediatrics, medicine, surgery, critical care, and mental health. According to Wright and Leahey, community health nurses have many opportunities besides the traditional home visit to engage the family in a family interview. Community health nurses are employed in ambulatory care centers, occupational health and school sites, housing complexes, day care programs, residential treatment and substance abuse programs, and other official and nonofficial agencies. In each of these sites,

community health nurses meet families and can assess and intervene at the family and community levels.

The community health nurse can implement preventive programs for family units. The family is particularly appropriate because it experiences similar risk factors (i.e., physiological, behavioral, and environmental). For example, in a classic study conducted by Manley and Graber (1977) in a community hospital, family members of patients with coronary heart disease were invited to attend preventive screening and educational programs. Family members were evaluated for hypertension, smoking, and triglycerides. Findings were similar to those in large epidemiological studies. For example, 25% had lipid abnormalities, 44% were overweight, 12% smoked, and 15.5% had previously undetected hypertension. Such programs can occur in community health settings and demonstrate the need to go beyond intervention with the individual family to groups of families, serving the population as a whole. A community health nurse working with Mexican-American families with diabetes could implement such a program basing assessment on both needs of the individual families and biostatistics that reflect populations at risk. For example, diabetes is found in Mexican-Americans at three times the rate found in whites and Mexican-Americans are less likely to see a physician (Council of Scientific Affairs, 1991).

Involving family members in newborn assessments can aid the community health nurse in determining the family's adjustment to the newborn and parenthood. The nurse can do this in the home, clinic, or other health care center. Family members should be involved during the first contact or visit, and if they do not attend, a telephone call explaining the nurse's interest in them should take place (Wright and Leahey, 1994).

More husbands and family members are becoming involved in the pregnancy and delivery phases of childbirth. The community health nurse in the well-baby clinic may often see parents for whom a family interview or home visit may be valuable. A general statement may introduce the commonality of hurdles faced by new parents. For example, "many new parents face similar problems, which usually last only a short period of time. We find that bringing all of the family members together is important because the entire family is affected when a new baby comes into the home."

HOME VISITS BY NURSES TO POOR, UNMARRIED, TEENAGE WOMEN PROMPT MORE RAPID RETURN TO SCHOOL, INCREASE EMPLOYMENT, AND RESULT IN FEWER SUBSEQUENT PREGNANCIES

A nursing home visit program provided comprehensive care to poor, unmarried, white teenagers bearing their first children in a semirural county in upstate New York. The study found that women who received home visits from the prenatal period through two years after the birth of their child were more likely to return to school more rapidly than women who did not receive home visits, increase the number of months they were employed, have fewer subsequent pregnancies, and postpone the birth of their second child.

Data from Olds DL et al: Improving the life-course development of socially disadvantaged mothers: a randomized trial of nurse home visitation, *Am J Public Health* 78:1436, 1988.

The community health nurse working with single-parent families may face particular challenges. Mothers in single-parent families report a higher incidence of children's academic and behavioral problems than mothers in two-parent families. For example, in the National Health Interview Survey of 1988, researchers found that children 3 to 17 years of age living with a formerly married mother were more than three times as likely to have received treatment for emotional or behavioral problems in the preceding 12 months (8.8%) as children living with both biological parents (2.7%) (Dawson, 1991). However, children living in a nuclear family who experience severe conflict may have as many problems as children from a disrupted household. Children in these families need a chance to express their concerns; the family interview is important in giving care to these families.

School Nurse
The school nurse has a unique opportunity to compare the child in the school system with the child in the family system. The school nurse is becoming increasingly involved in planning special programs in the schools. Astute assessment of children's needs within the context of their families in interviews at school or in the home can lead to innovative interventions such as leading support groups for children with chronic

illness. Other areas of assessment and intervention that benefit from a family approach include learning or behavioral problems and absenteeism (Wright and Leahey, 1994).

Occupational Health Nurse
The nurse in the occupational health setting can also use a family approach to care to improve the health of the worker and contribute to overall productivity. For example, alcohol and chemical abuse account for much absenteeism in the workplace. Effective intervention with these families has been demonstrated (Steinglass, 1985). Assessment of occupational hazards may involve conducting reproductive histories in an effort to determine the effects of a chemical or agent on the reproductive capacity of the couple (Swanson and Nies, 1997). Toxic agents can also transfer to family members from the workplace via clothes and equipment (Whorton, 1984).

An awareness and a high degree of suspicion about the risks of occupational hazards in community industry are necessary. Obtaining an occupational history from all family members who have entered the workplace and obtaining referrals for family members' screening and health education will contribute to unraveling occupational hazards and effects in the future. In addition, the community health nurse should be aware of the many family-related work issues that may trigger stress-related illness, such as promotion or loss of job and shift work.

Intervention in Cases of Chronic Illness
Perhaps as many as 80% of families are dealing with chronic illness in a family member (Vaughn-Cole et al., 1998). Also significant is the fact that resources, such as third-party reimbursement, caused most of these families to learn to manage the chronic problems with limited or infrequent intervention by health professionals. The community health nurse working with families coping with chronic illness in a child, adult, or older adult is aided by the family interview. As Glaser and Strauss state in their classic work on chronic illness (1975), chronic illness interjects change into various areas of family life.

> Sex and intimacy can be affected. Everyday mood and interpersonal relations can be affected. Visiting friends and engaging in other leisure time activities can be affected. Conflicts can be engendered by increased expenses stemming from unemployment and the medical treatment . . . different illnesses may have different

kinds of impact on such areas of family life, just as they probably will call for different kinds of helpful agents (p. 67).

Changes in family patterns, fears, emotional responses, and expectations of individual family members can be assessed in the family interview. Special needs of the primary caretaker (i.e., often the spouse, daughter, or daughter-in-law) can be assessed. The community health nurse making family visits to older adults and the terminally ill is able to assess intergenerational conflict and stress and influence family interaction positively (Wright and Leahey, 1994).

Moving from the Family to the Community

Dreher (1982) stated that the practice of public health nursing is distinct from that of other specialties in nursing because its scope and orientation to the care of the public differs, not because its practice setting differs. According to Dreher, preparation of the public health nurse cannot be limited to "'following a family in the community'—paltry preparation for a career in caring for the health of the public" (p. 509). The care of entire populations is the major focus, as stated by Freeman in her classic work (1963).

> The selection of those to be served . . . must rest on the comparative impact on community health rather than solely on the needs of the individual or family being served. . . . The public health nurse cannot elect to care for a small number of people intensely while ignoring the needs of many others. She must be concerned with the population as a whole, with those in her caseload, with the need of a particular family as compared to the needs of others in the community (p. 35).

The challenge to the community health nurse is to provide care to communities and populations and not to focus only on the levels of the individual and family. The community health nurse, who traditionally carries a caseload of families, extends practice in the field with families to include a focus on the community. To do so, an aggregate, community, and population focus must serve as a backdrop to the entire practice.

For example, families must be viewed as components of communities. The community health nurse must know the community. As stated in Chapter 5, a thorough community assessment is necessary to practice in the community. By way of review, the

nurse must remember that communities must be compared not only in terms of different health needs, but also in terms of different resources to effect interventions that influence policies and redistribute resources to ensure that community and family health needs are met. Dreher (1982) stated the following:

> Data gathered about the physical, social, and demographic variables of the population being served are essential to provide an empirical basis for the development and delivery of nursing services. Unless these data, however, are viewed within a larger context—across communities—they will never serve to develop either the more encompassing theories which explain the relationship between society and health or the policies which will be most effective in assuring health and health care (p. 508).

SOURCES OF DATA ABOUT THE COMMUNITY'S HEALTH

National data are available from resources such as the U.S. Census Bureau, U.S. Department of Commerce, NCHS, and CDC. The *Health Status of Minorities and Low Income Groups*, published annually by the U.S. Census Bureau (US Bureau of the Census, 1999), and the *MMWR*, published weekly by the CDC, are examples of data sources. State data are also provided in these publications. More in-depth data at the state level may be obtained from state department of health publications that give mortality and morbidity statistics. Local data are available from the census, city planners, and city or county departments of health.

Community health nurses must then compare city data with county data and then county data, state data, and national data. In addition, they may need to compare local census tract data and areas of a city or county with other areas of the city or county.

For example, community health nursing students in San Antonio, Texas, who were planning home visits to families of pregnant adolescents attending a special high school, compared local, state, and national statistics on infant mortality rates as a part of a community assessment. They found higher rates of infant mortality in San Antonio in census tracts on the south side of the city in which the population was predominantly Mexican-American. They also found the population to be younger, to have a higher rate of functional illiteracy among adults, to be less educated, to be more likely to drop out of high school, to have higher fertility rates, to have higher birth rates among adolescents, and to be more likely to be unemployed. They found that specific health needs varied among census tracts. Common major health needs of this subpopulation were identified from the community assessment, which assisted the students in planning care for these families. For example, their goals were broadened from carrying out interventions at the individual level to interventions at the family and community levels. In addition to targeting good perinatal outcomes for the individual teenage parent, nursing students planned to include assessments of functional literacy at the individual and family levels and arranged for group sessions in clinic waiting rooms that informed and referred individuals and family members to alternative resources to enable teenage parents to complete school, take classes in English as a second language, and use resources for family planning and employment at the community level.

In addition to the cross-comparison of communities, the community health nurse also cross-compares the needs of the families within the communities and sets priorities. As the students just mentioned found that specific health needs varied among census tracts, so too the nurse in the community finds that specific health needs vary among families. The nurse must account for time spent with families and choose those families on the basis of their needs compared with the needs of others in the community.

Delegation of Scarce Resources

Although the community health nurse serves the community or population as a whole, fiscal constraints hold the nurse accountable for the best delegation of scarce resources. Time spent on home visits has traditionally allowed the community health nurse to assess the environmental, social, and biological determinants of health status among the population and the resources available to them. Fiscal accountability, nevertheless, means setting priorities. In 1985, Anderson, O'Grady, and Anderson listed the factors that influence public health nursing practice, especially home visits, as "the need to justify personnel costs in a time of fiscal constraint, the increasing number of medically indigent who turn to local public health services for primary care, and the change in reimbursement mechanisms by the federal government and some states" (p. 146). In the shift to managed care, Anderson's observations still hold true.

Double Standard in Public Health

A double standard is tolerated in public health. Although the government is responsible for the maintenance of health, a minimal amount of health care is guaranteed to each person because public resources are limited. Smith (1985) stated the following:

> This prohibits discrimination based upon traits of persons that are not matters of free choice: for example, race, sex, and other congenital conditions; and wealth, poverty, or geographic location when these cannot be altered by the individual (p. 143).

A minimum is established for all; however, as demonstrated with Medicare and Medicaid (see Chapter 3) unequal care exists as a result of differences in income (i.e., Medicare) and geographical location (i.e., Medicaid). In a market system, the wealthy can purchase all the health care services they desire and the poor cannot afford these services. The few supplemental resources provided by the government to ensure a minimum for all vary among communities, states, administrations, and countries.

In a period of cost containment, the focus of community health nurses on prevention and health maintenance, which are difficult areas to justify, must carefully legitimate home visiting services by identifying aggregates in need of care. The following is stated in the definition of public health nursing by the Public Health Nursing Section of the APHA (APHA, 1981):

> Identifying the subgroups, or aggregates, within the population which are at high risk of illness, disability, or premature death and directing resources toward these groups is the most effective approach for accomplishing the goal of public health nursing (p. 4).

Prioritizing groups at highest risk and using home visits in conjunction with planning for larger aggregates' needs are necessary. Working for social and policy changes to alter the conditions that place these families at high risk goes hand-in-hand with this activity. Little research has been done on the necessity for home visits in conjunction with group instruction or other agency-based care. Anderson, O'Grady, and Anderson (1985) reported a study of the integration of public health nursing and primary care in northern California. They found that "the teaching component of primary care and the continuity of nursing care from hospital to clinic and home for patients served by county medical services was strengthened" (p. 146). Populations at high risk that may benefit from home visiting are being identified (Brooten

Ten-year-old Jean Wilkie was referred by her teacher to the school nurse. She was withdrawn, had no school friends, and was dropping behind in her schoolwork. The school nurse talked to Jean in her office. Jean said that she had no friends because the other girls stayed overnight with one another "all the time" and that she did not want to bring her friend's home because her father "drank all the time." The school nurse decided that Jean's problems needed assessment within the context of the family and arranged to visit the family at home. The father refused to participate in the family interview, but Jean's mother, her 13-year-old brother Peter, and Jean expressed concerns that the father had changed jobs several times in the past year, was frequently absent from work, and had been in two recent car accidents while "drinking." The school nurse was able to verify the family context as the basis of Jean's "problems," continue her family assessment, and plan for intervention at the family level. In addition, she was prompted to assess the community's preventive efforts directed toward drinking and the ability to provide ongoing care for families of alcoholics.

et al., 1986; Olds et al., 1988). Evidence indicates that costs are cut by home visits for high-risk infants in combination with other support systems such as social and medical services (Brooten et al., 1986).

APPROACHES TO FAMILY HEALTH

Many schools of thought regarding the approaches to meeting family health needs exist among community health, community mental health, and public health nursing professionals. Dreher (1982) stated that the traditional basis for community health nursing intervention has a focus that has long endorsed psychological and social-psychological theories to explain variations in health and patterns of health care, such as those set forth by Erikson (1963), Maslow (1970), and Duvall (1977). Dreher (1982) stated that what is needed are "more encompassing theories which explain the relationship between society and health [and] the policies which will be most effective in assuring health and health care" (p. 508). To help bridge this gap, three frameworks are presented (i.e., meeting family health needs through the application of family theory, systems framework, structural-functional conceptual framework, and developmental theory).

Family Theory

Many reasons exist for why the community health nurse should work with families. Friedman (1992) listed the following six reasons:

1. The belief that within the family unit any "dysfunction" (e.g., separation, disease, or injury) that affects one or more family members will probably affect other family members and the family as a whole.

2. The wellness of the family is highly dependent upon the role of the family in every aspect of health care, from prevention to rehabilitation.

3. The level of wellness of the whole family can be raised through care that reduces lifestyle and environmental risks by emphasizing "health promotion, 'self-care,' health education, and family counseling" (p. 5).

4. Commonalities in risk factors and diseases shared by family members can lead to case finding within the family.

5. A clear understanding of the functioning of the individual can be gained only when the individual is assessed within the larger context of the family.

6. The family as a vital support system to the individual member needs to be incorporated into treatment plans.

Nurses have relied heavily on the social and behavioral sciences for approaches to working with families. These approaches include psychoanalytical, anthropological, systems or cybernetic, structural-functional, developmental, and interactional frameworks (for reviews, see Friedman, 1992; Whall and Fawcett, 1991; Wright and Leahey, 1994). The use of a framework for assessing families is useful to help the nurse understand the health potential for the family. Three conceptual frameworks (systems, structural-functional, and developmental), often used by nurses in providing health care to families, are described. These models help the nurse empower the family in the process of family health promotion.

Systems Framework

The systems approach has been widely used in diverse areas such as education, computer science, engineering, and communication. **General systems theory** (von Bertalanffy, 1968, 1972, 1974) has been applied to the study of families. General systems theory is a way to explain how the family as a unit interacts with larger units outside the family and with smaller units inside the family (Friedman, 1992). The family may be affected by any disrupting force acting on a system outside the family (i.e., suprasystem) or on a system within the family (i.e., subsystem). Allmond, Buckman, and Gofman (1979) compared the family as a system with a piece of a mobile suspended from the air that is in constant movement with the other pieces of the mobile. At any time, the family, like any piece of the mobile, may be caught by a gust of air and become unbalanced, moving "chaotically" for a time; however, eventually, the stabilizing force of the other parts of the mobile will reestablish balance. Box 17-2 presents the major definitions from the systems approach.

Characteristics of Healthy Families

In a classic work, Pratt (1976) characterized healthy families as "energized families" in the following ways:

- Members interact with each other repeatedly in many contexts.
- Members are enhanced and fulfilled by maintaining contacts with a wide range of community groups and organizations.
- Members make efforts to master their lives by becoming members of groups, finding information and options, and making decisions.
- Members engage in flexible role relationships, share power, respond to change, support growth and autonomy of others, and engage in decision making that affects them.

Structural-Functional Conceptual Framework

With the structural-functional conceptual framework approach to the family, the family is viewed according to its structure, or the parts of the system, and according to its functions, or how the family fulfills its roles.

Structural

Wright and Leahey (1994) stated that three aspects of family structure can be examined (internal struc-

ture, external structure, and context). **Internal structure** of the family refers to the following five categories:

1. Family composition, the family members, and changes in family constellation
2. Gender
3. Rank order, or positions of family members by age and sex
4. Subsystem or labeling of the subgroups or dyads (e.g., spouse, parental, and interest) through which the family carries out its functions
5. Boundary, or who participates in the family system and how they participate (e.g., a single-parent mother who does not allow her 17-year-old son to have his girlfriend spend the night in their home)

ROLE RELATIONSHIPS

When Edna Smith, a 64-year-old client with severe arthritis, was diagnosed with diabetes, her longtime friend, Frank Gardens, a widower of several years, moved in with her and assumed a caregiver role. The community health nurse assessed the dietary habits of Mr. Gardens and Mrs. Smith and found that Mr. Gardens did the shopping and the cooking because Mrs. Smith's mobility was severely restricted from her arthritis. Mr. Gardens did the cooking; therefore he purchased canned fruits and vegetables rather than fresh or frozen. Mr. Gardens perceived cooking, which was a new role for him, as demanding. After several visits, he disclosed to the nurse that his resistance to preparing fresh or frozen fruits and vegetables came from "the time it takes to clean the darn things, cook 'em, store 'em, and clean up the 'fridge when they go bad on ya." He stated unequivocally that it was stressful caring for Mrs. Smith and that he wanted to do it, but it was "much easier" to just "open a can" and "heat it in a pan" than to take the time and energy that preparation of fresh or frozen foods would require. The shift in roles that is often required of couples when one is diagnosed with a chronic illness can have an influence on the health of the family. Miller (2000) provides additional reading about how couples manage with chronic illness.

BOX 17-2

Major Definitions from Systems Theory

- System: "A goal-directed unit made up of interdependent, interacting parts which endure over a period of time" (Friedman, 1992, p. 115). A family system is not concrete. It is made up of suprasystems and subsystems and must be viewed in a hierarchy of systems. The system under study at any given time is called the *focal, target,* or *system*. In this chapter, the family system is the focal system.

- Suprasystem: the suprasystem is the larger system of which the family is a part, such as the larger environment or the community (e.g., churches, schools, clubs, businesses, neighborhood organizations, and gangs).

- Subsystem: subsystems are the smaller units of which the family consists, such as sets of relationships within the family (e.g., spouse, parent-child, sibling, or extended family).

- Hierarchy of systems: the hierarchy comprises the levels of units within the system and its environment that in their totality make up the universe. Higher-level units are composed of lower level units (e.g., the biosphere is made up of communities, which are made up of families). Families are made up of family subsystems, and in turn, family subsystems are made up of individuals, who are made up of organs, which are made of cells, which are made of atoms.

- Boundaries: a boundary is an imaginary definitive line that forms a circle around each system and delineates the system from its environment. Auger (1976) conceptualized the boundary of a system as a "'filter' which permits the constant exchange of elements, information, or energy between the system and its environments. . . . The more porous the filter, the greater the degree of interaction possible between the system and its environment" (p. 24). Families with rigid boundaries may lack necessary information and resources pertinent to maintaining family health or wellness.

- Open system: an open system interacts with its surrounding environment and gives outputs and gets inputs necessary to survival. An exchange of energy occurs. All living systems are open systems. However, if a boundary is too permeable, the system may be too open to input new ideas from the outside and may be unable to make decisions on its own (Wright and Leahey, 1994).

- Closed system: a closed system theoretically does not interact with the environment. This is a self-sufficient system; no energy exchange occurs. Although no system has been found that exists in a totally closed state, if a family's boundaries are impermeable (i.e., less open as a system), needed input or interaction cannot occur. An example is a refugee family from Vietnam living in San Francisco; they may remain a closed family for some time because they have differences in culture and language.

- Input: input is information, matter, or energy that the open system receives from its environment that is necessary for survival.

- Output: output is information, matter, or energy dispensed into the environment as a result of receiving and processing the input.

- Flow and transformation: the system's use of input may occur in two forms. Some input may be used in its original state, and some input may have to be transformed before it is used. Both original and transformed input must be processed and flow through the system before being released as output (Friedman, 1992).

- Feedback: feedback is "the process by which a system monitors the internal and environmental responses to its behavior (i.e., output) and accommodates or adjusts itself" (Friedman, 1992, p. 117). The system controls and modifies inputs and outputs by "receiving and responding to the return of its own output" (Friedman, 1992, p. 117). Internally, the system adjusts by making changes in its subsystems. Externally, the system adjusts by making boundary changes.

- Equilibrium: equilibrium is a state of balance or steady state that results from self-regulation or adaptation. As with the concept of a system as a mobile in the wind, balance is dynamic and, with change, is always reestablishing itself.

- Differentiation: differentiation is the tendency for a system to actively grow and "advance to a higher order of complexity and organization" (Friedman, 1992, p. 117). Energy inputs into the system make this growth possible.

- Energy: energy is needed to meet a system's demands. Open systems will require more input through porous boundaries to meet high energy levels needed to maintain high levels of activity.

External structure refers to the extended family and larger systems (Wright and Leahey, 1994). It includes the following two categories:

1. Extended family, including family of origin and family of procreation
2. Larger systems, including work, health, and welfare

Context refers to the background or situation relevant to an event or personality in which the family system is nested (Wright and Leahey, 1994). It includes the following five categories:

1. Ethnicity
2. Race
3. Social class
4. Religion
5. Environment

Functional

Wright and Leahey (1994) also dichotomized *family functional assessment,* or how family members behave toward one another, into two categories (instrumental functioning and expressive functioning). **Instrumental functioning** refers to activities of daily living (e.g., elimination, sleeping, eating, or giving insulin injections). This area takes on important meaning for the family when one member of the family becomes ill or disabled and is unable to carry out daily functions and must rely on other members of the family for assistance. For example, an older adult may need assistance getting into the bathtub or a child may need to have medications measured and administered.

The second type of family functional assessment is **expressive functioning**, or affective or emotional aspects. This aspect has nine categories, which follow:

1. *Emotional communication:* Is the family able to express a range of emotions, including happiness, sadness, and anger?
2. *Verbal communication* focuses on the meaning of words. Do messages have clear meanings rather than distorted meanings? Wright and Leahey (1994) gave the example of masked criticism when a father states to his child, "Children who cry when they get needles are babies" (p. 83).
3. *Nonverbal communication,* which includes sounds, gestures, eye contact, touch, or inaction. An example is when a husband remains silent and stares out the window when his wife is talking to him.
4. *Circular communication* is commonly observed between dyads in families. A common example is the blaming, nagging wife and the guilty, withdrawn husband.
5. *Problem solving* refers to how the family solves problems. Who identifies problems? Someone inside or outside the family? What kinds of problems are solved? What patterns are used to solve and evaluate tried solutions?
6. *Roles* refer to "established patterns of behavior for family members" (Wright and Leahey, 1994, p. 88). Roles may be developed, delegated, negotiated, and renegotiated within the family. It takes other family members to keep a person in a particular role. Traditional roles are being challenged and are changing with economic and feminist changes; many women are entering the workforce outside the home. Formal roles, with which the larger community agrees, may come into conflict with roles set by family members and influenced by religious, cultural, and other belief systems.
7. *Influence* refers to methods used to affect the behavior of another. *Instrumental influence* refers to the use of reinforcement via objects or privileges (e.g., money and watching television). *Psychological influence* refers to the influence of behavior through the use of communication or feelings. *Corporal control* refers to use of body contact (e.g., hugging and spanking).
8. *Beliefs* refer to assumptions, ideas, and opinions that are held by family members and families as a whole. Beliefs shape the way families react to chronic or life-threatening illness. For example, if a family of a person with colon cancer believes in alternative treatments, then acupuncture may be a viable option.
9. *Alliances and coalitions* are important within the family. What dyads or triads appear to occur repeatedly in the family? Who starts arguments between dyads? Who stops arguments or fighting between dyads? Is there evidence of mother and father against child? When does this change to parent and child against the other parent? The balance and intensity of relationships between subsystems within the family are important. Questions may be asked regarding the permeability of the boundary. Does it cross generations?

SUMMARY OF FAMILY FUNCTIONAL ASSESSMENT

I. Instrumental functioning (i.e., activities of daily living)

II. Expressive functioning
   a. Emotional communication
   b. Verbal communication
   c. Nonverbal communication
   d. Circular communication
   e. Problem solving
   f. Roles
   g. Influence
   h. Beliefs
   i. Alliances and coalitions

Data from Wright LM, Leahey M: *Nurses and families: a guide to family assessment and intervention,* ed 2, Philadelphia, 1994, F.A. Davis.

Developmental Theory

Nurses are familiar with developmental states of individuals from prenatal through adult. Duvall (Duvall and Miller, 1985), a noted sociologist, is the forerunner of a focus on *family* development. In her classic work, she identified eight stages that normal families traverse from marriage to death.

FAMILY LIFE CYCLE

1. Beginning family (marriage)
2. Early childbearing family (eldest child is in infancy through 30 months of age)
3. Preschool children (eldest child is 2.5 to 5 years of age)
4. School-age children (eldest child is 6 to 12 years of age)
5. Teenage children (eldest child is 13 to 20 years of age)
6. Launching family (oldest to youngest child leaves home)
7. Middle-age family (remaining marital dyad to retirement)
8. Aging family (retirement to death of both spouses)

Data from Duvall EM, Miller BC: *Marriage and family development,* ed 6, New York, 1985, Harper & Row.

The community health nurse must comprehend these phases and the struggles that families go through during them to assess the family. Wright and Leahey (1994) called attention to the need to distinguish between "family development" and "family life cycle." They stated that the former is the *individual, unique* path that a family goes through, whereas the latter is the *typical* path many families go through.

The developmental categories listed in Box 17-3 outline the six stages of the middle-class North American family life cycle (Carter and McGoldrick, 1988; Wright and Leahey, 1994) and the tasks necessary for the family's resolution of each stage. Nurses may use the stages to delineate family strengths and weaknesses.

However, when reviewing these stages and tasks, the profiles of families living in North America and in many other parts of the world are changing dramatically from what they have been in the recent past, both in structure and form (Wright and Leahey, 1994). Language used in reference to the family should be inclusive of many kinds of "families," be they dual-career families, single parents, unmarried couples, gay or lesbian couples including children, or remarried couples. The nurse should no longer use terms such as *working mother, children of divorce,* or *fatherless home* when speaking of the family.

Alterations in Family Development: Divorce and Remarriage

Alterations to the life cycle occur as seen in previously reviewed statistics of separation, divorce, single-parent families, and remarriage. Carter and McGoldrick (1980, 1988) identified phases involved in the processes of divorce, postdivorce, and remarriage (Tables 17-1 and 17-2). The family must engage in emotional work as a result of divorce, a process that may occur suddenly or may be long and drawn out. In her classic study, Stern (1982a) interviewed stepfather families in their homes and conceptualized the integration of the blended family once remarriage occurs as the integration of two distinct family cultures. In addition, Stern (1982b) identified a set of affiliating strategies that families can learn to establish stepfather-child friendship.

ASSESSMENT TOOLS

Many tools exist for the community health nurse to use in assessing the family (Friedman, 1992; Wright

BOX 17-3

Stages and Tasks of Middle-Class North American Family Life Cycle

I. Launching: single young adult leaves home
   a. Coming to terms with the family of origin
   b. Development of intimate relationships with peers
   c. Establishment of self: career and finances
II. Marriage: joining of families
   a. Formation of identity as a couple
   b. Inclusion of spouse in realignment of relationships with extended families
   c. Parenthood: making decisions
III. Families with young children
   a. Integration of children into family unit
   b. Adjustment of tasks: childrearing, financial, and household
   c. Accommodation of new parenting and grandparenting roles
IV. Families with adolescents
   a. Development of increasing autonomy for adolescents
   b. Reexamination of midlife marital and career issues
   c. Initial shift toward concern for the older generation
V. Families as launching centers
   a. Establishment of independent identities for parents and grown children
   b. Renegotiation of marital relationship
   c. Readjustment of relationships to include in-laws and grandchildren
   d. Dealing with disabilities and death of older generation
VI. Aging families
   a. Maintenance of couple and individual functioning while adapting to the aging process
   b. Support role of middle generation
   c. Support and autonomy of older generation
   d. Preparation for own death and dealing with the loss of spouse and/or siblings and other peers

Data from Wright LM, Leahey M: *Nurses and families: a guide to family assessment and intervention*, ed 2, Philadelphia, 1994, F.A. Davis.

and Leahey, 1994). Reviewed here are the genogram, ecomap, family health tree, and a family health assessment.

Genogram

The **genogram** is a tool that helps the nurse outline the family's structure. It is a way to diagram the family (Fig. 17-1). Generally, three generations of family members are included in a family tree using symbols (Fig. 17-2) to denote genealogy. Children are pictured from left to right, beginning with the oldest child.

PERSONAL GOALS OF RECENTLY DIVORCED WOMEN

From divorce records in three counties, the authors identified recently divorced women with children. Of 528 women contacted by mail and by telephone, 252 completed questionnaires and interviews. The women described eight categories of personal goals. The most frequently cited goals were, in order of frequency, independence, employment, and education. Older women were more likely to choose employment and environmental goals over mental health goals than were younger women.

Data from Duffy ME, Mowbray CA, Hudes M: Personal goals of recently divorced women, *Image J Nurs Sch* 22:14, 1990.

The community health nurse may use the genogram during an early family interview, starting with a blank sheet of paper and drawing a circle or a square for the person initially interviewed. The nurse tells the family that he or she will ask several background questions to gain a general picture of the family. The nurse may draw circles around family members living in separate households.

For example, as depicted in the case study, the Chan family, a refugee family from Vietnam, is a nuclear family. Fig. 17-3 depicts a sample genogram of the Chan family. With the death of Mr. Chan upon the family's arrival in San Francisco three months before the first home visit, the family became a single-parent family. Although Mr. Chan is no longer physically present in the family, his presence is still felt because the nurse learns that the family has yet to express their loss appropriately. Some families may

TABLE 17-1

Dislocations of the Family Life Cycle Requiring Additional Steps to Restabilize and Proceed Developmentally

Phase	Emotional Process of Transition; Prerequisite Attitude	Developmental Issues
Divorce		
1. Decision to divorce	Acceptance of inability to resolve marital tensions sufficiently to continue relationship	Accepting own part in the failure of the marriage
2. Planning of the breakup of the system	Support of viable arrangements for all parts of the system	a. Working cooperatively on problems of custody, visitation, and finances b. Dealing with extended family about the divorce
3. Separation	a. Willingness to continue cooperative coparental relationship b. Work on resolution of attachment to spouse	a. Mourning loss of intact family b. Restructuring marital and parent-child relationships; adaptation to living apart c. Realigning relationships with extended family; staying connected with spouse's extended family
4. Divorce	More work on emotional divorce: overcoming of hurt, anger, and guilt	a. Mourning the loss of intact family: giving up fantasies of reunion b. Retrieving hopes, dreams, and expectations from the marriage c. Staying connected with extended families
Postdivorce Family		
1. Single-parent family	Willingness to maintain parental contact with ex-spouse and support contact of children and ex-spouse and ex-spouse's family	a. Making flexible visitation arrangements with ex-spouse and ex-spouse's family b. Rebuilding own social network
2. Single-parent (i.e., noncustodial)	Willingness to maintain parental contact with ex-spouse and support custodial parent's relationship with children	a. Finding ways to continue effective parenting relationship with children b. Rebuilding own social network

From Wright LM, Leahey M: *Nurses and families: a guide to family assessment and intervention,* Philadelphia, 1984, F.A. Davis, as adapted from Carter E, McGoldrick M: The family life cycle and family therapy: an overview. In Carter E, McGoldrick M: *The family life cycle: a framework for family therapy,* New York, 1980, Gardner Press.

be cooperative in helping the nurse fill out the genogram, freely relating significant information such as divorces and remarriages. Other families may be sensitive to such information, particularly when it is shown to recur with each generation.

Family Health Tree

The **family health tree** is another tool that is helpful to the community health nurse (Fig. 17-4). Based on the genogram, the family health tree provides a mechanism for recording the family's medical and health histories (Diekelmann, 1977; Friedman, 1992). The nurse should note the following on the family health tree:

- Causes of death of deceased family members
- Genetically linked diseases, including heart disease, cancer, diabetes, hypertension, sickle cell anemia, allergies, asthma, and mental retardation
- Environmental and occupational diseases
- Psychosocial problems such as mental illness and obesity
- Infectious diseases

Text continued on p. 429

TABLE 17-2

Remarried Family Formation: A Developmental Outline

Steps	Prerequisite Attitude	Developmental Issues
1. Entering the new relationship	Recovery from loss of first marriage (i.e., adequate "emotional divorce")	Recommitment to marriage and to forming a family with readiness to deal with the complexity and ambiguity
2. Conceptualizing and planning new marriage and family	a. Acceptance of own fears and those of new spouse and children about remarriage and formation of a stepfamily b. Acceptance of need for time and patience for adjustment to complexity and ambiguity of the following: • Multiple new roles • Boundaries: space, time, membership, and authority • Affective issues: guilt, loyalty conflicts, desire for mutuality, and unresolvable past hurts	a. Work on openness in the new relationships to avoid pseudomutuality b. Plan for maintenance of cooperative coparental relationships with ex-spouse(s) c. Plan to help children deal with fears, loyalty conflicts, and membership in two systems d. Realignment of relationships with extended family to include new spouse and children e. Plan of maintenance of connections for children with extended family of ex-spouse(s)
3. Getting remarried and reconstituting family	Final solution of attachment to previous spouse and ideal of "intact" family: acceptance of a different model of family with permeable boundaries	a. Restructure of family boundaries to allow for inclusion of new spouse-stepparent b. Realignment of relationships throughout subsystems to permit interweaving of several systems c. Room for relationships of all children with biological (i.e., noncustodial) parents, grandparents, and other extended family d. Sharing of memories and histories to enhance stepfamily integration

From Wright LM, Leahey M: *Nurses and families: a guide to family assessment and intervention,* Philadelphia, 1984, F.A. Davis, as adapted from Carter E, McGoldrick M: The family life cycle and family therapy: an overview. In Carter E, McGoldrick M: *The family life cycle: a framework for family therapy,* New York, 1980, Gardner Press.

FIGURE 17-1

Genogram (Redrawn from Wright LM, Leahey M: *Nurses and families: a guide to family assessment and intervention,* ed 2, Philadelphia, 1984, F.A. Davis).

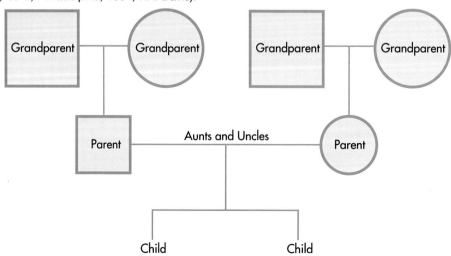

FIGURE **17-2**

Genogram and attachment symbols (Redrawn from Wright LM, Leahey M: *Nurses and families: a guide to family assessment and intervention,* ed 2, Philadelphia, 1984, F.A. Davis).

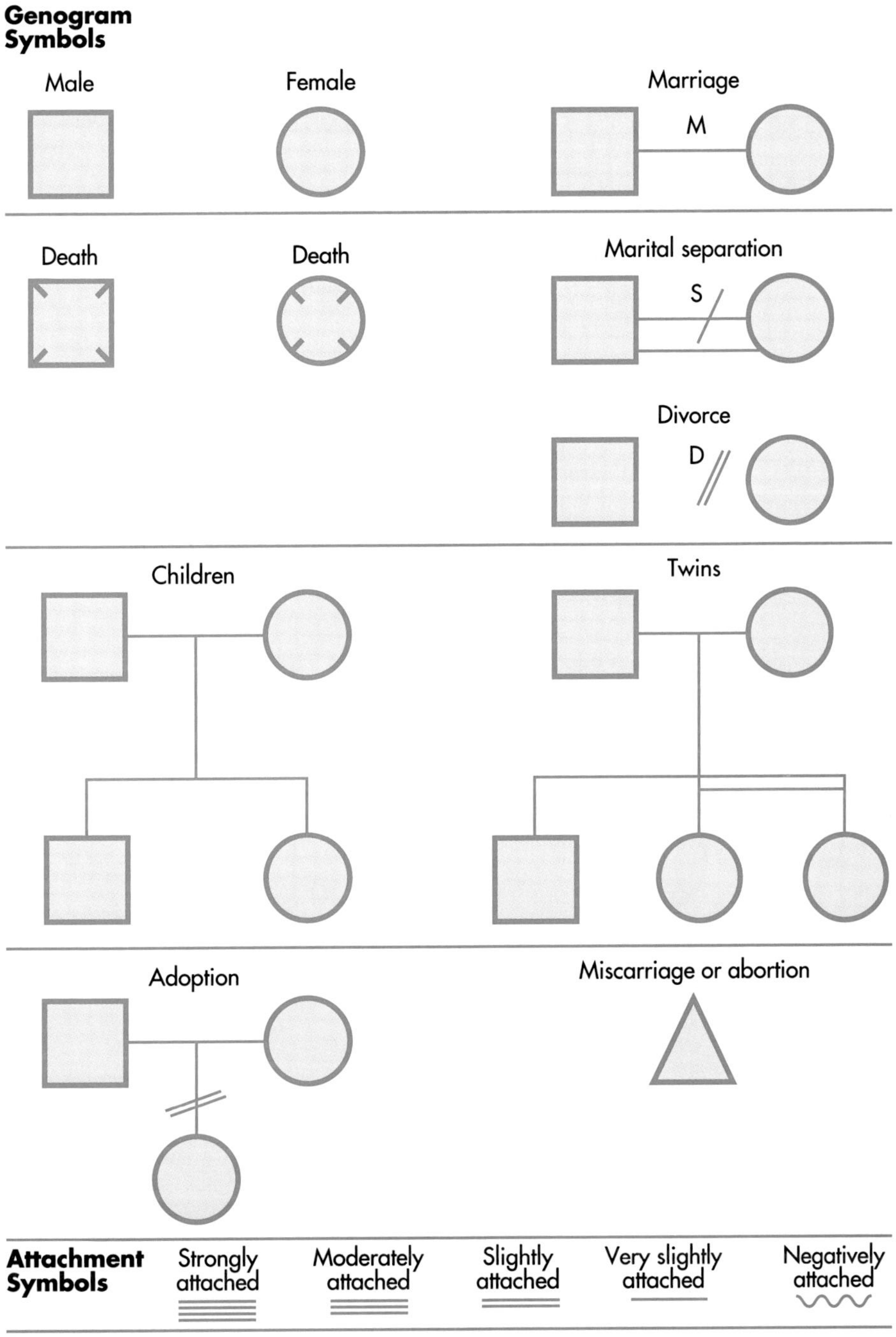

FIGURE 17-3

Sample genogram of the Chan family.

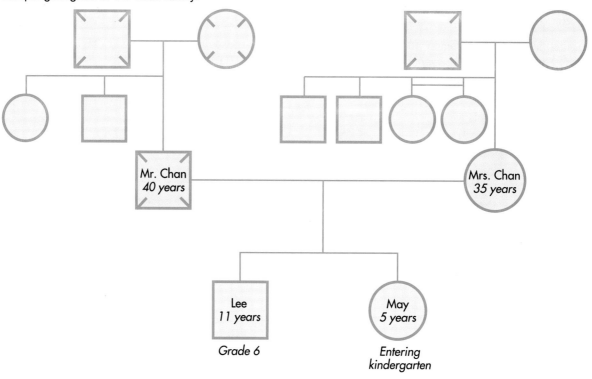

FIGURE 17-4

Chan family health tree (Modified from Diekelmann N: *Primary health care of the well adult,* New York, 1977, McGraw-Hill. Reproduced with permission).

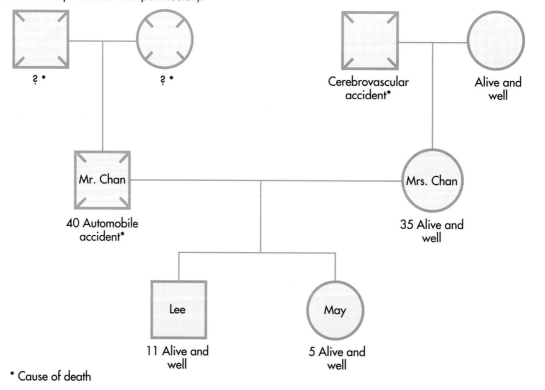

* Cause of death

- Familial risk factors from health problems
- Risk factors associated with the family's methods of illness prevention, such as having periodic physical examinations, PAP smears, and immunizations
- Lifestyle-related risk factors (i.e., by asking what family members do to "handle stress" and "keep in shape")

The family health tree can be used in planning positive familial influences on risk factors, such as dietary, exercise, coping with stress, or pressure to have a physical examination.

Ecomap

The **ecomap** (Fig. 17-5) is another classic tool that is used to depict a family's linkages to their suprasystems (Hartman, 1979; Wright and Leahey, 1994). As originally stated by Hartman (1978):

> The eco-map portrays an overview of the family in their situation; it depicts the important nurturant or conflict-laden connections between the family and the world. It demonstrates the flow of resources, or the lacks and deprivations. This mapping procedure highlights the nature of the interfaces and points to conflicts

to be mediated, bridges to be built, and resources to be sought and mobilized (p. 467).

As with the genogram, the nurse can fill out the ecomap during an early family interview, noting people, institutions, and agencies significant to the family. The nurse can use symbols used in attachment diagrams (see Fig. 17-2) to denote the nature of the ties that exist. For example, in Fig. 17-6, the Chan family ecomap suggests that few contacts occur between the family and the suprasystems. The community health nursing student was able to use the ecomap to discuss with the family the types of resources in the community and the types of relationships they wanted to establish with them.

The nurse can use these tools for family assessment with families in every health care setting. They help increase the nurse's awareness of the family within the community and help guide the nurse and the family in the assessment and planning phases of care.

Family Health Assessment

Many agencies in the community have developed guidelines for assessment of the family that help practitioners identify the health status of individual members of the family and aspects of family composition, function, and process. Often included in family health assessment guidelines is information about the environment, or community context, and information about the family. The Family Health Assessment (Fig. 17-7) is an example of a guideline that the nurse can use to assist in data collection and organization of the data collected from families over time.

Bergman and colleagues (1993) reviewed four key family characteristics that can influence how people recover from and function over time after health-related disruptions, which follow:

1. *Family cohesion,* or emotional bonding of family members and the degree of individual autonomy of each person in the family
2. *Family adaptation,* or the degree of flexibility evidenced by the ability to change roles, relationships, and power structures in response to stress
3. *Family social integration,* or the degree of social network with neighbors, friends, other family members, and religious or social organizations
4. *Degree of stress experienced by the family,* including combinations of stressors that may influence the family

FIGURE 17-5

Ecomap (Redrawn from Hartman A: Diagrammatic assessment of family relationships, *Social Casework* 59:469, 1978).

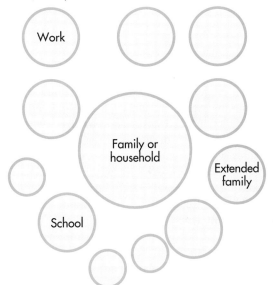

FIGURE 17-6

Sample ecomap of the Chan family.

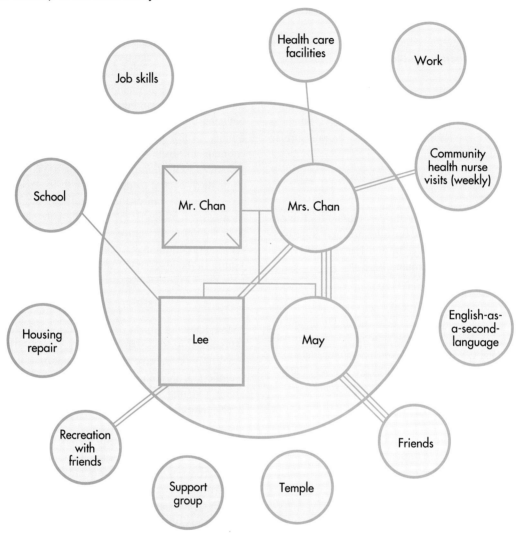

The nurse can obtain information for the Family Health Assessment through interviews of one or more family members individually, interviews of subsystems within the family (e.g., dyads of mother-child, parent-parent, and sibling-sibling), or group interviews with more than two members of the family. The nurse can also obtain information through observation of individual family members, dyads, and the entire family and observation of the environment in which the family lives, including housing, the neighborhood, and the larger community.

Family assessment tools have been developed by nurses and other professionals such as sociologists, SWs, and psychologists working with families to assess a range of dimensions of the family such as marital satisfaction, parental coping abilities, and family dysfunction (see Hanson and Mischke, 1996, for a review and listing of family assessment tools). An example is the Family Adaptability and Cohesion Evaluation Scale (FACES I), which assesses family interactions, cohesion, and adaptability (Olson, Sprenkle, and Russell, 1979). Observation of communication and behavior of the individual, dyad, or family can also provide important information. For example, a mother's self-report about her communication with her husband may be different from observation of interaction between the couple. The "ability to negotiate" is a characteristic that cannot be attributed

Text continued on p. 434

Continued

FIGURE 17-7

Family health assessment.

Family Health Assessment

Family surname: _____
Household members (name, age, and relationship to head of household): _____
_____
_____
_____

Famiy composition: _____
_____

Genogram:

Family health tree (include health problems of individual members):

Ecomap (for social and health agencies include hours of service, distance and transportation, availability of interpreters, and criteria for receiving services such as age, sex, and income barriers):

Family characteristics	Source(s) of information	Date
Extended family		
Relatives living outside household		
Location of relatives		
Frequency and duration of contact		
Means of communication		
Family mobility		
Length of time living in residence		
Location of previous residence		
Frequency of geographic moves		
Country/area of origin		
Family structure		
Educational experiences		
Employment history		
Financial resources		
Leisure time interests		
Division of labor		
Allocation of roles		
Distribution of authority and power		

Family health assessment.—cont'd

Family characteristics	Source(s) of information	Date
Family cohesion		
Emotional bonding of family members		
Degree of individual autonomy		
Family adaptation		
Flexibility in role change		
Flexibility in power structures		
Family processes		
How members communicate		
How decisions are made		
How problems are solved		
How conflict is handled		
Family social integration		
Language(s) and/or dialect(s) spoken; where		
Literacy; ability to read or write in language(s)		
Degree of racial or cultural identity		
Degree of social network with neighbors, friends, and other family members		
Network with religious organizations		
Network with social organizations		
Degrees of stress experienced by the family		
Combinations of stressors:		
1.		
2.		
3.		
Family health behavior		
Activities of daily living (how family spends typical day)		
Health history		
Health status (i.e., problems and priorities)		
Risk behaviors		
Self-care (health promotion and prevention)		
Health care resources		
Professionals and lay healers		
Working with family and agencies		
Family strengths		
Family priorities		

Family health assessment.—cont'd   *Continued*

Family characteristics	Source(s) of information	Date
Family–nurse contract(s)		

Family cultural influences
Values, attitudes, and beliefs about

Spirituality

Rituals (holidays and celebrations)

Customs

Dietary habits

Child-rearing practices

Health

Folk diseases and folk medicine

Cultural healers

Care of ill family member

Role of spiritual leader in care of ill family member

Family environment	Source(s) of information	Date
Family residence Adequacy of size		
Structurally safe		
Sanitation: water, sewage, and garbage		
Adequacy of sleeping arrangement		
Cooking and refrigeration		
Storage of medicines and cleaning agents		
Loose rugs		
Smoke alarm		
Emergency numbers		
Family neighborhood Location (e.g., urban or rural)		
Type (e.g., semicommercial)		
Age composition		
Safety Traffic patterns		
Lighting		
Security (i.e., police)		
Density (i.e., noise, crowding, poverty, and crime)		

FIGURE **17-7—cont'd**

Family health assessment.—cont'd

Family environment	Source(s) of information	Date
Modes of transportation		
Resources		
Grocery shopping		
Pharmacy		
Recreational (e.g., parks)		
Educational		
Religious		
Emergency (i.e., fire and hospital)		
Neighborhood interaction		
Family community		
Industry and business		
Leadership		
Government		
Migration (i.e., in and out of community)		
Community memberships/interaction		
Social services		
Health services		
Primary care		
Institutions (e.g., hospital or nursing home)		

to one person, but may be obvious from observation of the couple. "Conflict avoidance" may be obvious from observation of the entire family. However, the nurse must not attribute a characteristic of the entire family, such as "flexible," to each individual in the family because an individual family member, away from the family, is rigid (Copeland, 1990).

The **Family Health Assessment** addresses family characteristics, including structure and process and family environment (i.e., residence, neighborhood, and community). Not all dimensions on the Family Health Assessment will be appropriate for every

family; therefore the nurse should modify content of the assessment guideline and adapt it as necessary to fit the individual family. The guidelines should serve as a guide only, as a means to record pertinent information about the family that will assist the nurse in working with the family. The nurse should gather information in the assessment spontaneously over several contacts with the family and various members and dyads within the family. It should also include multiple forays into the community, neighborhood, and home in which the family resides. Several contacts with the family will be required to complete the Family Health Assessment.

Social and Structural Constraints

In addition to the tools just reviewed, an important aspect of family assessment and planning for intervention is the need to make note of the social and structural constraints that prevent families from receiving needed health care or achieving a state of health. These constraints explain why some families differ in mortality rates, ability to achieve "integrity" rather than "despair," or ability to "self-actualize." Social and structural constraints are usually based in social and economic causes, which affect a wide range of conditions associated with major health indicators (i.e., mortality and morbidity rates) such as literacy, education, and employment. Families most frequently served by the community health nurse are disadvantaged in that they are unable to buy health care from the private sector. However, constraints to obtaining needed health and social services by these families are well documented and may be from characteristics of health and social services rather than individual family limitations. The nurse can note these constraints on the ecomap because they influence each family's ability to interact with a specific agency. For example, in addition to noting the strength of the relationship between family and agency or institution, the nurse should note those constraints that prevent use or full use of the resource. Constraints include hours of service, distance and transportation, availability of interpreters, and criteria for receiving services such as age, sex, and income barriers. Specific examples include the different guidelines posed by each state for Medicaid and by each community for home-delivered meals to the homebound.

Helping families understand constraints and linking them to accessible resources is necessary, but intervention at the family level is not sufficient. The common basic human needs of families in a community add up and the community health nurse must tally structural constraints faced repeatedly by families and compare them with families in other communities. The nurse can then plan interventions and carry them out at the aggregate level. Muecke (1984) reported the process of community health nursing diagnosis carried out by undergraduate community health nursing students among households in Seattle of Mien refugees from Laos. The following section is an overview of how community health nurses can extend intervention at the family level to larger aggregates and social action.

EXTENDING FAMILY HEALTH INTERVENTION TO LARGER AGGREGATES AND SOCIAL ACTION

Institutional Context of Family Therapists

Many theories exist to help bridge the gap between the application of nursing and family theory to the family and broader social action on behalf of communities of families. Most family theorists view the family as a system that interfaces with outside suprasystems or institutions only when a problem is to be addressed, such as in the school or a courtroom. The following three approaches go beyond the family as a system to address the interaction between the family and the larger social system:

- ecological framework,
- network therapy, and
- transactional model.

Ecological Framework

The **ecological framework** is a blend of systems and developmental theory with an individual's understanding of his or her environment. This approach indicts the specialization and fragmentation seen in the social and health service structure based on Western concepts of time and space. This approach focuses on providing a more complex and flexible structure. Helping families transcend rigid boundaries and intake procedures of agencies that they need to maintain themselves in their environment is essential, as is changing the social and health service structure. For example, Koepke (1994), in a study investigating health care settings as resources for giving information to parents, found less than one third of 82 physicians' waiting rooms provide parenting information. However, a majority of the physicians agreed to display parenting pamphlets for a trial period; all found them helpful to patients and desired additional pamphlets. A simple intervention can aid families in a traditional health care setting.

Another example of a study using an ecological approach assessed health risk in homeless urban older adults and described various hazards within a single geographical area over a 24-hour period (Reilly, 1994). The spatial-temporal distribution of resources; factors in the natural environment, including temperature and patterns of daylight and dark; and factors in the human-created environment such as crime and traffic patterns were identified as hazards within the urban environment. Hazards of importance to homeless older adults also included the social milieu, the effects of aging, homelessness, and behavior (e.g., alcohol abuse). The interactive effect caused by the convergence of hazards and nursing interventions to reduce risk is presented.

Network Therapy

Network therapy involves changing the network of families, be it extended family or friends, who tend to maintain a dysfunctional status quo in the nuclear family. This is done by replacing the network with others from the wider system who would be able to provide more support and enhance the functioning of the family. Examples of network therapy are drawn from community mental health. In a study evaluating the social networks of 24 people with schizophrenia one year after social network therapy, 12 of the 24 people showed significant improvement in their social network (Gillies et al., 1993). In comparison with the unimproved group, the improved group had an increase in the number of reciprocal relationships, an increase in the number of confidants, and improvement in scales measuring psychotic symptoms, anxiety, and depression.

In Britain, a review of the literature about social networks of people with long-term mental illness showed that larger social networks are associated with a more favorable prognosis than smaller social networks (Brewer, Gadsden, and Scrimshaw, 1994). The Community Group Network model, a day care approach to care for people with long-term mental illness, is presented as advantageous to these people over other day care approaches. Biegel, Tracy, and Corvo (1994) described a model to aid mental health case managers who desire to increase the natural support systems of their clients through community resource development and building of community ties. Building support systems for vulnerable populations such as the chronically mentally ill remains a challenge in the community, but may be enhanced through social network therapy.

Transactional Model

In the transactional model, the term *transaction* refers to a system in process with a system that focuses on process as opposed to a linear approach. This may lead to blaming or labeling. The family

as an institution, along with other institutions (e.g., religious, educational, recreational, or governmental), is culturally anchored (i.e., each holds a distinct set of beliefs and values about the nature of the world and human existence). An awareness of culture (e.g., beliefs and values) as it is expressed in each system is important (i.e., as it is expressed in mainstream U.S. values vs. the value patterns of the family).

The following are examples of research using the transactional model. A study of parent influences on the self-esteem of children from economically disadvantaged families used data from both parents and their children and reported the influence of the parents on the child's self-concept and self-esteem, parental support, children's competencies, child-rearing practices, and family conflict (Killeen, 1993). A study of common stressors and coping strategies in rural adolescents defined *coping* as "a cognitive and transactional process between a person and the person's environment" (p. 50) and included events related to school, family, friendship, health, and transportation (Puskar, Lamb, and Bartolovic, 1993). In working with culturally and ethnically diverse families in particular, an awareness of the culture of origin, how the family's values are changing according to where they are in the process of acculturation, and the family's interpretation of mainstream U.S. values is essential to viewing the transaction of systems with each other.

Models of Social Class and Health Services

Social class places major limitations on access to medical care. In 1997, 15% of children had no health coverage of any kind. This accounts for 10.7 million children in the United States. The number of children covered by private insurance has decreased between 1979 and 1997 from 74% to 67%. In 1996, children receiving public assistance were twice as likely not to have a usual source of health care. Older children were more likely not to have a source of health care than younger children and 27% of adolescents on public assistance did not have a regular source of health care (US Department of Education, 1999).

Between 1980 and 1995, the age-adjusted percentage of people younger than 65 years of age without health care coverage increased from 12.5%

to 15% (NCHS, 1997). Those without health care coverage included people not covered by private insurance, Medicaid, Medicare, or military plans. In 1999, 8% of children lived in families with incomes of less than 50% of the federal poverty level, or $8200 for a family of four, and 30% lived in families with incomes less than 150% of poverty level, or $24,600 (US Census Bureau, 1999). For children residing with grandparents, the number of poor and uninsured increases significantly as illustrated in Fig. 17-8 (US Census Bureau, 1999).

Most children in poverty are white and non-Hispanic; however, the percentage of black or Hispanic children living in poverty are higher than that of white families. In 1997, 11% of white, nonHispanic children lived in poverty as compared with 37% of black children and 36% of Hispanic children (US Census Bureau, 1999). Among these groups, there are also differences in access to health

care. For example, in 1995, Hispanic people were more than twice as likely as white people to be without health care coverage (34% vs. 16%, respectively) (NCHS, 1997). Blacks were also less likely to have coverage than whites (23% vs. 16%, respectively). A greater proportion of people living in the southern part of the United States were less likely to have health care coverage (21.9%) than those living in the Midwest (11.9%), Northeast (14.3%), and West (19%).

Another difference in access affected by income is the setting in which people receive health care. In 1992, the location of visits where ambulatory care occurred was different for white and black people. About 16% fewer blacks used physicians' offices than whites (263 and 312 per 100 people, respectively) (NCHS, 1995). Use of hospital outpatient departments by blacks was double that for whites (40 vs. 20 visits per 100 people). Blacks were also more likely to receive ambulatory care in hospital emergency rooms than whites (55 vs. 34 visits per 100 people).

A classic theoretical perspective used to explain the reasons for these disparities was suggested three decades ago by medical sociologists as a **culture of poverty view** of life that discouraged self-reliance (Lewis, 1966). Reasons for lack of use of health services included a crisis orientation, a living-for-the-moment attitude, a low value of health, and a lack of psychological "readiness." Another explanation is the *structural view,* which considers constraints that limit use of medical care such as material constraints (i.e., money to buy services) and characteristics of health care settings for the poor in contrast to private office practices for the nonpoor (e.g., available hours, waiting time, transportation, block appointments, specialty clinics, and disease-oriented rather than preventive care).

Research has examined use of health care by using attitudes and beliefs to test the culture of poverty explanation and using financial and systems barriers to test the structural explanation (Riessman, 1984). Although studies have acknowledged some problems methodologically and with generalizability, evidence supports the findings that unequal use of health care is likely the result of the system of care rather than of individual characteristics of people seeking care. For example, Patrick (1992) compared health status and health care use of the insured and uninsured residents of Washington state and found that both health status and health care use were

FIGURE **17-8**

Percentage of children residing in different households types who are in poverty, uninsured, and receiving public assistance (From US Bureau of the Census: *Racial-ethnic and gender differences in returns to cohabitation and marriage: evidence from the current population survey,* Population Division Working Paper No 35, Washington, DC, May, 1999, The Author).

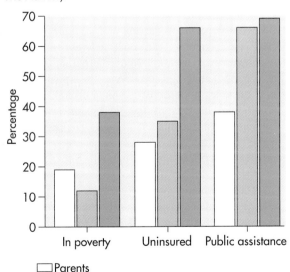

influenced by insurance coverage. The uninsured had more sinus problems than insured families after family characteristics were controlled for income, family size, education, and ethnicity. The uninsured also used health services less frequently because they made fewer ambulatory visits to health care providers and reported fewer hospitalizations. However, the uninsured reported more often that the emergency room was their usual source of care and even attributed limited health care access to cost barriers.

With recent cutbacks in services and the increased closing of public hospitals, increasingly more people are forced to attend overcrowded public clinics where professionals have little control over the nature of their work and little time to establish ongoing relationships with clients. Riessman (1984) stated that increasing clients' access to these kinds of services is not in itself sufficient. Instead, she noted changes called for by a new generation of medical sociologists (i.e., changes in the culture of medicine with its technological approach to human problems that separates the provider from the consumer and the consumer from a network of family and friends in society). Although managed care settings provide access to a primary care provider who will see the patient over time, the amount of time clinicians can spend with patients is usually closely regulated; also, the amount of control over their work and the ability of the provider to link the consumer to a network of family and friends has yet to be established.

Models of Care for Communities of Families

Models exist to guide the community health nurse in providing care to communities of families in special need of services that improve access, equality between consumer and provider, and sensitivity to human need. Riessman (1984) reviewed the following classic models:

1. The first model was Su Clinica Familiar, an alternative childbirth center initiated by consumer efforts. This center is located in the Rio Grande Valley in southern Texas. It is situated in a "family-oriented rural health clinic" and serves mostly low-income Mexican-American agricultural worker families. NMs performed 93% of the center's services between 1972

and 1979. Prenatal care and professionally assisted deliveries that encouraged family participation were made available to women who previously lacked access to care. Outcomes showed lower rates of prematurity than the state average, favorable birth weights, and positive Apgar scores.

2. A second model was initiated by a pediatrics department within an urban teaching hospital. This alternative delivery model offered home care for chronically ill children of poor, largely black, and Hispanic families in New York City. A team focus that involved home visits by pediatric NPs was compared with usual in-hospital care. No difference in influence on the family and functional status of the child existed between the families receiving home care and those receiving standard hospital care at six months. However, significant differences existed at 6 and 12 months for psychological adjustment of the child and the mother's satisfaction with medical care; the home care group was favored.

Riessman (1984) stated that these alternative programs were strategies to change the structural barriers that prevent access to care for low-income families. Professional role functions changed as nurses, rather than physicians, provided health care. Active self-care was promoted and health and medical knowledge was shared. Assistance by family and social networks was encouraged. However, Riessman warned that although both programs addressed aspects of the cultural critique of medicine, the programs did not "address the social determinants of disease." Neither program addresses the health-damaging conditions that poor people face, such as poor housing, malnutrition, and environmental hazards at the workplace and in the community. Although these programs represent steps in the right direction, changes in access to medical and health services are not enough. Social changes are also necessary.

The following are two health care delivery models initiated by community health nurses to promote access to care for families: the Block Nurse Program and the De Madres a Madres program.

Block Nurse Program

Community health nurses in St. Paul, Minnesota, initiated a block nurse program (Jamieson, 1990;

Jamieson and Martinson, 1983; Martinson et al., 1985). The program links RNs who live closest to families who have older adults in need of care with nursing services, medical supervision, and support services such as social work and volunteers. Based on a community needs assessment, census data showed that the one-square-mile geographical area of St. Anthony's Park had a population of 6969. Of this population, 12.5%, or 872, were 65 years of age or older. Of these older adults, more than 50% lived in family households, 33% lived in nonfamily households, and approximately 17% lived in "group quarters." Annual incomes for these households were below the poverty level ($7500) for 26%, which accounted for approximately 5.2% of all older adults living in the district.

More than 40 RNs lived in the same district and 18 signed up to assist their older adult neighbors. These nurses made nursing services available to them to keep them out of hospitals and nursing homes. They were also involved in prevention and case finding. The nurses became roster nurses for the Ramsey County Public Health Nursing Service and completed 60 hours of gerontological nursing courses. Services are covered by Medicare, Medicaid, third-party insurance, and private funds. Private funding was needed because many of the nursing services needed by people with chronic illness are not covered under current reimbursement guidelines. Careful documentation of services that are not covered will be useful to show the need for health policy and programs to cover services in the home that ultimately cut the cost of more expensive hospitalization and nursing home care.

With the projected increase of the older adult population and the early discharge from hospitals related to managed care and case management to cut costs, the need for nursing services for this aggregate of older adults is clear. Keeping people with chronic illness in the home is a priority for the future.

De Madres a Madres Program

A PHP was initiated in Houston, Texas by community health nursing faculty at the College of Nursing, Texas Women's University using Freire's empowerment education model (Freire, 1983; Mahon, McFarland, and Golden, 1991; McFarlane and Fehir, 1994). Funded by the Houston March of Dimes and the W.K. Kellogg Foundation, the program originally linked the general public, businesses, volunteer mothers, and a community health nurse with a targeted community of high-risk Hispanic mothers in need of early prenatal care, a major public health and community problem. The peer education program De Madres a Madres (i.e., from mothers to mothers), named by the volunteer mothers, trains volunteer Hispanic women to identify women at risk of late prenatal care in the community, provide culturally relevant information about resources in the community, and give social support. Methods of providing information in culturally acceptable milieus was a priority. Examples include group meetings in a food pantry in the community, the homes of the volunteers, or the homes of the women at risk.

During the first year of the program, 14 volunteer mothers contacted more than 2000 women at risk of delayed prenatal care. The program grew and eventually a home was rented, a volunteer mother was hired to manage the center, and two community health nurses were hired to assist in the development of the community coalition. The center became a hub of community activity and the source of empowerment of women as it responded to community needs such as the inaccessibility of eligibility cards for health care. Men and children came with the women and received information about health care, food, shelter, child care, legal aid, and employment. Outreach efforts extended to schools, banks, bakeries, and supermarkets within the community. By the end of the fifth year, the volunteers changed their mission statement from targeting prenatal care for high-risk pregnant women to providing support for families in the near north side of Houston.

The transfer of power from the professionals occurred as the professionals taught grant development skills, budgets, and networking with funding agencies to the volunteers. A grant from the Hogg Foundation for Mental Health was given to reach high-risk Hispanic families with a "parent-to-parent" support program. The volunteers have purchased the building, secured operating funds from foundations, and now have paid staff. They have also begun a business to create and market handicrafts to fund their outreach efforts. As necessary for true community empowerment, the professionals have left; they now serve as volunteers on the board of directors and the advisory board.

These programs initiated by community health nurses also represent steps in the right direction to overcome barriers to medical and health services among older adults and high-risk women and families. The need to address social determinants of health, such as poor housing, malnutrition, and poverty, call for such efforts and even more proactive social change programs by nurses, the community, and the country. For additional reports of action research by community health nurses at the community level, which address many of the social determinants of health, see Flick and colleagues' report (1994) of building a community for health and the 1994 report by Flynn, Ray, and Rider of their Healthy Cities projects.

APPLICATION OF THE NURSING PROCESS

Home Visit

Home visiting is increasing in popularity in some contexts and coming under increased scrutiny in others. Providing health care in the home to people with an identified health problem is cheaper than hospital care (Berg and Helgeson, 1984; Brooten et al., 1986). The shift in financial structure to proprietary or for-profit corporations in home health care poses difficult questions for community health nursing. Although the home health care client has the same basic human needs now as before the shift to a market system, the shift creates an ethical dilemma in the belief in market justice vs. social justice. Questions about cost-effectiveness of home visiting to well families in the face of limited public health resources have resulted in home visiting to largely high-risk populations. Setting priorities and visiting groups (i.e., families) in the community at high risk of illness, disability, or premature death is becoming necessary because the current focus is on cost constraints. Financial and other considerations are made in conjunction with an agency's policy regarding home visits (see Chapter 30).

This section presents the application of the nursing process to a family on a home visit. The example notes the use of the home visit to identify a high index of suspicion of needs in larger aggre-

gates within the community and consequent programs planned to meet those needs, which ultimately will benefit a population of families in the future.

The home visit is a crucial experience for the student and family (Warner et al., 1994). Important factors that may influence the home visit include the family's background experience with the health care system, the agency in which the student is working, the family's experience with previous students who have visited the family, and the student's background. For example, student characteristics may vary; the student brings differing levels of knowledge of medical and nursing practice, self, and the community.

The student brings previous learning about families, family-related theory, the growth and development of members of different ages within a family, disease processes, and access to the health care system. Curricula within schools of nursing vary; therefore some students will also bring preparation in all specialties—medical-surgical nursing, childbearing, parent-child nursing, and psychiatric and mental health nursing—to the experience. Others may be taking basic clinical courses such as pediatrics and psychiatric-mental health nursing concurrently with community health. Thus the need for review of appropriate theory, health education, and standard assessment tools for individuals and families will vary.

The student's knowledge of self, previous life experience, and values are also important. Research reveals that conflict related to culture exists in the delivery of health care (see Chapter 12) For example, in a study of community health nurses' conceptions of low-income black, Mexican-American, and white family lifestyles and health care patterns, Erkel (1985) found that respondents could not identify major health care delivery problems in giving care to different ethnic groups. However, only half of the respondents felt they could work equally well with each group. Students must recognize their strengths and weaknesses in these areas in preparation for entering a new community.

Knowledge of the community and level of comfort with a new environment (i.e., one outside the student's previous experience) are also important. Additional preparation by all students is necessary before the first home visit, depending on the content of the referral.

CASE STUDY

APPLICATION OF THE NURSING PROCESS

The first home visit is usually initiated by a referral. The source of a referral may be a clinic, school, private physician, or agency responsible for the care of a particular aggregate. Doris Wilson, a community health nurse, received a referral to visit the Chan family from the Intercultural Agency, a private agency responsible for follow-up with refugees from Southeast Asia. The referral traditionally lists family members, names, and ages; address; telephone number; identifying characteristics of family; reason for referral; and response to referral.

The Chan family consists of Mrs. Chan, aged 35; Lee, aged 11; and May, aged five years. The referral noted that the Chan family were from Vietnam and had been in the United States for three months. Mrs. Chan was recently widowed after her husband was killed in a hit-and-run automobile accident. Mrs. Chan spoke some English. The referral requested a home visit to assess health needs, immunization status, and knowledge of health care sources.

Doris reviewed previous learning in anticipation of her initial home visit and assessment of the family. She brought many skills such as interviewing, knowledge of pediatrics and adult health, and specific nursing care skills. She reviewed what was expected in terms of growth and development parameters for each family member. She also reviewed the grieving process, its effect on the widow and children, and supportive interventions. To provide anticipatory guidance to the family, she

needed to research areas in which she was lacking information or skill, such as immunization needs, school requirements, and nutritional needs. She carefully researched the cultural health beliefs, values, and practices of the Vietnamese. She collaborated with a Chinese community health nurse working in the health center for additional insight and guidance. She also investigated the health care resources and facilities available to refugee clients. She ensured that she had basic emergency telephone numbers to give the family for ambulance, fire, and police service in their neighborhood. She reviewed agency policy and university or college policy regarding safety (see Chapter 30).

Doris engaged in work on behalf of the family, known as *parafamily work,* to ready herself for the visit. If she had questions about the family that required answers (e.g., if the referral did not state the family's ability to speak English), she contacted the agency of referral. If necessary, she then sought an interpreter through the agency to make the initial appointment and accompany her on home visits. She also contacted agencies she was unfamiliar with that provided needed services to the family. She elicited information from them about criteria, location, available hours, and contact name for the family. Examples of such agencies for the Chan family included the local health department for immunizations, the medical center dental clinic for low-cost dental care, and several primary care clinics at public and private hospitals. She continued to

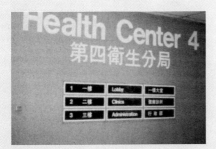

The Public Health Center is one setting in which community health nurses work.

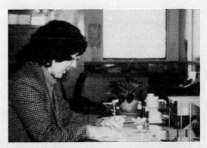

The community health nurse reviews a referral before making a home visit.

Continued

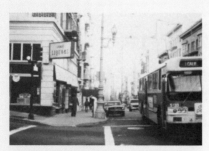

As the nurse enters the neighborhood of her clients, she observes the density of housing, the bus services, and other aspects of the community.

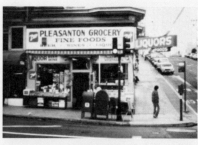

The nurse visits a neighborhood store to assess the types and prices of foods available.

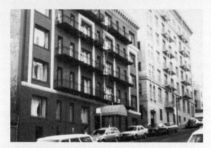

Arriving at the client's apartment building.

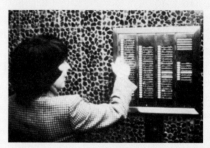

Many nationalities are represented here. If she has difficulty locating the family, the nurse may seek help from the apartment house manager.

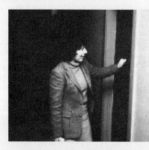

After knocking on the door, the nurse must announce who she is because some people will not respond to a knock on the door for safety reasons.

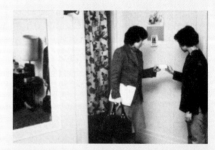

The nurse presents her card from the health department and states the purpose of her visit.

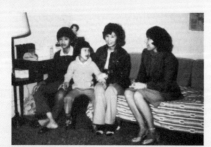

The importance of social talk in establishing a relationship and trust is understood by the nurse, and she takes time to chat with the family before beginning tasks.

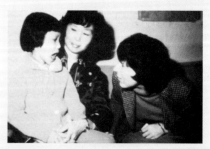

After first establishing a relationship with the adult, the nurse directs a question to a young child, who is far more comfortable on her mother's lap.

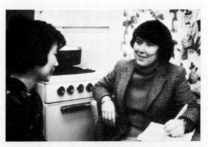

Periods of silence may be necessary while the client reflects on her thoughts and feelings.

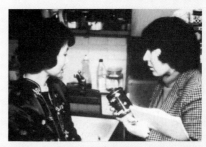

The nurse may observe folk health practices during a home visit, which helps her learn more about the family's health beliefs and needs.

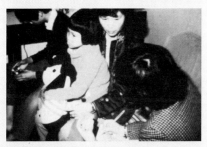

Keeping the daughter healthy was a mutually agreed-upon goal.

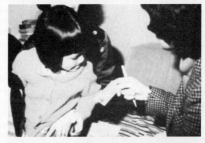

Finding a source of dental care is agreed upon as a first priority and a referral is made.

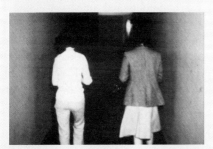

At the end of the home visit, the client accompanies the nurse to the elevator.

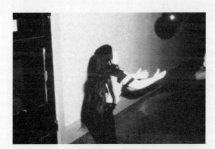

The nurse remains observant as she is leaving the client's apartment and notices children playing in a dark and poorly maintained hallway.

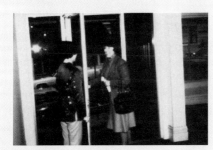

The client accompanies the nurse to the apartment building's front door.

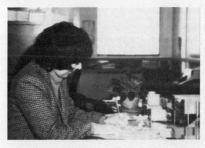

The community health nurse returns to the health center and records the visit. Charting objectively and promptly and according to agency policy is part of the responsibility of making a home visit.

Continued

do parafamily work throughout her visiting as she contacted the family and shared the exploration of resources.

Doris obtained a city map and rapid transit maps for the bus and subway. She familiarized herself with the Chan family's neighborhood; the nearest schools and hospitals; and the bus lines between the hospitals, other health care agencies, and the family home. She planned her own route and transportation method to visit the family. If possible, she planned to visit during the day, after school hours, when Lee and May should be home.

She visited the neighborhood, engaging in a "community walk" in which she used her five senses to observe and experience the community to familiarize herself before she made her visit. She noted the high density of apartment housing, the high number of cars, the bus services, and the ages and number of people on the sidewalks. She noted children playing on the street, which was on a steep hill. She noted that the busy, steep hill was the children's neighborhood, community, and playground (i.e., where they spend their time). She also observed groups of older men clustered at street corners and talking. She observed the availability of grocery stores, mostly "mom and pop" stores, and the lack of supermarkets. She entered one store near the Chan apartment and noted the availability and price of staples such as fresh produce, meat, rice, and milk; she planned to compare these prices with those in a suburban supermarket. She also noted the location of the nearest pharmacies, private physicians' offices, and clinics. The wide variety of entertainment available ranged from an elite theater to "adult" entertainment; she asked herself if these were the types of entertainment her family might choose or could afford to choose.

Initial Contact

Mrs. Chan had a telephone and spoke English; therefore Doris called for an appointment, announcing, "My name is Doris Wilson. I am a community health nursing student from the University, working with the San Francisco Health Department. The Intercultural Agency is concerned about how you and the children are doing and if you have found places to get health care. They have asked me to stop by and visit you. I would like to see Lee and May, too. I have time on Tuesday or Thursday at

3:00 PM. It would probably take about an hour. Could I visit at 3:00 PM after school is out?"

If families do not have telephones, the community health nurse may stop by the home and ask for an appointment for a later time that is convenient to the family. However, the nurse must be prepared for a visit even when "dropping by" with a note because the family may be receptive, invite the nurse in, and proceed with a visit. When the family is not home, the nurse should leave a card on the door from the agency with a message asking them to call the nurse or set a tentative time when the nurse will stop by again. Leaving personal cards or other messages in a mailbox is illegal. However, a note with a card may be mailed to the family.

If the family does not respond within one week, the nurse should return to the home and ask the apartment manager and neighbors if the family is still living in the residence. Apartment managers can aid in helping nurses locate families. Wright and Leahey (1994) reviewed the methods of dealing with family members who are reluctant or never present for a family interview, particularly men and fathers. Letting reluctant family members know that they have a unique and important view of the family, one only they can provide, is important. The nurse must also realize that some families will reject visits by not being at home at the arranged time, not answering the door, closing the door once the nurse identifies who is there, or asking the nurse not to return.

Gaining Entrée

Coordinating visits with bus schedules or parking meters is important to allow ample time for the nurse to devote complete attention to gaining entrée and carrying out a successful first home visit. Doris noted that many different names represent many different nationalities, including several families named "Chan," on the roster of the large apartment building. She was thankful that the apartment number was noted on the referral. When Mrs. Chan answered through the speaker system, Doris clearly announced who she was, that she spoke with Mrs. Chan on the telephone, and that she was there for the scheduled visit.

Finding her way to the elevators and through the apartment maze, Doris walked down a darkly lit hallway, yet she noticed a large hole in the hallway door with wooden splinters and made a mental note of this environmental hazard. Doris knocked on the door and stated, "Mrs. Chan, this is Doris Wilson, the community health nursing student." The nurse must announce who she is because, for safety reasons, some people will not respond to a knock on the door. Mrs. Chan took a moment to open the door and Doris heard the shifting of several latches, a cue that safety might be a concern to the family. Doris realized that she was a guest, said hello, shook Mrs. Chan's hand, and again stated who she was, showing Mrs. Chan her university identification card and a card from the agency. She again stated the purpose of her visit and set the approximate time limit for the visit.

> I am from the health department, and I am a community nursing student at the university. The Intercultural Agency asked me to visit with you to talk about your family's immunizations and where you and your family might go to see a physician, nurse, or dentist. Here is my card with my name and office telephone number. I can stay about an hour, if that is all right with you.

She reassured the family that in the United States nurses make visits in the home and that she was not from the Immigration and Naturalization Service.

Assessment

Throughout the visit and on each succeeding visit, Doris assessed and reassessed the family in its home environment within its particular neighborhood in the community. Doris used the conceptual framework of systems theory to organize her approach to the family. Her view of the community as a suprasystem and the family as a system composed of subsystems helped her organize the data she collected during the assessment phase and carry out the other steps of the nursing process at the individual, family, and community levels. In assessing the family as client, Doris was aware that she should collect data about the family from as many members of the family as possible, rather than from only one individual, to accurately reflect its situation.

Developing rapport and trust between the community health nurse and the family is essential (Wright and Leahey, 1994). The nurse may have a natural reluctance to enter the family's territory and to do so without "props," such as stethoscopes, blood pressure cuffs, and thermometers relied on so heavily in the acute care setting. The nurse may tend to immediately take the client's blood pressure so that he or she will feel more comfortable with something familiar. Wright and Leahey (1994) stated that the first stage of the interview is important; an alliance can begin to be established during this phase.

The importance of social talk in establishing a relationship and as a means of assessment cannot be overstressed. Kendall (1993) explored the extent to which clients participated in encounters with health visitors (i.e., British public health nurses) on home visits. The study found that participation by the client was rarely initiated by the client and rarely elicited by the health visitor. Morgan and Barden (1985) examined nurses' interactions with perinatal patients during home visits and found that the majority of the nurses' visits (53.8%) were categorized by nurse-observers as "asks for information" or "gives information." Few visits (7.9%) were reported as "seems friendly." However, patients agreed that the nurses were friendly to them and to others. Nurses appeared to be more critical of visits than patients. When focused on allowing the family to express itself, the social phase can cut down on the nurse asking for and giving information, promote friendly interaction, and elicit data appropriate to the assessment phase.

In a study by Berg and Helgeson (1984) of students' first home visits, time spent socializing during the first home visit ranged between 5% and 100%; 13 of 15 students reported obtaining important data during the socializing phase of the visit. The nurse can note important verbal and nonverbal cues (e.g., smiling, maintaining eye contact, shaking hands, and inviting the nurse to sit down). Environmental and behavioral cues, when noted and mentioned, can serve to elicit a family's history, biographical aspects, and biographical exchange between the nurse and the family. For example, noting family members' photographs, a record collection, or types of books, magazines, plants, or pets can serve as cues that elicit much information about the family. Such cues are based on the family's world and their response interprets the meaning of that world as the family sees it. That

Continued

does not discount health-related cues such as bottles of Alka-Seltzer or commercial soups for a family member on a low-sodium diet or herbal teas and folk treatments in an immigrant's home, but the nurse should concentrate on establishing a trusting relationship before discussing health-related topics.

Fostering the relationship involves letting the family express their concerns before introducing sensitive topics such as source of income. The nurse does not always need to complete agency assessment forms on the first visit; he or she can best complete them after the relationship is established. For example, Doris said hello to May, who was clinging to her mother, and to Lee, who was working on a puzzle. However, knowing the respect older adults in Asian cultures deserve, she directed her main conversation first to Mrs. Chan. The nurse may make comments about everyday topics such as the weather and the family. For example, "how long have you lived here?"; "where is the rest of your family?"; and "what are the neighbors like?" The social phase, which the nurse should repeat as an informal phase at the beginning of each visit, sets the stage for the rest of the visit. It is a way to informally check in with the family to find out what is happening in their world and it prepares the family for the more focused phase of the visit by giving them a chance to renew their acquaintance with the nurse and relax.

Having created a social footing on which the nurse and the family establish communication and rudimentary elements of trust, the focused phase of the visit allows the nurse and family to communicate more intensely around areas of concern to each and to determine needs, plans, and actions that need to be taken.

In this phase, the use of focused questions can elicit more details about the family important to assessment, such as the following: "tell me how you came San Francisco" (this may elicit a life review); "tell me, how do you spend your day?" (this may elicit activities of daily living or social interaction). This question is repeated at different times with other members of the family.

In addition to gaining the information just discussed, the community health nurse is able to observe family dynamics. This includes the relationships and patterns of communication among family members, roles that are taken, the division of labor or how things get done, and whether the family as a system is open or closed (see systems framework and structure-function framework sections in this chapter). The nurse uses the five senses in making an ongoing assessment, attending to what is seen, heard, felt, smelled, and, on occasion, tasted.

Doris asked May, "How old are you, May?" May sat on her mother's lap, grinned, and buried her face in her mother's shoulder without verbally responding. Mrs. Chan stated that May would start kindergarten in the fall. She expressed concern because May had not been to a dentist and she wanted to take her so she would be ready for school. In addition, neither Lee nor Mrs. Chan received dental hygiene. Mrs. Chan did not know whether May needed an immunization. Mrs. Chan invited Doris into the kitchen where she kept a shoe box full of papers. She showed Doris all of their immunization records. Doris, prepared for the visit, assessed that May needed her fifth diphtheria-pertussis-tetanus immunization (i.e., second booster) and needed it before school started.

A corner at the kitchen table in the small apartment gave Doris a chance to talk to Mrs. Chan alone. Doris asked, "How are *you* doing, Mrs. Chan?" Mrs. Chan was silent. Nursing students bring communication and psychiatric skills with them to the community setting. The community health nurse knows to allow periods of silence while the client reflects on her thoughts and feelings.

"My husband is gone . . ." Mrs. Chan said, covering her face with her hands.

"It must be hard to be alone . . . and with the children," Doris reflected. Mrs. Chan shook her head. "I don't want to talk right now," she said. Doris realized that support at a later date, once rapport is better established, was appropriate. A sensitive issue such as this cannot be pushed, but it must not be overlooked in the long term. Doris knew she should continue assessment on a following visit, perhaps when the children were in school. She noted mentally that she also needed to assess the children's response to their father's death.

Doris observed several unusual kinds of teas and asked Mrs. Chan if she used special medicines. Mrs. Chan showed Doris one of the special teas she used when May had an upset stomach. She detailed that each of the different teas had a use for a specific ailment. An important exchange occurred, and Doris had the opportunity to learn the family's folk health practices.

Doris observed the kitchen. In particular, she viewed the food storage techniques of new refugees. Many refugee families are unfamiliar with how to prepare foods for storage and are unaware of which foods need refrigeration. Assessment of these seemingly routine food-handling tasks and instruction requires tact and ingenuity.

Doris summarizes the following areas as appropriate to consider in her assessment of the Chan family:

Individual

- Language ability of individual members
- Sex-role–related behavior of family members
- Lifestyle patterns that place individuals at risk (e.g., poor diet, inadequate exercise, and use of alcohol or drugs)
- Patterns of self-care in health and illness
- How leisure time is spent
- Use of preventive health services (e.g., physical examinations, dental hygiene, and immunizations)

Family

- Family configuration; traditional beliefs and signs of acculturation
- Division of household labor and decision-making patterns
- Parenting patterns
- Ability of family members to disclose feelings to each other and to others
- Ability of family members to give emotional and physical support to each other during times of crisis and noncrisis
- Manner in which family members process grief
- Family history of death and illness
- Family interaction with groups in the neighborhood and community

Community

- Community resources available to the family, particularly to Asian refugee families, such as school, sports, or religious activities
- Physical environment of apartment, building, and neighborhood
- Resources in the community for recreation and leisure
- Neighborhood safety

Diagnosis

Doris made a mental nursing diagnosis for each individual in the family and a tentative diagnosis for the family as a whole and posed community diagnoses. Ross and Helmer (1988) stated that nursing diagnoses for the *individual* usually stem from using approaches such as lifestyle, activities of daily living, and symptomatology. They stated that nursing diagnoses for a *family* often differ from those for the individual and are developed using approaches such as a systems framework, structural-functional framework, problems in communication or roles, and value conflicts. Wright and Leahey (1994) preferred generating a list of family strengths and problems rather than diagnoses, noting that the list is limited to the perspective of one observer, not necessarily the "truth" about a family.

Individual

- Alterations in health maintenance related to lack of routine dental hygiene (May, Lee, and Mrs. Chan)
- Alterations in health maintenance related to lack of immunizations for age (Carpenito, 1984) (May)
- Grieving related to loss of husband (Mrs. Chan)
- Knowledge deficit related to language and cultural differences (Mrs. Chan)

Family

- Alterations in health maintenance related to failure to seek health care despite awareness that such health care is needed
- Risk of family crisis resulting from prolonged stress secondary to premature death of father
- Alteration in family processes related to situational cross-cultural relocation
- Potential accidental wound related to faulty maintenance of apartment building environment

Community

- Inadequate systematic programs for linking Asian refugee families to community resources
- Inadequate systematic programs for maintaining environmental safety of apartment dwellers as a result of faulty upkeep of buildings

Continued

For more information about formulating appropriate nursing diagnosis, refer to the list of sources of nursing diagnosis in the community at the end of this chapter.

Planning

In Morgan and Barden's (1985) study of nurse-client interactions on home visits, both nurses and clients "were uncertain as to whether or not they had agreed on goals to work toward" (p. 165). The authors concluded that the client should be more involved in the process of goal setting. Planning with the family is essential. Planning involves mutual goal setting between nurse and family; mutual setting of objectives to meet goals; prioritizing, or setting short- and long-term goals with the family; contracting, or establishing the division of labor between nurse and family that will meet the objectives; and evaluation of the process and outcome.

Contracting is "any working agreement, continuously renegotiable, between nurse and clients" (Sloan and Schommer, 1991, p. 306). The purpose of the contract is to jointly delineate the change needed and how it will come about. Joint contracting will involve the family as an active participant. In a study of contracting by senior community health nursing students, Helgeson and Berg (1985) found that contracts were rated as important to the majority of students and families, but were not appropriate to all. For example, written contracts were not appropriate for families who did not read or write. Written and oral contracts were not appropriate for families in crisis situations. In addition, some families did not grasp the idea of a contract and did not agree to its use.

Individual

Long-Term Goal
* Doris mentally noted the long-term need for teaching the importance of immunizations.

Short-Term Goals
Doris planned and contracted verbally with Mrs. Chan around the following mutually agreed-upon goal: keeping May healthy so that she would be ready for school. Receiving dental care for May was a priority for Mrs. Chan, who stated that she would seek the immunization after the source of dental care was found. Doris agreed to Mrs. Chan's plan, realizing that the dental care may have a more visible, concrete outcome for the family and would reinforce the benefits of the family's efforts in seeking care. Doris told Mrs. Chan about the dental clinic at the medical center. Mrs. Chan believed she could take May by bus to the clinic but asked if Doris would call for an appointment for her "because I'm still afraid to speak on the phone." Doris answered, "I'll be glad to call. It can be difficult until you practice. I'll make this call and then you can try the next call later for the immunizations." An informal contract was established with the nursing student calling first and giving Mrs. Chan support in her ability to try to make the second call later for the immunizations. Mrs. Chan and Doris then set a time frame in which Doris would call and make the appointment and inform Mrs. Chan, and Mrs. Chan agreed to keep the appointment time with May. A brief, reasonable, specific, and realistic contract is more likely to lead to the desired outcome. In addition, contracts must be continually reviewed, evaluated, and negotiated anew (Helgeson and Berg, 1985).

Family

Long-Term Goal
* Long-term plans included fostering the ability of the family to find and use appropriate support services for physical and mental care.

Short-Term Goal
* Short-term plans included assisting the family in expressing their feelings of loss in the grieving process.

Community

Long-Term Goal
Planning at the community level also included an investigation into the process of how to initiate responsibility for obtaining repairs to the inner-city apartment in which the Chan family lived.

Short-Term Goal
In addition to planning at the family level, Doris was aware that planning was needed at the commu-

nity level. For example, she planned to identify existing programs that specifically addressed the physical and mental health needs of Asian refugees and to see whether coordination of such programs included creating awareness of the programs in the referral systems of agencies such as the Intercultural Agency.

Intervention

Doris realized that many interventions must be carried out at the individual, family, and community levels.

Individual
An example of an intervention at the individual level is referral for preventive health examinations for each family member.

Family
At the family level, an example of an intervention is referral to a support group for the family's experience of grief.

Wright and Leahey (1994) categorized direct interventions offered by the nurse as those directed at family functioning at the following levels:

- Cognitive: new information is provided to the family, usually educational, that promotes problem solving by the family. An example is giving Mrs. Chan the location of a dental care resource and information regarding the immunizations May needed.
- Affective: families are encouraged to express intense emotions that may be blocking their efforts at problem solving. An example is Doris' planned validation of Mrs. Chan's emotions to allow her to work through the grieving process.
- Behavioral: tasks are negotiated to be carried out either during the family interview or as homework between visits. An example is May's dental appointment between visits.

The nurse may also counsel a family to stop doing something it is doing, using changes in the following three areas: providing information; encouraging the expression of affect that may be acting as a barrier, such as anger; and jointly assigning tasks.

Community
In addition, Doris realized she already used the referral process. She engaged in self-preparation and ongoing parafamily work to identify how the community was mobilized to provide physical and mental health care to refugee families. Does anyone at the dental clinic speak Chinese or Vietnamese? Are interpreters available there and at the health department or at the clinics and the hospitals? If any exist, where are they? Where do most refugee families receive health care and social support? Is anyone working with widows? Are classes on English as a second language available for Asians? Are job skills courses or programs available for women approaching midlife? Questions such as these bring up many areas of assessment that Doris will need to make with the Chan family and the community in the future, but her visit is over and she must plan ongoing evaluation and terminate the visit.

Evaluation

Evaluation includes taking note of progress made during the following phases: the ongoing process of carrying out the contract and the outcome at the termination of the relationship and the home visits (Helgeson and Berg, 1985).

Individual
Doris reviewed the basic informal contract with Mrs. Chan that led to an appointment and dental care for May. Doris evaluated the progress made during the next home visit with Mrs. Chan.

Family
Upon termination of the visit to the family, Doris evaluated the overall outcomes for the family in terms of changes in risk factors and health status. Using a systems approach, she evaluated each component of the system, individual family members, dyads within the family, and the family as a whole in terms of goal achievement. For example, she noted whether the family system was open or closed, the degree of equilibrium established, and the degree of change on the part of the family in finding and seeking care in the suprasystem.

Continued

Community

In addition to evaluating the family system, she also evaluated the ability of the suprasystem (i.e., the community) to provide culturally acceptable health resources and environmental safety the family needed and continued to intervene at the community level as needed to ensure that these resources were available to this and other families.

Terminating the Visit

At the end of the home visit, Doris reviewed the needs that were identified and summarized the plan that each would carry out. Doris asked the family whether they had any questions and instructed Mrs. Chan to call her at the number of the agency on the card she had given her upon entry to the home. They jointly agreed on a date and time for the next home visit and planned to meet earlier in the day before Lee was home from school. May would have a neighbor to play with to allow them more privacy. Doris also set realistic expectations to the visits by telling Mrs. Chan that she would be available to visit her over the course of the next 12 weeks.

When she left, Doris noticed that May and a friend were playing in a darkly lit hallway. The large hole in the hallway door with wooden splinters reminded her that nurses in the community need to be aware of the environmental conditions that their families are encountering. With this information, to which most other health professionals do not have access, the nurse can act as an advocate and collaborator in mobilizing the community to take action in addressing housing and environmental health concerns. Mrs. Chan accompanied Doris to the entrance of the apartment building as she left.

Postvisit

The community health nurse was not finished with the visit. She returned to the agency and recorded the visit. If Mrs. Chan called and needed a visit before she returned to the field the following week, the community health nurse on duty would know that a visit was made, what occurred, and future plans. The observations made should be recorded objectively and the charting should be carried out

according to agency format and policy. The dental clinic may need a written referral. The referral from the Intercultural Agency must be answered and returned.

As she considered future plans for her visits, Doris felt overwhelmed because she had only begun to assess the family. She believed that she needed to know much more about Mrs. Chan, May, and Lee. She also believed that she needed to carefully review how to assess the family as a whole. Are they a closed or an open system? How does Mrs. Chan get support? What kinds of friends does Lee have? What roles does he play in the family now that he is without a father? How do culture and the process of acculturation affect family functioning? What are the family's financial and social resources?

In addition to questions about the family, Doris had many questions about other families faced with similar conditions. Cues from the home visit triggered thinking about the needs of larger aggregates (i.e., single-parent refugee families; women in midlife without English-speaking skills, education, or job skills; and preteenagers and teenagers who enter U.S. schools with little English-speaking ability). What supports or group activities are available to meet their special needs?

Levels of Prevention

Society's expectations of the family are in transition. Application of the levels of prevention to families by the community health nurse must take into account the changing family configuration; the financial, emotional, and physical burdens often compounded in the single-parent family; and the lack of resources such as nonexisting health insurance or inadequate health insurance.

Primary

Examples of primary prevention for the Chan family are applied at the individual, family, and community levels.

Individual
- Assessment, teaching, and referral related to self-care behaviors such as immunization and dental hygiene

Family
* Teaching, role modeling, and reinforcing roles that allow family members to express feelings

Community
* Health centers in the community where culturally acceptable preventive services are readily available to Southeast Asian refugees

Secondary

Examples of secondary prevention for the Chan family are applied at the individual, family, and community levels.

Individual
* Screening for dental caries, cervical cancer, and alterations in growth and development

Family
* Screening for risk factors related to family dysfunction concerning how stress is processed by the family

Community
* Organization of screening programs in community centers and distribution of informative flyers in multiple languages in markets where nonEnglish-speaking people shop for native foods

Tertiary

Examples of tertiary prevention for the Chan family are applied at the individual, family, and community levels.

Individual
* Assistance to family members to express feelings related to grief in the loss of the father or husband; assistance to family members to seek repair of dental caries

Family
* Assistance to family members to deal with grief, assume flexible roles, and support each other in other ways

Community
* Assistance to community to provide support services for widows and families experiencing grief

SUMMARY

This chapter highlighted the community health nurse's work with families and identified the major family-related health care needs that the health care system has not adequately addressed. The nature of the family is changing and challenging traditional definitions and configurations. Approaches to meeting the health needs of families must go beyond that of the traditional health care system, which addresses the individual as the unit of care. Strategies are given for expanding notions of care from the individual to the family and from the family to the community. Nurses have traditionally relied on common theoretical frameworks used to guide intervention with families from the disciplines of psychology or social psychology. These frameworks often target individuals; frameworks are needed that go beyond the individual to the family and community and address social and policy changes needed to alter the social, economic, and environmental conditions under which families must function. Tools are provided for assessing the family and the family within the community. Provided are examples of the extension of family health intervention to larger aggregates, which involves social action to overcome constraints to accessing health services. Nonnursing and community health nursing models of care provided for communities of families are presented and critiqued. The nursing process is applied at the individual, family, and community levels on a home visit. Examples of interventions by the community health nurse at individual, family, and community levels are presented.

Families remain the core of society with diversity as the constant for families in the United States. Family nursing must be understood and practiced by community health nurses. An understanding of family theory provides a mechanism for assessing and intervening with families to improve their level of wellness and increase the health of the community as a whole.

LEARNING ACTIVITIES

1. Define the term *family* with a group of three colleagues. Compare definitions and list similarities and differences. Develop a list of criteria for being a member of a family.

2. Complete a personal genogram. What are the high-risk factors in the family history? Current risk factors? Categorize current risk factors into physical, interpersonal, and environmental. Identify needed health education and determine who needs the education. Identify sources of appropriate screening in the community for the identified risk factors.

3. Complete a personal ecomap. Is the family an "open" or "closed" family system? What resources do family currently use for mental, physical, emotional, social, and community health? What referrals are needed?

4. Identify family types or situations (e.g., families of different cultures, gay or lesbian families, or never-married mother families) that elicit "discomfort" in working situations. Identify ways to overcome barriers in working with these types of families.

RECOMMENDED READINGS

Austin JK: Assessment of coping mechanisms used by parents and children with chronic illness, *MCN Am J Matern Child Nurs* 15:98, 1990.

Bomar PJ: *Nurses and family health promotion: concepts, assessment, and interventions,* Philadelphia, 1996, W.B. Saunders.

Bomar PJ: Perspectives on family health promotion, *Fam Community Health* 12:12, 1990.

Bushy A: Rural determinants in family health: considerations for community nurses, *Fam Community Health* 12:29, 1990.

Cox R, Davis LL: Family problem solving: measuring the elusive concept, *J Fam Nurs* 5(3):332, 1999.

Denham SA: Family health in an economically disadvantaged population, *J Fam Nurs* 5(2):184, 1999.

Donnelly E: Family health assessment, *Home Health Nurse* 11:30, 1993.

Eddy LL: The impact of children with chronic health problems on marriage, *J Fam Nurs* 5(1):23, 1999.

Feeley N, Gottlieb LN: Nursing approaches for working with family strengths and resources, *J Fam Nurs* 6(1):9, 2000.

Feetham SL: The future in family nursing is genetics and it is now, *J Fam Nurs* 5(1):3, 1999.

Francis MB: Homeless families: rebuilding connections, *Public Health Nurs* 8:90, 1991.

Gennaro S et al: A sociodemographic comparison of families of very low-birthweight infants: 1982-1991, *Public Health Nurs* 11:168, 1994.

Gilliss CL et al: *Toward a science of family nursing,* Menlo Park, Calif, 1989, Addison-Wesley.

Hall WA: New fatherhood: myths and realities, *Public Health Nurs* 11:219, 1994.

Lauri S: Health promotion in child and family health care: the role of Finnish public health nurses, *Public Health Nurs* 11:32, 1994.

Reifsnider E: The use of human ecology and epidemiology in nonorganic failure to thrive, *Public Health Nurs* 12:262, 1995.

Robinson CA, Wright LM: Family nursing interventions: what families say make a difference, *J Fam Nurs* 1(3):327, 1995.

Seideman RY et al: Culture sensitivity in assessing urban Native American parenting, *Public Health Nurs* 11:98, 1994.

Solomon R, Liefeld CP: Effectiveness of a family support center approach to adolescent mothers: repeat pregnancy and school drop-out rates, *Family Relations* 47(2):139, 1998.

Stetz KM, Lewis FM, Houck GM: Family goals as indicators of adaptation during chronic illness, *Public Health Nurs* 11:385, 1994.

Swanson JM et al: Community health nurses and family planning services for men, *J Community Health Nurs* 7:87, 1990.

Swanson JM, Nies MA: *Community health nursing: promoting the health of aggregates,* ed 2, Philadelphia, 1997, W.B. Saunders.

Taylor C: Social threats to family health: redefining nursing's roles, *J Fam Nurs* 1:30, 1995.

Weeks SK, O'Connor PD: Concept analysis of family health a new definition of family health, *Rehabil Nurs* 19:207, 1994.

Wegner GD, Alexander RJ: *Readings in family nursing,* Philadelphia, 1993, J.B. Lippincott.

Zotti ME, Siegel E: Preventing unplanned pregnancies among married couples: are services for only the wife sufficient? *Res Nurs Health* 18:133, 1995.

ADDITIONAL READINGS ON GAY PARENTING

Benkov L: *Reinventing the family: the emerging story of lesbian and gay parents,* New York, 1994, Crown Publishers.

Bigner JJ, Jacobsen RB: Adult responses to child behavior and attitudes toward fathering: gay and nongay fathers, *J Homosex* 23:99, 1992.

Burke P: *Family values: two moms and their son,* New York, 1993, Random House.

Gold MA et al: Children of gay or lesbian parents, *Pediatr Rev* 15:354, 1994.

Martin A: *The lesbian and gay parenting handbook: creating and raising our families,* New York, 1993, Harper Perennial.

McIntyre DH: Gay parents and child custody: a struggle under the legal system, *Mediation Quarterly* 12:135, 1994.

Ricketts W: *Lesbians and gay men as foster parents,* Portland, Me, 1991, National Child Welfare Resource Center, Center for Child and Family Policy, Edmund S. Muskie Institute of Public Affairs, University of Southern Maine.

Tasker F, Golombok S: Adults raised as children in lesbian families, *Am J Orthopsychiatry* 65:203, 1995.

Zeidenstein L: Gynecological and childbearing needs of lesbians, *J Nurse Midwifery* 35:10, 1991.

SOURCES OF NURSING DIAGNOSIS IN THE COMMUNITY

The following resources are available to aid in the formulation of appropriate nursing diagnoses in the community:

Alex WM: Nursing diagnosis with the family and community. In Logan BB, Dawkins CE, editors: *Family-centered nursing in the community,* Menlo Park, Calif, 1983, Addison-Wesley.

Hamilton P: Community nursing diagnosis, *Adv Nurs Sci* 5:21, 1983.

Houldin A, Salstein S, Ganley K: *Nursing diagnoses for wellness,* Philadelphia, 1987, J.B. Lippincott.

Lee HA, Frenn MD: The use of nursing diagnoses for health promotion in community practice, *Nurs Clin North Am* 22:981, 1987.

Martin KS, Scheet NJ: *The Omaha system: a pocket guide for community health nursing,* Philadelphia, 1992, W.B. Saunders.

Muecke MA: Community health diagnosis in nursing, *Public Health Nurs* 1:23, 1984.

Neufeld A, Harrison M: The development of nursing diagnoses for aggregates and groups, *Public Health Nurs* 7:251, 1990.

Porter E: Administrative diagnosis—implications for the public's health, *Public Health Nurs* 4:247, 1987.

Porter E: The nursing diagnoses of population groups. In McLane A editor: *Classification of nursing diagnoses: proceedings of the Seventh Conference,* St. Louis, 1987, Mosby, 1987.

REFERENCES

Allmond BW, Buckman W, Gofman HF: *The family is the patient,* St. Louis, 1979, Mosby.

American Public Health Association: *The definition and role of public health nursing in the delivery of health care,* Washington, DC, 1981, The Association.

Anderson MP, O'Grady RS, Anderson IL: Public health nursing in primary care: impact on home visits, *Public Health Nurs* 2:145, 1985.

Auger JR: *Behavioral systems and nursing,* Englewood Cliffs, NJ, 1976, Prentice-Hall.

Beard M: Home nursing, *Public Health Nurs Q* 7:44-51, 1915.

Berg C, Helgeson D: That first home visit, *J Community Health Nurs* 1:207, 1984.

Bergman A et al: High-risk indicators for family involvement in social work in health care: a review of the literature, *Soc Work* 38:282, 1993.

Biegel DE, Tracy EM, Corvo KN: Strengthening social networks: intervention strategies for mental health case managers, *Health Soc Work* 19:206, 1994.

Brewer P, Gadsden V, Scrimshaw K: The community group network in mental health: a model for social support and community integration, *Br J Occupat Ther* 57:467, 1994.

Brooten D et al: A randomized clinical trial of early hospital discharge and home follow-up of very-low-birthweight infants, *N Engl J Med* 315:934, 1986.

Carpenito LJ: *Handbook of nursing diagnosis,* Philadelphia, 1984, J.B. Lippincott.

Carter E, McGoldrick M: The family life cycle and family therapy: an overview. In Carter E, McGoldrick M, editors: *The family life cycle: a framework for family therapy,* New York, 1980, Gardner Press.

Carter E, McGoldrick M, editors: *The changing family life cycle: a framework for family therapy,* ed 2, New York, 1988, Gardner Press.

Casper LM, Bryson KR: *Co-resident grandparents and their grandchildren: grandparent maintained families,* Washington, DC, 1999, Population Division, US Census Bureau.

Cohen PN: *Racial-ethnic and gender differences in returns to cohabitation and marriage: evidence from the current population survey,* Washington, DC, 1999, US Census Bureau.

Cook E: *The life of Florence Nightingale,* vol 2, London, 1913, Macmilian.

Copeland A: Behavioral differences in the interactions between type A and B mothers and their children, *Behav Med* 16:111, 1990.

Council of Scientific Affairs: Hispanic health in the U.S., *JAMA* 265:248, 1991.

Dawson DA: *Report on children with physical, mental, behavioral, and social problems, by family structure, 1988,* USDHHS Pub No PHS 91-1506, Washington, DC, 1991, US Government Printing Office.

Diekelmann N: *Primary health care of the well adult,* New York, 1977, McGraw-Hill.

Dreher MC: The conflict of conservatism in public health nursing education, *Nurs Outlook* 30:504, 1982.

Duffy ME, Mowbray CA, Hudes M: Personal goals of recently divorced women, *Image J Nurs Sch* 22:14, 1990.

Dunn HL: *High-level wellness,* Arlington, Va, 1961, R.W. Beatty.

Duvall EM: *Marriage and family relationships,* ed 5, Philadelphia, 1977, J.B. Lippincott.

Duvall EM, Miller BC: *Marriage and family development,* ed 6, New York, 1985, Harper & Row.

Eliason MJ: Lesbian and gay family issues, *J Fam Nurs* 2(1):10, 1996.

Erikson E: *Childhood and society,* ed 2, New York, 1963, W.W. Norton.

Erkel EA: Conceptions of community health nurses regarding low-income black, Mexican American, and white families: part 2, *J Community Health Nurs* 2:109, 1985.

Farber B: *Family and kinship in modern society,* Glenview, Ill, 1973, Scott, Foresman.

Flick LH et al: Building community for health: lessons from a seven-year-old neighborhood/university partnership, *Health Educ Q* 21:369, 1994.

Flynn BC, Ray DW, Rider MS: Empowering communities: action research through healthy cities, *Health Educ Q* 21:395, 1994.

Freeman R: *Public health nursing practice,* ed 3, Philadelphia, 1963, W.B. Saunders.

Freire P: *Education for critical consciousness,* New York, 1983, Continuum Press.

Friedman MM: *Family nursing: theory and assessment,* ed 3, East Norwalk, Conn, 1992, Appleton-Lange.

Gillies LA et al: Differential outcomes in social network therapy, *Psychosoc Rehabil J* 16:141, 1993.

Glaser B, Strauss AL: *Chronic illness and the quality of life,* St. Louis, 1975, Mosby.

Guyer B, Martin J: Annual summary of vital statistics-1999, *Pediatrics* 100(6):905, 1997.

Hanson S, Mischke KB: Family health assessment and intervention. In Bomar PJ, editor: *Nurses and family health promotion: concepts, assessment, and interventions,* ed 2, Philadelphia, 1996, W.B. Saunders.

Hartman A: Diagrammatic assessment of family relationships, *Social Casework* 59:465, 1978.

Hartman A: *Finding families: an ecological approach to family assessment in adoption,* Beverly Hills, 1979, Sage.

Helgeson DM, Berg CL: Contracting: a method of health promotion, *J Community Health Nurs* 2:199, 1985.

Helvie CO: *Community health nursing: theory and process,* New York, 1981, Harper & Row.

Jamieson M: Block nursing: practicing autonomous professional nursing in the community, *Nurs Health Care* 11:250, 1990.

Jamieson M, Martinson I: Comprehensive care built around nursing can keep the elderly at home, *Nurs Outlook* 33:271, 1983.

Johnson R: Promoting the health of families in the community. In Stanhope M, Lancaster J, editors: *Community health nursing: process and practice for promoting health,* St. Louis, 1984, Mosby.

Jordheim AD: Alternative life-styles and the family. In Reinhardt AM, Quinn MD, editors: *Family-centered community nursing: a sociological framework,* St. Louis, 1982, Mosby.

Kendall S: Do health visitors promote client participation? an analysis of the health visitor-client interaction, *J Clin Nurs* 2:103, 1993.

Killeen MR: Parent influences on children's self-esteem in economically disadvantaged families, *Issues Ment Health Nurs* 14:323, 1993.

Koepke JE: Health care settings as resources for parenting information . . . physicians' waiting rooms, *Pediatric Nurs* 20:560, 1994.

Kurdek L: The nature and correlates of relationship quality in gay, lesbian, and heterosexual cohabitating couples. In Green BY, Herek G, editors: *Lesbian and gay psychology,* Thousand Oaks, Calif, 1994, Sage.

Leahey M et al: The impact of a family systems nursing approach: nurses' perceptions, *J Cont Educ Nurs* 25(5):219-225, 1995.

Lewis O: The culture of poverty, *Sci Am* 215:19, 1966.

Mahon J, McFarland J, Golden K: De madres a madres: a community partnership for health, *Public Health Nurs* 8:15, 1991.

Manley M, Graber A: Coronary prevention program in a community hospital, *Heart Lung* 6:1045, 1977.

Martinson IM et al: The block nurse program, *J Community Health Nurs* 2:21, 1985.

Maslow A: *Motivation and personality,* ed 2, New York, 1970, Harper & Row.

McFarlane J, Fehir J: De madres a madres: a community, primary health care program based on empowerment, *Health Educ Q* 21:381, 1994.

McGoldrick M: Ethnicity and family therapy: an overview. In McGoldrick M, Pearce JK, Giordano J, editors: *Ethnicity and family therapy,* New York, 1982, Guilford Press.

Miller FM: *Coping with chronic illness: overcoming powerlessness,* Philadelphia, 2000, F.A. Davis.

Morgan BS, Barden ME: Nurse–patient interaction in the home setting, *Public Health Nurs* 2:159, 1985.

Muecke MA: Community health diagnosis in nursing, *Public Health Nurs* 1:23, 1984.

National Center for Health Statistics: *Health, United States: 1994,* Hyattsville, Md, 1995, PHS.

National Center for Health Statistics: *Health, United States: 1997,* Hyattsville, Md, 1997, PHS.

National League for Nursing: *A curriculum guide for schools of nursing,* New York, 1937, The Author.

Olds DL et al: Improving the life-course development of socially disadvantaged mothers: a randomized trial of nurse home visitation, *Am J Public Health* 78:1436, 1988.

Olson DH, Sprenkle DH, Russell CS: Circumplex model of marital and family systems. I: cohesion and adaptability dimensions, family types, and clinical applications, *Family Process* 18:3, 1979.

Patrick DL: Health status and use of services among families with and without health insurance, *Medical Care* 30:941-949, 1992.

Patterson CJ: Children of gay and lesbian parents, *Child Dev* 63:1025, 1992.

Patterson JM: Healthy American families in a postmodern society: an ecological perspective. In Green WH et al, editor: *Health and welfare for families in the 21st century,* Boston, 1999, Jones & Bartlett.

Pratt L: *Family structure and effective health behavior,* Boston, 1976, Houghton Mifflin.

Puskar KR, Lamb JM, Bartolovic M: Examining the common stressors and coping methods of rural adolescents, *Nurs Pract* 18:50, 1993.

Reilly FE: An ecological approach to health risk: a case study of urban elderly homeless people, *Public Health Nurs* 11:305, 1994.

Richardson BK: 7 ways to win your patient's trust, *Nurs* 17(3):44-45, 1987.

Riessman CK: The use of health services by the poor: are there any promising models? *Soc Policy* 14:30, 1984.

Robinson CA: Women, families, chronic illness, and nursing interventions: from burden to balance, *J Fam Nurs* 4(3):271, 1998.

Ross MM, Helmer H: A comparative analysis of Neuman's model using the individual and family as the units of care, *Public Health Nurs* 5:30, 1988.

Saluter AF: Marital status and living arrangements: March 1993. In US Census Bureau: *Current population reports,* Series P20, No 478, Washington, DC, 1994, The Author.

Singer BL: *Gay and lesbian stats: a pocket guide of facts and figures,* New York, 1994, New Press.

Sloan MR, Schommer BT: The process of contracting in community health nursing. In Spradley BW, editor: *Readings in community health nursing,* Philadelphia, 1991, J.B. Lippincott.

Smith JB: Levels of public health, *Public Health Nurs* 2:138, 1985.

Steinglass P: Family systems approaches to alcoholism, *J Subst Abuse Treat* 2:161, 1985.

Stern PN: Affiliating in stepfather families: teachable strategies leading to stepfather-child friendship, *West J Nurs Res* 4:75, 1982b.

Stern PN: Conflicting family culture: an impediment to integration in stepfather families, *J Psychosoc Nurs Ment Health Serv* 20:27, 1982a.

Stuart M: An analysis of the concept of family. In Whall A, Fawcett J, editors: *Family theory development in nursing: state of the science and art,* Philadelphia, 1991, F.A. Davis.

Swanson JM, Nies MA, *Community health nursing: promoting the health of aggregates,* ed 2, Philadelphia, 1997, W.B. Saunders.

US Bureau of the Census: *Co-resident grandparents and their grandchildren: grandparent maintained families,* Population Division Working Paper No 26, Washington, DC, March 1998, The Author.

US Bureau of the Census: *How we're changing: demographic state of the nation 1997,* Series P23-193, Washington, DC, March, 1997, The Author.

US Bureau of the Census: *Racial-ethnic and gender differences in returns to cohabitation and marriage: evidence from the current population survey,* Population Division Working Paper No 35, Washington, DC, May, 1999, The Author.

US Department of Commerce: *Current population reports,* Series P23-193, Washington, DC, March 1997, The Author.

US Department of Education: *America's children, 1999: forum and child and family statistics,* Washington, DC, 1999, The Author.

Vaughn-Cole B et al: *Family nursing practice,* Philadelphia, 1998, W.B. Saunders.

Von Bertalanffy L: *General systems theory: foundations, development, applications,* New York, 1968, George Braziller.

Von Bertalanffy L: General systems theory and psychiatry. In Arieti S, editor: *American handbook of psychiatry,* New York, 1974, Basic Books.

Von Bertalanffy L: The history and status of general systems theory. In Klir G, editor: *Trends in general systems theory,* New York, 1972, Wiley.

Wald L: The family as a unit of care: a historical review, *Public Health Nurs* 3:427-428, 515-519, 1904.

Warner M et al: The teamwork project: a collaborative approach to learning to nurse families, *J Nurs Educ* 33:5, 1994.

Whall AL: The family as a unit of care: a historical review, *Public Health Nurs* 3:240-249, 1981.

Whall AL, Fawcett J, editors: *Family theory development in nursing: state of the science and art,* Philadelphia, 1991, F.A. Davis.

Whorton MD: Environmental and occupational reproductive hazards.In Swanson J, Forrest K, editors: *Men's reproductive health,* New York, 1984, Springer.

Wright LM, Leahey M: Maximizing time, minimizing suffering: the 15-minute (or less) family interview, *J Fam Nurs* 5(1):259, 1999.

Wright LM, Leahey M: *Nurses and families: a guide to family assessment and intervention,* ed 2, Philadelphia, 1994, F.A. Davis.

18

Senior Health

Melanie McEwen and Lucille Davis

Upon completion of this chapter, the reader will be able to do the following:

1. Identify major indicators of senior health.
2. Describe problems associated with aging.
3. Discuss the factors that promote senior health.
4. Coordinate support services for older adults.
5. Plan appropriate nursing care for seniors in the community.
6. Discuss allocation of resources for senior health.

Alzheimer's disease
assistive devices
centenarians
cognitive impairment
disability
elder abuse
incontinence
institutionalization
Older Americans Act
Research On Aging Act
Social Security Act
thermal stress

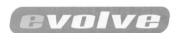

http://evolve.elsevier.com/Nies/

As stated in *Healthy People 2010*, a major goal for the health of the nation is to increase the years of healthy life (YHL) for all Americans. This supports a new paradigm in aging (i.e., shifting the focus from an illness and disease perspective to one focused on prevention and wellness). This change is significant because many of the chronic conditions that affect older adults are best managed within a framework of lifestyle changes, which emphasize healthy environments (USDHHS, 2000).

For older adults, the achievement of *Healthy People 2010* objectives is confirmed by the visibility of active elders who continue to make valuable contributions to all aspects of community life. Failure to meet the goal is demonstrated by an exponential increase in the number of older adults whose lives are restricted by physical and mental handicaps before succumbing to a premature death. Although older adults are living longer than in the past, provisional data show that these increased years of life are not necessarily "quality" years of life, referred to as YHL.

One of the primary goals of *Healthy People 2010* is not simply to increase life expectancy, but to increase the YHL, or the number of years that older adults can live independently and participate in activities that are personally important and rewarding (USDHHS, 2000). Many of the *Healthy People 2010* objectives were developed to meet this goal. Table 18-1 lists a few of the objectives specifically addressing the health of seniors.

Health care for older adults requires a team approach and the nurse is a key individual in the coordination of these services. Numerous challenges

TABLE 18-1

Healthy People 2010 and Selected Objectives for Senior Health

Objective	Baseline (1998)	Target (%)
2-9: Reduce the overall number of cases of osteoporosis.	10%	8%
2-10: Reduce the proportion of adults who are hospitalized for vertebral fractures associated with osteoporosis.	14.5 per 10,000 population 65 years of age and older	11.6 hospitalizations per 10,000 population 65 years of age and older
3-12a: Increase the proportion of adults 65 years of age and older who have received a fecal occult blood test within the preceding two years.	34%	60%
7-12: Increase the proportion of older adults who have participated during the preceding year in at least one organized health promotion activity.	12%	90%
12-6b: Reduce hospitalizations of adults between 75 and 84 years of age with heart failure as the principal diagnosis.	26.9 per 1000	13.5 per 1000
14-5b: Reduce invasive pneumococcal infections in adults 65 years of age and older.	62 per 100,000	42 per 100,000
14-29a: Increase the proportion of noninstitutionalized adults 65 years of age and older who are vaccinated annually against influenza.	63%	90%
15-28a: Reduce hip fractures among females 65 years of age and older.	1121 per 100,000	491 per 100,000
28-7: Reduce visual impairment resulting from cataracts.	NA	NA
28-15: Increase the number of people who are referred by their primary care physician for hearing evaluation and treatment.	NA	NA

and opportunities exist for community health nurses to improve the health of seniors. This chapter presents an overview of the older adults' population, a discussion of the major age-related problems, and a review of some solutions directed to the goal of an improved QOL in old age.

HEALTH NEEDS OF OLDER ADULTS: A GLOBAL PERSPECTIVE

In April 1999, the WHO warned that the growth of global older adult populations and the health consequences of aging need to be taken seriously. WHO estimated that 580 million people worldwide are 60 years of age or older, 355 million of whom live in developing countries. Furthermore, by 2020, one billion people worldwide will be older adults.

The growing older adult population leads to more cases of hearing and vision deficits, mental health problems, arthritis, and oral or dental ailments. Currently, care in developing countries focuses on communicable diseases and little attention is paid to the needs of older adults. Health personnel need information and skills to manage the needs of older adults. To this end, the WHO has urged governments to develop policies and programs to support modification of health priorities and service delivery to strengthen the family and community base to support health needs of older adults (Kumar, 1999).

CONCEPTS AND THEORIES OF AGING

Concept of Aging

Aging is defined by chronological age. As an aggregate, older adults are people 65 years of age and older. These ages are arbitrary and were originally defined to facilitate the administration of social programs. For example, in 1884, Germany identified 65 as the entrance to old age for the purpose of establishing a national pension program. Other nations subsequently followed Germany's lead.

Dramatic changes have occurred in health and longevity over the past century. At the beginning of the twenty-first century, society is characterized by rapid growth in technology and knowledge. Correspondingly, the norms and definitions related to age have undergone significant change. With increasing longevity, the life cycle and the concept of aging must be redefined. Ebersole and Hess (1998) categorized older adults as follows:

- very young-old (56 to 64 years of age),
- young-old (65 to 75 years of age),
- middle-old (76 to 84 years of age),
- old-old (85 to 99 years of age), and
- elite-old (100 years of age and older).

Older adults are not a homogeneous group and their health needs and resources are not the same. For example, the health needs and resources for the very young-old will be different from those of the middle-old or old-old.

Selected Theories of Aging

Nurses and other health care providers should review theoretical perspectives describing the aging process and older adults. An understanding of theories of aging can provide direction for assessment, planning interventions, and anticipatory guidance. A few social theories of aging are described, as follows:

- Activity Theory: the key to successful aging is the maintenance of optimal levels of activity from the middle years of life. This theory led to the establishment of many activity centers.
- Disengagement Theory: as people age, their needs change from active involvement to withdrawal for contemplation about the meaning of life and impending death. In addition to the withdrawal of the individual from society, withdrawal of society from the aged occurs. This theory caused great controversy.
- Socioenvironmental Theory: this theory responded to the limitations of disengagement and activity theories. As a holistic theory, it integrates older adults and their social and environmental contexts. The theory has the following basic components:
  - Normative component: involves behavior expectations shared by older adults in social situations.
  - Individual component: based on the amount of behavioral flexibility that older adults have in terms of resources (i.e., health and money).

- Personal component: older adults consider the meanings that norms have for themselves and their interactions with others.

- Loss of Major Life Roles Theory: this theory challenged the disengagement theory by claiming that disengagement was forced by denying older adults societal roles (e.g., mandatory retirement from the workforce). This led to the establishment of government programs to provide volunteer and work opportunities.

- Continuity Theory: the unique personality and lifelong behavioral characteristics and habits of an individual continue into old age. This theory is an attempt to balance the extremes of the activity and disengagement theories.

- Socially Disruptive Events Theory: if life is severely disrupted in several ways in a brief period of time (e.g., by retirement or loss of a spouse), social withdrawal becomes an appropriate response. This response should reverse with time; however, if disengagement becomes established, it becomes difficult to reverse.

- Reconstruction Theory: negative labeling of older adults by society and self-labeling after negative life events led to a view of older adults as incompetent and helpless.

- Age Stratification Theory: this theory assumes that societies are inevitably stratified by age and class. The relative inequality of older adults at any given time or situation depends on their typical life course experiences and is due mostly to the physical and mental changes that take place and the history of the time (e.g., wars) through which the cohort lived.

- Modernization Theory: loss of social status among older adults is a universal experience in all cultures in which modernization processes, which mostly affect the young and often involve new technology, are occurring.

- Wear and Tear Theory: this theory focuses on degenerative aspects of aging and the various multiple rates of degeneration. It is based on the idea that the essential ingredients of the life process essentially "run out."

- Autoimmune Theory: this theory is based on the premise that as age increases, mutations in cell divisions increase and the body responds to these mutations as foreign matter. In an attempt to neutralize the mutations, antibodies are produced, resulting in an autoimmune response. Although autoimmune responses are intended to be adap-

tive, over time these responses result in the body destroying itself.

DEMOGRAPHIC PATTERNS OF THE ELDERLY POPULATION IN THE UNITED STATES

The aggregate of older adults is the most rapidly expanding section of the U.S. population. In 1900, people older than 65 years of age made up just 4% of the population. The graying of America is reflected in the dramatic increase in the number and percentage of older adults. By 2000, more than 34 million Americans were 65 years of age and older, accounting for 13% of the U.S. population; of these, four million were 85 years of age or older. The aging of the "baby boomers" (i.e., those born between 1946 and 1964) began in 1999, with the first group turning 50 years of age. By 2030, the number of Americans over 65 years of age will grow to an estimated 77 million (NCHS, 1999). Furthermore, the greatest growth will occur in the group aged 85 years and older, whose numbers are expected to triple (USDHHS, 2000).

Variation exists on the number of older adults based on race because minorities make up a smaller percentage of older Americans. Some 15% of nonHispanic whites are 65 years of age or older as compared with 8% of blacks, 7% of Asians, 7% of Native-Americans, and 6% of Hispanics (American Association of Retired Persons [AARP], Administration on Aging [AoA], 1999).

Demographically, the largest number of older adults live in California (over 3.5 million). Florida and New York each have more than 2.4 million older adults, and more than one million older adults live in Pennsylvania, Texas, Illinois, Ohio, Michigan, and New Jersey. Florida has the highest percentage of older adults, with 18.3% of the population over 65 years of age. Agricultural states including Iowa, West Virginia, Arkansas, and Nebraska have high proportions of older adult residents and people 65 years of age and older are less likely to live in metropolitan areas than younger people (AARP and AoA, 1999; Ebersole and Hess, 1998).

The increase in longevity is largely attributed to the control of communicable diseases in the first half of the 1900s and a decrease in mortality rates among the middle-age and older adult populations in the second half of the century. The implications of the growth in the number of seniors present a great challenge to future government policy makers because older adults are the greatest users of health services and, with advancing age, are in increasing need of various systems of support.

EXPONENTIAL GROWTH IN NUMBER OF CENTENARIANS

The number of **centenarians**, or people aged 100 years or older, in the United States is growing rapidly. During the 1990s, the number of centenarians nearly doubled from 37,000 at the start of the decade to more than 70,000 in 2000. Furthermore, analysts at the U.S. Census Bureau believe that this per-decade doubling trend may continue with the centenarian population possibly reaching 834,000 by 2050. Centenarians share many characteristics that may prove helpful in planning for their future needs:

■ More than 80% of centenarians are women.

■ Approximately 78% of centenarians are white, but that is expected to decrease to about 55% by 2050, with corresponding increases in the number of older blacks, Hispanics, and Asians.

■ Only about 50% of centenarians in 1990 had completed some high school compared with 80% of people 65 to 69 years of age. This increase in education should influence the health of these older adults.

■ Centenarians are concentrated on the U.S. coasts with about 10% living in California and 8% living in New York.

■ Iowa has the highest percentage of centenarians, followed by South Dakota.

From National Institutes of Health, National Institute on Aging: *New census report shows exponential growth in number of centenarians,* News Release, June 16, 1999.

Mortality Rate

Humans appear to have a natural life span of between 85 and 100 years (Fries, 1980). In the United States, life expectancy at birth has increased from 47.3 years in 1900 to 78.9 years for those born in 1995. In addition, a 65-year-old American can expect to live an average of 18 more years and those 75 years of age can expect to live an average of 11 more years (USDHHS, 2000). Despite the dramatic improvement

in longevity, Americans lag behind residents of most industrialized countries as shown in Table 18-2. Fig. 18-1 illustrates that life expectancy varies by gender, age, and race.

In all ethnic groups, it is true that women tend to live longer than men do and this is attributable to biological, environmental, and lifestyle differences. Life expectancy also varies by racial or ethnic group. In the United States, Asian and Pacific Islanders have the greatest life expectancy at birth. They are followed in descending order by Hispanics, Native-Americans (especially women), nonHispanic whites, and blacks (USDHHS, 2000).

Differences in life expectancy are reduced with decreases in socioeconomic variability. Higher incomes usually mean longer life and better health than lower incomes among all racial or ethnic groups. Current trends to a wider gap between rich and poor in the United States may result in increases in the difference in life expectancy between people at different socioeconomic levels. More research is needed on other lifestyle variables to determine their influence on longevity (Bradsher, 1995).

Causes of Death

Although the leading cause of death for all people older than 65 years of age is heart disease, considerable variation exists based on age. For example, for those 65 to 74 years of age, the leading causes of death in descending order are cancer, heart disease, COPD, stroke, and pneumonia and influenza. For those 75 to 84 years of age, the rank order is heart disease, cancer, stroke, COPD, and pneumonia and influenza. For those 85 years of age and older, the leading causes of death are heart disease, cancer, stroke, pneumonia and influenza, and COPD (NCHS, 1999).

At present, heart disease causes about 35% of all deaths among older men, but overall, mortality rates from heart disease and stroke have fallen since the 1980s. Conversely, mortality rates from cancer have continued to rise. The following are other statistics related to causes of death among older adults (NCHS, 1999):

■ The proportion of deaths resulting from stroke increase with age to 10% after 85 years of age.

■ Pneumonia and influenza are responsible for 7% of all deaths for people 85 years of age and older.

■ Chronic lung diseases account for about 7% of all deaths in older adults.

TABLE 18-2

Life Expectancy at Birth by Gender: Selected Industrialized Countries, 1995

Female		Male	
Country	**Life Expectancy**	**Country**	**Life Expectancy**
United States	78.9	United States	72.5
Japan	82.9	Japan	76.4
France	82.6	Sweden	76.2
Switzerland	81.9	Israel	75.3
Sweden	81.6	Canada	75.2
Spain	81.5	Switzerland	75.1
Canada	81.2	Greece	75.1
Australia	80.9	Australia	75.0
Italy	80.8	Norway	74.9
Norway	80.7	Netherlands	74.9
Netherlands	80.4	Italy	74.4
Greece	80.3	England and Wales	74.3
Finland	80.3	France	74.2
Austria	80.1	Spain	74.2
Germany	79.8	Austria	73.5

From US Department of Health and Human Services: *Healthy people 2010,* conference edition, Washington, DC, 2000, US Government Printing Office.

FIGURE 18-1

Life expectancy at birth, 65 years of age and 85 years of age, by sex and race: United States, 1997 (From Centers for Disease Control and Prevention, National Center for Health Statistics: *Health United States, 1999,* PHS 99-1232, October 13, 1999d, Hyattsville, Md, US Government Printing Office).

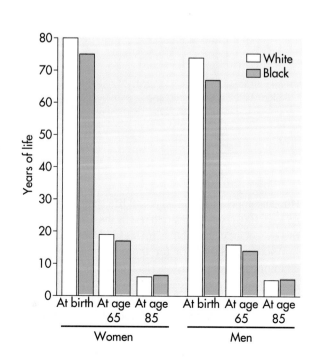

■ Diabetes was the third leading cause of death among older Native-Americans and the fourth leading cause of death among older Hispanics.

■ Alzheimer's disease is the sixth leading cause of death among white women 85 years of age and older.

Morbidity

Morbidity statistics show where the U.S. population ranks on the wellness-illness continuum. These statistics can help the nurse focus on areas of health risk and the need to promote better health for older adults. Most older adults in the community describe their health as good to excellent. However, in a national survey conducted in 1996, some 28% of those 65 years of age and older reported their health as only fair or poor (NCHS, 1999; USDHHS, 2000).

Chronic, degenerative diseases are common with aging, with some 79% of Americans 70 years of age and older reporting they have at least one chronic condition. Although not all chronic disease are life threatening, they create a substantial burden on the health and economic status of individuals, their families, and the nation as a whole (NCHS, 1999). Arthritis affects almost one half of the older adult population. Hypertension, heart disease, and hearing and vision difficulties afflict between one fourth and one third of older adults. Other disabling conditions are orthopedic impairment, chronic sinusitis, cataracts and other vision problems, and diabetes (NCHS, 1999; USDHHS, 2000). When planning for the health needs of older adults, the community health nurse should consider the following (NCHS, 1999):

■ 63% of women over 70 years of age have arthritis.

■ 33% of adults over 70 years of age have hypertension.

■ 25% of adults over 70 years of age have heart disease.

■ 11% of adults over 70 years of age have diabetes.

■ 18% of older adults are visually impaired as a result of cataracts, glaucoma, or macular degeneration.

■ 33% of older adults suffer from hearing loss.

Older women report occurrences of acute and chronic conditions more often than older men; the only exception is for conditions that involve limitation of major activity. This inconsistent finding that the longer-living female sex is also the less healthy

sex is interpreted in the following three ways (US Senate Special Committee on Aging, 1991):

1. The diseases reported by men are more often chronic diseases that cause death, whereas diseases reported by women are more often acute diseases that respond to treatment.

2. Male injuries and illnesses are not fully reported and occur more often than the data show.

3. Women are more likely to seek medical help when ill.

Frequently, older adults must be hospitalized for acute episodes of chronic conditions; they are often hospitalized repeatedly for the same disease. Hospitalization is most often from neoplasms or from cardiac, cerebrovascular, or respiratory diseases. Osteoporosis is particularly problematic because some 90% of women and 54% of men aged 85 years and older have a measurable reduction of hipbone density. Fractures of all sites are an important cause of hospitalization among women older than 75 years of age. Hip fractures contribute to some 300,000 hospitalizations each year and 80% of them are in women (NCHS, 1999).

CHARACTERISTICS OF OLDER ADULTS

Several characteristics of older adults have an influence on their health and well-being. A few of these characteristics are described in this section, including health status; income and poverty; literacy and education; marital status, relationships, and living arrangements; and religion.

CHARACTERISTICS OF OLDER ADULTS

Older adults are not:

■ Phony
■ Well, but worried
■ Chronically fatigued
■ Reckless
■ Crybabies

Older adults are:

■ Punctual
■ Flexible
■ Polite
■ Responsible
■ Postmenopausal

Adapted from Anderson EG: Reflections on a practice going geriatric, *Geriatrics* 44:91, 1989.

Health Status

In 1998, 27% of older adults stated that their health is fair or poor (compared with 9.2% of all people). Little difference existed between the sexes, but older blacks (41%) and older Hispanics (35%) were much more likely to rate their health as fair or poor than older whites (26%) (AARP and AoA, 1999). Additionally, those reporting fair or poor health were less likely to have supplemental health insurance than people reporting good to excellent health although they were more likely to need extra insurance to pay for health care.

Medicare populations with problems of access to care include minorities, residents of high-poverty urban areas, and residents of health care professional shortage areas (HPSAs). These populations neglect preventive services such as mammograms and influenza vaccines, rely heavily on hospital emergency rooms and outpatient departments for primary care services, and have longer hospital stays and higher mortality rates (Physician Payment Review Commission, 1994).

Income and Poverty

In 1998, the median income for older adults was $18,000 for males and $10,500 for females. For families headed by an older adult, the median income was $31,500 that same year. Variation existed based on race or ethnic group because the median income was $32,400 for older whites, $22,100 for blacks, and $22,000 for Hispanics (AARP and AoA, 1999).

Social Security benefits are the major source of income for older adults. Social Security benefits account for 40% of aggregate income for older adults and provide more than half of the total income for the majority of recipients. About 25% of recipients derive almost all of their income from this source. Earnings, interest on savings, and pension plans from other organizations provide other income (AARP and AoA, 1999; US Census Bureau, 2000).

Poverty rates for older adults have been declining during the past three decades because older adults benefit from Social Security and Medicare. In 1959, 35% of people 65 years of age and older lived in poverty compared with 11% in 1997 (NCHS, 1999). In 1998, some 3.5 million Americans over 65 years of age lived in poverty and another 2.1 million (6.3% of older adults) were classified as near poor (i.e., income between the poverty level and 125% of this level) (AARP and AoA, 1999; US Census Bureau, 2000).

Poverty is most likely to occur in households headed by women (12.8%) and in minorities. Some 26.4% of older black adults and 21% of older Hispanic adults are considered impoverished (AARP and AoA, 1999). Fig. 18-2 graphically depicts poverty in older adults by sex, race, and ethnicity.

Although a substantial number of older adults live fairly close to the poverty level, most of them are not considered poor. Reduction in family size as children leave home, lower taxes with lower income, and fewer or no work-related expenses may allow relatively more disposable income.

Many older adults want to work after retirement, but they usually prefer part-time work. The companionship of other people and a feeling of purpose may be as important as the extra income. In 1986, age-based mandatory retirement for most workers was abolished, but older adults still face

FIGURE **18-2**

Percentage in poverty among persons 65 years of age and over by sex, race, and Hispanic origin: United States, 1997 (Note: Figures are based on the civilian noninstitutionalized population. The race groups white and black include persons of both Hispanic and nonHispanic origin. Persons of Hispanic origin may be of any race. From Dalaker J, Naifeh M, US Census Bureau: *Poverty in the United States, 1997: current population reports,* Series P60-201, Washington, DC, 1998, US Government Printing Office).

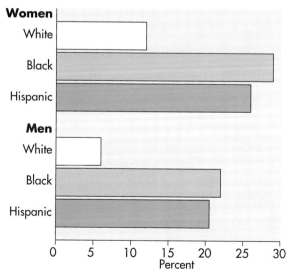

discrimination when competing with younger workers for jobs.

Literacy and Education

Educational attainment depends on prevailing attitudes and opportunities in various time periods. As an aggregate, older adults have had less formal schooling than later generations, but this is changing. Between 1970 and 1998, the percentage who completed high school rose from 18% to 67%. Furthermore, approximately 15% of older adults had a bachelor's degree or more in 1998. Among older adults, whites achieved higher educational levels than nonwhites. In 1998, 69% of whites, 43% of blacks, and 30% of older Hispanic adults had completed high school (AARP and AoA, 1999).

Functional illiteracy, which is the inability to read and write at an eighth grade level (i.e., the level of most newspapers and below the level of most government forms and health promotion material), is present in 20% to 25% of the population and may be higher in older adults, especially the oldest old, who have had fewer opportunities for formal schooling. Nurses must be sure that older adults can read written instructions, or they must find other ways of conveying information.

Marital Status, Relationships, and Living Arrangements

Women live longer than men; there are approximately 143 women for every 100 men 65 years of age and older. Therefore the fact that most older men are married (75% in 1998) and many older women are widowed (45%) is not surprising (AARP and AoA, 1999).

Most older adults (approximately 80% of men and 58% of women) live in a family setting. This proportion decreases with age; only 45% of those 85 years of age and older live in a family setting. About 31% of noninstitutionalized older adults live alone (41% of women and 17% of men) (AARP and AoA, 1999). The living arrangements of older adults reflect their health status and familial and cultural ties. Older nonmarried people who live alone are generally in better health than nonmarried people who do not live alone.

Many older adults live in an extended family situation. About 70% have one or more surviving children, 57% live fairly close to at least one child,

and most have frequent contact with their child or children. Increasing numbers of the very old are dependent on children who are also older adults. Young family members may find themselves caring for two older generations. This can become an impossible burden and the larger community may be increasingly called upon to provide support.

Only a small proportion of the noninstitutionalized older population live with nonrelatives. Among women 65 years of age and older, 2% live with nonrelatives. Among men, the percentage living with nonrelatives was 3% for those 65 to 84 years of age (NCHS, 1999).

Most older adults own their own home, but an increasing number (currently about 21%) rent living space. A significant number of older adults cling tenaciously to inadequate housing. Many do not have a telephone, which can be a lifeline in case of emergency. Only 4.2% of those 65 years of age and older live in nursing homes, but the percentage increases dramatically with age, ranging from 1.1% for people 65 to 74 years of age to 4.2% for people 75 to 84 years of age and 19.8% for people 85 years of age and older (AARP and AoA, 1999).

Religion

As people age, they become more committed to religious beliefs and participate more in church activities. Church membership is claimed by 73% of women and 63% of men older than 50 years of age, although fewer attend regularly. Women are more likely to attend than men and attendance increases with age.

Churches are resources for social networks, safety and reassurance programs, and counseling. Religious institutions have responded well to the needs of older adults in their congregations and in the community. They provide many services to help them continue living at home and participate in community activities. The parish nurse role is expanding steadily (see Chapter 29).

HEALTH CARE USE BY ELDERS

In the United States, patterns of health care use vary greatly by age and gender. The very young, childbearing women, and older adults are the most frequent consumers of health care. This section presents data on older adults' health care use patterns, focusing on hospital care, ambulatory health care, and home health care.

Hospitalization

People 65 years of age and older are the major consumers of inpatient care. In 1997, an estimated 31 million discharges of inpatients (i.e., excluding newborn infants) from short-stay hospitals occurred in the United States. Despite representing only 13% of the population, people 65 years of age and older accounted for 39% of all discharges. Hospitalizations increase with age; people 85 years of age and older have more than twice the rate of hospital discharges than those 65 to 74 years of age (NCHS, 1999). Overall, the most common reasons for hospitalization are as follows (CDC and NCHS, 1999a):

- heart disease (4.2 million),
- delivery (3.8 million),
- malignant neoplasms (1.3 million),
- pneumonia (1.3 million),
- psychoses (1.2 million),
- cerebrovascular disease (one million), and
- fractures (one million).

For people 65 years of age and older, the most common health complaint leading to hospitalization is heart disease. In 1997, 802 discharges per 10,000 population occurred with diagnoses of heart disease, with an average length of stay of 5.1 days. Some variation exists in hospitalization based on gender, which is illustrated in Fig. 18-3. The most commonly reported procedures for older adults are cardiac procedures (i.e., catheterization, coronary artery bypass, removal of coronary artery obstruction, and insertion of stents), intestinal endoscopy, and orthopedic procedures (CDC and NCHS, 1999a).

After the dramatic changes in health care financing beginning in the mid1980s and continuing throughout the 1990s, patterns of hospital use have changed dramatically. The length of stay in hospitals for sick older adults decreased substantially for virtually all conditions. In 1997, the average length of stay was 5.1 days (5.5 for males and 4.8 for females). This was down from nine days in 1990 (HCFA, 2000).

Rehospitalization for chronic health conditions and/or multiple health problems is not unusual in older adults and becomes increasingly common with age. From an in-depth review of medical records, Marcantonio and colleagues (1999) discovered five factors that were associated with hospital readmission, which follow: individuals 80 years of age and older, previous admission within 30 days, five or more medical comorbidities, history of depression, and lack

of documented patient and/or family education. The authors concluded that older adults, particularly those with comorbidities and functional impairments, are at the greatest risk of suffering poor outcomes from shortened lengths of hospital stay. Nurses working in both acute care settings and community settings, particularly home health, should be aware of these risk factors and develop interventions to address the health risks.

Ambulatory Health Care

Use of ambulatory medical services by older adults has been monitored for two decades. Americans average three visits per person to physicians and other ambulatory care providers each year. This is an increase from 2.6 in 1975. Rates increase with age after 24 years of age, and people 75 years of age and older have the highest rate at 6.5 visits per person. In addition, women made 60% of all office visits in 1997 (CDC and NCHS, 1999b). Fig. 18-4 shows these data. The source of payment for most ambulatory health care visits is private insurance, which accounts for 53% of all payments. Medicare is the second most common source of payment at 20.7% (HCFA, 2000).

For those 65 years of age and older, the major reasons for ambulatory care visits are routine chronic problems (39.5%), acute problems (26.8%), presurgery or postsurgery follow-up (11%), flare-up of a chronic problem (10.6%), and nonillness care (10%). The most common diagnoses for all ages are acute upper respiratory infections, essential hypertension, routine infant or child health check, normal pregnancy, arthritis, general medical examination, diabetes, otitis media, and cancer (CDC and NCHS, 1999b).

Home Health Care

Community and hospital health care systems have a responsibility to provide services to ensure a smooth transition from hospital to home. Bull (1994) showed that predischarge functional ability and age can predict the need for home care services and suggested that older adults who receive home health care services are less likely to suffer hospital readmission.

In conjunction with the attempts to control health care costs through prospective payment schedules for Medicare recipients, hospitals are pressured to dis-

FIGURE 18-3

Hospital discharge rates in nonFederal short-stay hospitals for selected first-listed diagnoses among persons 65 years of age and over by age and sex: United States, 1996 (Note: Rates are based on the civilian population as of July 1, 1996. From Centers for Disease Control and Prevention, National Center for Health Statistics: *1997 summary: national hospital discharge survey,* Pub No 308, Hyattsville, Md, August 19, 1999, US Government Printing Office).

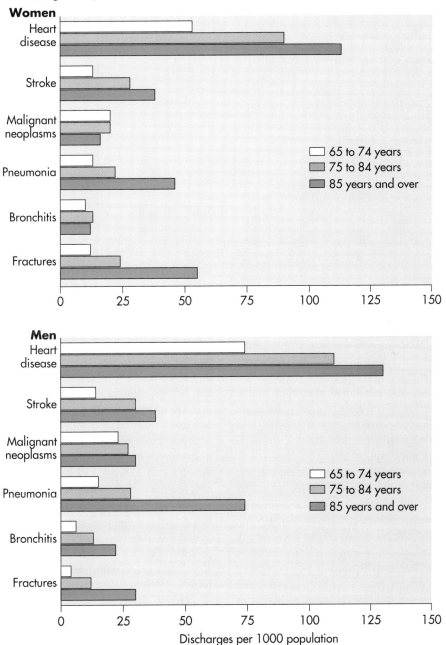

FIGURE 18-4

Annual rate of visits to office-based physicians by patient's age and sex: United States, 1997 (From Centers for Disease Control and Prevention, National Center for Health Statistics: *National ambulatory medical care survey: 1997 summary,* USDHHS Pub No 99-1250, Rockville, Md, 1999b, The Authors).

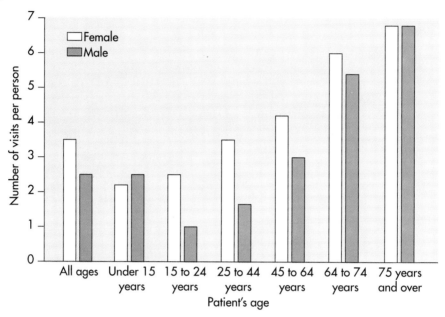

charge patients quickly, which means that more severe degrees of illness are now experienced by clients who are at home. This can severely strain the physical, financial, and emotional resources of the family. Home health nurses assist not only the client but also the family or household in understanding and complying with required treatment and the management of often complex equipment.

Home health care has grown rapidly over the past decade and the estimated number of people served by home health care agencies rose from 1.2 million in 1992 to 2.4 million in 1996 (CDC and NCHS, 1999c). In a detailed report, the NCHS noted that home health patients were predominately women (70%), 75 to 84 years of age (47%), nonHispanic (65%), widowed (47%), living in private residences (92%), and living with family members (50%). The average length of service was 107 days, but 70% of older adults used home health services for 60 days or less.

The most frequent primary admission diagnoses for home health services for men are diseases of the circulatory system and diseases of the respiratory system. Diseases of the circulatory system, injury, and poisoning are the most frequent reasons for women to receive home health care. Cancer is the primary diagnosis for 11% of men and 7% of women (CDC and NCHS, 1999c).

The purpose of home health care is to provide services to individuals and their families in their place of residence to promote, maintain, or restore health, or to maximize the level of independence and minimize the effects of disease and disability. Several services are provided by home health agencies. Nursing services are the most common, being used by 85% of home health patients. The second most common are household services, used by 28% of home health patients. Physical therapy (19.8% of patients) and social services (10.6%) are also common (CDC and NCHS, 1999c).

Other than skilled nursing care, the most frequent help received from home health agencies are assistance with activities of daily living (ADLs) and assistance with instrumental activities of daily living (IADLs). Table 18-3 lists the most frequently reported assistive tasks delivered by home health personnel.

TABLE 18-3

Most Frequent Assistance by Home Health Agencies

ADLs	Percentage Receiving Assistance by Home Health Personnel	IADLs	Percentage Receiving Assistance by Home Health Personnel
Bathing or showering	53%	Shopping for groceries	84%
Dressing	46%	Doing light housework	39%
Transferring to or from a bed or chair	30%	Taking medications	23%
Using the toilet	23%	Preparing meals	23%

From Centers for Disease Control and Prevention, National Center for Health Statistics: *Characteristics of elderly home health care users: data from the 1996 National Home and Hospice Care Survey,* USDHHS Pub No 2000-1250, Rockville, Md, 1999c, The Authors.

HEALTH PROBLEMS OF OLDER ADULTS

Most problems associated with aging arise from the deterioration of physical or mental abilities. Blomquist (1993) stated that happiness in aging is "someplace to live, someone to love, and something to do," which implies the ability to live and function effectively in society and to exercise self-determination. The inability to do these things is perceived as a problem. This section examines several potential sources for health problems among older adults, including nutrition, disability, accidents, hearing and vision impairment, depression and cognitive impairment, oral and dental problems, and incontinence.

Nutrition

Recommended dietary allowances (RDAs) of nutrients for older adults are different from those for young and middle-aged adults. As people age, their caloric needs typically decrease and vitamin and mineral requirements remain the same. Older adults must balance their nutritional intake to maintain optimum health. Table 18-4 presents dietary guidelines for senior adults.

As many as 50% of older adults living alone have specific nutritional deficiencies, and about 24% of all Medicare beneficiaries fall in a high-risk group for inadequate nutrition. Those most at risk are the oldest old, minorities, the poor, and those with Alzheimer's disease or other dementias. The signs of malnutrition are often confused with the signs of aging and misdiagnosis results in premature death and increased

cost to the health care system (Adequate Nutrition for the Elderly, 1992).

If food is not appealing and the person has no desire to eat, nutrition is not likely to be adequate. Even if prepared meals are delivered, the person may not eat them if food symbolizes family gatherings to a person now living alone or if cultural or religious tradition dictates that the ingredients would have been prepared differently. Loneliness, depression, grief, and anxiety are common reasons for altered eating habits. Too many older adults exist on coffee and donuts and sink into malnutrition because such food satisfies hunger and is easily available when feelings of low self-esteem sap the energy required for the preparation of more nutritious food.

The nurse is challenged to identify the nutritional adequacy of food consumed by older adult clients and piece together the resources available to meet deficiencies in the broad categories of the ability to obtain, prepare, eat, digest, absorb, and eliminate food. If the nurse suspects nutritional inadequacy, he or she should request a conference with a registered dietitian. Consistent, good nutrition is probably the greatest single contribution to physical and mental health and gives the greatest return for the money and time invested. Malnutrition resulting from involuntary fasting leads to the following:

- delay in any healing process;
- lowering of the metabolic rate, body temperature, pulse rate, and blood pressure;
- dry and itchy skin;
- anemia;

- ulcerated mouth;
- abnormal heart rhythm;
- erosion of bone mineral;
- difficulty walking;
- loss of sight and hearing;
- speech impairment;
- coma; and
- death.

The nutrition checklist presented in Table 18-5 lists warning signs and risk factors of poor nutritional health.

TABLE 18-4

Dietary Guidelines for Senior Adults*

Nutrient	Women	Men
Calories	1800	2400
Protein	50 g	63 g
Vitamin A	4000 IU	5000 IU
Vitamin C	60 mg	60 mg
Thiamin	1.0 mg	1.2 mg
Riboflavin	1.2 mg	1.4 mg
Niacin	13 mg	15 mg
Calcium	800 mg	800 mg
Iron	10 mg	10 mg
Phosphorus	800 mg	800 mg
Fat	No more than 30% of total calories	
Cholesterol	Not to exceed 300 mg daily	
Sodium	Limit to 1100 to 3300 mg daily	
Fiber	Limit to 20 to 30 g daily, not to exceed 35 g	

Data from National Research Council: *Recommended dietary allowances,* ed 10, Report of the Subcommittee of the Tenth Edition of the RDAs, Food and Nutrition Board, Commission on Life Sciences, Washington, DC, 1989, National Academy Press. Sodium recommendation from the American Heart Association. Fiber recommendation from the National Cancer Institute.
*RDAs for daily intake for moderately active people 50 years of age or older.

Disability

A central theme of senior health is maintaining the mental and physical functional ability to perform the daily activities necessary for a healthy, independent life. Any limit to these activities is a **disability**. Older adults maintain their independence and eliminate expensive caregiving services by shopping for themselves, cooking their own meals, and bathing and dressing themselves. Disability turns these routine ADLs (e.g., bathing, eating, and dressing) and IADLs (e.g., making meals, shopping, and cleaning) into time-consuming challenges and is a source of constant irritation as mobility and communication with the outside world are affected.

Activity limitations increase with age and women are more likely than men to have physical limitations. About 20% of those over 70 years of age have difficulty performing at least one ADL and 10% have difficulty performing at least one IADL. Blacks report higher levels of disability than whites and women are more likely to report disabilities than men (NCHS, 1999). Arthritis is the most commonly reported condition associated with disability; about 11% cite it as one of the primary causes of difficulty performing ADLs (USDHHS, 2000). Fig. 18-5 documents data on disabilities in older adults.

Assistive devices such as hearing aids, diabetic and respiratory equipment, canes, and walkers are useful in managing health problems and prolonging independent living. Of those 70 years of age and older, 39% report using assistive devices. The proportion of older adults using these devices increases with age and people 85 years of age and older are twice as likely to use three or more devices than people 70 to 74 years of age. Mobility aids (e.g., canes and walkers) are the most commonly used devices, followed by hearing aids, respiratory equipment, and diabetic equipment (NCHS, 1999).

POTENTIAL PROBLEMS OF EVERYDAY LIFE FOR OLDER ADULTS

- Opening medicine packages
- Reading product labels
- Reaching items located on high shelves
- Fastening buttons, snaps, or zippers

- Vacuuming and dusting
- Going up and down stairs
- Cleaning bathtubs and sinks
- Washing and waxing floors
- Putting on clothes over the head
- Putting on socks, shoes, or stockings
- Carrying home purchases
- Using tools
- Suffering accidents or trauma at home that are unnoticed by others
- Using the shower or bathtub
- Tying shoelaces, bows, and neckties
- Moving around the house without slipping or falling

Data from Gallup Organization: *Survey of new product needs among older Americans,* Princeton, NJ, 1983, The Author.

Accidents

Reduced sensory perception, increased reaction time, circulatory changes resulting in dizziness or loss of balance, and confusion associated with dementia combine to make older adults accident prone. Walker (1998) outlined the most common reasons for falls, which follow:

- poor vision,
- poor mobility (i.e., gait posture and balance),
- loss of muscle strength and flexibility,
- medications and alcohol (e.g., dizziness, weakness, and sleepiness),
- chronic disease (e.g., arthritis, Parkinson's disease, and diabetes),
- dementia, and
- fear of falling.

Assessment of the environment and interventions to avoid accidents are typical primary prevention

TABLE 18-5

Nutrition Checklist: Warning Signs of Poor Nutritional Health

Health Threat or Problem	Possible Consequence Related to Nutrition
The nutrition checklist is based on the following warning signs using the word *determine:*	
D = Disease	Any disease or chronic condition that changes the way the individual eats or makes it difficult to eat (e.g., depression or diabetes) can result in inadequate nutrients.
E = Eating poorly	Eating too little, eating too much, eating the same foods day after day, and not eating fruits and vegetables can lead to poor health.
T = Tooth loss	Missing, loose, or rotten teeth or dentures that do not fit well make it hard to eat.
E = Economic hardship	Low income and choosing to spend less than $25 to $30 per week for food make it difficult to get the foods needed.
R = Reduced social contact	Living alone may negatively influence nutritional health.
M = Multiple medicines	The more medicine taken, the greater the chance for disease effects such as increased or decreased appetite, change in taste, constipation, weakness, drowsiness, diarrhea, or nausea.
I = Involuntary weight loss or gain	Losing or gaining a lot of weight is an important warning sign.
N = Need assistance	Many older adults have trouble shopping, buying, and cooking food.
E = Eighty plus	As age increases, health problems increase.

From American Association of Retired Persons: *Determine your nutritional health,* 2000, The Author, www.aarp.org/contfacts/health/nutrithealth.html.

FIGURE 18-5

Percentage of persons 70 years of age and over who have difficulty performing one or more physical activities, activities of daily living, and instrumental activities of daily living by age and sex: United States, 1995 (Note: Based on interviews conducted between October 1994 and March 1996 with noninstitutionalized persons. From Centers for Disease Control and Prevention, National Center for Health Statistics: *1994 national health interview survey: second supplement on aging,* Atlanta, 1996, The Authors).

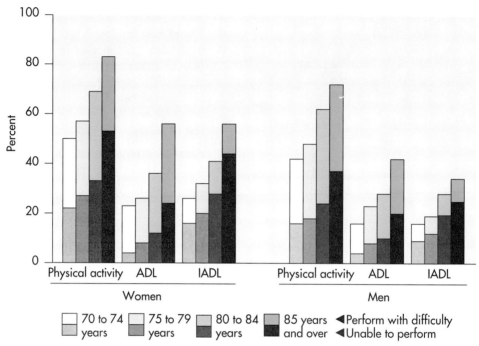

strategies in community health care for both old and young clients. Simple measures that prevent accidents include removing throw rugs, reducing the water heater setting to 120° to 125° F, checking the kitchen stove, and providing accessible fire extinguishers near fire hazards and a plan to escape in case of fire. A smoke detector should be installed in every home, but many older houses do not have them.

SOME CAUSES OF ACCIDENTS IN OLDER ADULTS

- Altered vision
- Aortic stenosis
- Cardiac arrhythmias
- Diabetes mellitus
- Generalized debility

- Hypothyroidism
- Medication reactions
- Nutritional deficiencies
- Orthostatic hypotension
- Peripheral vascular disease
- Sensory loss

From Escher JE, O'Dell C, Gambert SR: Typical geriatric accidents and how to prevent them, *Geriatrics* 44(5): 54, 1989.

ACCIDENT PREVENTION AT HOME

Think **ACCIDENTS**:

- **A**ctivities of daily living
- **C**ognition
- **C**linical findings
- **I**ncontinence
- **D**rugs
- **E**yes, ears, and environment
- **N**eurological deficits
- **T**ravel history
- **S**ocial history

Do the following:

- Remove all loose rugs.
- Tack down carpet edges.
- Install secure handrails in the bathroom and wherever else needed.
- Use a nonslip mat in the shower or bathtub.
- Check stairs for stability, uniformity, and safety.
- Eliminate clutter.
- Avoid slippery floors.
- Check the furnace and all heating devices, including the stove, to maintain proper functioning.
- Lower hot water temperatures.
- Label hot and cold water outlets and appliances with directions.
- Install and maintain smoke detectors.
- Check for proper storage of household chemicals, especially flammable substances.
- Increase artificial lighting in all rooms.

From Escher JE, O'Dell C, Gambert SR: Typical geriatric accidents and how to prevent them, *Geriatrics* 44(5):54, 1989.

The telephone is literally a lifeline for the older adult because help can be summoned directly and assistance can be sent if a scheduled call is not answered. Lifeline, an innovative telephone program, was instituted in the mid1970s and is currently the leading provider of personal emergency response service. Supported by the Red Cross, Lifeline is a 24-hour electronic monitoring service that allows older adults and those with physical limitations to continue living in their own homes and avoid institutionalization. It is available on a subscription basis. For more information about this service,

access a link to Lifeline's web page through the WebLinks section on the book's SIMON website at SIMON www.wbsaunders.com/simon/nies/. The Red Cross also works collaboratively with other agencies (e.g., churches) to provide the service for those who are unable to pay for it.

Similar to Lifeline, many churches provide frequent, regular telephone calls to people in the area regardless of whether the recipient is a member of that particular congregation. Advanced permission is obtained and provision is made for notifying a third person or entering the home if a call is not answered when expected.

SPECIAL TELEPHONE SERVICES FOR OLDER ADULTS

- Speakerphones for hands-free conversations
- Big-button telephones for easy dialing
- Memory telephones for one-touch dialing
- Telephones compatible with hearing aids
- "Signalman" control unit, which flashes a lamp for incoming calls
- Telecommunication Device for the Deaf (TDD) equipment

Dental Problems

Poor oral health in older adults may be caused by malnutrition, aging, diabetes, poor dental hygiene, or faulty dental restoration, which can create irritation by improperly fitted bridges or dentures. The dental needs of older adults are frequently neglected. Despite an increased need with age, older adults are less likely to visit a dentist than those younger than 65 years of age, usually because finances limit them. Many older adults never visit the dentist, which often results in the loss of all teeth. Over 50% of those over 65 years of age have lost some teeth from tooth decay or periodontal disease and some 26% of Americans 65 to 74 years of age have had all of their teeth extracted. A notable difference exists by race and SES; 30% of blacks, 24% of Hispanics, and 48% of low-income older adults have lost all of their teeth (USDHHS, 2000).

Shay (1994) reported that the dental needs of senior adults may be very complex from comorbidities in addition to their dental history. Many of those without teeth need dental care to ensure properly fitting dentures. Loss of teeth leads to poor nutrition and causes a change in body image that leads to lower self-esteem and withdrawal from supportive social networks.

Signs of poor oral health include mouth odor, gum swelling, redness and bleeding, loose teeth, and tooth loss. Management includes removing the irritating factor (e.g., plaque or faulty dentures) and promoting good oral hygiene, regular dental checkups, and smoking cessation. Antibiotic therapy may be indicated in severe cases. The nurse should be prepared to refer an older adult to a dentist or agency to receive partial or full dentures.

The nursing home and homebound older adults in particular need comprehensive dental assessment. A survey of institutionalized and homebound older adults gave similar results for both groups. More than 90% of those surveyed had dental caries, 31% to 50% were not satisfied with their dentures, and almost 50% had not been to the dentist in more than five years (Henry and Ceridan, 1994).

Hearing Impairment

Some 33% of individuals 65 years of age and older and more than half of those over 85 years of age have some degree of hearing impairment (USDHHS, 2000). Hearing loss in older adults can contribute to social isolation, depression, and exacerbation of coexisting psychiatric problems. The following are the most common types of hearing loss and associated factors (National Institute on Aging [NIA], 1999a):

- *Presbycusis,* most common in older adults, results from changes in the inner ear with aging and is manifested by slow decline in hearing ability.
- *Tinnitis* is a symptom that results in auditory ringing or roaring. It may be caused by cerumen, infection, aspirin, certain antibiotics, or a nerve disorder.
- *Conductive hearing loss* results from fluid in the middle ear, abnormal bone growth, or middle ear infection.
- *Sensorineural hearing loss* results from damage to parts of the inner ear or auditory nerve. This damage is caused by birth defects, head injuries, tumors, illnesses, certain prescription drugs, hypertension, or stroke.

Older adults with hearing problems should be encouraged to seek care from an otolaryngologist and

---

BOX 18-1

Working with Older Adults with Hearing Difficulties

- Face the person and speak clearly.
- Stand where there is good lighting and low background noise.
- Speak clearly, naturally, and at a reasonable speed.
- Do not hide or cover mouth, eat, or chew gum.
- Use facial expressions or gestures to give useful clues.
- Rework statements if needed.
- Be patient and stay positive and relaxed.
- Ask if there are ways to help the listener.
- Include the hearing-impaired person in all discussions to prevent feelings of isolation.
- Use pencil and paper if necessary.

From National Institute on Aging: *Hearing and older people,* 1999a, The Author, www.nih.gov/nia/health/agepages/hearing.htm.

---

an audiologist for evaluation and management. Several assistive devices can be helpful, including hearing aids. Box 18-1 contains tips for health care providers who work with older adults with hearing difficulties to promote effective communication.

Vision Impairment

Vision loss in adults is common and its prevalence increases with age. More than 90% of older adults require the use of corrective lenses. Furthermore, approximately 18% of people 70 years of age and older are visually impaired. Other than presbyopia, the most common eye problems in older adults are cataracts and glaucoma; more than 25% of people 70 years of age and older have cataracts and 8% have glaucoma (NCHS, 1999). Other frequent health problems that result in vision disturbances are floaters, macular degeneration, diabetic retinopathy, retinal detachment, and corneal diseases (NIA, 2000a).

A comprehensive eye examination, including screening for visual acuity and glaucoma, should be performed every one to two years for individuals 65 years of age and older. To determine the influence of visual impairment, the nurse should question the patient about activity limitations associated with poor vision. Determining whether the patient is using visual assistive devices such as glasses, contact lenses, magnifying lenses, or large print books can be beneficial in recognizing the degree of adaptation (McEwen, 1998).

The community health nurse should be aware of resources to help older adults get needed eye care and assistive devices. Organizations include the National Eye Institute, the American Foundation for the Blind, the Lighthouse National Center for Vision and Aging, and the National Society to Prevent Blindness. Additional information for these and other resources can be obtained through the WebLinks section on the book's SIMON website at 🅢🅘🅜🅞🅝 www.wbsaunders. com/SIMON/nies/.

Mental Disorders

Although some degree of **cognitive impairment** is common among older individuals, growing older does not necessarily result in a decline in mental health comparable with that in physical health. In the absence of disease, the lack of growth and challenge may predispose to a decline of health and premature death.

An estimated 25% of older adults experience specific mental disorders that are not part of normal aging, such as depression, anxiety, substance abuse, and dementia. Screening for depression and cognitive function should be a routine component of health examinations. Screenings should assess orientation, short-term memory, receptive and expressive language ability, attention, visual-spatial ability, and depression. If the nurse notes cognitive impairment or depression, consultation with family members and referral to a specialist may be indicated.

In general, older adults with mental health problems are neglected. The large unmet need for treatment of mental disorders among older adults is attributed to patient, provider, and health system barriers. Patient barriers may include tendency to under- or over-emphasize somatic problems and reluctance to disclose psychological symptoms. Provider barriers include lack of awareness of the manifestations of mental disorders, complexity of treatment, and reluctance to inform patients of a diagnosis. Mental health delivery system barriers include time pressures and reimbursement policies (USDHHS and National Institute of Mental Health [NIMH], 1999).

Community mental health resources for older adults are rarely sufficient to meet needs. Some home health agencies provide psychiatric services for clients with third-party reimbursement. Government programs intended to provide mental health services to older adults have been weakened and underfunded to the point of being largely ineffective. Even if services are available, many older adults may be reluctant to seek them owing to ignorance of the services offered, distrust, fear of being labeled mentally ill, or a belief that their condition is appropriate for their age.

Alzheimer's Disease

Alzheimer's disease is the most common form of dementia and one of the principal reasons for the institutionalization of older adults. Alzheimer's disease is a particularly devastating degenerative disease that affects approximately four million Americans and is costly in terms of personal and financial resources. Consider the following:

- Approximately 14 million Americans will have Alzheimer's disease by the year 2050 unless a cure or prevention is found.
- One in 10 people over 65 years of age and nearly half of those over 85 years of age have Alzheimer's disease.
- People with Alzheimer's disease live an average of eight years from onset of symptoms.
- Alzheimer's disease costs the United States $7 billion annually in health and long-term care.
- More than 70% of people with Alzheimer's disease live at home and most are cared for by family members and friends.
- Half of all nursing home patients suffer from Alzheimer's disease or a related disorder, which costs between $42,000 and $70,000 per person per year.
- The average lifetime cost of Alzheimer's disease per patient is $174,000.

Alzheimer's disease usually begins after 65 years of age and the risk grows with age. Risk factors are age and family history. Other possible risk factors include a serious head injury and lower levels of education. Other potential contributing factors are inherited factors, environmental factors (e.g., aluminum, zinc, and other metals have been identified in the brain tissue of people with Alzheimer's disease), and viruses. Symptoms are progressive and include memory loss, disorientation, confusion, problems with reasoning and thinking, agitation, anxiety, delusions, depression, hallucinations, insomnia, and wandering. Eventually, most patients need total care.

Management of people with Alzheimer's disease must be comprehensive and family centered. A treatment plan should include the following:

- Referral to appropriate structured activities (e.g., exercise, recreation, and adult day care service).
- Treatment of medical conditions.
- Treatment of behavior problems and mood disorders using nonpharmacological approaches (e.g., environmental modification, task simplification, and appropriate activities).
- Referral to social service agencies or support organizations.
- Medication if clinically indicated.

ESTROGEN REPLACEMENT THERAPY NOT EFFECTIVE FOR TREATMENT OF ALZHEIMER'S DISEASE IN SOME WOMEN

Estrogen replacement therapy (ERT) does not appear to improve the memory or function of women with mild to moderate Alzheimer's disease. A large, longitudinal clinical trial showed that estrogen should not be used to treat dementia once the disease is established. However, scientists who conducted the study emphasized that ERT may help fight the onset of Alzheimer's disease at an earlier point in the disease process; several epidemiological studies have indicated that estrogen may prevent or delay Alzheimer's disease. Additional research is currently under way to examine the possible preventive effects of estrogen.

From National Institutes of Health: *Estrogen replacement therapy not effective for treatment of Alzheimer's disease in some women,* NIH News Release, Feb 22, 2000, The Author, www.nih.gov/nia/news/pr/2000/02-22.htm.

Depression

Depression in older adults causes distress and suffering and leads to mental and physical impairments and social isolation (USDHHS and NIMH, 1999). Although common, depression in older adults is often missed, untreated, or undertreated because, as a person ages, the signs of depression are likely to be dismissed as "crankiness" or "grumpiness." Confusion or attention problems caused by depression can mimic Alzheimer's disease or other brain disorders. In addition, mood changes and other signs of depression can be caused by medications (NIA, 2000b).

Depression is one of the most prevalent conditions among older adults, and symptoms include feelings of despair, irritability, fatigue, and loneliness (Phillips, 2000). Although all older adults in the community are at risk for depression, depression rates are much higher among older adults who have a physical health problem. Findings indicate that 8% to 20% of older adults in the community and up to 37% in primary care settings experience symptoms of depression (USDHHS and NIMH, 1999). Risk factors for depression among older adults include widowhood, physical illness, educational attainment less than high school, impaired functional status, and heavy alcohol consumption (USDHHS and NIMH, 1999).

Symptoms of depression and management of depression in older adults are similar to those of the general population. Older adults should be evaluated for the following (NIA, 2000b):

- feelings of sadness and anxiety,
- tiredness and lack of energy,
- loss of interest in everyday activities,
- sleep problems,
- problems with eating and weight,
- crying,
- difficulty focusing,
- remembering and making decisions,
- feelings of helplessness,
- irritability, and
- thoughts of death or suicide.

Counseling and antidepressants can assist in alleviating many of the symptoms of depression. However, the nurse should manage medication with great care because side effects, drug-drug interactions, comorbidities, and barriers to compliance may exist (USDHHS and NIMH, 1999).

Suicide

It is well documented that depression is a foremost risk factor for suicide in older adults. Older adults have the highest rates of suicide in the United States; suicide rates increase with age, and older white men have a suicide rate more than six times that of the general population. The suicide rate for individuals 85 years of age and older is the highest (USDHHS and NIMH, 1999). Furthermore, suicide rates are

BOX 18-2

Suicide and Older Adults: 1997

- Suicide was the eighth leading cause of death in the United States in 1997.
- Comprising only 13% of the population, individuals 65 years of age and older account for 20% of suicides.
- The highest suicide rates were for white men over 85 years of age (65 per 100,000).
- Men account for 84% of all suicides among people 65 years of age and older.
- Risk factors for suicide among older adults include depression and social isolation.
- Suicide rates among older adults are highest for those who are divorced or widowed.
- Older adults make fewer suicide attempts per completed suicide.
- Firearms are the most common method of suicide by both males and females 65 years of age and older (78% of male and 36% of female suicides).
- Many older adults who commit suicide have visited their primary care provider close to the time of the suicide (20% on the same day, 40% within one week, and 70% within one month of the suicide).

From National Institute of Mental Health: *Suicide facts,* 1999, The Author, www.nimn.hin.gov/research/suifact. htm; National Institute of Mental Health: *Older adults: depression and suicide facts,* 1999, The Author, www. nimh.nih.gov/publicat/elderlydepsuicide/cfm.

MENTAL HEALTH OF ELDERS

Positive:
- Good relationships
- Friends
- Participation in activities
- Goals for the future
- Enjoyment of life

Negative:
- Depression
- Isolation
- Confusion
- Disorientation
- Dementia

Rule out:
- Poor nutrition
- Wrong use of medication
- Drug reaction or interaction
- Perception of "elderly role"
- Illness

increasing for older adults. Box 18-2 presents relevant facts on suicide (NIH and NIA, 1999).

Prevention of mental illness in older adults is vitally important. Several preventive approaches may be beneficial. The nurse should make efforts to continue to research the etiology, risk factors, pathogenesis, and course of mental illness to stimulate prevention interventions. Prevention of depression may include grief counseling for widows and widowers. Participation in self-help groups can ameliorate depression and improve social adjustment and counseling and pharmacological treatment can also be effective.

For people with long-term or recurrent mental health problems, efforts to prevent relapse or recur-

rence are essential. Prevention of side effects and adverse reactions for medications and prevention of disability are also important. A primary goal should be prevention of premature institutionalization (USDHHS and NIMH, 1999).

Incontinence

Incontinence (i.e., the involuntary loss of urine) is a common problem in older adults. Approximately 10% to 15% of people 65 years of age and older suffer from incontinence that ranges from mild leakage to total loss of bladder control (NIH and NIA, 1999). Incontinence contributes to social isolation, embarrassment, feelings of loss of control, and low self-esteem (Lashley, 1995).

Despite the prevalence of urinary incontinence, it is widely underdiagnosed and underreported. Reasons cited include lack of education about the condition on the part of health care providers and shame or embarrassment on the part of the patient (USDHHS and AHCPR, 1992). The following are the most common types of urinary incontinence:

- Stress incontinence (most common): involuntary loss of urine associated with movements that put pressure on the bladder (e.g., exercise, coughing, sneezing, laughing, and lifting heavy objects).

- Urge incontinence: involuntary urine leakage before reaching a toilet; most often found in those with enlarged prostate, diabetes, infection, stroke, dementia, Parkinson's disease, multiple sclerosis, or those taking certain pharmaceuticals.
- Overflow incontinence: involuntary urine leakage from an overdistended bladder; usually from urethral obstruction in older men and uterine prolapse in older women.
- Functional incontinence: urine leakage that occurs in older adults who have a hard time getting to the toilet from restricted mobility such as arthritis (NIH and NIA, 1999).

A thorough health history should include questions regarding elimination patterns. Diagnosis includes physical examination, measurement of postvoid residual volume, and urinalysis. Blood testing is also recommended to assess renal function and rule out diabetes. Treatment options are related to etiology and include behavior techniques, pharmacological therapy, surgery, or a combination of these.

Thermal Stress

When people age, their bodies lose the ability to efficiently maintain core temperature. The ability to respond to **thermal stress** is impaired in older adults. A comfortable indoor climate can be maintained through air conditioning or heating. However, the degree of thermal stress is often a function of socioeconomic factors because older adults may not be able to afford air conditioning or heat.

Heat-Related Problems

Older adults are vulnerable to heat exhaustion and mortality rates increase with age, outside temperature, and duration of a heat wave. Environmental temperatures do not have to be excessive to put the individual at risk. Risk factors include poor circulation; heart, lung, and kidney disease; hypertension; inability to perspire (i.e., may be caused by medications including diuretics, sedatives, and tranquilizers); being overweight or underweight; and drinking alcoholic beverages (NIA, 1999b).

The nurse should encourage people who live in a home without fans or air conditioners to open windows at night, create cross-ventilation by opening windows on two sides, cover windows exposed to direct sunlight, and keep curtains or shades drawn during the hottest part of the day. If possible, the nurse should encourage the individual without fans or air conditioners to go to shopping malls, movie houses and libraries, or the homes of friends or relatives during times of extreme heat. The nurse should also warn them against overdressing.

Emergency treatment may be indicated. If the nurse suspects heat-related problems, he or she should take the person out of the sun and into a cool place. The nurse should offer fluids, but avoid alcohol and caffeine, encourage a bath or shower, and urge the person to lie down and rest in a cool place. Symptoms of heat stroke include confusion, combativeness, bizarre behavior, faintness, staggering, tachycardia, flushed skin, lack of sweating, and in severe cases, delirium or coma.

Hypothermia

Older adults are also at risk of hypothermia, which may occur with an environmental temperature of 65° F or below. Hypothermia may occur after accidents in older adults, especially if a fall occurs at night when the victim wears only lightweight nightclothes, is unable to call for help, and must wait until someone arrives.

Signs of hypothermia include change in behavior, confusion, sleepiness, clumsiness, slurred speech, and shallow breathing. A temperature below 96° F will not register on many oral thermometers. If the reading is at or below 96° F, the emergency medical system should be called. The following are recommendations of the NIA to prevent hypothermia (NIA, 1999c):

- Dress warmly in layers of clothing.
- Wear warm clothing to bed and use blankets.
- Ask friends or neighbors to check in once or twice daily.
- Use alcohol moderately, if at all.
- Eat hot foods and drink hot liquids to keep warm.
- Set the thermostat to at least 68° to 70° F in living or sleeping areas.
- Use fuel-assistance programs (through local utility companies).

Funding exists to help pay winter fuel bills for low-income older adults, but it is much less frequently available for summer cooling. Local utility companies and human resource offices are good sources of information. If transportation is not a problem, the nearest enclosed shopping mall can provide an agreeable climate and social stimulation. However, this is only a temporary solution. Resources for climate control can be identified by discussion with the affected individual, family, or community.

HEALTH PROMOTION FOR OLDER ADULTS

Although health promotion and illness prevention interventions for older adults can be beneficial in reducing death and disability and improving QOL, the health care system has not systematically encouraged or provided preventive health services for this population. Most older adults seek medical care only in response to illness and are unlikely to see health care providers when they have no symptoms. They rely on health care professionals to recommend preventive tests and screening. Older patients may be unaware of activities that would improve their heath and well-being; therefore providers must seek opportunities to provide health teaching, perform screenings, and encourage other preventive services.

This section presents information on health promotion and illness prevention strategies that will work to improve the health of older adults. Described are preventive service guidelines, immunizations, and teaching on medication usage.

Clinical Preventive Guidelines

Access to clinical preventive primary care is an important component of *Healthy People 2010*. Preventive care involves routine timely screenings, counseling, and immunization. Box 18-3 presents recommendations for screening and counseling for older adults from the U.S. Preventive Services Task Forces.

Health providers, who work with older patients, should be prepared to perform the suggested assessments, laboratory tests, counseling, and immunizations as appropriate. Health professionals or specialists for referral should be determined in advance, and mechanisms for timely, systematic, and streamlined care by specialists through interagency and interdisciplinary collaboration and communication should be strongly encouraged (McEwen, 1998).

Immunization

Pneumonia and influenza are two infectious diseases that result in increased mortality rates in older adults. Vaccines are available for both diseases and are widely encouraged, especially for frail older adults. Medicare beneficiaries are not required to pay for

---

BOX 18-3

Clinical Preventive Services for Older Adults

Immunizations:
- Influenza
- Pneumonia
- Tetanus
- Hepatitis B

Screening:
- Cancer screening
    - Breast (clinical examination and mammography)
    - Colorectal (occult blood stool and sigmoidoscopy)
    - Cervix and uterus (clinical examination, PAP smear, and endometrial biopsy)
    - Prostate (clinical examination, ultrasonogram, and laboratory tests)
    - Skin (clinical examination)
- Blood pressure measurement
- Vision examination and glaucoma screening
- Hearing tests
- Cholesterol measurements
- Diabetes screening
- Thyroid screening
- Asymptomatic coronary artery disease (exercise stress test)
- Osteoporosis (developing techniques)
- Dental health assessment
- Mental status and dementia
- Depression screening
- Multiple health risks and appraisal and assessment
- Functional status assessment

Education and Counseling:
- Nutrition
- Weight control
- Smoking cessation
- Home safety and prevention of injury
- Stress management
- Appropriate use of medications
- Exercise

From Office of Technology Assessment: *The use of preventive services by the elderly: preventive health services under Medicare (paper 2),* Washington, DC, 1989, Health Program, Office of Technology Assessment, Congress of the United States.

influenza and pneumococcal vaccinations, but almost half have not received them. Those who do not receive an influenza vaccination are largely unaware of the need and have misconceptions about their safety and efficacy. Some 62% of Medicare recipients received an influenza vaccination in 1996, but more than one-third did not. The most common reason for not receiving a vaccination was lack of knowledge about necessity (CDC, 1999).

Current levels of immunization coverage among adults vary widely among age, risk, and racial and ethnic groups. Older white adults have the highest rates (57%), followed by older Hispanic adults (44%) and older black adults (36%). For noninstitutionalized adults 65 years of age and older, only 62% received an influenza vaccination in 1997 and only 40% had been vaccinated for pneumococcal disease. In some but not all cases, those in high-risk groups (e.g., those with diabetes, heart disease, or cancer) were slightly more likely to have been vaccinated (USDHHS, 2000).

Whether all older adults should be immunized against pneumonia and influenza is an ethical and economic consideration. Although minimal, immunization itself carries risks and the decision of whether to be immunized should be made by informed individuals. However, in times of epidemic, the immunization costs to society are far less than the treatment costs and their associated complications.

Continuing education of providers and the community is needed to increase the awareness and demand for adult vaccinations. To improve immunization rates among older adults, a national commission recommended the following (Jancin, 1999):

- provider reminder and recall systems (e.g., messages in charts to alert providers),
- patient notification and reminder systems (e.g., mailed or telephone reminders),
- feedback to providers about immunization rates, and
- standing orders.

IMMUNIZATION SCHEDULE FOR ADULTS 65 YEARS OF AGE AND OLDER

- All people in this age group should receive an influenza vaccine each year (contraindication: history of allergic reactions to eggs).
- All people in this age group should receive pneumococcal vaccine. Revaccination should be considered every six years.
- All older adults should be evaluated for completion of the primary series of vaccination against diphtheria and tetanus and receive booster doses of combined toxoids at 10-year intervals (contraindication: history of severe reaction to previous dose).
- The lifestyle, occupation, and special circumstances (including travel plans) of older adults should be assessed for consideration of other vaccines.

From Centers for Disease Control and Prevention: Adult immunizations, *Morb Mortal Wkly Rep* 44:741, 1995.

Medication Use by Elders

Americans over 65 years of age take about 25% of all prescription drugs. In addition to being substantial consumers of prescription drugs, they also use many over-the-counter medications and traditional, or "folk," remedies. Historically, the FDA has not included older adults in clinical trials; therefore the effect of different drugs on the aging population is unknown and drug dosage is achieved through trial and error. Furthermore, little attention is given to possible drug-drug or drug-food interactions.

Even if the most appropriate medications are prescribed, they are often not used as directed. Medications may not be taken unless the person feels ill, they may be over-consumed because the person believes that more is better, they may be taken erratically because the person has memory loss and lack of a system, or they may never be purchased if money is needed for other things. An estimated 5% to 30% of all geriatric hospital admissions have been associated with inappropriate drug administration (Eliopolus, 1996). Nurses who work with older adults should be aware of factors that contribute to medication noncompliance and should anticipate and recognize potential problems and be prepared to intervene.

Monitoring drug therapy in the home is an important challenge for community health nurses. Pharmacists and nurses have a common interest in medication compliance and in providing ways to help older adults understand how to take medications.

Hussey (1994) recommended tailoring interventions to the individual client and finding success with both verbal teaching and color-coded methods among people with low literacy levels. Mackowiak and colleagues (1994) surveyed client preference among four devices to assist in compliance and found strong preference for simple, easy-to-use devices such as a medication organizer tray.

Ten times as many deaths from accidental poisoning occur among older adults than among children younger than 15 years of age (USDHHS, 2000). In older adults, poisoning results from the combined effect of drugs and alcohol or from an unintentional drug overdose after confusion or forgetfulness. To prevent accidental poisoning, the older adult should not keep medications by the bedside; he or she should flush outdated medications down the drain and the nurse should devise a plan to assist the client in taking medications only as prescribed. The nurse should consider including poisoning prevention education and interventions when giving medication instruction.

Other Issues Related to Care of Older Adults

Caring for older adults is dynamic and complex. Several issues warrant review, consideration, and discussion, including transitions in later life, family issues, institutionalization, death and bereavement, abuse, and crime. Community health nurses who work with older adults should be aware of each of these issues and be prepared to intervene as necessary.

Transitions in Later Life

Later life is a time of multiple transitions such as relocation, retirement, chronic illness, widowhood, and caregiving roles. As adults age, they move from one life phase to another and experience many role transitions (e.g., parent to grandparent or worker to retiree). These processes can be disruptive and require new skills, relationships, and coping strategies. Transitions can be developmental or related to a crisis such as illness.

Responses can vary depending on whether they are positive and anticipated or negative and unanticipated. For example, if an older adult chooses to retire and has planned for it, then it is positive. On the other hand, if retirement is forced, resulting from poor health or "company policy," then it is not viewed as positive. Another example includes the grandparent

TABLE 18-6

Comparison of Healthy and Unhealthy Transitions

Healthy Transitional Processes	Unhealthy Transitions
Redefining meaning and awareness	Resisting new meanings
Modifying expectations	Maintaining unrealistic expectations
Developing new knowledge and skills	Avoiding new knowledge and skills
Maintaining continuity	Experiencing unnecessary continuity
Creating new choices	Limiting new choices
Finding opportunities for growth	Refusing opportunities for growth

role, which may be welcomed or seen as "premature" and not one that the person sees as positive. Table 18-6 compares healthy transitions and unhealthy transitions.

Several nursing interventions are available to assist older adults with transitions, including the following:

- Assess the nature of the transition and provide ongoing support during the transitional period.
- Identify resources needed to acquire new skills and knowledge.
- Assist with mobilization of formal and informal resources (e.g., family, friends, or church).

Institutionalization

Institutionalization usually refers to the placement of people in a nursing home or care facility when they cannot care for themselves any longer and they cannot return to an independent life in the community. Only about 5% of the older adult population live in nursing homes, but the proportion increases rapidly with age, from 1% of people 65 to 74 years of age, to 6% of those 75 to 84 years of age, to more than 20% of those 85 years of age or older (NCHS, 1995). The use of nursing homes increases as limitations in ADLs increase. Nursing home residents are most likely to be older, female, and white and to have been living alone with an income below poverty level. Almost 80% of nursing home residents have some type of mental disorder.

Institutionalization is often a last resort when the care of an older relative has exhausted a family. Insurance policies for long-term care are becoming available, but they are expensive and do not help those who are already old. Medicare does not provide for institutionalization, but when resources are spent, the resident becomes eligible for Medicaid. The issue of long-term care is of great concern to older adults at this time.

Family Issues

Generally, most older adults up to 75 years of age do more for their children than their children need to do for them. However, if or when physical frailty becomes a problem, parent-child roles tend to become reversed, which can be a major source of stress for the family. Daughters or daughters-in-law usually become the primary caregivers (Brakman, 1994), which is sometimes at considerable financial and emotional cost. Lost wages are compounded by the loss of job-related benefits such as Social Security, a company-related pension, or medical insurance.

Although older caregivers may not have the role conflicts or strain of younger caregivers, they have a lesser physical capacity. Usually, a long relationship has existed between the caregiver and the person requiring care and siblings may show amazing mental strength and devotion. However, they are often frail and vulnerable physically, they have their own chronic diseases or life-threatening illness, and they are at great risk for additional health problems from the stress and burdens of caregiving. Community support services should be used to relieve strain. An older caregiver is only one accident or health incident away from institutionalization for himself or herself and the person requiring care.

The QOL for the frail older adult may be substantially increased when a family member gives care. The older adult often feels wanted, comfortable, and in familiar surroundings. He or she has more freedom and personal control with family than in an institution. With the increase of home health services, including house calls by physicians, accessible advice and treatment are more easily available, which satisfies both the client and caregiver.

For the caregiver, benefits can include the personal satisfaction of fulfilling a family obligation and the avoidance of guilt for refusing to care for a parent or grandparent. Unfortunately, the benefits for the caregiver can be outweighed by the physical and emotional costs of caring for a sick older adult who can only become more dependent until death is seen as a release for everyone. The caregiver is three times more likely to report symptoms of depression than the recipient of care and four times more likely to report anger. Other expressed feelings include guilt, frustration, and sometimes desperation because the needs of the older adult may conflict with and take precedence over the caregiver's needs. Family caregivers may feel powerless in the situation or may feel like victims of circumstance. Stress arises from the following:

- increased workload;
- intrafamily conflicts and social embarrassments caused by the older adult's confused behavior;
- increased vigilance, worry, and concern over being responsible for someone who could hurt himself or herself or others; and
- interference in the marital, family, work, and community responsibilities of the caregiver caused by the older adult's care.

Many families care for their elders with little outside support and a lack of awareness about existing social programs. Family members are often so isolated from support systems that they are not aware that support is needed until they become exhausted. The literature strongly encourages extension of existing programs, creation of new programs, and tax credits or financial reimbursement to support the care of frail elders by family members.

Death and Bereavement

Old age is a time of adjusting to loss. In the natural order of things, loss of parents is followed by loss of spouse, siblings, friends, contemporaries, and ultimately, the individual's own death. A new phenomenon is the loss of adult children who have become aged. The effects of bereavement in older adults may not be expressed for some months after the death of a spouse or loved one and may continue for several years.

Many older adults turn to churches, synagogues, and other religious institutions at this time. Ministers, priests, rabbis, and other religious leaders have much experience helping people through the grief process. Support groups for widows and widowers are often provided by religious organizations and are usually available for anyone in need. Other resources include secular support groups, private groups, or individual therapy.

Elder Abuse

Elder abuse is present throughout the United States and it affects two million older adults each year (Berliner, 1999). This figure will undoubtedly increase as the numbers of older adults rise. Elder abuse occurs in private homes and in institutional settings.

Mistreatment or *abuse* is defined as acts of commission through infliction of harm or acts of omission through neglect. Abuse generally falls into the following five categories (Berliner, 1999):

1. Physical abuse: beatings, burns, rape, misuse of restraints, and misuse of sedatives.
2. Psychological abuse: threats, isolation, insults, and fear.
3. Financial abuse: theft of money or property or mismanaging assets.
4. Neglect: not providing food, health care, medications, and assistance with personal care.
5. Violation of personal rights: not letting the older adult make his or her own decisions.

Most states have laws requiring the mandatory reporting of elder abuse often based on child abuse statutes. However, these laws are often minimally enforced. Elder abuse is less likely to be reported than child abuse, but public and professional awareness of the problem is growing. Studies have shown that older adults are very unlikely to report abuse and only 8% to 25% of cases are reported. Reasons cited for underreporting include love for the abuser, shame or embarrassment, and a desire to protect the abuser. Furthermore, older adults may fear retaliation or nursing home placement, or they may think no one will believe them (Berliner, 1999).

In most cases the abuser is a caregiver who is either a close family member or provider in a nursing home. Several situations may lead to abuse. Stress of the caregiver is often cited because providing care may lead to exhaustion, anger, and frustration. Financial problems may compound the stress. The caregiver also frequently has a history of drug and alcohol use or a personal or family history of abuse. Risk factors include the victim's dependency on the caregiver, confusion, incontinence, frailty, illness, and mental disabilities (McEwen, 1998).

Detection of elder abuse is often difficult. The signs of abuse may be subtle and hard to identify. The following are possible indicators of elder abuse (Campbell and Landenburger, 2000):

- unexplained or repeated injury;
- discrepancies between injury and explanation;
- inappropriate use of medications (i.e., overuse or underuse);
- fear of the caregiver;
- untreated wounds;
- evidence of poor care, withdrawal, and passivity;
- failure to seek appropriate medical care;
- contractures resulting from immobility or restraints; and
- unwillingness or inability of the caregiver to meet the patient's needs.

Time spent observing the interaction between an older adult and a caregiver and a personal interview alone with the older adult can aid in the assessment process. A nurse suspecting abuse may be placed in a difficult ethical and legal position if the older adult requests that the abuse not be reported.

Prevention is important in cases of elder abuse. When possible, the nurse should work to promote older adults' independence and family functioning to support positive interactions and relationships. The nurse should identify older adults and families at risk and promote maximum functioning and coping of both the older adult and the family. This may include referral to appropriate community agencies for respite care to help alleviate caregiver stress. In known or suspected cases of elder abuse, the nurse must intervene to protect the older adult and prevent reoccurrence of abuse.

ABUSE ASSOCIATED WITH INCREASED RISK OF DEATH FOR OLDER ADULTS
A groundbreaking study by researchers from Cornell University and Yale University compared mortality rates of abused older adults with those of a matched control of nonabused older adults. The findings indicate that although no older adults in the study died directly as a result of abuse, a general increased risk of death existed in mistreated older adults.

Continued

In the study, people seen for mistreatment or self-neglect had poorer survival rates and an increased risk of death. Specifically, mistreated older adults had a risk of dying 3.1 times greater than those with no reported mistreatment. The self-neglected group had a risk of dying 1.7 times greater. The study noted that the increase in risk takes into account factors associated with death in older adults, including dementia, depression, chronic disease, functional problems, and SES.

From National Institute on Aging: *Abuse associated with increase risk of death for older people,* NIH New Release, August 4, 1998, The Author, www.nih.gov/nia/news/pr/1998/08-04.htm.

Crime and Older Adults

Although older adults are the least likely of all age groups in the United States to experience crime, crime is a concern to this population. Each year about two million older adults are crime victims. They are particularly vulnerable to fraud, robbery, personal theft, and burglary (NCHS, 1999). Older adults are easy targets for crime because physical frailty and mental confusion make them less likely to fight back. Also, many older adults reside in deteriorating neighborhoods with high crime rates.

Recovery from being a victim of crime takes a long time. Physical injuries in older adults take longer to heal than in younger people and the emotional scars may last forever. The fear of being victimized is often enough to precipitate withdrawal, isolation, and depression. Economic and property loss may never be regained. Older adults can take the following steps to reduce the threat of becoming a crime victim (NIH and NIA, 1999):

■ Lock doors and windows with substantial locks.
■ Have monthly pension or Social Security checks sent by direct deposit.
■ Do not carry a lot of cash; try not to carry a purse.
■ Do not wear good jewelry, furs, and other valuables in questionable areas.
■ Do not take money from a bank account based on request or advice of a stranger because many scams and con games use variable approaches.
■ Stay away from deals that ask for money up front and promise success.

■ Check with the Better Business Bureau before investing.
■ Do not give a credit card or bank account number over the phone to people selling a product or asking for a contribution.
■ Do not be taken in by quick cures for health problems.
■ Report suspected crimes to local police.

PUBLIC POLICY AND LEGISLATION AFFECTING OLDER ADULTS

Legislation, bills, and amendments to previously passed legislation affecting older adults takes innumerable forms. The acts discussed here have the most direct influence on the health of older adults and the health care system.

Social Security Act

Originally passed in 1935, the **Social Security Act** has been amended many times. It is administered by agencies within the USDHHS and includes the SSA and the HCFA. Most employed people are enrolled automatically in the Social Security program, which is financed by contributions from employers, employees, and the self-employed.

Part of the Social Security contribution is designated for Medicare, which is the world's largest health insurance program and provides health services for 39 million Americans. Medicare provides health insurance for those 65 years of age and older, those who are disabled, and those with end-stage renal disease (HCFA, 2000). Medicare is divided into the following three parts:

1. *Medicare Part A* covers inpatient hospital services, short-term care in skilled nursing facilities, postinstitutional home health care, and hospice care. Part A costs are met through payroll taxes; it is automatic for most people and covers most of the cost of hospital care and certain kinds of care after discharge. The patient must pay a large deductible ($776 per each benefit period in 2000) and coinsurance ($194 per day for the sixty-first through the ninetieth day per benefit period) for hospital coverage (access www.hcfa.gov/stats/mdedco00.htm).
2. *Medicare Part B* covers physician services, outpatient hospital services, home health care not covered by Part A, and a variety of other medical

services such as diagnostical tests, durable medical equipment, and ambulance needs. Part B
requires a monthly premium ($45.50 in 2000), a
deductible of $100 per year, and coinsurance of
20% of the approved amount for the service
provided (HCFA, 2000).
3. *Medicare Part C* (i.e., Medicare+Choice) is the
newest component of Medicare. It was established by the Balanced Budget Act of 1997 and is
composed of managed care and other health plan
choices for beneficiaries through an open enrollment process. Under Part C, benefits are available
through coordinated care plans, medical savings
accounts plans, and private fee-for-service plans
(HCFA, 2000).

Poor older adults are eligible for Medicaid
coverage for Medicare Part B premiums and the
deductibles and copayments if treatment is needed.
The criteria vary from state to state and may be
obtained from state Medicaid offices through the
Qualified Medicare Beneficiary (QMB) program. For
people who exceed the QMB limits, options are
Medicare supplement (i.e., Medigap) insurance policies or joining an HMO or competitive medical plan
(CMP), which receives Medicare payments in exchange for providing care.

Older Americans Act

Signed into law by President Johnson in 1965, the
Older Americans Act established the Administration
on Aging (AoA) within the USDHHS. The AoA's
purpose is to identify the needs, concerns, and
interests of older adults and coordinate available
federal resources to meet those needs. Amendments to
the Act in 1973 established area agencies on aging to
provide local planning and control of programs,
which must include nutrition services either as
home-delivered meals or in communal settings. Mul-
tipurpose senior centers nationwide are sites for not
only nutrition programs but also recreational, social,
and health programs; housing assistance; counseling;
and information services, which are all mandated by
the Act (Title III).

Other requirements of the Act are the development of employment opportunities for low-income
older adults by means of the community service
employment programs (Title V) and the establishment of programs for training personnel and supporting research (Title VI). Amendments passed in

1984 instruct area agencies on aging to plan for
community-based programs to help older adults
remain in their homes and provide supportive services to people with Alzheimer's disease and their
families.

National priority services for older adults include
transportation, home services, legal and other counseling services, and residential repair and renovation
programs. The target population is people older than
60 years of age with the greatest economic or social
needs, especially low-income minorities, but the
provisions of the Act benefit all older adults through
response to community needs.

Research on Aging Act

The **Research on Aging Act** (1974) created the
National Institute on Aging (NIA) within the NIH.
The Act's purpose is to conduct and support biomedical, social, and behavioral research and training
related to the aging process and the diseases and other
special problems and needs of older adults. The
philosophy of the NIA is to view aging as a
fundamental human process about which much more
knowledge is needed and to reduce current rates of
morbidity and institutionalization. The NIA is a
source of grant funding for nurses conducting research on problems of aging, which is discussed in the
next section.

Other Legislation

A maze of legislation has had an influence on
people as they age. Two important acts address
people still in the workforce, but have implications
for older adults. The Age Discrimination in Employment Act (1967) provided workers 40 to 65
years of age with the same opportunities as younger
employees for participation in employee benefit
plans. In 1978, amendments raised the mandatory
retirement age to 70 years. In 1986, mandatory
retirement at any age was abolished for almost all
workers.

Employee pension rights in private pension
plans were safeguarded by the Employee Retirement
Income Security Act (1974), which set minimum
federal standards for private plans. The Retirement
Equity Act (1984) increased protection for the
surviving spouse or former spouse of pension-
eligible workers and the Tax Reform Act (1986)
reduced vesting requirements for pension eligibil-

ity. These provisions are expected to eventually maintain the income of many older adults. Public sector pension plans are subject to a somewhat different set of rules and have a complexity of variables that may leave employees and spouses a lesser claim to benefits.

RESEARCH ON AGING

Research focusing on older adults and the process of aging is desperately needed. The NIA set research priorities for aging-related study and divided them into four general areas (biology, neuroscience and neuropsychology, behavior and social research, and geriatrics). Box 18-4 shows specific topics currently funded by the NIA in each of these general areas.

Nursing research on various aspects of health care needs and issues of older adults are supported by the NINR and other government and private

agencies. The following are published focus areas for funding for 2000 by the NINR:

■ chronic illness or conditions (i.e., enhancing adherence to diabetes self-management behaviors and care of children with asthma),
■ behavioral changes and interventions (i.e., bio-behavioral research for effective sleep in health and illness and disparities of infant mortality rates), and
■ response to compelling public health concerns (i.e., end of life and palliative care research, collaborative clinical trials network, and training and career development).

Research areas specific to older adults funded by the NINR include studies on cultural and ethnic issues related to aging and health care delivery, caregivers, effective nursing intervention, and medication compliance. Box 18-5 lists recent research studies funded by the NINR pertaining to senior health.

BOX **18-4**

National Institutes of Aging: Examples of Research Priorities

Biology
■ Cell biology: membranes and membrane receptors, growth factors, skin and cartilage, and intercellular communication
■ Endocrinology: age-related changes in hormone production, metabolism, and action; biology of menopause; and age-related changes in control of prostate growth
■ Genetics: characterization of longevity assurance genes, genetics of aging, and longevity
■ Immunology: regulation of immune specificity, response of immune system to biochemical stimuli, and autoimmune diseases
■ Nutrition and metabolism: nutritional factors in age-related diseases
Behavioral and Social Research
■ Cognitive functioning and aging: behavior genetics, cognition interventions, and memory strategies
■ Personality and social psychological aging: gender, race, and SES and health
■ Demography of aging: socioeconomic differentials in mortality rates; changes in age structure of populations
■ Older people in society: consequence of cultural and social institutions; intergenerational relationships
Neuroscience and Neurobiology
■ Fundamental neuroscience: mechanisms of neural cell death
■ Sleep and biological rhythms: pathogenesis of sleep disorders of older people
■ Motor function: movement disorders in aging
■ Clinical studies: diagnosis, treatment, and management of patients with Alzheimer's disease
Geriatrics
■ Osteoporosis: clinical research to identify age-associated process in bone loss and osteoporosis
■ Endocrinology: physiological processes and sequelae of menopause
■ Cardiovascular/pulmonary/renal: research on alterations in blood pressure regulation, orthostatic hypertension, changes with age in kidneys, and pulmonary function

ROLES OF THE COMMUNITY HEALTH NURSE IN CARING FOR OLDER ADULTS

A primary role of the community health nurse is to act as an advocate and a resource for health care of older adults and their families. Other important roles include educator for the client and community, case manager, facilitator, data collector, researcher, case finder, coordinator of care between agencies, and provider of clinical nursing care. Nurses should also seek to be board members of organizations that affect their clients and be political lobbyists. Given the constraints of working for government agencies, within which most community health employment lies, this may require ingenuity, a valuable characteristic of community health nurses.

BOX **18-5**

Recent Research Studies Funded by the NINR

Cost Impacts of Enhancing Alzheimer's Disease Caregiving (Harrow, 1999)

This was a study of interventions of the Resources of Enhancing Alzheimer's Caregiver Health (REACH) project to measure the cost of community-based caregiving for Alzheimer's disease across ethnically and geographically diverse populations and calculate and compare the cost-effectiveness ratios for two interventions with technology components.

PREP: Family-Based Care for Frail Older Persons (Archbold, 1999)

This was a randomized controlled efficacy trial of PREP and a home health intervention designed to increase preparedness, enrichment, and predictability in family care for frail older adults. PREP has the following three parts: family and nurse working together, 24-hour PREP advice line, and follow-up contact by the nurse.

Nonkin Caregivers to Dependent Older Adults (Barker, 1999)

This involved exploration of the dynamics between aged community-dwelling care receivers and their nonkin caregivers recruited from probate court, home care agencies, voluntary organizations, and other individuals in the general community.

Testing a geriatric advance practice nurse (GAPN) Care Model for Elders with Hip Fracture (Krichbaum, 1999)

This was a test of a model of time, sequence, and coordination of health care given to people over 65 years of age who fractured a hip. Interventions include use of a care management protocol for improving recovery outcomes in older adult clients and use of a gerontological advanced practice nurse as case manager.

Behavioral Interventions for Insomnia in Older Adults (Epstein, 1999)

This was a study to evaluate and compare the efficacy of single interventions (i.e., stimulus control instructions or sleep restriction therapy) and multicomponent intervention (i.e., stimulus control instructions and sleep restriction therapy) for sleep maintenance insomnia in community dwelling older adults.

Alzheimer's Caregivers: An Attribution Analysis (Lilly, 1999)

This was an examination of the relationships between caregiver controllability attributions, affect, and response behaviors of caregivers of people with Alzheimer's disease.

Relocation of Ethnic Elders: Decisions Sequelae (Johnson, 1999)

This was a cross-sectional, descriptive study to delineate the differences across ethnic groups in formal and informal support sources used before and during relocation. Factors were promotion and prevention of relocation and the decision-making process of relocation.

Teaching Resourcefulness to Chronically Ill Elders (Zauszniewski, 1999)

This was research to test the effectiveness of two interventions in a randomly selected group of older adults in assisted living facilities. The study evaluates learned resourcefulness training and help-seeking behavior training.

APPLICATION OF THE NURSING PROCESS

As described throughout this book, the nursing process can be used to plan and deliver care at the individual, family, aggregate, or community level. The principles of assessment, planning, implementation, and evaluation apply to whichever level is required. The following section demonstrates how the nursing process can be applied in directing health care for seniors.

Assessment

Data collection should be complete and systematic. A standardized form is often helpful, but the nurse must understand the reasoning, or theory base, behind the form to be able to adapt it to a situation outside the norm. The following common approaches are often helpful:

- Systems theory: with systems theory, the nurse examines a system, its subsystems and suprasystems, and its relationship with other systems. For example, if the primary focus is on the client as the system, the nurse may examine the client's biological, psychological, and social subsystems and the client's suprasystems, such as family interaction and neighborhood environment. The nurse is a part, or subsystem, of the health care system that has a relationship with the client. The interaction between the client and the health care system provides data for evaluating and planning desired outcomes.
- Epidemiological triad: in the epidemiological approach, the nurse analyzes the host, agent, and environment. This method is more easily used for one problem at a time. The client is the host, a particular problem is examined as the agent, and the environment includes all causes and possible solutions for the problem that affects the host.
- General problem solving: a third method is a problem-solving approach, which identifies strengths and weaknesses and compensates for weaknesses.

In practice, the nurse uses many theories concurrently. The principles of systems theory and the epidemiological triad can be identified in the case study at the end of this chapter.

Assessment of older adults must take aging changes into account and the nurse must measure data against norms for older adults. Assessment of older adults should include the following:

- medical history,
- physical examination,
- laboratory tests (e.g., blood and urine),
- functional assessment of vision and hearing,
- bowel and bladder control,
- nutrition,
- mental abilities (i.e., thinking, remembering, and reasoning),
- ADLs,
- gait and balance, and
- sleep habits.

The assessment should also include evaluation of emotional status, economic resources, and the need for community services (Norrgard, 1999). Nursing diagnoses stem from validated data.

Planning

Planning care and interventions are based on the assessment data and should consider all three levels of prevention. In community health, the nurse must set short- and long-term goals that are congruent with the desired outcomes of the client. A community health nurse works in the environment of the client, which adds complexity to the process. The nurse may have the patient's attention and respect, but compliance may not be good unless the patient sees value in outcomes desired by the nurse. The client, family, and the environment of the client will control the speed and depth of implementation of the nursing care plan.

Evaluation

Evaluation, as with every other step of the nursing process, is a joint activity of the client and nurse. It measures movement toward or away from specified goals and gives ongoing feedback that affects planning and intervention. Older adults may be slow to achieve progress because they suffer from one of many chronic health problems. In addition, chronic illness has a long-term time frame and the standard for evaluation may be the prevention of deterioration as opposed to a "cure." Community problems may have an even longer time frame, or they may be solved fairly quickly if a general problem affects a small group and the solution is inexpensive.

CASE STUDY

APPLICATION OF THE NURSING PROCESS

Mrs. Darren, a 75-year-old widow, was referred to the community health nurse by her physician, who did not believe she could care for herself sufficiently. Her diagnoses were hypertension, mild congestive heart failure, arthritis, and occasional confusion after transient ischemic attacks.

During the initial home visit, the nurse observed that Mrs. Darren lived in a run-down house in an inner-city neighborhood. The roof leaked and the house had no functioning heat unit. A rat was scrambling in the garbage. Mrs. Darren told the nurse that she did not have children and her only relative was a sister who lived with her family in another state. She was used to the neighborhood and knew her neighbors, but she was frightened of the teenagers who lingered when she took the bus to the supermarket to cash her Social Security check.

Mrs. Darren had Supplemental Security Income, Medicare, Medicaid, and food stamps. She ate mostly bread and butter and drank coffee, but she enjoyed fried chicken and oranges after going to the supermarket. Constipation was sometimes a problem and she took a laxative every night. She said she did not always remember whether she took her medication and held out a small bottle containing an assortment of pills of different colors, shapes, and sizes.

Assessment

With Mrs. Darren as the system, or central planning focus, the nurse identified her biopsychosocial subsystem strengths and weaknesses and looked for actual or potential connections to her family and community suprasystems. Considering aging theories, the nurse believed Mrs. Darren was undergoing disengagement from her physical and social circumstances and decided that this might reverse if her health could be maintained and her links to the community strengthened. On a practical level, the nurse also checked with Mrs. Darren's physician regarding the prescriptions and identified the assortment of pills by taking them to the pharmacist who filled the prescriptions.

By means of a problem-solving approach for data gathering, Mrs. Darren's assets were identified as the following:

- being basically able to care for herself,
- receiving medical treatment,
- receiving income from various sources, and
- being accustomed to the neighborhood and knowing her neighbors.

Her liabilities were more extensive, as follows:

- inadequate nutrition;
- confusion with medications and improper use of laxatives;
- condition of the house, which was not supportive of health;
- threat of violence in neighborhood and possibility of attack for her Social Security money;
- physical impairment resulting from age and illness;
- no children or other family living nearby;
- probable progression of confusion; and
- possibility of a major stroke at home while unattended.

Diagnoses and Planning

Diagnoses and related short- and long-term goals address Mrs. Darren's situation. The nurse wrote plans at the three levels of prevention for the diagnoses and included suggestions for intervention with families.

Individual
Diagnosis: Altered nutrition of less than body requirements, which was related to difficulty or inability to procure food

Short-Term Goal
Mrs. Darren will improve her diet to include an RDA of nutrients, including fiber and fluids as evidenced by diet recall and report regular bowel habits without use of laxatives.

Continued

Long-Term Goals

- Mrs. Darren will maintain a nutritionally adequate diet through self-care and use of community programs as evidenced by a steady weight and normal tests for nutritional status during physical examinations.
- Mrs. Darren will avoid inconsistency in her medication regimen related to forgetfulness and mild confusion.

Short-Term Goal

Mrs. Darren will identify medications and know when to take them as evidenced by demonstration to a nurse.

Long-Term Goal

Mrs. Darren will continue to take medications as ordered as evidenced by stabilization of disease processes and intermittent demonstration to a nurse.
Diagnosis: Potential for injury related to inadequate housing, possibility of robbery for Social Security money, aging, and progression of disease.

Short-Term Goal

Mrs. Darren will improve her home to allow healthy habitation, avoid robbery by varying her routine and using banking services, expand her social network, and maintain health care appointments.

Long-Term Goal

Mrs. Darren will explore sheltered housing for older adults and continue contact with a community health nurse and neighborhood friends.

Family
Diagnosis: Potential for injury to family unit related to unanticipated loss of interaction with Mrs. Darren because her health is declining and her residence is distant.

Short-Term Goal

The family's addresses are included in Mrs. Darren's record to facilitate emergency contact.

Long-Term Goal

Mrs. Darren will maintain family contact by mail, telephone, or possible visits.

Community
Diagnosis: Knowledge deficit of nutritional services related to lack of publicity of available nutritional programs for older adults.

Short-Term Goal

Identify existing community programs.

Long-Term Goal

Promote publicity campaign to advertise nutrition services for older adults in the community.
Diagnosis: Lack of support programs for medication consistency related to unrecognized need.

Short-Term Goal

Identify existing programs and memory aids for consistency with medication regimen.

Long-Term Goals

- Support community pharmacists in the campaign to increase public awareness of the need to take medications as prescribed.
- Identify and support programs that will assist with provision of prescribed medications for people who have difficulty obtaining prescriptions from a lack of insurance, money, transportation, or other problems.

Diagnosis: Lack of programs and resources for older adult residents of limited income related to cost of services and competition for limited funds.

Short-Term Goal

Identify existing programs for older adults in the community.

Long-Term Goal

Community groups work together to maximize use of resources.

Intervention

When the nurse discussed the nursing diagnoses and plans with Mrs. Darren, Mrs. Darren agreed with the short-term goals, but she was not sure that she wanted to leave her home for other housing or meet other people through community activities. However, she agreed that she would try.

During the course of the next few visits, the nurse explained basic nutritional principles and helped make a shopping list and menus for one week. Together they developed a plan to assist with medication scheduling. Referrals initiated by the nurse resulted in a greatly improved living situation. A financial advisor from the city's Supportive Services to the Elderly program encouraged Mrs. Darren to open a bank account for the direct deposit of her checks and showed her how to use it. A home health aide from the same program came for half a day each week to assist with shopping and cleaning. The sanitation department of the health district exterminated the rats, the local Area Agency on Aging fixed the roof, and a church-sponsored group painted the house and cleaned the yard. A small heater was purchased from the Salvation Army store and application was made to the utility company for help with bills during the winter months.

The nurse encouraged Mrs. Darren to talk about her earlier life during the nurse's visits. She had been widowed soon after her marriage when her husband was killed serving the army overseas and she had never remarried. She lived in the neighborhood where she grew up, although it had deteriorated over the years. She had worked as a secretary until her retirement and had no pension plan.

With this information, the nurse planned to increase Mrs. Darren's social contacts by introducing her to a group that met frequently and offered several activities she might enjoy. If she was unexpectedly absent, the group would check on her. A neighbor invited her to a senior center, where she became involved in a domino-playing group. Mrs. Darren allowed her name to be put on the waiting list for an apartment for older adults. With the other changes, the apartment was no longer a priority and Mrs. Darren could make a decision when an apartment became available.

Evaluation

With the nurse as intermediary and coordinator of community services, Mrs. Darren easily accepted help with the problems related to security and survival. When her home improvements were completed, Mrs. Darren was able to maintain herself more comfortably with the help of the weekly visit from the home health aide. The establishment of orderly routine, the companionship at the nutrition site, and safer financial arrangements increased Mrs. Darren's feelings of belonging and self-esteem. The nurse reduced her home visits, but maintained contact with Mrs. Darren during her visits to the health clinic for blood pressure checks and preventive health care to supplement her medical care.

Discussion with the home health aide informed the nurse of proposed funding cuts to the city's Supportive Services to the Elderly program, which would result in reduced services. The nurse spoke to the president of the district branch of the professional nurse's association, who notified the state level of the association to monitor funding on the state level. The association also assisted the nurse in working with other local agencies for older adults to establish a publicity campaign against proposed funding cuts through writing letters to the editors of local newspapers, speaking at public hearings on the city budget, and speaking at city council meetings. Although funds were reduced, the cuts were much less severe than they would have been without the campaign, and most services were able to continue, although with increased waiting time for admission of new clients.

Levels of Prevention

Primary
Goal: Promote good nutrition.

Individual
- Instruct about nutritional needs.
- Plan a shopping list and menus incorporating a prescribed diet for health problems.

Family
Instruct about nutritional needs of family members by age, sex, or special needs.

Community
Increase nutrition information where food is sold.
Goal: Promote safety and prevention of injury.
Continued

Individual
- Provide immunizations as appropriate.
- Provide community services for assistance to maintain property and prevent deterioration.
- Encourage a network of friends and family members.

Family
- Provide services of community health nurse or case manager.
- Provide counseling.
- Provide respite care.

Community
- Provide community education programs for older adults.
- Be aware of potential hazards for older adult residents and provide intervention as needed.

Secondary
Goal: Assess and treat nutrition-related disorders.

Individual
- Provide referral for assessment of possible nutrition-related disorders.
- Provide hospitalization or prescribed nutritional supplements for illness resulting from inadequate nutrition.

Family
Provide referral for nutritional assessment and counseling.

Community
Encourage emergency food supplies.
Goal: Diagnose and treat medication-related injuries.

Individual
- Provide referral for apparent overmedication or undermedication symptoms.
- Diagnose and treat drug or food reactions.

Family
Reassess the patient's understanding of medications.

Community
- Provide a 24-hour poison hotline.
- Provide an emergency department with 24-hour response.
- Provide medical services.

Tertiary
Goal: Maintain improved nutrition.

Individual
Encourage use of community services.

Family
- Encourage exchange of family recipes.
- Encourage attendance of home economics classes.

Community
- Provide campaigns for nutritional awareness and healthy eating.
- Encourage the eating of healthy snacks in food machines.
- Encourage use of funding of community food services for aggregates or emergencies.
- Encourage use of services providing access to food (e.g., food banks, MOW, and food stamps).
- Encourage use of transportation to grocery stores or nutrition services.

Goal: Be consistent with prescribed medications and prevent medication error.

Individual
- Provide written and oral instructions when medications are dispensed at the level of understanding and in the language of the client.
- Have the client repeat instructions to the health care provider.

Family
Have the client repeat instructions to family members.

Community
Provide a community education program about understanding medications.

SUMMARY

This chapter has taken a broad approach to describe the health care needs of older adults. Increased longevity coupled with aging Baby Boomers will cause the number of older adults to continue to rise dramatically. Community health nurses must be aware of characteristics of older adults that may either be beneficial to their health or put them at risk for poor health. The nurse can then work to modify those characteristics for the best possible outcome.

In addition, the nurse should understand common health problems and be aware of health promotion or illness prevention measures to address these potential problems. Finally, he or she should be aware of community resources and legislation that can positively influence the health of older adults.

LEARNING ACTIVITIES

1. In small groups, review the case history of Mrs. Darren presented in this chapter. Discuss assessment using different theories. What other information would be helpful? What other services may she need (e.g., dentistry)? Where are these services located in the community? What interventions could have taken place earlier in her life to prevent or delay some of her problems now? What changes should be made in the health system to improve access at all stages of life? What would a comprehensive health system look like?

2. Read the local newspaper and a weekly news magazine. Keep a scrapbook of articles about legislation that affects older adults. How many articles or advertisements highlight information of specific interest to older adults (e.g., products and services)?

3. Talk to police officers in small towns or incorporated cities about older adults in their communities. Ask what facilities are available for older adults. Be prepared to discuss needs and offer solutions. Look for community strengths and weaknesses.

4. Talk to a minister, priest, rabbi, imam, or other religious leader in the community. Ask about contributions to the congregation and the community made by older members and programs provided for older adults. Look for resource networking.

5. Visit a private retirement community. Talk to the social director and arrange to interview and record the reminiscences of some residents. Prepare a journal of interviews and give copies to those interviewed. Do the same in a public-funded housing community for older adults. Note the similarities and dissimilarities of the stories. Ask a community librarian for local history related by older adults.

6. Investigate activity and exercise programs in senior congregate housing. Evaluate or design and implement a program for its effectiveness in keeping all residents active and able to live independently.

REFERENCES

Adequate Nutrition for the Elderly: *Hearing before the Select Committee on Aging, House of Representatives, July 30, 1992,* Comm Pub No 102-890, Washington, DC, 1992, US Government Printing Office.

American Association of Retired Persons: *Determine your nutritional health,* 2000, The Author, www.aarp.org/contfacts/health/nutrithealth.html.

American Association of Retired Persons, Administration on Aging: *Profile of older Americans,* Washington, DC, 1999, The Author.

Anderson EG: Reflections on a practice going geriatric, *Geriatrics* 44:91, 1989.

Archbold PG: *Family-based care for frail older persons,* Grant No 1R01AG17909-01, 1999, NINR, www.nih.gov/ninr/1999grants/pdf/geron/geron_parchbold.pdf.

Barker JC: *Nonkin caregivers to dependent older adults,* Grant No 5R01NR04278-04, 1999, NINR, www.nih.gov/ninr/1999grants/pdf/geron/geron_jbarker.pdf.

Berliner H: Abuse of older adults, *Clinical Reference Systems* August 1, 5, 1999.

Blomquist KB: Prevention: older adults. In Knollmeuller RN, editor: *Prevention across the life span,* Washington, DC, 1993, ANA.

Bradsher K: Gap in wealth in U.S. called widest in West, *New York Times* 1A, April 17, 1995.

Brakman SV: Adult daughter caregivers, *Hastings Center Report* 24:26, 1994.

Bull MJ: Use of formal community services by elders and their family caregivers 2 weeks following hospital discharge, *J Adv Nurs* 19:503, 1994.

Campbell J, Landenburger K: Violence and human abuse. In Stanhope M, Lancaster J: *Community health nursing: promoting the health of aggregates, families, and individuals,* ed 5, St. Louis, 2000, Mosby.

Centers for Disease Control and Prevention: Adult immunizations, *Morb Mortal Wkly Rep* 44:741, 1995.

Centers for Disease Control and Prevention: Reasons reported by Medicare beneficiaries for not receiving influenza and pneumococcal vaccinations: United States, 1996, *Morb Mortal Wkly Rep* 48(Oct 8):886, 1999.

Centers for Disease Control and Prevention, National Center for Health Statistics: *1994 national health interview survey: second supplement on aging,* Atlanta, 1996, The Authors.

Centers for Disease Control and Prevention, National Center for Health Statistics: *1997 summary: national hospital discharge survey,* USDHHS Pub No 99-1250, Rockville, Md, 1999a, The Authors.

Centers for Disease Control and Prevention, National Center for Health Statistics: *National ambulatory medical care survey: 1997 summary,* USDHHS Pub No 99-1250, Rockville, Md, 1999b, The Authors.

Centers for Disease Control and Prevention, National Center for Health Statistics: *Characteristics of elderly home health care users: data from the 1996 National Home and Hospice Care Survey,* USDHHS Pub No 2000-1250, Rockville, Md, 1999c, The Authors.

Centers for Disease Control and Prevention, National Center for Health Statistics: *Health United States, 1999,* PHS 99-1232, October 13, 1999, Hyattsville Md, 1999d, US Government Printing Office.

Dalaker J, Naifeh M, US Census Bureau: *Poverty in the United States, 1997: current population reports,* Series P60-201, Washington, DC, 1998, US Government Printing Office.

Ebersole P, Hess P: *Toward healthy aging,* St. Louis, 1998, Mosby.

Eliopolus C: *Gerontological nursing,* ed 4, Philadelphia, 1996, J.B. Lippincott.

Epstein DR: *Behavioral interventions for insomnia in older adults,* Grant No 5R29NR04951-02, 1999, NINR, www.nih.gov/ninr/1999grants/pdf/sleep/sleep_depstein.pdf.

Escher JE, O'Dell C, Gambert SR: Typical geriatric accidents and how to prevent them, *Geriatrics* 44(5): 54, 1989.

Fries JF: Aging, natural death, and the compression of morbidity, *N Engl J Med* 303:130, 1980.

Gallup Organization: *Survey of new product needs among older Americans,* Princeton, NJ, 1983, The Author.

Harrow BS: *Cost impacts of enhancing Alzheimer's disease caregiving,* Grant No 5R29NRO4350-03, 1999, NINR, www.nih.gov/ninr/1999grants/pdf/neuro/neuro_bharrow.pdf.

Health Care Financing Administration: *A profile of Medicare,* Rockville, Md, 2000, USDHHS, HCFA.

Henry RG, Ceridan B: Delivering dental care to nursing home and homebound patients, *Dent Clin North Am* 38:537, 1994.

Hussey LC: Minimizing effects of low literacy on medication knowledge and compliance among the elderly, *Clin Nurs Res* 3:132, 1994.

Jancin B: Raising the elderly's immunization rate, *Family Practice News* 29:1, 1999.

Johnson RA: *Relocation of ethnic elders: decisions sequelae,* Grant No 7R29NR04435-02, 1999, NINR, www.nih.gov/ninr/1999grants/pdf/geron/geron_rjohnson.pdf.

Krichbaum KE: *Testing a GAPN care model for elders with hip fracture,* Grant No 5K01NR00094-03, 1999, NINR, www.nih.gov/ninr/1999grants/pdf/arthritis/arthritis_kkrichbaum.pdf.

Kumar S: World Health Organization sets the agenda for care of the elderly, *Lancet* 353(9161):1339, 1999.

Lashley ME: Elderly persons in the community. In Smith CM, Mauer FA, editors: *Community health nursing: theory and practice,* Philadelphia, 1995, W.B. Saunders.

Lilly ML: *Alzheimer's caregivers: an attribution analysis,* Grant No 5F31NR07402-02, 1999, NINR, www.nih.gov/ninr/1999grants/pdf/neuro/neuro_mlilly.pdf.

Mackowiak ED et al: Compliance devices preferred by elderly patients, *Am Pharm NS* 34:47, 1994.

Marcantonio ER et al: Factors associated with unplanned hospital readmission among patients 65 years and older in a Medicare managed care plan, *Am J Med* 107(1):13, 1999.

McEwen M: *Community-based nursing practice,* Philadelphia, 1998, W.B. Saunders.

National Center for Health Statistics: *Health, United States: 1999,* Hyattsville, Md, 1999, USDHHS, NCHS.

National Center for Health Statistics: *Trends in the health of older Americans: United States, 1994,* Analytic and Epidemiologic Studies, Series 3, No 30, Hyattsville, Md, 1995, The Author.

National Institutes of Health: *Estrogen replacement therapy not effective for treatment of Alzheimer's disease in some women,* NIH News Release, Feb 22, 2000, The Author, www.nih.gov/nia/news/pr/2000/02-22.htm.

National Institutes of Health, National Institute on Aging: *New census report shows exponential growth in number of centenarians,* News Release, June 16, 1999, The Author, www.nih.gov/nia/news/pr/1999/16-16.htm.

National Institute of Mental Health: *Older adults: depression and suicide facts,* 1999, The Author, www.nimh.nih.gov/publicat/elderlydepsuicide/cfm.

National Institute of Mental Health: *Suicide facts,* 1999, The Author, www.nimh.nih.gov/research/suifact.htm.

National Institute on Aging: *Abuse associated with increase risk of death for older people,* NIH New Release, August 4, 1998, The Author, www.nih.gov/nia/news/pr/1998/08-04.htm.

National Institute on Aging: *Aging and your eyes,* 2000a, The Author, www.nih.gov/nia/health/agepages/eyees.htm.

National Institute on Aging: *Depression: a serious but treatable illness,* 2000b, The Author, www.nih.gov/nia/health/agepages/depresti.htm.

National Institute on Aging: *Hearing and older people,* 1999a, The Author, www.nih.gov/nia/health/agepages/hearing.htm.

National Institute on Aging: *Hyperthermia: a hot weather hazard for older people,* 1999b, The Author, www.nih.gov/nia/health/agepages/hyperthe.htm.

National Institute on Aging: *Preventing hypothermia,* 1999c, The Author, www.nih.gov/nia/health/agepages/hypothe.htm.

National Research Council: *Recommended dietary allowances,* ed 10, Report of the Subcommittee of the Tenth Edition of the RDAs, Food and Nutrition Board, Commission on Life Sciences, Washington, DC, 1989, National Academy Press.

Norrgard C: Geriatric assessment, *Clinical Reference Systems* No 628, July 1, 1999.

Office of Technology Assessment: *The use of preventive services by the elderly: preventive health services under Medicare (paper 2),* Washington, DC, 1989, Health Program, Office of Technology Assessment, Congress of the United States.

Phillips SC: Preventing depression: a program for African American elders with chronic pain, *Fam Community Health* 22(4):57, 2000.

Physician Payment Review Commission: *Annual report to Congress,* Washington, DC, 1994, The Commission.

Shay K: Identifying the needs of the elderly dental patient: the geriatric dental assessment, *Dent Clin North Am* 38:499, 1994.

US Census Bureau: *Poverty 1998,* 2000, The Author, www.census.gov/hhes/poverty/poverty98/pv98est1.htm.

US Department of Health and Human Services: *Healthy people 2010,* conference edition, Washington, DC, 2000, US Government Printing Office.

US Department of Health and Human Services, Agency for Health Care Policy and Research: *Urinary incontinence in adults: clinical practice guidelines,* HCPR Pub No 92-0038, Rockville, Md, 1992, AHCPR.

US Department of Health and Human Services, National Institute of Mental Health: *Mental health: report of the Surgeon General,* Rockville, Md, 1999, USDHHS, SAMHSA, CMHS, NIH, NIMH.

US Senate Special Committee on Aging: *Aging America: trends and projections,* Pub No LR 3377 [991]-D12198, Washington, DC, 1991, USDHHS.

Walker BL: Preventing falls, *RN* 61(5):40, 1998.

Zauszniewski JA: *Teaching resourcefulness to chronically ill elders,* Grant No 5R01NR04428-02, 1999, NINR, www.nih.gov/ninr/1999grants/pdf/chronic/chronic_jzauszniewski.pdf.

19

Populations Affected by Disabilities

Linda L. Treloar and Barbara Artinian

Linda L. Treloar and Barbara Artinian

OBJECTIVES

Upon completion of this chapter, the reader will be able to do the following:

1. Differentiate between medical model and sociopolitical or social construct definitions for disability.
2. Describe historical attitudes and perspectives surrounding disability that have contributed to devaluation and disempowerment of people with disabilities.
3. Compare and contrast short- and long-term, health-related, disabling conditions.
4. Discuss key federal legislation applicable to people with disabilities.
5. Identify selected health care and social issues that influence people with disabilities' ability to live and thrive in the community.
6. Apply a nursing model that integrates a holistic focus promoting the health and well-being of people with disabilities and their families.

KEY TERMS

activities of daily living (ADLs)
Americans with Disabilities Act (ADA)
disability
handicap
impairment
Individuals with Disabilities Education Act (IDEA)
instrumental activities of daily living (IADLs)
Intersystem Model
reasonable accommodations
Work Incentives Improvement Act (WIIA)

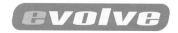

http://evolve.elsevier.com/Nies/

After developing an incomplete spinal cord injury following an automobile accident, a 29-year-old man named Jim progressed from visible physical disability and paralysis to continued disability without the use of a wheelchair. Jim explained his progression, which follows:

> You know it's really weird. In some ways it's hard to enter into that wheelchair life, to go into that life and then come back out of it again. I entered into a whole other realm [life with paralysis] that I'd only observed. I stepped into the unknown and pulled back out of it again. Yet, one foot is still in that world
>
> (Treloar, 1999c, p. 189).

According to Jim, disability may create a "whole other realm," or an "unknown" world. Like Jim, most people lack awareness of the divergence of perceptual worlds that disability creates and the historical, sociopolitical context and culture that surrounds disability. Nurses may think they understand disability, but this may not be true. Attitudes toward disability influence people's responses to and care for others; therefore nurses should consider the following self-assessment.

SELF-ASSESSMENT: RESPONSES TO DISABILITY

What comes to mind when you think of *someone with a disability?* Focus on those sights, sounds, and smells. What are your thoughts and feelings? List characteristics using adjectives or short phrases to describe people with disabilities. What values, customs, and traditions are promoted or blocked by members of the group?

Picture yourself as a *person with a disability.* What do you notice? What concerns you? How do others respond to you? Who or what kinds of supports can you rely on for help? What do you wish others understood about disability?

Now imagine living in a *family affected by disability.* How does disability affect you and your family? What types of activities does your family engage in that are associated with disability? What kinds of family or personal activities does disability make difficult to perform? How do people respond to your disability or your family member's disability? What do you wish others understood about living in a family affected by disability? What kinds of social and personal supports do you have? What kinds of supports do you wish were available to families like yours?

Think about your health as a *person with a disability.* What are your health care concerns and needs? What has been your experience with the health care system and its providers? What do you want nurses and others to understand about living with disability? How might health care professionals devalue and disempower you? How can nurses and other health care providers care for you in a way that conveys respect and concern for you as a person?

What is the experience of *living with disability within your community?* What social or environmental barriers related to disability exist? How can nurses intervene to reduce or eliminate these barriers? What major roles can nurses perform in working within an interdisciplinary team model that forms alliances with the patient and family affected by disability? What implications exist for health care policy and research related to disability?

Health care professionals are taught to assess and provide interventions that promote health and they usually believe they know what people with disabilities need. However, the actions of health care professionals may convey different messages to people with disabilities and their families. Regardless of their professional experience or familiarity with disability, patients may ask how they can understand disability if they are not themselves disabled.

Disability affects people irrespective of class, culture, race, or economic level. Depending on the term's definition, disability affects approximately 20% of Americans. Disability increases with age and it is estimated that 50% of all Americans will probably have some form of disability at some time. This chapter provides content that community health nurses can use in a variety of settings to provide knowledgeable, appropriate care for people with disabilities and their families.

DEFINITIONS AND MODELS FOR DISABILITY

According to the International Classification of Impairments, Disabilities, and Handicaps (ICIDH) (Pope and Tarlov, 1991), a **disability** involves any restriction on, or lack of ability to perform an activity in a normal manner or within the normal range. An anatomical, mental, or psychological loss or another abnormality is an **impairment**. A **handicap** is a disadvantage resulting from impairment or disability. In comparing these concepts, an impairment affects a human organ on a micro level; disability affects a

TABLE 19-1

Terminology for Impairment, Disability, and Handicap

Characteristic	Impairment	Disability	Handicap
Definition	Physical deviation from normal structure, function, physical organization, or development	Restricted ability to perform an activity in normal or expected manner; what activity the person cannot perform	Disadvantage imposed by impairment or disability related to environment
Measurability	Objective and measurable	May be objective and measurable	Not objective or measurable; is an experience related to the responses of others
Illustrations	Spina bifida, spinal cord injury, amputation, and detached retina	Cannot walk unassisted; uses crutches and/or a manual or power wheelchair; blindness	Reflects physical and psychological characteristics of the person, culture, and specific circumstances
Level of analysis	Micro level (e.g., body organ)	Individual level (e.g., person)	Macro level (e.g., societal)

person on an individual level; and a handicap involves society on a macro level of analysis (Batavia, 1993). Table 19-1 compares and contrasts these definitions related to disability.

A similar framework for disability is described by the Nagi model, which uses functional limitations to determine disability. Whether or not a disability becomes a handicap depends on how the person functions in the community. Impairments do not necessarily result in disabilities and disabilities do not necessarily produce handicaps. Although the ICIDH and Nagi frameworks recognize that a person's ability to perform a socially expected activity reflects characteristics of the individual and the larger social and physical environment, they are commonly criticized for their medical emphasis and definitional inconsistencies (Pope and Tarlov, 1991).

National Agenda for Prevention of Disabilities Model

The Committee on a National Agenda for the Prevention of Disabilities (NAPD) conceptualized a model for disability (Fig. 19-1) that extends the ICIDH and Nagi frameworks. In the NAPD model, disability occurs when a person's physical or mental limitations, in interaction with physical and social barriers in the environment, prevent the person from taking equal

part in the normal life of the community (Pope and Tarlov, 1991). Furthermore, disability develops through a complex, interactive process involving biological, behavioral, and environmental (i.e., social and physical) risk factors and QOL. In this social model for disability, *bodily impairments and functional limitations are not necessarily accompanied by disability.* Disability may be preventable and preventive measures can promote an improved QOL and reduce costs related to dependence, lost productivity or unemployment, and medical care.

Risk Factors

Three categories of risk factors for disability are identified in this model. These include *biological* (e.g., Rh type), *environmental* (e.g., access to care and lead paint), and *lifestyle and behavioral* characteristics (e.g., overeating or smoking) that influence health-related conditions.

The Disabling Process

The model provides an alternative framework for viewing four related and distinct stages in the disabling process. *Pathology* at the *cellular and tissue level* may produce an *impairment* in structure or function at the *organ level.* An individual with an impairment may experience a *functional limitation,* which restricts his or her ability to perform an action

FIGURE **19-1**

Model of disability (Reprinted with permission from Pope AM, Tarlov AR, editors: *Disability in America: toward a national agenda for prevention,* Washington, DC, 1991, IOM, National Academy Press. Copyright 1991 by the National Academy of Sciences. Courtesy of the National Academy Press, Washington, DC).

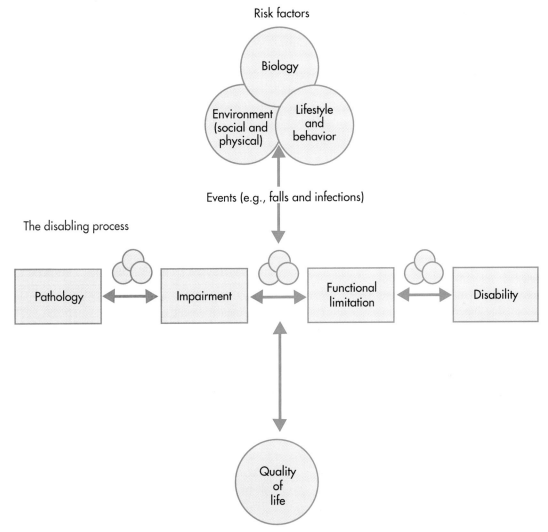

within the normal range. The functional limitation may result in a *disability* when certain socially defined activities and roles cannot be performed.

Although the model appears to indicate unidirectional progression from pathology, to impairment, to functional limitation, to disability, step-wise or linear progression may not occur. Disability prevention efforts can address any of the risk factors or stages in the disabling process. Health promotion efforts include primary prevention of disability, secondary

reversal of disability and restoration of function, and tertiary prevention of complications.

Quality of Life Issues in Disability

QOL perspectives cannot be separated from considerations related to the disabling process. Enabling or disabling influences created by environmental and social barriers commonly affect QOL for people with disabilities. However, people who establish hope and

Cathy sought repair of her broken eyeglasses, but first she required an eye exam. She is a grade school teacher and requires intact vision to properly supervise her students. Cathy has a neuromuscular disease that creates a mobility impairment from generalized muscular weakness and must use a motorized wheelchair. Her functional limitations necessitate help with all ADLs and many IADLs.

Cathy sought an eye exam at an optical center in a local department store where she did much of her shopping. Although the receptionist advised her that no one could see her for several months, she noted that the woman in line behind her received an appointment for the following day. Cathy left the store feeling puzzled and angry. She called several optical offices and advised them that unless their equipment could accommodate her motorized wheelchair, someone would need to lift her into the examining chair and hold her upright throughout the eye exam. The limitations of the optical equipment required someone to assist Cathy during the exam. After she contacted several potential providers, Cathy finally obtained an appointment.

One optometrist chose to see Cathy when the others failed. Physically disabled himself, the optometrist had a mobility impairment as evidenced by a limp. Although his functional limitations and the extent of his disability were much less severe than Cathy's, he also experienced societal bias and discrimination related to disability. Unfortunately, when people saw Cathy's wheelchair or heard about her potential need for accommodation, their attitudes may have transformed her disability into a handicapping condition.

meaning in their lives may choose to positively reframe the difficulties associated with functional limitations that others may find intolerable (Treloar, 1999c). The above clinical example illustrates concepts and definitions related to disability.

DISABILITY: A SOCIALLY CONSTRUCTED ISSUE

Much of the complexity in defining disability stems from its socially constructed nature. If disability were a fixed medical or social fact, it could be relatively easily determined. However, *since disability is more usefully conceptualized as the inability to perform important life functions, it becomes a product of interaction between health status and the demands of one's physical and social environment.* Thus using a wheelchair is disabling in a work place with steps and narrow doorways, but much less so in one with ramps and wide passageways. Similarly, cultural beliefs and attitudes shape the extent to which an impairment is disabling, and the extent to which people with physical or mental impairments are able to function in jobs and more broadly in public life

(Scotch, 1994, p. 172).

CHARACTERISTICS OF DISABILITY

Whether or not someone has a disability depends on the measurement criteria. The Americans with Disabilities Act (ADA) of 1990 and the Rehabilitation Act of 1973 defined a disability according to the limitations in a person's ability to carry out at a major life activity. Physical disabilities, sensory disabilities (e.g., being deaf or blind), intellectual disabilities (i.e., contemporary terminology for mental retardation), serious emotional disturbances, learning disabilities, significant chemical and environmental sensitivities, and health problems such as AIDS and asthma are examples of disabilities that may substantially limit at least one major life activity. A major life activity includes the ability to breathe, walk, see, hear, speak, work, care for oneself, perform manual tasks, and learn (Wehman, 1993).

Sources of Disability Data

Measures for disability differ, which makes it difficult to determine the number of Americans with disabilities. The two best known data sets vary in their definitions and measurement parameters for disability (Kraus, Stoddard, and Gilmartin, 1996).

The Survey of Income and Program Participation (SIPP), conducted by the U.S. Bureau of the Census (1997b), considers limitations in functional activities (e.g., seeing, hearing, talking, walking, climbing stairs, and lifting items), **activities of daily living**

(ADLs) (e.g., bathing, dressing, eating, or toileting), and **instrumental activities of daily living** (IADLs) (e.g., shopping, banking, light housecleaning, and preparing meals). It includes people who use an adaptive mobility device (i.e., wheelchair, cane, crutches, or walker) for six or more months; have a mental or emotional disability or mental retardation; or have an impairment that produces on-the-job limitations or the inability to perform housework.

The National Health Interview Survey (NHIS), conducted by the NCHS, measures disability according to limitations in activity associated with chronic health conditions and particular age groups. Levels of severity also vary (Kaye et al., 1996). The SIPP focuses on an inability to perform physical activities and the NHIS measures the need for assistance in daily activities.

Despite a lack of uniform data sets for disability, it is clear that the proportion of the U.S. population with disabilities that cause activity limitations has risen during the past quarter century (Kaye et al., 1996). This is accompanied by two distinct trends (i.e., demographic shifts associated with an aging population and increasing numbers of children and young adults with disabilities). Since 1990, there has been a growth in the prevalence of children with activity limitations. This may be associated with increasing rates of asthma, mental disorders (i.e., attention deficit disorder), intellectual disabilities, and learning disabilities (Kaye et al., 1996). Rates of orthopedic impairments and mental and nervous disorders increased during the same period for young adults.

Prevalence of Disability

The 1992 NHIS data indicated that about 15% of the noninstitutionalized U.S. population, approximately 38 million people, experience some activity limitation from chronic health conditions or impairments (LaPlante and Carlson, 1996). However, the 1994 to 1995 SIPP data estimated that 20.6% of the noninstitutionalized general population, nearly 54 million people, has a disabling condition that interferes with life activities (US Bureau of the Census, 1997b). Furthermore, approximately half of these people, about 26 million people, have a severe disability.

A person with a "severe" disability is an individual who fits the following criteria:

- aged 15 years or older,
- unable to perform one or more functional activities, or

TABLE 19-2

Selected Disability Data, SIPP, 1994 to 1995

Disability: A Common Experience Nearly 54 Million People in the United States (i.e., 1 out of 5) are Disabled. About 26 Million People (i.e., 1 out of 10) are Severely Disabled.	
Limitation	**Numbers**
Use a wheelchair	1.8 million; aged six years and older
Use a cane, crutches, or walker	5.2 million; used for six months or longer
Difficulty seeing	8.8 million; aged six years and older
Unable to see	1.6 million; aged six years and older
Difficulty hearing	10.1 million; aged six years and older
Unable to hear	1.0 million; aged six years and older
Need ADL(s) assistance	4.1 million; aged six years and older
2.2 million of these were aged 65 years and older
Unable to perform one or more functional activities	15.3 million; aged 15 years and older
Need IADL(s) assistance	Nine million; aged 15 years and older
4.9 million of these were aged 65 years and older

From US Bureau of the Census: *Current population reports: Americans with disabilities: 1994-1995,* August 1997b, The Author, www.census.gov/prod/3/97pubs/p70-61.pdf.

- depends on others' help to perform one or more ADLs or IADLs, or
- uses an assistive device on a long-term basis.

In addition, people with Alzheimer's disease or a developmental disability, those aged 16 to 67 who are unable to do housework or work at a job or business, or those who receive federal disability benefits meet the criteria for a severe disability. Table 19-2 provides selected data on disability.

Causes of Disability

Overall, heart disease is the leading cause of activity limitation for adult males and females, followed by back disorders and arthritis (LaPlante and Carlson, 1996). Table 19-3 lists the 15 highest prevalence conditions that cause activity limitations in adults.

TABLE 19-3

Conditions with Highest Prevalence, All Causes of Limitation, NHIS, 1992

	All Causes	
Condition Causing Limitation	**Number**	**%**
All listings	61,047	100
Heart disease	7932	13
Deformities, orthopedic impairments, and spine and back disorders	7672	12.6
Arthritis and allied disorders	5721	9.4
Orthopedic impairment of lower extremity	2817	4.6
Asthma	2592	4.2
Diabetes	2569	4.2
Mental disorders excluding learning disability and mental retardation	2035	3.3
Eye disorders	1577	2.6
Learning disability and mental retardation	1575	2.6
Cancer	1342	2.2
Visual impairments	1294	2.1
Orthopedic impairment of shoulder and/or upper extremities	1196	2.0
Other unknown and unspecified causes	1188	1.9
Hearing impairments	1175	1.9
Cerebrovascular disease	1174	1.9

Data from LaPlante MP, Carlson D: *Disability in the United States: prevalence and causes*, 1996, Disability Statistics Rehabilitation Research and Training Center, Institute for Health and Aging, School of Nursing, University of California, http://dsc.ucsf.edu/UCSF/pub.taf?_function=search&recid=65&grow=1.

However, causes of activity limitation vary considerably based on age. According to the NHIS (LaPlante and Carlson, 1996), the five leading causes of activity limitation for children and adolescents under 18 years of age include the following: asthma (19.8% of all limiting conditions), learning disability and mental retardation (19.2%), mental illness (8.8%; roughly two thirds is related to hyperkinetic syndrome of childhood), speech impairments (6.7%), and hearing impairments (3.8%).

For adults aged 18 to 44 with activity limitations, back disorders rank first (21.9%), followed by orthopedic impairments of the lower extremity (7.8%), mental illness (5.5%), asthma (5.1%), and orthopedic impairments of the shoulder or upper extremity (3.9%). The prevalence rates shift for those aged 45 to 69, with heart disease ranking first (17.1%), followed by back disorders (13.7%), arthritis (11.1%), diabetes (5.6%), and lower extremity orthopedic impairments (4.2%). From 70 years of age and older, heart disease is the most frequent cause of activity limitation; arthritis, back disorders, diabetes, vision disorders and impairments, and dementia take on increasing importance (LaPlante and Carlson, 1996).

Although estimates for mental retardation range from 0.67% to 3.0% based on age and the definition used, the most commonly accepted estimates indicate that 1% of the noninstitutionalized U.S. population (2.5 million people) have mental retardation. In addition, approximately 695,000 people with mental retardation lived in residential settings, nursing homes, and other institutions in 1995 (Kraus, Stoddard, and Gilmartin, 1996).

Estimates for people disabled by mental and emotional disorders vary widely for a number of reasons. These include a lack of standard measurement criteria for the disorders and their associated limitations and underreporting related to stigma associated with mental illness and substance abuse. Mental and emotional disorders are sometimes described as "hidden" disabilities because observation alone often cannot detect these disorders. However, whether or not a mental disorder is disabling depends on how disability is defined.

According to Jans and Stoddard (1999), the National Health Interview Survey on Disability (NHIS-D) estimated that, in 1994 and 1995, 23.5 million people in the United States had mental disorders. The findings suggested that approximately 70% of people with mental disorders have a functional disability, a work limitation disability, a perceived disability, and/or receive some kind of governmental support services (e.g., Social Security Disability Income [SSDI], Supplemental Security Income [SSI], a disability pension, or special education services).

TABLE **19-4**

Status of Children Aged 6 to 14 Years, SIPP, 1994 to 1995

Limitation and/or Characteristic	Proportion
Some type of disability	12.7%
Classified as severely disabled	1.9%
Difficulty with regular schoolwork	6.2%
Classified as learning disabled	4.5%
Developmental disability*	1.3%
Personal assistance needed with ADL	0.8%

From US Bureau of the Census: *Current population reports: Americans with disabilities: 1994-1995,* August 1997b, The Author, www.census.gov/prod/3/97pubs/p70-61.pdf.
* Includes conditions of mental retardation, autism, and cerebral palsy.

Disability Prevalence Differences by Gender, Age, and Race

According to SIPP estimates, 53% of the population with disabilities are female (Jans and Stoddard, 1999). In contrast, among children aged 21 years and younger, boys have a higher disability prevalence rate than girls. Overall, females are more likely to be disabled than males, which is related to females' greater average longevity. An estimated 28.6 million women and girls have disabilities, which comprises 21.3% of the female population. An estimated 25.3 million men and boys (19.8% of American males) appear to be disabled.

During 1994 and 1995, an estimated 2.6% of U.S. children under age three had a developmental condition for which he or she received therapy or diagnostic services (US Bureau of the Census, 1997b). For children aged three to six years old, 4.1% had a developmental condition and 1.9% had difficulty walking, running, or using the stairs. The proportion with either type was 5.2%. For the 35 million children aged 6 to 14 years, the percentage of children with some type of disability increased to 12.7% as noted in Table 19-4. For adolescents and young adults aged 15 to 21 years, 12.1% had some type of disability and 3.1% had a severe disability (US Bureau of the Census, 1997b).

Comorbid chronic health problems associated with aging increase the likelihood of developing a disability (Jans and Stoddard, 1999). Table 19-5

TABLE **19-5**

Disability Prevalence by Age, SIPP, 1994 to 1995

Age Range	Proportion with a Disability	Number with Disability	Proportion with Severe Disability
6 to 14 years old	12.7%	4.5 million	1.9%
15 to 21 years old	12.1%	3.05 million	3.2%
22 to 44 years old	14.9%	14.1 million	6.4%
45 to 54 years old	24.5%	7.4 million	11.5%
55 to 64 years old	36.3%	7.5 million	21.9%
65 to 79 years old	47.3%	11.6 million	27.8%
Aged 80 or older	71.5%	4.9 million	53.5%

From US Bureau of the Census: *Current population reports: Americans with disabilities: 1994-1995,* August 1997b, The Author, www.census.gov/prod/3/97pubs/p70-61.pdf.

illustrates that people who live longer are more likely to have a severe disability. About half of seniors aged 65 years and older (16 million of an estimated 31 million people) reported having a disability from 1994 to 1995. Further, the proportion of people with disabilities is expected to increase as the population ages. If current trends continue, people aged 65 years and older in the United States will increase from 12% to approximately 20% of the population by the year 2030; the numbers with disabilities will rise proportionately (US Bureau of the Census, 1997a).

Although age is the main factor that influences the likelihood of having a disability, prevalence rates vary according to race and ethnicity within age groups (US Bureau of the Census, 1997b). In comparing rates of severe disability for whites, Hispanics, and African-Americans within the group aged 22 to 44 years, the prevalence of severe disability is least among whites and greatest among African-Americans (US Bureau of the Census, 1997b) as noted in Table 19-6. Within the group aged 45 to 54 years, the severe disability rate was also least among whites (10.5%) and higher for African-Americans (18.4%) and people of Hispanic origin (15.7%).

Native-American populations appear to have the highest overall rate of disability. Indeed, approximately one of every four Native-Americans has some form of disability (Kraus, Stoddard, and Gilmartin, 1996). Compared with other women, Native-American and African-American women have the highest rates of disability (Jans and Stoddard, 1999).

A variety of socioeconomic and cultural variables likely influence differences in the disability prevalence rates related to race, ethnicity, and gender. The community health nurse who cares for culturally diverse populations must carefully assess people's perceptions of the disability experience. Sociocultural biases and traditions may influence the personal and family meaning of disability. Ultimately, the personal belief system of the individual and the family will influence their participation in health care related to the disability.

COSTS ASSOCIATED WITH DISABILITY

Disability is associated with costly medical, social, public health, and moral issues (Pope and Tarlov, 1991). Specific impairments and their accompanying limitations often are of minor importance to people with disabilities when compared with societal issues of exclusion, blocked access, discriminatory practices, educational segregation, poverty, and unemployment. Although the past 10 years has evidenced noteworthy improvements for people with disabilities, they continue to lag behind nondisabled Americans in many of the most basic aspects of life. These include gaps in employment, income, education, access to transportation, health care, frequency of socializing, entertainment, attendance at religious services, and political participation (National Council on Disability, 1999; National Orga-

TABLE 19-6

Disability Prevalence by Selected Race and Ethnic Origin, SIPP, 1994 to 1995

Racial and Ethnic Group	Age Range	Disability Type	% Distribution
NonHispanic whites	22 to 44 years	Severe	5.6%
Any race of Hispanic origin	22 to 44 years	Severe	6.7%
Blacks	22 to 44 years	Severe	11.8%
NonHispanic whites	45 to 54 years	Severe	10.5%
Any race of Hispanic origin	45 to 54 years	Severe	15.7%*
Blacks	45 to 54 years	Severe	18.4%*

From US Bureau of the Census: *Current population reports: Americans with disabilities: 1994-1995*, August 1997b, The Author, www.census.gov/prod/3/97pubs/p70-61.pdf.
*The difference is not statistically significant.

nization on Disability and Louis Harris and Associates, 2000). According to an IOM publication, *Enabling America,* disability consumes an estimated 4% of the gross domestic product, approximating an annual aggregate cost of $300 billion, which includes medical care expenditures and lost productivity costs (Brandt Jr. and Pope, 1997).

Employment and Earnings

People with severe disabilities have one of the highest unemployment rates of any minority group, which is commonly cited at around 70% (Presidential Task Force on Employment of Adults with Disabilities, 1998). A national survey performed by Louis Harris and Associates (National Organization on Disability and Louis Harris and Associates, 2000) found that working-age adults with disabilities made only limited employment gains compared with 10 years previous. The Harris Survey also indicated that only 32% of disabled people aged 18 to 64 worked full or part-time compared with 81% of the non-disabled population. Among working age Americans with disabilities, two out of three of those unemployed said they would prefer to work. These findings are comparable to SIPP data for 1994 and 1995, which estimated the employment rate for people aged 21 to 64 at 82.1% for nondisabled people, 76.9% for those with a nonsevere disability, and 26.1% for those with a severe disability (US Bureau of the Census, 1997b). In comparing gender differences, women face "double jeopardy," because they are less likely to participate in the workforce and they receive lower earnings (Jans and Stoddard, 1999).

Many people with disabilities live at or near the poverty level (Jans and Stoddard, 1999). Nearly one third (29%) of the adults with disabilities in the Harris Survey (National Organization on Disability and Louis Harris and Associates, 2000) reported living in households having a total income of $15,000 or less, compared with only 10% of those who are nondisabled. This income gap has not narrowed appreciably since a similar survey in 1986. Table 19-7 compares incomes of disabled and nondisabled men and women. It is important to note that although 77.4% of disabled people aged 22 to 64 do not receive public assistance, about half the people who received government cash, food, or rent assistance in 1994 and 1995 were disabled (US Bureau of the Census, 1997a).

Long-Term Care and Personal Assistance Support

Of the 9.3 million people aged 15 and older who require assistance in performing ADLs or IADLs, family members commonly provide about 80% of the personal assistance support (US Bureau of the Census, 1997a). Nearly half of these primary helpers live with the person who has a disability (US Bureau of the Census, 1997a, 1997b). Not surprisingly, the need for assistance increases with age. However, despite the high rate of disability among people aged 80 years and older (i.e., 71.5% had a disability and 53.5% had a severe disability), only 34.1% receive personal assistance.

U.S. public policy is limited by the absence of an affordable system for long-term services and supports for individuals and families affected by disabilities. An institutional bias exists in the Medicaid statute; therefore nursing home care is mandatory in every state and home and community-based care is optional. Institutional services receive approximately 80% of the funding for long-term services and supports (National Council on Disability, 1999). Although the vast majority of people with disabilities and their families prefer that services are delivered in the "most integrated" home- and community-based settings, the current system offers few real choices for people with disabilities who need long-term support.

Health Insurance

People with disabilities are more likely to participate in public health programs (e.g., Medicare and Medicaid) compared with nondisabled people. In addition, they are less likely to have private health insurance (Table 19-8).

TABLE 19-7

Median Monthly Earnings, SIPP, 1994 to 1995

Disability Status	Men	Women
No disability	$2190	$1470
Nonsevere disability	$1857	$1200
Severe disability	$1262	$1000

From US Bureau of the Census: *Current population reports: Americans with disabilities: 1994-1995,* August 1997b, The Author, www.census.gov/prod/3/97pubs/p70-61.pdf.

TABLE 19-8

Health Insurance Coverage, People Aged 22 to 64 years, SIPP, 1994 to 1995

Insurance Coverage	No Disability	Nonsevere Disability	Severe Disability
Private	79.9%	71.1%	43.7%
Government only	3.0%	6.1%	39.6%
Not covered	17.1%	22.7%	16.7%*

From US Bureau of the Census: *Current population reports: Americans with disabilities: 1994-1995,* August 1997b, The Author, www.census.gov/prod/3/97pubs/p70-61.pdf.
*Not statistically different from the noncoverage rate for nondisabled people.

HEALTHY PEOPLE 2010 AND THE HEALTH NEEDS OF PEOPLE WITH DISABILITIES

People with disabilities experience increased health concerns and are more likely to develop secondary conditions (e.g., medical, physical, social, emotional, spiritual, or societal). Disability increases the population's need for fully accessible health care that promotes health and well-being, prevents secondary conditions, and provides support for long term health conditions. One of the 26 major goals of *Healthy People 2010* is to promote the health of people with disabilities, prevent secondary conditions, and eliminate disparities between people with and without disabilities and the U.S. population (USDHHS, 2000). Table 19-9 lists selected *Healthy People 2010* objectives for people with disabilities and secondary conditions.

TABLE 19-9

Selected *Healthy People 2010* Objectives for People with Disabilities and Secondary Conditions

Objective	Baseline (i.e., 1998)	% Target
6-2: Reduce the proportion of children and adolescents with disabilities who are reported to be sad, unhappy, or depressed.	31%	17%
6-5: Increase the proportion of adults with disabilities reporting sufficient emotional support.	70%	79%
6-6: Increase the proportion of adults with disabilities reporting satisfaction with life.	87%	96%
6-7: Reduce the number of people with disabilities in congregate care facilities, consistent with permanency planning principles.	NA	NA
6-8: Eliminate disparities in employment rates between working-aged adults with and without disabilities.	52%	82%
6-9: Increase the proportion of children and youth with disabilities who spend at least 80% of their time in regular education programs.	45%	60%
6-10: Increase the proportion of health and wellness and treatment programs and facilities that provide full access for people with disabilities.	NA	NA
6-11: Reduce the proportion of people with disabilities who report not having the assistive devices and technology needed.	NA	NA
6-12: Reduce the proportion of people with disabilities reporting environmental barriers to participation in home, school, work, or community activities.	NA	NA

US Department of Health and Human Services: *Healthy people 2010,* Updated November 10, 2000, Office of Disease Prevention and Health Promotion, USDHHS, www.health.gov/healthypeople.

A disabled person's ability to perform a socially expected activity reflects the characteristics of the individual and the larger social and physical environment; therefore considerations for each of these elements must be incorporated into community health programs that serve people affected by disability. For example, nurses may consider how to promote access to food and medication labeling for people with visual disabilities. Nurses must be sensitive to environmental and social barriers that could prohibit any person's participation in health promotion activities. For example, current estimates indicate that women with functional limitations are less likely to participate in preventative screening for breast and cervical cancer (Jans and Stoddard, 1999). Community health nurses might ask the following:

Can a woman who uses a wheelchair obtain mammography for breast cancer screening, or is the lack of adaptive equipment a barrier to her participation?

What is the availability and cost of accessible transportation to the screening site?

Although this chapter focuses on health promotion for people with disabilities, primary prevention of disability for nondisabled people must not be minimized. Prevention of osteoporosis in nondisabled women, or in women who are mobility impaired from a physical disability, may prevent secondary health problems such as hip and spine fractures that produce significant morbidity and mortality in older women. The health care concerns of nondisabled people may differ from those of people with disabilities. They may be accentuated or minimized. Epidemiological studies are needed to augment information on health promotion strategies specific to people with disabilities.

Health care for people with disabilities must incorporate remedies that address issues surrounding access to health care and the removal of environmental and social barriers that prevent full participation in society. Nurses who practice holistic nursing will recognize that caring for people affected by disabilities requires a perspective that transcends the individual. The community health nurse will use a range of support systems that promote the health of the person with a disability and that of his or her family. Fig. 19-2 illustrates these support systems. The importance of governmental public policies, including disability legislation and financial support, cannot be overemphasized. It is only when the nurse considers a broad

approach to disability that he or she can realize the objectives of *Healthy People 2010*.

A HISTORICAL CONTEXT FOR DISABILITY

Current models and definitions for disability cannot be understood apart from their historical-sociopolitical context. As cultures changed, and with them images of beauty and value, "exceptional" people have experienced a wide range of treatment. They have been loved as mascots and fascinating freaks. In other cases, people with disabilities have been isolated, ridiculed, and discriminated against, or worse yet, marked for extermination (Bogdan, 1986). The following section explores some of the images and attitudes that surround people with disabilities.

Early Attitudes toward People with Disabilities

Societal bias toward people with disabilities has ancient roots (Gartner and Joe, 1987). Since the beginning of recorded history, people with disabilities were *set apart* from others and viewed as different or unusual.

Carvings on the walls of Egyptian tombs contain pictures of dwarfs and blind or disabled musicians and singers. Early Greek and Roman cultures emphasized bodily and intellectual perfection. Babies who were sick, weak, or born with obvious disabilities were typically killed or left to die (Barnes, 1996). In Biblical times, many people with disabilities were outcasts. Commonly viewed as unclean and/or sinful, people with disabilities were frequently isolated and separated from others. However, the Jewish culture prohibited infanticide based on sanctity of life beliefs. In European history, people with disabilities served as royal court pets, entertainers, circus performers, and sideshow exhibitions.

Attitudes toward People with Disabilities in the Eighteenth and Nineteenth Centuries

In the absence of a scientific model for understanding and treating disability, people saw disability as an irreparable condition caused by supernatural agency (Longmore, 1987). People with disabilities were viewed as sick and helpless. They were expected to participate in whatever treatment was deemed neces-

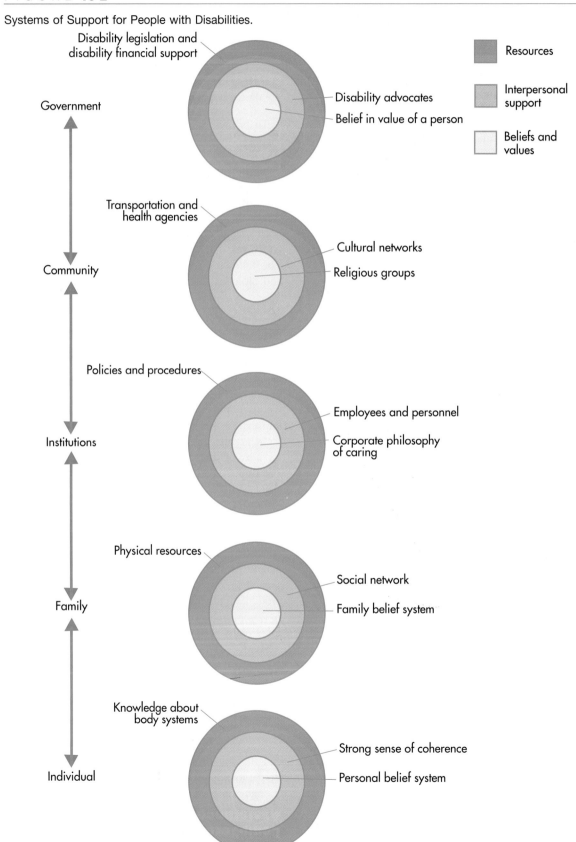

FIGURE **19-2**

Systems of Support for People with Disabilities.

Disability legislation and
disability financial support

Government

Disability advocates

Belief in value of a person

Resources

Interpersonal
support

Beliefs and
values

Transportation and
health agencies

Community

Cultural networks

Religious groups

Policies and procedures

Institutions

Employees and personnel

Corporate philosophy
of caring

Physical resources

Family

Social network

Family belief system

Knowledge about
body systems

Individual

Strong sense of coherence

Personal belief system

sary to cure or produce a reasonable level of social and/or vocational performance. This treatment typically followed the emerging "medical model" (Gartner and Joe, 1987). Although contemporary perspectives for disability in Western civilizations do not support these ancient views, they continue to persist, varying across cultures and within populations.

During the nineteenth century, the Industrial Revolution stimulated a societal need for increased education. Those who could not reach the minimum educational level (i.e., equivalent to a contemporary third-grade education) were labeled as "feeble-minded" (Pfeiffer, 1993). Although this included people with mental disabilities, soon the label transferred to those with sensory and communication disorders (e.g., vision, hearing, and speech) and mobility impairments.

Schools for people who were deaf and blind were established in the early 1800s. In 1849, Dr. Samuel Gridley Howe established the Massachusetts School for Idiotic Children and Youth in Boston. Although these early efforts demonstrated that people with disabilities could be educated and integrated into society, institutionalization and segregation of people with disabilities was the norm (Pfeiffer, 1993; Shapiro, 1993).

Disability in the Twentieth Century

World War I stimulated application of economic concepts surrounding disability (Hahn, 1985). The first federal vocational rehabilitation legislation for veterans with disabilities in 1918 and for civilians in 1920 focused on limitations in the amount or type of work that people with disabilities could perform (Longmore, 1987). Special interest groups for this population developed at about the same time. For example, the Association for Retarded Citizens (ARC) used its collective power to advocate for the needs of people with intellectual disabilities (Turnbull III, 1990).

In the early 1900s, Social Darwinism and the eugenics movement promoted involuntary sterilization of those with intellectual disabilities (Pfeiffer, 1993; Shapiro, 1993). Hitler's attempts to exterminate "inferior" people in World War II, including those who were disabled or weak, are well known. These activities confirmed the medical model view of disability as undesirable and abnormal person-centered pathology (Hahn, 1985).

By the 1950s and 1960s, many groups worked on behalf of people with disabilities and focused on the delivery of needed services. In the 1960s and 1970s, parents' groups and professionals worked together to improve institutional care and establish community-based independent living centers (Longmore, 1987; Shapiro, 1993). However, professionals and parents, rather than people with disabilities, commonly assumed leadership roles within these groups. The public retained the predominant assumption that people with disabilities were *dis*-abled. In classic sociological writings on stigma and social identity, Goffman (1963) associated stigma with blemish and moral inferiority. In the social deviance model of disability, the stigmatized person was "not quite human," which necessitated avoidance by others.

Contemporary Conceptualizations of People with Disabilities

Common stereotypical images of people with disabilities are found in contemporary literature and the media. These portrayals range from pitiful and pathetic, to sinister and/or evil, to laughable or curious, and to a burden or heroic figure (e.g., "super crip") (Friedberg, Mullins, and Sukiennik, 1985). People with disabilities are seldom presented with a full range of personalities and abilities. Even when the media portrays people with disabilities as fully functioning, integral members of society, society may perceive this as unusual or unexpected rather than normal and expected.

A survey was performed to determine the changes in media portrayals of people with disabilities (Martin and Catlett, 1999). The study examined the content from 191 articles for themes associated with disability issues. Table 19-10 describes the findings from the study and suggests that media images appear to be changing positively following the passage of the ADA of 1990. A continuing emphasis on inclusion, normalization, and deinstitutionalization of people with disabilities appears to have contributed to this change. Although pathos or pity remains the predominant societal response, the lives and stories of people with disabilities are increasingly viewed as "normal."

Common responses toward people with disabilities range from ambivalence and avoidance to pity and paternalism. Some reported responses follow:

> Being deaf is an accident of nature. Being indifferent is very often a deliberate choice of mankind. Of these two wounds in our society, one is at least curable
>
> (Nanette Fabray cited in Friedberg, Mullins, and Sukiennik, 1985).

TABLE 19-10

Changing Media Portrayals of People with Disabilities

Logical Fallacy	Frequency	%	Reliability
Pathos or pity	69 articles	36.1%	92.7%
Normalization	44 articles	23%	77%
Super human	26 articles	13.6%	100%
Challenging the system	22 articles	11.5%	91%
Devaluation	16 articles	8.3%	81.6%
Non sequitur (i.e., cause and effect does not necessary follow)	11 articles	5.6%	100%

Data from Martin SS, Catlett SM: *Same window, new view: print media and persons with disabilities,* Unpublished paper presented at 1999 TASH Conference, Chicago, Ill, 1999.

Society does not value our bodies, which makes it difficult for us to value ourselves. We constantly hear that we are faulty, malformed, broken and sick. Many people with disabilities respond in kind, hating their bodies and their disabilities, wishing they were different

(Creamer, 1995, p. 68).

In a society focused on activities, on doing and on fixing, people with chronic illnesses and disabilities are an enigma. We cannot be fixed. We find that generally people want to *do* something when what we need is someone just to be near, to accompany us. Some are willing to help for a while, but usually people expect us to get better and get discouraged when we do not

(Caron, 1996, p. 24).

Stigmatizing influences continue to influence our perceptions surrounding disability (Marinelli and Orto, 1991; Nagler, 1993). Johnson and Johnson (1995) coined the word "disaphobia" to describe the "prejudice, ignorance, fear and anxiety that persons feel in their interaction with the disabled, based on societal stigmatization" (p. 31). Murphy, an anthropologist, reports the following in *The Body Silent*:

One cannot. . . shelve a disability or hide it from the world. A serious disability inundates all other claims to social standing, relegating to secondary status all the attainments of life, all other social roles, even sexuality. It is not a role; it is an identity, a dominant characteristic to which all social roles must be ad-

justed. And just as the paralytic cannot clear his mind of his impairment, society will not let him forget it

(Murphy, 1990, p. 106).

Murphy's description sharpens an understanding of the marginalized status often attributed to people with disabilities. People using wheelchairs are commonly noticed by others, but are seldom acknowledged. Parents often teach their children not to look at a person who is obviously disabled, which reinforces "deviance disavowal" of disability. A community health nurse describes societal stigma experienced by the families of children with disabilities, which follows:

It's a huge amount. The teasing in schools. Kids are brutal to normal kids. We try to run some groups on teasing and how to cope with that. . . Families talk about going to the grocery store and being sick of answering questions or having people stare at the child. I don't know that any of the families really always know how to deal with that

(Treloar, 1999e).

Contemporary language and actions may convey a lack of respect for people with disabilities (Blaska, 1993). For example, people continue to use the term handicap improperly to refer to people with disabilities whether or not these people are handicapped by their environments (Batavia, 1993). Table 19-11 provides further information on uses of language related to disability. To help the reader understand this aggregate, Table 19-12 lists common misconceptions surrounding disability. Finally, Table 19-13 notes

TABLE 19-11

Language Usage Surrounding Disability

Less Desirable Language	More Desirable Language
Confined to a wheelchair; wheelchair-bound	Uses a wheelchair
Afflicted with or suffers from cerebral palsy	Has cerebral palsy
The blind, the deaf, and the disabled	People who are blind, deaf, or disabled
Mentally handicapped or mentally retarded	People with intellectual disabilities
Handicapped students and normal classmates	Students who are disabled and nondisabled or students with and without disabilities
The spinal-cord injury in Room 232	John, in Room 232, has a spinal cord injury

TABLE 19-12

Misconceptions Surrounding Disability

Disability = cannot have fun	Wheelchair = hard of hearing
Disability = want to be pitied	Wheelchair = blind
Disability = cannot live in the community	Wheelchair = mentally retarded
Disability = menace to society	Learning disabled = mentally retarded
Clear voice = clear mind	Mentally retarded = cannot learn
You can always tell if someone has a disability by looking at the person	People with disabilities do not know when someone makes fun of them
All parents want to keep a child with a disability	Most disabilities and disabling diseases are contagious

TABLE 19-13

Do's and Dont's for Interactions with People with Disabilities

Don't	Do
Assume anything or offer expert advice or assistance based on what you think the person needs or can do	Ask if the person needs help and how to assist; listen and follow his or her instructions; allow him or her to do what he or she can
Ignore or exclude the person Be afraid of joking with or offending the person	Treat him or her like any other person or friend; approach and include him or her
Be afraid to ask questions	Recognize that educating others helps remove attitudinal barriers; children who ask are less likely to be afraid of people with disabilities
Focus on differences	See the person as able; accept differences and be patient; seek out similarities and shared interests
Lean on or move the person's wheelchair	Respect a wheelchair as part of the person's personal space; sit or kneel at eye level when communicating with the person
Assume that a person who is blind knows who is speaking or who is present	Inform the person of who is present; say good-bye when leaving
Grab the arm of a person who is blind	Let the person take your arm so he or she does not lose balance

Continued

TABLE 19-13—cont'd

Do's and Dont's for Interactions with People with Disabilities—cont'd

Don't	Do
Become impatient and complete the speech or the action of the person	Acknowledge that the person has something important to say or do; take time to listen and understand
Repeat loudly what you want to say	Face the person; speak distinctly and slightly more slowly (this is particularly important for the person who lip reads)
Pet a working dog; there are service dogs for people with physical, hearing, or visual disabilities	Ask for permission to pet the dog; better yet, don't interrupt the dog's work
Assume that the person can participate	Consider possible environmental obstacles (e.g., sensory, architectural, colognes or fragrances for people with chemical sensitivities)
Assume that "bad" parenting explains children's behavior	Recognize that autism and other invisible disabilities influence behavior
Assume that disability and failure to be healed reflects unresolved sin and lack of faith in God	Recognize that humans as holistic beings benefit from interventions that address spiritual meaning for disability

reminders that promote effective interactions between people with and without disabilities.

DISABILITY AND PUBLIC POLICY

Since the 1980s, parallels have been drawn between people with disabilities and other groups who have been subjected to discrimination and oppression. Disability has been reconceptualized as a socially constructed and stigmatized role (Hahn, 1985; Longmore, 1987; Pfeiffer, 1993). Gartner and Joe (1987) wrote the following:

> Persons with disabilities are not treated seriously because they have limited power and are seen as neither whole nor equal. And they are seen that way because they have limited power. Work then needs to be carried out on both sides of the equation: in changing the images and in changing the opportunity structure. At present, the disabling images constrain opportunities and the resulting limited achievements confirm the images. It can be different. (p. 208).

Redefinition of disability, the disability rights movement, and growing recognition of disability's impact on the U.S. economy and population have contributed to the development of Disability Studies as an emerging discipline. Practitioners and scholars from a broad interdisciplinary base share concerns about disability policy and issues that affect people

BOX 19-1

Public Policy Values Related to Disability

Equal protection: All deserve equal protection under the law.

Egalitarianism: Regardless of differences in abilities, all people should receive equal treatment through equal opportunities.

Normalization: People with disabilities should be treated like nondisabled people, minimizing differences wherever possible.

with disabilities. Box 19-1 contains foundational values and ideologies that underlie public policy related to people with disabilities.

Disability policy attempts to minimize disadvantages related to impairments and disabilities and it maximizes opportunities for people with disabilities to live productively in their communities (Batavia, 1993). According to DeJong (1994), disability policy includes civil rights protections (e.g., Title 504 of the Rehabilitation Act and the ADA), skill enhancement programs (e.g., special education and vocational rehabilitation), and income and in-kind assistance programs (e.g., Social Security Disability Insurance, Medicare, and Medicaid).

People with disabilities use disproportionately more health care services than those who are nondisabled; therefore public health perspectives related to epidemiology and disability prevention have assumed increasing importance (DeJong, 1994). People's health and well-being reflects the resources available to them; therefore community health nurses must be knowledgeable about public health and social support programs that affect a disabled person's ability to live in the community.

Legislation Affecting People with Disabilities

Consistent with historical and social changes and the recognition of barriers and discrimination, key federal legislation has passed that supports the rights of people with disabilities. The following section presents three of the most significant Acts.

The Education for All Handicapped Children Act

The Education for All Handicapped Children Act (EHA) of 1975 (20 USC 1401 or PL 94-142), later renamed the **Individuals with Disabilities Education Act** (IDEA), was a vital piece of legislation for children with disabilities. The EHA was enacted in 1975 following other legislation and court cases ruling that children with disabilities should receive access to public education. Since this legislation, exclusionary or discriminatory practices by schools have spurred a multitude of judicial remedies designed to protect the rights of children with disabilities (Turnbull III, 1990). The IDEA Amendments of 1997 strengthened the provisions of the previous Act (US Department of Education, 1999), which provided procedural safeguards to protect the rights of children with disabilities and their parents.

Addressing special education needs requires appropriate evaluation services. The Act helped eligible children receive free, appropriate public education in the least restrictive environment for their individual needs (US Department of Justice, 2000). Parents, students, and professionals participate in decision making, particularly through the development of an Individualized Education Program (IEP) that includes special educational goals and related services for the child.

The Americans with Disabilities Act

The most comprehensive civil rights legislation for people with disabilities, the **Americans with Disabil-**

ities Act (ADA) (PL 101-336), became law in July 1990; most provisions took effect in January 1992 (Wehman, 1993). This landmark civil rights legislation provided a clear and comprehensive mandate against discrimination toward people with disabilities in everyday activities (US Department of Justice, 2000). The ADA uses the authority of the federal government to guarantee *equal opportunities* for people with disabilities related to employment, transportation, public accommodations, public services, and telecommunications. In addition, it provides protections to people with disabilities similar to those provided to any person on the basis of race, color, sex, national origin, age, and religion.

The ADA refers to a *qualified individual with a disability* as a person with a physical or mental impairment that *substantially limits* one or more *major life activities,* a person with a record of such an impairment, or a person who is regarded as having such an impairment. The ADA also prohibits discrimination against people based on a known association or relationship with an individual with a disability (US Department of Justice and Commission and US Equal Employment Opportunity Commission, 1996).

A qualified individual with a disability must meet legitimate skill, experience, education, or other requirements of an employment position. The person must be able to perform the *essential functions* of the job, such as those contained within a job description, with or without *reasonable accommodation.* Provided that the person is qualified under these conditions, except for limitations caused by a disability, the employer must consider whether the person could perform these functions with reasonable accommodation (US Department of Justice and Commission and US Equal Employment Opportunity Commission, 1996).

Reasonable accommodations are necessary to allow a qualified person to participate in an educational program (Treloar, 1999a) or an employment setting at a level equal to nondisabled people. These include modifications of equipment or instructional materials; job restructuring or placement in an available, alternate job; altered work schedules; providing readers, interpreters, or note takers; and other activities that promote architectural accessibility of the physical environment. The organization must provide reasonable accommodations unless it can demonstrate that the accommodation will cause significant difficulty or expense, producing an *undue hardship* (US Department of Justice and Commission and US Equal Employment Opportunity Commission, 1996). A number of factors influence whether an accommodation may be burdensome. Possible remedies may involve other funding sources (e.g., through the state vocational rehabilitation office) and other financial incentives that could include tax credits and deductions for small businesses.

The ADA is landmark legislation that confirms U.S. leadership in protecting the rights of people with disabilities (Jones, 1991). Continuing refinements and interpretations of this and other legislation will shape future disability policy. Rather than attempt to become an expert on disability law, the community health nurse should develop a resource network that includes disability resource center specialists, public interest law firms, and legal advocacy groups. High priority interventions include helping the person with a disability learn about his or her rights and empowering the person to act on his or her own behalf.

The ADA addresses the civil rights of people with disabilities. The United States needs other public policies to help assure that all Americans, disabled or not, have equal opportunities to become productive citizens. Historically, national public policy has defined disability as the inability to work. Typically, people with disabilities could only qualify for benefits like health care, income assistance programs, and personal care attendant services if they chose not to work.

THE DILEMMA OF CHOOSING EMPLOYMENT VS. HEALTH CARE AND COMMUNITY SUPPORT ASSISTANCE

John uses a power wheelchair because he has what he calls "spastic quadriplegia" from cerebral palsy. John is college educated and chooses not to work. John weighed his options and acknowledged that if he worked, he would lose the state supported social service benefits that provide his health care services and attendant caregiver services. Unfortunately, until public policy provides adequate health and social support programs, John's disability will remain a handicapping condition (Treloar, 1999c).

Work Incentives Improvement Act

In 1998, President Clinton created a Task Force on Employment of Adults with Disabilities (Presidential Task Force on Employment of Adults with Disabili-

ties, 1998). The purpose of this Task Force was to create a national policy that brought adults with disabilities into employment at the approximate rate of nondisabled Americans. In December 1999, Congress passed the bipartisan Jeffords-Kennedy-Roth-Moynihan **Work Incentives Improvement Act** (WIIA) and signed it into law.

Among other provisions, this legislation removes guidelines that typically result in the termination of Medicaid and Medicare benefits for people with disabilities when they return to work. In addition to other state incentives, the WIIA modernizes the employment services system for people with disabilities. The passage of the WIIA signals a shift in how the population views public health care programs such as Medicare and Medicaid; these programs become "tools rather than barriers" as people with disabilities seek opportunities for employment and increased self-sufficiency (Young, 1999). Successful implementation of the WIIA at federal and state levels will offer people with disabilities increased options in reentering the workforce.

RECONCEPTUALIZING HEALTH CARE FOR PEOPLE WITH DISABILITIES

Disability rights advocates and scholars commonly criticize the medical model of disability for its assumptions about people with disabilities (Hahn, 1985; Hahn, 1991; Oliver, 1996). They argue that this perspective has done the following:

> Played a role in the segregation of people with disabilities, and in the labeling of those people—often as aberrant, deviant, or contaminated, and certainly as abnormal. . . has discouraged full citizenship for people with disabilities
>
> (Monaghan, 1998, p. A15).

In the medical model, the health professional prescribes interventions designed to remedy or ameliorate functional limitations of the ill person. Social, psychological, economic, or political factors receive limited attention. This perspective focuses on problems and solutions related to the individual rather than from an environmental or societal perspective. Although patient autonomy receives increasing attention, professionals who operate from the medical model tend to disempower the person with a disability (Northway, 1997). Table 19-14 summarizes these contrasting perspectives.

TABLE **19-14**

Disability Paradigm Influences Policy and Actions

Defining Characteristic	Medical Model	Social Construct
Framework or paradigm	Disability as pathology; emphasizes functional limitations; physical limitations are primary source of problems	Disability as expected (i.e., normal); emphasizes minority-group model (i.e., discrimination and oppression related to social attitudes and other barriers
Focus of concern	Person	Environment
Problem	Personal deficits (e.g., an impairment, lack of a vocational skill, poor adjustment, or lack of motivation)	Environmental barriers (e.g., attitudinal, architectural, sensory, economic, and inadequate social supports)
Person with a disability	Patient in need of professional help	Person is expert, knowledgeable about self, may or may not seek professional assistance
Role of the health professional	Expert and expects advice to be followed	Collaborating partner; mutually negotiated role reflects needs and desires of person and resources of professional
Perspective of discipline	Medicine, nursing, rehabilitation, medical sociology and psychology, special education, and allied health	Disability studies and disability policy
Model for decision making	Hierarchical (i.e., professional on top)	Collaboration for empowerment of person
Plan of care	Professional centered	Person centered
Desired outcomes	Reflect professionals' goals	Reflect person's goals

The social construct paradigm for disability differs from that the health sciences, rehabilitation, medical sociology, special education, and related fields traditionally use. Disability may not be pathological or require disease management. Functional limitations do not necessary result in a handicapping condition. This model implies the following:

Disability stems from the failure of a structured social environment to adjust to the needs and aspirations of disabled citizens rather than from the inability of a disabled individual to adapt to the demands of society . . . The devaluation of disabled persons has not resulted from a lack of economic productivity or from their alleged biological inferiority . . . this inequality has resulted from the reluctance of society to recognize their dignity and worth as human beings or to grant them civil rights as members of a political community (Hahn, 1985, p. 93).

Rather than emphasize personal deficits like the medical model, contemporary *sociopolitical perspectives for disability* focus on the modification of attitudinal, architectural, sensory, and economic barriers in the environment. According to Pfeiffer (1993), perceived problems emphasize inadequate support services to overcome barriers and may include overdependence on professionals and others. Solutions include self- and system-advocacy, removal of barriers, and control by the person with a disability based on desired outcomes.

Nursing education and practice must move beyond the traditional rehabilitation model to incorporate the social construction of disability. According to Woodill, nurses who are disability-conscious can speak out against oppression when they encounter it, use their nursing skills to provide needed support and services for organizations of persons with disabilities, and make others aware of issues and concerns that affect persons with disabilities. However, as able-bodied persons, nurses must first "learn to see the world from the perspective of a person with a disability" (Woodill, 1994, p. 47).

Richardson (1997) urged nurses to establish working alliances with families affected by disabilities and develop goals and interventions that address disabling environmental and social barriers. Turnbull and Turnbull III (1996) stated that nurses must work with families affected by disabilities to promote "collaboration for empowerment," which combines an increased control over an individual's life with the dynamic process of connecting families' resources within an empowering context to make decisions collectively. This requires the nurse to view people with disabilities and their families as collaborators and enable them to move beyond a position limited to decision making or receiving professionals' expert judgments. Such collaboration promotes self-determination and allows choices that promote personal values and preferences.

THE PERSONAL EXPERIENCE OF DISABILITY

Olkin (1999) stated that "persons with disabilities constitute the largest minority in the United States" (p. 16). In fact, most people whose lives do not end abruptly will experience disability. Although there are many types of diseases and conditions that result in disability, many experiences are common to the disability experience. However, the personal experience (i.e., the personal meaning of disability) differs significantly for those who develop disability from different events or disease processes. Table 19-15 summarizes the difference between short-term disability and long-term conditions characterized by disability.

It is clear that those who develop a temporary disability from a sprained or broken ankle have a very different experience than those who are permanently disabled. Although they may experience all the frustrations of immobility that necessitate the use of a wheelchair or crutches, they do not enter the world of people with disabilities because they know they will soon reenter society able bodied. They often do not develop the skills of living with a disability such as walking on crutches expertly, obtaining a disabled parking placard, and learning to perform daily activities with a disability. They view it as a temporary problem and a temporary setback.

In contrast, those who develop a permanent disability from an accident or disease process such as a stroke must learn to incorporate the modifications required for living into their daily living and identity. Silvers, Wasserman, and Mahowald (1998) describe their situation in the following way: "Their difference from other people is inescapable and can be concealed—if at all—only at formidable cost to their energy and self esteem" (p. 2).

Two people who have not attempted to conceal their disabilities and are nationally recognized for their creative response to disability are Joni Eareckson Tada and Christopher Reeve. Although cure is unlikely, their impairments do not prohibit their ability to perform useful work. Their disabilities become a challenge and an obstacle to overcome. Their disabilities are visible and definitive; therefore they did not make a decision about disclosing disability or deciding to use assistive devices.

People who become disabled from the progressive decline of a chronic illness often put off accepting the assistive devices that would make life easier for them. They believe that accepting the device would mean accepting the label of disabled. In one study of people with COPD (Artinian, 1995), many patients reported continuing to work without using oxygen, long after adequate oxygenation was necessary, to avoid the associated stigma. Others reported reluctance to use a cane or wheelchair because they did not want to appear disabled. Others reported reluctance to use a disabled parking placard because they appeared physically fit and did not want people to accuse them of abusing the placard.

In many progressive diseases, a benchmark event forces the person to accept the label of disabled (e.g., failure to wean from the ventilator, a driving accident caused by failing eyesight or mental capacity, a leg amputation from diabetic complications, or a fall when a degenerative disease such as multiple sclerosis impairs mobility). For these people, their bodies have become unreliable. They can no longer plan daily activities and expect to accomplish them. Although some young adults experience this type of disability, many of the elderly have chronic illnesses that end in disability.

THE INTERSYSTEM MODEL

The community health nurse working with patients from any of these groups must look beyond the actual limitations to the meaning these limitations hold for

TABLE **19-15**

Conceptualization of Chronic Health Conditions

	Short-Term Conditions	Long-Term Conditions		
Dimension		**Model Case**	**Related Case**	**Contrary Case**
	Acute illness	Chronic illness	Disabling condition	Life-threatening illness
Cellular	Inflammation	Inflammation; degeneration	Destruction or atrophy	Proliferation
Time	Short	Long	Long	Short or long
Purpose of Rx	Rx to remove problem (i.e., cure)	Rx to alleviate symptoms	Rx to improve functioning	Rx to kill cancer cells (i.e., cure)
Examples of immediate effect of treatment	Severe pain of surgery; immobility	Weight gain of prednisone therapy; dietary restrictions	Discomfort of splinting; pain of retraining muscles	Loss of hair, nausea, and weight loss
Anticipated outcome	Cure expected	Cure not expected	Cure not expected	Cure hoped for or death feared
Trajectory	Short	Exacerbations and remissions; slow progressive decline; shortened life span	Steady	Remission or cure or death
Effect on ADL	Severe during Rx or none after	Regimen required	Modifications required	Severe during Rx or none during remission or cure
Mental outlook	Temporary problem	Depression or challenge	Stigma or challenge	Fear or hope
Metaphorical interpretation	A temporary setback	Chain binding; a prisoner of uncertainty because body is unreliable	Obstacle to overcome	Sword hanging over head; a sentence

the patient. The **Intersystem Model** (Artinian and Conger, 1997) provides a framework that assists the nurse in understanding the patient's knowledge about the disability, the values the person has regarding life with the disability, and the skills the person has for managing the disability. Taylor (1997) used this model to design a program for patients with spinal cord injuries based on health-related principles in contrast to pathogenic principles. Each person in the rehabilitation team was a teacher and the patient was an active participant in the process. The program focused on partnership as it helped people live with disability.

The Intersystem Model (Artinian and Conger, 1997) focuses on the interaction between the nurse and the patient or client who is faced with a stressor that cannot be resolved without nursing assistance. The goal of the interaction is to establish a joint plan of care that is congruent with the values and beliefs of the client to increase his or her Situational Sense of Coherence (SSOC) in relation to the defined problem. SSOC is measured on the basis of comprehensibility (i.e., knowledge about the problem), motivation (i.e., the willingness to work on the problem), and resources to manage the problem. Each aspect can be scored on a scale of one to three (one being low and three being high).

The interaction begins with a clear definition of the nature of the problem that concerns the patient or nurse. The client can be an individual, a family, an institution, or a community. Each has a biological subsystem, a psychosocial subsystem, and a spiritual subsystem. Problems can arise from any of these subsystems and a problem in one subsystem can affect other subsystems. The nurse assesses the patient's subsystems, including beliefs, values, past experiences, coping mechanisms, support systems, religious preferences, physical conditions, and current needs. A strength of the model is that the nurse assesses both the patient and himself or herself in terms of their knowledge about the problem, the values they hold in relation to the problem, and the resources they bring to the situation.

Both patient and nurse are active participants in the process. Collaboration is required to develop a plan of care that both the patient and nurse find acceptable. Sometimes the nurse must be flexible in his or her expectations. In the final analysis, the patient will only accomplish what he or she agrees to accomplish. This model produces a shift from an authoritarian relationship to a collaborative and supportive relationship between the patient and nurse. Fig. 19-3 presents a summary of the decision-making process in this model. Nurses who use the Intersystem Model in working with patients or their families describe their interactions in the following way:

> The first thing is sensitivity. It's being able to listen, being able to hear families, being able to respond to where they're at. Not your own agenda, and that's real hard for nurses. You have such an agenda, what you think you need to do for health care and you really lose track of where the family is and put all kinds of things onto family that are experts in their child's own care. They may not do it the way we want, but they're experts in their own child's care
>
> (Treloar, 1999e).

Another nurse who works with the frail elderly in a rural community said the following: "I give them many options, but they need to decide what will work best for them because they know what their situation is and what they have already tried" (Artinian, 1999).

A nurse who works with newborns and children

up to three years old helps families who are just learning about their children's disabilities navigate "the system." She states that although many parents become very capable, they do not know what to do about the disability in the beginning (Treloar, 1999e).

These examples illustrate how patients and their families interact with the community health nurse from very different perspectives. In one case, a patient has been living with disability for a long time and has become sensitive to the needs of his or her body. This patient wants the nurse to listen to these concerns and may benefit from a referral to health-related resources. However, *this patient does not need to be told how to manage the disability*. Fig. 19-4 describes this patient as the "knowledgeable patient." The nurse must ask the patient what works best for him or her and what goals the patient is pursuing. In contrast, the newly diagnosed patient can use the nurse's information regarding the disability itself and the available community and governmental resources for the patient and family. Fig. 19-4 describes this as the "knowledgeable nurse."

If the nurse attempts to tell the "knowledgeable patient" what to do, the patient may become angry with the health care system and seek help from other sources. If the nurse is unable to help a newly diagnosed patient learn how to manage the disability and accept himself or herself as disabled, the nurse may lose the opportunity to help the person come to terms with the disabled state. For example, the staff at a clinic for congenital amputees believed it was important to contact the family before friends and relatives could present a negative image of the child.

STRATEGIES FOR THE COMMUNITY HEALTH NURSE IN CARING FOR PEOPLE WITH DISABILITIES

Nurses who partner with people with disabilities and their families provide nursing care using a number of strategies in a variety of community-based sites. The individual, his or her family, and the community may be the primary client.

People affected by disabilities have health care needs and resources common to nondisabled people; others are unique to disability. In comparing disabled and nondisabled people, the person with a disability is both the same as a nondisabled person and different (Treloar, 1999b). The nurse's role should reflect the needs and resources of the patient and his or her

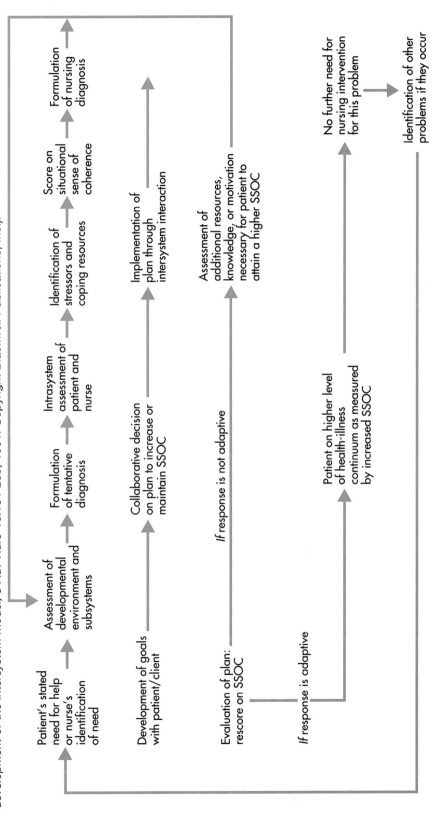

FIGURE 19-3

A summary of the clinical decision making process used to implement the Intersystem Model (Reprinted with permission from Artinian BM: *The development of the intersystem model, J Adv Nurs* 16:164-205, 1991. Copyright Blackwell Publications, Inc.).

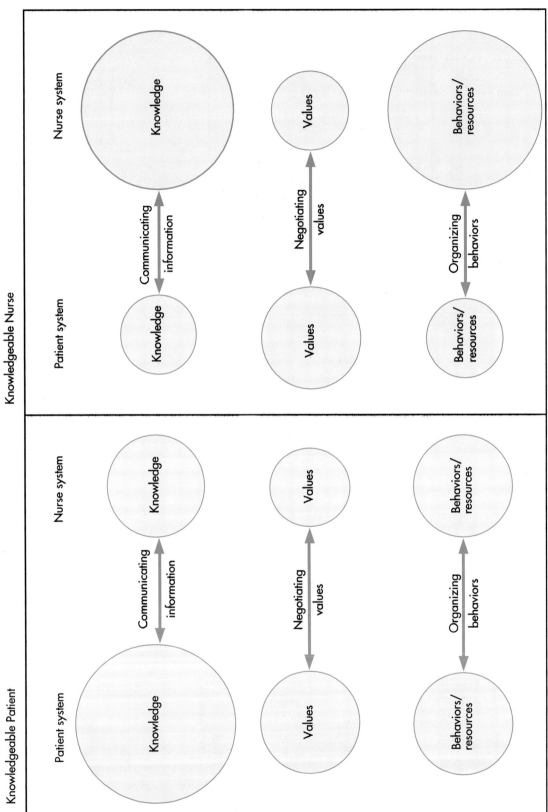

FIGURE 19-4

Knowledgeable Patient and Knowledgeable Nurse in the Intersystem Model.

family. Data from interviews conducted with nurses who provide care to this population and people with physical disabilities illustrate the following guiding principles (Treloar, 1999e):

- **Don't assume anything:** The nurse should collect data from the perspective of the person and family with a disability. A nurse case manager for families with disabled children explains the following:

  Look at each person, patient, family, each situation as a totally new and different one. Not assuming anything. Not lumping people into categories. I know we learn cultural things, we learn stereotypes. You have to put that out of your mind. There are cultural things that you would want to respect. But, don't assume anything . . . And then, listen to what isn't said. I watch people . . . You go into a home and you can learn a tremendous amount by not even asking any questions at times.

- **Adopt the patient's perspective:** If the nurse operates from his or her agenda or personal cultural norms rather than from those of the patient, less productive and satisfactory outcomes will result. More importantly, the nurse will fail to establish a relationship that respects the patient as expert in his or her own health status. Recognize that people's situations may not exist as expected or as they appear. Further, what appears to be a barrier or a limitation may not reflect the true situation or the patient's perspective. Another nurse comments, which follows:

  There can be very good families that are taking excellent care of their children in poverty situations. That doesn't mean that's a bad place for that child. I think we become very quick to pull children out of what visually is not good from our perspective. It may be the most loving thing that child is going to ever have.

- **Listen and learn from the patient:** Gather data from the perspective of the patient and family. If the patient has severe mental disabilities and cannot offer reliable information, ask the family or caregiver. Nurses must establish relationships that are responsive to the person's methods and the family's methods for dealing with disability. One adult who uses a wheelchair said the following about the difficulties she experienced with health care providers:

  Health care providers who have training of some sort, at whatever level, already have set ideas of how things

are supposed to be done. I prefer someone that has no idea what they are supposed to do . . . They do it exactly how they're being told, to the best of their ability, and they do it like a human being instead of like a robot that's going by a list of instructions.

An experienced nurse explained that she does not consider herself the "expert," which follows:

That parent or caretaker is the one that's there for that child all the time. They know that child far better. I may know something medical that they don't know. How can we share that information? That's where you get down to sharing those kinds of things. Teach me. I'm always there to learn.

- **Care for the patient and the family, not the disability:** The style and intent of patient and provider communication influences the acceptability of the interaction. A "conversational" style that establishes an equal partnership with the patient is preferable to an "open up the textbook" approach that tells the patient "here's what you need to do." The nurse should ask what the patient needs help with, what the patient is capable of doing, what the patient would like to do, and how he or she can help. This approach is dramatically different from saying, "Okay, I can see that you cannot do this, this, and this. This is what I'm going to do."

A community health nurse illustrates these ideas in working with families of children with disabilities, which follows:

Are they able to develop a health care plan of their own for their child? Which again, may not be ours [plan]. Are they able to follow through on the important pieces of health care for their child, or at least identify that they don't have the resources to do that? . . . At times we make families feel that if they don't follow our plan, then they're bad parents. So then they don't talk to us about the fact that they can't follow our plan or it's not their plan.

- **Be well informed about community resources:** Learning about resources by reading a community manual is less helpful than meeting with the staff and agencies in person. People often respond differently to requests by someone they know and respect; therefore it may be beneficial for the community health nurse to contact agency personnel about a patient and family need. A nurse explains the following:

[When the nurse understands the community resources, she can direct families to] the better systems . . . Help them identify who the crucial people in those systems are to perhaps help them through them. [She can assist families to] positively interface with systems and get support so that they don't become so embittered.

■ Become a strong advocate: The community health nurse's advocacy for the person affected by a disability extends beyond a resource and referral coordinator role or speaking on the other's behalf. People with disabilities want to speak for themselves. They want to be in control of their lives and their health care. One person with a disability stated the following:

They [health care providers who act in an advocacy role] provide the information, but they leave the choice up to the person. And then even if the person chooses against what has been suggested, they still provide the same support.

According to this person with a disability, advocacy implies that the community health nurse's support continues even when the patient or family's health care decisions conflict with the health care provider's recommendations.

The community health nurse's perspective on disability will influence the nursing role and the level of care he or she provides to people with disabilities and their families. A variety of systems ranging from government, community, institutions, family, and the individual (see Fig. 19-2) influence the experience of living with a disability. Whether or not the nurse chooses to work in a setting that specializes in health care services for people affected by disabilities, disability is a common experience that all practicing nurses will encounter.

ETHICAL ISSUES FOR PEOPLE AFFECTED BY DISABILITIES

People with disabilities and their families are concerned about the same contemporary ethical and legal issues that concern nondisabled people. However, some of the associated issues carry particular interest for people with disabilities and their families, including questions and problems surrounding definitions of personhood, respect for human beings, and the rights of people with disabilities.

Associated issues include abortion when prenatal screening suggests the presence of impairments and health problems and the determination of appropriate medical care for infants, children, and adults with disabilities. Differences in QOL and justice perspectives intersect with concerns about the control of health care costs. For example, people with disabilities and their families may be concerned with how many and what kind of health care services they should be entitled to receive and whether or not these expenditures should be capped, and if so, under what criteria.

New genetic technologies offer hope for the prevention and cure of disease. However, people with disabilities wonder if these scientific advances will serve to eliminate people with disabilities, similar to Hitler's attempts to exterminate undesirable peoples in World War II. Disability advocacy groups, including "Not Dead Yet," have taken a strong stance against physician-assisted suicide (Burgdorf Jr., 1997) fearing it will lead to the early and/or forced death of people with disabilities. Parents who seek cochlear implants for their deaf children often encounter opposition by deaf advocacy groups. These groups argue that people should accept deafness because deafness is not abnormal. Similarly, the use of Ritalin and other stimulant medications for children or adults with attention deficit hyperactivity disorder carry pro and con arguments that include ethical considerations. An emphasis on self-determination, the deinstitutionalization movement, and the accompanying expansion of community-based independent living centers and other residential settings for people with disabilities create other legal and ethical issues.

Like any ethical problem, issues related to disability do not have easy solutions. However, societal attitudes and bias toward people with disabilities may negatively influence policies and decisions related to the interests and fair treatment of people with disabilities. Disability rights proponents worry that the devaluation of people with disabilities may promote their unnecessary and untimely deaths (Burgdorf Jr., 1997). Ethical decision making cannot separate from discussions that include the meaning associated with life and life's accompanying challenges.

SUMMARY

To address these issues, community health nurses must recognize that there are a variety of personal and societal perspectives on disability with accompanying moral or ethical issues. They should practice holistic nursing care that incorporates mind, body, and spiritual care considerations into the health care practice (Treloar, 1999d). To this end, nurses can do the following:

■ Become familiar with a variety of ethical frameworks for decision making and learn a strategy to analyze ethical problems related to health care for people with disabilities.

■ Help the patient and family access needed information from the health care team to make informed decisions that reflect their interests.

■ Help educate the public on health care issues within the nurse's scope of practice and knowledge and skill level.

■ Participate in the development of institutional policies and procedures for ethical and legal issues related to disability.

■ Take a position on an ethical issue with political implications.

■ Work to influence governmental policies and laws related to disability.

LEARNING ACTIVITIES

1. Interview a person with a disability or a family with a disabled family member about their experiences with health care providers and the health care "system."

2. Shadow a nurse in a community-based health clinic that serves children with disabilities. Observe the roles and the interactions of the multidisciplinary team members. Follow a family through clinic. If possible, meet the family at their home before clinic and observe their preparations prior to coming to clinic. Accompany them from clinic check-in until their departure. After returning to their home, ask them for their thoughts on the clinic experience.

3. Interview a community resident who has a serious disability. How does he or she view himself or herself? What challenges or concerns does the resident mention? Interview a caregiver about the caregiving experience.

4. Ask an experienced nurse about his or her encounters with people with disabilities. Listen to his or her language and perceptions of disability. Compare these to the perspectives reflected in the social construct model for disability.

5. Visit with the residents and staff in a community-based living environment for people with disabilities. Assist with caregiving for the residents.

6. Visit one or two community-based agencies that provide services to people with disabilities. How do families gain access to services and what services are offered? How do available services and resources address the needs of people affected by disabilities?

7. Spend time in the home of a family who has a child with intellectual disabilities. Note the family relationships. Interview the parents and siblings about their experiences with a child with special needs. Spend time with the child.

REFERENCES

Artinian B: *The process of regaining control: outcome of a pulmonary rehabilitation program for patients with advanced COPD,* Paper presented at the California Society of Pulmonary Rehabilitation, San Francisco, Calif, 1995.

Artinian B: Unpublished interviews, 1999.

Artinian BM, Conger M, editors: *The intersystem model: integrating theory and practice,* Thousand Oaks, Calif, 1997, Sage.

Barnes C: Theories of disability and the origins of the oppression of disabled people in western society. In Barton L, editor: *Disability and society: emerging issues and insights,* New York, 1996, Longman.

Batavia AI: Relating disability policy to broader public policy: understanding the concept of "handicap," *Policy Stud J* 21(4):735-739, 1993.

Blaska J: The power of language: speak and write using "person first." In Nagler M, editor: *Perspectives on disability: text and readings on disability,* Palo Alto, Calif, 1993, Health Markets Research.

Bogdan R: Exhibiting mentally retarded people for amusement and profit: 1850-1940, *Am J Ment Deficiency* 91(2):120-126, 1986.

Brandt EN Jr, Pope AM, editors: *Enabling America: assessing the role of rehabilitation science and engineering,* Washington, DC, 1997, Committee on Assessing Rehabilitation Science and Engineering, IOM, National Academy Press.

Burgdorf RL Jr: *Assisted suicide: a disability perspective position paper,* March 24, 1997, Updated September 14, 1998, National Council on Disability, www.ncd.gov/publications/suicide.html.

Caron C: Making meaning out of the experiences of our lives, *Womens Educ des femmes* 12(2):22-25, 1996.

Creamer D: Finding God in our bodies: theology from the perspective of people with disabilities, part II, *J Religion Disabil Rehabil* 2(2):67-87, 1995.

DeJong G: Toward a research and training capacity in disability policy, *Policy Stud J* 22(1):152-160, 1994.

Friedberg JB, Mullins JB, Sukiennik AW: *Accept me as I am: best books of juvenile nonfiction on impairments and disabilities,* New York, 1985, RR Bowker Company.

Gartner A, Joe T, editors: *Images of the disabled, disabling images,* New York, 1987, Praeger.

Goffman E: *Stigma: notes on the management of spoiled identity,* Englewood Cliffs, NJ, 1963, Prentice-Hall.

Hahn H: Theories and values: ethics and contrasting perspectives on disability. In Marinelli RP, Orto AED, editors: *The psychological and social impact of disability,* ed 3, New York, 1991, Springer.

Hahn H: Toward a politics of disability: definitions, disciplines, and policies, *Soc Sci J* 22(4):87-105, 1985.

Jans L, Stoddard S: *Chartbook on women and disability in the United States,* 1999, Updated July 21, 1999, Department of Education, National Institute on Disability and Rehabilitation Research, www.infouse.com/disabilitydata.

Johnson AF, Johnson LS: Shame and spirituality: taboo topics in the disability community, *J Religion Disabil Rehabil* 2(3):29-38, 1995.

Jones NL: Essential requirements of the act: a short history and overview, *Milbank Q* 69(1):25-54, 1991.

Kaye HS et al: *Trends in disability rates in the United States: 1970-1974,* Disability Statistics Abstract 17, November 1996, Disability Statistics Rehabilitation Research and Training Center, Institute for Health and Aging, School of Nursing, University of California, http://dsc.ucsf.edu/UCSF/pub.taf?_UserReference=990250451A6B1392BC11FF67&_function=search&recid=63&grow=1.

Kraus LE, Stoddard S, Gilmartin D: *Chartbook on disability in the United States,* 1996, An InfoUse Report, Updated November 12, 1998, US National Institute on Disability and Rehabilitation Research, www.infouse.com/disabilitydata/chartbook.choices.html.

LaPlante MP, Carlson D: *Disability in the United States: prevalence and causes,* 1996, Disability Statistics Rehabilitation Research and Training Center, Institute for Health and Aging, School of Nursing, University of California, http://dsc.ucsf.edu/UCSF/pub.taf?_function=search&recid=65&grow=1.

Longmore PK: Uncovering the hidden history of people with disabilities, *Rev Am History* 15(3):355-364, 1987.

Marinelli RP, Orto AED, editors: *The psychological and social impact of disability,* ed 3, New York, 1991, Springer.

Martin SS, Catlett SM: *Same window, new view: print media and persons with disabilities,* Unpublished paper presented at 1999 TASH Conference, Chicago, Ill, 1999.

Monaghan P: Pioneering field of disability studies challenges established approaches and attitudes, *Chron High Educ* XLIV(20):A15-16, 1998.

Murphy RF: *The body silent,* New York, 1990, Henry Holt.

Nagler M, editor: *Perspectives on disability: text and readings on disability,* Palo Alto, Calif, 1993, Health Markets Research.

National Council on Disability: *National disability policy: a progress report: November 1, 1997 to October 31, 1998,* February 16, 1999, The Author, www.ncd.gov/publications/policy97-98.html.

National Organization on Disability, Louis Harris and Associates: *N.O.D./Harris 2000 survey of Americans with disabilities,* 2000, The Author, www.nod.org/attitudes.html.

Northway R: Disability and oppression: some implications for nurses and nursing, *J Adv Nurs* 26(4):736-743, 1997.

Oliver M: A sociology of disability or a disablist sociology? In Barton L, editor: *Disability and society: emerging issues and insights,* New York, 1996, Longman.

Olkin R: *What psychotherapists should know about disability,* New York, 1999, The Guilford Press.

Pfeiffer D: Overview of the disability movement: history, legislative record, and political implications, *Policy Stud J* 21(4):724-734, 1993.

Pope AM, Tarlov AR, editors: *Disability in America: toward a national agenda for prevention,* Washington, DC, 1991, IOM, National Academy Press.

Presidential Task Force on Employment of Adults with Disabilities: *Recharting the course: first report of the presidential task force on employment of adults with disabilities,* November 15, 1998, The Author, www.dol.gov/dol/_sec/public/programs/ptfead/rechart.html.

Richardson M: Addressing barriers: disabled rights and the implications for nursing of the social construct of disability, *J Adv Nurs* 25(6):1269-1275, 1997.

Scotch RK: Understanding disability policy: varieties of analysis, *Policy Stud J* 22(1):170-175, 1994.

Shapiro JP: *No pity: people with disabilities forging a new civil rights movement,* New York, 1993, Times Books.

Silvers A, Wasserman D, Mahowald MB: *Disability, difference, discrimination: perspectives on justice in bioethics and public policy,* Lanham, Mass, 1998, Rowman & Littlefield, Inc.

Taylor D: *The implications of sense of coherence for the early treatment of people who have had a traumatic spinal cord injury,* Unpublished doctoral dissertation, University of Wollongong, Wollongong, Australia, 1997.

Treloar LL: Lessons on disability and the rights of students, *Community College Rev* 27(1):30-40, 1999a.

Treloar LL: People with disabilities—the same, but different: implications for health care practice, *J Transcult Nurs* 10(4):358-364, 1999b.

Treloar LL: *Perceptions of spiritual beliefs, response to disability, and the church,* Unpublished doctoral dissertation, The Union Institute, Cincinnati, Ohio, 1999c.

Treloar LL: Spiritual care: assessment and intervention, *J Christian Nurs* 16(2):15-18, 1999d.

Treloar LL: Unpublished interviews, 1999e.

Turnbull AP, Turnbull HR III: *Families, professionals, and exceptionality,* Upper Saddle River, NJ, 1996, Merrill.

Turnbull HR III: *Free appropriate public education: the law and children with disabilities,* Denver, Colo, 1990, Love.

US Bureau of the Census: *Census brief 97-5: disabilities affect one-fifth of all Americans,* December, 1997a, The Author, www.census.gov:80/prod/3/97pubs/cenbr975.pdf.

US Bureau of the Census: *Current population reports: Americans with disabilities: 1994-1995,* August 1997b, The Author, www.census.gov/prod/3/97pubs/p70-61.pdf.

US Department of Education: *Twentieth annual report to congress on the implementation of the Individuals with Disabilities Education Act,* December 7, 1999, The Author, www.ed.gov/offices/OSERS/OSEP/OSEP98AnlRpt.

US Department of Health and Human Services: *Healthy people 2010,* Updated November 10, 2000, Office of Disease Prevention and Health Promotion, USDHHS, www.health.gov/healthypeople.

US Department of Justice: *A guide to disability rights laws,* Pub No 466-728/20269, Pueblo, Colo, 2000, Consumer Information Center.

US Department of Justice and US Equal Employment Opportunity Commission: *The Americans with Disabilities Act: questions and answers,* Pub No 412-943/50507, Pueblo, Colo, 1996, Consumer Information Center.

Wehman P, editor: *The ADA mandate for social change,* Baltimore, Md, 1993, Paul H. Brookes.

Woodill G: The role of an able-bodied person in a disability movement, *Disabil Stud Q* 14(2):48, 1994.

Young J: Personal communication, November 21, 1999.

Homeless Populations

Nellie S. Droes and Diane C. Hatton

Upon completion of this chapter, the reader will be able to do the following:

1. Discuss two meanings of the term *homeless*.
2. Describe the scope of homelessness in the United States.
3. Analyze factors that contribute to homelessness.
4. Identify major health problems among various homeless aggregates.
5. Discuss access to health care for the homeless.
6. Analyze the health problems of the homeless using upstream thinking and a social justice perspective.
7. Apply knowledge about the homeless when planning community health services for this aggregate.

acceptability
accessibility
accommodation
affordability
availability
disconnectedness
dual diagnosis
homeless
market justice
social justice

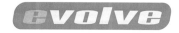

http://evolve.elsevier.com/Nies/

Since the 1980s, the number of homeless people has surpassed that of the Great Depression (US Department of Housing and Urban Development [HUD], 1994). Not only have the numbers of homeless individuals increased, but the demographic profile of this population has also changed. Joining the "traditional" homeless predominantly composed of single males are the "new homeless," which include families (Wright, Rubin, and Devine, 1998). Projections indicate that in the near future the majority of the homeless in the United States will be single mothers with children (Bassuk, Browne, and Buckner, 1996; Rog and Gutman, 1997; Wright, Rubin, and Devine, 1998).

The purpose of this chapter is to define *homelessness* and describe the scope of this problem. The authors analyze factors that contribute to homelessness, discuss the consequences of such an existence on health, and describe the health status of various aggregates of the homeless population. The authors address issues of health care access, explore conceptual approaches to understanding health among the homeless, and propose community health nursing strategies for the primary, secondary, and tertiary prevention of homelessness and its associated problems.

DEFINITIONS AND PREVALENCE OF HOMELESSNESS

Many meanings exist for the term **homeless**. Some view the term *home* as a synonym for the place where an individual's family resides. People without family ties, such as those living in single-room-only hotels (SROs) without family contacts, are, from this perspective, "homeless" (Jencks, 1994). However, government agencies' definitions of *homeless* focus on living quarters, or more specifically sleeping places, and not family ties. Current government reports continue to use the definition put forth by the Stewart B. McKinney Homeless Assistance Act of 1987, which defined *homeless* as follows:

1. An individual who lacks a fixed, regular, and adequate night-time residence and;
2. An individual who has a primary night-time residency that is the following:
   ■ A supervised publicly or privately operated shelter designed to provide temporary living accommodations (e.g., welfare hotels, congregate shelters, and transitional housing for the mentally ill);

■ An institution that provides a temporary residence for individuals intended to be institutionalized; or
■ A public or private place not designed for or ordinarily used as a regular sleeping accommodation for human beings.
3. This term does not include any individual imprisoned or otherwise detained under an Act of Congress or a state law

(Burt et al., 1999, p. 5).

However, many Americans use another definition of *homelessness*. This colloquial usage reflects the more traditional view of the homeless as the shabbily dressed people they notice in public places during the day (O'Flaherty, 1996). Homeless advocates argue that it is also important to consider those who are poor and tenuously housed. This includes those who are without their own shelter but have "doubled up" with a family member or friend. An estimate of this population is difficult at best. Definitions of *homelessness* vary and consequently give rise to many interpretations and confusion regarding research findings and policy implications (Shinn and Baumohl, 1999).

Demographic Data

The homeless are intrinsically difficult to count (Breakey and Fischer, 1990; Jencks, 1994; Lindsey, 1989; Vladeck, 1990; Wright, Rubin, and Devine, 1998). The U.S. Census Bureau has attempted to collect data on the homeless population. On "Shelter and Street Night," or "S-Night" (i.e., the evening of March 20 and the early morning hours of March 21, 1990), enumerators counted people in preidentified locations. Data from the S-Night count revealed 178,638 people living in emergency shelters for homeless people, 49,734 people visible in street locations, and 11,768 people in shelters for abused women. Furthermore, the breakdown of these data revealed that, in these three categories, males numbered 123,358, 39,255, and 2533, respectively. Females numbered 55,280, 10,479, and 9235, respectively (US Department of Commerce, 1992).

The U.S. Conference of Mayors (1999) provides another source of data on the homeless in their annual reports. Their survey of 26 major cities in the United States revealed that during 1999, requests for emergency shelter increased overall by 12%. Requests from homeless families increased by 17%, and estimates indicate that 25% of the requests by

F I G U R E **20-1**

Breakdown of people seeking shelter (From US
Conference of Mayors: *A status report on hunger
and homelessness in America's cities,* Washington,
DC, 1999, The Author).

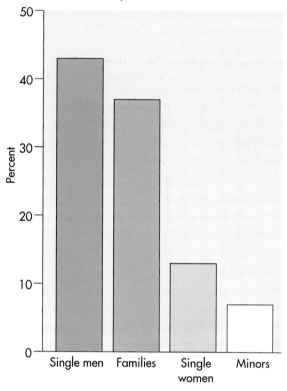

F I G U R E **20-2**

Breakdown of people seeking shelter by ethnicity
and race (From US Conference of Mayors: *A status
report on hunger and homelessness in America's
cities,* Washington, DC, 1999, The Author).

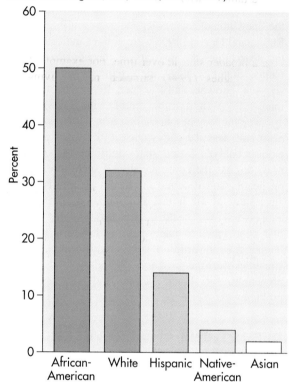

B O X **20-1**

**Twenty-Six Major Cities Included in U.S.
Conference of Mayors Survey (1999)**

Boston	Norfolk
Charleston	Philadelphia
Chicago	Portland
Cleveland	Providence
Denver	Salt Lake City
Detroit	San Antonio
Kansas City	San Diego
Los Angeles	San Francisco
Miami	San Juan
Minneapolis	Seattle
Nashville	St. Louis
New Orleans	St. Paul
New York City	Trenton

homeless people overall and 37% of requests by
families went unmet. About 54% of the cities
indicated that the amount of time people remain
homeless increased during the year, with people
remaining homeless an average of seven months.

The U.S. Conference of Mayors (1999) survey
found that single men comprised 43% of the homeless; families with children comprised 37%; single
women comprised 13%; and unaccompanied minors
comprised 7% (Fig. 20-1). Ethnic composition of the
population reported was as follows: blacks 50%,
whites 31%, Hispanics 13%, Native-Americans 4%;
and Asians 2% (Fig. 20-2). Box 20-1 lists the 26 cities
the survey included.

Although the data from both the U.S. Census
Bureau and the U.S. Conference of Mayors are useful,
they have limitations. The count provided by the U.S.
Census Bureau is a "point prevalence" count of the
total homeless population (i.e., it represents one point

in time) (HUD, 1994). Wright, Rubin, and Devine (1998) estimated that the Census Bureau's count included only one of three of the nation's literally homeless. Data from the U.S. Conference of Mayors provide information only on those homeless individuals and families who sought shelter in 26 major cities during 1999.

To obtain a more thorough understanding, some researchers have attempted to estimate the population from a broader sample over time. For example, Link and colleagues (1994) sampled people living in households with telephones and asked subjects whether there was a time in their lives when they considered themselves homeless. The researchers also asked whether subjects had been homeless during the five-year period between 1985 and 1990. To determine the nature of the homeless experience, interviewers asked whether the subject had slept in a park, abandoned building, street, or train or bus station; slept in a shelter; or slept in a friend's or relative's home because they were homeless. The investigators considered answers of "yes" to item one or two as examples of "literal" homelessness.

The findings indicate that, among the 1507 subjects, the prevalence of homelessness of any type was 14% and the five-year prevalence of any type of homelessness was 4.6%. On the basis of these lifetime prevalence rates, the researchers "estimate that about 13.5 million (7.4%) adult residents of the U.S. have been literally homeless at some time during their lives"; and using the five-year prevalence rates, "5.7 million of these have been homeless" in the span between 1985 and 1990 (Link et al., 1994, p. 1910). Moreover, these figures probably underestimate the problem because the sample excluded households without telephones (i.e., about 7% of the U.S. population). The latter may tend to be poor and more likely to experience homelessness. The estimates also exclude those living in institutions such as prisons and mental hospitals. These individuals are more likely to have experienced homelessness than a domiciled sample.

Ringwalt and colleagues (1998) studied the extent of homelessness among adolescents between 12 and 17 years of age in the United States. They concluded that a 5% annual prevalence rate was a low estimate of homelessness in this young population. They suggested that homelessness among adolescents is more common than generally believed.

In a more recent study, Phelan and Link (1999) reviewed published homeless research to assess the extent to which the use of point prevalence samples bias conclusions drawn about homeless people. Their findings suggest that point prevalence studies, which provide useful information about long-term homeless people and their characteristics, do not provide useful information about people who have experienced homelessness at some point in their lives but are not currently homeless. These researchers note that the characteristics of formerly homeless and currently homeless are different. More than 75% of currently homeless were men, in contrast to about 50% of the formerly homeless. Racial and ethnic minorities made up 54% to 70% of the currently homeless and they comprised only 20% of the formerly homeless. The currently homeless were less likely to have completed high school and were more likely to have histories of psychiatric hospitalization, incarceration, and detoxification than the formerly homeless.

For the reader attempting to grasp the various nuances involved in counting the homeless, Wright, Rubin, and Devine (1998) offer the following helpful metaphor:

> Given the episodic nature of much homelessness, trying to count the homeless is a little like trying to count the number of flies in a house whose windows and doors are wide open. At any one moment, there is a definite number of flies in the house and that number is theoretically countable. Practically speaking, however, the rapid movement of flies in and out means that no count can be definitive or even very useful. Likewise, while there is some finite and theoretically countable number of literally homeless people in the United States at any one time, they are but a fraction of a much larger number of persons who are at risk of homelessness and who are destined to be homeless at some other time. In this sense, the number of flies or of homeless people is a less pertinent question than the transition probabilities that govern movement in and out of the condition being counted (p. 63).

The homeless population is difficult to define and count. However, recent research findings that attempt to estimate homelessness over time from a broad sampling of households have revealed that the magnitude of the problem is greater than believed in the past (National Coalition for the Homeless, 1999b). However, despite attempts to count the homeless more accurately, Kozol (1988) argued the following:

> We would be wise . . . to avoid the numbers game. Any search for the "right number" carries the assumption

that we may at last arrive at an acceptable number. There is no acceptable number. Whether the number is 1 million or 4 million . . . there are too many homeless people in America (p. 10).

FACTORS THAT CONTRIBUTE TO HOMELESSNESS

Conditions in larger society that contribute to homelessness include poverty, lack of affordable housing, and changes in the labor market. The United States experienced continued economic growth between 1993 and 1998 and a decline of the poverty rate to 12.7% in 1998. The reduction in poverty has contributed to a decrease in unemployment and a rise in the wages of low paid workers. Political leaders of all parties claimed this as evidence of the success of welfare reform instituted in 1996 (CBPP, 1999; Sherman et al., 1998).

However, a critical review of the data reveals an increase in extreme childhood poverty, a proliferation of inadequately paid employment, and indicators of increased hardships for many families leaving welfare. Between 1994 and 1998, the percentage of poor children whose families received cash assistance and food stamps fell from 62% to 43% and 94% to 75%, respectively (Sherman et al., 1998).

Over the past 15 to 20 years, the growing shortage of affordable rental housing and an increase in poverty are two trends largely responsible for the increase in homelessness. The U.S. Department of Housing and Urban Development (HUD) operates federally funded programs that provide assistance to low-income families. Between 1995 and 1998, a net increase did not occur in the supply of federally subsidized housing for low-income families; the number of households receiving such subsidies declined during this period for the first time in the program's history (Sard and Daskal, 1998). Between 1998 and 1999, the number of families on waiting lists to obtain public housing or Section 8 housing vouchers increased by 10% to 25%. In addition, waiting list time increased substantially between 1996 and 1998; public housing waiting time was 11 months in 1998, and waits for Section housing vouchers were 28 months (HUD, 1999; National Coalition for Homeless, 1999a).

The shift of goods production to services over the past 25 years contributed to changes in the labor market that have consequences for increased joblessness and homelessness. Labor markets have also demanded a highly educated workforce. The consequences of these economic conditions (i.e., decreased job opportunities and extreme poverty) exist in rural and urban centers. Homeless clients reported that insufficient income and lack of employment prevented them from leaving homelessness (Burt et al., 1999).

Within the context described previously, additional factors contribute to homelessness including lack of affordable health care, domestic violence, mental illness, and addiction disorders (National Coalition for the Homeless, 1999c).

A survey of homeless clients of shelters and other homeless services conducted in 1996 reported that 55% had no medical insurance compared with 16% for all American adults (Burt et al., 1999). A serious illness or disability can lead to a downward spiral into homelessness as a result of job loss, use of savings to pay for care, and inability to pay rent. As mentioned previously, changes in welfare programs and a robust economy have affected low-income families. Fewer low-income parents are receiving welfare and the Medicaid coverage that typically accompanies welfare. More of these parents are working at low-wage jobs that offer no health insurance coverage (National Coalition for the Homeless, 1999a).

Several organizations concerned with homelessness purport that domestic violence is a contributing factor to homelessness (Health Care for the Homeless, 1999; National Coalition for the Homeless, 1999f; Rosenheck et al., 1999; US Conference of Mayors, 1999). The information that these organizations provide addresses women who leave abusive situations without alternatives other than shelters. However, issues exist concerning the emphasis on women as victims and men as batterers and the reluctance to address men as victims and women as batterers (Clark, 1999). Information regarding the relationship of domestic violence and homelessness as it concerns men who left abusive situations is lacking.

A disproportionate number of homeless people are mentally ill. Data suggest that this is not from the deinstitutionalization of the mentally ill that occurred in the 1950s and 1960s because the vast increase in homelessness occurred in the 1980s. However, concerns exist that a new wave of deinstitutionalization and denial of services or premature and unplanned discharge brought about by an underfunded mental health system and the more recent move to managed care arrangements contribute to the continued presence of people with serious mental illness within the homeless population (Drake and Wallach, 1999; National Coalition for the Homeless, 1999d).

Past surveys of homeless people, particularly men, reveal a disproportionate prevalence of drug and alcohol addiction among the homeless compared with the nonhomeless. However, most drug and alcohol addicts never become homeless. More recent studies have questioned these results because they were based on long-term shelter users and single men and used lifetime rather than current measures of addiction. Currently, no generally accepted numbers describe prevalence of addictive disorders among the homeless. Changes in eligibility that deny SSI and SSDI to people whose addictions contribute to their disability are feared to increase homelessness among this subpopulation (National Coalition for the Homeless, 1999e).

One factor alone does not force an individual or family into homelessness. Rather, multiple factors that reflect conditions in society interact with vulnerability-enhancing factors found among certain individuals and families to increase the probability of homelessness. Jencks (1994) noted that "it is a combination of personal vulnerability and political indifference that has left people in the streets" (p. 48).

HEALTH STATUS OF THE HOMELESS

As discussed in Chapter 1, the WHO has defined *health* from a broad perspective. This classic definition, which purports that health is "a state of complete physical, mental, and social well-being and not merely the absence of disease or infirmity" (WHO, 1958, p. 1), is particularly useful when considering the health status of the homeless. For these individuals, a continual interaction exists between these three dimensions (physical, mental, and social) that have enormous consequences for health. The boundaries of these dimensions overlap; therefore it is difficult if not impossible to address health among the homeless without a concomitant analysis of physical, mental, and social dimensions. Therefore this text addresses the health status of various homeless aggregates from this broad WHO interpretation. Specifically, the subgroups discussed include men, women, children, and adolescents. Special groups considered are homeless families and homeless people in the community with mental health and substance abuse problems.

Homeless Men

Reporting on the results of the Health Care for the Homeless Project, Wright (1990b) and Wright, Rubin, and Devine (1998) related that homeless men experience acute physical health problems, respiratory infections, trauma, and skin disorders at higher rates than men in the general population. Chronic disorders including hypertension, musculoskeletal disorders, gastrointestinal problems, peripheral vascular disease, COPD, neurological disorders including seizures, and poor dentition are also more prevalent among homeless populations. In addition, HIV and AIDS, TB, and STDs occur at higher rates than in the general population (Douglass et al., 1999; IOM, 1988; Sachs-Ericsson et al., 1999; Stratigos et al., 1999).

Burt and colleagues (1999) relate that homeless people reported physical acute and chronic health problems similar to those identified by health care providers. They also note that clients' self-reports may be underestimated because there is a lack of knowledge of medical conditions or reluctance to admit to some conditions.

Many of these acute and chronic conditions are exacerbated by alcoholism, which occurs more frequently among homeless than nonhomeless men; alcoholism may be the single most prevalent health problem among the homeless. Likewise, serious mental illnesses occur more frequently among the homeless than in the general population. In addition, minor emotional problems (e.g., personality disorders) are also more frequent among homeless than nonhomeless men. Drug abuse, like alcohol abuse, occurs more frequently among the homeless and considerable overlap exists among alcohol and drug abuse. Men are more likely than women to report alcohol abuse (Glasser, 1994; IOM, 1988; Wright, 1990b; Wright, Rubin, and Devine, 1998).

Studies comparing homeless and housed poor people indicate that homeless adults are more likely to be male and have veteran status than the housed poor. Homeless adults are more likely to be unemployed, or if employed, the job is temporary or at a low wage and without benefits. Consequently, their income is insufficient to maintain housing costs. Although a lack of monetary resources is a variable related directly to becoming and remaining homeless, additional deficits in social resources contribute to the condition. Many of the homeless have relied on social support from families and friends to provide housing. Homelessness results when both monetary resources and social support are exhausted (Wright, Rubin, and Devine, 1998).

Data from the National Health Care for the Homeless Program, an initiative funded by the RWJ Foundation and the Pew Charitable Trust Fund in the late 1980s, are the basis of much of the information available on the health status of men. Although dated, these data nevertheless stand as major sources of information on the health status of the homeless population.

Homeless Women

Homeless women experience health problems of enormous complexity and lack general health maintenance (Adkins and Fields, 1992; Gelberg, Doblin, and Leake, 1996). These women have limited communication with health professionals and tend to conceal stigmatizing health problems, especially those related to violence, substance abuse, and mental illness (Hatton and Fisher, 1999). They are unlikely to have preventive care; therefore homeless women often seek their health care in costly emergency rooms when problems have become acute and more difficult to manage (Hatton, 1997).

Research evidence indicates that homeless women have more physical health problems (e.g., asthma, anemia, and ulcers) than do their domiciled counterparts. In addition, homeless women rate their overall physical functioning lower than women in the general population (Bassuk et al., 1996).

The incidence of STDs among homeless women is about twice that of women in the general ambulatory population. Data indicate that the pregnancy rate among homeless women is 10.1% compared with 7.1% in a general ambulatory population of women (Wright, 1990a). Pregnancy is extraordinarily difficult for homeless women because living conditions make eating well, managing morning sickness, and keeping dry and clean virtually impossible. In addition, homeless women often experience UTIs and often neglect signs of complications (Killion, 1995).

A considerable stigma accompanies women who are without a home or family in the United States (Burroughs et al., 1990) and inevitably homelessness disrupts an individual's sense of identity and feelings of self-worth and self-efficacy (Buckner et al., 1999). These conditions compound mental-health–related problems in this subgroup. Many experience the psychological sequelae of violence including anxiety, panic disorders, major depression, substance abuse, somatization, eating disorders, self-mutilation, suicidal behaviors, and other risk-taking behaviors (Bassuk, Melnick, and Browne, 1998). In addition, homeless women report significantly more hospitalizations for emotional problems or substance abuse than housed women (Bassuk et al., 1996).

Epidemiological studies suggest that approximately 20% of homeless women suffer from alcohol problems and 10% to 20% suffer from other drug problems (Fischer, 1991). In their sample, Bassuk and colleagues (1996) found that four times as many homeless women as housed women reported injecting drugs at least once. Also, a portion of homeless women have a dual diagnosis of psychiatric and substance use disorders. These women represent extreme vulnerability; they are difficult to treat and are especially susceptible to residential instability and homelessness (Buckner, Bassuk, and Zima, 1993).

Inadequate social support can affect homeless women's ability to take care of health concerns. Often they experience **disconnectedness**, which is an inability to connect with family and friends. Disconnectedness has roots in the transience and abuse that often begins in childhood and continues into adult life (Anderson, 1996). These women frequently have fewer people in their social networks and the people they encounter often experience emotional distress and have high-risk behaviors (Bassuk, Browne, and Buckner, 1996; Nyamathi, Flaskerud, and Leake, 1997).

Although their problems are likely to be more intense, more frequent, and more apt to occur in concert, homeless women suffer from the same problems that impede many women in the United States. Often homeless women have limited education, earning power, and fragmented support networks. Trapped by this lack of economic and social opportunities, they profoundly experience society's inequalities (Bassuk, 1993).

Homeless Children

Wright, Rubin, and Devine (1998) noted that pediatricians in New York City identified a "homeless child syndrome" (p. 158), which consisted of "poverty related health problems, immunization delays, untreated or under-treated acute and chronic illnesses, unrecognized disorders, school, behavioral and psychological problems, child abuse and neglect" (p. 158). Although not all homeless children exhibit all aspects of this syndrome, they occur more commonly among homeless children than in children in the general poverty-level population.

Mothers of homeless children frequently lack prenatal care and sufficient nutrition and are more likely to deliver low-birth-weight infants. Infant mortality rates are higher for infants born to homeless women than for those born to women in public housing. More homeless children experience immunization delays, upper respiratory tract and ear infections, asthma, skin disorders, diarrhea, and anemia than housed poor children. In addition, more homeless children than domiciled poor children are apt to go without sufficient food because they lack money (Bassuk and Weinreb, 1993; Rafferty and Shinn, 1991; Wright, Rubin, and Devine, 1998).

Among the homeless children in the Health Care for the Homeless Initiative funded by the RWJ Foundation and the Pew Charitable Trust Fund, acute disorders were more common and chronic disorders were less common in children than in adults (Wright, Rubin, and Devine, 1998). Other studies have documented similar problems (Menke, 1998; Menke and Wagner, 1997; Weinreb et al., 1998).

In addition to physical health problems, homeless children experience mental health problems and developmental delays at greater rates than low-income housed children. These children frequently experience stressful life events including placement in foster care. Homeless children tend to experience depression and anxiety more often than housed children from poverty groups (Bassuk et al., 1997; Buckner et al., 1999).

Research findings reveal that when children under age five years are screened using the Denver Development Screening Test (DDST), homeless children are more likely to lack personal and social skills, language skills, and gross and fine motor skills than poor housed preschoolers. Among the homeless children, delays in personal, social, and language areas occur more frequently than delays in motor skill areas (Rafferty and Shinn, 1991). Using different measurements to assess infant and toddler development, Coll and colleagues (1998) found that homeless and low-income housed children did not differ in their cognitive and motor skills. However, older children tended to score lower than younger children, which suggested that the cumulative effects of poverty gather over time.

Notwithstanding the paucity of research on the educational achievement of homeless children, Rafferty and Shinn (1991) noted that the few studies undertaken indicate that homeless children score poorly on standardized reading and mathematics tests compared with the general school population. Zima, Wells, and Freeman (1994) demonstrated that sheltered homeless children are four times more likely to score at or below the tenth percentile in vocabulary and reading levels than children in the general population. Studies comparing homeless children with housed poor children reveal that homeless schoolchildren are more likely to repeat grades. Moreover, homeless children miss more days of school than poor housed children. Poor children miss school primarily because they are ill; homeless children miss school because their family is transient (Rafferty and Shinn, 1991).

Most research studies related to health status focus on homeless children in emergency shelters. Many of the instruments used to assess developmental and mental health are not standardized for poor and minority children. Developmental problems may be underestimated because the DDST is a conservative screening instrument. Assessing the mental health of children is problematic because available instruments are inadequate, privacy or space to conduct interviews is lacking, and parents are concerned with daily living rather than the interview. Although the nurse must be careful generalizing across studies because there are frequent small sample sizes, lack of comparison groups, and differences in administration, the studies to date reveal that poor children in general face multiple physical, mental, and social problems (Rafferty and Shinn, 1991; Weinreb et al., 1998; Wright, Rubin, and Devine, 1998; Zima et al., 1999; Zima, Wells, and Freeman, 1994).

Homeless Adolescents

The following section describes the health problems of adolescents in general, the health problems of homeless adolescents, and the health problems of homeless adolescent subpopulations. In their extensive review of homeless youths, Robertson and Toro (1999) note that the literature on homeless adolescents is limited and lacks rigorous research. A large majority of the studies were conducted in metropolitan areas and many areas were located on the West Coast. The age group varied; some studies included young adults up to 24 years of age.

An increasing number of adolescents from all sectors of society face serious health problems including unintended pregnancy, STDs including HIV and

AIDS, alcohol and drug abuse, depression, and suicide. However, homeless adolescents experience these problems at higher rates than the general adolescent population (AMA, 1992; Diamond and Buskin, 2000; Forst, Jonathan, and Goddard, 1993; Grunbaum et al., 1999; Kann et al., 1998; Lock and Steiner, 1999; Walters, 1999).

Homeless adolescents experience STDs, physical and sexual abuse, skin disorders, anemia, drug and alcohol abuse, and unintentional injuries at higher rates than adolescents in the general population. Depression; suicidal ideation; and disorders of behavior, personality, or thought also occur at higher rates among homeless adolescents. Family disruption, school failures, prostitution or "survival sex," and involvement with the legal system indicate that homeless adolescents' social health is severely compromised (Busen and Beech, 1997; Cohen, Mackenzie, and Yates, 1991; Ennett, Bailey, and Federman, 1999; Ennett et al., 1999; Forst, Jonathan, and Goddard, 1993; Reuler, 1991; Smart, 1991; Yates et al., 1991b).

Homeless adolescents who are pregnant, engage in prostitution, or identify themselves as gay experience more health problems than other homeless adolescents. Pregnant homeless adolescents have more severe mental health problems and use alcohol and drugs more than nonpregnant homeless adolescents. Not surprisingly, they have higher rates of negative pregnancy outcomes than nonhomeless adolescents (Ennett, Bailey, and Federman, 1999; Ennett et al., 1999; Greene, Ennett, and Ringwalt, 1999; Pennbridge, Mackenzie, and Swofford, 1991; Ringwalt, Greene, and Robertson, 1998).

Runaway or homeless adolescents, both female and male, make up a large percentage of all youth involved in prostitution. Many become involved because they need money to meet subsistence needs, which is the source of the term *survival sex.* These adolescents are more likely to have serious mental health problems and to be actively suicidal. Alcohol and drug use occurs at higher rates among this group than among homeless adolescents not engaged in prostitution. Youths involved in prostitution are more likely to report histories of physical and sexual abuse (Ringwalt, Greene, and Robertson, 1998; Yates et al., 1991b).

Rates of attempted suicide are higher among gay homeless adolescents. A large majority of males involved in survival sex identify themselves as gay or bisexual. Many of these youths are on the streets resulting from the effects of homophobia and preju-

dice. Facing problems similar to other homeless adolescents, gay-identified youth face an additional set of problems as a result of the rejection and low self-esteem from their sexual orientation (Kruks, 1991; Yates et al., 1991a).

The previously cited studies are quantitatively descriptive of samples of various sizes and locations of homeless youths. These types of studies are an important part of the literature on homeless youth; however, they lack the poignancy and detail found in qualitative case-study types of research. Finley and Finley (1999) present homeless youth "in their own voices" in a research story entitled *"Sp'ange,"* the street term for "spare change." Their account includes themes of "formation by homeless youth of family like structures, the use of cocaine and heroin, early use of alcohol and primacy of alcohol as the drug of choice, and attitudes toward government economic structures and work" (p. 313), thereby bringing the life of throwaway youth into sharp focus.

Finley and Finley (1999) relate the following account:

> There's the one [story] about pregnant girls dancing for dollars at private parties in New Orleans for men whose fetish is pregnancy—'the more pregnant you are, the more money you make.' A related story is the one about the toddler whose development is delayed probably because his mother never stopped using drugs and drinking alcohol while she was pregnant. (She did, however, make enough money dancing while pregnant to finance an apartment for the first year of the child's life.) Then, there's the one about the 17 year old boy who used to prostitute around New York, but who is now 'too old' to earn much money in that way (p. 332).

Adolescents in the general population are at risk, homeless adolescents are at even higher risk, and the special subgroups of adolescents including those who are gay identified, those who are pregnant, and those who are practicing survival sex, are particularly vulnerable. Health for many of these youths is severely jeopardized.

Homeless Families

Homeless families make up approximately 37% of the homeless population. During 1999, requests for shelter from this aggregate increased by an average of 17% in cities that the United States Conference of Mayors (1999) surveyed and estimates indicate that 37% of family requests for shelter were not met. In many cases, families seeking shelter have to separate from one another to find accommodations; moreover, they may have to leave the shelter during the day because emergency facilities are often open only in the evening.

The high-risk conditions under which homeless families live "contradict the essence of what we often think of as family life—a stable, secure, and sheltered place for nurturing children" (Hausman and Hammen, 1993, p. 358). Earlier in this chapter, the authors described the health consequences for homeless children and women; single mothers most often head homeless families with children. Moreover, many of the factors that make parents more vulnerable for becoming homeless also impair their functioning as parents. Therefore homeless families deal with a double crisis in experiencing the trauma of losing a home and losing the parent's capacity to function as a caregiver (Hausman and Hammen, 1993). The following paragraphs present selected studies that relate to homeless families.

In a study of 80 families living in shelters in Los Angeles County, McChesney (1992) concluded that homeless families are a heterogeneous group. Using source of income as a basis, McChesney identified the following four types of families at risk of becoming homeless: "(1) unemployed couples, (2) mothers leaving relationships, (3) AFDC mothers, and (4) mothers who have been homeless teenagers" (p. 246).

In a study of homeless and low-income domiciled mothers, Wagner and Menke (1991) reported similarities and differences between the two groups. Both groups report using similar coping behaviors. However, homeless mothers are "slightly older, have more children to care for, are not as educated, and are less likely to be employed" (p. 82). Additionally, the homeless women have more stressors "in the areas of intra family stress, marital strain, and financial difficulties" (p. 82).

Findings from a study of 80 homeless families in Massachusetts indicate that homeless mothers had relationships with men characterized by instability, conflict, and violence. Approximately one third leave their parental homes and unstable family relationships and enter relationships with men who batter them. More than 40% of the women noted that their most recent male partner was a substance abuser, and two thirds link battering to alcohol use (Bassuk, 1992).

With their histories of abuse, it is not surprising that some of these mothers may perpetuate the cycle of violence. In Bassuk's 1992 study, the Department of Social Services investigated 23% of the mothers for child abuse or neglect or both. Other clinical problems such as mental illness exacerbate these situations. Bassuk reported that 71% of the mothers in her sample had a diagnosis of personality disorder.

Comparing the social support of homeless and housed mothers, Letiecq, Anderson, and Koblinsky (1998) also examined differences in the type of housing among emergency shelters, transitional housing, and "doubling up" (i.e., living with relatives or friends). Mothers in emergency and transitional shelters had smaller social support networks than permanently housed mothers.

Exploring the relationship among self-efficacy and time perspective on coping strategies in obtaining housing and employment, Epel, Bandura, and Zimbardo (1999) employed a sample of adults with at least one child who resided in family shelters. The sample was comprised of newly homeless; 76% reported that it was their first episode of homelessness. Results suggest that self-efficacy and future orientation predicted proactive search behaviors but not in obtaining stable housing. However, a present temporal perspective was a predictor of obtaining temporary housing. The authors note that a present orientation is necessary in times of acute crisis (e.g., finding some type of place to live as the time limits on the shelter stay expire).

Despite adversities inherent in homeless circumstances, Hodnicki and Horner (1993) reported that homeless mothers describe caring behaviors toward their children including "sacrificing, struggling with limitations, guarding from harm, and seeking answers" (p. 352). Hodnicki and Horner concluded that the mothers in their study actively sought ways to overcome crises and improve the well-being of their families. Managing children and homelessness is an enormous task for these mothers and it has consequences for their health. Anecdotal evidence indicates that homeless mothers rarely tend to their health problems and prolong seeking health care until they are so acutely ill that they need emergency treatment (Berne et al., 1990).

Homeless People with Mental Health and Substance Abuse Problems

This section describes problems that homeless people experience with mental health and substance abuse and examines inherent risks for health status. Wright, Rubin, and Devine (1998), in a substantial review of multiple studies on homelessness and the mentally ill, note that the rate of psychiatric disorder is higher among the homeless compared with the domiciled population. Estimates of mental illness among homeless people have varied from 10% to 90%. In a 1996 national survey of clients of homeless service providers, 45% of respondents self-reported experiences with mental health problems in the previous year (Burt et al., 1999).

Variations in rates of mental illness are attributed to different measurement methods (Bellavia and Toro, 1999; Buckner, Bassuk, and Zima, 1993). For example, using hospitalization rates does not consider those homeless who have not entered the hospital; samples consisting of service provider clients exclude those who do not use such services. Consequently, these estimates may be at the low end. Conversely, many of the measurements employed fail to consider the context of homelessness. Unhappiness, discouragement, worry, and tiredness are components of frequently used measurements of mental health. These feelings are common among the homeless. As Wright, Rubin, and Devine (1998) note, if homeless people were happy about their circumstances, their "grasp on reality" (p. 107) would be in doubt. Lay people frequently label behaviors that are necessary for survival (e.g., rummaging in garbage cans and urinating in public) as crazy or abnormal. However, when the homeless lack money for food or lack access to public restrooms, such behaviors may demonstrate survivability.

Wright, Rubin, and Devine (1998) allege that the estimated rate of alcohol abuse exceeds 40% among the nations' homeless and is near 50% among homeless men. An extensive study of the homeless in New Orleans estimated that 75% of the city's homeless abuse alcohol and more than half abuse other drugs (i.e., mostly crack). Substance abuse was a critical factor in determining homelessness because those with more resources consumed more drugs and those with fewer resources consumed fewer drugs. The nature of the disorder prevented these homeless people from using the resources that they had for improved social or housing alternatives (Wright, Rubin, and Devine, 1998). In the previously mentioned 1996 national survey (Burt et al., 1999), 46% of the adult respondents reported problems with alcohol and 38% reported problems with other substances within the previous year.

Moreover, for a sizable proportion of the homeless, severe mental illness exists concomitantly with the problems of alcohol or other drug use, which is a phenomenon known as *comorbidity* or **dual diagnosis** (USDHHS, 1992). In a review of epidemiological studies, Fischer (1991) concluded that 10% to 20% of homeless single adults suffer from this combination of a psychiatric disorder and substance use, or comorbidity. Among homeless adults in Los Angeles, Koegel and colleagues (1999) found that 77% of people with a severe or chronic mental disorder were also chronic substance abusers. They also note that this rate was nearly a twofold increase compared with a study they conducted 10 years earlier. Homeless individuals with a dual diagnosis may represent the most vulnerable and the most difficult to treat among the homeless; they are especially vulnerable to residential instability because they are less able to compete for scarce housing resources.

Substance abuse carries considerable health risks. Alcohol abuse and dependence are associated with a wide range of health problems involving the liver, nervous system, and heart. The loss of economic productivity, vulnerability to accidents, and victimization are common outcomes. Drug use involving intravenous administration carries risks of infections (e.g., hepatitis) and STDs (e.g., HIV) and significant social, legal, and economic problems (Goldfinger et al., 1999; McMurray-Avila, Gelberg, and Breakey, 1999).

This section outlined the health status of various aggregates of homeless people including men, women, children, adolescents, families, and people with mental illness and/or substance abuse. These aggregates experience more acute and chronic health problems than people in the general population. In addition, these groups of homeless experience considerable difficulty in accessing health care services.

ACCESS TO HEALTH CARE FOR THE HOMELESS

Proposing to clarify "access" as it relates to health care services, Penchansky and Thomas (1981) noted that access is a general concept that represents the "degree of 'fit' between the clients and the system" (p. 128). Furthermore, the general term *access* summarizes the following five specific areas of "fit between the patient and the health care system" (p. 128):

1. **Availability** refers to the relationship between the amount (i.e., number of providers and facilities) and type of health care services to the amount and type of client needs.
2. **Accessibility** connotes the relationship between the location of the services and the clients' location.

3. **Accommodation** indicates the relationship between how services are organized (e.g., hours of operation and appointment systems) and the client's ability to accommodate to these factors. The client's perception of the appropriateness of these factors is a component of accommodation.
4. **Affordability** refers to the price of provider services or payment requirements and the client's ability to pay.
5. **Acceptability** represents the relationship between the client's attitudes about providers and providers' attitudes about acceptable client characteristics.

These five factors are used as a framework for exploring problems in accessing health care by people who are poor but housed, homeless people in general, and special aggregates of the homeless.

Poor but housed people experience considerable problems related to each of the five access dimensions; however, the primary problem is affordability. Many poor people lack any form of health insurance including Medicaid. For those who do meet Medicaid eligibility requirements, the low reimbursement rate discourages or prohibits health care providers from participating. A consequence of the inability to afford the services of a market-driven system, those who are excluded from the private fee-for-service arrangement must rely on public hospital systems' outpatient clinics, emergency rooms, and inpatient services. Heavy demands on these less-than-adequate facilities frequently result in less-than-desirable or appropriate accommodations. Long waits for services in overcrowded, uncomfortable settings may discourage people from seeking care at an earlier and more easily treated stage.

Notwithstanding such difficulties, these facilities are frequently situated some distance from the client's shelter or work. Although the inner-city resident may access such facilities through a public transportation system, those individuals who reside in rural areas lack such services and must find other resources (e.g., relatives, neighbors, and friends) or do without health care. Providers in many public systems are under considerable stress working in less than optimal conditions with heavy workloads and find it difficult to provide care to poor clients who frequently have complex problems and different cultural and language expectations. Consequently, these clients may find such services unacceptable and may fail to seek care until illnesses are intolerable (Aday, 1992; IOM, 1988; Wright, 1990b).

Like people who are poor but housed, homeless people experience considerable difficulty accessing the health care system. However, the homeless face more severe problems than the housed poor. Eligibility for many services frequently requires forms of documentation that homeless people find difficult to provide because they are homeless. Lacking secure storage space makes it difficult to protect personal papers from loss, theft, or weather. Frequently, homeless people must walk to service sites because use of public transportation is too costly. Consequently, accessibility is even more problematic for the homeless than for those who are housed and have a more intact system of transportation (e.g., transportation vouchers, relatives, neighbors, and friends). Without a permanent mailing address or message center, accommodating a health care system that relies on mailed notification of appointments or results of health care procedures is unlikely. Furthermore, the hours of service may force the homeless to choose between obtaining health care and obtaining food and shelter (Aday, 1992; IOM, 1988; Wright, 1990b).

Special aggregates within the homeless population experience additional problems in obtaining health care services. The following section describes the problems of homeless people who are chronically mentally ill and homeless pregnant women.

Although physical health services available to the poor are inadequate, mental health services are even less available. Koegel and colleagues (1999) examined the use and predictor of mental health and substance abuse treatment among a community-based sample of homeless adults. Only 20% of those with chronic mental illness or substance abuse reported receiving treatment within the 60 days before being interviewed. Koegel and colleagues stress that attention to systems-level features is necessary to provide access for this especially vulnerable group of homeless people. The historic conditions of deinstitutionalization, whereby community-based mental health services failed to materialize, and the current policy, whereby Medicaid and managed care plans reimburse less for mental health services than for physical health services, cause the need for mental health services for homeless mentally ill clients to far exceed the supply.

The homeless mentally ill also require physical health services. Obtaining such care from these two disconnected and complex systems requires considerable skill in negotiation. The nature of the illness frequently compromises this skill. Notwithstanding the lack of services, the chronically mentally ill, from the intrinsic nature of their health problems, frequently experience significant problems related to dimensions of accommodation and acceptability. Frequently distrustful of established institutions, the chronically mentally ill find the traditional services provided by mental health agencies inappropriate. Many providers find their bizarre manner of dress, lack of personal hygiene, and inappropriate physical appearance difficult to accept (Aday, 1992; IOM, 1988; USDHHS, 1992).

Given the conditions of homelessness and the necessity of obtaining food and shelter, pregnant homeless women frequently find seeking early prenatal care a lesser priority. Compounding the lower priority are the problems of obtaining prenatal and obstetric care. Some obstetric providers refuse to see or limit the number of women on Medicaid they will see because low reimbursement rates, complex billing requirements, and increased risk associated with malpractice suits exist. Consequently, the availability of prenatal and obstetric services is severely compromised. Long waits for initial appointments and long waits at each visit impose considerable stress in obtaining prenatal care. Many providers find the unhealthy lifestyles, lack of compliance with provider advice, and failure to keep appointments unacceptable (Aday, 1992; Curry, 1989; IOM, 1988). Multiple complex factors reduce access to health care for this vulnerable, underserved aggregate.

CONCEPTUAL APPROACHES TO HEALTH OF THE HOMELESS

The following discussion provides a conceptual and theoretical framework for exploring health care of the homeless and outlines the market justice and social justice approaches to the distribution of benefits and burdens. It provides an explanation of social justice as the absence of structural violence and discusses upstream vs. downstream approaches to homeless health care.

Models of justice provide a blueprint for considering the health problems of the homeless. Beauchamp (1979) distinguished between the two types of justice that influence public health policy in the United States (i.e., market justice and social justice). **Market justice** has been the dominant model and purports that people are entitled to valued ends (i.e., status, income, and happiness) according to their own individual efforts. Moreover, this model stresses individual responsibility, minimal collective action,

and freedom from collective obligations other than respect for another person's fundamental rights. In contrast, under a **social justice** model, all people are equally entitled to key ends (i.e., access to health care and minimum standards of income). Consequently, all members of society must accept collective burdens to provide a fair distribution of these ends. Moreover, social justice is a foundational aspect of public health (Krieger and Birn, 1998).

Additional explication of social justice is found in Galtung's analysis of violence. Distinguishing between physical and structural violence, Galtung (1969) defined *violence* as "present when human beings are being influenced so that their actual somatic and mental realizations are below their potential realization" (p. 168). The difference is between the actual and the possible. He further distinguished between physical and structural violence according to whether a person who acts is present. Galtung noted that when an actor is present who commits the violence, this is personal or direct violence. In contrast, structural violence is indirect because it lacks an actor. More specifically, the violence is built into the social structure and is displayed as unequal power and unequal life chances. Stated differently, resources are unevenly distributed (e.g., access to medical services from ability to pay or from location). Presence of structural violence is also known as social injustice. Conversely, its absence is social justice.

Butterfield discusses McKinlay's (1979) use of the metaphor depicting illness as a river; health workers focus exclusively on pulling people out of the river rather than going upstream to find out why people are in the river. Hence, the predominant mode of approaching societal problems is a downstream mode of intervention.

As McKinlay and Marceau (2000) note, a social philosophy that is focused on an individualistic approach is the dominant approach to public health problems in the United States. In this approach, individual people are the center of concern. Collectivism is a contrasting approach that focuses on "categories (age, sex, social class, race/ethnicity) or places and social positions in society" (p. 26), which is the more dominant theme in Europe.

The authors argue that the market justice model, accompanied by an individualistic social model, results in a downstream approach to problems and contributes to structural violence. This model holds individuals responsible for their own conditions and negates the responsibility of all individuals and groups to share in the burdens of prevention. In contrast, the social justice model, which seeks to reduce the structural conditions contributing to the problem through collective action, supports upstream thinking.

Building on McKinlay's "river" metaphor, the authors suggest conceptualizing homelessness as the river and the people in the river as the homeless. The authors purport that government and private efforts to address homeless health care problems largely focused on "pulling the bodies out of the river of homelessness." Such downstream interventions aimed at treating or alleviating health care problems such as physical disease and mental illnesses are worthy and needed. However, these interventions are far less adequate in alleviating homeless people's social health problems. To improve the social health of the homeless, it is necessary to go upstream and focus on the primary contributors to homelessness itself (i.e., lack of access to affordable housing and an adequate income).

Some purport that affordable housing and income support are sufficient to relieve homelessness (Timmer, Eitzen, and Talley, 1994). Timmer and colleagues argued that the homeless are not different from other people in physical and mental health status. The research reviewed here does not support these conclusions; it indicates that the homeless have more health problems than the poor who are housed. Although the authors of this text agree that the primary mode of preventing homeless health problems is to prevent homelessness, they also believe that secondary and tertiary types of interventions are necessary.

RESEARCH AND THE HOMELESS

Many factors make conducting research among the homeless complex. The transient nature of the population makes it difficult to locate and maintain study participants. The presence of alcoholism, mental illness, and other acute and chronic conditions can impede data collection procedures and the researcher may find it difficult to locate a safe and appropriate place for data gathering. Other barriers to data collection include language and cultural differences between researcher and study participants and often questionnaires and other instruments assume a level of literacy inappropriate for this aggregate (Christensen and Grace, 1999).

Homeless individuals may be reluctant to participate in research for fear of reprisal or negative consequences that may occur because they revealed information during a study (Vredevoe, Shuler, and Woo, 1992). They may also be reluctant to ask questions to clarify their roles in the study and give their informed consent (Anderson and Hatton, 2000).

Researchers can use several strategies to enhance investigations with the homeless including the recruitment and retention of participants. Negotiating entry into an agency where homeless people congregate can be critical to the success of a research project. Developing relationships with staff members who in turn introduce the researcher to homeless clients can increase a researcher's effectiveness. In addition, staff members can encourage the homeless to ask questions about a study and about their risks and benefits as potential participants (Anderson and Hatton, 2000).

Despite the obstacles, a considerable body of research from a variety of disciplines, including nursing, exists within this aggregate. Nursing research has focused on families of origin among homeless women (Anderson, 1996), health practices (Flynn, 1997), and health promotion (Alley et al., 1998). Dr. Adeline Nyamathi and colleagues at UCLA have examined drug and alcohol use, supportive people, and AIDS education among homeless women (Nyamathi et al., 1998, 1999; Nyamathi, Keenan, and Bayley, 1998). Although these studies reflect the heterogeneity of slightly different homeless subgroups throughout the United States, all provide evidence of diverse and complex health needs.

Nurse scientists can pool their clinical and research perspectives to enhance investigations; therefore they have extraordinary expertise to conduct research with the homeless. These combined perspectives provide insight into such complex phenomena as family interactions and parenting within an emergency shelter (Droes, 1993; Droes and Hatton, 1991; Hatton and Droes, 1991). In the latter grounded theory study, data analysis revealed several family constellations and interactions that had consequences for parenting and health-seeking behaviors. Particularly important were families in which the male parent dominated the interaction and focused attention on himself for a clinically minor concern rather than on a seriously ill child. Women in these families had relatively little voice in the family's health care decisions.

Findings from another qualitative grounded theory study of single women with children living in transitional shelters indicated that for these women health care decision making was problematic. During in-depth interviews, these women revealed their reluctance to seek health care and to discuss problems openly with providers. This reluctance stemmed from a variety of sources including shame, fear, lack of information, and eligibility for services (Hatton, 1997). In these instances, shelter staff members played a critical role in the identification and management of health needs, yet staff members often had little health-related knowledge and intervened based on their personal experiences and intuition. They frequently focused attention on health problems such as head lice and chickenpox. They generally did not perceive the importance of dealing with the more "invisible" problems that had more serious consequences from a clinical perspective. The latter included TB and HIV infection (Hatton et al., in review; Hatton et al., in press).

Hatton's most recent study, funded by the NINR (Hatton, 1999), builds on the above qualitative investigations. The aims of this ongoing research project are to increase homeless women's health maintenance behaviors, improve their general health, and decrease their use of costly emergency room visits. Using an experimental design, the investigator tests the effectiveness of an intervention that includes social support sessions with homeless women living in a transitional shelter. The intervention helps women develop the necessary skills for managing health and helps them establish communication with health professionals. Findings from this study will provide community health nurses with increased knowledge about how to improve health outcomes among homeless women.

Future nursing research must continue to address the issues facing community health nurses and their practice with the homeless. Potential inquiries include the following:

- What interventions will give homeless individuals a voice in their health care interactions?
- How can researchers conceptualize and measure parenting and health care decision making as outcomes for homeless parents?
- What interventions with shelter staff members will provide them with the expertise to deal with health problems in their settings?
- What interventions most effectively prevent homelessness in a community?

Nurse scientists need to consider multiple factors in their investigations such as poverty, affordable housing, and available resources that influence health outcomes among the homeless. Nurses do not deliver care to homeless clients in isolation; they work with others such as shelter staff members, social workers, and physicians. Future studies incorporating an interdisciplinary focus that allows the perspectives of each discipline to interact and enhance the research process (Olesen et al., 1990) will provide the broad knowledge necessary for effective community health nursing practice.

CASE STUDY

APPLICATION OF THE NURSING PROCESS

Community health nurses have contact with homeless individuals and families in a variety of settings including schools, jails, emergency departments, community clinics, and shelters. Nurses practicing in these settings have a unique opportunity to address the health needs of this aggregate. Many nurses are highly skilled in risk reduction and illness treatment, but caring for vulnerable populations such as the homeless requires a new and emerging set of nursing knowledge and skills that includes providing resources. Although many nurses do not have these skills, they have long been within the domain of public health nurses (Flaskerud, 1999).

The following case study provides an illustration of a nurse working with the homeless in a county health department and demonstrates the nursing process at the individual, family, and aggregate levels. As the case demonstrates, Butter field's use of the "upstream thinking" metaphor provides a useful perspective for considering primary, secondary, and tertiary prevention. The case also demonstrates how nurses must work to provide resources for the homeless at the individual and aggregate levels.

Connie Boiley, a nurse working with a county health department, received a referral from a local homeless shelter. Staff members requested that she assess Ruth Smith, a client, and assist her in adapting to the shelter's communal living situation. The referral form indicated that Ruth was a white woman aged 29 with eight children. She only had custody of her newborn daughter. Her other seven children resided in foster homes.

Assessment

When Connie visited the shelter, Ruth told her she had a history of hospitalization for "mental health problems." Ruth had difficulty focusing on their conversation and told Connie that she heard voices. Ruth said that after the birth of her daughter, her obstetrician recommended that she stop all medications because she wanted to breast feed the infant. Ruth also informed Connie that she had a long history of crack cocaine use.

Shelter staff members reported that Ruth's behavior was disruptive to the other shelter residents and they were unable to manage clients with psychiatric problems. Generally, the shelter does not allow clients requiring psychiatric medications to stay because they are unable to adequately monitor them. Staff members decided to give special consideration to Ruth because she had a newborn. However, difficulties among Ruth, the staff members, and other clients escalated. Connie understood from experience that the community did not have other facilities that offered shelter to mothers with psychiatric problems.

Diagnosis

Individual
Altered health maintenance

Family
- Impaired home maintenance management
- Alteration in parenting

Community
- Lack of mental health services for women with children
- Lack of affordable housing

Planning

Connie discussed the priority for managing Ruth's mental health problems with Ruth and the shelter staff members. She also consulted with colleagues in her community who had experience working with homeless mentally ill people and identified treatment resources. Connie explored the community resources for ongoing well-baby care and family planning services.

Intervention

For psychiatric evaluation and treatment, Connie referred Ruth to a community mental health agency that provided services to low-income and homeless people. This agency had services especially designed for individuals with a dual diagnosis (e.g., a substance use disorder and mental illness). The shelter's staff members facilitated Ruth's care by helping her reestablish her Medicaid eligibility and begin to explore her eligibility for disability benefits. Ruth began to leave the newborn in the shelter's day care facility for short periods and attended a day treatment program at the community mental health agency. She also resumed taking her medications and began bottle feeding her baby.

Connie worked with the shelter's staff members to develop strategies for caring for Ruth and her newborn in the shelter. Ruth attended parenting classes with other shelter residents on a regular basis. Staff members clearly identified expectations for Ruth in the shelter including household tasks, management of her illness, and care of her newborn. As Ruth gradually adapted to shelter living, Connie referred her to a nearby community clinic for family planning services and well-baby care.

Evaluation

Connie developed specific guidelines with the staff members to monitor Ruth's progress in the shelter. Ruth, Connie, and staff members met on a biweekly

Continued

basis to review the overall situation and analyze emerging problems.

Levels of Prevention

As noted in the discussion about conceptual approaches to the health of the homeless, efforts to address homeless health care problems have focused on downstream interventions. In Ruth's case, Connie helped pull her out of the "river of homelessness." As McKinlay (1979) argued, health professionals are so busy pulling the bodies to the shore that they have no time to go upstream and see who is pushing them in. To consider an "upstream" intervention, or in this case primary prevention, community health nurses must address the primary contributors to homelessness itself (i.e., the conditions in society that influence homelessness and the vulnerability-enhancing factors among individuals and families).

Primary Prevention

To address the problem of homelessness at this level, community health nurses must deal with the economic and political institutions in the United States. Nursing has a long history of responding to public need. The Henry Street settlement nurses provide such an example. These nurses saw that their work was different from that of a hospital where infants were cured when they were sick. Instead, the Henry Street settlement nurses sought to care for infants before they became sick and to keep them well (Portnoy and Dumas, 1994).

Similarly, contemporary community health nurses work with individuals and families who experience vulnerability-enhancing factors such as mental illness, substance use problems, violence, and weakened family ties to prevent homelessness. At an aggregate level, community health nurses play a role by influencing policy that has consequences for homelessness in the United States.

Rosenheck (1994) summarized the seriousness of homelessness and its implications for public policy action in the following:

> Homelessness is a symptom of much deeper and more serious changes in American society. How we would reverse these changes is not easy to specify in policy recommendations that are both empirically based and politically acceptable. Effective action is urgently needed in the areas of housing, health care, employment, and education. The alternative of continued social disintegration will have grave consequences for the national health and welfare and makes this a problem on which we cannot turn our backs (p. 1886).

Secondary Prevention

At the level of secondary prevention, community health nurses can provide outreach programs for homeless individuals and families. Again, at the aggregate level, the influence on policy for programs for the homeless is critical. Maurin (1990) argued that nurse researchers can work with health care providers to provide research data about the homeless and their health problems to local community leaders to improve resources available to meet their needs.

Tertiary Prevention

At the level of tertiary prevention, the community health nurse can work with clients such as Ruth Smith. In this instance, Ruth's social and mental health problems escalated. The community health nursing goal is to facilitate management and prevention of further deterioration of her mental illness. At an aggregate level, the community health nurse again works within the political arena to improve resources available to meet the needs of the homeless. In cases such as Ruth's, facilities are necessary that offer housing and psychiatric services to women with children.

SUMMARY

Homelessness evolves from the interaction of complex factors at the societal level and among vulnerable individuals. Consequently, these individuals and families find themselves living in the streets, abandoned buildings, other public places, and shelters. Homeless people are heterogeneous, difficult to count, and suffer from a variety of complex health problems. Their access to health care is problematic at best and interventions to deal with this enormous problem represent largely downstream endeavors. Future research with members of this aggregate, which will explore the complexity of their lives from a variety of methodological perspectives, will generate the knowledge necessary for more upstream community health nursing interventions.

LEARNING ACTIVITIES

1. Explain the difference between the U.S. Census Bureau count of the homeless and surveys that measure lifetime prevalence rates of homelessness. What are the advantages and disadvantages of these approaches for estimating the number of homeless persons in the United States?
2. Analyze at least three or four factors that contribute to homelessness in the United States.
3. Discuss common health problems found among homeless men, women, children, and adolescents.
4. Identify two special subgroups of the homeless and describe their health problems.
5. Describe the five specific areas of access identified by Penchansky and Thomas (1981). What is the significance of these areas for community health nursing practice with homeless individuals and families?
6. Analyze how the United States has approached the health problems of the homeless using a market justice model and a social justice model.

REFERENCES

Aday LA: *At risk in America: the health and health care needs of vulnerable populations in the United States,* San Francisco, 1992, Jossey-Bass.

Adkins CB, Fields J: Health care values of homeless women and their children, *Fam Community Health* 15:20, 1992.

Alley N et al: Health promotion: lifestyles of women experiencing crises, *J Community Health Nurs* 15(2):91, 1998.

American Medical Association: *Guidelines for adolescent preventive services,* Chicago, 1992, The Association.

Anderson D: Homeless women's perceptions about their families of origin, *West J Nurs Res* 18(1):29, 1996.

Anderson DG, Hatton DC: Accessing vulnerable populations for research, *West J Nurs Res* 22(2):244, 2000.

Bassuk EL: Social and economic hardships of homeless and other poor women, *Am J Orthopsychiatry* 63:340, 1993.

Bassuk EL: Women and children without shelter: the characteristics of homeless families. In Robertson MJ, Greenblatt M, editors: *Homelessness: a national perspective,* New York, 1992, Plenum Press.

Bassuk EL, Browne A, Buckner JC: Single mothers and welfare, *Sci Am* 275(4):60, 1996.

Bassuk EL et al: Determinants of behavior in homeless and low-income housed preschool children, *Pediatrics* 100(1):92, 1997.

Bassuk EL et al: The characteristics and needs of sheltered homeless and low-income housed mothers, *JAMA* 276(8):640, 1996.

Bassuk EL, Melnick S, Browne A: Responding to the needs of low-income and homeless women who are survivors of family violence, *J Am Med Wom Assoc* 53(2):57, 1998.

Bassuk EL, Weinreb L: Homeless pregnant women: two generations at risk, *Am J Orthopsychiatry* 63:348, 1993.

Beauchamp DE: Public health as social justice. In Jaco EG, editor: *Patients, physicians, and illness,* New York, 1979, Free Press.

Bellavia CW, Toro PA: Mental disorder among homeless and poor people: a comparison of assessment methods, *Community Ment Health J* 35(1):57, 1999.

Berne AS et al: A nursing model for addressing the health needs of homeless families, *Image J Nurs Sch* 22:8, 1990.

Breakey WR, Fischer PJ: Homelessness: the extent of the problem, *J Soc Issues* 46:31, 1990.

Buckner JC, Bassuk EL, Zima B: Mental health issues affecting homeless women: implications for intervention, *Am J Orthopsychiatry* 63:385, 1993.

Buckner JC et al: Homelessness and its relation to the mental health and behavior of low-income school-age children, *Dev Psychol* 35(1):246, 1999.

Burroughs J et al: Health concerns of homeless women. In Brickner PW et al, editors: *Under the safety net: the health and social welfare of the homeless in the United States,* New York, 1990, Norton.

Burt MR et al: *Homelessness: programs and the people they serve: a summary report of the findings of the National Survey of Homeless Assistance Providers and Clients,* Washington, DC, 1999, HUD.

Busen NH, Beech B: A collaborative model for community-based health care screening of homeless adolescents, *J Prof Nurs* 13(5):316, 1997.

Center on Budget and Policy Priorities: *Low unemployment, rising wages fuels poverty decline,* October, 1999, The Author, www.cbpp.org/9-30-99pov.htm.

Christensen RC, Grace GD: The prevalence of low literacy in an indigent psychiatric population, *Psychiatric Serv* 50(2):262, 1999.

Clark C: *Ceasefire! why women and men must join forces to achieve true equality,* New York, 1999, Free Press.

Cohen E, Mackenzie RG, Yates GL: HEADSS, a psychosocial risk assessment instrument: implications for designing effective intervention programs for runaway youth, *J Adol Health* 12:539, 1991.

Coll CG et al: The developmental status and adaptive behavior of homeless and low-income housed infants and toddlers, *Am J Public Health* 88(9):1371, 1998.

Curry MA: Nonfinancial barriers to prenatal care, *Women Health* 15:85, 1989.

Diamond C, Buskin S: Continued risky behavior in HIV-infected youth, *Am J Public Health* 90(1):115, 2000.

Douglass RL et al: Health care needs and services utilization among sheltered and unsheltered Michigan homeless, *J Health Care Poor Underserved* 10(1):5, 1999.

Drake RE, Wallach MA: Homelessness and mental illness: a story of failure (editorial), *Psychiatr Serv* 50(5):589, 1999.

Droes N: *Family interactions in a homeless shelter: use of dimensional analysis (abstract),* Communicating Nursing Research 26, Boulder, Colo, 1993, Western Institute for Nursing.

Droes N, Hatton D: *Family interactions in a homeless shelter,* presented at the meeting of the Western Social Science Association, Reno, Nev, 1991.

Ennett ST, Bailey SL, Federman EB: Social network characteristics associated with risky behaviors among runaway and homeless youth, *J Health Soc Behav* 40(1):63, 1999.

Ennett ST et al: HIV-risk behaviors associated with homelessness characteristics in youth, *J Adol Health* 25(5):344, 1999.

Epel ES, Bandura A, Zimbardo PG: Escaping homelessness: the influences of self-efficacy and time perspective on coping with homelessness, *J Appl Soc Psychol* 23(3):575, 1999.

Finley S, Finley M: Sp'ange: a research story, *Qualitative Inquiry* 5:313, 1999.

Fischer PJ: *Alcohol, drug abuse, and mental health problems among homeless persons: a review of the literature, 1980-1990,* Rockville, Md, 1991, National Institute on Alcohol Abuse and Alcoholism.

Flaskerud JH: Emerging nursing care of vulnerable populations, *Nurs Clin North Am* 34(2):xv, 1999.

Flynn L: The health practices of homeless women: a causal model, *Nurs Res* 46(2):72, 1997.

Forst ML, Jonathan H, Goddard PA: A health-profile comparison of delinquent and homeless youths, *J Health Care Poor Underserved* 4:386, 1993.

Galtung J: Violence, peace, and peace research, *J Peace Res* 16:167, 1969.

Gelberg L, Doblin BH, Leake BD: Ambulatory health services provided to low-income and homeless adult patients in a major community health center, *J Gen Intern Med* 11(1):156, 1996.

Glasser I: *Homelessness in global perspective,* New York, 1994, GK Hall.

Goldfinger AM et al: *HIV, homelessness and serious mental illness: implications for policy and practice,* 1999, National Resource Center on Homelessness and Mental Illness, Policy Research Associates, Inc, www.prainc.com/nrc/papers/hiv/hiv_toc.shtml.

Greene JM, Ennett ST, Ringwalt CL: Prevalence and correlates of survival sex among runaway and homeless youth, *Am J Public Health* 89(9):1406, 1999.

Grunbaum JA et al: United States: youth risk behavior surveillance—National Alternative High School Youth Risk Behavior Survey, 1998, *Mor Mortal Wkly Rep* 48(SS07), 1999, www.cdc.gov/mmwr/indss_99.html.

Hatton DC: *Improving health outcome among homeless women,* Grant No R15-NRO497-01, 1999, NIH, NINR, www.nih.gov/ninr/1999grants/1999NINRgrants_womens.htm.

Hatton DC: Managing health problems among homeless women with children in a transitional shelter, *Image J Nurs Sch* 29(1):33, 1997.

Hatton DC et al: Homeless women and children's access to health care: a paradox, *J Community Health Nurs* in press.

Hatton DC et al: *The health work of homeless shelter staff,* in review.

Hatton DC, Droes NS: *The nature of families and family interaction in a homeless shelter,* Paper Presented at the 11th Annual Florida VA Nursing Research Conference, Gainesville, Fla, 1991.

Hatton DC, Fisher A: Strategies for managing health problems among homeless women: three case studies, *Nurs Case Manag* 4(11):19, 1999.

Hausman B, Hammen C: Parenting in homeless families: the double crisis, *Am J Orthopsychiatry* 63:358, 1993.

Health Care for the Homeless Information Resource Center: *The face of homelessness,* 1999, Policy Research Associates Inc, www.prainc.com/hch/intro/face.html.

Hodnicki DR, Horner SD: Homeless mothers' caring for children in a shelter, *Issues Ment Health Nurs* 14:349, 1993.

Institute of Medicine: *Homelessness, health, and human needs,* Washington, DC, 1998, National Academy Press.

Jencks C: *The homeless,* Cambridge, Mass, 1994, Harvard University Press.

Kann L et al: Youth risk behavior surveillance: United States 1997, *Morb Mortal Wkly Rep* 45(SS-3):1, 1998.

Killion CM: Special health care needs of homeless pregnant women, *Adv Nurs Sci* 18(2):44, 1995.

Koegel P et al: Utilization of mental health and substance abuse services among homeless adults in Los Angeles, *Med Care* 37(3):306, 1999.

Kozol J: *Rachel and her children: homeless families in America,* New York, 1988, Fawcett Columbine.

Krieger N, Birn AE: A vision of social justice as the foundation of public health: commemorating 150 years of the spirit of 1848, *Am J Public Health* 88(11):1603, 1998.

Kruks G: Gay and lesbian homeless/street youth: special issues and concerns, *J Adol Health* 12:515, 1991.

Letiecq BL, Anderson EA, Koblinsky SA: Social support of homeless and housed mothers: a comparison of temporary and permanent housing arrangements, *Family Relations* 47:415, 1998.

Lindsey A: Health care for the homeless, *Nurs Outlook* 37:78, 1989.

Link BG et al: Lifetime and five-year prevalence of homelessness in the United States, *Am J Public Health* 84:1907, 1994.

Lock J, Steiner H: Gay, lesbian, and bisexual youth risks for emotional, physical, and social problems: results from a community-based survey, *J Am Acad Child Adol* 38(3):297, 1999.

Maurin JT: Research utilization in the social-political arena, *Appl Nurs Res* 3:48, 1990.

McChesney KY: Homeless families: four patterns of poverty. In Robertson MJ, Greenblatt M, editors: *Homelessness: a national perspective,* New York, 1992, Plenum Press.

McKinlay JB: A case for refocusing upstream: the political economy of illness. In Jaco EG, editor: *Patients, physicians, and illness,* ed 3, New York, 1979, Free Press.

McKinlay JB, Marceau LD: To boldy go . . . public health matters, *Am J Public Health* 90(1):25, 2000.

McMurray-Avila M, Gelberg L, Breakey WR: Balancing act: clinical practices that respond to the needs of homeless people. In Fosburg LB, Dennis DL, editors: *Lessons learned,* Washington, DC, 1999, HUD, US Department of Health.

Menke EM: The mental health of homeless school-age children, *J Child Adol Psychiatr Nurs* 11(3):87, 1998.

Menke EM, Wagner JD: A comparative study of homeless, previously homeless, and never homeless school-aged children's health, *Issues Compr Pediatr Nurs* 20:153, 1997.

National Coalition for the Homeless: *Fact sheet #1: why are people homeless?* June 1999a, The Author, www.nch.ari.net.

National Coalition for the Homeless: *Fact sheet #2: how many people experience homelessness?* February 1999b, The Author, www.nch.ari.net.

National Coalition for the Homeless: *Fact sheet #3: who is homeless?* February 1999c, The Author, www.nch.ari.net.

National Coalition for the Homeless: *Fact sheet #5: mental illness and homelessness,* June 1999d, The Author, www.nch.ari.net.

National Coalition for the Homeless: *Fact sheet #6: addiction disorder and homelessness,* April 1999e, The Author, www.nch.ari.net.

National Coalition for the Homeless: *Fact sheet #8: domestic violence and homelessness,* April 1999f, The Author, www.nch.ari.net.

Nyamathi A et al: Effectiveness of a specialized vs. traditional AIDS education program attended by homeless and drug-addicted women alone or with supportive persons, *AIDS Educ Prev* 10(5):433, 1998.

Nyamathi A et al: Perceived factors influencing the initiation of drug and alcohol use among homeless women and reported consequences of use, *Women Health* 29(2):99, 1999.

Nyamathi A, Flaskerud J, Leake B: HIV-Risk behaviors and mental health characteristics among homeless or drug-recovering women and their closest sources of social support, *Nurs Res* 46(3):133, 1997.

Nyamathi A, Keenan C, Bayley L: Differences in personal, cognitive, psychological, and social factors associated with drug and alcohol use and nonuse by homeless women, *Res Nurs Health* 21(6):525, 1998.

O'Flaherty B: *Making room: the economics of homelessness,* Cambridge, Mass, 1996, Harvard University Press.

Olesen V et al: The mundane ailment and the physical self: analysis of the social psychology of health and illness, *Soc Sci Med* 30:449, 1990.

Penchansky R, Thomas JW: The concept of access: definition and relationship to consumer satisfaction, *Med Care* 19:127, 1981.

Pennbridge J, Mackenzie RG, Swofford A: Risk profile of homeless pregnant adolescents and youth, *J Adol Health* 12:534, 1991.

Phelan JC, Link BG: Who are "the homeless?" reconsidering the stability and composition of the homeless population, *Am J Public Health* 89(9):1334, 1999.

Portnoy FL, Dumas L: Nursing for the public good, *Nurs Clin North Am* 29:371, 1994.

Rafferty Y, Shinn M: The impact of homelessness on children, *Am Psychol* 46:1170, 1991.

Reuler JB: Outreach health services for street youth, *J Adol Health* 12:561, 1991.

Ringwalt CL et al: The prevalence of homelessness among adolescents in the United States, *Am J Public Health* 88(9):1325, 1998.

Ringwalt CL, Greene JM, Robertson MJ: Familial backgrounds and risk behaviors of youth with thrownaway experiences, *J Adol* 23:241, 1998.

Robertson MJ, Toro PA: Homeless youth: research, intervention, and policy. In Fosburg L, Dennis MA, editors: *Practical lessons: the 1998 National Symposium on Homelessness Research,* 1999, The Author, www.aspe.os.hhs.gov/progsys/homeless/symposium/toc.htm.

Rog DJ, Gutman M: The homeless family program: a summary of key findings. In Isaacs SL, Kindman JR, editors: *To improve health and healthcare 1997: the Robert Wood Johnson Foundation anthology,* San Francisco, 1997, Jossey-Bass.

Rosenheck R: Homelessness in America (editorial), *Am J Public Health* 84:1885, 1994.

Rosenheck R, Bassuk E, Salomon A: Special populations of homeless Americans. In Fosburg LB, Dennis DL, editors: *Lessons learned,* Washington, DC, 1999, HUD, US Department of Health.

Sachs-Ericsson N et al: Health problems and service utilization in the homeless, *J Health Care Poor Underserved* 10(4):443, 1999.

Sard B, Daskal J: *Housing and welfare reform: some background information,* Washington, DC, 1998, CBPP.

Sherman A et al: *Welfare to what: early findings on family hardship and well-being,* Washington, DC, 1998, Children's Defense Fund, National Coalition for the Homeless.

Shinn M, Baumohl J: Rethinking the prevention of homelessness. In Fosburg LB, Dennis DL, editors: *Lessons learned,* Washington, DC, 1999, HUD, US Department of Health.

Smart DH: Homeless youth in Seattle, *J Adol Health* 12:519, 1991.

Stratigos AJ et al: Prevalence of skin disease in a cohort of shelter-based homeless men, *J Am Acad Dermatol* 41(2 Pt 1):197, 1999.

Timmer DA, Eitzen S, Talley KD: *Paths to homelessness: extreme poverty and the urban housing crisis,* Boulder, Colo, 1994, Westview Press.

US Conference of Mayors: *A status report on hunger and homelessness in America's cities,* Washington, DC, 1999, The Author.

US Department of Commerce: *1990 census of population: general population characteristics, United States,* 1990 CP-1-1, Washington, DC, 1992, US Government Printing Office.

US Department of Health and Human Services, National Institute of Mental Health: *Outcasts on main street: report of the Federal Task Force on Homelessness and Severe Mental Illness,* ADM 92-1904, Washington, DC, 1992, Interagency Council on Homeless.

US Department of Housing and Urban Development: *Priority home! the federal plan to break the cycle of homelessness,* HUD-1454-CPD[1], Washington, DC, 1994, US Government Printing Office.

US Department of Housing and Urban Development: *Waiting in vain: an update on America's rental housing crisis,* March 1999, The Author, www.huduser.org/publications/affhsg/waiting.html.

Vladeck BC: Health care and the homeless: a political parable for our time, *J Health Polit Policy Law* 15:305, 1990.

Vredevoe DL, Shuler P, Woo M: The homeless population, *West J Nurs Res* 14:731, 1992.

Wagner J, Menke EM: Stressors and coping behaviors of homeless, poor, and low-income mothers, *J Community Health Nurs* 8:75, 1991.

Walters AS: HIV prevention in street youth, *J Adol Health* 25:187, 1999.

Weinreb L et al: Determinants of health and service use patterns in homeless and low-income housed children, *Pediatrics* 102(3 Pt 1):554, 1998.

World Health Organization: *Chronicle of WHO,* New York, 1958, WHO.

Wright JD: Poor people, poor health: the health status of the homeless, *J Soc Issues* 46:49, 1990b.

Wright JD: The health of homeless people: evidence from the National Health Care for the Homeless Program. In Brickner PW et al, editors: *Under the safety net: the health and social welfare of the homeless in the United States,* New York, 1990a, Norton.

Wright JD, Rubin BA, Devine JA: *Beside the golden door: policy, politics and the homeless,* New York, 1998, de Gruyter.

Yates GL et al: A risk profile comparison of homeless youth involved in prostitution and homeless youth not involved, *J Adol Health* 12:545, 1991a.

Yates GL et al: The Los Angeles system of care for runaway/homeless youth, *J Adol Health* 12:555, 1991b.

Zima BT et al: Psychosocial stressors among sheltered homeless children: relationship to behavior problems and depressive symptoms, *Am J Orthopsychiatry* 69(1):127, 1999.

Zima BT, Wells KB, Freeman HE: Emotional and behavioral problems and severe academic delays among sheltered homeless children in Los Angeles County, *Am J Public Health* 84:260, 1994.

21

Rural and Migrant Health

Doris Henson, Kathleen Chafey, and Patricia G. Butterfield

OBJECTIVES

Upon completion of this chapter, the reader will be able to do the following:

1. Describe features of the health care system and population characteristics common to rural aggregates.
2. Explain why rural populations and geographical areas must be defined specifically.
3. Discuss the impact of structural barriers vs. personal barriers on the health of rural aggregates.
4. Identify factors that place farmers and migrant workers at risk for illness and accidents.
5. Discuss the importance of the informal care network to rural health and social services.
6. Describe the characteristics of rural community health nursing practice.
7. Apply an upstream perspective to health promotion, illness prevention, and premature death and disability.

KEY TERMS

acute pesticide poisoning
Community-Oriented Primary Care (COPC)
frontier
informal care systems
metropolitan
migrant workers
National Health Service Corps (NHSC)
rural
seasonal workers

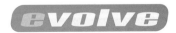

http://evolve.elsevier.com/Nies/

RURAL UNITED STATES

One in four Americans, approximately 61 million people, lives in rural America in both farm and non-farm residences. The 1990 census data reported that rural Americans make up 25% of the nation's population, 21% of the nation's children, 15% of the nation's elderly, and 50% of the nation's poor. Although the urban growth rate has been steadily climbing since 1890, with numbers of urban dwellers surpassing those in rural areas around 1920, the actual number of rural residents is the highest in the country's history (Ricketts, Johnson-Webb, and Randolph, 1999).

Stereotypically, rural residents have long been considered farmers and ranchers who make a living through produce, grain, or livestock. However, the 1990 census classified 8% of the rural population (less than 2% of the total U.S. population) as farmers, compared with 62% in 1920 (Ricketts, Johnson-Webb, and Randolph, 1999). Many farms are now sustained by one or more family members' off-farm jobs. Despite the shrinking number of farmers, agriculture continues to be an important part of the rural and U.S. economy.

Agriculture currently generates 17% of the GNP. By 2005, the projected figure will be 25%. Although agriculture is one of the fastest growing industries of the 1990s, only 40% of farms currently have the potential to make a profit. In the middle and late 1990s, field crop and cattle prices fell to a 40-year low. The low prices especially affected sparsely populated rural western states, although farm and ranch financial conditions showed wide regional variation. According to the United States Department of Agriculture (USDA), these western farmers and ranchers earned only 11% of their incomes from the land in 1997. Forty percent of farmers and ranchers are over age 65 and only 13% of farm property remains in a family more than three generations (Kohl, 1995). Changing demographic and economic conditions are transferring agriculture from family farm ownership to large agribusiness corporations.

Farm owners are selling long-time family farms when they retire. The younger generation does not want to invest in a business known for small profits and long hours. Generations ago, many families began farming when they came to the United States as European immigrants. In the 1990s, new immigrants began buying and operating their own small family farms. Between 1992 and 1997, the number of immigrant Hispanics who owned small farms doubled. Like those before them, these immigrants want something for themselves. Former migrant workers believe that farming is a difficult way to make a living, but say that now "we [the family] have something for ourselves." They work with their families and feel they are safely removed from dangerous chemicals. As one man interviewed said, "I'm like a fish in the water, not making money but having a lot of fun" (Arnold, 1999).

Nonfarm families have always played an important role in the rural community. Traditional nonfarm occupations include mining, government employment, and manufacturing. In rural America, 70,000 small- and medium-sized industrial firms exist (Mayer, 1993). The ratio of nonfarm to farm residents continues to increase in most communities. Currently, manufacturing and service industry employees exceed agricultural workers in rural America (Ricketts, Johnson-Webb, and Randolph, 1999). Recent demographic changes have included an influx of retirees and escapees from urban areas who are able to live in rural areas and conduct business through modern telecommunication and airline travel (Purdy, 1999).

Definitions of Rural Populations

Multiple definitions of rural populations have been formulated to understand the characteristics of low population density areas. The U.S. Census Bureau classifies those people who live in towns with a population of less than 2500 or in open country as **rural**. This definition is further differentiated into subcategories of farm and rural nonfarm. A similar classification developed by the U.S. Census Bureau categorizes counties as metropolitan or nonmetropolitan. **Metropolitan** counties or "metrocounties" contain an urban population center of 50,000 or more; all other counties are nonmetropolitan. In 1990, the latter included 2444 of the United States' 3088 counties (Ricketts, Johnson-Webb, and Randolph, 1999). A third classification of interest uses the term **frontier** for geographical areas with less than six people per square mile (Elison, 1986). Many counties of the Great Plains and West, including Alaska, are designated frontier.

A more refined classification scheme arranges residence into nine categories (see Box 21-1). These range from core and fringe areas, with a minimum of one million people, to nonmetropolitan, to nonadjacent counties with the smallest place having less than 2500 people (Farmer, Clark, and Miller, 1993). Farmer and colleagues used infant mortality data and

BOX **21-1**

Residence Categories

1. Core and fringe: 1 million plus
2. Core and fringe: 500,000 to 999,999 population
3. Core and fringe: 50,000 to 499,999 population
4. Nonmetropolitan adjacent largest place: 10,000 to 50,000 population
5. Nonmetropolitan adjacent largest place: 2500 to 9999 population
6. Nonmetropolitan adjacent largest place: <2500 population
7. Nonmetropolitan nonadjacent largest place: 10,000 to 49,999 population
8. Nonmetropolitan nonadjacent largest place: 2500 to 9999 population
9. Nonmetropolitan nonadjacent largest place: <2500 population

From Farmer F, Clark L, Miller M: Consequences of differential residence designations for rural health policy: the case of infant mortality, *J Rural Health* 9:17-26, 1993. Used with permission.

this nine-category classification scheme to show the heterogeneity of rural areas. Infant mortality, a major health status indicator, varies greatly by geographical area. Mortality for white infants in rural areas adjacent to a population center less than 2500 varied from a high of 9.85 per 1000 in the South to 6.46 per 1000 in the West. This difference is not apparent if a cruder classification is used. This provides some insight into the heterogeneity of rural populations and shows why a health status indicator such as infant mortality can be misleading for a particular area.

In summary, the concept of rural is multidimensional; to provide the most useful information, rural populations and corresponding health status indicators should be examined using the most refined classification scheme available. Unfortunately, government agencies often do not provide figures for more specific categories.

Rural populations differ in complex geographical, social, and economic areas. Although older, poorer, and less educated people are overrepresented in nonmetropolitan areas, this may not apply to all rural areas or to everyone in a given location. Remembering that there are many "rural Americas in rural America" is paramount to a successful community health nursing practice (Miller, Farmer, and Clarke, 1994).

COMMUNITY AND STATISTICAL INDICATORS OF RURAL HEALTH STATUS

Rural communities vary in economic and cultural resources, employment patterns, population density, relative isolation, age distribution, and ethnic composition. The literature suggests that rural residents more often assess their health as fair or poor, have a higher prevalence of chronic illness and disability, and have more disability days associated with acute conditions than their urban counterparts. A disproportionate number live in poverty, lack health insurance, and experience a lack of available health care providers and access to health care (Braden and Beauregard, 1994). This section of the chapter discusses some of the disparities in the health status of rural vs. urban dwellers and the nature of some of the common barriers to primary health care in rural America.

Using Statistical Data

The health profiles discussed below are shared by rural areas in general and may be contrasted with overall patterns of health, health habits, and health care in urban settings. However, the reader should note that there are difficulties associated with interpreting differences between urban and rural health. First, statistically significant differences between urban and rural health indicators may seem small when data are aggregated to "rural areas" in general. The differences tend to become larger when data are available for particular rural areas (e.g., certain counties) or particular rural subgroups (minorities) or specific characteristics (e.g., percentage of uninsured children). Second, heterogeneity of race, age, economic status, regional distribution, and cultural groupings makes health data for "the rural population" useful only as estimates of individual health. For example, an AARP publication lists the U.S. poverty level for 1995 to 1996 as 13.8%. This publication also provides state-by-state data. During this period, Montana, a rural western state, had a poverty level of 16.2%. In Oregon, a state with both urban and rural areas, 11.5% of the population was at or below the poverty level and Mississippi, another rural state, had a poverty rate of 22%, among the highest in the nation (Lamphere et al., 1998).

Because population numbers are small, rural data can only provide suggestions about the health needs of a particular area; therefore it may be useful to examine aggregate data across rural populations. Program planners will still need to determine whether certain health or health care delivery problems apply to their specific geographical areas. Useful data sources might include county statistics, community-level data gathered from health care providers, local records, focus groups, and older residents who know the area's history.

A list of helpful resources at the end of this chapter provides a rich source of current geographical, demographic, and health-related data for many different political locales and regions in the United States. These resources contain the latest available data that can help identify current potential health care problems and assist with planning health care delivery at the state, county, or local level.

Structural and Financial Barriers to Care

Regardless of their diverse demographic and geographical attributes, rural groups share certain health patterns and difficulties and delays in obtaining health care. Structural, financial, and personal barriers to accessing health care services exist in all environments (IOM, 1993). However, rural residents are unique in how they experience structural barriers. Availability of services, distance, isolation, low population density, and lack of transportation all contribute to these barriers. These structural problems vary from state to state, but they tend to be most serious in regions with the lowest population densities and per capita incomes (Hicks, 1992).

WHAT IS THE "POVERTY RATE?"

In concept, the poverty line is the minimum income level needed by a family or individual to just meet basic needs of food, shelter, clothing, and other essential goods and services. Official poverty lines adjusted for family size and composition are set by the Office of Management and Budget (OMB) for use by all Federal agencies. They are adjusted each year for inflation. In 1996, the poverty line was $15,911 for a family of two adults and two children, $10,815 for a family of one adult and one child, and $8163 for a single individual. Each household's cash income (including pretax income and cash welfare assistance, but excluding in-kind welfare assistance, such as food stamps and Medicare) is compared to the poverty line for the household. The poverty rate for an area or for a category of people is the percentage of persons in households with income less than the poverty line for their household (p. 81).

From Nord M: Rural poverty rate unchanged, *Rural Cond Trends* 9(2):81-84, 1999.

Financial barriers to adequate health care also exist in both urban and rural areas; however, in the aggregate, rural dwellers have lower educational levels, higher unemployment, longer unemployment periods, higher poverty rates, and lower income levels (Hicks, 1992). In 1990, the Office of Technology Assessment (OTA) reported that rural incomes were 77% of urban incomes. By 1996, the USDA calculated that the disparity had grown to 71%; overall, current poverty rates among rural people are 16% compared with 13% for urban people; this trend has remained stable since 1992 (Ghelfi, 1999).

In nonmetropolitan America, 63% of the poor are whites. The remaining one third of this population consists of blacks (21%), Hispanics (11%), and Native-Americans (4%). "Other" groups make up the remaining 1%. In metropolitan settings, roughly 40% of the poor are whites and 60% are minorities.

Among nonMetropolitan Statistical Areas (nonMSAs), the highest rates of poverty and unemployment are in certain counties of the Southeast, the Southwest, and the Northern Plains states. In these counties, three minority groups (i.e., blacks, Hispanics, and Native-Americans) make up one third or more of the rural population (Cook, 1999). "Poverty rates [in 1996] among rural minorities were nearly three times as high as that of rural whites and substantially higher than those of urban minorities" (Nord, 1999). Of the three minority groups, rural blacks have the highest rates of poverty followed by Native-Americans and Hispanics.

Racial and ethnic minorities and people of color, who account for only 15% of the total rural population, comprised approximately 37% of the rural poor in 1999 (Nord, 1999). Blacks are less likely than whites to have private health insurance, but are most likely to be publicly insured. Hispanics are both the least likely to be insured (nearly 3 in 10 Hispanic children have no health insurance) and are the least likely to get private health insurance through their jobs (Kass, Weinick, and Monheit, 1999). With a history of higher rates of poverty and unemployment, lower levels of education, and higher levels of food insecurity and hunger, these groups are overrepresented among disadvantaged segments of rural America (Cook, 1999) and among rural dwellers who need better access to health care and adequate nutrition.

Health insurance coverage influences health patterns and may pose financial barriers to adequate health care for rural dwellers. Rural people are often employed in industries characterized by economic uncertainty, decline, high unemployment risk, and occupational accidents and death (e.g., agriculture, mining, forestry, and fisheries). Employment in these industries contributes to the increased and increasing number of uninsured rural families. Self-employed farm families need to purchase private health insurance; however, in periods of hardship they often cannot afford the increasingly high premium costs. Farm families tend to be two-parent households; therefore they are unlikely to qualify for Medicaid. In fact, fewer than 6% of farm families with incomes below the federal poverty level could qualify for Medicaid according to the OTA's 1990 report.

Although Medicare recipients are more apt to live in rural than in urban areas, Medicare spends less on rural beneficiaries. This may be because rural beneficiaries use fewer health care services than their urban peers and providers receive lower reimbursement rates. Finally, 46% of the Medicare population in rural counties vs. 31% of Medicare recipients in urban counties lack any form of prescription drug coverage (Harriman, 1999).

Health insurance is a major issue for the health of the nation. During 1995 and 1996, 17.6% of the nation were people under age 65 (Lamphere et al., 1998; Morgan et al., 1999). From 1992 to 1997, there was a 7.3% national increase in the percentage of people of all ages who were uninsured by any source (e.g., Medicare or Medicaid and employer-provided or private insurance). By 1999, the percent of uninsured dropped to 15.5%, the first decline in 18 states since 1987. Some states had higher uninsured rates than others (e.g., 24.1% in Texas) and the uninsured rates also varied by age, ethnicity, and income, although poor children are less likely to be insured than children with higher incomes. The percent of uninsured children has fallen to 13.9% in 1999. Over one third of Hispanics were uninsured in 1999 and, overall, 48% of poor workers were without health insurance. These figures released by the U.S. Census Bureau in 2000 dramatize the disparities in health care coverage in the Unites States (US Census Bureau, 2000).

Public health professionals and health planners are most concerned with the impact of increasing numbers of uninsured children. In 1998, 21% of rural children vs. 14% of urban children were uninsured (Dunbar and Mueller, 1998). These figures vary widely from state to state and are influenced by employment patterns, the percentage of children in the population, state Medicaid policies, poverty levels, and other factors (e.g., numbers of migrant or seasonal farmworkers). In Texas and Arizona, which have large numbers of migrant workers, over one third of children were uninsured during 1995 and 1996 (35.6% and 35.4%, respectively). These rates continue to rise.

In the absence of health insurance, poverty becomes an even more powerful predictor of poor health for all age groups (i.e., particularly for children). A national initiative to insure children known as CHIP is now underway to redress this alarming situation. See the "Legislation and Programs Affecting Public Health in Rural Americas" section in this chapter.

Problems Related to Demographic, Personal, and Geographical Health Patterns

In addition to structural and economic differences, rural communities vary in demographic and personal characteristics, population density, relative isolation, age distribution, and ethnic composition. For example, on the basis of census and health survey data, rural residents are more likely to be white, married, and older than 65 years or younger than 18 years than their urban counterparts. There are also aggregate differences in health and lifestyle. Rural adults, particularly minorities, have reported their health status as fair or poor more frequently, as excellent less often, and have a greater prevalence of diagnosed chronic conditions than those in core metropolitan populations (Harriman, 1999; Hicks, 1992).

Overall mortality rates are lower among rural populations, but there are two notable exceptions. Infant mortality is slightly higher and deaths from unintentional injuries were approximately 63% higher in nonmetropolitan than metropolitan counties in 1994. The highest rates were in the more rural counties. Unintentional injuries leading to death and disability include drowning, occupational injuries, and motor vehicle crashes. Native-Americans die in motor vehicle accidents about twice as often as whites or blacks. Suicides are also highest among Native-American males aged 44 and younger and among white males in older age groups. The CDC (1998b) reported that the combined rates for all suicides are highest in nonmetropolitan areas and in the Western states. In addition, rural residents have greater levels of injury disability.

Geography, health care costs, and lack of available services are structural problems that keep many rural adults and children from obtaining needed primary, secondary, and tertiary preventive services. A good example is the lack of mental health services available for rural dwellers of any age. In a report by James Ciarlo, Ph.D., he stated, "The availability of mental health services in the frontier [areas he defines as having a population density of between 2 and 20 people per square mile] is vastly inferior to other areas. . ." (Ricketts, 1999, p. 174). Although need approximates 80% to 85% of the rate for more densely settled areas, availability of psychiatrists and child psychiatrists in 1994 was less than 10% of the per capita rate for other areas. Rather than mental health specialists, primary care doctors, nurses, and PAs provide most of the mental health care.

Health Habits

Health habits also vary along the rural-urban continuum and within rural populations by geographical area. Researchers with the NHIS concluded that adults in nonmetropolitan areas use seat belts less often and are less likely to use preventive screening, but this trend is confounded by access problems. Rural residents in the Southern states are more likely to be obese, smoke more heavily if they do smoke, use smokeless tobacco, and engage in sedentary lifestyles. In the rural West, smoking, seat belt use, and obesity are lower and alcohol and smokeless tobacco use are higher (CDC, 1998b, 1999). In addition to health concerns related to socioeconomic and geographical patterns, rural populations, like urban populations, reflect health patterns and problems related to demographic characteristics such as age and gender, occupation, race and ethnicity, and health care access.

These patterns are related to and sometimes confounded by structural and financial factors. Structural factors may include availability of health information, preventive and illness services, sewage and water systems, and transportation systems. Financial factors are affected by local economic conditions and employment patterns. Demographic and personal characteristics such as age distribution, population size and density, language, culture, and education round out the examples of factors that affect health and may serve as barriers to available services and access to existing services (Braden and Beauregard, 1994).

Age

Age is an important consideration in planning health care services for rural communities. According to demographer Carolyn Rogers (1999), one quarter of all older Americans live in rural areas. The elderly, the majority of whom are women, make up 18% of the rural population compared with 15% of the urban population (Rogers, 1999). Elderly women live at or near the poverty level and achieve poverty status twice as often as men. Along with educational attainment, this is a critical indicator of well-being for the elderly and the young. The elderly poor tend to be isolated and lack access to support services, health care, adequate nutrition, and transportation.

In contrast, although white residents of rural areas are in the majority, their birth rates are lower than those of rural minority groups; over one third of the rural population were under age 18 in 1997 (Swanson, 1999). Evidence suggests that fetal, infant, and maternal mortality are slightly higher in nonmetropolitan than metropolitan areas and that care in the later prenatal stages is problematic. According to 1996 data, nonmetropolitan children, like adults, are more likely to live in poverty. In 1990, housing with incomplete plumbing disconnected from public water or sewer systems far exceeded that in metropolitan areas (Ricketts, 1999). Rural children are involved in farm and highway accidents and deaths. In fact, data from a 1992 report by the National Vital Statistics System revealed that "fatal injuries were 44% higher among rural children aged 1 to 19 years compared with their urban counterparts" (Ricketts, 1999, p. 155). Among younger children aged 1 to 14, death rates for all races were at least 20% higher than in urban areas. The death rates were higher in urban areas only among blacks aged 15 to 19. The latter disparity is largely due to homicides; however, suicide rates and deaths from motor vehicle crashes among rural youth are comparable. Finally, a 1993 Vital Statistics of the United States Report titled "Access to Health Care," revealed that attributed cost, poor insurance coverage, and lack of access to care caused rural children to go without corrective treatment for orthopedic, dental, speech, hearing, visual, and cosmetic problems more often (Ricketts, 1999).

Youth substance use and abuse are problems in rural America. Lisnerski and colleagues (1991) reported on the use of smokeless tobacco by elementary school children in a rural southeastern state. In this study, roughly one third of male first graders experimented with smokeless tobacco; by the seventh grade, 70% of these rural males had experimented with or were regular users of smokeless tobacco. Use was attributed to "perceived flavor" but was also predicted by "self-concept and presentation to peers" and "family influence." Furthermore, Long and Boik (1993) reported that nearly 60% of sixth and seventh graders in their rural sample reported using alcohol.

Education

Recent research on the socioeconomic determinants of health has revealed a strong positive correlation between health and length of schooling (Fuchs, 1998). As Swanson (1999, p. 2) discussed, "Demographic characteristics of a minority group both affect and result from their economic and social status. Age structure and education combine as an indication of the level of employment a group might be able to enjoy." For the aged and for ethnic and racial minorities, a pattern of lower educational attainment and unfavorable economic circumstances emerges with increasing rurality. Although the education picture is changing, many elderly women in their 70s and 80s grew up before public education was mandatory. Families could not afford to send them to school or simply expected them to learn to read and write, seek employment, and marry. Education, with its links to economic and health variables, is still a serious problem for rural America. Low education and employment levels characterize all rural minority groups except Asians. "Children of all racial and ethnic groups who live in precarious economic conditions have additional challenges to doing well in school and remaining in school through high school graduation" (Swanson, 1999, p. 4).

Occupation

Occupation plays a significant role in rural health; rates of disabling injuries and injury-related mortality are dramatically higher in the rural population (OTA, 1990). In 1997, logging was the most dangerous occupation in the country followed by fishing and water transportation occupations. In addition to mechanical, chemical, and thermal injuries and many job-related fatalities, farmers reportedly suffer from psychological stress and high suicide rates. Miners also work in hazardous conditions and suffer from a variety of acute and chronic problems including "trauma, respiratory illness, vascular problems and malignancy" (Weinert and Burman, 1994, p. 72).

According to a government report in 1990, the private-sector work-related death rate for the United States was 5.5 per 100,000 workers. For the same year in Wyoming and Montana, work-related deaths were 18 per 100,000 workers and 13 per 100,000 workers, respectively (OTA, 1990). The national average in the mid1990s was 5.0 deaths per 100,000. At this time, deaths in Montana dropped to 12 per 100,000 and in Wyoming deaths dropped to 14 per 100,000, which is almost three times the national average.

Another occupational at-risk rural population consists of subgroups that support fruit and vegetable production. In general, Migrant and Seasonal Farmworkers (MSFW), Native-Americans, and Alaska-Natives may have the poorest health of any aggregate in the United States, yet they have the least access to affordable health care. Eighty-five percent of the MSFW are Hispanic or black. The remainder are largely white seasonal workers who follow the harvests to drive combines or haul crops from the fields to storage, market, or seaports. These populations, estimated between three and five million people each year, are vulnerable to a host of health problems and diseases that center on occupational and environmental hazards and other health correlates as described in the section about agricultural workers.

Gender

Rural men and women in the aggregate exercise fewer preventive behaviors, have less contact with physicians, and often have less access to care than people with similar problems in urban areas. For example, although rural populations are at lower risk for cancer in most anatomic sites, rural cancer patients experience more late-stage cancers that are unstaged at diagnosis (Monroe, Ricketts, and Savitts, 1992). Lack of cancer screening is a particularly serious problem for minorities and the elderly, especially women. According to National Health Survey data reported in 1994, 60.9% of women aged 40 years and over reported receiving mammograms in the two previous years (CDC, 1999). The percentage was higher for black, nonHispanic women (64.4%) and lower for Hispanic women 40 years of age and over (51.9%) for the same reporting period. Health objectives for the year 2000 called for at least 80% of American women aged 40 and older to have received a mammogram and clinical breast exam in the previous two years (IOM, 1993). The highest level achieved by 1994 was among women aged 50 to 64 who had incomes at or above poverty level (70.3%). Hispanic women, women over 65, and all women living below poverty level are less likely to have mammograms. The percentage of poor women over 65 who had a mammogram in the previous two years was 43.2% (CDC, 1999). Likewise, poor, elderly, and less educated women in general and minority women in particular are less likely to receive PAP smears on a regular basis, if ever (IOM, 1993). The number of Native-American and Alaskan Native women who had PAP tests actually decreased from 1993 to 1994 and 43% of elderly minority women reported never having a PAP test. Like breast cancer screening, the percentage of women who reported receiving a PAP test as of 1990 was related to both race and income (Calle et al., 1993; IOM, 1993; National Women's Health Information Center, 1999).

Rural-dwelling men suffer the long-term effects of poor health habits, lack of consistent primary health care, and participation in hazardous occupations as mentioned previously. In rural areas, particularly the Mountain West, men (i.e., especially older white men and younger American-Indian men) have the highest suicide rates of any group (Pickle et al., 1996).

Race and Ethnicity

Problems that affect certain races or ethnic groups are the most illustrative barriers to rural health care. A 1993 IOM study drew attention to the glaring and growing disparities in access between whites and ethnic minorities. Black and Native-American children have higher rates of poverty than the population as a whole. Children of migrant workers live in families with incomes of approximately $7500 per year and usually do not receive government assistance. By almost any measure or index (e.g., AIDS, birth weight, blood pressure, cholesterol, cancer, and substance use), blacks are less healthy than whites and the disparity is often exaggerated by rurality and poverty. For example, Johnson and colleagues (1994) concluded that living in a rural area and being black significantly increased the likelihood for higher total fat, saturated fat, cholesterol, and sodium intake in children aged 1 to 10 years *regardless* of household income and availability of additional food resources. Hispanic women and older black women underuse both mammography and PAP test screening in rural areas.

Perhaps no other group better illustrates the many problems that characterize rural health care than Native-Americans. The following are excerpts from a special report compiled by faculty and students from the University of Montana School of Journalism entitled "A Health Crisis:"

- In Montana, Indians die prematurely at a rate almost twice that of the general population.
- Death rates among Indians as a result of heart disease, cancer, accidents, cirrhosis, suicide and diabetes are higher for Indians than for other citizens of this state.
- This terrible toll afflicts Native-Americans from the moment of their birth. The state's infant mortality rate for Indian babies is 43 percent higher for Montana Indian infants than for babies born of other ancestry.
- Montana Indians live in poverty at a rate three times that of their fellow residents. Half of those Indians who are poor are children and adolescents and they are more than three times more likely to come from homes where a mother is the only parent present. Yet Indians get free health care, so why are they so sick?

Because, as the American Indian Health Care Association found, Indians face significant barriers to getting that health care. Only enrolled tribal members living on a reservation can get full health care benefits supplied by the federal government. And that health care is rationed. Many Indians live long distances from Indian Health Service facilities. That becomes a factor when studies show that more than twice as many Montana Indians than white people have no access to a vehicle. And almost half the Indians in the state are without a telephone. A third of tribal and Indian Health Service facilities in Montana have no emergency and ambulance services, a critical need on Montana's large and rural reservations

(School of Journalism, 1993, p. 1).

Hispanics will become the largest minority group in the United States within the next 50 years and are already the largest in the rural West. Hispanics have a diverse culture, history, and socioeconomic and health status. The largest Hispanic subgroups are of Mexican, Cuban, and Puerto Rican descent, although Mexican is the largest by far (63% of the Hispanic population living in the United States). In nonmetropolitan areas, Hispanics, who made up only 3.8% of the population in 1990, increased to 19.2% as of March 1999 (US Census Bureau, 1999). As emphasized in earlier paragraphs, this growing segment of the population continues to be overrepresented among the rural poor. In 1999, the U.S. Census Bureau reported that just over 25% of Hispanics live below the federal poverty level compared with 8.2% of the white, nonHispanic population. Of those under age 18, the percentage living below the poverty level was 34% for Hispanics vs. 10.6% of white, nonHispanics. The elderly were also two and one half times more likely to live below the poverty line than white, nonHispanics. Hispanics are most likely to report barriers in obtaining needed health care and are least likely to have a usual source of care for those blacks and Hispanics reporting a usual source of care, the source is most likely to be hospital-based (Kass, Weinick, and Monheit, 1999).

Minority Health and *Healthy People 2010*

Healthy People 2010, like its predecessor *Healthy People 2000,* represents the health promotion and disease prevention agenda for the nation (USDHHS, 2000). Additionally, *Healthy People 2010* is the United States' contribution to WHO's "Health for All" strategy. The framework for *Healthy People 2010,* developed through public consensus, builds upon the national health program established since the 1980s. It includes the broad goals of increasing QOL and YHL, reducing disparities in health among different population groups and increasing access to preventive health services.

Healthy People 2012 is based on the premise that the health of the individual is "almost inseparable from the health of the larger community and that the health of every community in every State and territory determines the overall health status of the Nation" (USDHHS, 2000, p. 2). The new 10-year plan takes a bold step forward by presenting only one set of standards for the health of all racial, ethnic, income, gender, and age groups. The new goal aims to eliminate health disparities, achieve access to preventive health services, and add YHL for all groups.

Nearly all the states have developed their own Healthy People plans built upon national objectives, but they have tailored them to each state's particular needs and population configurations. To eliminate disparities among different population groups, the health care system will need to undertake programs that seek dramatic improvements in the health of minority groups on no fewer than 93 health indicators that show a 25% or greater disparity in health statistics based on race and ethnicity, SES, gender, age, and geographical location. Rural states, often struggling with structural and economic deficits, will face daunting challenges in meeting the 2010 targets. The challenges are great, but public health professionals and planners in every state will have a plan to direct and guide their efforts. Fig. 21-1 presents a diagram of the 2010 approach to health improvement.

SPECIFIC RURAL AGGREGATES

Agricultural Workers

Agriculture and its impact on human health are a central focus of rural nursing. Despite the shrinking proportion of farm to nonfarm families since the 1980s, agriculture continues to have an impact on the health status of most rural communities. Much of the country's heritage has been strongly associated with agriculture; beliefs that humans can and should settle undeveloped land and make it productive are deeply rooted in its history. Although the belief that "humans triumph over nature" has evolved considerably in the past century, a number of agricultural myths continue to permeate citizens' beliefs about health and health risks.

The myth that farming is a safe and innately healthful activity has helped perpetuate the notion that farmers and their families, because they have a relationship with nature, are in some way protected from the health dangers and threats of contemporary society. In reality, health risks of farming are different, as opposed to fewer, than those encountered in metropolitan areas. Agriculture, along with construction and mining, shares the highest rates of worker fatality of any U.S. industry (US Department of Labor, 1989). Children bear a disproportionately high risk of fatal injury; an estimated 300 pediatric fatalities occur annually (Rivara, 1985). In addition to fatalities, farmers and their families have high risks for conditions such as hearing loss, respiratory illness, nonfatal accidents, and illnesses associated with chemical hazards.

Accidents and Injuries

Working in highly variable environmental conditions (i.e., temperature extremes, a wide variety of work tasks, and unpredictable circumstances) is associated with an increased frequency of accidents and fatalities. Farm-related activities are extremely heterogeneous and vary significantly with the season, types of crops produced, and types of machinery used. Farmers are located in geographically isolated areas and often work alone. This constellation of factors places farmers and their families at increased risk for accidental injury and delayed access to emergency or trauma care.

The 1996 rate of fatal injury for those employed in agricultural crop production was 31 per 100,000

FIGURE **21-1**

Diagram of the *Healthy People 2010* Approach to Health Improvement (From US Public Health Service: *Healthy people 2010: healthy people in healthy communities,* Washington, DC, 1997, US Government Printing Office).

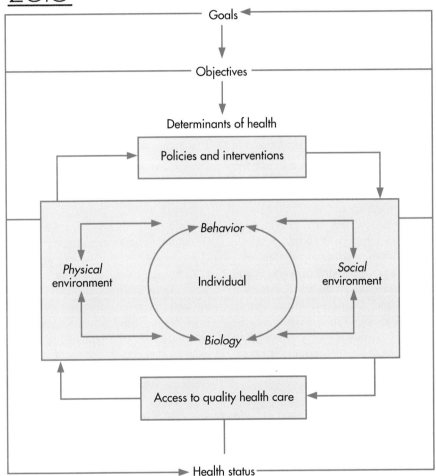

Healthy People in Healthy Communities
A Systematic Approach to Health Improvement

Goals

Objectives

Determinants of health

Policies and interventions

Behavior

Physical environment

Individual

Social environment

Biology

Access to quality health care

Health status

workers, compared with a rate of 5 per 100,000 for all types of U.S. workers. Farming activities accounted for 9% of all job-related fatalities during 1996 and transportation incidents accounted for almost half those deaths (Toscano and Windau, 1998). According to the National Institute for Occupational Safety and Health (NIOSH) (1992), agricultural machinery is the most common cause of fatalities and nonfatal injuries of U.S. farmers. Tractor-related accidents are the most frequent events associated with loss of life (Etherton et al., 1991). NIOSH released an alert warning of an increase in scalping-type accidents associated with tractor drive shafts, referred to as power takeoffs (NIOSH, 1994). It is easy to see why accident prevention programs for farm children and families have focused heavily on tractor safety awareness.

Acute and Chronic Illnesses
Several types of farming activities are associated with higher than expected occurrences of acute and chronic respiratory conditions. People with long-term exposure to grain dusts, such as grain elevator workers,

have diminished respiratory function and increased frequency of respiratory symptoms such as cough or phlegm production (Cotton et al., 1989). Occupational asthma and more exotic fungal or toxic gas-related conditions also occur in higher frequency in agricultural than nonagricultural populations (Warren, 1989). Community health nurses, who are familiar with local farming practices in rural areas, often make links between farm work and respiratory symptoms. In such situations, the role of the nurse is to refer patients to appropriate health care providers and provide support and education for affected people and their families.

Exposure to pesticides, herbicides, and other chemicals is a major concern for farmers and their families. From an occupational perspective, farming is unusual because the home and the work site are the same. Exposure risks to children and spouses may be heightened when farmers wear contaminated clothing and boots into the home. Homes are often located in close proximity to fields and animal containment facilities, which are treated with a variety of chemicals.

Nurses in rural emergency rooms or other ambulatory care settings may be the first providers to encounter farmers and others with acute pesticide poisoning. During discussions with farmers, ranchers, or other high-risk groups (e.g., nursery workers and tree planters), community health nurses may note a pattern of headaches and nausea that occur during planting or spraying seasons. In such an instance, the nurse can serve as an important resource by obtaining a careful history of signs and symptoms, the temporal nature of symptom occurrence, and the types of pesticides and personal protection used (e.g., respirators and protective clothing). When evidence suggests pesticide-related illness, appropriate referral and follow-up are imperative to ensure the safety of the affected person and the family.

Signs and symptoms of **acute pesticide poisoning** are fairly clear and most health providers in rural communities should recognize them. Although there are exceptions, it frequently follows exposure to insecticides classified as organophosphates or carbamates. These products, which are sold under a wide variety of trade names (e.g., Parathion, Vapona, Sevin, and Dursban), kill insects by inhibiting the enzyme acetylcholinesterase; this leads to an accumulation of acetylcholine in the neuromuscular junction (EPA, 1989). Common symptoms include headache, dizziness, diaphoresis, nausea, and vomiting. If left untreated, those affected may experience a progression

of symptoms including dyspnea, bronchospasm, and muscle twitching. Deaths are relatively uncommon, but they do occur.

Overall, farmers have a lower rate of CVD than nonfarmers; the physically demanding nature of farm work may help protect them against heart disease. In addition, the prevalence of smoking in farmers is generally lower than in the general population (Blair and Zahm, 1995). National and international data addressing cancer risks in farmers provide evidence that farmers have lower rates of some cancers and elevated rates of other cancers. Generally, rates of lung, bladder, and esophageal cancers are lower in farmers. Higher than expected rates of nonHodgkin's lymphoma, prostate cancer, leukemia, brain tumors, multiple myeloma, and cancer of the lip have been observed by cancer epidemiologists in the United States and Canada (Blair and Zahm, 1995; Gabos, Fincham, and Berkel, 1995; Morrison et al., 1995).

Migrant and Seasonal Farmworkers

Although the discussion of agricultural issues has focused primarily on farmers and farm families, it is important to understand the role of **migrant workers** (i.e., migrate to find work) and **seasonal workers** (i.e., reside permanently in one place and work locally when farm labor is needed) farmworkers in U.S. agricultural production and the health risks to this population. Older references to farmworkers often referred to three "migrant streams," in which workers entered the country through Mexico and migrated north. The present reality is that migrant workers enter the country through a variety of access points and follow any route necessary to obtain work. Seasonal workers permanently reside in agricultural areas and take various farm jobs during harvesting times. For example, a seasonal worker may be employed in restaurant work during the winter and may spend the summer months picking apples or working in a local apple shed or cannery.

MSFW comprise a vulnerable population in regard to health risks because they have low income and migratory status. In many rural areas, community health nurses form the central link between farmworkers and health services. Through standing or mobile clinic sites, nurses have established a leadership role in the provision of episodical and preventive services for workers and their families. Lacking access to many types of preventive services, farmworkers often visit a migrant clinic with any number of health problems including severe dental problems, unresolved communicable diseases, and untreated injuries. In addition to the direct provision of care, nurses in many communities have served as important advocates on behalf of farmworkers and have worked to ensure health care access to those traveling through their areas.

Cultural, linguistic, economic, and mobility barriers all contribute to the nature and magnitude of health problems observed in farmworkers. Cultural and linguistic barriers are the most overt because many of the communities where farmworkers work consider them outsiders. In many settings, migrant workers live isolated from the agricultural communities they serve. Although some workers travel in extended family groups and have the support that comes with being together, other workers leave their families at home. Often these are male workers who work and live together. A common misconception among U.S. health care providers is that these farmworkers are from Mexico and Spanish is their primary language. Farmworkers originate from many communities in Mexico, the Caribbean, Central and South America, and speak the language of their home country, English, or several languages.

Health Needs and Opportunities for Preventive Care

Similarities in exposure and work practices make some of the farmworkers' health needs similar to those of farmers and their families. Generally, these health needs reflect the increased rates of accidents and injuries, dermatological conditions, and pulmonary problems observed in both populations. However, there are additional challenges in both the identification and treatment of farmworkers with health problems. One of the biggest problems that nurses face in designing health programs is understanding the full magnitude of their problems. Many farmworkers who become ill eventually return to their countries of origin to obtain treatment and to be with family. This phenomenon makes it difficult to get complete, reliable numbers about disease rates. A variety of public health indicators are likely to undercount farmworkers as a group, ranging from tumor registries to workers' compensation injuries (Schenker, 1995). In addition, farmworkers may be less likely to seek treatment for health problems that do not require emergency treatment or surgery.

Studies of farmworkers' health status have provided data indicating that farmworkers are less likely to receive preventive care from any health source (Schenker, 1995). Preventive needs include dental care, vision screening and treatment, and gynecological and breast exams. In addition, children of farmworkers are likely to receive incomplete sets of immunizations by age five (Schenker, 1995). Many farmworkers, because they move from community to community, are often unaware of clinical and social services they could receive at reduced or no cost to low-income families.

Contact with herbicides, insecticides, and fertilizers may put farmworkers at increased risk for acute and chronic health problems associated with exposure to these chemical agents. There is some evidence that, like farmers, farmworkers have elevated rates of multiple myeloma and cancers of the prostate, stomach, and testes. A few smaller studies indicate that rates of oral, lung, and liver cancer may also be elevated in farmworkers (Zahm and Blair, 1993). However, it is important to remember that studies that collect data from tumor registry files may lead to biased results from incomplete case finding. To improve the incomplete science that characterizes cancer rates in farmworker populations, Zahm and Blair (1993) recommend additional research that quantifies exposure dose to specific farm products and studies that track workers as they move from town to town over an extended period of time.

Hearing Farmworkers' Voices

Several studies and pilot projects have used focus groups, community meetings, or other qualitative research methods to listen to farmworkers' concerns and give these concerns a voice through publication and advocacy. Several years ago, the Farmworker Justice Fund brought female farmworkers together in a national effort to give them a forum for their concerns and their impressions of health needs. The women identified priority concerns in the areas of child and family issues, health care services, workplace issues, and empowerment. The group's recommendations in the area of health care included the following directives: keep clinics open during evening hours, provide transportation to clinics, increase access through mobile health units, provide social and health services in one building, increase home visits by students, encourage careers in farmworker health, enhance nutrition education to families, teach first aid, enforce farm labor health laws, and give farmworkers a copy of the record after each clinic visit (Wilk, 1995). It is interesting to note that a group of baccalaureate nursing students in Georgia documented similar concerns. During an immersion course, the students listened to and documented the concerns of farmworker families. The need to restructure health services was a predominant theme voiced by the workers, who noted the importance of health care worker field visits and evening home visits (Bechtel and Davidhizar, 1999).

APPLICATION OF RELEVANT THEORIES AND "THINKING UPSTREAM" CONCEPTS TO RURAL HEALTH

Upstream and prevention-oriented approaches have several implications for nurses in rural practice settings. Three strategies for upstream interventions follow: attack community-based problems at their roots, emphasize the "doing" aspects of health, and maximize the use of informal networks.

Attack Community-Based Problems at Their Roots

Upstream approaches to community health problems direct the nurse toward an understanding of the precursors of poor health within populations of interest. Individual nurses can be effective forces in uncovering and enhancing community awareness of health-endangering situations. Environmental health issues in rural communities, such as pesticide exposure or health hazards from point-source factory emissions, are more effectively assessed and remedied on a community level than on a case-by-case basis. Nurses' involvement in helping people understand health problems in a larger context can be the genesis of change. Nurses and other community members can take social action on behalf of those affected. For example, by heightening awareness of sulfur dioxin levels from a local refinery and the relationship of those emission levels to respiratory problems in vulnerable populations, nurses can help citizens gain an understanding of the collective rather than individual burden of the refinery on their community's health.

Emphasize the "Doing" Aspects of Health

There are consistent differences between the way rural and nonrural residents perceive health. The primary one may be the relative importance of "work" and "being able to work" in self-reported

definitions of health (Weinert and Long, 1987). Rural attitudes generally emphasize the "doing" aspects of health by functioning and performing the daily activities fundamentally important in their daily lives. The high value placed on "being able to do" can provide astute nurses with intervention opportunities for both families and communities. Examples of nursing intervention strategies that capitalize on this include accident prevention programs for children, exercise and nutrition programs for seniors, and local industry participation in risk reduction programs for workers. Active involvement of the target population in all phases of program planning and implementation is key to the success of these programs.

Maximize the Use of Informal Networks

Recognizing and using informal networks in the community is essential to the "doing" concept of prevention programs. The name used, such as empowerment models or community action models, is less important than soliciting the involvement of informal networks and local leaders in planning health interventions. As most people who have been involved in community empowerment programs will attest, the involvement of these important entities is not easy or straightforward. Turf issues and collateral agendas can sometimes seem to obstruct rather than facilitate change. However, failure to elicit community involvement in population-based health interventions will result in unfavorable consequences; frequently, superimposed change tends to fit poorly with the community it is intended to serve. Rural change strategies will be short-lived unless members understand it and invest in their own well-being.

RURAL HEALTH CARE DELIVERY SYSTEM

In the past, rural illness care was modeled after urban areas. Urban models emphasize specialist providers and in-hospital acute care with many high-tech, expensive procedures. Many rural hospitals can no longer compete with the larger facilities. This brief overview discusses past and present characteristics of the system and how many community members, providers, and health policy analysts believe it should be changed.

In the 1980s, rural health was focused almost exclusively on hospitals, with the emphasis on making them financially viable. Health administrators and health policy analysts, who recommended that the community hospital become the community's health center, examined the rural small hospital crisis. To many public health professionals, this appeared to be a contradiction of terms. Public health providers assert that hospitals deliver treatment for illness and ignore health promotion and disease prevention. Providers and institutions delivering acute care and those promoting public health have long mistrusted one another. Public health, with its commitment to disease prevention, health promotion, and universal access to community-oriented primary health care, had little in common with cure-oriented hospitals.

In the late 1980s and 1990s, many hospitals developed wellness programs and some additional increased services. For example, at the request of the county government, a small frontier hospital surmounted the barrier between the hospital and public health by taking over the following basic public health

services: home visits, school nursing, and immunization clinics. Hospital-employed nurses make school visits for health education and screening and home visits for prenatal follow-up. The shift toward public health orientation served to broaden the hospital's commitment to the community (Clancy, 1992).

The new century dawns on substantial changes within rural hospitals and in their communities. Numerous hospitals have elected to provide a full continuum of care ranging from preventive services to long-term care. Many are joining networks and merging or affiliating with other rural hospitals, physicians, advance practice nurses, and other providers. Some find a viable option in opening outpatient clinics or long-term care units while providing a small number of beds for acute inpatient care as in the limited service hospitals model (Fig. 21-2) (Rural Health News, 1997). These adaptations may change a community's health, the organization of its social services, and its financial base. Rural health research will be necessary to provide information about how these changes affect the health of rural communities.

FIGURE 21-2

Potential Configurations for the Small Rural Hospital (From Rural Health News: Ready or not: rural hospitals are changing, *Rural Health News* 4(1):1-3, 1997. Used with permission).

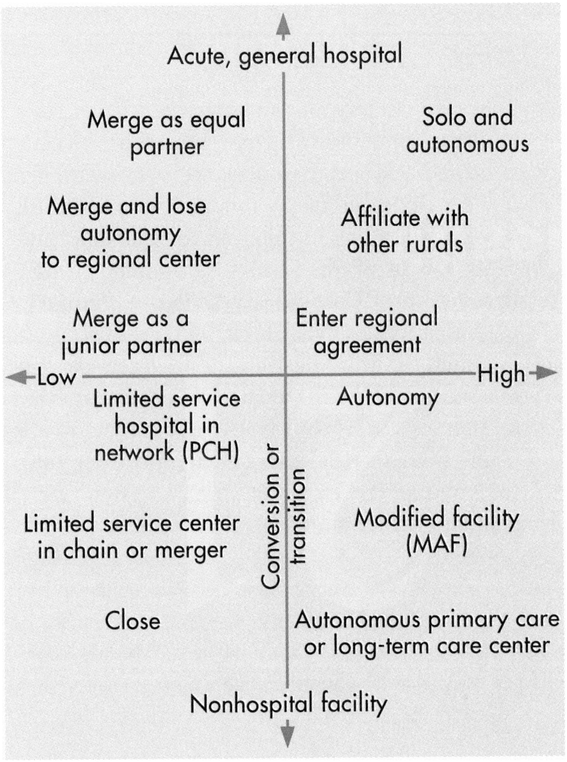

LIMITED SERVICE HOSPITALS

During a five-year period (1987 to 1991), 193 rural hospitals closed nationally. Fortunately, the trend toward rural hospital closure did not continue through the 1990s. They numbered 28 from 1994 through 1997 (Ricketts and Heaphy, 1999). In the more populated rural areas, another hospital was often available within 20 miles. However, for populations in frontier counties, there were very real problems with finding basic primary care. In the United States, 11% of rural hospitals are in frontier areas. These hospitals serve a wide geographical area (46% of the total U.S. land area) where 1% of the U.S. population resides.

Closure of the local hospital can result in the loss of physicians and other providers and the reduction or curtailment of primary care services and emergency medical services. To adapt to the realities of health care management and to improve access to care in frontier areas, new rural hospital models are being developed.

The first alternative model that the HCFA funded was the Montana Medical Assistance Facility (MAF) (Office of the Inspector General, *Continued*

USDHHS, 1993). This and other demonstration models developed between 1987 and 1998 provided the impetus for a nationally legislated program for the development of limited access hospitals. Limited access facilities are called critical access hospitals. This legislation is moving rural America, especially frontier areas, toward development and maintenance of local primary care networks and emergency medical services. A study of rural communities' decisions to convert threatened local hospitals to limited access facilities reported that the need for local emergency service and improvement of recruitment and retention of primary care providers were the most important factors in the determination to change (Shreffler et al., 1999).

Health Care Provider Shortages

The shortage of health care professionals is a barrier to care delivery. In actual numbers, the shortage has been growing since 1990. Although approximately 25% of the U.S. population lives in nonmetropolitan counties, only 18% of RNs practice there. In addition, the supply of PAs, NPs, and physicians has not equaled service need in rural areas. The percentage of rural PAs has increased only slightly from 19.9% in 1989 to 20.2% in 1997. Approximately 20% of NPs (Baer and Smith, 1999; Ricketts, 1994) and less than 11% of physicians practice in rural areas. The recommended 2000:1 ratio in HPSA would require twice as many physicians (National Rural Health Association [NRHA], November 1998). Rehabilitative services provided by speech therapists, occupational therapists, and PTs are in short supply. There is little effort ensuring that these services are available to rural residents (Jones and Brand, 1995).

The growing nursing shortage will affect all of America. This is both a supply and a demand shortage. Declining school enrollments, retirement of current nurses, and the increased need for care of an aging population make the situation especially critical (Sigma Theta Tau International, 1999). A survey by the American Organization of Nurse Executives (AONE) found that in small hospitals, usually located in rural areas, it takes significantly longer time to fill vacancies than in larger urban facilities

(Beyers, 1999). Rural nurses earn less than their urban counterparts, which compounds recruitment difficulties. Nurses with baccalaureate and masters degrees, other than masters prepared NPs, are compensated less for this additional education (Pan, Straub, and Szigeti, 1998).

A solution proposed for the shortage of health care providers is for rural communities to "grow their own." A rural community, a group of small communities, or a county could support local students attending college and recruit students currently attending professional schools. The students make a commitment to work in the community in return for monetary support for their educations (Jones and Brand, 1995). Tuition reimbursement and access to distance learning programs can assist practicing nurses. Continuing education and baccalaureate and masters degrees are available through email, Internet-based courses, interactive video classes, and by-mail videos. Some programs are provided exclusively via the Internet. Nebraska rural communities are enthusiastic about the University of Nebraska College of Nursing Internet courses. The program is helping them grow their own nurses. Research shows that nurses educated in rural communities are more apt to stay and work there than those who move away to attend school (Pullen, 1998).

Community-Wide Health Care Systems

To cope with provider shortages and fewer acute care facilities, community members, rural health care planners, and health care professionals are recommending the development of a community-wide health care system with the hospital as one component. The central focus of this system is community-based care in the form of **Community-Oriented Primary Care (COPC)** services (Van Hook, 1992). COPC is a model in which for-profit health care providers can function in concert with public agencies. There is an axiom that all politics are local. It is also appropriate to consider health care as a local affair. Rohrer provides guidelines for building the local health care system within the context of community.

- The delivery system needs to enhance the health of the community.
- The system should be frugal, because communities do not appreciate ostentatiousness or wasted resources.

- The critical health care delivery organization is not a physical institution, such as a hospital, nursing home . . . but is a local system of primary care (e.g., a community network).
- The mission of the local health care system must be optimization of the community's health. The emphasis is on primary care, health promotion and prevention, and coordination with public health agencies.
- Some key concepts for health systems based on "community" are community governance, population-based planning, information systems, accountability, and community-oriented primary care

(Rohrer, 1999, p. 22).

Primary care is first-line care a provider (e.g., physician, nurse, NP, PA, mental health counselor, or other health care professional) gives in an office or clinic setting. A recommended model for rural communities combines the primary care model with that of COPC services. COPC is often called primary *health* care. A primary health care model assumes that providers address the health and illness concerns of not just the clients they see in the clinic or office, but of the community as a whole using an epidemiological orientation. Providers integrate aspects of public health, health promotion, and disease prevention into their primary care practices. This model moves the provider's orientation from individual clients in the office or clinic practice to population health. For example, this community-oriented, or upstream, approach to prevention will help providers establish a community education program on farm safety and provide the immediate cleaning and suturing of a client's hand lacerated by a piece of farm machinery (Butterfield, 1990; IOM, 1983).

The formation of a community health care system that includes primary care and a community-oriented primary health care focus may bring accessible and affordable illness care to "the country." This system bases health promotion and disease prevention on the needs of the community. Bringing a holistic and integrated approach to both health and illness care, it appears to resemble a nursing model rather than a medical model (Van Hook, 1992). This approach is cooperative rather than market driven and competition based. The community-oriented model complements the public health philosophy of optimal allocation of limited resources and the social justice ethic of equitable access to health and illness care.

Rural communities struggle to define what illness care services they need, want, and can afford. Although outsiders are not always trusted, some communities have successfully enlisted trained facilitators to help develop and execute an effective, practical plan for maintaining or eliminating local services. These facilitators help communities determine how much and what kinds of services to implement. This process is a type of community organization model that includes community participation, needs assessment, and leadership training (Amundson, 1993).

Rural and frontier community health nurses, with their knowledge of advocacy, community assessment, aggregates, and community involvement strategies, can be an excellent local resource for the planning process (Shreffler, 1996). Currently, most planning is related to illness care. Involvement by community health nurses and other local and state health department personnel is integral to a community-wide health care system. Community-based care is central to the development of such a system (ANA, 1996). Optimal models for reformed rural health care systems are those in which the community is the central organizing and sponsoring group for the system. The essential feature of these models is a community-primary care orientation under local leadership (NRHA, February 1998).

Managed Care in the Rural Environment

Managed care has recently changed health care delivery in the United States. In rural areas, health care delivery networks with managed care elements are being developed. An NRHA Issue Paper has identified potential benefits and risks of managed care to rural areas. Possible benefits include the potential to lower primary care costs, improve the quality of care, and help stabilize the local rural health care system. Risks are also apparent including probable high start-up and administrative costs and the volatile effect of large, urban-based for-profit managed care companies (NRHA, 1995).

Managed care has yet to become a major presence in much of rural America because small, disperse populations, few visits per individual, and large numbers of elderly on Medicare with low-level reimbursements do not make the aggregate financially attractive to a MCO. Providers in rural markets face severe financial constraints as HMOs increasingly cope with smaller enrollee and continue to decrease provider reimbursement. The NRHA recommends that "communities or networks develop community health plans, combining delivery and financing systems at the local level. Assuming responsibility for the financing of care for prepaid enrollees is accomplished either by rural communities obtaining their own HMO licenses or by establishing strategic partnerships with HMOs or insurance companies that allow local assumption of financial risk" (NRHA, February 1998, p. 4). In frontier communities, a partnership to reach a critical mass of enrollees would be the most appropriate strategy for meeting the challenge of managed care. Communities that make the most progress toward partnerships or integration are those whose local leaders and providers have strong incentives to work together and are motivated to bring about change to the health care system (Fasciano et al., 1999). Authorities in rural health and managed care report that it is too soon to know whether managed care will become a significant way of delivering health care in rural areas like it has become in urban America (Voelker, 1998).

COMMUNITY-BASED CARE

In the mid1990s, the phrase "community-based care" became a popular term for the myriad of services provided outside the walls of an institution. Examples of these services include home health care, in-home hospice care, nutrition programs, home visits to high-risk pregnant women, community mental health, and adult day care. The concept also includes community participation in decisions about health care services, a focus on all three levels of prevention, and an understanding that the hospital is no longer the exclusive health care provider.

Home Care and Hospice

Home health and hospice programs vary in structure. Larger communities may support a hospital-based home care agency with hospice service, a free-standing, full-service agency, or both. In sparsely populated rural locations, these services are often contracted from a larger regional agency, if they are available at all. The larger agency may hire a nurse from the local area to serve it. A successful Utah model for hospice service development combines external resources based in a city with those of a small community. The large urban-based facility provides administrative support for local nurses hired to work in the hospice program (Memmott, 1991).

A study by Buehler and Lee (1992) reported that family caregivers for cancer patients in the most rural areas believed they had limited formal resources. Nurse case management and development of local resources, using the county extension services as a bridge for outreach services, can improve home care for these patients and provide support for their families. A partnership between the county health nurse and county extension service could provide support and information groups and caregiving classes for the important informal provider network.

Faith Communities and Parish Nursing

Faith communities in rural America have a long and positive legacy; therefore rural residents trust them and they reflect the local customs (Griffin, 1999). They are places of health and healing (Marty, 1999). For these reasons, they can be valuable partners in improving overall community health.

In the past 15 years, RNs have developed a role as parish nurses throughout the United States. Over 3000 nurses are estimated to be working as paid and unpaid staff in both urban and rural centers such as synagogues, churches, or mosques. Professional nursing and parish nursing are based on health and healing (ANA, 1998a).

The parish nurse can be influential in engaging members of a congregation in a partnership. A partnership might consist of an informal network of lay volunteers and the home care nurse. These lay volunteers often visit parish members who are confined to home and may need or receive home care. Parish nurses direct or participate in health promotion and disease prevention activities and work with the lay visitors. Collaboration between the agency and faith community can help extend limited rural community health resources.

When developing this partnership, the parish nurse should define what is meant by health and healing in the context of the partnership, be clear about what resources the agency or institution can contribute, what the congregation will contribute, and identify one person who will be a liaison with the congregation (Wylie and Solari-Twadell, 1999). Chapter 29 provides an in-depth discussion of parish nursing.

Informal Care Systems

Limited availability and accessibility of formal health care resources in rural areas combined with self-reliance and self-help traits of rural residents have resulted in the development of strong rural community informal care and social support networks. Rural residents are more apt to entrust care to established informal networks than to new formal care systems (Weinert and Long, 1987, 1990). One study reported that rural residents sustain a higher level of social health than urban residents. They attributed this social health to their higher level of family and community involvement (Eggebeen and Lichter, 1993), which may contribute to the formation and use of informal systems.

Informal care systems or networks include people who have assumed the role of caregiver based on their individual qualities, life situations, or social roles. People who participate in these networks may provide direct help, advice, or information. They may also serve as a channel of communication within the community (Human Services in the Rural Transition, 1989). Rural residents identify family members, friends, and neighbors as the informal providers of care (Magilvey and Congdon, 1994).

It is important that both institution- and community-based professional health care providers recognize the strengths and positive contributions of informal care systems, which are valuable community resources. It is especially significant that community-based providers identify and combine informal services with formal systems (Weinert and Long, 1987, 1990).

Rural Public Health Departments

There are approximately 3200 local health departments in the United States, but some provide only limited public health services (Pickett and Hanlon, 1990). *Healthy People 2000* objective 8.14 set a goal that a local health department that effectively accomplished the core functions of public health by the year 2000 would serve 90% of Americans (USPHS, 1990). Chapter 1 addresses the three core functions of public health (i.e., assessment, policy development, and assurance). Data from 1993 suggest that a local health department that meets this standard served less than 40% of urban and rural Americans (Turnock et al., 1994).

Less than 4% of all money spent on health care in the United States is spent on public health. It is unlikely that this will improve given limited public resources, the aging of the population with the subsequent need for acute illness care, and changing Medicaid from public to private providers. A recent report of 1992 to 1993 survey data illustrates the circumstance in which public health finds itself. The average annual per person expenditure was $26.00, or less than 10 cents per day for local health departments that support essential public health services (Gordon, Gerzoff, and Richards, 1997).

Many rural counties are either too small to support a health department staffed by adequately trained personnel or have insufficient financial resources to support the needed services. The tax base of a county of fewer than 10,000 residents cannot support a full-service health department. A sanitarian, nurse, and clerk may comprise the entire staff. A local physician often serves as a part-time, unpaid health officer (Pickett and Hanlon, 1990). Often, these small facilities can only offer federally funded programs with few locally funded services.

Local health departments aren't the only entities delivering public health services. Others include Rural Health Clinics (RHCs), Migrant Health Centers (MHCs), public schools, parish nurses, family planning centers, Head Start programs, and public hospitals. To develop the most comprehensive services possible for the population, rural community health nurses need to develop relationships with all sorts of agencies.

Rural Mental Health Care

The economic crisis that affected much of the rural population in the 1980s contributed to mental health problems (American Psychological Association, 1995). Natural disasters such as drought and flood and economic downturns in the late 1990s have contributed to continuing chronic stress. Those affected are most apt to work in the traditional ranching, farming, mining, forestry, and fishing industries. They have not enjoyed the good economic times generated by the information and technology age (NRHA, 1999). A lack of understanding regarding the importance of diversity in rural America has resulted in research studies that ignore the differences within the population. A simple rural-urban division does not provide discrete information to base decisions about the extent of mental illness within various rural groups. Clearly, large sections of at-risk rural populations are without mental health care (NRHA, 1999; Wagenfield, 1990).

A survey by the American Psychological Association (1995) found major barriers in residents' lack of acceptance of mental health care professionals and their lack of awareness of problems within the rural community. Rural mental health care providers also face problems similar to those confronted by other primary health care workers. These include a more diverse practice, fewer opportunities for ongoing education, and fewer professionals to consult than their colleagues in urban practice.

The number of mental health care providers in rural America is insufficient. The most recent figures show that only 79.5% of rural counties have mental health services (NIMH, 1991). Clearly, it is a serious challenge for community health nurses to find providers who will accept a referral for a client needing a mental health assessment.

Emergency Services

Emergency medical services (EMS) in rural areas become increasingly important when hospitals close. Many small rural communities have a volunteer EMS response team, but do not have a local hospital or medical clinic. EMS has become a vital component of community-based care.

Rural EMS teams face the same financial pressures as providers serving a sparsely populated area. Private for-profit organizations find it unprofitable to locate in these areas. Consequently, most EMS units consist of dedicated local volunteers (Garnett, 1991). In medically underserved areas, EMS systems play an increasingly important role in decreasing the morbidity and mortality of individuals needing emergency care. Getting patients from the place of injury to the trauma center within the "golden hour" is frequently not possible in rural areas because distance, terrain, climatic conditions, and communication methods produce barriers. Some rural facilities are more than two hours away by air from the nearest trauma center or tertiary care hospital (Furlow, 1999).

Problems among rural EMS systems include a shortage of volunteers, a lower level of training than among urban providers, training curricula that often do not reflect rural hazards (e.g., farm equipment trauma), lack of guidance from physicians, and lack of physician training and orientation to the EMS system. Low population density, large, isolated, or inaccessible areas, severe weather, poor roads, and lower density of telephones or other communication methods contribute to difficult public access for emergency care. These problems make the challenges of developing EMS in rural and frontier areas substantial (NRHA, 1997; OTA, 1989).

Rural and frontier residents depend on EMS because they encounter many serious injuries and the distance from acute care facilities increases the morbidity and mortality associated with trauma and medical emergencies. Federal policy-making agencies currently recommend that the overall system of care in rural areas incorporate EMS into the system (NRHA, 1997). Public health agencies must ensure that this vital tertiary prevention component is accessible to geographically isolated populations.

LEGISLATION AND PROGRAMS AFFECTING PUBLIC HEALTH IN RURAL AREAS

Public health legislation and programs derive their legitimacy from the Preamble to the Constitution, which declares a fundamental purpose of government to "promote the general welfare." Furthermore, the Constitution invests Congress with the power "to lay and collect taxes . . . and provide for the common defense and general welfare" (Pickett and Hanlon, 1990, p. 166). Before 1912, the federal government was involved in the public's health to a very limited extent and was primarily concerned with the health of merchant marines and protecting the public from communicable diseases that overseas immigrants might bring into America. The Children's Bureau was established in 1912 through the efforts of Lillian Wald.

Maternal and child advocates continued to bring their concerns for the health, welfare, and mortality of mothers and children to national attention. In 1922, in response to concerns about rural maternal and child care, the Sheppard-Towner Act passed. It encouraged states to develop programs to address these problems. The act moved federal funding into personal health services for the first time and shifted the orientation of public health "from disease prevention to promotion of overall health" (IOM, 1988, p. 66). Grants-in-aid to the states provided incentives to establish the programs and became the model for federal-state partnerships. In the 1960s, block grants for federally prioritized public health programs replaced the grants-in-aid program.

During the Great Depression, Congress recognized the special health problems of rural areas. Hunger and poverty evidenced the alarming increases in infant mortality, which was the most sensitive index of overall population health. The Social Security Act of 1935, passed during this era, carried the legacy of earlier maternal and child care provisions and added grants-in-aid for public health training and programs. Maternal and child care and benefits for the poor and elderly were also covered in the Social Security Amendments of 1965, which created direct federal aid to individuals in the Medicare and Medicaid sections of that act.

Health Care Programs for Rural Areas

Federal- and state-funded health care programs continue to impact the availability and provision of rural health care services. Government insurance, in the form of Medicare and Medicaid, benefits people through individual and programmatic assistance and funds a significant portion of rural health care. When other federal programs that finance or provide direct health care (e.g., Department of Veterans Affairs and IHS) are added to Medicare and Medicaid, the impact of the federal and state government on rural health care is substantial, but major gaps in health care delivery remain. One of these gaps has been adequate coverage for uninsured or underinsured individuals or groups (e.g., elderly people who cannot afford prescription drugs).

In 1996, approximately 28% of uninsured children (3.1 million) lived in rural or frontier areas, and as discussed earlier, 21% of rural children are uninsured (Office of Rural Health Policy, 1999b). In 1999, the HCFA approved plans by each of the 50 states, territories, and the District of Columbia to implement CHIP. The program provided the largest increase in federal funding for children's health insurance since the passage of Medicaid in 1965. The initiative was designed to reach the nearly 11 million uninsured American children. Many of these children came from working families with incomes too high to qualify for Medicaid and too low to afford private health insurance.

Before the enactment of CHIP, about 5.7 million children, or 65% of all uninsured children, were ineligible for Medicaid and more than 33% of uninsured children were eligible for Medicaid but not enrolled (Reschovsky and Cunningham, 1998). According to Reschovsky and Cunningham, children go without health insurance because they have limited access to employer-sponsored health insurance, parents are offered employer-sponsored insurance but decline because there are associated costs, there are gaps in the coverage of public insurance such as Medicaid, and parents fail to enroll children in Medicaid although they are eligible. Language barriers, stigma, and eligibility hassles are frequently cited reasons. With a larger percentage of uninsured children in rural and frontier states, a growing percentage of Hispanics, and a shortage of health and welfare

services, these states are likely to realize the smallest reductions in the percentage of children who remain uninsured. The new program will help fill the gap; an estimated 33% of all uninsured children who do not qualify for Medicaid will be eligible for insurance under CHIP, but 31% of all uninsured children (some 2.7 million) will remain ineligible for federally-supported health insurance (Reschovsky and Cunningham, 1998). Under this legislation, block grants are made for states that have designed programs to expand Medicaid, subsidize private insurance, or combine the two approaches. Under federal guidelines, states have considerable discretion in setting Medicaid eligibility levels. The program is particularly beneficial to rural families because an estimated 28% of all uninsured children live in rural or frontier areas (Office of Rural Health Policy [ORHP], 1999b; Reschovsky and Cunningham, 1998). Additional information about this new program and the chances of its success is available on the ORHP website. See the Resources Box at the end of this chapter.

A second category of federal programs provides federal block grants to the states. The block grants fund the following three major programs: maternal and child health, preventive health and health services, and alcohol, drug abuse, and mental health program administration. Block grants have been marked by shifts in locus of responsibility for funding and they struggle for domination in formulating health policy.

A third category of federal programs for rural health care services identified in the 1990 OTA report comprises those "whose primary purpose is to augment the health resources available to underserved areas and populations" (p. 61). These programs were established through federal legislation and are designed to increase personnel, facilities, and planning resources. Most programs are administered through the USDHHS and HRSA.

With every new administration and Congress, the availability of federal funding and the sharing of power among the three levels of government change, which makes continuity in public health programming and administration profoundly difficult. Furthermore, the burden of providing public services grows in areas that have experienced in-migration, immigration, and other forms of population growth. General economic decline intensifies the difficulties, particularly in the rural West where the cost of delivering services is exacerbated by the problem of low population density, vast distances, and a shortage of health care personnel. The trend toward cost shifting from the federal government to the states will continue to place an increasing share of the burden on the states as it has with financing health care for Medicaid; for example, the state contribution for Medicaid nearly doubled between 1975 and 1990 and by 1996, for every dollar spent on Medicaid, the states paid 40 cents, on average, although the contribution is much higher in some rural states (Ricketts, 1999; Straub and Walzer, 1992).

Programs that Augment Health Personnel

One of the greatest disparities between rural and urban health care is the supply of health care personnel. Over 22 million rural Americans live in areas designated primary care HPSAs (Division of Shortage Designation, Bureau of Primary Health Care, 1998). Data from the Sixth National Sample Survey of RNs and the American Academy of Physician Assistants show that approximately 20% of midlevel providers delivered primary care to rural and frontier areas (Baer and Smith, 1999). Programs such as the **National Health Service Corps** (NHSC) and Area Health Education Centers encourage health professionals to practice in HPSAs through volunteer, scholarship, and loan repayment programs (i.e., in the case of the NHSC). They also attract and retain primary care providers in shortage areas where only 1 of 10 physicians practiced in 1998 (AMA, 2000; Office of Rural Health Policy, 2000).

Other programs attract health professionals to shortage areas through grants to educational institutions, school construction grants, and student assistance programs. Special programs are also available to support education for advance practice nurses and minority and disadvantaged students preparing for health professional careers (OTA, 1990). NPs and PAs, some of whom come through the NHSC program or receive federal traineeships, are helping meet the needs for rural primary care in increasing numbers.

Programs that Augment Health Care Facilities and Services

Several programs are particularly important to meeting the public health needs of rural people. One is the Community Health Centers (CHC) program, administered by the PHS. The CHC benefit underserved areas and populations by providing primary health care and, in some cases, supplemental secondary and tertiary health care such as hospital care, long-term home health care, and rehabilitation. RHCs are designed to improve access to primary care. As an incentive to

rural communities to apply for RHCs, Medicare and Medicaid are reimbursed at a higher rate than usual. As a result, their numbers more than quadrupled during the 1990s.

The MHC program and the Migrant Health Program (MHP) also come under the Division of Community and Migrant Health and HRSA. The MHC program provides comprehensive nursing and medical care and support services to MSFW and their families. The centers provide culturally sensitive care to a racially and culturally diverse farm labor force from many countries in Latin America and the Caribbean. Bilingual, bicultural health personnel including lay outreach workers use culturally appropriate protocols for providing primary care, preventive health care, transportation, dental care, pharmaceuticals, and environmental health. The MHCs must provide the same services as the CHC and may also offer supplemental services such as environmental health services, infectious disease and parasite control, and accident prevention programs. The MHP administers the MHC program and provides grants to public and private nonprofit organizations that develop and operate some 390 of these centers in 35 states and Puerto Rico.

Medicare's new Rural Hospital Flexibility (RHF) grant program replaces earlier demonstration programs administered by the HCFA during the 1990s (McNeely, 1992). It provides funding to states to establish limited-service hospitals that can obtain designation as Critical Access Hospitals (CAH) in rural communities. Grants are awarded for planning, implementing, and establishing networks of care and improving EMS. The ORHP and HRSA administers this program (Office of Rural Health Policy, 1999a).

Primary care cooperative agreements facilitate the development of primary care services and attract primary care providers to rural HPSAs. Special legislation for HPSAs has also created programs to provide acute care facilities and services. The Rural Transition Grants Program, administered by HCFA, helps small rural communities with nonprofit hospitals adjust to changes in clinical practice patterns and in-hospital use, shifts from hospital- to community-based care, and changes in emergency care delivery patterns.

Programs that Assist with Health Care Policy, Planning, and Research

The AHRQ includes health research in its mandate in addition to demonstration and evaluation of the effectiveness of rural health care services (OTA, 1990). The ORHP is part of HRSA and serves in an advisory capacity on diverse rural health issues including availability and access to health professionals and care. The advisory committee also offers advice on the prioritization and financing of rural health care services. The ORHP manages the Rural Health Research Center grant program and serves as a clearinghouse for information about research findings of interest to providers (OTA, 1990).

Most of these federal programs provide competitive grants for research studies, demonstration and evaluation programs, and training and recruiting of health professionals. With the exception of CHC and MHC, they do not provide direct services. Direct health care services to Medicaid recipients and public health programs are increasingly the burden of state and local governments because rural economies are declining and the demand for services is increasing in many areas.

Until the early twentieth century, responsibility for health care policy, programs, and financing was largely a local government matter. Now the responsibility is shifting back from the federal government to the state and from the state to local governments. The extent and quality of public health programming may vary again with the ability and willingness of citizens to invest increasingly scarce resources in minimum protections. The conclusions of a 1998 IOM study were pessimistic about progress in solving public health problems, not withstanding great strides forward in scientific discovery, social reforms, and government activities. Likewise, a study by the IOM in 1992 described the current state as stagnant with little improvement in access to care over the previous decade and stated that "underlying most of the indicators is a growing division between the haves and the have-nots in our society" (IOM, 1992, p. 3).

RURAL COMMUNITY HEALTH NURSING

Perhaps a more accurate title than rural community health nursing would be "community health nursing along the rural continuum." Nonmetropolitan areas adjacent to a population center of 50,000 are at one end of the continuum; towns of less than 2500 people with the open country of farms and ranches are at the most rural end.

Practice in a rural area may require working as the only nurse at a health department in a remote Western Great Plains frontier county with a population of 6000, at a full-service health department in a town of 50,000, or at a large health department in a rural area next to an urban population. A practice in a rural area adjacent to a large metropolitan area often appears to have more in common with the urban end of the continuum in terms of agency size, distances, and resources. For the purposes of this discussion, the practice setting is at the more "rural" end of the continuum.

The following definition illustrates the broad-based, generalist focus of the modern rural community health nurse. It includes the important geographical and cultural environment where community health practice is implemented and helps define appropriate nursing interventions.

> Rural nursing is the practice of professional nursing within the physical and sociocultural context of sparsely populated communities. It involves the continual interaction of the rural environment, the nurse, and his or her practice. Rural nursing is the diagnosis and treatment of a diversified population of people of all ages and a variety of human responses to actual (or potential) occupational hazards or actual or potential health problems existent in maternity, pediatric, medical/surgical and emergency nursing in a given rural area (Bigbee, 1993, p. 132).

Nursing Roles in Community Health Practice

The nature of community health nursing is broad-based and generalist. Strong generalists, these nurses are professionals who can move into a selected specialty area or provide care across specialty areas (Turner and Gunn, 1991). They need strong decision making skills to practice where minimal professional support and supervision may be available (Lassiter, 1985). Components of this role include educator, direct care provider, case manager, coordinator, and administrator.

Nurses who practice in rural areas are held accountable for the same scope and standards of practice as their urban counterparts. The ANA Standards of Clinical Nursing Practice (ANA, 1998b) outline competent levels of nursing care and professional performance universal to all nurses active in clinical practice. Scope and standards for nursing specialties are built upon these general ones and are outlined in ANA publications. These define the specialties for public accountability. The specialties most common in rural settings that have ANA-published standards are the following: community health, home health, gerontology, mental health, nurse administration, nursing staff and professional development, oncology, and parish nursing. The Code for Nurses with Interpretive Statements also directs the rural nurse's practice (ANA, 1985). All nurses in the United States must be licensed in the state where they practice. By law, nurses are required to follow the scope of practice outlined by the rules and regulations in their respective states.

Characteristics of Rural Nursing

Dolphin (1984) reported that the several positive aspects of rural nursing were "ability to give holistic care, to know everyone well, and to develop close relationships with the community and with coworkers." Autonomy, professional status, and being valued by the agency and community are reported components of positive job satisfaction (Davis and Droes, 1993; Dunkin et al., 1992). Public health nurses report slightly higher job satisfaction than home health nurses. In general, salary was consistently rated as least satisfying and professional status as most satisfying (Juhl et al., 1993). On the negative side of rural practice are physical and professional isolation, problems related to scarce resources (e.g., low salary and few positions and personnel), problems within the work environment, role diffusion, and lack of anonymity (Davis and Droes, 1993; Dolphin, 1984; Dunkin et al., 1992; Long and Weinert, 1989; Movassaghi et al., 1992; Scharff, 1998). Some nurses viewed "in-depth interpersonal knowledge of clients" (Davis and Droes, 1993, p. 166), a wide variety of necessary skills, a diversity of client problems, and the slower pace of rural life as negative components and some viewed them as positive (Bigbee, 1993).

Of those components identified as negative, agencies and professional organizations are most actively addressing professional isolation. Distance learning is moving training and education out to rural nurses. The technology ranges from basic telephone lines to full-motion interactive two-way video. Web-based Internet university degree programs and continuing education are rapidly becoming available. Not only does distance learning help currently employed nurses improve skills and network with other nurses, its presence also assists in attracting new personnel (ANA, 1996; Crandall and Coggan, 1994).

Scharff (1998) discussed the distinctive nature of the rural nurse's practice. She found that the rural nurse is a generalist and generalist is not synonymous with boring. Interviews with rural nurses show that they feel an "intensity of purpose" that makes rural nursing distinctive. Nurses living and practicing in the same place have a strong sense of integration and continuity between practice and community.

> The newcomer practices nursing in a rural setting, unlike the old-timer, who practices *rural nursing*. Somewhere between these extremes lies the transitional period of events and conditions through which each nurse passes at her or his own pace. It is within this time zone that nurses experience rural reality and move toward becoming professionals who understand that having gone rural, they are not less than they were, but rather, they are more than they expected to be. Some may be conscious of the transition, and others may not, but in the end, a few will say, "I am a rural nurse"
>
> (Scharff, 1998, p. 38).

Rural community health nursing is rewarding and challenging. Services can include prenatal care, infant and child care in clinics and homes, home care for acute and chronic disease, hospice care for all ages, school health, parish nursing, and mental health. The nurse practicing with the autonomy common in rural practice brings knowledge and competence in other clinical specialties. The work requires a discriminating, solid practitioner who can perform general nursing at a skill level beyond that of the outdated "mile wide and inch deep" general nursing. The rural nurse must be an "expert generalist."

Knowledge Base of the Expert Generalist in Rural Community Health Nursing

Personal barriers to health care include culture, language, attitudes, acceptability, education, and income (IOM, 1993). The interaction of personal barriers with structural and financial barriers is complicated and often difficult to understand. For example, the presence of a new primary health care provider in a small town does not necessarily mean the residents find this newcomer acceptable. They may prefer to see an established NP in a town 40 miles away. In this scenario, personal preference causes people to travel for care although no structural barrier, or lack of a local provider, exists.

Health care preferences and health perceptions must be assessed when planning care that is acceptable to individuals, families, aggregates within the community, and the community as a whole. To know what interventions and implementation strategies will work, the community health nurse must comprehend how the people perceive health, health care, and illness. Reports of studies can be helpful. Understanding and applying this information will decrease personal barriers by making interventions more acceptable and more likely to achieve a positive outcome.

Many small rural communities are insular and reluctant to accept assistance from outsiders or outside experts. They often prefer to receive care from someone they know rather than from a provider who is new to the community. Weinert and Long (1987) documented the distrust of "outsiders" or "newcomers." Rural families' resistance to "outside experts" and change was reportedly a major obstacle in establishing a primary prevention program about health and safety risks (Posey, 1995). In another example, small rural community EMS were not initially welcomed because community members perceived that if they accepted federal money, they would relinquish local control (OTA, 1989).

These examples show resistance to outside influence and a preference for local control. Outsider nurses, physicians, teachers, and ministers can unknowingly pose a threat to the community, especially if they persist in trying to share knowledge (Norris, 1993). A new nurse who enthusiastically provides health information may encounter resistance that is unexpected, misunderstood, and quite discouraging.

Independence and self-reliance, characteristics of rural people, influence their understanding of health and their reactions to illness (Lee, 1985). Rural residents identify themselves as healthy if they can do their usual work. Although they may be in pain while working, they don't identify themselves as ill because they can do the work (Weinert and Long, 1987). A group of elderly women described self-reliance related to aging and health as the ability to care for themselves, to make choices and decisions, and to assert themselves in realizing their personal goals (Chafey, Sullivan, and Shannon, 1998).

Hardiness is a personality characteristic that influences coping and adaptation when stressful life events occur. Rural families identified as hardy are more able to respond to stress as a strengthening experience rather than one that weakens the family. A study about rural family hardiness reported that work, lifestyle, and daily pressures related to occupation play a primary role in the perception of physical ailment and family conflict (Carson et al., 1993). Lee (1991), in a study about hardiness and its relationship to perceived health in rural adults, reported that control and commitment were components of hardiness

whose presence predicts positive health. For the nurse, the implications of these findings are that rural clients will react to interventions more positively if they have as much control as possible. Commitment to work is also very important. Therefore when planning activities for individuals, families, or communities, consider the importance of the seasonal nature of many of rural America's occupations (e.g., farming, ranching, logging, firefighting, and forest service work).

Rural women perform more traditional marriage and family roles than their urban counterparts. They are described as "keepers of the culture" and "carriers of collective healing" (Battenfield, Clift, and Graubarth, 1981). They facilitate role socialization of children (i.e., the keepers of the culture) and self-care related to health care needs (i.e., carriers of collective healing). Most often in rural families the women monitor family members' health and encourage them, especially the men, to seek care (Lee, 1993). Little economic opportunity and few child day care facilities are two reasons rural women continue to carry out their traditional primary child care responsibilities. Economic conditions have caused some women to seek employment, although available jobs in rural areas are limited, especially for women (Bushy, 1990).

The isolation found in much of rural America can be intensified for victims of domestic violence. Rural people resist reporting domestic violence. Police sometimes are family and friends, or the police or providers are of a culture other than that of the victim. For nonEnglish speaking migrant workers, language and cultural barriers worsen the situation. Anything that inhibits people from making contact with providers can bring disadvantages and dangers to them (Carrick, 1998).

Researchers who studied 820 low-income Hispanic farmworkers reported that 17% had been physically or sexually abused by a spouse, boyfriend, or family member. Drug and alcohol use by a woman's partner and pregnancy were the significant predictors of abuse (Van Hightower and Gorton, 1999). The community health nurse must realize that domestic abuse is a personal and cultural issue. Care programs for victims and curricula for educating providers must factor into the existing cultural norms of the people who receive care (Rural Health News, 1999).

Community health nurses can be more effective educators and caregivers if they recognize the pivotal role of women in the health care of rural families. Community and health status indicators, economic factors, and beliefs influence outcomes. Clinical practice is carried out when the nursing process is applied to individuals, families, and aggregates within a community. Nursing and public health theories are combined to deliver a broad range of services in numerous settings. Nursing care becomes holistic by integrating the following into the nursing process: rural health information, rural residents and their communities, community health nursing, and the prevention-oriented upstream approach to population-based health.

RURAL HEALTH RESEARCH

Community-Based Health Care: Nursing Strategies, a report by the Priority Expert Panel of the NINR, affirms that the rural health research foundation is inadequate and studies are infrequently repeated. This situation exists because rural health is not studied as frequently as urban health (NINR, 1995). If rural Americans are to attain equity in health care cost, access, and quality, high-caliber research must be available to provide a clear picture of individuals, family, and community health care needs.

Nurses working in the field have identified research priorities (Bushy, 1991, 1992; Ide, 1992; Long, 1998; Long and Weinert, 1989). The NRHA's Research Conference (Hersh and Van Hook, 1989) and the NINR (1995) have also identified research priorities. Broadly stated, these priorities focus on the development of rural nursing theory and the refinement of rural nursing practice models, health care policy, rural health care delivery systems, and nursing approaches using community-based interventions directed at the three levels of prevention.

Rural nursing theory and practice models are in the early stages of development. The work by Long and Weinert (1989) and Weinert and Long (1990) on developing a foundation for rural nursing theory helps in guiding research, rural community nursing practice, and education. The work done by Drs. Long and Weinert at Montana State University-Bozeman provides a substantial descriptive theory of rural nursing. The theory emphasizes the importance of comprehending the rural resident's definition of health. For example, rural people value the ability to work and are more apt to reject the sick role than urban residents. If they can do their work, they do not consider themselves ill. Concepts related to nursing are lack of anonymity (i.e., knowing many people in the rural community in both work and social roles), outsider-insider, and old-timer–newcomer. In relation to outsider-insider and old-timer–newcomer, a rural

community is less likely to accept a community health nurse if he or she is new to the area than if he or she grew up in or lived in that community for 20 years (Weinert and Long, 1987). Three future directions for rural nursing theory research include assembling the key concepts into a clear theory; replicating research in other geographical areas and with other cultures; and additional translating, applying, and testing of the theory (Long, 1998).

Ide (1992) developed a rural nursing practice model that includes ideas garnered from current rural literature and includes needs and priorities synthesized from graduate student's community health assessments. This model outlines the ways in which the health status, beliefs, and behaviors of rural dwellers and nursing practice are influenced by their environment. The extensive discussion of environmental effects provides helpful direction to nurses, teachers, and researchers for planning health care delivery and initiating scholarly inquiry.

Bushy (1991), in a review of the rural family health literature, identified the need for more research addressing the relationships of life events such as marriage, unemployment, business foreclosure, and rural location.

The NRHA research agenda outlined in 1989 remains relevant in 1999. Research still focuses on the following: maternal child health, rural hospitals, alternative delivery systems (e.g., HMOs and MCOs), the poor and underserved, the elderly, and primary care. Problems related to research needs that are important to all the listed issues are the need for government agencies to standardize definitions considering the differences of rural populations; the need for secondary analysis of existing data and reporting of aggregate data by small, geographical regions to ensure that important regional differences are not overlooked; dilemmas related to recruitment, retention, and health care provider training in rural communities; the negative affect of professional liability on providers; transportation obstacles (e.g., distance, terrain, climatic conditions, poor roads, and nonexistent public transit system) that limit access to health care; and outcome measurements of quality health care (Hersh and Van Hook, 1989).

A research agenda specific to the needs of the community and Migrant Health Center program is divided into in the following three general categories: outcomes research, managed care applications including finance issues, and delivery of service (Mueller et al., 1998). A detailed listing of the 15 major research priorities is available on the Nebraska

Center for Rural Health Research website, which can be accessed through the SIMON website at ⟨SiMON⟩ www. wbsaunders.com/SIMON/nies/.

Community-Based Health Care: Nursing Strategies identifies three essential research topics at the primary and secondary intervention levels (i.e., unintentional injuries, maternal and child health with a focus on infant mortality, and lifestyle or personal actions that contribute to premature mortality). At the tertiary level of rehabilitation and supportive care, formal and informal support and chronic illness are identified as the essential subjects of research (NINR, 1995).

Previously, this chapter described rural residents as self-reliant, independent, and distrustful of outsiders. Shreffler (1999) reported that these characteristics could pose challenges to outside investigators if insiders believe researchers are encroaching on privacy and meddling in local issues. She identified the need for research methods that are sensitive to rural culture and communities. Also, she described adaptations that researchers can make to conventional survey methods that improve the rate of return and show respect for the study participants' culture.

Well-designed qualitative and large-scale quantitative studies are needed to improve rural research. Nurses must collaborate with researchers in describing problems and gathering data. Additionally, the need to disseminate findings to nurses and other rural health care providers in clinical practice is of paramount importance (Bushy, 1992). Without that critical link to the clinician, research is an academic exercise and does not serve the needs of individuals, families, and communities.

RESOURCES FOR THE RURAL COMMUNITY HEALTH NURSE

To obtain information about the various health care organizations that deal with rural health issues, visit the book's SIMON website, at ⟨SiMON⟩ www. wbsaunders.com/SIMON/nies/.

Videos

Opening Doors: Public Health Nursing in its 100th Year (1994)
TS Media
16212 Bothell Way SE
Mill Creek, WA 98012
(800) 876-6334

On the Frontier: The Challenges and Rewards of Rural Nursing (1995)
Glaxo, Inc.
Research Triangle Park, NC 27709
Cost: no charge

Parish Nursing in Montana (1999)
Parish Nursing Center, Carroll College
16 N Benton Ave
Helena, MT 59625-0002
(406) 447-5494
Cost: no charge

CD-ROMs

Domestic Violence
(for emergency medical providers)
Critical Illness and Trauma Foundation
(406) 585-2669

EMS for Children
Pediatric Programs (five CD-ROMs)
(703) 905-1203
Developed by the Critical Illness and Trauma Foundations and the Montana State Emergency Medical Systems Agency.

Partners for a Safer Community
(Special Project of the National Future Farmers of America Foundation)
Safety program includes video, CD-ROM, and program guides. Call this phone number to find out about training programs in your state: (203) 773-0644.

Written Resources

Call for Health: Newsletter from the National Migrant Resource Program
To order call (512) 328-7682.

Lee H, editor: *Conceptual basis for rural nursing,* New York, 1998, Springer Publishing.
To order contact Springer Publishing, (212) 431-4370.

Norris K: *Dakota, a spiritual geography,* New York, 1993, Ticknor and Fields.
Available in bookstores, libraries, and from the publisher.

Rothenberg, David: *With these hands: the hidden world of migrant farmworkers today,* St. Louis, 1999, Harcourt Brace.
To order contact Harcourt Brace: (800) 543-1918.
Continued

The resources listed below can be ordered from the National Highway Traffic Safety Administration: (202) 493-2052.
Protecting Your Newborn

Kids Aren't Cargo
Sudden Impact
Three Ways to Keep a Friend Alive
National Standard Curriculum for Bystander Care

CASE STUDY

APPLICATION OF THE NURSING PROCESS

All three levels of prevention (i.e., primary, secondary, and tertiary) are reflected in rural practice. These are applied to individuals, families, and aggregates. The generalist nature of the rural community health practice gives the nurse an excellent opportunity to assess health needs and help improve health status at all levels of prevention. The following case study includes short-term individual and family approaches. It also focuses on upstream interventions developed to handle the identified problems. Upstream interventions focus on population and prevention. They deal with political, economic, and environmental factors that are precursors to health problems.

At 4:30 PM on a hot fall day, RN Mary Fieldson drove up a narrow gravel township road 40 miles from her office in the county courthouse. She had just completed her sixth home health visit. By the time Mary returned home, she traveled more than 150 miles, but she enjoyed the drive. She worked in a rural county of 6000 where she grew up. She made a skilled visit to Joe Lingh, the father of a high school friend. On her way home, she traversed the valley where she once lived. She recently returned "home" after a 15-year absence to live, work, and raise her 12-year-old daughter.

When she approached the Connelly farm, Mary saw Eliza Connelly standing by the road waving her down. Mary stopped to say hello. Mrs. Connelly said, "I called Ruth Lingh and she said you had just left. How is Joe's leg?" Mary was aware that this was a friendly inquiry about a neighbor of 40 years, but she was mindful of the need for confidentiality. Mary told Mrs. Connelly that Joe was glad to be

home from the hospital. Mrs. Connelly asked whether Mary heard about her husband's accident Monday evening. He "cut his hand up in the silage chopper and is in the hospital in Spring City," she told Mary tearfully. "I just knew something was going to happen someday. I worry so much about them working with all that machinery and the men work in the fields alone so much. I feel about ready to fall apart. Thank God Jim [their son] was working with him when it happened!"

Mary had a cup of coffee with Eliza, who regained her composure. Eliza continued to talk about long-standing fears for the safety of her family in doing the farm work. She asked Mary to stop by and check on her husband, Austin, when he returned home the following week. Mary told Eliza to request a referral from the primary care physician so insurance would pay for the visits. At 5:30 PM Mary began the drive back to her office in Wolsey, the county seat.

Monday afternoon Mary received a telephone call from Dr. Lobban, the local primary care physician. He requested weekly skilled nursing visits for Austin for the next three weeks to check for infection and monitor recovery. Austin was discharged from the Spring City hospital the following day, six days after the injury. Dr. Lobban sent Mary the emergency room records and the hand specialist's discharge summary.

Assessment

The medical records provided the following information. The first finger was severed at the metacarpophalangeal joint (i.e., the third joint) and reattached. The second, third, and fourth fingers were severed distal to the proximal interphalangeal joints (i.e., between the first and second joints). The severed portions of the second, third, and fourth fingers could not be reattached because they were too badly mangled. At discharge, infection was not evident. The injuries were healing well.

The Connelly family provided additional information about the circumstances of the accident. At approximately 6:30 PM, Austin and his son, Jim, were chopping oats for silage. Seeing rain clouds on the horizon, Jim and Austin hurried to finish before rain fell on the unchopped grain. The silage chopper was not working well. Austin shut it off and hurriedly reached into the inspection hole. The still-turning blades caught his right hand, severing the fingers. Jim wrapped his father's hand tightly in his shirt, retrieved the fingers, and drove his father to their house two miles away. Jim went back to the field to finish chopping the oats. Eliza drove her husband 23 miles to the primary care hospital emergency room. The family physician cleaned and dressed Austin's hand, gave him medication for pain, and packed the severed fingers for transport to the hand specialist in Spring City. A family friend and his son drove Mr. and Mrs. Connelly 150 miles to the Spring City hospital where Austin was admitted and underwent surgery. Eliza went home with their friend and his son after the surgery. She spoke to Austin by telephone daily and drove to Spring City on Tuesday to bring him home.

On her first home visit Mary assessed the following:

- Individual client, Mr. Connelly, for signs and symptoms of infection, pain control, and functional positioning
- Eliza's comfort level and knowledge of dressing changes and signs and symptoms of infection (i.e., she is the primary caregiver)
- Stress and grief processing of all family members
- Ability of family members to provide physical and emotional support during crisis resolution
- Risk-taking behaviors, especially those related to work, of all family members
- Assessment of neighborhood groups and neighbors who can provide support and help the family with the fall harvest work

Diagnosis

Individual
- At risk for infection, pain, and loss of hand function (Austin)
- At risk for grief related to loss of fingers, some use of hand, and decreased ability to do farm work (Austin)
- Anxiety related to ongoing fear of injury of family members (Eliza)
- Stress related to new responsibilities for farm management (Jim)

Family
- At risk for family crisis related to instability caused by the injury

Community
- Inadequate programs for farm injury prevention
- Nonexistent EMS or first-response service

Planning

A plan of care is developed at the individual, family, and community levels. Mutual goal setting and contracting are essential if the outcomes are to be optimal.

Individual

Long-Term Goal
- Client will experience successful rehabilitation.

Short-Term Goals
- Client will remain free of infection.
- Individual family members will be able to express grief.

Family

Long-Term Goals
- Family will demonstrate coping skills appropriate to the crisis.
- Family will identify risky behavior related to farm work.

Short-Term Goals
- Identify support to help with farm work.
- Identify ways to keep in contact with each other when family members are working alone in the fields.

Continued

Community

Long-Term Goal

- Program will be established for farm injury prevention education for populations at risk.

Short-Term Goals

- Begin the health planning process to put into place a farm injury primary prevention program.
- Explore the potential for a volunteer EMS response team.

Intervention

Mutual goal setting between Mary Fieldson and the Connelly family made it possible for them to carry out interventions collaboratively.

Individual

Mary taught Eliza how to change dressings and monitor Austin's hand for infection and function. Austin was involved in his care during healing and was able to monitor and manage the pain. He was most concerned about rehabilitation. He especially wanted to know when he could return to work and how disabled he would be. The local physician monitored Austin's progress. With Austin and Eliza present, the local physician consulted with the hand specialist by two-way interactive video conferencing. This enabled them to confer, thereby eliminating a 150-mile trip to Spring City. The home care PT visited the farm once to set up a program of hand exercises. Austin, who plays the piano, wanted to know if piano playing would be a good exercise. "Playing 'Moonlight Serenade' would sure stretch that right hand," he told the therapist. The therapist told him that he should play three times a day as part of the rehabilitation care plan.

Family

Mary worked with the family to find ways to finish the fall work. They decided to hire part-time help, and two workers helped full-time until the crop was harvested. While in the hospital, Austin was able to assist his son by supporting his ability to make the necessary decisions about farm management. After discharge, he also was able to participate in the process. The family identified the need for more awareness about the dangers of farm work. They

immediately purchased a cellular phone to take to the field. Eliza felt this would relieve her anxiety about being out of touch with Austin and Jim and not knowing why they were later than expected for meals. There was much discussion about the cost of the telephone and service. Eliza convinced the men that her peace of mind was worth the cost.

The stress and grief reactions were minimal. Most of the stress centered on getting the fall farm work done and seeing that Austin recovered enough to work "the way he is used to doing." Support from neighbors and the rehabilitation program helped them deal with stress and grief.

Community

When an accident happens in a small rural community, it brings home the dangerous nature of farm work. People begin recalling their own "close calls" and remembering friends and family members who have been injured. This period of high awareness is an excellent time to bring people together to discuss accident prevention. During the annual fall 4-H Achievement Days, Mary Fieldson set up an information booth in the exhibit hall and asked for volunteers to plan and implement a farm safety program in the county.

Austin's accident was handled appropriately by the family without EMS intervention. However, others had recently required trained personnel at the site to stabilize the injured person and minimize damage during transport to the primary care hospital. For Mary, her home care visits to farm families reinforced the need for EMS in these remote areas. She met with the county health department, local physicians, and county commissioners to investigate the feasibility of establishing an EMS.

Evaluation

Individual

Individual members of the Connelly family used the home care nurse, PT, and local physician appropriately as evidenced by Austin's successful healing and rehabilitation. Austin returned to work with minimum disability. During a drop-in visit by Mary three months after the accident, Austin treated her to a rousing piano rendition of "Stars and Stripes Forever."

Family

With Mary's guidance, the family wrote down a list of hazards and strategies to improve safety on the farm. Interestingly, one of the items was to wear seat belts in the car and truck. The family installed seat belts in a 40-year-old farm truck still in regular use. They purchased the cellular phone and used it to keep Eliza in touch with Austin and Jim while they were in the field. This has proven so successful that several neighbors have also bought cellular phones.

The family continued to demonstrate good coping skills as Austin progressed in his rehabilitation. Communication between father and son was excellent after the initial concern that Austin would feel like his position as farm manager was being usurped. He became involved with daily decision making as soon as he returned home from the hospital. The family effectively solved the problem of getting the fall work done by requesting the help of friends and neighbors. They borrowed money from the bank to hire a part-time farm hand until Austin could work again.

Community

Mary's information booth at the 4-H Achievement Days attracted the attention of several women from the County Extension Club. As a result of their interest, the club made farm safety education their service project for the following year. Lack of community support halted development of a volunteer emergency medical first-response team.

Levels of Prevention

The following are examples of the three levels of prevention as applied to the individual, family, and community.

Primary Prevention

- Assessment and teaching about farm accident prevention to family
- Initiation of a program of farm safety information at the community level
- Use of a cellular telephone to decrease anxiety about family members' location and well-being

Secondary Prevention

- Infection prevention and pain management of injured hand
- Screening at family and community level for farm hazards (i.e., a component of the overall primary prevention education program)

Tertiary Prevention

- Rehabilitation of Austin to limit disability
- Assessment and counseling to help family and injured individual cope with stress and grief reactions
- Attempted development of an EMS system to facilitate stabilization and safe transport

SUMMARY

This chapter provides an overview of rural and migrant health. People who live in rural areas make up 61 million, or approximately 25%, of the U.S. population. The reader must not assume that all rural people are similar; diversity exists in age, ethnicity, income, education, and geography.

Not all rural residents are disadvantaged. The data show that, in some ways, they are penalized as a whole no matter how diverse the rural population. Health care access and income levels are areas where disadvantages generally exist. Provider shortages, an ineffective health care system, hospital-based and community-based care, and little health promotion and disease prevention services represent a marginal health care network. One half of the poor in the United States live in rural areas. The combination of poor health care access and low-income level results in higher morbidity and mortality rates in rural populations. The high-risk nature of occupations such as farmworkers, miners, and loggers also contribute to disability and death rates. This chapter describes the structural, financial, and personal barriers contributing to poor health care access.

Nurses who work with rural people must assess each aggregate's characteristics. A ranching community in Wyoming will have different needs than a migrant community in Arizona. Demographic information, aggregate morbidity and mortality data, emerging rural nursing theory, knowledge of barriers, and rural health care research are all necessary to plan appropriate upstream community health nursing interventions. Integrating these concepts gives nurses the tools to improve the health of rural people.

LEARNING ACTIVITIES

1. University libraries commonly subscribe to newspapers published within the state. Visit the library and select three to four small town or rural county newspapers. Read them for information about health care activities and concerns related to the health of the individuals, families, and community.
   - Report findings to the class about rural health concerns and activities.
   - Identify one priority problem that could be researched in the community and has relevance to rural community health nursing practice.

2. Select a rural community health nurse (i.e., public health or home care) and conduct an interview in person or by telephone if distance prohibits a face-to-face meeting.
   - Identify what the nurse sees as the pros and cons of rural nursing.
   - If negative aspects of rural nursing are identified, discuss how the nurse deals with them.
   - Ask the nurse to discuss the three highest priority efforts related to his or her rural practice.

3. Choose one of the major causes of morbidity and mortality in migrant populations.
   - On the basis of risk factor and natural history, specify interventions for primary, secondary, and tertiary prevention of this problem.
   - Identify which of these interventions are examples of upstream thinking.

4. Locate a telephone book or community resource directory from a rural community.
   - List and evaluate the resources that are available for prevention, assessment, intervention, and follow-up care for the major cause of mortality and morbidity identified in Learning Activity 3.
   - Would it be necessary to go outside the rural town or county for any of the needed resources? Which ones? Where might they be located?

REFERENCES

American Medical Association: *Trends in the distribution of nonfederal physicians in metropolitan and nonmetropolitan areas for selected years 1980-97: physician characteristics and distribution in the U.S.,* Chicago, Ill, 2000, The Association.

American Nurses Association: *Code for nurses with interpretive statement,* Washington, DC, 1985, The Association.

American Nurses Association: *Rural/frontier nursing: the challenge to grow,* Washington, DC, 1996, The Association.

American Nurses Association: *Scope and standards of parish nursing practice,* Washington, DC, 1998a, The Association.

American Nurses Association: *Standards of clinical nursing practice,* Washington, DC, 1998b, The Association.

American Psychological Association, Office of Rural Health: *Caring for the rural community,* Washington, DC, 1995, The Association.

Amundson B: Myth and reality in the rural health service crisis: facing up to community responsibilities, *J Rural Health* 9:176-187, 1993.

Arnold C: *The new family farm,* Morning Edition, November 29, 1999, National Public Radio.

Baer LD, Smith LM: Nonphysician professionals and rural America. In Ricketts TC, editor: *Rural health in the United States,* Cecil Sheps Center for Health Services Research, University of North Carolina-Chapel Hill, 1999, Oxford University Press.

Battenfield D, Clift E, Graubarth R: Patterns for change: rural women organizing for health. In Bushy A, editor: *Rural nursing,* vol 1, Newbury Park, Calif, 1991, Sage Publications.

Bechtel GA, Davidhizar R: Community health strategies: an innovative education strategy in a migrant farm community, *Nurs Educ* 24(1):23-24, 1999.

Beyers M: The new nursing shortage, *JONA* 1(3):22-24, 1999.

Bigbee J: The uniqueness of rural nursing, *Nurs Clin North Am* 28:131-144, 1993.

Blair A, Zahm SH: Epidemiologic studies of cancer among agricultural populations. In McDuffie H et al, editors: *Agricultural health and safety: workplace, environment, sustainability,* Boca Raton, Fla, 1995, CRC Press.

Braden J, Beauregard K: *Health status and access to care of rural and urban populations,* AHCPR Pub No 94-0031, National Medical Expenditure Survey Research Findings 18, Rockville, Md, February, 1994, PHS.

Buehler J, Lee H: Exploration of home care resources for rural families with cancer, *Cancer Nurs* 15:299-308, 1992.

Bushy A: Rural determinants in family health: considerations for community nurses. In Bushy A, editor: *Rural nursing,* vol 2, Newbury Park, Calif, 1991, Sage Publications.

Bushy A: Rural nursing research priorities, *J Nurs Adm* 22:50-56, 1992.

Bushy A: Rural US women: traditions and transitions affecting health care, *Health Care Women Int* 11:503-513, 1990.

Butterfield P: Thinking upstream: nurturing a conceptual understanding of the societal context of health behavior, *Adv Nurs Sci* 12:1-8, 1990.

Calle EE et al: Demographic predictors of mammography and Pap smear screening in US women, *Am J Public Health* 83:53-60, 1993.

Carrick P: Cultural isolation. In Lee HJ, editor: *Conceptual basis for rural nursing,* New York, 1998, Springer.

Carson D et al: Hardiness as a mediator of the effects of stressors and strains on reported illnesses and relational difficulties in farm and ranch families, *J Rural Health* 9:215-226, 1993.

Centers for Disease Control and Prevention: Guidelines for school health programs to promote lifelong healthy eating, *Mor Mortal Wkly Rep* 45(RR-9):1-42, 1996.

Centers for Disease Control and Prevention: Projected smoking-related deaths among youth: United States, *Mor Mortal Wkly Rep* 45:971-974, 1996.

Centers for Disease Control and Prevention: Tobacco use among high school students: United States, 1997, *Mor Mortal Wkly Rep* 47(12):229-233, 1998a.

Centers for Disease Control and Prevention, National Center for Health Statistics: *Health, United States, 1998 and socioeconomic chartbook,* Hyattsville, Md, 1998b, The Authors.

Centers for Disease Control and Prevention, National Center for Health Statistics: *Health, United States, 1999 with health and aging chartbook,* Hyattsville, Md, 1999, The Authors.

Chafey K, Sullivan T, Shannon A: Self-reliance: characterization of their own autonomy by elderly rural women. In Lee HJ, editor: *Conceptual basis for rural nursing,* New York, 1998, Springer.

Clancy F: Rural rx, *Harrowsmith Country Life* 2:31-37, 1992.

Cook PF: Recent indicators send mixed signals about rural economic performance, *Rural Cond Trends* 9(2):63-66, 1999.

Cotton DJ et al: Effects of grain dust exposure on respiratory symptoms and lung function. In Dosman JA, Cockcroft DW, editors: *Principals of health and safety in agriculture,* Boca Raton, Fla, 1989, CRC Press.

Crandall LA, Coggan JM: Impact of new information technologies on training and continuing education for rural health professionals, *J Rural Health* 10:208-215, 1994.

Davis D, Droes N: Community health nursing in rural and frontier counties, *Nurs Clin North Am* 28:159-169, 1993.

Division of Shortage Designation, Bureau of Primary Health Care: Selected statistics on health professional shortage areas: as of December 31, 1998, Bethesda, Md, 1998, Health Resources and Services Administration, USDHHS.

Dolphin N: Rural health. In Logan B, Dawkins C, editors: *Family centered nursing in the community,* Menlo Park, Calif, 1984, Addison-Wesley.

Dunbar J, Mueller C: Anticipating the 1997 state children's health insurance program: what's current in five rural states? Bethesda, Md, January 1998, The Project HOPE Walsh Center for Rural Health Analysis.

Dunkin J et al: Job satisfaction and retention of rural community health nurses in North Dakota, *J Rural Health* 8:268-275, 1992.

Eggebeen D, Lichter D: Health and well-being among rural Americans: variations across the life course, *J Rural Health* 9:86-98, 1993.

Elison G: Frontier areas: problems for delivery of health care services, *Rural Health Care* 8:1-3, 1986.

Environmental Protection Agency: Recognition and management of pesticide poisonings, ed 4, EPA Pub No 540/9-88-001, Washington, DC, 1989, US Government Printing Office.

Etherton JR et al: Agricultural machine-related deaths, *Am J Public Health* 81:766-768, 1991.

Farmer F, Clark L, Miller M: Consequences of differential residence designations for rural health policy: the case of infant mortality, *J Rural Health* 9:17-26, 1993.

Fasciano MK et al: Preparing rural communities for managed care: lessons learned, *J Rural Health* 15(1):78-86, 1999.

Federal Office of Rural Health Policy: *Facts about rural physicians,* Rockville, Md, 2000, HRSA, USDHHS.

Fuchs VR: *Who shall live? health, economics and social choice,* River Edge, NJ, 1998, World Scientific Publishing.

Furlow L: Crisis in the country: addressing the challenges of rural trauma care, *Texas J Rural Health* 17(1):4-6, 1999.

Gabos S, Fincham S, Berkel J: The interaction between farming occupation and exposure to smoking in squamous carcinomas of the lip. In McDuffie H et al, editors: *Agricultural health and safety: workplace, environment, sustainability,* Boca Raton, Fla, 1995, CRC Press.

Garnett G: Challenges of serving as the director of an emergency medical service in Alaska. In Bushy A, editor: *Rural nursing,* vol 2, Newbury Park, Calif, 1991, Sage Publications.

Ghelfi LM: Rural per capita income grows slightly faster than urban, *Rural Cond Trends* 9(2):63-65, February 1999.

Gordon RL, Gerzoff RB, Richards TB: Determinants of US local health department expenditures, 1992-1993, *Am J Public Health* 87(1):91-95, 1997.

Griffin J: Parish nursing in rural communities. In Solari-Twadell PA, McDermott MA, editors: *Parish nursing: promoting whole person health within faith communities,* Thousand Oaks, Calif, 1999, Sage Publications.

Harriman J: *Facts about the rural population of the United States,* Beltsville, Md, 1999, Rural Information Center Health Service, National Agricultural Library.

Hersh A, Van Hook R: A research agenda for rural health services: a rural health services research agenda, *Health Serv Res* (special issue, conference summary) 23:1053-1064, 1989.

Hicks LL: Access and utilization: special populations-special needs. In Straub LA, Walzer N, editors: *Rural health care: innovation in a changing environment,* Westport, Conn, 1992, Praeger Press.

Human Services in the Rural Transition: *A training packet: Great Plains staff training and development for rural mental health,* Lincoln, Neb, 1989, Department of Psychology.

Ide B: A process model of rural nursing practice, *Texas J Rural Health* 38:30-38, 1992.

Institute of Medicine: *Access to health care in America,* Washington, DC, 1993, National Academy Press.

Institute of Medicine: *Community oriented primary care,* Washington, DC, 1983, National Academy Press.

Institute of Medicine: *The future of public health,* Washington, DC, 1988, National Academy Press.

Johnson RR et al: Characterizing nutrient intakes of children by sociodemographic factors, *Public Health Rep* 109:414-420, 1994.

Jones HP, Brand MK: Providing rehabilitative services in rural communities: report of a conference, *J Rural Health* 11(2):122-127, 1995.

Juhl N et al: Job satisfaction of rural public and home health nurses, *Public Health Nurs* 10(1):42-47, 1993.

Kass BL, Weinick RM, Monheit AC: Racial and ethnic differences in health, 1996, MEPS Chartbook No 2, Pub No 99-0001, Rockville, Md, 1999, Agency for Health Care Policy and Research.

Kohl DM: Cattlewomen's column, *Times Clarion,* Harlowton, Mont, p. 7, April 13, 1995.

Lamphere J et al: *Reforming the health care system state profiles: 1998,* Washington, DC, 1998, AARP Public Policy Institute.

Lassiter P: Rural practice: how do we prepare providers? *J Rural Health* 1:23-26, 1985.

Lee H: Health perceptions of middle, "new middle," and older rural adults, *Fam Community Health* 16:19-27, 1993.

Lee H: *Relationship of ecological rurality to current life events, hardiness, and perceived health status in rural adults,* dissertation, Austin, Tex, 1985, University of Texas-Austin.

Lee H: Relationship of hardiness and current life events to perceived health in rural adults, *Res Nurs Health* 14:351-359, 1991.

Lisnerski DD et al: Demographic and predictive correlates of smokeless tobacco use in elementary school children, *Am J Health Promotion* 5:426-431, 1991.

Long K: Future directions for rural nursing theory. In Lee HJ, editor: *Conceptual basis for rural nursing,* New York, 1998, Springer.

Long K, Boik R: Predicting alcohol use in rural children: a longitudinal study, *Nurs Res* 42:79-86, 1993.

Long K, Weinert C: Rural nursing: developing the theory base, *Sch Inq Nurs Pract* 3:113-127, 1989.

Magilvey J, Congdon J: Circles of care: rural home care for older adults, *Rural Clin Q* 4:3-4, 1994.

Marty ME: Introduction. In Solari-Twadell PA, McDermott, MA, editors: *Parish nursing: promoting whole person health within faith communities,* Thousand Oaks, Calif, 1999, Sage Publications.

Mayer LV: Agricultural change and rural America. In Gahr WE, editor: Rural America: blueprint for tomorrow, *Ann Am Acad Polit Soc Sci* 529:80-91, 1993.

Memmott R: Developing hospice programs in frontier communities. In Bushy A, editor: *Rural nursing,* vol 2, Newbury Park, Calif, 1991, Sage Publications.

Miller M, Farmer F, Clarke L: Rural populations and their health. In Beaulieu J, Berry D, editors: *Rural health services: a management perspective,* Ann Arbor, Mich, 1994, AUPHA Press, Health Administration Press.

Monroe AC, Ricketts TC, Savitts LA: Cancer in rural vs. urban populations: a review, *J Rural Health* 8:212-220, 1992.

Morgan R, Morgan S: *Health care: state rankings,* 1999, Lawrence, Kan, 1999, Morgan Quitno Press.

Morrison HI et al: Mortality among Canadian fruit and vegetable farmers. In McDuffie H et al, editors: *Agricultural health and safety: workplace, environment, sustainability,* Boca Raton, Fla, 1995, CRC Press.

Movassaghi H et al: Nursing supply and characteristics in the nonmetropolitan areas of the United States: findings from the 1988 national sample survey of registered nurses, *J Rural Health* 8:276-282, 1992.

Mueller KJ et al: Building a research agenda: responding to

the needs of community and migrant health centers, *J Rural Health* 14(4):289-294, 1998.

National Center of Farmworker Health: *Facts about farmworker health,* Austin, Tex, 1999, The Center.

National Institute of Mental Health: *Fact sheet rural mental health,* June 1, 1999, The Author, www.nimh.nih.gov/publicat/ruralresfact.cfm.

National Institute of Nursing Research: *Community-based health care: nursing strategies.* A report of the Priority Expert Panel, Pub No 95-3917, October 1995, USDHHS, PHS, NIH.

National Institute for Occupational Safety and Health: *Alert: preventing scalping and other severe injuries from farm machinery,* NIOSH Pub No 94-105, Cincinnati, Ohio, 1994, The Author.

National Institute for Occupational Safety and Health, Division of Safety Research: *National traumatic occupational fatalities surveillance system: in house analyses,* Morgantown, W Va, 1992, The Author.

National Rural Health Association: *A vision for health reform models for America's rural communities,* Issue paper, Kansas City, Mo, February 1998, The Association.

National Rural Health Association: *Managed care as a service delivery model in rural areas,* Issue paper, Kansas City, Mo, April 1995, The Association.

National Rural Health Association: *Mental health in rural America,* Issue paper, Kansas City, Mo, May 1999, The Association.

National Rural Health Association: *Physician recruitment and retention,* Issue paper, Kansas City, Mo, November 1998, The Association.

National Rural Health Association: *Rural and frontier emergency medical services toward the year 2000,* Issue paper, Kansas City, Mo, May 1997, The Association.

National Women's Health Information Center: *Putting prevention into the context and continuum of women's lives,* New Brunswick, NJ, 1999, National Women's Health Resource Center.

Nord M: Rural poverty rate unchanged, *Rural Cond Trends* 9(2):81-84, 1999.

Norris K: *Dakota: a spiritual geography,* New York, 1993, Ticknor and Fields.

Office of Rural Health Policy, Health Resources and Services Administration: *Rural hospital flexibility program,* Rockville, Md, 1999, USDHHS.

Office of Rural Health Policy, Health Resources and Services Administration: *Why is ruralism important? enrolling rural children in CHIP and Medicaid,* The Rural Workgroup of the Interagency Task Force on Children's Health Insurance Outreach, Rockville, Md, 1996, USDHHS.

Office of Technology Assessment, Congress of the United States: *Health care in rural America,* Pub No OTA-H-434, Washington, DC, September 1990, US Government Printing Office.

Office of Technology Assessment, Congress of the United States: *Rural emergency medical service,* Pub No OTA-H-445, Washington, DC, November 1989, US Government Printing Office.

Office of the Inspector General, US Department of Health and Human Services: Medical assistance facilities, Pub No OEI-04-92-00731, Washington, DC, 1993, USDHHS.

Pan S, Straub L, Szigeti E: Factors influencing nurses to practice in rural areas, *Texas J Public Health* 16(2):5-14, 1998.

Pickett G, Hanlon J: *Public health: administration and practice,* St. Louis, 1990, Mosby.

Pickle LW et al: *Atlas of United States mortality,* Hyattsville, Md, 1996, CDC, NCHS.

Posey S: *Dissemination of farm health and safety information,* Poster presented at the Seventh Session of the Rural Nursing Conference, Greely, Colo, 1995, University of Northern Colorado, School of Nursing.

Pullen C: Modern technology brings nursing education into rural students' homes, *Rural Clinician Q* 8(3):3-5, 1998.

Purdy J: The new culture of rural America, *The American Prospect,* pp. 26-31, December 20, 1999.

Reschovsky JD, Cunningham PJ: *CHIPing away at the problem of uninsured children,* Issue Brief No 14, Washington, DC, August 1998, Center for Studying Health System Change.

Ricketts TC: Health care professionals in rural America. In Beaulieu J, Barry D, editors: *Rural health services: a management perspective,* Ann Arbor, Mich, 1994, AUPHS Press, Health Administration Press.

Ricketts TC, Heaphy P: Hospitals in rural America. In Ricketts TC, editor: *Rural health in the United States,* New York, 1999, Cecil Sheps Center for Health Services Research, University of North Carolina-Chapel Hill, Oxford University Press.

Ricketts TC, Johnson-Webb KD, Randolph RK: Populations and places in rural America. In Ricketts TC, editor: *Rural health in the United States,* New York, 1999, Cecil Sheps Center for Health Services Research, University of North Carolina-Chapel Hill, Oxford University Press.

Rivara FP: Fatal and nonfatal farm injuries to children and adolescents in the United States, *Pediatrics* 76:567-573, 1985.

Rogers CC: Socioeconomic circumstances of minority elderly differ from those of white elderly, *Rural Cond Trends* 9(2):35-41, 1999.

Rohrer JE: *Planning for community oriented health systems,* ed 2, Washington, DC, 1999, APHA.

Rural Health News: Domestic violence is a rural health issue, Maine Rural Health Research Center, University of Southern Maine, Portland, Me, *Rural Health News* 5(2):1,9, 1999.

Rural Health News: Ready or not: rural hospitals are changing, *Rural Health News* 4(1):1-3, 1997.

Scharff KE: The distinctive nature and scope of rural nursing practice: philosophical bases. In Lee HJ, editor: *Conceptual basis for rural nursing,* New York, 1998, Springer.

Schenker MA: General health status and epidemiologic considerations in studying migrant and seasonal farmworkers. In McDuffie H et al, editors: *Agricultural health and safety: workplace, environment, sustainability,* Boca Raton, Fla, 1995, CRC Press.

School of Journalism, University of Montana: *A health crisis,* Missoula, Mont, 1993, The Missoulian.

Shreffler MJ: An ecological view of the rural environment: levels of influence on access to health care, *Adv Nurs Sci* 18(4):48-59, 1996.

Shreffler MJ: Culturally sensitive research methods of surveying rural/frontier residents, *West J Nurs Res* 21(3):426-435, 1999.

Shreffler MJ et al: Community decision-making about critical access hospitals: lessons learned from Montana's medical assistance facility program, *J Rural Health* 15(2):180-188, 1999.

Sigma Theta Tau International: *Facts on the nursing shortage,* July 1, 1999, The Author, www.nursingsociety. org/media/facts_nursingshortage.html.

Straub LA, Walzer N: Financing the demand for rural health care. In Straub LA, Walzer N, editors: *Rural health care: innovation in a changing environment,* Westport, Conn, 1992, Praeger Press.

Swanson LL: Minorities represent growing share of tomorrow's work force, *Rural Cond Trends* 9(2):1-5, 1999.

Toscano GA, Windau JA: Profile of fatal work injuries in 1996, *Compensation Working Conditions* Spring:37-44, 1998.

Turner T, Gunn I: Issues in rural health nursing. In Bushy A, editor: *Rural nursing,* vol 2, Newbury Park, Calif, 1992, Sage Publications.

Turnock B et al: Local health department effectiveness in addressing the core function of public health, *Public Health Rep* 109:653-658, 1994.

US Bureau of the Census: *Census of population,* Washington, DC, 1990, Department of Congress.

US Bureau of the Census: *Health insurance coverage: 1999-highlights,* Washington, DC, March 2000, The Bureau.

US Department of Labor, Bureau of Labor Statistics: *Occupational injuries and illnesses in the US by industries,* Bulletin No 2379, Washington, DC, 1989, US Government Printing Office.

US Department of Health and Human Services: *Healthy people 2000: national health promotion and disease prevention objectives,* Washington, DC, 1991, PHS.

US Department of Health and Human Services, National Center for Health Research: *Healthy people 2000 review 1998-99,* Hyattsville. Md, 1999, PHS.

US Department of Health and Human Services, Office of Disease Prevention and Health Promotion: Putting prevention into the context and continuum of women's lives, *Prev Rep* 12(3):1-4, 1997.

US Department of Health and Human Services, Public Health Service: *Healthy people 2010: volume I understanding and improving health,* Washington, DC, 2000, PHS.

Van Hightower NR, Gorton J: A predictive model of domestic violence among Latina farmworkers, *Texas J Rural Health* 17(4):45-56, 1999.

Van Hook R: Foreword. In Straub L, Walzer N, editors: *Rural health care: innovation in a changing environment,* Westport, Conn, 1992, Praeger Press.

Voelker R: Does managed care fit for rural America? *Adv RWJ Newsletter,* Princeton, NJ, Issue 4, 1998.

Wagenfield MO: Mental health and rural America: a decade review, *J Rural Health* 6:507-522, 1990.

Warren CP: Overview of respiratory health risks in agriculture.In Dosman JA, Cockcroft DW, editors: *Principals of health and safety in agriculture,* Boca Raton, Fla, 1989, CRC Press.

Weinert C, Burman M: Rural health and health seeking behaviors. In Fitzpatrick JJ, Stevenson JS, editors: *Annual review of nursing research,* vol 12, New York, 1994, Springer.

Weinert C, Long KA: Rural families and health care: refining the knowledge base, *J Marriage Fam Rev* 15:57-75, 1990.

Weinert C, Long KA: Understanding the health care needs of rural families, *Fam Relations* 36:450-455, 1987.

Wilk VA: Reducing health risks: farmworker women working together. In McDuffie H et al, editors: *Agricultural health and safety: workplace, environment, sustainability,* Boca Raton, Fla, 1995, CRC Press.

Wylie JL, Solari-Twadell PA: Health and the congregation. In Solari-Twadell PA, McDermott MA, editors: *Parish nursing: promoting whole person health within faith communities,* Thousand Oaks, Calif, 1999, Sage Publications.

Zahm SH, Blair A: Cancer among migrant and seasonal farmworkers: an epidemiologic review and research agenda, *Am J Ind Med* 24:753-766, 1993.

Special Needs in Community Mental Health

22 Mental Health

23 Violence in the Community

24 Substance Abuse

22

Mental Health

Jill Powell

OBJECTIVES

OBJECTIVES

Upon completion of this chapter, the reader will be able to do the following:

1. Describe the role of mental health nurses in the community.
2. Discuss the influence of deinstitutionalization on mental health aggregates.
3. Discuss the influence of managed care on selected aggregates.
4. Identify four elements of comprehensive community mental health assessment.

KEY TERMS

Benjamin Rush
Community Mental Health Act
deinstitutionalization
Dorthea Dix
marginalization
Mental Health Equitable Treatment Act
mental illness
Program of Assertive Community Treatment (PACT)

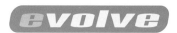

Community health nurses will continue to face the challenge of providing mental health services to an increasing number of clients with fewer resources. Historically, people with mental illness have been treated in acute care settings and are now living in the community with little or no access to mental health services (National Advisory Mental Health Council [NAMHC], 1998). Across the nation, acute care settings have downsized, private insurance reimburses fewer mental health services, and waiting lists in publicly funded mental health centers grow longer. This state of affairs is a result of the following four factors: decreased state and federal funding, managed care, discriminate private insurance coverage, and the influence of deinstitutionalization (Torrey, 1997). The purpose of this chapter is to illuminate critical issues that affect the mental health of communities and explore the potential influence that nurses have on these issues. This chapter explores these factors and their environmental, biological, social, and political dynamics.

Words used to describe people with **mental illness** have been a source of social and political debate, particularly since the 1990s. Historically, words and labels assigned to people with mental illness have been a source of discrimination and stigma (Corrigan, 1999). For example, *crazy, insane,* and *deranged* conjure images of violence, fear, and intellectual inadequacy. The stigma and discrimination many people diagnosed with mental illness experience are unfounded and based on faulty assumptions and misinformation (Roman, 1981). People diagnosed with mental illness are neighbors, colleagues, and family members. Most people diagnosed with mental illness are productive members of every community and they all have meaningful lives. Words have been harmful to people with mental illness; therefore they must be chosen carefully. Throughout this chapter, the concepts of mental health and mental illness are used frequently. Mental illness is used to describe a person with a diagnosed neurobiological brain disorder (NBD). Mental illness and NBDs are used interchangeably in this chapter. Mental health describes the absence of NBDs or the state that occurs when the symptoms of NBDs are controlled and do not interfere with an individual's life experience.

OVERVIEW AND HISTORY OF COMMUNITY MENTAL HEALTH

Since recorded history, communities have been both formally and informally caring for members with mental illness. The evolution of community mental health is discussed in the following five phases: Age of Confinement, mental health reform, medicalization of mental illness, deinstitutionalization, and Decade of the Brain. Identification of people with mental illness in communities has generally been based on the ability to characterize individual behavior or personality as different from the social norm.

Age of Confinement

During the Age of Confinement, individuals who behaved in ways inconsistent with social norms were labeled "mad," separated from their communities, and placed in the custodial care of the state. Poverty, homelessness, alcoholism, seizure disorders, and mental illness were all illnesses or life conditions that created rationale for placement in asylums. Conditions in the early asylums were often deplorable. Individuals residing in these asylums were often restrained, whipped, ill fed, unwashed, and treated with bloodletting, purgatives, and other "curative" therapies. In addition, madness was attributed to idleness; therefore treatment included forced labor. The early asylums became places of harborage and indentured servitude for individuals labeled with mental illness. Those confined were commonly required to bear the labor of public works. The same places that confined the mentally ill served as places of incarceration for those who committed crimes against the state (Foucault, 1965; Hunter, 1963).

Mental Health Reform

By the end of the eighteenth century, inhumane conditions and treatment in houses of confinement gained the attention of philanthropists and humanists. In 1796, an English Quaker merchant family, headed by William and Samuel Tuke, opened the York retreat in England to demonstrate that humane treatment could abate mental illness. Pinel and Tuke sought to liberate individuals with mental illness from confinement and create a milieu of human kindness and moral treatment. Humanistic person-centered principles replaced indentured servitude and confinement (Grob, 1991).

In the middle of the nineteenth century, **Dorthea Dix** took up the cause of reform in the United States. Aided by changed attitudes toward suffering and social welfare, she gained American hospital and prison reform. She established Saint Elizabeth's Hospital, a federal hospital, in 1885 and eventually 32 state mental hospitals (Grob, 1983).

Medicalization of Mental Illness

After treatment reform in the middle to late 1800s, societies convened to govern conduct at asylums. The American Society of Superintendents of Mental Institutions of the Insane became the American-Medico-Psychological Association in the late 1800s. Its membership included neurologists, psychologists, and asylum-trained psychiatrists and nurses. The association of psychiatry with neurology proved to be a seminal event in the historical development of psychiatry and community mental health. Neurologists had publicly chastised psychiatry as an inexact science without empirically based standards for which other branches of medicine were held accountable. In response, psychiatrists attempted to formulate associations between insanity and biological or organic causes. **Benjamin Rush**, an American physician, proposed the first physiologic etiology of insanity in 1835. Rush believed the cause of insanity was positioned primarily in the vessels of the brain. Rush theoretically linked mental illness to other physical ailments involving arterial abnormalities (Grob, 1983). In 1845, Griesinger published *Pathology and Therapy of Mental Diseases,* which established psychiatry as a medical specialty specifically concerned with diseases of the brain (Grob, 1983). During the late 1800s, insanity was also linked to the ingestion of intoxicating substances, trauma to the brain, and neuritis. Scientific and political respectability for psychiatry depended on a biomedical perspective.

Numerous somatic treatments for mental illness followed biomedical theories. Those treatments included lobotomy, electroconvulsive therapy (ECT), insulin shock therapy, and hydrotherapy (Deutsch, 1949). As discussed by Grob (1983), Moniz, a Portuguese neurologist and neurosurgeon, introduced prefrontal lobotomy in 1935 for the treatment of mental illness. Moniz assumed that the synapse was the organic foundation of thought; therefore normal psychic thought was dependent upon proper functioning of the synapse and mental disorders were a result of synaptic derangement. Moniz believed it was necessary to alter these synaptic paths to modify corresponding ideas and force thought into different channels. Insulin shock therapy, hydrotherapy, and ECT were thought to have the same organic outcome. Moniz won the Nobel Prize in 1949 for the therapeutic use of prefrontal lobotomy (Grob, 1994). It was not until the early 1950s that the antipsychotic medication thorazine was discovered to alleviate some of schizophrenia's most troubling symptoms of mental illness in a more humane fashion (Deutsch, 1949; Grob, 1991).

Community Mental Health and Deinstitutionalization

Treatment reform was based largely on the premise that people were not bad or morally flawed, but sick and in need of treatment. The Great Depression of the 1930s continued to force the issue of treatment reform based primarily on financial concerns. States could no longer afford the vast expense of the custodial and institutional care for people diagnosed with mental illness. Caregivers, families, and communities became viable alternatives to costly institutional care. The **Community Mental Health Act** of 1963 mandated **deinstitutionalization** and produced a mass exodus of individuals from institutions across the nation. Often after many years of institutionalization, patients returned to families and communities who were ill prepared to care for them. In addition, alternative community mental health resources were not established when deinstitutionalization occurred (Grob, 1994). With ill-prepared families and minimal community services, many individuals with mental illness found themselves homeless, in shelters, or in prisons or jails. In the mid1970s, the federal government acknowledged the relative inadequacies of the Community Mental Health Act and made recommendations to link community mental health services with informal community support services. The 1980s marked the beginning of major financial health care reform and funding and services began to dwindle (NAMHC, 1993; Torrey, 1997).

The Community Mental Health Act and subsequent legislation improved environmental conditions in institutions, but the medical treatment for mental illness remained relatively unchanged since the accidental discovery of thorazine in 1952. A physician in a military hospital prescribed thorazine for nausea to a patient who was also hearing voices. After the administration of thorazine, the voices dissipated. Thorazine was reclassified as an antipsychotic medication and used extensively for decades to treat individuals diagnosed with mental illnesses such as schizophrenia (Grob, 1994).

Decade of the Brain

The development of neuroimaging in the 1980s provided new data on the anatomical and neurochemical nature of the brain (Buchsbaum, 1982). These data rendered the foundation for developing pharmacological agents to treat mental illness that had a mechanism of action different from thorazine. Given the advances in technology, the NAMHC recommended that the Decade of the Brain be initiated for the 10 years preceding the year 2000 (USDHHS, 1999c). The annual research budget of the NIMH increased and much of the funding was allocated to research aimed at uncovering the biomedical etiology of schizophrenia and continuing to develop new pharmaceuticals. At the close of the Decade of the Brain, several new psychiatric medications were developed that have vastly improved the QOL for those diagnosed with mental illness (Barr, 1994; DeLisi, 1992; Kandel, 1998).

PREVALENCE AND INCIDENCE OF MENTAL ILLNESS IN THE UNITED STATES

The influence of untreated mental illness on communities and their social structure has been vastly understated. Mental illness accounts for 15.4% of the disease burden in global market economies, which is second only to all forms of cardiac disease. In the United States, the most recent estimated cost of mental illness was $148 billion (Murray, 1996). This section discusses mental illnesses with a neurobiological origin (i.e., depression, bipolar affective disorder, schizophrenia, and anxiety disorders).

Depression is the most frequently diagnosed mental illness in the United States. Approximately 19 million adults will become depressed in any given year. In developed nations, depression is the leading cause of disability among people aged five years or older. In addition, depression is often a complication of serious physical disorders such as heart attack, stroke, diabetes, and cancer. Women are affected by depression at two times the rate of men (Murray, 1996; NIMH, 1998).

Bipolar affective disorder of manic-depressive illness affects men and women equally. Bipolar affective disorder affects about 1% (2.3 million) of the population in the United States. Approximately 20% of individuals with bipolar affective disorder end their life by suicide.

Schizophrenia affects more than two million American adults. Schizophrenia is the most costly mental illness and accounts for $32.5 billion of the GNP annually. No gender difference is present in the prevalence of schizophrenia. Men tend to be affected in their late teens, whereas symptoms of schizophrenia rarely appear in women until their twenties or early thirties. Schizophrenia is a deadly illness. Approximately 10% of all individuals diagnosed with schizophrenia commit suicide.

In the United States, anxiety disorders affect another 16 million adults with a diagnosed mental illness. In 1990, anxiety disorders accounted for $46.6 billion of the GNP. Anxiety disorders include obsessive-compulsive disorder, posttraumatic stress disorder, social phobias, and generalized anxiety disorder.

Undoubtedly, the greatest cost of mental illness in the United States is measured in human lives. Almost all people who commit suicide have a diagnosable mental illness (i.e., depression is most common). In 1996, the third leading cause of death among those aged 15 to 24 was suicide. In any given year, approximately 31,000 people will die as a result of suicide in the United States (Murray, 1996).

HEALTHY PEOPLE 2010 AND MENTAL HEALTH

Healthy People 2010 is the third generation of health initiatives aimed at improving the overall QOL and longevity of individuals and communities. *Healthy People 2010* identified indicators of a healthy community. These indicators include but are not limited to preventable deaths, poverty, physical activity, substance abuse, and health care access. The following are three select examples of community mental health indicators consistent with *Healthy People 2010*: suicide reduction, increased accessibility to mental health care in communities, and implementation of assertive community mental health treatment.

Suicide Reduction

In 1999, the USDHHS and the Office of the Surgeon General identified suicide as a primary public health problem of the new millennium. Consistent with the select aims of *Healthy People 2010,* the Surgeon General's Call to Action attempts to "put into place national strategies to prevent the loss of life and the suffering suicide causes" (USDHHS, 1999b, p. 7) through increased public awareness, expansion of mental health services, and continuation of support of research aimed at understanding and preventing suicide in the United States.

Risk and protective factors are identified in relation to suicide prevention. Risk factors include previous suicide attempts, mental illness, substance abuse, and barriers to accessing mental health treatment. Protective factors may decrease the risk of suicide and include appropriate mental health care, easy access to treatment, community support, and continuing support from medical and mental health care providers.

Increased Accessibility of Mental Health Services

The accessibility of mental health service is pivotal in promoting and maintaining the health of aggregates. In the age of financial health care reform, privatization of mental health services, and managed care; community mental services have been deemed the "second wave of deinstitutionalization" (Pickens, 1998). Decreased funding for services, managed care limitations on mental health coverage, and the inequality of coverage by the insurance industry have caused downsizing or forced closure in the traditional places of treatment such as community mental health and community hospitals. In most cases, the decrease in acute care services has not been balanced by an increase in community mental health services (USDHHS, 1999b). Consequently, the accessibility to community mental health services has become an issue of significant concern. In addition, the symptoms of mental illness often interfere with an individual's ability to access services. Alterations in thoughts and perceptions, anxiety, and decreased energy are all common symptoms of mental illness and all interfere with negotiating the complex systems that currently surround mental health service provision (USDHHS, 1999b).

Implementation of Assertive Mental Health Care

The National Alliance for the Mentally Ill (NAMI) recently released the Omnibus Mental Illness Recovery Act (ORA) as an "initiative to expand and improve public mental health systems" (Ross, 1999, p. 5). Traditionally, clinical contacts or episodes of care measure the use of mental health services. NAMI has taken the position that measuring episodes of care cannot be "directly related to the number of persons served and thus it becomes impossible to discern if those with the most serious mental illness are those receiving services" (Ross, 1999). The ORA is aimed at linking otherwise fragmented mental health services. The ORA includes seven components (Box 22-1) and is based on the following principles: consumer and family participation in treatment, equitable health care coverage for mental illnesses, and assertive community mental health treatment (Ross, 1999).

BOX 22-1

Omnibus Mental Illness Recovery Act

1. Enactment of equitable health care coverage, including parity for mental illness
2. Access to new medication by allowing medically necessary medication despite formulary restrictions and ensuring that prescribing physicians practice evidence-based medicine
3. Expansion of assertive community treatment programs, including the evidence-based PACT model
4. Creation of work incentives for people with severe mental illness by allowing health insurance coverage for people formerly on income assistance who obtain meaningful employment
5. Reductions in life-threatening and harmful actions by significantly reducing the use of restraint and seclusion and limiting such use to only emergency safety situations
6. Reduction in the criminalization of mental illness through a multipronged strategy of activities, including jail diversion programs
7. Increase in access to permanent, safe, and affordable housing with appropriate community-based services

From Ross EC: NAMI campaign, policy team launch Omnibus Mental Illness Recovery Act, *NAMI Advocate* 20(4):1, 1999.

The **Program of Assertive Community Treatment** (PACT) (Box 22-2), in existence since the late 1960s, has become the exemplar of community mental health treatment models. The PACT program moves the traditional 24-hour treatment model of acute care settings into the community and serves people with mental illness in a highly individualized fashion (Becker, 1999; McGrew, 1995; Solden, 1999). The PACT model provides around-the-clock supportive therapy, mobile crisis intervention, psychiatric medications, hospitalization, education, and skill teaching for consumers and their families. PACT brings service to the consumer and is considered the model of effective community mental health treatment of the future. Currently only six states have statewide PACT programs and 19 have at least one pilot project. A NAMI PACT initiative proposes that all states have assertive community treatment by 2002 (Ross, 1999).

BOX 22-2

Key Features of the Program of Assertive Community Treatment

- Psychopharmacological treatment
- Individual supportive therapy
- Mobile crisis intervention
- Hospitalization
- Substance abuse treatment
- Behaviorally-oriented skill teaching
- Supported employment
- Support for resuming education
- Collaboration with families and assistance to clients with children
- Direct support to help clients obtain legal and advocacy services

FACTORS INFLUENCING THE MENTAL HEALTH OF AGGREGATES

Biological Factors

The explosion of research since 1990 indicates that the biological foundation of mental illness involves complex and evolving concepts. Although several key studies have led to fundamental changes in the way mental illness is comprehended, science has yet to explain its biological basis. Contemporary views on the biological etiology of mental illness can be grouped into the following three areas: genetic factors, neurotransmitters, and structural brain abnormalities (Weinberger, 1997).

Genetic Factors

The success of the Human Genome Project in mapping the structure of deoxyribonucleic acid (DNA) markers has made it possible to examine human genes to investigate sites potentially linked to mental illness. For example, several gene linkage studies have been performed with families that have a high prevalence of schizophrenia (Wienberger, 1997).

Other studies show variation associated with mental illness in genes at specific neurotransmitter receptor sites in the brain. The actual mechanism associated with variations and its contribution to mental illness is unknown (Barron, 1996). A key question remaining in the search for a genetic basis for mental illness is how genes that convey greater susceptibility

for mental illness actually produce specific symptoms. A synthesis of the genetic research on NBDs suggests that multiple genes convey a small amount of genetic susceptibility. The role of genetics in schizophrenia remains poorly understood (Weinberger, 1997).

Neurotransmitters

Before the advent of neuroimaging, the role of amino acids and neurotransmitters in NBDs was poorly understood (Henn, 1982). Recently, several neurotransmitters and amino acids have been implicated in NBDs. For example, the dopamine hypothesis suggests that schizophrenia is associated with an excess of dopamine neuronal activity in the brain. This conclusion is based on research demonstrating that medications that decrease dopamine activity have antipsychotic effects and medications that increase dopamine activity cause psychotic symptoms (Weinberger, 1997).

Several theories about NBDs emphasize the primary role of amino acid neurotransmitters. The principal neurotransmitters implicated in NBDs are glutamate and gamma-aminobutyric acid (GABA) (Olney, 1995; Taber, 1996; Toru, 1994; Tsai, 1995).

Structural Brain Abnormalities

In the Decade of the Brain, identifying abnormalities in brain development as a factor in NBDs became an increasingly popular topic for research. Evidence indicates that structural brain abnormalities seem to occur more often in those with NBDs. An increase in ventricular spaces and cortical volume deficits in the cerebral cortex are associated with NBDs. Research concerning the association with general structural abnormalities in schizophrenia suggests a decrease in brain volume in the left temporal and right frontal regions of the brain (Lim, 1996; Marsh, 1994).

Although many theories of the etiology of NBDs have been developed from research during the Decade of the Brain, many have not been replicated. Information from studies to date is insufficient to establish a definitive biological NBD. Many scholars have concluded that NBDs are multifactoral, complex physiological phenomena and that one or more of the current theories may play a role (Davis, 1991; Weinberger, 1997).

Social Factors

Throughout history, the symptoms of NBDs have been perceived as permanent, dangerous, frightening, and shameful. People diagnosed with an NBD have been described as lazy, idle, weak, immoral, irrational, and feigning illness. Based on these characterizations and assumptions, many people diagnosed with a mental illness have experienced widespread social rejection (Durant and Durant, 1961; Hanson, 1998; Holiday, 1996). People with an NBD experience stigmas and discrimination. In this chapter, the concept of **marginalization** (Hall, Stevens, and Meleis, 1994) is used as the framework to discuss the response of the dominant social groups to individuals with mental illness. Marginalization is the process of social and political peripheralization of individuals or groups based on real or perceived differences from the majority. Marginalization makes access to the goods and services of a community more difficult (Hall, Stevens, and Meleis, 1994).

Although mental illness is assumed to have a biological basis, it is also a complex and abstract cultural construct. The myths associated with mental illness have historical, political, economic, and social roots. Individuals diagnosed with mental illnesses are shunned, less likely to be hired, and less likely to be accepted as neighbors (McCrae, 1996). To combat marginalization, many myths must be dispelled. When individuals have personal experience with an individual with mental illness, fear, discrimination, and stigmas are decreased (Penn, 1994). Attempts to reduce marginalization through education alone have not been successful, but one recent study demonstrated that education was more beneficial if it directly targeted the association between dangerousness and mental illness (Penn and Martin, 1998).

When episodes of violence are associated with NBDs, they are generally highly publicized, which furthers the marginalization of people with NBDs. A survey of literature (Torrey, 1999a) about the relationship between violence and mental illness dispels myths about mental illness and provides the following conclusions: individuals with severe NBD *who are taking* medication are not more dangerous than the general population and individuals with severe NBD who *are not taking* medication are more dangerous than the general population (Penn and Martin, 1998; Steadman, 1998). These findings again point to the ultimate importance of adequate community treatment for people with severe NBDs.

During the time of deinstitutionalization, many people with NBDs left state institutions to live in communities that were ill prepared to provide treatment. Consequently, many individuals with NBDs are homeless, incarcerated, or living in residential boarding homes. With the ongoing decrease in community services, this trend continues, leaving people with mental illness vulnerable to victimization. In the Western world, a disproportionate number of people with NBDs are physically and/or sexually assaulted. A single element links violence by and against people with NBDs (i.e., the failure or inability to receive treatment).

Political Factors

Primary in the politics of mental illness is parity in health care coverage. *Parity* refers to equal access to health care for physical and mental illnesses. For example, mental and physical illness affecting the same physiological symptoms is often treated with disparity.

Although both illnesses affect the same neurotransmitter (i.e., dopamine), a person diagnosed with Parkinson's disease might have full insurance coverage and a person diagnosed with schizophrenia might have no coverage (NIMH, 1998).

On April 13, 1999, legislation was introduced to Congress to end disparity in health care coverage. The **Mental Health Equitable Treatment Act** of 1999 (SB 796) would require equal health care benefits for individuals diagnosed with severe NBDs. Explicit in this legislation is a prohibition on limits on lifetime and annual mental health benefits, inpatient hospital stays, outpatient visits, and inequitable copayments. Cost analysis of mental health parity indicates an increase of less than 1% of total health care cost annually (National Mental Health Council, 1988; NIMH, 1998). Although parity in mental health coverage would increase accessibility of services, it does not ensure increased use of mental health services. As indicated in the recent *Surgeon General's Report on Mental Health* (USDHHS, 1999c), an estimated 50% of people experiencing NBDs do not seek treatment because a stigma is attached.

In addition to disparity in mental health care coverage, a recent audit of the NIMH found that only 36% of the NIMH's annual research budget was allocated to study about severe mental illness (Table 22-1). Only 11.9% of NIMH-funded research addresses clinical or treatment issues for severe mental illness, whereas 14.2% of the total budget funded research about HIV illness and another

TABLE 22-1

National Institute for Mental Health Funding, Fiscal Year 1997

Disease Category	Number of Research Grants Targeting Disease	Percentage of Total NIMH Research Grants (n=2029)	Total Amount of Funds (Millions of Dollars) Going to Grants Targeting that Disease	Percentage of NIMH Research Grant Funds (Total $422.5 Million)
Schizophrenia	235	11.6	57.1	13.5
Bipolar disorder	71	3.5	21.9	5.2
Major depression	279	13.8	76.9	18.2
Obsessive-compulsive disorder	30	1.5	8.8	2.1
Panic disorder	58	2.9	15.4	3.6

From Torrey EF: *The failure of the National Institute of Mental Health to do sufficient research on severe mental illness,* 1999b, NAMI, www.NAMI.org/pressroom/failsummary.html.

3.6% funded research about Alzheimer's disease (Torrey, 1999b).

ROLE OF THE COMMUNITY MENTAL HEALTH NURSE

During and shortly after deinstitutionalization, mental health service could be accessed through the following distinct points of contact: inpatient facilities, community mental health centers, and community support programs. Community mental health services have become more complex. Services are currently provided in diverse settings that often are not in direct communication with one another (USDHHS, 1999c).

To understand the mental health needs of an aggregate, nurses must consider several divergent factors that affect the mental health of aggregates such as genetic inheritance, life experience, and temperament. In addition, mental health and mental illness are not static concepts. Mental health is subject to multiple influences. Consequently, mental illness and mental health must also be assessed in the context of social environments that include family, community, peer reference groups, and physical and cultural surroundings. Formal and informal sources of community mental health support are equally important. Consumers and their families have been a valuable and often overlooked community resource. For example, NAMI's Family-to-Family Education Program includes peer support and intensive educational programs about mental illness offered by the families of consumers to the families of consumers (Ross, 1999).

Community mental health nursing roles can be conceptualized as two-dimensional (e.g., educator and activist or practitioner and coordinator). As an educator and activist, the community mental health nurse is charged with improving public awareness of effective treatments and existing community resources. Community mental health nurses as educators and activists can dispel myths and provide accurate information about mental illness. In addition, the educator and activist responsibility includes influencing policy and legislation to empower and advocate for the rights of those with mental illness.

As practitioner and coordinator, the nurse works directly with individuals, groups, and families. Unlike the acute care setting, the community mental health environment is generally the consumer's home. Besides intervening to assist consumers in controlling or alleviating the symptoms of mental illness, the practitioner and coordinator also helps the consumer "navigate" within the segmented web of agencies and other service providers. Community mental health nurses do not merely take action to solve an immediate problem. They plan and intervene within parameters that ensure safety, continuity, and quality of care for consumers. Therefore the practitioner and coordinator role requires skills in anticipating and evaluating the actions of other providers and communicating with consumers, families, rehabilitation services, and government or social agencies.

Within this aspect of community mental health nursing, individual-, family-, and community-level crises are anticipated, prevented, and failing these, contained. For example, as practitioner and coordinator, nurses might organize people taking psychotropic medications to share experiences about interacting with a psychiatrist. Consumers might understand all of their options and maximize the benefits of medications. This is proactive in preventing crises resultant from sudden self-discontinuation of medication. In the practitioner and coordinator role, community mental health nurses work toward matching consumers and families with culturally appropriate and sensitive providers to achieve the "best fit."

RESEARCH IN MENTAL HEALTH

Kane, DiMartino, and Jimenez explored the differences between two short-term multifamily group intervention programs for relatives of hospitalized chronic schizophrenics in a nonequivalent comparison group design. A psychoeducational intervention consisted of interactive instructional activities and the support group intervention consisted of nonstructured discussions. The analysis of covariance on adjusted posttest means indicated a differential treatment effect for depression and satisfaction for the psychoeducational groups. The authors' findings suggest that the process of a support group may not be compatible with a short time frame.

From DiMartino E, Jimenez M: A comparison of short-term psychoeducational and support groups for relatives coping with chronic schizophrenia, *Arch Psychiatr Nurs* 4:343, 1990.

Taft and Barkin explored the use and misuse of psychotropic drugs in care for patients with Alzheimer's disease. The authors noted that family caregivers often report feelings of guilt associated with administering psychotropic drugs and may attribute the use of these to their own inability to cope. The role of the nurse is to establish and monitor therapeutic goals, assess the incidence and severity of predictable side effects, and provide a safe, supportive environment that reduces the need for pharmacologic interventions.

From Taft LB, Barkin RL: Drug abuse: use and misuse of psychotropic drugs in Alzheimer's care, *J Gerontol Nurs* 16:4, 1990.

CASE STUDY

APPLICATION OF THE NURSING PROCESS

The nursing process is used uniquely in community mental health nursing. Assessment is a synthesis of diverse information that is used to understand the particular mental health needs of individuals or aggregates. Diagnosis uses the synthesized information to identify points for intervention. Interventions are actions developed mutually with consumers, families, or communities. Evaluation is the process of reflecting on the outcome of interventions.

At 9:02 AM on April 19, 1995, a bomb destroyed the Alfred P. Murrah Federal Building in Oklahoma City, Oklahoma. Multiple lives were lost, survivors of the explosion were traumatized, and significant others were plunged into a state of grieving. The blast was felt across the state. The personal accounts of more than 1000 survivors, rescuers, nursing staff members, medical staff members, counselors, volunteers, and children have been shared. The residual effects of this tragedy remain in the hearts and minds of those left behind. Nursing played an important role during the disaster relief efforts. On the day of the bombing, nurses assisted in rescue efforts by caring for the injured and dying. Nurses set up on-site triage units, administered tetanus shots to rescue workers, provided mental health counseling, served as supplemental hospital staff for emergency care, provided support to families,

Continued

assisted temporarily displaced homeless people, and cared for victims' significant others and fellow disaster workers.

When examining this case, the nurse should consider the following questions related to the nursing process:

- What community mental health services are available to care for victims and families?
- How might resources be mobilized?

- What is the cultural expectation for expression of grief?
- Does the community embrace or reject difference?
- Have other crises occurred? How did the community respond?
- What are the short- and long-term points of intervention?
- How will you measure "success" at points of intervention?

SUMMARY

The depiction of community mental health nursing is a "slice in time" in an ever-changing health care environment. In the next millennium, conditions for those with mental illness may drastically improve, although exploration of historical factors in this chapter evidences long-standing stigmatization and marginalization, especially of those with what are now considered "major mental illnesses." The Decade of the Brain is coming to a close and signs of hope exist in the pharmacological realm. Nevertheless, medication has always proved to be only a partial means of addressing a whole person with a mental illness. Hopefully, the framework for community mental health nursing presented in this chapter will prove useful in improving the lives of individuals, families, aggregates, and communities regardless of how the future unfolds.

LEARNING ACTIVITIES

1. Reflect on personal experience interacting with individuals with mental illness. What thoughts or feelings did this experience produce?
2. Locate the NAMI chapter in the community. What services do they offer? How might those services be helpful in the community mental health nursing role?
3. List five ways to act as an educator and activist for mental health issues in the community.

REFERENCES

Barr CL: Linkage studies of susceptibility locus in the autosomal region, *Schizophr Bull* 20:277, 1994.

Barron M: Linkage results in schizophrenia, *Am J Med Genet* 67:121, 1996.

Becker RF: Employment outcomes for clients with severe mental illness in a PACT model replication program, *Psychiatr Serv* 50(1):104, 1999.

Buchsbaum MS, Haier RJ: Functional and anatomical brain imaging, *Schizophr Bull* 14:383, 1982.

Corrigan PW, Penn DL: Lessons from social psychology on discrediting psychiatric stigma, *Am Psychol* 54:765, 1999.

Davis KL: Dopamine in schizophrenia: a review and reconceptualization, *Am J Psychiatry* 149:1474, 1991.

DeLisi JK: Left ventricular enlargement associated with diagnostic outcome in schizophrenia, *Biologic Psychiatry* 32:199, 1992.

Deutsch A: *The mentally ill in America: a history of their care and treatment from colonial times,* New York, 1949, Columbia University Press.

DiMartino E, Jimenez M: A comparison of short-term psychoeducational and support groups for relatives coping with chronic schizophrenia, *Arch Psychiatr Nurs* 4:343, 1990.

Durant W, Durant A: *The story of civilization: part VII. the age of reason begins,* New York, 1961, Simon and Schuster.

Foucault: *Madness and civilization,* New York, 1965, Random House.

Grob GN: *From asylum to community: mental health policy in modern America,* Princeton, NJ, 1991, Princeton University Press.

Grob GN: *Mental illness and American society, 1875-1940,* Princeton, NJ, 1983, Princeton University Press.

Grob GN: *The mad among us: a history of the care of America's mentally ill,* New York, 1994, Free Press.

Hall JM, Stevens PE, Meleis AI: Marginalization: a guiding concept for valuing diversity in nursing knowledge development, *Adv Nurs Sci* 13(3):16, 1994.

Hanson KW: Public opinion and the parity debate: lessons from the survey literature, *Psychiatr Serv* 49:1059, 1998.

Henn F: Dopamine: a role in psychosis or schizophrenia. In Henn F, Nasrallah AH, editors: *Schizophrenia as a brain disease,* New York, 1982, Oxford.

Holiday SG: *Schizophrenia: breaking down the barriers,* Manchester, England, 1996, Wiley.

Hunter RA: *Three hundred years of psychiatry: 1535-1800,* London, 1963, Oxford University Press.

Kandel ER: A new intellectual framework for psychiatry, *Am J Psychiatry* 155:457, 1998.

Lim KO: Gray matter volume deficits in young onset schizophrenia, *Biologic Psychiatry* 40:4, 1996.

Marsh L: Medial temporal lobe structures in schizophrenia: relationship of size to duration of illness, *Schizophr Res* 11:25, 1994.

McCrae CN: *Stereotypes and stereotyping,* New York, 1996, Guilford Press.

McGrew JH: Critical ingredients of assertive community treatment: judgments of the experts, *J Ment Health Adm* 223(2):13, 1995.

Murray CL: *The global burden of disease,* Cambridge, Mass, 1996, Harvard University Press.

National Advisory Mental Health Council: Health care reform for Americans with severe mental illnesses, *Am J Psychiatry* 150:1447, 1993.

National Advisory Mental Health Council: *Parity in financing mental health services,* Washington, DC, 1998, US Government Printing Office.

National Institute for Mental Health: *Parity: the equivalence of mental illness with general medical illness,* Washington, DC, 1998, US Government Printing Office.

National Mental Health Council Report to Congress on the Decade of the Brain: *Approaching the 21st century: opportunities for NIMH neuroscience research,* USDHHS Pub No 89-1580, Rockville, Md, 1988, NIMH.

Olney JE: Glutamine receptor dysfunction and schizophrenia, *Arch General Psychiatry* 52:998, 1995.

Penn DL: Dispelling the stigma of schizophrenia: what sort of information is best? *Schizophr Bull* 20:567, 1994.

Penn DL, Martin J: The stigma of severe mental illness: some political solutions for a recalcitrant problem, *Psychiatr Q* 69:235, 1998.

Pickens J: Formal and informal care of people with psychiatric disorders: historical perspectives and current trends, *J Psychosocial Nurs* 36(1):37, 1998.

Roman PM: Social acceptance of psychiatric illness and psychiatric treatment, *Soc Psychiatry* 16:21, 1981.

Ross EC: NAMI campaign, policy team launch Omnibus Mental Illness Recovery Act, *NAMI Advocate* 20(4):1, 1999.

Solden J: The benefits of assertive community treatment, *Nurs Times* 98(16):50, 1999.

Steadman HJ: Violence by people discharged from acute psychiatric inpatient facilities and by others in the same neighborhoods, *Arch Gen Psychiatry* 55(5):393-401, 1998.

Taber MT: Glutamate receptor agonist decrease extracellular dopamine in the rat nucleus accumbens in vivo, *Synapse* 24:165-172, 1996.

Taft LB, Barkin RL: Drug abuse: use and misuse of psychotropic drugs in Alzheimer's care, *J Gerontol Nurs* 16:4, 1990.

Torrey EF: *Out of the shadows: confronting America's mental illness crisis,* New York, 1997, John Wiley & Sons.

Torrey EF: *Survey of scientific studies demonstrating the connection between violence and untreated severe mental illness,* Washington, DC, 1999a, Treatment Advocacy Center Publication.

Torrey EF: *The failure of the National Institute of Mental Health to do sufficient research on severe mental illness,* 1999b, NAMI, www.nami.org/pressroom/failsummary.html.

Toru M: Excitatory amino acids: implications for psychiatric disorders, *Life Science* 66:1683, 1994.

Tsai G: Abnormal excitatory neurotransmitter metabolism in schizophrenic brains, *Arch Gen Psychiatry* 37:694-701, 1995.

US Department of Health and Human Services: *Healthy People 2010 leading health indicators final report,* Washington, DC, 1999a, US Government Printing Service.

US Department of Health and Human Services: *Surgeon General's report: a call to action for suicide prevention,* Washington, DC, 1999b, US Government Printing Office.

US Department of Health and Human Services: *Surgeon General's report on mental health,* Washington, DC, 1999c, US Government Printing Office.

Weinberger DR: The biological basis of schizophrenia: new directions, *J Clin Psychiatry* 58(10):22, 1997.

Violence in the Community

Alice Pappas and Kathy Lee Dunham Hakala

OBJECTIVES

Upon completion of this chapter, the reader will be able to do the following:

1. Describe the concept of *community violence*.
2. Identify long-term effects of violence on society.
3. Identify at-risk populations for violence and the role of public health in dealing with the epidemic of violence.
4. Describe the role of the nurse in primary, secondary, and tertiary prevention of violence.
5. Identify protection measures necessary for nurses and others working in situations where violence is prevalent.

KEY TERMS

cycle theory of violence
date rape drugs
dating violence
domestic violence
elder abuse
emotional abuse
emotional neglect
intentional injuries
intimate partner violence (IPV)
physical abuse
physical neglect
sexual abuse
shaken baby syndrome
violence

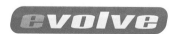

http://evolve.elsevier.com/Nies/

Two adolescent males ambushed their high school classmates with guns, killing 13 and wounding many others before they killed themselves. A young woman who complained to the police about being stalked was killed when she opened a package delivered to her apartment. A deranged man opened fire on a Jewish preschool. A black male was dragged to death by three white supremacists. A distraught mother murdered her two children after a bitter custody battle. A drunken driver killed five family members as they returned home from church on Christmas Eve. Terrorists bombed a federal building to retaliate for perceived governmental injustices. Two college women visited a rape crisis center suspecting they were sexually assaulted by their dates who tainted their drinks with a date rape drug. A six-year-old boy shot and killed a six-year-old girl because she yelled at him the day before.

The last four U.S. Surgeon Generals have declared violence as a national public health epidemic. When viewed from a public health perspective, violence is clearly a learned behavior that can be changed and prevented.

The purpose of this chapter is to explore the influence of violence from a public health perspective as it relates to individuals, families, and communities. Included in this chapter are discussions of the effects of violence on society in terms of death, illness, and injury; homicide and suicides among emerging high-risk groups; death and injury resulting from use of firearms; the direct influence of violence on individuals and society; public health interventions to reduce violence; the roles and responsibilities of the community health nurse in dealing with those experiencing violence; and measures to increase awareness of violence in the workplace.

OVERVIEW OF VIOLENCE

Violence is the intentional use of physical force against another person or against oneself, which results in or has a high likelihood of resulting in injury or death. Violence includes suicidal acts and interpersonal violence such as psychological, sexual, and/or physical abuse (Rosenberg, O'Connell, and Kenneth, 1992). In public health, injuries from violence are referred to as **intentional injuries**. Violence threatens the health and well-being of many people of all ages across the United States. On an average day, approximately 53 people die from homicide and a minimum of 18,000 survive interpersonal assaults. Furthermore,

84 people commit suicide and as many as 3000 attempt suicide on a daily basis (USDHHS, 2000).

The reasons for the high rate of violence in society are complex. "Alvin Toffler in his book *Powershift* identifies violence or the threat of violence as one of the three fundamental sources of all human power, the other two are money and knowledge. Of the three, violence is the lowest form of power because it can only be used to punish" (Koop and Lundberg, 1992, p. 3075).

The five most frequently cited underlying causes of or risk factors for violence are as follows:

1. Access to firearms
2. Drug and alcohol abuse
3. Poverty and unemployment
4. Specific personal characteristics of victims and perpetrators (e.g., between 15 and 34 years of age, 65 years of age or older, urban dweller, dependent upon caregivers, or socially isolated)
5. Having been a witness to violence (i.e., particularly as a child witnessing family violence)

Other causes mentioned less frequently include racism, lack of academic opportunity, gang membership, neural chemical imbalances, absence of moral and behavioral guidance for young people, and exposure to media violence (Winett, 1998).

Research has demonstrated a link between violence in television shows that children watch and heightened aggressive behavior. Watching violent behavior on television makes it harder for children to distinguish between reality and fantasy. Access to firearms is easy and even children are carrying guns to elementary schools to protect themselves. A high level of violence is associated with the sale of illegal drugs. Killings, either execution-style shootings or drive-by shootings, are often the result of a failed drug deal.

Anger abounds in society among individuals who have not been taught how to control or deal with anger in a nonaggressive fashion. Adolescents and children are increasingly using violence as a means of resolving conflicts. Many studies link abuse during childhood with violent behavior in adult life. Children are often brutalized by a parent or other family member or they may witness one parent beating the other. Research shows a strong correlation between childhood abuse and risk for exhibiting abusive behavior as an adult. A study of adult male prisoners convicted of first-degree murder found that two thirds had experienced "continuous, remorseless brutality during childhood" (Mason, 1991).

HISTORY OF VIOLENCE

Violence is not limited to the present day or to the United States. Since the beginning of time, humans have dealt violently with other humans. Cain killed his brother Abel out of jealousy and anger. Infanticide, or the killing of unwanted newborn children, has been practiced throughout history. For example, children were left to die from exposure or some other means when they were born a female, a twin, sickly, or deformed. Children, especially first-born children, were often sacrificed for religious reasons. Infanticide was not condemned until early in the fifth century; however, this did not protect children in many societies. Children were the property of the father and he could do whatever he wanted with them (Campbell and Humphreys, 1993).

Throughout the ages, corporal punishment has been used as a means of controlling children. Biblical reference to corporal punishment has often been used as a justification for some types of child abuse. To some parents, "spare the rod and spoil the child" (Proverbs, 13:24) implies an imperative to abusively discipline an errant child. Physical child abuse has also been included in the education process. The idea of "beating some sense into him" was considered necessary to ensure that the lesson was learned. In 1874, the first legal protection against child abuse in the United States occurred when the Society for the Prevention of Cruelty to Animals (SPCA) intervened to protect an eight-year-old girl. As a result of the notoriety associated with this case, the New York Society for the Prevention of Cruelty to Children was organized later that year (Campbell and Humphreys, 1993).

Even nursery rhymes that adults read to small children seem to condone violence against them. Consider the following Mother Goose nursery rhyme:

> There was an old woman who lived in a shoe,
> She had so many children she didn't know what to do.
> She gave them some broth without any bread,
> And whipped them all soundly and sent them to bed
> (*Mother Goose Nursery Rhymes*, p. 195-196, 2000).

Wife beating was legal in the United States until 1824. Wives were seen as their husbands' chattel and could be beaten for such offenses as "nagging too much." In fact, the common phrase "rule of thumb" was derived from English law that allowed a man to beat his wife with a cane no wider than his thumb. Biblical interpretation of "wives be subject to your husband" (Ephesians, 5:22) still provides some males with a faulty rationalization for wife beating.

The silence that long surrounded domestic violence is derived from a historical perspective of women as their husbands' property. The problem of assault against women was not explored in America until the Civil Rights Movement of the 1960s. Marital rape was not considered an offense in the United States until 1980; marital rape is still not an offense in some states. In the last two decades, additional cultural issues have surfaced in the United States regarding domestic abuse. These include female circumcision and genital mutilation, abuse between gay partners, and the reality that men are also victims of domestic violence.

Elder abuse is also a problem that is not new. In preindustrial Europe, legal documents were commonly drawn to allow the older parent to continue to sit at the family table and use the front door. The problem is of greater magnitude now because people are living longer, which results in more older adults. Elder abuse frequently goes undetected because there is a lack of awareness on the part of health care professionals and society. The exact prevalence of elder abuse is unknown because there is a lack of mandatory reporting in all states.

SCOPE AND PATTERNS OF ABUSE AND VIOLENCE

Homicide

One of America's greatest public health challenges is violence reduction. According to the CDC, the United States ranks first in the industrial world in violent death rates. Murder and suicide together claim the lives of over 50,000 individuals each year. An additional 2.2 million people are injured in violent assaults (CDC, 1995). Furthermore, more than 70% of homicides are committed with a firearm. Many states and the District of Columbia report more deaths caused by firearms than motor vehicle accidents.

Homicide claimed the lives of almost 20,000 people in 1997. Certain populations are at greater risk for death by homicide. These include young people, women, and black and Hispanic males. Although only 13% of U.S. residents are black, 50% of all murder victims are black (USDHHS, 2000). In 93% of cases, blacks killed other blacks (Elders, 1994).

Homicide and Youths

Homicide is the second leading cause of death among Americans aged 10 to 24 years and the *leading* cause of death among black males aged 15 to 34 years. This homicide rate is eight times greater than for whites of comparable age (CDC, 1999b). Children are not only victims of homicide, but increasingly younger children are committing murder. Incidents of school-related homicide have increased dramatically since 1990. In a news conference, the Council on Crime in America warned that by 2005, the skyrocketing rise in violent crime among teenagers and the 23% increase in males aged 14 to 17 years will require governments to attach more importance to preventing young people from becoming criminals (Butterfield, 1996).

The United States has the dubious distinction of having the highest youth homicide rate among the 26 wealthiest nations (Palestra, 1999). In January 1999, the American Academy of Pediatrics labeled the incidence of violence in children an "epidemic," which was the first time a U.S. medical association identified violence as a health issue.

Women and Homicide

Homicide is the fourth leading cause of death from injury among females; the rate is substantially higher among black females than among white females. Homicide is the leading cause of death from injury and the leading cause of death from all causes in black women aged 15 to 34 years (Dannenberg, Baker, and Li, 1994). Domestic violence is the leading cause of homicide among women in all ethnic groups. Murder-suicide is a relatively common form of violence against women. About 50% to 75% of murder-suicides in the United States involve a male who abused and murdered his girlfriend or wife and then committed suicide (Loring and Smith, 1994).

Suicide

Often ignored or overlooked, suicide is the eighth leading cause of death for all Americans. More people die from suicide than from homicide in the United States; suicide took the lives of 30,500 people in 1997 (11.4 per 100,000).

Suicide is becoming common in increasingly younger age groups. For young people aged 15 to 24 years, suicide is the third leading cause of death behind unintentional injury and homicide. In 1997, more teenagers and young adults died from suicide than from cancer, heart disease, AIDS, stroke, pneumonia, and chronic lung disease *combined* (CDC and National Center for Injury Prevention and Control [NCIPC], 2000b). Suicide among the

young is particularly problematic because young people do not completely fit the depression profile. Suicide is often an impulsive act that results from trouble at home, in school, or with the police; combined with weapons in the home, this creates a deadly combination.

Other high-risk populations include white males, who account for 72% of all suicides (83% of suicides among people aged 65 years or older); Native-Americans (i.e., particularly young male Native-Americans), whose rates are 1.5 times the national incidence; and unmarried jail inmates (CDC and NCIPC, 2000b). Suicide rates among black teens have grown dramatically since 1990. In 1995, suicide was the third leading cause of death among black youths aged 15 to 19 years; high-school–aged blacks were as likely as whites to attempt suicide (CDC, 1998).

Nearly 60% of all suicides are committed with a firearm (CDC and NCIPC, 2000b). Research indicates that suicidal individuals are five times more likely to kill themselves if a gun is in the home (Kellerman et al., 1992).

Violence against women is also responsible for high rates of female suicides. About 50% of all black women and 25% of all white women who attempt suicide do so to escape domestic violence (Sassetti, 1993). Further research is needed to determine the risk for other racial groups.

Nonhomicide and Nonsuicide Abuse

Each year, more than 500,000 Americans visit emergency rooms for violent injury (Blow and Gest, 1993). Assault, primarily in the context of marital or dating relationships, is a major source of injury among females. Studies of college (White and Koss, 1991) and high school (Gray and Foshee, 1997) students suggest that both males and females inflict and receive dating violence in equal proportion. However, the motivation for violence by women is more often for defensive purposes.

The 1998 National Violence Against Women Survey indicated that 1.5 million women are raped or physically assaulted by an intimate partner each year in the United States (Tjaden and Thoennes, 1998). Between 22% and 35% of all women seeking treatment in emergency rooms are abused. Annual estimates of the influence of injuries from family violence on health care are 21,000 hospitalizations that total 99,800 days, 39,000 physician visits, and 28,700 emergency room visits for a total medical cost of $44,393,700 (Loring and Smith, 1994).

Influence of Firearms

Approximately 192 million privately-owned firearms exist in the United States and 65 million are handguns. In 1997, almost 20,000 people were murdered in the United States; firearms were used in two out of three of those murders (USDHHS, 2000).

People may feel that they need a handgun in their home for protection; however, statistics do not reflect the logic of keeping a gun at home because the risk for gun accidents and violence in the home far outweighs the protective factor. Guns kept in the home for self-protection are 43 times more likely to kill a family member or a friend than an attacker. The presence of a gun in the home triples the risk of homicide in the home and increases the risk of suicide fivefold (CDC, 1999a).

In 1997, 32,436 Americans were killed with firearms (homicides, suicides, and accidents), which made gun-related injuries the second leading cause of death from injury in the United States after motor-vehicle–related incidents (CDC, 1999a). In comparison, 33,651 Americans were killed in the Korean War and 58,148 Americans were killed in the Vietnam War. In 1994, the firearms injury death rate among males aged 15 to 24 years was 32% higher than the motor vehicle death rate. In 1996, comparison of death by handguns in the United States with other industrialized nations showed the following (Palestra, 1999):

- New Zealand: 2 deaths
- Japan: 15 deaths
- Great Britain: 30 deaths
- Canada: 106 deaths
- Germany: 213 deaths
- United States: 9390 deaths

On an average day, over 700 Americans are shot; of these 700 Americans, 30 are children and 65 die. Three of four homicide victims and two of three suicide victims die of gunshot wounds. More than 50% of the victims are under 25 years of age and 85% are males (Blow and Gest, 1993).

Guns do not *cause* violence, but they greatly raise the severity of the health consequences. Major trauma centers report that between 20% and 25% of nonfatal gunshot wounds cause permanent neurological impairment. The violence produced by guns is more severe and more likely to lead to death instead of injury alone.

The cost of violence from guns is enormous. In 1990, firearm injuries cost over $20.4 billion in direct costs for hospital and other medical care and in indirect costs for long-term disability and premature death. Hospitalization for each firearm injury costs $32,000 (Max and Rice, 1993). Tax dollars fund at least 80% of the economic costs of treating firearm injuries because the overwhelming majority of hospital treatment for firearm injuries is unreimbursed care (Elders, 1994).

Discussion regarding firearms often evokes a heated response from opponents of gun control who see violence as the work of aberrant individuals. According to their view, the focus on guns as a major public health threat is misdirected in comparison with other health issues. Many opponents of gun control cite their constitutional "right to bear arms" and interpret efforts to control guns as an assault on their personal freedom. They believe that "law-abiding citizens" have a right to protect themselves despite the hazards of private gun ownership.

VIOLENCE AND SELECTED AGGREGATES

Youth-Related Violence

Violence is taking a toll on youth as an aggregate population. Violent crimes among youth are increasing and crimes such as homicide, rape, robbery, and aggravated assault are much more prevalent among adolescents than adults. In 1998, violence among adolescents took place twice as often than among the general population. Assaults are significantly higher among adolescent males, higher for black than white teens, and higher for those with lower household incomes (USDHHS, 2000).

The average age of homicide offenders and victims has decreased in recent years. Most of the increased homicide rates among American youth are attributable to death caused by firearms. Teens are more likely to die from gunshot wounds than from all natural causes combined (Palestra, 1999). Table 23-1 lists risk factors for youth-related violence.

Violence among youth exists across the United States. It is not a only problem of minority communities and inner cities, although it is more concentrated there. It also puts a disproportionate burden on minority communities. Shooting or killing someone has become the symbol of a new rite of passage and the bestowing of manhood among some segments of society (Ozmar, 1994). Minority youth are particularly influenced and violence among them is a large,

TABLE 23-1

Risk Factors for Youth-Related Violence*

Risk Factor	Comment
Poverty	The most closely correlated risk factor with youth violence is low family income.
Repeated exposure to violence	Children in inner-city neighborhoods are often exposed to chronic and extreme violence, enough that inner-city children often exhibit the same symptoms of posttraumatic stress as children living in war-torn countries.
Drugs	Not only does a pharmacological connection exist between aggressive behavior and consumption of drugs and alcohol, but there is also a financial connection between the drug trade and violence.
Easy access to firearms	About 50% of all households in the United States have a gun.
Unstable family life	About 70% of juvenile offenders come from single-parent homes. Single-parent homes correlate with elevated rates of school dropout, which correlates with elevated violent crime rates.
Family violence	Juvenile delinquency has been found to correlate with a history of childhood abuse and neglect. Alcohol and/or drug use is closely associated with domestic violence.
Delinquent peer groups	Gangs are using more lethal weapons to engage in increasingly violent behavior.
Media violence	By the time a child reaches seventh grade, he or she has witnessed 8000 murders and more than 100,000 other acts of violence on television. Witnessing violence increases short- and long-term aggression, desensitization, and fear in children.

Adapted from Ruttenberg H: The limited promise of public health methodologies to prevent youth violence, *Yale Law* 103:1885, 1994.
*Multiple risk factors have a cumulative effect.

complex problem. The toll of homicide and assault among young minority men, both black and Hispanic, is well known.

Adolescents and children increasingly use violence to handle disputes. Many children are not taught nonviolent ways of resolving differences. Schools have become a common site for violence (Box 23-1). Factors influencing this include the availability of guns and drug trafficking on campus and the unfortunate reality of remote or absentee parents. A profile of a student who kills includes the following (Stewart, 1998):

- Male
- Unstable family environment
- Poor peer relationships, but a strong need for group belonging
- Deeply identified with violence

Retribution for perceived wrongs from peers has also been cited as a cause of school violence.

Fighting is a prominent cause of injuries among high school students and often precedes homicides. Studies have indicated that homicide or suicide by youths is almost always an impulsive act that is immediately regretted. Unfortunately, in the case of suicide, the impulsive act destroys one life; in homicide, it destroys two lives.

Many young people have become immune to violence and believe they are invincible. They experience tremendous peer pressure to experiment with guns. Their impulsiveness and immaturity results in tragedy, which changes their lives forever.

Domestic Violence

Domestic violence is a pattern of coercive behaviors that are perpetrated by someone who is or was in an intimate relationship with the victim. These behaviors include battering resulting in physical injury, psychological abuse, and sexual assault. These acts result in

BOX 23-1

Violence in Schools

A national study on school violence was conducted in the late 1990s. Deaths were reported in 25 states and happened in both primary and secondary schools and communities of all sizes. Among the findings were the following:

- Less than 1% of all homicides among school-age children (i.e., 5 to 19 years of age) occur in or around school grounds or on the way to or from school.
- 65% of school-associated violent deaths were students, 11% were teachers or other staff members, and 23% were community members killed on school property.
- 83% of school homicide or suicide victims were males.
- 28% of fatal injuries happened inside the school building, 36% occurred outdoors on school property, and 35% occurred off campus.

From Centers for Disease Control and Prevention: Youth risk behavior surveillance: national alternative high school youth risk behavior survey, United States, 1998, *Morb Mortal Wkly Rep* 48(SS07):1, 1999b.

progressive social isolation, deprivation, and intimidation of the victim. Abuse is typically repetitive and often escalates in frequency and severity.

Battering, spousal abuse, wife abuse, and *domestic violence* are terms used to describe violence within an intimate relationship. The CDC now uses the term **intimate partner violence** (IPV), which is defined as the intentional, emotional, or physical abuse by a spouse or ex-spouse, boyfriend or girlfriend, ex-boyfriend or ex-girlfriend, or date (CDC and NCIPC, 2000a). This term is more inclusive and may replace *domestic violence.* Partners do not need to be married; violence may begin in casual or dating relationships.

More than one million incidents of nonlethal IPV occur each year and men direct violence against women approximately 85% of the time (CDC and NCIPC, 2000a). Violence may also be directed by women against women in lesbian relationships, men against men in homosexual relationships, and by women against men in a small but growing percentage of cases.

IPV cuts across all ethnic, racial, socioeconomic,

and educational lines. About 25% of women and 8% of men report being raped and/or physically assaulted by a current or former spouse, cohabiting partner, or date at some point in their life (CDC and NCIPC, 2000a). The strongest predictor of IPV is likely a history of alcohol abuse in the male partner (*Journal of Psychosocial Nursing and Mental Health,* 1999). The following are risk factors for IPV (CDC and NCIPC, 2000a):

- Female between 19 and 29 years of age
- Family with income below $10,000
- Women who were abused as children
- Alcohol or drug use by the perpetrator (75% of the time alcohol or drugs were used at the time of the assault)
- Being stalked by a current or former husband or cohabiting partner

Domestic violence is the least reported crime in the United States and is the single greatest cause of injury to women. These physical injuries are frequently borne in silence and/or accepted as a transgenerational pattern of normative behavior. When children witness abuse between parents, they learn that violence is a means of control. Male perpetrators of IPV are abusive because "they can and it works" (Hakala, personal communication, November 20, 2000).

Sexual abuse occurs in almost half of the battered population. Often abusive partners believe it is their right to have sex whenever they want. Women may report that they were subjected to forced intercourse when they were ill or had recently given birth. They also report forced anal intercourse and other violent sexual acts.

IPV often increases in frequency and severity and one study found that 42% of abused women are killed by their male partners (Stein, 1994). In 1996, about 5000 women were murdered and 85% were killed by someone they knew. Of these, approximately half were murdered by a husband, ex-husband, or boyfriend (USDHHS, 2000). In recent years, well-publicized cases have been reported of battered women who have killed their partners. Although their legal appeal has been "self-defense," it is a controversial issue, which is often difficult to prove.

Dating Violence

Dating violence has become a national concern. **Dating violence** refers to the perpetration or threat of an act of violence (e.g., sexual assault, physical violence, or verbal or emotional abuse) by a member of an unmarried couple on the other member within the context of dating or courtship. A national study of college students found that 27.5% of women suffered rape or attempted rape at least once since age 14 years. Between 80% and 95% of rapes that occur on college campuses are committed by someone the victim knows (Gray and Foshee, 1997).

Victims of dating violence are typically women aged 12 to 18 years (i.e., women are six times more likely than men to experience violence at the hands of an intimate partner), have been associated with female peers who have been sexually victimized, have lower church attendance, have a greater number of dating partners, show acceptance of dating violence, and experienced a previous sexual assault. Perpetrators of dating violence are males with sexually aggressive peers; are heavy drug or alcohol users; show acceptance of dating violence; assume the male's roles of initiating the date by driving and paying expenses; show miscommunication about sex; had previous sexual intimacy with the victim; and have an interpersonal history of violence (CDC and NCIPC, 2000a).

A particularly alarming type of dating abuse involves the use of the **date rape drugs** such as gamma-hydroxybutyrate (GHB) and Rohypnol to reduce inhibitions and promote anesthesia or amnesia in the victim. GHB is odorless, tasteless, and can easily be made at home. Instructions are available in libraries and on the Internet, which may explain the drug's rapid rise in popularity. Although illegal in the United States, it has become popular in many nightclubs where it is available in clear liquid form. GHB has been touted as an aphrodisiac and an anesthetic. It is actually a depressant that slows down the respiratory system and has been responsible for at least one death and numerous overdoes. When mixed with alcohol, it can be deadly.

Rohypnol, classified as a benzodiazepine, has been compared to Quaaludes, the "love drug" of the 1960s and 1970s. Like GHB, Rohypnol is not legal in the United States, but many reports have been received of its use at fraternity parties, at other college gatherings, and in gay bars on both coasts. The ability to provide a quick, cheap high with long-lasting effects may explain its popularity. Combined with alcohol, serious side effects including death have been reported (Lyman, Hughes-McLain, and Thompson, 1998).

Abuse During Pregnancy

Pregnancy does not exclude women from the danger of abuse. Pregnancy may increase stresses within the family and provoke the first instances of battering. The reported incidence of battering during pregnancy varies from 3% to 17% (Curry, Doyle, and Gilhooley, 1998). This high incidence is a public health concern because it may outrank diabetes and pregnancy-induced hypertension in common complications in selected populations. Societal awareness of IPV during pregnancy is a relatively recent phenomenon; the mention of abuse during pregnancy began to appear in the health literature in the 1980s. The image of a woman being battered during pregnancy shatters the idealized image of pregnancy as a time for nurturing and protection.

All pregnant women and adolescents should be routinely screened for abuse because pregnancy is a risk factor for battering. Studies have shown that detection of abuse is more likely to occur when the health care provider routinely asks about abuse more than once during each prenatal visit. Abused pregnant women report blows to the abdomen, injuries to their breasts and genitalia, and sexual assault. Such violence can result in spontaneous abortion, stillbirths, preterm deliveries, and lower-birth-weight infants (Nichols and Zwelling, 1997).

Abusive Pattern

The **cycle theory of violence** was developed by Walker (1979) and explains a common abusive pattern of domestic violence. Depicted in Fig. 23-1, this theory contains the following three phases: tension, explosion, and contrition (commonly known as the *honeymoon phase*).

During the *tension phase,* minor battering incidents may occur, such as slapping, kicking, and spitting. External influences that the batterer reacts to inappropriately (e.g., problems at the batterer's job, heavy traffic, or crying children) may trigger these minor incidents.

The second and most dangerous phase is the *explosive phase.* The explosive phase is inevitable as tension builds and is characterized by uncontrolled rage. The batterer may only stop when he or she becomes exhausted or is stopped by a third party (e.g., the police or other family member). Physical injuries occur during this phase; therefore the victim may seek health care. However, unless the injury is severe, the victim may not seek medical help because he or she feels shame and/or the need for secrecy.

Some women who have been through the violence cycle actually report provoking the batterer into the explosive phase. Such behavior, although startling to others, seems logical to the victim who has been

FIGURE 23-1

Walker's "Cycle of Violence" (From Rawlins P, Williams S, Beck C: *Mental-health psychiatric nursing: a holistic life-cycle approach,* St. Louis, 1993, Mosby).

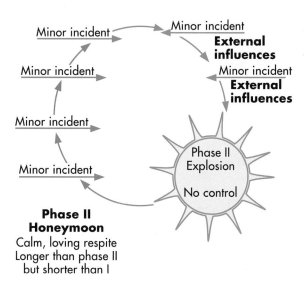

**Phase I
Tension building**
Limited control

Minor incident
Minor incident
External influences
Minor incident
Minor incident
External influences
Minor incident
Minor incident
Minor incident

Phase II
Explosion

No control

**Phase II
Honeymoon**
Calm, loving respite
Longer than phase II
but shorter than I

through this before. By provoking the batterer into the inevitable explosive phase, the cycle can be completed and the tension relieved for a time.

The *honeymoon phase* is characterized by promises that the abuse will never happen again. The victim may be initially lulled into a sense of security as he or she receives apologies and the showering of gifts. This phase may also include pleas for forgiveness and a promise to seek counseling on the part of the batterer. The cycle of violence is characterized by the following (Sonkin and Durphy, 1997):

1. The more times the cycle is completed, the less time it takes to complete.
2. The longer the cycle goes uninterrupted, the worse the violence gets.
3. The longer the cycle goes uninterrupted, the shorter the third stage becomes.

Like many forms of violence, domestic violence is a learned behavior that is often modeled from transgenerational patterns. Children, especially males, who have witnessed their mothers being abused are at high risk for imitating this behavior as adults with their own partners. Although they may have tried to

protect their mother from the abuse as children, they subconsciously learn that violence is a means of control. Lacking role models for developing healthy emotional relationships, these children often become adults who batter. Domestic violence is about control, not anger; therefore the objective of the abuse is to exert power and control over the victim. The victim may have also been exposed to domestic violence as a child. In these cases, the learned response may be one of helplessness that implies passivity and acceptance of abuse.

The Domestic Abuse Intervention Project in Duluth, Minnesota, has developed a wheel of violence that depicts the types of power and control that are used. This includes emotional abuse and intimidation, minimization, denial and blaming, coercion and threats, isolation, economic abuse, and use of children. Male privilege is another excuse often given by men for abuse. They may cite Biblical reference to rightful male authority over women or exploit cultural gender bias. Fig. 23-2 depicts the power and control wheel.

Effects of Domestic Violence

Chronic stress characterizes the lives of people in relationships with violent partners. When subject to repeated abuse, the abuse victim experiences a variety of responses including shock, denial, confusion, withdrawal, psychological numbing, and fear. He or she lives in anticipatory terror and often suffers chronic fatigue and tension, disturbed sleeping and eating patterns, and vague gastrointestinal and genitourinary complaints. Health care providers frequently overlook or misdiagnose this pattern of obscure symptoms. In many instances, providers may label the abuse victim as hypochondriacal or clinically depressed, which results in a sense of guilt, extreme passivity, and helplessness. Few victims spontaneously disclose that they are being abused; therefore the failure of health care professionals to assess for abuse in all emergency and routine health care visits significantly contributes to the missed diagnosis of abuse.

Fear, helplessness, and lack of knowledge regarding resources are primary reasons that many victims do not readily leave an abusive situation. The legal system is cumbersome and often inadequate. Victims who seek help through restraining orders or other judicial means find that such methods do not provide real safety or solutions. For example, after reporting abuse to the police, the partner may be jailed and given bail within 24 hours or less and return home, unannounced, to deliver another beating. After attempting to use the judicial system as a solution and

FIGURE **23-2**

Power and control wheel developed by the Domestic Abuse Intervention Project, 206 West Fourth Street, Duluth, Minnesota 55806. Used by permission.

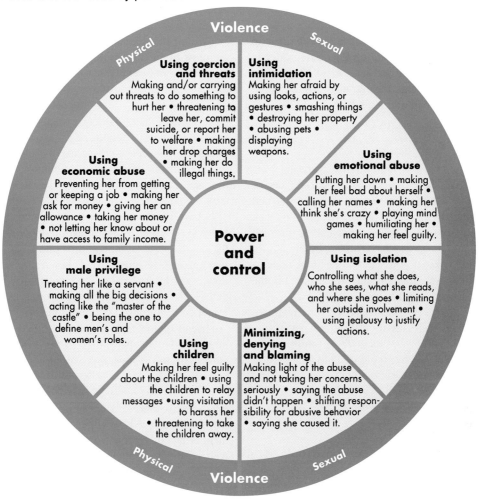

experiencing its failure, the victim is unlikely to consider the legal system as a source of safety. He or she may also fear that legal intervention might be a threat to custody of his or her children.

Other factors that keep a victim in an abusive situation are culture, religion, and economics. Victims with few marketable skills who leave an abusive situation face serious economic problems and may fall into poverty. When children are involved in such economically dependent relationships, the victim may choose to remain in the setting as a means of economic survival for his or her children. Health care providers, including nurses, often ask the victim, "Why don't you just leave?" or "What did you do to deserve this?" These misdirected questions often re-

inforce the victim's sense of helplessness and guilt regarding his or her abusive situation. These questions reflect a lack of understanding regarding the dynamics of abuse and a lack of sensitivity toward the victim.

Victims who are most likely to leave a battering situation include the following (Campbell and Humphreys, 1993):

1. Those who have resources such as money, friends, family, and support
2. Those who have power (e.g., a job, credit cards, and status outside the family)
3. Those without children
4. Those who were not abused as children
5. Those who did not see their mothers beaten

6. Those involved in battering situations that are frequent or severe
7. Those whose partner begins to beat children in the family

The most dangerous time for the victim is when he or she leaves or attempts to leave the relationship because it is seen as an assault on the abuser's desire to control the victim. The victim is more likely to be killed at this time than at any other time in the relationship (Campbell and Humphreys, 1993).

Child Abuse

Patterns of child abuse within families vary. In some family situations, all children are equal targets of abuse. In other families, one child might be selected as the designated recipient of abuse. The child may be singled out by a particular physical characteristic such as hair color or resemblance to another family member who evokes negative emotions in the abusive parent. Child abuse, like domestic violence, is often a learned transgenerational behavior.

About 984,000 victims of child maltreatment lived in the United States in 1997 (13.9 per 1000). About 1196 fatalities resulted from child abuse (USDHHS, 2000). The five types of child abuse are as follows:

1. Physical abuse
2. Physical neglect
3. Emotional abuse
4. Emotional neglect
5. Sexual abuse

Physical Abuse

Physical abuse is an intentional injury inflicted by other than accidental means on a child by another person and accounts for 25% of child abuse cases (USDHHS, 2000). The most common type of physical abuse is beating, which can result in cuts, bruises, burns, and fractures. The type of physical injury varies only with the adult's imagination. Parents often select a method of meeting what they see as the child's disobedience. This may produce a "patterned" injury, which gives some clue to how the child was injured by leaving an imprint of the object on the child's skin. For example, a child who walks where he or she is not supposed to might have his or her feet dipped in scalding water; the burns would cover the stocking area of the foot. A child who touches a light cord or

light plug might be beaten with it, producing a looped or linear pattern. A child who plays with matches or the stove might have his or her hand placed in the flame. A crying child or a child who talks back might have hot pepper or Tabasco sauce poured into his or her mouth or might be suffocated with a pillow.

Young children between two and five years of age are most frequently injured by physical abuse. This is most commonly explained by developmental behavior such as the "terrible twos" and efforts toward physical autonomy and independence (e.g., toilet training and feeding issues). Parents who abuse have unreasonable expectations of their children and misinterpret the child's behavior as threats to their parental self-esteem and need to control. Infants are in the greatest danger of severe injury or death because they are small and helpless.

An example of extreme infant abuse is **shaken baby syndrome**. In this situation, violent shaking of the infant causes trauma at the brain stem-spinal cord junction and the morbidity and mortality rates for this injury are high. Serious and potentially permanent damage may occur including retinal hemorrhages, spinal cord injuries, and brain injuries. The spouse or boyfriend of the mother usually inflicts this type of injury. A female babysitter is the next most likely person to inflict this type of injury (Wolfner and Gelles, 1993).

Physical Neglect

Physical neglect is negligent treatment or maltreatment of a child by a person responsible for the child's welfare and is the most common form of child abuse, which accounts for 56% of all cases (USDHHS, 2000). The term includes acts of omission and commission on the part of the responsible person and includes failure to provide a nurturing environment for a child to thrive, learn, and develop. Physical neglect includes the failure to provide basic needs including safety, food, clothing, and shelter. In addition, failure to provide for the health needs of a child can also be construed as neglect.

Emotional Abuse

Emotional abuse accounts for approximately 6% of all child abuse cases and refers to willfully inflicting unjustifiable mental suffering on a child, which causes the child to be emotionally damaged (USDHHS, 2000). The behavior evident in the child may demonstrate a substantial impairment in a normal range of performance and behavior such as an overly compliant or passive child or the child who is very aggressive and apt to fly into a rage. These children frequently do not progress with the normal rate of physical, intellectual, and emotional development. Emotional abuse is almost always done in the home and is not witnessed by others and the symptoms displayed by the child can occur in children who are not abused; therefore treatment of these children is difficult. Examples of emotional abuse include locking a child in a closet for a prolonged period of time, tying a child to a bedpost, or engaging in bizarre acts of torture. Subtle abuse might include name calling such as "you're stupid," "you're a slut," or "you're bad or evil." Name calling can irreparably harm a child's self-concept.

Emotional Neglect
Emotional neglect is the failure to nurture a child in developmentally appropriate ways. Some examples of emotional neglect are failure to cuddle and/or physically stimulate a newborn, failure to give positive feedback, failure to pay attention to the overall emotional needs of a child, or deliberate withholding of affection.

Sexual Abuse
Sexual abuse refers to any sexual activity between an adult and a child, including use of a child for sexual exploitation, prostitution, or pornography. Approximately 12.5% of child abuse cases are sexual abuse (USDHHS, 2000). Sexual abuse can also involve an older child with a younger child, usually defined as five or more years of age between the two. *Incest* is the term used for sexual relations between close family members such as father and daughter, mother and son, or siblings within the family. The most common form of incestuous relationship is a stepfather with his stepdaughter (Campbell and Humphreys, 1993).

Sexual abuse often involves a person known to the child (i.e., a relative or friend). A growing concern is the sexual exploitation of children by Internet pedophiles who prey upon unsuspecting and naïve targets through chat rooms. It may occur over a prolonged period of time and threats to the child may be used to ensure secrecy.

Although most of the research has focused on females as victims of sexual abuse, recent reports indicate that males are also targets. The incidence of male sexual abuse in unknown. The victim may refrain from reporting such abuse because they are ashamed and because cultural values expect males to be assertive and capable of self-defense. The aftermath of sexual abuse may predispose the victims to low self-esteem, psychiatric illness, depression, suicide ideation, drug and alcohol addiction, negative sexual esteem and sexual maladjustment, delayed developmental processes, and planned pregnancy to escape an abusive situation (CDC, 1997). Table 23-2 describes physical and behavioral indicators of child abuse and neglect.

Elder Abuse

Child abuse and IPV have been public health policy issues since the 1980s, but in many areas of the United States **elder abuse** lags far behind as a social and health care issue because society fails to recognize the inhumanity many older adults experience. As a result, the exact number of abused older adults is unknown because elder abuse is underreported more often than child abuse. However, estimates indicate that 1% to 10% of the older adult population suffers some form of maltreatment. Reasons for this underreporting include shame on the part of the victim, social and physical isolation from resources, and the failure of health care providers to routinely assess for abuse and neglect during points of contact. The most likely victims of elder abuse are women over 70 years of age who are in poor physical or mental health and dependent upon others for physical or financial support (Wolfe, 1998).

The five commonly described types of abuse and neglect of older adults are as follows:

1. Physical abuse (i.e., purposeful infliction of physical pain or injury or unnecessary physical restraint)
2. Psychological-emotional abuse (i.e., verbal assault, threats, provoking fear, or isolation)
3. Sexual abuse (i.e., unwanted sexual contact)
4. Physical neglect (i.e., withholding of personal care, food, medications, or intimidation or humiliation)
5. Financial exploitation, theft, and misuse of money or property

Elder abuse tends to escalate in incidence and severity over time. When an older adult cannot care for himself or herself because he or she experiences the physical or mental infirmities of age, what happens to that person may depend on whether relatives can provide care or whether the person has financial resources to purchase care in his or her own home, a retirement home, or a residential care facility. If none

TABLE **23-2**

Physical and Behavioral Indicators of Child Abuse and Neglect

Physical Indicators	Behavioral Indicators
Physical Abuse	
Unexplained bruises and welts in various stages of healing that may form patterns	Wary of adult contacts
	Apprehensive when other children cry
Unexplained burns by cigars or cigarettes or immersion burns (e.g., socklike, glovelike, or on buttocks or genitalia)	Constantly on alert
	Exhibiting extremes of behavior; aggressive or passive and withdrawn or overly friendly to strangers
Rope burns	
Unexplained lacerations or abrasions	Frightened of parents
Unexplained fractures in various stages of healing; multiple or spiral fractures	Afraid to go home
	Reporting injury by parents
Unexplained injuries to mouth, lips, gums, eyes, or external genitalia	
Physical Neglect	
Hunger	Begging or stealing food
Poor hygiene	Alone at inappropriate times or for prolonged periods
Poor or inappropriate dress	Delinquent
Lack of supervision for prolonged periods of time	Stealing
Lack of medical or dental care	Arriving early to and departing late from school
Constant fatigue, listlessness, or falling asleep in class	Reporting having no caretaker
Sexual Abuse	
Difficulty in walking or sitting	Exhibiting negative self-esteem
Torn, stained, or bloody underwear	Exhibiting inability to trust and function in intimate relationships
Genital pain or itching	
Bruises or bleeding from the external genitalia, vaginal, or anal areas	Exhibiting cognitive and motor dysfunctions
	Exhibiting deficits in personal and social skills
Venereal disease	Exhibiting bizarre, sophisticated, or unusual sexual behavior or knowledge
Drug and alcohol abuse	
Developmental delays	Delinquent or a runaway
	Exhibiting suicide ideation
	Reporting sexual assault
Emotional Maltreatment	
Failure to thrive	Exhibiting behavior extremes from passivity to aggression
Lags in physical development	Exhibiting habit and conduct disorders (e.g., antisocial behavior and destructiveness)
Speech disorders	
Developmental delays	Exhibiting neurotic traits
	Attempting suicide

of these possibilities exist, the older adult may continue to live alone. This may be an unsatisfactory way of dealing with the problem because safety is an issue.

The caregivers are often adult children, nieces or nephews, or another relative of the older adult. This generation of individuals in their forties, fifties, and sixties are often called the *sandwich generation* because they begin by caring for their children and end by providing care for their parents. As parents age, the role reversal is often painful and demanding on the part of the older adult and the caregiver.

Care of an aging parent may require more sacrifice and commitment than their children's care required. When providing care for children, their dependency on the caregiver usually lessens as the child grows older. However, when caring for an aging parent or relative, they become more dependent and may become cognitively or physically impaired, which may be a factor in the likelihood of abuse. Older adults may not know who they are or may suffer changes in personality that make it difficult for their adult children to care for them. They may need to be lifted, which may be difficult for someone with limited strength. They may need assistance walking, toileting, or eating, which takes time that the caregiver may not feel he or she has. Another factor that can come to bear on aging parents is the care that they gave their children when they were young. If they were abusive to their children, adult children may use the older adult's dependency as an opportunity to finally respond in an abusive manner to them.

All of these factors cause stress, which is closely associated with abuse. This is especially true in families in which violence is a response to stress. Stress in the primary caregiver can be caused by the needs of the older adult exceeding the family's ability to meet them or personal stresses of the caregiver such as the interference with their job, illness, or other family problems.

In many ways, a helpless older adult is in the same vulnerable position as an abused child because he or she is dependent upon others to intervene. Until society becomes sensitized to this problem, elder abuse is likely to increase. The population of the United States is aging and the number of frail older adults (i.e., over 85 years of age) is the fastest growing demographic segment with increasing dependency needs. Recognition of possible indicators helps the professional become aware of possible abusive situations. None is conclusive in itself; however, they alert the professional to the need for careful and complete assessment. Table 23-3 lists the indicators of possible abuse of older adults.

VIOLENCE FROM A PUBLIC HEALTH PERSPECTIVE

Dealing with violence has traditionally been the U.S. criminal justice system's responsibility. However, violence has been called a *public health epidemic* and efforts have been made to prevent and manage it using public health strategies. Violence has a tremendous influence on morbidity and mortality rates and on QOL and health care resources. Violence is a problem of such magnitude that it has reached beyond criminal justice methods of protecting the public. Public health has been challenged to go beyond its traditional work to embrace programs to decrease poverty, illiteracy, environmental degradation, and violence. Many of these problems are interrelated; therefore a highly-coordinated approach should be used to address the issues (Foege, 1998).

Healthy People 2010 and Violence

Violence was one of the areas addressed by *Healthy People 2000* and again in *Healthy People 2010.* Several objectives regarding violence and abuse prevention have been established for *Healthy People 2010.* Table 23-4 lists a few of these (USDHHS, 2000). These objectives are intended to continue targeting causes of violence and abuse, improve national data collection and analysis, provide input for legislative funding, facilitate research efforts, and concentrate public health efforts on models that demonstrate effectiveness.

Many of the *Healthy People 2010* objectives are difficult to achieve because there are complex barriers. Some of these barriers include lack of comparable data sources, standardized definitions, resources to adequately establish consistent tracking systems, and resources to fund promising prevention programs. The achievement of positive change in 13 of the original 19 objectives indicates that coordinated national efforts can bring about progress.

PREVENTION OF VIOLENCE

The nurse who cares for people experiencing violence must be a skilled clinician who is knowledgeable about the problem and resources available in the community. The nurse may also be in a position of dealing with individuals and families before abuse has occurred. He or she can educate families in the care and nurturing of family members, the growth and development of children, and the needs of older adults. Table 23-5 provides components of a comprehensive program to reduce violence in the community.

Primary Prevention

One goal of primary prevention of violence is the promotion of optimal parenting and family wellness. Education plays a major part of primary prevention from educating children in grade schools regarding a

TABLE 23-3

Indicators of Possible Elder Abuse

Physical Indicators	Behavioral Indicators
Any injury that has not been cared for properly	Fear
Any injury incompatible with the history	Withdrawal
Lack of care for injuries	Depression
Evidence of inadequate care	Helplessness
Evidence of inadequate or inappropriate administration of medicine	Resignation
	Hesitation to talk openly
Poor skin hygiene	Implausible stories
Hemorrhage beneath the scalp	Confusion or disorientation
Signs of confinement (e.g., tied to furniture, bathroom fixtures, or locked in room)	Ambivalence; contradictory statements not caused by mental dysfunction
	Anger
	Denial
	Nonresponsiveness
	Agitation or anxiety

Family or Caregiver Indicators of Possible Elder Abuse	Financial Indicators of Possible Elder Abuse
Unwillingness to let the older adult speak for himself or herself or see others without presence of the caregiver	Unusual activity in bank accounts
Aggressive behavior	Concern by relatives that too much money is being spent for the care
Attitude of indifference or anger	Refusal to spend money on the care of the older adult
Blaming of the older adult for things beyond his or her control such as incontinence	Unexpected change in power of attorney
Problems with alcohol or drugs	Recent will change when the older adult is incapable of making a will
Conflicting accounts of incidents by the family and victim	Recent acquaintances expressing undying affection for a wealthy older adult
Unwillingness or reluctance to comply with service providers in planning care of the older adult	Recent change of title of house in favor of a "friend" when the older adult is incapable of understanding the nature of the transaction
Indications of inappropriate sexual relationship	Isolation of older adult from friends and family causing the older adult to become alienated
Withholding affection	Promises of lifelong care in exchange for willing or deeding of all property or money to the caregiver
Lack of amenities such as grooming items and clothing when the estate can afford to buy it	Checks and documents signed when the older adult cannot write
	Missing personal belongings such as art, silverware, or jewelry
	Placement outside the home not commensurate with the financial ability of the older adult
	Signatures on checks that do not resemble the older adult's signature

Adapted from Carlton L: *Elder abuse prevention protocol,* San Francisco, 1983, San Francisco Task Force.

healthy family life and nonviolent methods of conflict resolution, to educating professionals to increase their awareness of violence and facilitate case detection and provision for early treatment. Community services are needed to provide care for families before serious injury occurs to any member. Nurses can be in the forefront in communities and act as an advocate for those in need of services. The nurse can work in the community to educate citizens about the problem of violence, potential causes of violence, and the community services that are necessary to serve those in need. Reduction of violence in the media and control of handguns and assault weapons are also essential.

Proposed changes range from an outright ban on private ownership of certain types of guns (i.e., especially assault rifles and small, cheap, poorly made handguns called *Saturday Night Specials*) to an increase in manufacturers' and dealers' liability and holding gun owners responsible for the injury and loss of life caused by their weapons. More stringent measures include enforcement of sales restrictions to "high-risk" individuals, higher sales taxes for guns and ammunition, tighter federal dealer licensing standards, limits on the number of guns a person may

purchase within a month, and new gun designs intended to reduce their lethality. Such design modifications include load indicators, magazine safety devices, push button locks, fingerprint or voice recognition chips, and a magnetic ring worn by the shooter that enables the gun to be fired (Palestra, 1999).

Primary prevention of abuse against women must begin at a societal level, helping to change attitudes toward violence and women. Children should be taught that no one has the right to beat another person or touch another person inappropriately. Each child has a right to be free from abuse. Children who witness their mothers being abused are at particular risk. Boys are at risk to grow to adulthood and abuse women with whom they have an intimate relationship. Girls are at risk for developing low self-esteem and ending up in an abusive relationship. Primary prevention must focus on stopping the transgenerational aspect of abuse.

Primary prevention to prevent child abuse must include education about parenting. In a nation preoccupied by the need for education to meet the challenge of technological change, many people still do not value education for effective parenting. Par-

TABLE 23-4

Violence and *Healthy People 2010 Objectives*

Objective	Baseline (1998)	Target
15-32: Reduce homicides	6.2 per 100,000	3.2 per 100,000
15-33a: Reduce maltreatment of children under 18 years of age	13.9 per 1000	11.1 per 1000
15-33b: Reduce child maltreatment fatalities for children under 18 years of age	1.7 per 100,000	1.5 per 100,000
15-34: Reduce the rate of physical assault by current or former intimate partners for children 12 years of age and older	4.5 per 1000	3.6 per 1000
15-35: Reduce the annual rate of rape or attempted rape for children 12 years of age and older	0.9 per 1000	0.7 per 1000
15-36: Reduce sexual assault other than rape for children 12 years of age and older	0.6 per 1000	0.2 per 1000
15-37: Reduce physical assaults for children 12 years of age and older	31.1 per 1000	25.5 per 1000
15-38: Reduce physical fighting among adolescents grades 9 to 12	37%	33%
15-39: Reduce weapon carrying by adolescents on school property for grades 9 to 12	8.5%	6%

TABLE **23-5**

Components of a Comprehensive Program to Reduce Violence for Individuals, Families, and the Community

Individuals	Family	Community
Primary Prevention—Goal: Promotion of Optimal Parenting and Family Wellness		
Family life education in schools, churches, and communities	Parenting classes in hospitals, schools, and other community agencies	Community education concerning family violence
Education of children on methods of conflict resolution	Provision of bonding opportunities for new parents	Reduction of media violence
Birth control services for sexually active teens	Referral of new families to community health nurses after early discharge from the hospital for follow-up services	Development of community support services such as crisis lines, respite placement for children, respite care for families with dependent older adult members, shelters for battered women and their children
Child care education for teens who babysit	Social services for families	Handgun control
Preventive mental health services for adults and children		
Training for professionals in early detection of violence		
Secondary Prevention—Goal: Diagnosis of and Service for Families in Stress		
Nursing assessment for evidence of family violence in all health care settings	Social services for individuals or families	All health professionals skilled in assessment of violence and equipped with protocols for dealing with the victim to help ensure their safety
A well thought-out safety plan for victims	Referral to self-help groups in the community	Hospital emergency rooms and trauma centers with 24-hour response, reporting, case intake, coordination with legal and medical authorities, coordination with voluntary agencies who have services, coordination with social services departments for provision of services
Knowledge of legal options to help ensure safety	Referral to community agencies that provide services for victims	Death review teams to review deaths from injury, especially for infants and children
Shelter or foster home placement for victims		Public authority involvement by police, district attorneys, and courts
		Epidemiological tracking and evaluation of violence
		Handgun control
Tertiary Prevention—Goal: Reeducation and Rehabilitation of Violent Families		
Empowerment strategies for battered women	Parenting reeducation (i.e., formal training in childrearing)	Foster homes, shelters, and care for older adults
Professional counseling services for individuals	Professional counseling services for families	Public authority involvement
	Self-help groups	Follow-up care for known cases of abuse
		Gun control

enting is the most difficult job that most individuals will undertake, yet there is a widespread myth that parenting "comes naturally." Reality and the disturbing statistics of abuse show that this is not true. Classes for parents should focus on more than preparation for labor and physical care of the infant. The realities of parenthood, the effect of fatigue on a new mother, the need for support from a significant other or family member, and fears and questions of new parents must be addressed.

Changes in the health care delivery system cause nurses in the hospital to have far less time than they once did to help new mothers learn basic newborn care before discharge. Hospitals and public health agencies must provide follow-up to ensure that new parents can adequately care for their infant. This is especially true of any person deemed to be high risk, including teenage mothers, mothers without supportive others, or women with a history of spousal abuse.

Support for caregivers can help in the primary prevention of abuse of older adults. Education about the needs of older adults and the need for respite care for the caregiver should be available to those who face the care of aging parents. Just as a parent does not know everything about parenting simply by having a baby, an adult who may not have intimate contact with anyone of advanced age must be educated about the developmental processes and needs of the aging. Support groups for caregivers have been shown to be an effective outlet to vent frustration and receive needed counseling. Caregiving is frequently a 24-hour responsibility. Institutional abuse occurs in a setting where workers provide care in shifts, but the stress for those who do not have that relief is much greater. Nurses need to help the caregivers care for themselves.

Secondary Prevention

The goal of secondary prevention related to violent behaviors is to provide assessment of and service to families in stress, which facilitates early diagnosis and treatment. Safety of family members is critical. Family violence is not just a nine-to-five event during weekdays; around-the-clock assistance is crucial. Women who do not have money must have access to legal options. Shelters should be available to offer sanctuary to a victim and to shield a woman and her children from danger. A shelter can temporarily provide safety while the woman plans for her future. In the United States, there are more animal shelters than shelters for abused women.

Public health surveillance is important to obtain accurate numbers for intentional injuries of all individuals. Forming review teams can play an important part by analyzing the incidence of death from injury to determine whether the injury was intentional or unintentional. Removing guns from the hands of children and violent individuals is also an important facet in reducing deaths from violence. Some states have initiated gun "buy-back" programs to encourage community involvement in these efforts.

Secondary prevention begins with assessment of

a battered victim. Consistent assessment of all women during health care visits will increase case finding and provide opportunities for earlier intervention. This is particularly crucial during pregnancy. Women should be interviewed in private when they are asked about battering. Questions should be asked in a matter-of-fact way and the health care provider should not show shock or dismay at their response. The Nursing Research Consortium on Violence and Abuse has developed a simple three-question abuse assessment screen (Table 23-6).

These three questions should be asked of *all* women at *each visit*. If the woman responds "yes" to the questions about physical battering, she should be handed a pencil and allowed to mark the areas on the body where she has been injured. If the nurse observes injuries, careful and detailed charting should be done. This screening tool may be reproduced and used for assessing women in a wide variety of settings. After disclosure of abuse, the nurse's response should include the following three statements:

1. "I am sorry this happened to you."
2. "This is not your fault."
3. "What is happening to you is illegal."

These three statements offer support and educate the victim about the dynamics of abuse (Hakala, personal communication, November 20, 2000).

By law, the victim must be offered resources that may increase his or her safety once the existence of a violent situation is known. However, the victim may not be ready to leave the situation and it is wise to explore available options so that he or she can plan ahead. The victim should have knowledge of legal options and how to access them. The nurse should ask the victim about what resources he or she has, including friends and family, and if he or she could enlist their support if needed.

Some states that have mandatory reporting laws for spousal abuse have developed protocols for nurses who deal with the victims. Review of these protocols can help the nurse become familiar with the questions to ask the client and the suggestions that he or she should make to help the victim make a safety plan. A safety plan is essential in providing comprehensive care. The nurse should discuss it with the victim in privacy and place it in the victim's hands if it is safe. Table 23-7 is a sample of a safety plan that the nurse can use to help a victim explore his or her options.

Secondary prevention of child abuse begins with

TABLE 23-6

Abuse Assessment Screen

1. WITHIN THE LAST YEAR, have you been hit, slapped, kicked, or otherwise physically hurt by someone?	YES	NO
If YES, by whom?		
Total number of times		
2. SINCE YOU'VE BEEN PREGNANT, have you been hit, slapped, kicked, or otherwise physically hurt by someone?	YES	NO
If YES, by whom?		
Total number of times		
MARK THE AREA OF INJURY ON THE BODY MAP. SCORE EACH INCIDENT ACCORDING TO THE FOLLOWING SCALE:		SCORE
1 = Threats of abuse including use of a weapon		
2 = Slapping, pushing; no injuries and/or lasting pain		
3 = Punching, kicking, bruises, cuts, and/or continuing pain		
4 = Beating up, severe contusions, burns, broken bones		
5 = Head injury, internal injury, permanent injury		
6 = Use of weapon; wound from weapon		
If any of the descriptions for the higher number apply, use the higher number.		
3. WITHIN THE LAST YEAR, has anyone forced you to have sexual activities?	YES	NO
If YES, by whom?		
Total number of times		

From McFarlane J, Parker B: Preventing abuse during pregnancy: an assessment and intervention protocol, *MCN Am J Matern Child Nurs* 19(6):321-324, 1994.
Developed by the Nursing Research Consortium on Violence and Abuse. Readers are encouraged to reproduce and use this assessment tool.

the discovery that the child has suffered from dysfunctional parenting or has been injured. The community health nurse in the home or school may be the one to discover the injured child and initiate the mandatory report to child protective or emergency services. The nurse can continue to support and educate the parent even though a report must be made. The primary focus should be obtaining a safe environment for the child.

In secondary prevention of abuse of older adults, the nurse's focus should be on the client and his or her needs. *Each time* an older adult is seen in the health care system, the nurse must make an opportunity to screen for the possibility of abuse. Elder abuse remains grossly unreported across the United States; therefore routine screening can begin to change attitudes and provide earlier intervention. A suggested screening protocol, such as the one shown in Fig. 23-3, can provide an algorithm that the nurse can use in a variety of health care settings. Nurses can help raise professional and societal consciousness of elder abuse by participating in political activities to create or strengthen mandatory reporting laws and fund support groups for at-risk families.

The nurse must establish a trusting relationship when treating any person experiencing violence. A
Text continued on p. 617

TABLE 23-7

Planning for Safety

You can choose to leave or to stay with an abusive person. It is your choice and your choice alone. We all have the right to say and do what we want and to feel safe. Also, we all have the right to want to save an important relationship. We have the right to protect ourselves and our children while we maintain the relationship.

If You Choose to Leave

Here are some things to consider as you plan to leave the abuser.

Support

We all need support people. Do you have people in your life who want to help you and who are able to help?

	Yes	No
Parents?		
Brothers and/or sisters?		
Friends?		
Other relatives?		
Counselors?		
Support group members?		
Others? (specify)		

Have these people helped you with past difficulties? Under what circumstances do you think you could call on them for help? What kinds of help do you think you could ask from them?

Basic Survival Needs

We all have different ideas about where and how we want to live. Do you have a plan that suits you?

	Yes	No
Do you have a place to live?		
Do you have furniture?		
Do you have money for food?		
Do you have medical care?		
Do you have a regular income that is large enough to live on?		
Do you have transportation?		
Do you have safe, reliable child care?		

If you answer no to any question, how would you solve that problem? Can your support people help?

From Mid-Valley Women's Crisis Service: *Safety plan,* March, 2000, The Author, www.mvwcs.com.   *Continued*

Planning for Safety—cont'd

Legal Protection		

Abusers use different threats to control victims. Many use divorce and custody battles, continued violence, and manipulation. Do you have a plan to deal with these potential problems?

	Yes	No
Will the abuser use legal battles?		
Will he try to steal the children?		
Will he abuse you if he finds you?		
Do you need a restraining order?		
Do you need a lawyer?		

If you answer yes to any of these questions, how can you solve these problems? Can your support people help?

If You Choose to Stay		

Here are some things to consider as you plan to return to your partner.

Support		

We all need support people. Do you have people in your life who want to help you and who are able to help?

	Yes	No
Parents?		
Brothers or sisters?		
Friends?		
Other relatives?		
Counselors?		
Support group members?		
Others? (specify)		

Have these people helped you with past difficulties? Under what circumstances do you think you could call on them for help? What kinds of help do you think you could ask from them?

Basic Survival Needs		

We all need a safe place to go in a crisis. Do you have a plan you can carry out?

	Yes	No
Do you have a safe place to go?		
Do you have money or a way to get money?		
Do you have transportation or a way out?		

If you answer no to any question, how would you solve that problem? Can your support people help?

From Mid-Valley Women's Crisis Service: *Safety plan,* March, 2000, The Author, www.mvwcs.com.

T A B L E 23-7—cont'd

Planning for Safety—cont'd

Legal Protection		
Abusers use different threats to control victims. Do you have a plan for handling legal problems?		
	Yes	**No**
Do you recognize when he is getting abusive?		
Will you get out while you are still safe?		
Do you know how to get a restraining order?		
Will you call the police for protection?		
Do you need a lawyer?		
If you answer no to any question, how would you solve that problem? Can your support people help?		

nurse working with the client over a long period of time can promote the most favorable climate for improved care. Time is required to gain an older adult client's confidence and to build a trusting relationship.

As individuals age, they confront ongoing losses. One of the most significant of these is the threat of losing their living arrangement. The feelings of grief and loss associated with this threat may influence an individual to tolerate abusive behavior from the caregiver to stay in their own home or apartment. The nurse must be aware of this need for independence because it may seem bewildering to others why an older adult would tolerate such behavior. As long as the client can make competent decisions, he or she has the legal autonomy to do so.

The nurse should also work with all family members or caregivers who provide care for the older adult client and help promote healthier relationships. Stress is a contributing factor to abuse. Helping the caregiver deal with stress by finding respite care, a home health aide, or counseling may help. Most older adult victims live with the offender and are dependent on them; consequently, to help the victim, the nurse must also help the offender deal with the stresses that are causing or contributing to the abuse. The caregiver may also have problems such as mental illness or drug or alcohol abuse. Until the nurse deals with these problems, the abuse will most likely continue.

The nurse should respect the patient's right to privacy and confidentiality. However, in states with mandatory reporting laws for the abuse of children,

women, or older adults, the nurse *must* comply with the law. Nurses must be familiar with community resources for the client and family. The clinical issue of abuse is rarely managed by nursing alone, but rather in combination with other disciplines, which may include physician, child and/or adult protective services, social worker, probation officer, chaplain, and police. The nurse should use an interdisciplinary approach whenever possible for optimal outcomes.

Precise charting is a crucial aspect of providing help to all victims of abuse and complying with medicolegal requirements. The nurse should record observations fully and completely and refrain from opinions and interpretations. This is especially important because court proceedings may use documentation that may have direct bearing on the victim's welfare.

When dealing with abuse, competing interests of the family, community, or institution often surface, such as the following:

- Financial dependency of caregivers upon the older adult
- Myths that an intact family is the ideal, children are better off in a two-parent home, and family problems should stay within the family
- Institutional short staffing that does not ensure the safe care of older adults

The nurse has the moral and legal obligation to prioritize the needs of the victim before all others.

FIGURE **23-3**

Clinical decision-making tree for detecting and treating elder abuse (From Hakala KLD: *Clinical decision making tree for detecting and treating elder abuse,* unpublished manuscript, 1999).

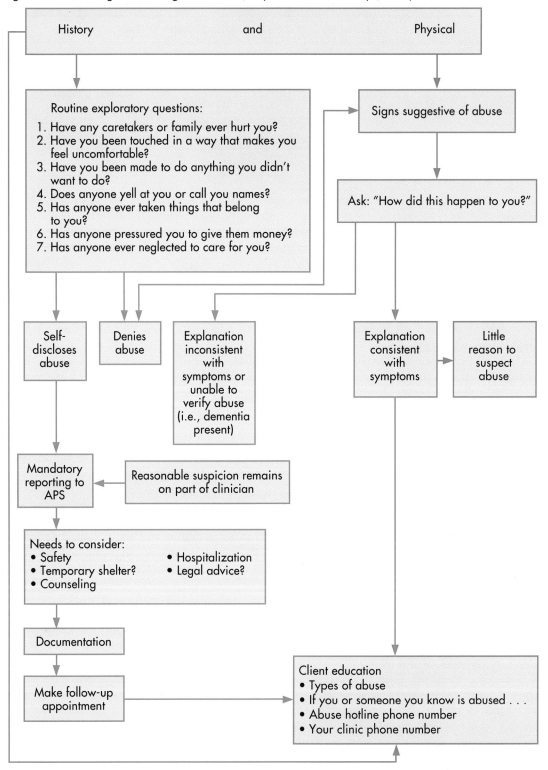

Depending upon the circumstances, this may require considerable courage and commitment.

Tertiary Prevention

The goal of tertiary prevention is to provide rehabilitative services to violent families. Involvement of a social service agency or local law enforcement members will be necessary if an injury has resulted in a report. Prosecution and punishment of the abuser or court-ordered removal of the victim from the family situation may occur. Professional counseling services and self-help or court-ordered groups can be helpful to the family. Long-term follow-up and supervision may be necessary as in any rehabilitative situation.

Tertiary prevention is aimed at the rehabilitation of a victim who has been severely beaten. When dealing with an abused victim, the nurse should focus on the person first. Accepting the victim and developing a trusting relationship is important for the patient and nurse to work together. The nurse should make community resources available to the patient. Telephone numbers for crisis lines and shelters need to be posted throughout the community in such areas as health clinic waiting rooms, public restrooms, bus stations, churches, and grocery stores. Nurses can carry cards in their pockets with referral numbers and give them to victims for future use.

Long-term care is necessary for an abuse victim. Maintaining contact with the individual and continuing support is essential for therapeutic nursing intervention. Support in the victim's ability to make decisions, even small ones, can help empower the abused victim. Many victims make the decision to remain in an abusive relationship; therefore health care providers may experience helplessness and possible anger toward the client. The nurse must understand the dynamics underlying the victim's decision to stay. The victim may take months or years to feel empowered to leave the situation. During this time, the nurse can provide crucial support and continue to offer resources. The nurse will be frustrated not knowing when or if these resources will be used; however, the nurse is most effective if he or she remains diligent in his or her support despite apparent lack of progress.

Tertiary care for a victim of child abuse usually entails a family involved in the court system. The courts or a local government agency such as protective services may refer the family to the community health nurse. The nurse may work with the parents while the child is in foster care after severe abuse; when a child is returned to his or her family, the nurse may provide ongoing care and supervision. The public health nurse must work with other health care providers and community agencies such as social workers, probation officers, and school nurses to provide coordinated care.

Tertiary prevention is important for children and adolescents who were sexually abused. Psychotherapy is usually necessary to resolve emotional problems that result from sexual abuse. These can be numerous and include anxiety, anger, eating disorders, and somatic complaints such as headaches, abdominal distress, and concern with the genitourinary tract in younger children. Older girls are at increased risk for substance abuse, sexual promiscuity, pregnancy, and prostitution. They may become truants or run away from home. This behavior should be viewed as a way to escape the dysfunctional family situation and not as a means of normal adolescent rebellion.

Tertiary prevention may continue in the treatment of the adult woman who was sexually abused as a child. Sexuality issues often surface when these individuals require gynecological or mental health services. All of these patients require sensitivity during physical examinations and procedures. Some of the women may benefit from seeing a female practitioner to increase their comfort level. Depression and sleep disorders are common complaints. These women often experience anxiety and low self-esteem and may have chronic sexual problems dealing with fear of intimate relationships. Self-destructive behavior and substance abuse may also be evident. The first step to receiving treatment is the recognition of the problem; nurses play an important role in recognition. After the nurse identifies the problem, he or she should refer the patient to a mental health professional for specific assistance. The nurse should remain available and in a supportive relationship with the patient.

Many obstacles may be present for the nurse in tertiary prevention of abusive situations in older adults. These include the reluctance to report the abuse, limited access to the client in his or her home, lack of consistent mandatory reporting laws, or lack of verifiable evidence. An additional factor is that the client is an adult and should be able to control his or her life as much as possible. An adult should be able to live in the manner that he or she chooses freely and safely. Care should not overly restrict the individual's freedoms.

Just as care is not forced on a battered woman, care cannot be forced on an older adult. Older adults who are deemed mentally incompetent have legal protection in many states similar to that provided for abused children. More research is necessary to develop appropriate care for older adult citizens because this is the fastest growing segment of the population. Increased momentum for the protection of older adults is building as consumer groups such as the

AARP and the Gray Panthers advocate for change. The aging of the baby boomers is also expected to accelerate political advocacy for protection of older adults.

SAFETY OF THE HEALTH PROFESSIONAL

Nonfatal workplace violence tends to be higher (over 85%) in certain service-oriented work environments including health care (Elliott, 1997). Such

---

BOX **23-2**

Safety Issues for the Community Health Nurse

Plan Ahead
- Know the area you are visiting.
- Schedule the visit ahead of time and get the correct address, directions, and information about who will be in the home.
- Tell the office where you will be and check in regularly.
- Carry a small amount of money and change for pay telephones and keep other items to a minimum.
- Dress for function and mobility and wear a name tag.
- Ensure that the vehicle you drive is in good repair, has a full gas tank, and has emergency equipment. Always carry two sets of car keys.

Approaching the Home
- Notice the environment, animals, fences, activity, indicators of crime, and places you could go for assistance if necessary.
- Walk with confidence and maintain a professional attitude.
- Listen for signs of fighting before knocking. If you hear sounds of fighting, leave!
- Do not enter a home if you suspect an unsafe situation.

In the Home
- Be aware of who is in the home and what is going on. If angry people are in the home, use your professional and social skills. Do not expect the client to protect you.
- Note the exits and sit between the client and an exit of the home. Be prepared to leave quickly if the situation changes suddenly.
- If someone in the home is violent, leave and call 911.

Handling a Tight Situation
- Do not show fear; control your breathing.
- Speak calmly and in a soothing manner. Be assertive but not aggressive.
- Repeat the reason for your visit and find a reason to leave.

Leaving the Home
- Take all of your belongings and keep your car keys in your hand.
- Watch for cars following you when you leave. Do not stop. If you feel that you are in danger, go to the nearest police station or well-lighted business and ask for help.

Trust Your Instincts. Never Forget Your Own Safety.

Adapted from Oregon Public Health Association, Public Health Nursing Section, Seattle-King County Department of Public Health, Washington State Public Health Association: *Public health nursing domestic violence protocol (booklet),* Seattle, Wash, and Salem, Ore, 1993, The Authors.

violence is widely believed to be underreported, perhaps in part from beliefs that it is an expected part of the job, especially in some specific settings (e.g., mental health and emergency departments). In recent years, workplace violence has gained increased attention because more dramatic incidents (e.g., shootings) and frequency have occurred. Nurses who work in public health roles are not immune to such risks because their work may bring them in contact with individuals prone to violent behavior. Identification of risk factors may offer some protection to the worker.

Simonowitz (1993) identified the following three risk factors for workplace violence that are applicable to the situation of the nurse in dealing with violence in the family and community:

1. Environment: The nurse who works in the community must be aware of his or her environment because a health care worker making home visits has little control over conditions of the community or the home. The nurse will sometimes find himself or herself in homes where violence is the rule.
2. Work practices: The greatest protection for the nurse is in careful work practices. Many involve common sense; others involve careful preparation. Preparing for the home visits, keeping the office aware of where he or she is at all times, and having emergency equipment such as a cellular telephone or a beeper should be standard.
3. Victim's and perpetrator's profiles: Knowledge of previous violence by a member of a household may be the best indicator of the future potential for violence in that family. Interviewing a victim of violence, where the secrecy is broken, may put the nurse at risk if the perpetrator is on the premises or suddenly returns. In situations of suspected danger, the nurse should ask for a police escort. Box 23-2 offers safety tips for public health nurses.

SUMMARY

Violence is a major public health issue in the United States and affects individuals across the life cycle. Morbidity and mortality statistics indicate that violence is epidemic in many communities. Violence at home, in the neighborhood, and at school affects countless numbers of individuals in the United States who live in fear for their lives. The easy access to and proliferation of handguns in the United States has been a major contributor to violence.

Violence can become transgenerational if the cycle of violence is not broken. This cycle causes indescribable pain to children, women, and older adults, who are the primary victims. The abuser is also a victim and the ultimate victim is society, who must care and pay for the results of violent acts.

Violence has been declared a public health epidemic; therefore national objectives for reducing violence have been identified. The efforts of public health have been mobilized to help stop this epidemic and bring healing to the nation. Health for all includes freedom from intentional injuries caused by violence. The core public health functions of needs assessment and surveillance, policy development, and assurance are useful methods of combating this epidemic.

The public health nurse can be a crucial member of the team confronting violence. Commitment to caring about the problem is a first step. Careful assessment of all clients for evidence of injury is a second step. Teaching alternate methods of dealing with stress, improved parenting relationships, and considerate care of older adults is the essence of primary prevention. If an upstream approach of discovering the problem and then preventing it from occurring is used, ultimately the transgenerational cycle will be broken and society as a whole will be healthier.

LEARNING ACTIVITIES

1. Determine professional responsibilities in the state by securing a copy or reviewing the reporting laws for child abuse, women battering, spousal rape, and elder abuse.
2. Using the telephone directory, find three public or private community agencies in the community that provide help for victims of violence. Make a list of the telephone numbers.
3. Call a child abuse hotline in the community and ask them what services they provide.
4. Call a battered women's shelter and determine the procedure in securing shelter placement for a battered victim and children.
5. Visit a respite center for older adults and observe the clients and the activities that are provided for them. What observed behaviors would contribute to stress in the caregiver?

6. Follow the newspapers for one month and clip articles that deal with violence. Determine how many individuals were killed or injured during that period in incidents of violence. How many of them were gun related and what type of weapon was used?

7. Find out what types of support groups exist in the community for older adult caregivers.

REFERENCES

Alcohol abuse and violence against women, *J Psychosoc Nurs Ment Health* 36(8):9, 1999.

Blow R, Gest E: A social disease: violence, *Mother Jones* 18:26, 1993.

Butterfield F: Crime panel fears new wave of violence, *San Francisco Chronicle* A7, January 6, 1996.

Campbell J, Humphreys J: *Nursing care of survivors of family violence,* St. Louis, 1993, Mosby.

Carlton L: *Elder abuse prevention protocol,* San Francisco, 1983, San Francisco Task Force.

Centers for Disease Control and Prevention: Nonfatal and fatal firearm-related injuries: United States, 1993-1997, *Morb Mortal Wkly Rep* 48(45):1029, 1999a.

Centers for Disease Control and Prevention: Perceptions of child sexual abuse as a public health problem, Vermont, September 1995, *Morb Mortal Wkly Rep* 46(34):801, 1997.

Centers for Disease Control and Prevention: Suicide among black youths: United States, 1980-1995, *Morb Mortal Wkly Rep* 47(10):193, 1998.

Centers for Disease Control and Prevention: Suicide among children, adolescents, and young adults: United States, 1980-1992, *Morb Mortal Wkly Rep* 44(15):289-291, 1995.

Centers for Disease Control and Prevention: Youth risk behavior surveillance: national alternative high school youth risk behavior survey, United States, 1998, *Morb Mortal Wkly Rep* 48(SS07):1, 1999b.

Centers for Disease Control and Prevention, National Center for Injury Prevention and Control: *Fact sheet on dating violence,* March 1, 2000a, The Author, www.cdc.gov/ncipc/dvp/yvpt/datviol.html.

Centers for Disease Control and Prevention, National Center for Injury Prevention and Control: *Suicide in the United States,* March 1, 2000b, The Author, www.cdc.gov/ncipc/factsheets/suifacts.html.

Curry MA, Doyle BA, Gilhooley J: Abuse among pregnant adolescents: differences by developmental age, *Am J Matern Child Nurs* 23(3):144, 1998.

Dannenberg A, Baker S, Li G: Intentional and unintentional injuries in women, *Ann Epidemiol* 4:133, 1994.

Elders J: Violence as a public health issue for children, *Childhood Educ* 70:260, 1994.

Elliott PP: Violence in health care: what nurse managers need to know, *Nurs Manage* 28(12):38, 1997.

Foege WH: Global Public Health: targeting inequities, *JAMA* 279(24):1931, 1998.

Gray HM, Foshee V: Adolescent dating violence: differences between one-sided and mutually violent profiles, *J Interpersonal Violence* 12(1):126, 1997.

Hakala KLD: *Clinical decision making tree for detecting and treating elder abuse,* unpublished manuscript, 1999.

Hakala KLD: *Personal communication,* November 20, 2000.

Kellerman AL et al: Suicide in the home in relation to gun ownership, *N Engl J Med* 327:467, 1992.

Koop C, Lundberg G: Violence in America: a public health emergency, *JAMA* 267:3075, 1992.

Loring M, Smith R: Health care barriers and interventions for battered women, *Public Health Rep* 109:328, 1994.

Lyman SA, Hughes-McLain C, Thompson G: 'Date-rape drugs:' a growing concern, *Health Educ J* 29(5): 271, 1998.

Mason J: Prevention of violence: a public health commitment, *Public Health Rep* 106:265, 1991.

Max W, Rice DP: Shooting in the dark: estimating the cost of firearm injuries, *Health Affairs* 12(4):171, 1993.

McFarlane J, Parker B: Preventing abuse during pregnancy: an assessment and intervention protocol, *MCN Am J Matern Child Nurs* 19(6):321-324, 1994.

Mid-Valley Women's Crisis Service: *Safety plan,* March, 2000, The Author, www.mvwcs.com.

Mother goose nursery rhymes, Bath, England, 2000, Robert Frederick Publishing.

Nichols FH, Zwelling E: *Maternal-newborn nursing: theory and practice,* Philadelphia, 1997, W.B. Saunders.

Oregon Public Health Association, Public Health Nursing Section, Seattle-King County Department of Public Health, Washington State Public Health Association: *Public health nursing domestic violence protocol (booklet),* Seattle, Wash, and Salem, Ore, 1993, The Authors.

Ozmar B: Encountering victims of interpersonal violence, *Crit Care Nurs Clin North Am* 6:515, 1994.

Palestra: *An epidemic of violence,* July, 1999, The Author, www.oclc.org.

Rawlins P, Williams S, Beck C: *Mental-health psychiatric nursing: a holistic life-cycle approach,* St. Louis, 1993, Mosby.

Rosenberg M, O'Carroll P, Kenneth E: Let's be clear: violence is a public health problem, *JAMA* 267:3071-3072, 1992.

Ruttenberg H: The limited promise of public health methodologies to prevent youth violence, *Yale Law* 103:1885, 1994.

Sassetti M: Domestic violence, *Primary Care Clin Office Pract* 20:289, 1993.

Simonowitz J: *Guidelines for security and safety of health care and community service workers,* San Diego, 1993, Medical Unit, Division of Occupational Safety and Health, Department of Industrial Relations.

Sonkin DJ, Durphy M: *Learning to live without violence: a handbook for men,* ed 4, Volcano, Calif, 1997, Volcano Press.

Stein A: Will health care reform protect victims of abuse? treating domestic violence as a public health issue, *Human Rights* 21:16, 1994.

Stewart M: RNs confront causes and consequences of school violence, *Am Nurs* 30(5):16-17, 1998.

Tjaden P, Thoennes N: *Prevalence, incidence and consequences of violence against women: findings for the National Violence Against Women Survey,* Washington, DC, 1998, US Department of Justice, CDC.

US Department of Health and Human Services: *Healthy People 2010,* Washington, DC, 2000, USDHHS, PHS.

Walker LE: *The battered woman,* New York, 1979, Harper & Row.

White JS, Koss MP: Courtship violence: incidence in a national sample of higher education students, *Violence Vict* 6(4):247, 1991.

Winett LR: Constructing violence as a public health problem, *Public Health Rep* 113:498-507, 1998.

Wolfe S: As America ages: look for signs of abuse, *RN* 61(8), 1998.

Wolfner G, Gelles R: A profile of violence toward children: a national study, *Child Abuse Neglect* 17:97, 1993.

Substance Abuse

Erika Madrid and Joanne M. Hall

Upon completion of this chapter, the reader will be able to do the following:

1. Discuss the historical trends and current conceptions of the cause and treatment of substance abuse.
2. Describe the current social, political, and economic aspects of substance abuse.
3. Describe the ethical and legal implications of substance abuse.
4. Detail the typical symptoms and consequences of substance abuse.
5. Identify issues related to substance abuse in various populations encountered in community health nursing practice.
6. Apply the nursing process to substance abuse problems.

abuse
addiction
codependency
continuation stage
dependence
dual diagnosis
gateway drugs
harm reduction
initiation
mutual help groups
professional enablers
substance abuse
transition stage

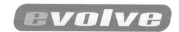

http://evolve.elsevier.com/Nies/

Perhaps no other health-related condition has as many far-reaching consequences in contemporary Western society as substance abuse. These consequences include a wide range of social, psychological, physical, economic, and political problems. Health problems and disability associated with substance abuse total approximately $276 billion annually. It costs an estimated $1000 per person for health care, law enforcement, accidents, treatment, and lost productivity related to substance abuse. More deaths, illnesses, and disabilities are attributed to substance abuse than any other preventable health condition in the United States (USDHHS, 2000).

Considering the social consequences of substance abuse, many offenders commit crimes while under the influence of drugs or alcohol or both. At least half the people arrested for homicide, theft, and assault used illicit drugs near the time of their arrest (Horgan, 1993).

All aggregates in society are potentially affected by substance abuse problems. Infants are born addicted to alcohol, stimulants, or opiates and are at risk for developmental problems because they are exposed in utero. Indirect social effects of substance abuse include relationship conflicts, divorce, spousal and child abuse, and child neglect (Campbell and Landenburger, 1995; Scherling, 1994). Although well intended, many local and national efforts to fight substance abuse are often inadequate and ineffective (Drucker, 1999).

In the past, alcoholism and drug addiction were problems of the urban poor; society and most health professionals virtually ignored them. Substance abuse problems now pervade all levels of U.S. society and awareness has increased. Community health nurses must be aware of substance abuse because it is a problem that frequently intertwines with other medical and social conditions.

This chapter focuses on helping community health nurses recognize substance abuse in their clients and the larger community. The chapter reviews historic trends, the causes of substance abuse, the most common symptoms of these disorders, and treatment options. The authors suggest nursing interventions appropriate for assisting substance abusers to provide the community health nurse with tools for addressing these problems.

HISTORIC TRENDS IN THE USE OF ALCOHOL AND ILLICIT DRUGS

During the twentieth century, fluctuations in the use of alcohol and illicit drugs were influenced by shifts in public tolerance and political and economic trends. In

general, alcohol use gained more social acceptance than other drug use. Alcohol consumption in the United States was higher during World War I and II and decreased during Prohibition and the Great Depression. Alcohol use was highest during the 1980s when states lowered the drinking age to 18 years of age. Lawmakers became alarmed at the increased rate of drinking and the increased number of alcohol-related deaths among 18- to 25-year-olds after lowering the drinking age and thereby reversed the decision. During the late 1980s, alcohol use declined after the minimum drinking age was reinstated to 21 years of age. The decline in alcohol consumption in the 1990s is attributed to less tolerant national attitudes toward drinking, increased societal and legal pressures and actions against drinking and driving, and increased health concerns among Americans (National Institute on Alcohol Abuse and Alcoholism, 1997).

Public attitudes and governmental policies have also influenced the history of illicit drug use. Although nineteenth-century physicians prescribed morphine for a large variety of ailments, the discovery of the addictive properties of cocaine and opiates led to increased governmental regulation at the beginning of the twentieth century. The Harrison Narcotic Act of 1914, and subsequent laws, lessened the medical profession's control over the use of addicting drugs; the legislation specified that the physician could prescribe these drugs only in the course of general practice and not to maintain an addiction (Brecher, 1972). This limitation on the physician's power to prescribe and dispense addictive drugs and restrictions on the importation of narcotics limited the supply of these drugs until the 1950s and 1960s. At that time, an increase in illegal drug trafficking caused heroin use to become a problem in inner cities.

By the 1970s, drugs were increasingly available and the younger population adopted a more positive attitude toward drug use. The use of heroin and other illicit drugs spread beyond urban drug subcultures to the general population. Alarmed by the social and personal consequences of this change, public tolerance decreased and prevention and treatment programs were given more attention and resources. After peaking in 1979, illicit drug use decreased among most segments of the population throughout the 1980s and 1990s (Drucker, 1999).

To combat concerns of the physical, social, and psychological impact of drug abuse and dependence, federal drug policy has emphasized law enforcement and interdiction to reduce the supply of illicit drugs. Despite the large amounts of money spent toward

TABLE 24-1

Reported Substance Use by Age and Racial and Ethnic Group: 1996

	White		Hispanic		African-American	
	All Ages	**12 to 17**	**All Ages**	**12 to 17**	**All Ages**	**12 to 17**
Alcohol	68.0%	34.4%	*	34.6%	*	26.6%
Cigarettes	33.3%	27.4%	28.6%	20.1%	32.9%	16.7%
Any illicit drug	10.8%	17.1%	9.6%	16.5%	13.4%	15.9%
Marijuana	8.6%	13.3%	7.0%	13.0%	11.1%	13.0%
Cocaine	1.7%	1.3%	2.4%	2.0%	2.4%	0.6%
Inhalants	1.3%	4.9%	0.7%	2.8%	0.5%	0.8%
Heroin	0.2%	*	0.2%	*	0.2%	*

From Substance Abuse and Mental Health Services Administration, Office of Applied Statistics: *National household survey on drug abuse: population estimates 1996,* USDHHS Pub No SMA, Rockville, Md, 1996, USDHHS, PHS.
*Not available.

reaching this goal, this strategy has been less than effective (Drucker, 1999). Trends have shown renewed interest in prevention and treatment efforts to decrease the amount of illicit drug use in society and lessen its impact (National Institute on Drug Abuse [NIDA], 1997).

PREVALENCE OF SUBSTANCE ABUSE

The U.S. National Household Survey on Drug Abuse (SAMHSA, 1998) reported that 6.2% of the general U.S. population over age 12 years were illicit drug users and used at least once in the 30 days before the survey. Additionally, approximately 52% of the U.S. general population used alcohol in the previous 30 days. Binge drinkers (i.e., those who consumed more than five drinks on one occasion during the previous 30 days) accounted for 15.7% of this total and heavy drinkers (i.e., those who consumed five or more drinks five or more times during the previous 30 days) accounted for 5.9% of the group.

Marijuana was the most commonly used illicit drug, especially among teens. Of those aged 12 to 17 years, 9.8% used marijuana in the month before the survey. The nonmedical use of prescription medications (e.g., tranquilizers, sedatives, analgesics, and stimulants) were the second most commonly misused drugs and 1.1% of the U.S. general population ingested them. During this time, 0.8% of the U.S.

population used cocaine. Other drugs, such as heroin, hallucinogens, stimulants, and inhalants, were used by less than 1% of the U.S. population (SAMHSA, 1998).

Demographic correlates in the 1998 SAMHSA survey showed some regional, gender, and racial differences related to individuals using alcohol and illegal substances. People living in the West had the greatest percentage of drug use at 7.3%, compared with 6.7% for those in the North Central Region, 5.8% for those in the Northeast, and 5.5% for those in the South. Table 24-1 provides information about substance abuse among various racial and ethnic groups for 1996 and Table 24-2 lists information specific to alcohol use and abuse for 1998.

In terms of gender related to drug use, the 1998 SAMHSA Household Survey reported that 8.1% of males used illicit drugs during the month before the survey compared with 4.5% of females. Individuals between 18 and 20 years of age had the highest prevalence of drug use (19.9% of the population). Prevalence among those aged 16 to 17 years was 16.4% and prevalence among those aged 21 to 25 years was 13.5%. Use percentages declined further as age increased.

There are distinctly different patterns for alcohol problems in women. In the 1998 Household Survey, 59% of men and 45% of women consumed alcohol in the 30 days before the survey. Concurrently, 23.2% of men were binge drinkers compared with 8.6% of women and 9.7% of men were heavy drinkers

TABLE 24-2

Alcohol Use by Race and Ethnic Group: 1998

	Percent Use in Previous 30 Days	Binge Drinking	Heavy Drinking
Caucasian	55.3%	16.5%	6.0%
African-American	45.4%	15.7%	6.5%
Hispanic	39.8%	11.4%	4.9%

From Substance Abuse and Mental Health Services Administration, Office of Applied Statistics: *National household survey on drug abuse: population estimates 1998,* USDHHS Pub No SMA, Rockville, Md, 1998, USDHHS, PHS.

compared with 2.4% of women (SAMHSA, 1998). Although the majority of adult women drank alcohol occasionally, the group that drank the most was between 21 and 34 years of age. This is supported by other literature that verifies drinking decreases as women age (Wilsnack et al., 1995).

HEALTHY PEOPLE 2010 OBJECTIVES AND SUBSTANCE ABUSE

The USDHHS and PHS, has set new goals and objectives for substance abuse in *Healthy People 2010: National Health Promotion and Disease Prevention Objectives.* The objectives consist of norms and targets for the decade for health conditions for the U.S. population. These new objectives for substance abuse were largely determined by the progress of the previous objectives set for *Healthy People 2000.*

On review, there were mixed results related to progress toward the year 2000 objectives regarding substance abuse (USDHHS, 2000). Alcohol-related motor vehicle deaths per 100,000 declined from 8.9 in 1990 to 6.5 in 1996 (target was 5.5 per 100,000). Cirrhosis deaths declined for the total population from 9.2 per 100,000 in 1987 to 7.6 per 100,000 in 1995 (target was 6.0 per 100,000) (USDHHS, 2000).

Conversely, drug-related deaths increased from 3.6 per 100,000 in 1990 to 5.1 per 100,000 in 1995 (target was 3.0 per 100,000). Drug abuse-related emergency department visits also increased from 175.8 per 100,000 in 1991 to 207 per 100,000 in 1996 (target was 140.6 per 100,000) (USDHHS, 2000).

Use by adolescents and young adults between 12 and 17 years of age declined for some substances and increased for others. Although use of alcohol declined from 21.6% to 18.8% in 1995, marijuana use rose from 6.0% in 1994 to 8.2% in 1995 before declining to 7.1% in 1996. Cocaine use rose from 0.3% in 1994 to 0.6% in 1996. Cigarette use dropped slightly from 18.9% in 1994 to 18.3% in 1996. In 1995, heavy drinking during the past two weeks remained relatively stable in high school seniors and college students. Thirty percent of seniors reported heavy drinking, which nears the 28% target. Fifty percent of college students reported drinking heavily (USDHHS, 2000). Table 24-3 presents selected objectives from *Healthy People 2010* related to substance abuse.

CONCEPTUALIZATIONS OF SUBSTANCE ABUSE

Conceptualizations of substance abuse and dependence have changed over the years, more often for political and social reasons than for scientific reasons. Some conceptualizations focus on the phenomenon of **addiction**, which is manifested by compulsive use patterns and the onset of withdrawal symptoms when substance use is abruptly stopped. Other views focus on the problems resulting from the substance use itself, regardless of whether an addictive pattern is present. Problematic consequences of substance abuse include intoxication, psychological dependence, relational conflicts, employment or economic difficulties, legal difficulties, and health problems. For example, addiction need not be present for individuals to experience legal consequences of illicit drug use, driving while intoxicated, or alcohol- or drug-related domestic violence.

Drawing fine distinctions among ideas of dependence, addiction, and abuse concerning substance use may seem irrelevant if there is evidence that the substance use has become problematic (Widiger and Smith, 1994). However, broadly labeling all habitual or compulsive behavior patterns as "addiction" or

TABLE 24-3

Healthy People 2010: Selected Objectives for Substance Abuse

Objective	Baseline (1998)	Target
13-3: Reduce the number of new AIDS cases among females and males who inject drugs	12,099 new cases in 1998	9075
16-17a: Increase reported abstinence from alcohol in the past month by pregnant women	86%	94%
18-10: Increase the proportion of persons with co-occurring substance abuse and mental disorders who receive treatment for both disorders	NA	NA
26-1a: Reduce alcohol-related deaths in motor vehicle crashes	6.1 per 100,000	4 per 100,000
26-3: Reduce drug-induced deaths	5.1 per 100,000	1 per 100,000
26-6: Reduce the proportion of adolescents who report that they rode, during the previous 30 days, with a driver who had been drinking	37% (grades 9 to 12)	30% (grades 9 to 12)
26-9c: Increase the proportion of high school seniors never using alcoholic beverages	19%	29%
26-11b: Reduce the proportion of college students engaging in binge drinking of alcoholic beverages	39%	20%
26-20: Increase the number of admissions to substance abuse treatment for injection drug use	167,960	200,000
26-25: Extend legal requirements for maximum blood alcohol concentration levels of 0.08% for motor vehicle drivers aged 21 years and older	16 states	All states and the District of Columbia

From US Department of Health and Human Services: *Healthy people 2010: conference edition,* Washington, DC, 2000, PHS.

"dependence" may obscure the fact that very specific interventions may be needed for each separate "addictive problem," such as overeating, and gambling.

Definitions

The term **substance abuse** came into common usage in the 1970s. Earlier conceptualizations generally focused on either alcoholism or drug addiction as singular addictive disorders. Currently, most substance abuse theories identify core commonalties that occur in regard to use of a variety of different substances or in relation to compulsive behavior syndromes (Leshner, 1997). There is also an emphasis on relapse prevention that may include moderate use goals and abstinence (Larimer and Marlatt, 1990).

There remains debate about how substance use and abuse should be defined and what substances should be included under this heading. Traditional conceptualizations of substance abuse focus solely on alcohol and illicit street drugs. Other conceptualizations include prescription medications such as tranquilizers or analgesics as abusable substances. In eating disorders such as bulimia and compulsive overeating, food is viewed as the abused substance. Table 24-4 shows a classification scheme for commonly abused substances.

In addition to varying in their abuse potential, substances vary in their degree of potential harm to those who use them and to others in the immediate environment. Tobacco is an example of a substance that is unsafe to the smoker and to those who inhale secondhand smoke. Those who abuse alcohol may also harm others by driving under the influence or

T A B L E 24-4

Classification of Commonly Used and Abused Substances

Substance	Desired Effect	Possible Withdrawal Symptoms
CNS Depressants		
Alcohol Barbiturates Sedative-hypnotics (e.g., benzodiazapines [Rohypnol]) Tranquilizers (e.g., GHB)	Euphoria, disinhibition, and sedation Retrograde amnesia Sedation and amnesia (e.g., "date rape" drug)	Anxiety, irritability, seizures, delusions, hallucinations, and paranoia
CNS Stimulants		
Amphetamines (e.g., methamphetamine) Cocaine Nicotine Caffeine	Euphoria, hyperactivity, omnipotence, insomnia, and anorexia	Depression, apathy, lethargy, and sleepiness
Narcotics-Opioids		
Codeine Meperidine and acetaminophen (e.g., Demerol) Hydromorphone (e.g., Dilaudid) Fentanyl Heroin Methadone Morphine Opium Oxycodone (e.g., Percodan)	Euphoria and sedation	Anxiety; irritability; agitation; runny nose, watery eyes; chills, sweating; nausea and vomiting; diarrhea; tremors; and yawning
Hallucinogens		
Mescaline LSD PCP (e.g., Ketamine) STP and MDA (e.g., "Ecstasy") Psilocybin (e.g., mushrooms)	Hallucinations, illusions, and heightened awareness PCP: violent dissociative and anesthetic effect	Depression
Cannabis		
Marijuana Hashish and THC	Relaxation, euphoria, and altered perceptions	Restlessness, insomnia, and anxiety
Inhalants		
Gasoline Toluene acetate Cleaning fluids Airplane cement Amyl nitrate	Euphoria	Restlessness, anxiety, and irritability

Adapted from Faltz B, Rinaldi J: *AIDS and substance abuse: a training manual for health care professionals*, San Francisco, 1987, Regents of the University of California. Used with permission.
CNS, central nervous system; *MDA,* methylene-dioxy-phenyl-iso-propanolamine; *PCP,* phencyclidine; *STP,* 2,5,dimethoxy,4,methyl amphetamine; *THC,* tetrahydrocannabinol.

by engaging in violent activities (e.g., domestic violence).

Integrating the various opinions regarding the diagnosis of substance abuse, the American Psychiatric Association (APA) has classified substance use disorders as either "dependence" or "abuse" (APA, 1994). The APA focused on the following psychoactive substances that affect the nervous system: alcohol, amphetamines, cannabis, cocaine, caffeine, hallucinogens, inhalants, nicotine, opioids, phencyclidine, sedatives, and hypnotics or anxiolytics. Substance use disorders can also be categorized as being in partial or full remission.

The criteria for the diagnosis of **dependence** include a cluster of cognitive, behavioral, and physiological symptoms that indicate continued use of the substance despite significant substance-related problems. A pattern of repeated, self-administered use results in tolerance, withdrawal, and compulsive drug-taking behaviors, which are frequently accompanied by a craving or strong desire for the substance.

In contrast, a diagnosis of substance **abuse** indicates a maladaptive pattern of substance use that is manifested by recurrent and significant adverse consequences related to repeated use of a substance. This may be a precursor of substance dependence. These adverse consequences include failure to fulfill major role obligations, repeated use in physically hazardous situations, multiple legal problems, and recurrent social and interpersonal problems. Boxes 24-1 and 24-2 list the criteria for diagnosis of substance dependence and substance abuse, respectively.

Etiology of Substance Abuse

Substance abuse has an impact on virtually every aspect of individual and communal life and many institutions and academic fields have addressed it. Several theories attempt to explain the cause and scope of these problems and offer solutions. Some theories address individual physiological, spiritual, and psychological factors. Others deal with social influences involving family, ethnicity, race, access to drugs, environmental stressors, economics, political status, culture, and sex roles. In most theories, a combination of factors is the underlying impetus for substance abuse.

Although physiological, medical model theorists have defined alcoholism as a loss of control over drinking or an individual malfunction; the cause of the disease of alcoholism was ambiguous in the past (Brown, 1969; Keller, 1972). Research has clearly

---

B O X   24-1

Diagnosis of Psychoactive Substance Dependence

A maladaptive pattern of substance use leading to clinically significant impairment or distress as manifested by three or more of the following occurring at any time in the same 12-month period:

1. Tolerance, as defined by either of the following:
   a. A need for markedly increased amounts of the substance to achieve intoxication or desired effect
   b. Markedly diminished effect with continued use of the same amount of the substance
2. Withdrawal, as manifested by either of the following:
   a. The characteristic withdrawal syndrome for the substance
   b. The same, or closely related, substance is taken to relieve or avoid withdrawal symptoms
3. Substance is often taken in larger amounts or over a longer period than intended
4. A persistent desire or unsuccessful efforts to cut down or control substance use
5. Much time is spent in activities necessary to obtain the substance, use the substance, or recover from its effects
6. Important social, occupational, or recreational activities are given up or reduced from substance use
7. Substance use is continued despite knowledge of having a persistent or recurrent physical or psychological problem that is likely to have been caused or exacerbated by the substance
8. Specify if with or without physiological dependence (e.g., tolerance or withdrawal).

Adapted with permission from American Psychiatric Association: *Diagnostic and statistical manual of mental disorders,* ed 4, Washington, DC, 1994, The Association.

---

identified genetic factors that increase a person's overall risk for alcohol abuse; there is strong evidence that alcoholism runs in families and genetic factors play an important role (Kendler and Prescott, 1998; NIDA, 1997).

BOX **24-2**

**Diagnosis of Psychoactive
Substance Abuse**

A. A maladaptive pattern of substance use leading to clinically significant impairment or distress as manifested by one or more of the
following occurring within a 12-month period:
1. Recurrent substance use resulting in a failure to fulfill major role obligations at work,
school, or home
2. Recurrent substance use in situations in
which it is physically hazardous
3. Recurrent substance-related legal problems
4. Continued substance use despite persistent or recurrent social or interpersonal
problems caused or exacerbated by the
effects of the substance
B. The symptoms have never met the criteria for
substance dependence for this class of
substance.

Adapted with permission from American Psychiatric
Association: *Diagnostic and statistical manual of mental
disorders,* ed 4, Washington, DC, 1994, The Association.

Individual and environmental factors also contribute to an increased risk for alcohol abuse. On the
individual level, a person's inherited sensitivity to
alcohol is a predictor for the development of alcohol
abuse. Two broad personality dimensions are also
associated with an increased risk for alcohol abuse.
One dimension is behavioral "under control," behavioral disinhibition, or deviance proneness marked by
unconventionality, overactivity, aggression, and impulsivity. The second personality dimension is "negative emotionality," which is marked by anxiety and
depression. Alcohol expectancies (i.e., beliefs about
anticipated consequences of drinking) are also a
predictor of alcohol abuse.

Medical models of alcoholism and other substance abuse conditions may not provide an understanding of commonalties among addictive behaviors
(e.g., excessive drinking, gambling, eating, drug use,
and sexual behavior). Cross-addiction, or multidrug
use, is more prevalent now than in the past and more
studies point to the presence of both automatic and
nonautomatic factors in addictive behavior. Specific

biological medical models are giving way to multicausal models.

In the biopsychosocial model, addiction is
thought to develop from an interplay of many factors.
Risk factors interact with protective factors to develop a predisposition toward drug or alcohol use.
This predisposition is then influenced by exposure
to the substance, availability, and the quality of the
first experience (e.g., pleasant or unpleasant). Continued availability of the substances and a social
support system that enables or supports their use is
also necessary. These factors combine to determine
whether addiction develops and is maintained.

SOCIOCULTURAL AND POLITICAL ASPECTS OF SUBSTANCE ABUSE

Within community settings, substance abuse problems
are not always easy to identify. For example, the
consequences of the sale and use of crack cocaine in
an inner-city, African-American neighborhood may
be apparent through media attention. However, the
silent ravages of alcohol abuse among elderly women
receive much less attention. Nurses must incorporate
the sociocultural and political dimensions of these
phenomena into caring for clients in the community
and being critical of media trends and biases.

Although there are subcultures with different
norms, the dominant culture drinking norms in the
United States are relatively permissive. Traditional
ceremonial and symbolic substance use patterns vary
significantly across cultures. Past cultural definitions
of "appropriate" use of alcohol and drugs may have
been dulled, leaving a void regarding social expectations. These cultural conditions create ambiguity in
clearly determining when a substance abuse problem exists. Furthermore, each subculture may define
abuse differently.

In addiction, a particular drug experience can be
understood as an interaction between the individual's
subjective mood and the actual pharmacological effects of the drug. This interaction does not take place
in a vacuum. Rather, the expectations of a drug's effect
are shaped by the user's culture and involve the adoption of roles taught by more experienced users and reinforced by other social groups, including health care
providers in some cases (Montagne and Scott, 1993).

Substances are also given economic value and are
bought and sold as commodities in a variety of social
arenas. The ways in which drugs, including medications and alcohol, are produced and distributed among

the various segments of the population are determined largely by economic, cultural, and political conditions. For example, the economic realities of the poor Colombians and Peruvians who rely on the growth and production of the coca leaf for financial survival can be understood as a confluence of larger society-level and individual-level factors. These individuals are involved in the drug trade for their financial survival. The drug trade is very lucrative for some; it raises their societal status, gives them access to material things, and provides an enhanced sense of power in that society. Among urban poor minority youth in the United States, the fact that drug trafficking often *precedes* drug use underscores the need for status and economic power (Greenberg and Schneider, 1994).

These changes in power can have other consequences on the subgroups within the culture who attain this new status. A group without cultural values, or with competing cultural values, suffers from chaos and disorganization. Competing value systems lead to cultural disintegration and a sense of powerlessness and hopelessness. The group becomes susceptible to forces that further threaten the group's ability to survive. Unable to organize or determine a collective direction because values conflict, the group and its members are separated and disempowered. The history of cocaine abuse and dependence among people of color is a good example of how these conditions are interrelated. Although cocaine use was epidemic in the 1980s, with crack cocaine most prevalent in poor communities, its use has declined markedly in recent years (Office of National Drug Control Policy, 1997).

Virtually all major theories of the origins of adolescent substance abuse agree that the perceived acceptance of problematic drug-using behavior among family, peers, and society is an important influence on an individual's decision to use or not use alcohol, tobacco, and drugs. The perception that alcohol use is socially acceptable correlates with the fact that more than 80% of American youths consume alcohol before their twenty-first birthday and the lack of social acceptance of other drugs correlates with comparatively lower rates of use. Similarly, widespread societal expectations that young people will engage in binge drinking may encourage this highly dangerous form of alcohol consumption (USDHHS, 2000).

TYPICAL COURSE OF ADDICTIVE ILLNESS

Perhaps the best approach to understanding the behavioral course and patterns of addictive illness is to view it on a continuum from initiation to dependency. However, it is necessary to note that not everyone who initiates drug or alcohol use will progress to dependency or display behaviors commonly associated with dependency. For example, data from surveys of high school seniors reveal that clear evidence does not exist proving that all cocaine users or other substance users will progress to addiction. This supports the idea that neither addiction nor dependency is a unitary phenomenon with a single isolated cause; it is the result of interactions among a host of variables.

Genetic and environmental vulnerabilities play important roles in the progression from initiation to continuation, transition, abuse, and, finally, addiction and dependency. Individuals often describe a progression that began with socially mediated use, which is **initiation**. Such use appears to meet usual expectations and occurs in the context of social interactions. For some, the substance and setting will be reinforcing and primes the individual for a pattern of use. For others, the experience will be unpleasant enough to prevent further use. In the case of stimulants such as cocaine, the drug produces such strong feelings of euphoria, alertness, control, and increased energy that future use is enticing, especially when the drug is easily accessible (Breiter et al., 1997).

The **continuation stage** of substance abuse is a subsequent period in which substance use persists but does not appear to be detrimental to the individual. In stimulant abuse, continued use often occurs in a binge pattern. Individuals are able to exercise some control over use, but use becomes more frequent. Neither the individual nor the social network views use during this stage as problematic.

A critical point is the **transition stage** from substance use to substance abuse. There may be evidence to both the users and their social networks that the use of the substance is having adverse effects. During this stage, users begin to use more often and in more varied settings. Rationalizations for use are commonly constructed during this stage to deny the seriousness and consequences of the substance use.

A user's social network may play a role in allowing the substance abuse to continue. Spouses may call work to report that their partner is "sick." Social network members may compensate for the fact that the student is absent from school, the car payment is late, or an important appointment is canceled or forgotten. These distress signals are common but often go unrecognized because periods of use are often interspersed with periods of abstinence. This reinforces the individual's, and often the significant other's, perceived sense of control over the substance use.

Changes in the individual's physical response to the drug play a significant role in the progression of susceptible individuals from abuse to dependency. In cocaine, heroin, and alcohol dependency, abstinence symptomatology plays a significant role in the progression from use to abuse and to dependency and addiction. Indeed, abstinence in the stimulant abuser can result in symptoms such as depression, lethargy, and anhedonia (i.e., inability to feel pleasure). These symptoms determine the pattern of withdrawal from the drug. The depression experienced by the user when not using stimulants is contrasted with the recalled euphoria produced by the use of the drug. These factors, coupled with associated cues, help initiate the vicious cycle of binge use with increased craving and continued self-administration to relieve symptoms.

The development of *addiction* or *dependency* is marked by changes in both behavior and cognition. There is an increasing focus on the substance and a narrowing of interests, social activities, and relationships. The process of becoming dependent or addicted requires the individual to deny or ignore evidence or information that may challenge the behavior or the rationalization of the behavior. There is a preoccupation with the substance and its procurement during this stage, even in the face of negative consequences. Table 24-5 outlines the stages in the process of stimulant addiction. Dependency on other substances such as alcohol or narcotics usually takes a similar course.

LEGAL AND ETHICAL CONCERNS OF SUBSTANCE ABUSE

For the past 25 years, the United States has pursued a drug policy based on prohibition and the active application of criminal sanctions against the use and sale of illicit drugs. During this time, the number of criminal penalties for drug offenses has climbed to 1.5 million offenses in 1996. There has also been a tenfold increase in imprisonment for drug charges since 1979 despite an overall decline in drug prevalence (Drucker, 1999).

This increase in drug-related imprisonment, especially in the 1980s, is a result of harsher enforcement policies and longer mandatory sentences for possession of smaller quantities of drugs. Although

TABLE **24-5**

Typical Course of Addictive Illness: Stages in Continuum from Initiation to Dependency

Stage	Characteristics
Initiation	First use of the substance
	Exposure frequently through family or friends
Continuation	Continued, more frequent use of substance
	Usually social use only, with no detrimental effects
Transition	Beginning of change in total consumption, frequency, and occasions of use
	More than just social use, with beginning of loss of control
Abuse	Adverse effects and consequences to substance use
	Rationalizations for continued use and denial of adverse effects present in user and significant others
	Unsuccessful attempts at control of use
Dependency and addiction	Physical or psychological dependence, or both, on the substance; marked by behavioral and cognitive changes
	Preoccupation with the substance and its procurement despite negative consequences
	Narrowing of interests, social activities, and relationships to only those related to the substance use

some individuals are in prison for violent crimes or major drug trafficking, the vast majority of drug offenders are arrested for small-scale drug deals made to support their personal use (US Department of Justice, Bureau of Justice Statistics, 1992.)

Alcohol use and abuse are different issues because the possession and sale of alcoholic beverages is only illegal if the individual involved is a minor. Concerns arise when individuals are intoxicated during work, while driving, or in situations that may affect the welfare of others. Legal penalties have increased for driving under the influence of alcohol because groups such as Mothers Against Drunk Driving (MADD) influence legislation.

Drug testing, as part of preemployment assessment and random testing during employment, is a phenomenon that has become more commonplace. Beginning in 1986, federal legislation such as the Drug-Free Workplace Act and the Omnibus Transportation Employee Testing Act has authorized drug and alcohol testing and required certain job classifications to participate in testing. Although employees' attitudes toward workplace drug testing are mixed, it has been shown to have a positive effect (Sweeney and Penner, 1997). There is evidence that the most effective deterrent to drug abuse in workers is a comprehensive program combining testing with an employee assistance program, supervisory training, employee education, and a clearly written substance use policy (Quazi, 1993).

Ethical issues regarding substance use and abuse relate to behaviors that present a risk to self, co-workers, or the public. A health care worker stealing medicine from a patient, thereby depriving the patient of pain relief, is both unethical and illegal (Dabney, 1995). Other ethical areas of concern include property theft or damage and the general welfare of others.

One area that has also received the attention of the legal system is the use of substances by pregnant women that put their fetus at risk for long-term developmental and behavioral problems. Pregnant addicts have been imprisoned and forced into treatment and their children have been removed from their custody after birth. Many treatment providers and patient advocates view this approach as punitive and counterproductive to assisting these women and their children. Some providers believe such sanctions are more likely to prevent addicted women from seeking treatment for fear of legal consequences (Chavkin et al., 1998; Paone and Alpern, 1998).

Heavy maternal use of alcohol during pregnancy can cause permanent birth defects, including fetal alcohol syndrome. Although alcohol-related defects are entirely preventable, the factors associated with maternal use of alcohol during pregnancy are complex and often resistant to change. The University of Washington has implemented a primary prevention and intervention program for those women identified as being "at risk" for producing children affected by prenatal alcohol exposure. Women identified as being at risk are referred to a multidisciplinary diagnostic clinic staffed by a physician, psychologist, language pathologist, occupational therapist, and social worker to facilitate diagnosis and comprehensive intervention for both the mother and affected children. This approach increases the potential for primary prevention of fetal alcohol syndrome by avoiding exposures and is a major protective factor in preventing conditions among affected children (CDC, 1998).

MODES OF INTERVENTION

Correlating with the numerous theories about substance abuse are a wide variety of intervention strategies incorporating all levels of prevention. At the community level, legislative measures have limited access to potentially addictive pharmaceuticals and illicit street drugs. The growing social demand for smoke-free environments in public buildings, restaurants, airplanes, and similar areas exemplifies how perceptions of tobacco and its risks have changed over the past 50 years. Alcohol taxes, zoning schemes for liquor outlets, a legal drinking age, and legal sanctions on driving while intoxicated are other examples of community efforts to prevent or contain substance abuse.

Educational programs administered through schools and penal institutions have also been developed to prevent or foster early recognition of substance abuse. Television and radio provide public service communications about the risks of substance abuse and the availability of treatment for these problems.

The formation of national associations, such as the National Council on Alcoholism, and the establishment of federal research entities, such as NIDA and the National Institute on Alcohol Abuse and Alcoholism, have facilitated centralized efforts in the areas of education, research, and treatment. At the state level, there have also been legislative provisions to fund substance abuse treatment and rehabilitation.

Prevention

In keeping with a public health model, community health nurses as client advocates should focus on primary prevention. Primary prevention in the community includes working with other providers to identify high-risk situations and potential problems that threaten the integrity of the community and its inhabitants. A community assessment can help identify macro-level and micro-level factors that predispose individuals to alcohol and drug problems.

On the federal level, prevention efforts have been overshadowed by the ongoing "war on drugs." A significant amount of fiscal resources has been allocated to law enforcement; interdiction; crop eradication; and harsh, punitive laws to prosecute drug users and manufacturers. At both the state and federal governmental levels, debate continues regarding the cost-benefit ratio of drug legalization or decriminalization (Grinspoon and Bakalar, 1994; Kleber, 1994). Supporters of legalization and decriminalization argue that to do so would lead to a reduction in crime and would move the drug problem out of the realm of moral failings of individuals toward more humane treatment approaches.

Opponents argue that decriminalization and legalization of drugs would do little to abate crime related to drug manufacture, sale, and use (Kleber, 1994). Further, problems associated with use (e.g., domestic violence and drunk driving) would potentially increase. Kleber (1994) argues that until society can effectively deal with the serious effects of two lethal but legal drugs (i.e., alcohol and nicotine), the argument for adding more is difficult to accept and to justify.

However, programs such as needle exchanges, which appear to support the proponents of legalization and decriminalization, have had some success. Needle exchange programs may not lead the intravenous drug user to abstinence, but they do, in fact, serve to break the link in the deadly chain of AIDS transmission and exposure (Bowersox, 1994). Other prevention efforts should target susceptible aggregates (i.e., women, adolescents, ethnic minorities, and the aging population).

Prevention efforts in the African-American community and other minority groups have produced results that are only marginally successful. Possible reasons are that treatment programs fail to incorporate culturally sensitive and appropriate interventions and strategies. The demand for culturally specific approaches is evidence that previous approaches and the assumptions that underlie them are insufficient for understanding and explaining the etiology of substance abuse among members of minority groups. Successful prevention efforts are usually not focused solely on alcohol and drug abuse, but are community controlled and work toward improving individuals' general competencies, communication skills, and self-esteem.

Community health nurses may be the first to identify or suspect an alcohol or drug problem in the clients and families with whom they are working. Nurses in all care contexts should routinely assess substance use patterns when performing client histories. The client history is a critical assessment and screening tool that can identify those at risk. Using current knowledge and theories about substance abuse etiology and risk factors should help identify those individuals predisposed to alcohol and drug use.

Treatment

Inpatient and outpatient are the two main types of treatment programs for substance abuse. Each of these programs may or may not include a detoxification component. Treatment programs also differ in the following ways: they may be voluntary vs. compulsory and pharmacologically based vs. drug free. In general, although treatment is intricately tied to the concept of recovery, disciplinary philosophy guides specific treatment approaches. There are a variety of treatment approaches and models, which are sometimes contradictory. The treatment models vary by such factors as the composition of staff and the philosophical approach (i.e., social vs. psychological vs. medical models) to substance abuse problems.

Inpatient treatment isolates individuals from the external world and provides an opportunity to focus only on substance abuse issues. However, outpatient treatment is appropriate for those who do not require such structure and protection and those with strong supportive social networks and high levels of motivation.

The severity of the individual's alcohol or drug problems and pertinent cultural factors determine the necessity and type of treatment. Therefore the assessment process is of primary importance and begins with an accurate social and medical history. The history taking begins with more general questions about lifestyle, employment, relationships, and self-perception. This general line of questioning permits the development of a therapeutic relationship with the client.

A therapeutic relationship based on trust is essential to collecting information about sensitive issues such as drug and alcohol use. The assessment should then proceed to determining risky behavior patterns and stressors. The interviewer assesses dietary practices; prior health problems; allergies; hospitalizations including psychiatric disorders; and family history of similar problems including drug- and alcohol-related problems. This general line of questioning can be followed by more specific questions about harmful behaviors such as smoking, drinking, and illicit drug use. This ordering of questions progresses from the more socially-sanctioned behaviors to more "socially-disapproved" behaviors and from the general to the more specific. Positive responses to questions about drug and alcohol use should be probed in a nonjudgmental, direct way to determine pattern, frequency, and timing.

Screening tools such as the CAGE test (Box 24-3) are brief and simple and allow health providers to talk about substance abuse by incorporating relevant questions into the interview and history

---

B O X 24-3

CAGE: An Alcoholism Screening Test

- Have you ever felt that you should *cut down* on your drinking?
- Have people *annoyed* you by criticizing your drinking?
- Have you ever felt bad or *guilty* about your drinking?
- Have you ever had a drink, or an *eye-opener*, first thing in the morning to steady your nerves or get rid of a hangover?

Two positive responses to these questions are considered a positive test and indicate that further assessment is warranted.

Adapted from Ewing JA: Detecting alcoholism: the CAGE questionnaire, *JAMA* 252:1905-1907, 1984.

(Ewing, 1984). A positive response to any of the CAGE questions does not constitute a diagnosis of alcohol or drug dependence, but should raise a high index of suspicion and mandate further investigation (Cherpitel, 1997).

A physical examination is another valuable tool in evaluating the client for potential or actual alcohol and drug problems. Although at-risk clients may not have physical signs of alcohol and drug problems and may even deny obvious consequences of such, certain physical findings warrant further investigation. Complaints such as vague, nonspecific abdominal pain, insomnia, depression, chronic fatigue, back pain, chronic anxiety, and night sweats require more intensive investigation. Clients with hypertension unaccounted for by specific pathogenesis, or refractory to pharmacotherapeutic intervention, should be questioned about alcohol consumption. Spider angiomata on the thorax or face may be the result of long-term alcohol use. Although laboratory tests may not yield clues to drug or alcohol use, certain laboratory findings (e.g., abnormal liver function), in the absence of other etiologic agents, may increase the index of suspicion.

Brief intervention strategies frequently begin with information about the effects of alcohol and drugs and a discussion of the solutions to substance abuse-related problems. This initial educational approach can defuse frequently-encountered barriers to intervention such as shame, denial, guilt, fear, and the client's erroneous perceptions and attitudes about alcohol and drug problems. Presenting information and solutions in a nonjudgmental and clear manner may help minimize defensiveness. Reframing interventions within the context of health maintenance or health promotion and education can be less threatening. Confronting myths about alcohol and drug problems may help clients change their attitudes and minimize the potential for serious consequences.

Ambivalent clients may respond to education and decide to abstain from substances or seek treatment. Other clients however, even when confronted with legal, financial, physical, and psychological consequences of substance abuse, may resist treatment offers. Therefore the clinician must continue to work with clients and involve important members of their social network to remove internal and environmental barriers and move clients toward readiness for change and treatment. Barriers such as fear of discrimination in group settings and logistical problems such as lack of child care are part of the resistance to treatment.

At the local level, much of the effort for substance abuse treatment has been invested in detoxification, residential, and outpatient treatment programs. *Detoxification* is best described as a short-term treatment intervention designed to manage acute withdrawal from the substance. It involves medical management to reduce the adverse side effects of the substance and help stabilize the client.

Addressing acute withdrawal symptoms is of utmost importance in detoxification, particularly in the case of the cocaine abuser who may experience extreme depression with suicidal ideation. Such feelings may cause the individual who is withdrawing from treatment to begin the vicious cycle of abuse again. Alcohol detoxification may have life-threatening medical consequences. Detoxification is one of the most crucial periods in the recovery process. Some detoxification programs are not medically supervised, but are administered by volunteers recovering from addiction. Clinicians should be aware of the level of services offered in any detoxification program to make appropriate referrals.

Outpatient and inpatient treatment programs vary, but they usually include group and individual therapy and counseling, family counseling, education, and socialization into 12-step mutual self-help groups. Some programs also use disulfiram, or Antabuse, therapy; methadone maintenance; hypnosis; occupational therapy; psychoanalysis; confrontation; assertiveness training; cognitive therapy; blood alcohol level discrimination training; and other behavior modification approaches. Relapses are common; therefore most effective treatment programs incorporate some form of relapse prevention as a part of the healing process. NIDA (1999) published a research-based guide to drug addiction treatment. Important points from this publication are listed in Box 24-4.

Having a substance abuse problem does not mean that problems are always attributable to the addiction. Many substance-abusing clients also have other psychiatric problems such as schizophrenia, depression, bipolar affective disorder, dissociative disorder, and posttraumatic stress syndrome. Likewise, many of these clients have chronic medical problems. In cases with compounding problems, specialized attention involving a case management approach is warranted.

Research on treatment programs demonstrates that some treatment is better than no treatment. Treatment evaluation also depends on the criteria used to measure effectiveness and the period of time over which the assessment takes place (Carroll, 1997).

Examples of criteria that have been used include the following:

- Number of days abstinent
- Number of days without negative consequences of substance use
- Employability or work attendance
- Self-image improvement
- Spouse's assessment of client's functionality
- Regular attendance at 12-step group meetings
- Compliance with follow-up appointments
- Absence of overt psychiatric symptoms such as depression or anxiety
- Self-reports of progress
- Evidence of personal satisfaction and growth

It is clear that treatment programs vary and that certain programs will be more culturally appropriate and effective than others for particular aggregates of individuals.

Pharmacotherapies

In the search for successful treatment of those susceptible to drug and alcohol problems, several pharmacotherapeutic adjuncts to formalized treatment have been discovered. Medications include either those drugs used to assist in the initiation and maintenance of abstinence, or those drugs used as a substitute for illegal drug use. This section discusses pharmacotherapies treatment providers currently use. Good clinical judgment and patient motivation should guide the use of any pharmacotherapy.

Disulfiram, or Antabuse, is sometimes used as an adjunct to treatment in those individuals with alcohol problems that do not respond successfully to treatment. Disulfiram, when combined with alcohol, produces the classic disulfiram ethanol reaction (DER) (i.e., flushing, tachycardia, nausea, headache, chest tightness, and chest pain). The DER is thought to be the result of a disturbance in alcohol metabolism. The response, which typically begins within minutes after alcohol consumption, is dose dependent and highly variable. Significant risks of the DER are cardiovascular symptoms of tachycardia, hypotension, dysrhythmia, and shock. Preexisting cardiac disease is an absolute contraindication. Emergency treatment of the DER is symptomatic.

Disulfiram is not a complete form of treatment of alcohol problems. A select group (i.e., those who are relapse prone, those who have supportive networks, and those who have histories of abstinence) may

BOX **24-4**

Guidelines for Drug Abuse Treatment

1. A single treatment is not appropriate for all individuals. Treatment should be tailored to the specific needs of the individual because not all addicts and alcoholics are the same.
2. Treatment must be readily available when people who are addicted are ready for treatment.
3. Effective treatment attends to the multiple needs of the individual, not just his or her substance use. It must address associated medical, psychological, social, vocational, and legal problems. Treatment should stress the importance of interaction with family or significant others and attempt to engage important social network members in the process.
4. An individual's treatment and services plan must be assessed continually and modified as necessary to ensure that the plan meets the individual's changing needs.
5. Remaining in treatment for an adequate time is crucial for treatment effectiveness. For most patients, the threshold of significant improvement is reached in about three months.
6. Individual or group counseling and other behavioral therapies are critical components of effective treatment for addiction.
7. Medications are an important element of treatment for many patients, especially when com-
bined with counseling and other behavioral therapies.
8. Addicted or drug-abusing individuals with coexisting mental disorders should have both disorders treated in an integrated way.
9. Medical detoxification is only the first stage of addiction treatment and does little to change long-term substance abuse.
10. Treatment does not need to be voluntary to be effective.
11. Possible drug use during treatment must be monitored continuously.
12. Treatment programs should provide assessment for HIV and AIDS, hepatitis B and C, TB, and other infectious diseases and should provide counseling to help patients modify or change behaviors that place themselves or others at risk for infection.
13. Recovery from drug addiction can be a long-term process and commonly requires multiple episodes of treatment. Relapses can occur, but participation in mutual help groups or self-help groups and ongoing support is helpful to maintain abstinence. Treatment is not recovery, but it is part of the recovery process and experience. Treatment programs must address the aftercare needs of the client to maintain the gains made in treatment.

From National Institute on Drug Abuse: *Principles of drug addiction treatment: a research-based guide,* Government Printing Office No 99-4180, Rockville, Md, 1999, USDHHS, www.nida.nih.gov.

benefit from short-term use. Requests for disulfiram should not be granted in the absence of treatment and supportive relationships.

Naltrexone is a long-acting narcotic antagonist currently used as an adjunct in the treatment of opiate dependence. It blocks the effects of opiates via competitive binding, but it does not block the effects of other substances such as benzodiazepines, cocaine, and alcohol. The National Institutes on Alcohol Abuse and Alcoholism recently published preliminary findings of a study detailing naltrexone's use in alcohol-dependent clients. This information indicates that naltrexone reduces craving, rates of relapse to alcohol, and severity of alcohol-related problems. Other clinical studies are ongoing (Gordis, 1995).

Methadone and buprenorphine deserve special mention as therapeutic aids in drug and alcohol treatment. Varying philosophical opinions about abstinence vs. sanctioned use is reflected in the debate over the use of methadone, a long-acting oral opioid. For a select group of opiate-dependent individuals, methadone has facilitated their return to normal functioning.

Traditionally, methadone has been used as either a detoxifying agent or a maintenance drug. As a detoxification agent, methadone is dispensed over a 21-day period in a tapering dose. Dosage is dependent on the degree of opiate withdrawal symptoms present. Dose reduction typically occurs gradually over one to two days. Methadone maintenance is more controversial because the individual remains dependent on the drug. It is dispensed under medical supervision as part of a treatment program. Maintenance may minimize or abate illegal activity, eliminate the infection hazards of injection drug use, reduce social disruption typically seen with opiate use, and facilitate increased levels of functioning. A myth about maintenance programs is that methadone produces an euphoric "high" and is therefore merely a legal substitute for heroin. Levo-alpha-acetylmethadol (LAAM) is a methadone-like drug that is longer acting and taken several times a week rather than daily (NIDA, 1999).

Buprenorphine is an opioid agonist-antagonist that has been used in the treatment of opiate-dependent clients and those with concurrent cocaine dependence. Buprenorphine does not produce severe withdrawal on abrupt cessation, which is an advantage over methadone. Its antagonist component helps reduce the possibility of lethal overdose. Clinical studies support the use of buprenorphine in reducing the frequency of heroin and cocaine self-administration.

Other Intervention Approaches

Substance abuse problems are socially defined and frequently attributed to sufferers who do not recognize their substance use as a problem. Furthermore, the substance abuse treatment system has increasingly taken on social welfare and criminal justice tasks (Drucker, 1999). In this sense, substance abuse differs from many other health-related problems. Most states have laws pertaining to involuntary treatment of substance abusers. Employers and families are often enlisted to assist or coerce the identified client into accepting treatment. This aspect of substance abuse as a health concern raises some crucial questions for health care providers in terms of the encroachment of therapeutic intervention on individual rights to privacy, informed consent, and self-determination.

On the individual level, substance abuse is treated in regards to cultural and educational background, resources of the person, the attitudes of significant others, the degree of invasiveness of the effects of the substance use, and the existence of alternatives. Interventions have been developed to assist some individuals in achieving moderation. Additionally, some research has shown that a small percentage of individuals who recognize a harmful pattern of substance use are able to stop using the substance or to achieve a controlled, nonpathological pattern of use. There are those who, because they experience an important life

change such as graduating from college or getting married, appear to change from excessive use to social alcohol use.

Nevertheless, many people exhibit serious problems related to their use of mood-altering substances. These individuals are usually not able to stop or control their use without outside intervention. Research on identified problem drinkers' ability to return to social alcohol use is still inconclusive. Consequently, most scientists and health care providers advocate abstinence from alcohol as a cornerstone of recovery. Serious criminal implications are involved in the use of illicit drugs; therefore moderate or social use is not usually considered.

Abstinence is difficult to maintain on a long-term basis. Therefore an important area of continuing research is relapse prevention (i.e., a behavioral approach that aims to prepare the client for the relapse situation in the hope of preventing it or minimizing its impact on recovery). Relapse prevention models can be applied to alcohol, drug, and behavioral addictive problems (e.g., overeating and compulsive gambling) and can have either controlled use or abstinence as their goal. In relapse prevention, cognitive reframing, role-playing, and plans for coping with negative mood states are done in preparation for meeting the challenge of craving and potential relapse.

Mutual Help Groups

Mutual help groups are associations that are voluntarily formed, are not professionally dominated, and operate through face-to-face supportive interaction focusing on a mutual goal. Many mutual help groups exist and they are usually organized by recovering substance abusers or those recovering from compulsive behavior patterns. The first mutual help group was Alcoholics Anonymous (AA), founded in 1935. Initially, a small group of male alcoholics found a way to stay sober "one day at a time" through meeting regularly with others like themselves. The early AA members developed 12 steps to guide the recovery process (Kurtz, 1979). The process can be summarized as follows (Kurtz, 1979):

- Admission of defeat and surrender to a higher power
- Inventory of past shortcomings and strengths
- Spiritual practices (e.g., prayer and meditation)
- Willingness to change
- Making amends
- Extension of this process into daily life

AA has been viewed as relatively successful. It is nonprofessional and is an ongoing source of assistance; therefore it is an invaluable resource to the community. However, not all of those with alcohol problems find AA comfortable, culturally relevant, and socially supportive. Predominantly in large cities, women, members of racial and ethnic minority groups, and gay men and lesbians with alcohol problems have formed their own AA groups and other mutual help organizations for support in recovery. Realities of social discrimination and regional variation in customs exist; therefore AA should not be considered a universal form of assistance for alcohol problems, but many individuals from diverse social backgrounds find acceptance and support in AA.

Other 12-step programs have developed through the adaptation of AA's approach to similar addictive problems. Narcotics Anonymous, Gamblers Anonymous, Debtors Anonymous, Cocaine Anonymous, Overeaters Anonymous, and Sex and Love Addicts Anonymous are examples. They became organized more recently than AA; therefore these groups may not be as well known or as widely available and they may not exhibit as much diversity among their membership as AA. The 12 steps have also been applied to the syndromes of compulsive behavior and other difficulties experienced by the children, partners, and close associates of substance abusers. Al-Anon, Codependents Anonymous, and Adult Children of Alcoholics are examples of these groups. Although these groups initially had a predominance of female members, the trend is moving toward participation by equal numbers of men and women.

AA meetings are not standardized. Customs shaping the actual format and sequence of the meeting vary according to region, group size, ethnic and sex composition, and other cultural biases of the members. In general, 12-step meetings follow one of the following formats:

- Uninterrupted talks by one or more speakers about "what it was like, what happened, and what it is like now"
- Each person at the meeting has the opportunity to speak briefly during discussion
- A combination of the first two options

At least two mutual help groups have developed in response to their founders' negative experiences in AA, or their failure to succeed in AA. Women for Sobriety was organized in 1976 to replace or augment AA for women; it addresses women's needs to overcome depression, guilt, and low self-esteem. Secular Sobriety Groups were organized to meet the needs of individuals who are unable to accept the concept of or to depend on a "higher power" in their recovery from alcohol problems. Additional information about these groups can be obtained through the WebLinks section of the book's website at *evolve* http://evolve.elsevier.com/Nies/.

Other mutual help groups that do not follow the 12 steps are available for a variety of addictive problems. AA does not require dues or fees, but some groups such as Weight Watchers require monetary commitment. Other groups such as Recovery Incorporated have more professional involvement. Any of these groups might also be resources for selected people with substance abuse problems.

The organization and proliferation of mutual help groups may be one of the most important social developments of the twentieth century. The groups make up the most important human and ideological resource readily available to communities for the purpose of managing substance abuse. In the future, mutual help groups may begin to address prevention and become more involved with professional and governmental entities in the war on substance abuse. An example of such involvement can be seen in neighborhood organization strategies, such as "Fighting Back," devised by those whose immediate environment has become highly unsafe, flooded with illicit drugs, and subject to the effects of gang warfare (RWJ Foundation, 1992). In this scenario, recovery has been redefined as a community reclaiming living space through collective action. This is often achieved one building and one block at a time.

To be effective, interventions for substance abuse take place at multiple levels and involve a number of individuals, activities, policies, and substances. Table 24-6 summarizes some of the many interventions for substance abuse at various levels.

Harm Reduction

New approaches have been proposed for substance use problems that are not amenable to traditional approaches. Some of these have been grouped under the general term **harm reduction**. Harm reduction consists of individual and collective approaches to the treatment of substance use that are not primarily aimed at complete abstinence from all substances. Instead, *incremental change* is sought, which involves elimination of the more harmful effects of substance use through behavior and policy modifications. Harm reduction is a process rather than a static approach or an end in itself. It is used in various ways, depending on the context and the needs of individual clients (Erickson, 1999; MacCoun, 1998).

Harm reduction strategies remain controversial (Erickson, 1999; Hamilton, 1999; Wild, 1999). Nevertheless, they are often the only options that will preserve a therapeutic relationship when people continue to use or drink problematically. An early example of harm reduction is the substitution of methadone for heroin. Although they are still using an opiate, this process allows individuals to be functional without getting "high" and without the need to engage in criminal activity for drugs.

Another example of harm reduction is exemplified in the case of the therapist who agrees to see a client who is still using substances as long as the client abstains for 24 hours before the therapy appointment. In some cases harm reduction is an end in itself; in other cases it is hoped that abstinence will eventually occur.

Harm reduction has been used in response to alcohol, illicit drugs, and tobacco (Berridge, 1999; Hughes, 1999). In the case of alcohol, harm reduction might involve decreasing the number of drinks, decreasing the number of days in which drinking occurs, or avoiding drinking when driving. On a community level, harm reduction may include attempts to legislate for decreased access to alcohol or raising the legal age for drinking. More controversial public health projects aimed at harm reduction are legalization of some illicit drugs and needle exchange programs (Lifson, 1998).

Viewed from a community health perspective, harm reduction involves planned social and policy changes. The goal of these changes is to decrease safety and health risks consequent to alcohol and other drug use among specific aggregates (Kearney, 1999; Wodak, 1995). Although harm reduction strategies are not usually sanctioned by lay support systems (e.g., 12-step groups), they can have an important impact. Community health nurses using harm reduction strategies can help reduce drug- and alcohol-related social problems by advocating for programs that "bridge the gap" for those who cannot immediately reach the goal of abstinence.

TABLE 24-6

Modes of Intervention for Substance Abuse

Level	Intervention
Individual and family levels	Education
	Treatment: detoxification, inpatient, outpatient, and residential
	Mutual help groups (e.g., AA, Narcotics Anonymous, Cocaine Anonymous, Al-Anon, and Narcanon)
Community level	Law enforcement measures to limit access to and distribution of addictive substances (e.g., street drugs)
	Alcohol taxes and zoning schemes for liquor outlets
	Legal drinking age and legal sanctions on driving while intoxicated
	Education programs at schools and penal institutions
	Television and radio public service communications concerning the risks of substance abuse and the availability of treatment
State and federal levels	Formation of national associations such as the National Council on Alcoholism
	Establishment of federal research entities such as NIDA and the National Institute on Alcohol Abuse and Alcoholism to centralize research, education, and treatment efforts
	Legislative provisions at the state level to fund substance abuse treatment and rehabilitation

People who drive while impaired by alcohol or other drugs are a public health hazard to themselves and others. During 1998, almost 16,000 deaths and approximately 305,000 injuries were from alcohol- or drug-related motor vehicle accidents. Reduction in alcohol-involved motor vehicle-related fatalities requires a variety of interventions to change drinking and driving behaviors. These include altering drivers' perceptions of risk to themselves and to others riding with them; increasing efforts to screen for alcoholism among people convicted of driving while intoxicated; and changing public policy to deter adult drinking and driving (CDC, 1999).

SOCIAL NETWORK INVOLVEMENT

Family and Friends

The social network of the substance abuser can either be highly influential in helping the individual alter behavior or aid and abet the substance abuser in self-destruction. There is evidence for both positive and negative effects of social support in either mitigating or supporting the behaviors of substance abusers (Ellis, Zucker, and Fitzgerald, 1997; Roberts and Leonard, 1997).

Particularly among adolescents and young adults, evidence suggests that substance use and abuse often occur in the context of social interactions. Adolescents may use alcohol and other substances as a social lubricant during an often-troubled developmental period (Sussman, Dent, and Galaif, 1997). Family treatment is considered essential in substance abuse because the family can enable continued substance abuse by protecting and supporting the individual during using and inactive using. In addition, the family has suffered the effects of substance abuse emotionally, socially, economically, physically, and spiritually. The family's wounds must be acknowledged and treated for the substance abuser to return to an environment supportive of recovery.

A term that deserves particular attention is **codependency**. *Codependency* is a common but ambiguous term and is used differently by various disciplines and segments of the lay population. Subby (1984) offered a comprehensive definition, stating that codependency is "an emotional, psychological and behavioral condition that develops as a result of an individual's prolonged exposure to, and practice of, a set of oppressive rules; rules which prevent the open expression of feelings as well as the direct discussion of personal and interpersonal problems" (p. 26).

Codependency is a newer term for an interactional pattern that was recognized decades ago; it was determined that definite and identifiable patterns of interaction describe the alcoholic or addicted family system (Jackson, 1954). These behaviors help maintain the family in a pattern that supports substance abuse and addiction. Other early researchers (Stanton et al., 1978; Steinglass, 1985) supported the existence of these patterns in the family of the substance abuser and alcoholic.

There are mutual help groups for addressing codependency that are founded on the principles of AA and provide opportunities to discuss the issues germane to the alcoholic or addicted family system or network. Families participating in treatment should also be encouraged to participate in these mutual help groups.

Codependency cannot be concretely defined the same way in each culture. Cultural groups vary in the degree to which individuals are expected to anticipate the needs of others and care for them. The danger in applying a rigid definition of codependency in all cases is that it might unfairly and inappropriately label it as a disease in some cultures that value interdependency over individualism.

The nurse should identify the important members of the social network for each client and the ways in which these individuals provide support for the client. The nurse must also recognize that the concept of family refers not only to nuclear families, but also includes alternative family systems. Whatever the constellation of family, significant others should be included in the treatment and intervention. Substance abuse, addiction, and recovery do not occur in a vacuum and many relapses are precipitated by interpersonal conflicts.

Effects on the Family

Substance abuse has been called a family disease because it affects the entire family system and holds potential adverse psychological and physical consequences for the family members in addition to the abuser. Family theorists view families, whether the traditional nuclear form or an alternative, as social systems that try to stay in balance (Minuchin, 1974; Satir et al., 1975). They see families as either functional or dysfunctional depending on how well they fulfill the social tasks expected of them by society. Substance-abusing families are frequently observed to be dysfunctional in clinical terms. However, cultural and political factors should also be considered because families may have developed these patterns for historical reasons rather than as the effects of substance abuse.

A functional family system is open and flexible and allows its members to be themselves. In the nuclear family model, the parents model intimacy for the children; differences are negotiated, boundaries are defined and maintained, and communication is consistent and clear. In functional family systems, whether the traditional nuclear family or other nontraditional forms, there is trust, individuality, and accountability among family members. All family members are able to have their needs met in a reasonable way.

On the other hand, dysfunctional families are closed systems with fixed, rigid roles. In the case of substance abuse, a major purpose of the system is to deny the substance abuse of the affected family member and keep it a "shameful" family secret. When a parent is the substance abuser, there may only be the appearance of intimacy between the parents. Generally, ego boundaries between the family members are weakened or nonexistent, with enmeshment of the members and an intolerance of individual differences. Rules are rigid and communication is unbalanced; the dynamics are either always conflicting or always superficially pleasant. Children may become involved in a "role reversal" in which they act as caretakers of their parents.

When one or more family members are substance abusers, family functions revolve around the substance abuser and accommodate or compensate the abuser's behavior (Brown, 1985). The individual needs of other family members are often unmet. Denial is central to a "dysfunctional" family system. The spouse of the substance abuser may gradually take over that person's role, functions, and control of the family. The children are cast into various roles (e.g., hero, junior parent, scapegoat, peacemaker, or caretaker) in their struggle for survival in this environment.

Adult children from dysfunctional families often carry these roles and coping mechanisms into adult life. Many become substance abusers or partners of substance abusers. The children of alcoholics are four to nine times more likely to experience alcohol use disorders than children of non-alcoholics, with varying estimates according to sampling methods, (Windle, 1997). They are also more likely to develop problematic behavior patterns that can have serious consequences in their adult lives (Jacob and Johnson, 1997). Frequently, they have difficulties with intimacy and parenting. Many have lifelong problems with depression and anxiety and physical illnesses often associated with depression and anxiety such as ulcers, colitis, migraine headaches, and eating disorders.

In addition to psychological burdens that substance abuse places on families, there are the financial burdens related to medical costs, loss of income from job difficulties or unemployment, and the financial losses attributable to divorce. Further, spousal violence and child abuse and neglect are strongly associated with substance abuse (Horgan, 1993).

Professional Enablers

Health care professionals can also contribute to the initiation and continuation of substance abuse and dependency in various ways, becoming **professional enablers**. One obvious way is the physician's role in prescribing psychoactive medications. The medical model advocates the treatment of symptoms by medication. The relief of pain, anxiety, and insomnia are not exceptions. The addictive potential of narcotic analgesics and antianxiety agents is often ignored if quick symptom relief is the main goal. Long-term goals for the treatment of medical problems and nonmedication management of pain and anxiety are more thoughtful approaches. However, undermedication or refusal to use "addictive" medicines can lead susceptible clients to self-medicate with illegal drugs or alcohol.

Physicians and nurses are often the first to see the physical effects of substance abuse and are in an excellent position to intervene. By focusing on the health consequences of substance abuse, they can often form trusting relationships, provide information, and refer patients to the appropriate treatment. Too often, this opportunity is missed because the health care professional is reluctant to bring up this taboo subject. This reluctance may be based on professionals' inability to examine their own drinking or drug-taking behaviors, or those of significant others, or concerns of negative responses by clients.

In the past, many psychiatrists and psychotherapists have focused on the reasons why the person uses substances rather than on the dependency itself. The assumption was that insight would lead to a change in behavior. This approach has usually not proved to be effective, especially if the psychiatrist is concurrently prescribing other potentially addictive antianxiety medications or hypnotics. Complete abstinence from all mood-altering medication is a model for preventing the cross-addiction common in substance abusers (i.e., substituting one substance for another such as a benzodiazepine for alcohol). Exceptions to this approach are patients with serious medical conditions requiring pain medication and those who also have a second psychiatric disorder that requires medication such as schizophrenia, depression, or bipolar affective disorder. Recovering substance abusers often need support when they must take medication for these psychiatric conditions because others may criticize the use of any medication and place the client in a difficult situation.

Caregivers have become more aware of signs of client substance abuse. Some providers are willing to begin therapy with a nonabstinent client under the stipulation that if therapeutic gains are not made, the client will be referred for treatment or the caregiver will withdraw services. Clients who lack social support may succeed using this strategy, which allows the formation of a trusting relationship before taking the "leap" to abstinence. Clinical wisdom and research continue to point toward more tailored, individualized approaches to substance abuse (Hall, 1993).

VULNERABLE AGGREGATES

Substance abuse problems viewed from a community perspective clearly affect some populations more severely than others. Some groups are more susceptible to experiencing substance abuse problems, may tend to deteriorate more quickly in the process, or may have fewer sources of support for recovery compared with middle-class, European-American, heterosexual men. These groups are termed *vulnerable aggregates* and require special attention in terms of prevention, intervention, and rehabilitation strategies.

Current resources for prevention, treatment, and mutual support may not be flexible enough to meet the needs of various vulnerable aggregates who are at risk of experiencing substance abuse problems and are often excluded or alienated from services by policies, provider attitudes, economic constraints, and social isolation. This section describes the issues of substance abuse with several vulnerable aggregates, including adolescents, the elderly, women, and racial and ethnic minorities.

Adolescents

Adolescents often use substances for the first time during this period of transition and social stress. Substance abuse patterns may begin during this time because there are combined influences of peer pressure, the user's physiological immaturity, social role pressures, a risk-taking orientation, and lack of other recreational alternatives. Experimentation often begins early. By eighth grade, 70% have tried alcohol; 10% have tried marijuana; 2% have tried cocaine; and 44% have smoked cigarettes. By twelfth grade, 88% have used alcohol; 37% have used marijuana; 8% have used cocaine; and 63% have smoked cigarettes (USDHHS, 2000).

Adolescents try cigarettes and alcohol before illicit drugs such as marijuana, hallucinogens, or cocaine; therefore they are considered **gateway drugs** and are increasingly the focus of prevention efforts. In a 1998 study, youths aged 12 through 17 who smoked cigarettes were 11.4 times more likely to use illicit drugs and 16 times more likely to drink heavily (SAMHSA, 1998). The younger the age for the initiation of drug or alcohol use, the more likely the individual will use heavily when he or she becomes older (Horgan, 1993).

Overall, there has been a decline in the use of drugs by adolescents, especially among the middle class. Adolescent substance abusers are more receptive to treatment and are effectively using AA and other self-help modalities. However, among poor socioeconomic groups, there may be minimal or no access to affordable care. The adolescents in these groups tend to face multiple problems related to social and family conditions and need effective treatment. There has been a decrease in funding for substance abuse treatment by insurance companies and other third-party payers in general, with less availability of resources. Unfortunately, this comes at a time when the problems of adolescent substance abusers are becoming more complex.

Adolescent substance abuse is more of a behavioral problem than a disease because it is linked to developmental issues, especially the task of forming an identity. Adolescents entering treatment tend to have more problems that complicate the process of forming an adequate identity than in previous years. Problems such as severe learning disorders; borderline personality disorders; and physical, sexual, and emotional abuse and neglect are common. These problems faced by adolescent substance abusers are frequently related to inadequate parenting and the presence of alcoholism or other addictions in family members (Morrison et al., 1993). Conversely, negative parental attitudes toward illicit drug use, absence of substance-abusing role models, and the existence of an extended family support system are deterrents against illicit drug abuse, especially in high-risk minority group adolescents (Gfroerer and de la Rosa, 1993).

Prevention efforts for adolescents that focus on drug education with an abstinence philosophy (e.g., "Just Say No") have not been as effective as hoped. A more practical approach emphasizes harm reduction as a goal and advocates using low-risk behaviors (e.g., not sharing needles). Increasingly, drug education in schools is focusing on the choices of adolescents and the consequences associated with these choices.

The increasingly sophisticated technology used to prepare for athletic competition has been a significant factor in the self-administration of performance-enhancing substances and associated risky injection practices. These substances include steroids and over-the-counter stimulant drugs and herbs, with steroids the most common. Nonmedical use of steroids poses serious problems because use is both illegal and dangerous. Behavioral and health problems that have been noted with steroid use include suicides, homicides, liver damage, and heart attacks.

Many substance abuse researchers believe that attempts to enhance athletic performance with steroids and other substances reduce the perceived negative consequences of substance abuse and increase the likelihood of using illicit drugs for other purposes. In addition, limited access to needles and other equipment results in a high rate of needle sharing among adolescent teammates who inject substances to enhance their performance (USDHHS, 2000).

Elderly

Elderly men and women are considered vulnerable to substance abuse problems because they have diminished physiological tolerance, increased use of medically prescribed drugs, and cultural and social isolation. Alcohol and drug abuse is the third most common mental health problem among Americans 55 years of age and older and constitutes 10% of admissions in geriatric mental health facilities. Although the overall prevalence of alcohol abuse in the elderly population is 10%, which is the same as in the younger population, the health consequences are worse and the use of effective interventions is more limited (King et al., 1994).

Illicit drug use is not common among the elderly, but it is expected to increase as young and middle-aged addicts grow older. However, prescription drug abuse is common among elderly women, especially with narcotic analgesics, sedatives, and hypnotics. The elderly of both sexes use many over-the-counter

medications that may have synergistic or interactive effects with their other medications. Professionals contribute to prescription drug problems when they fail to assess all the medications an elderly person is already taking before prescribing more. The complicated medication schedules required by many elderly patients demand full alertness to avoid inadequate doses or unintentional overdoses.

Part of early intervention efforts is thorough assessment and appropriate diagnosis. This can be difficult with the elderly because they do not manifest problems with substance abuse in the same ways as younger people. Moos and colleagues (1994) identified the following points to remember in assessing the elderly for substance abuse problems:

- One third of elderly people with alcohol problems do not have onset of symptoms until after age 60 years.
- There is a wide fluctuation in symptoms over time among elderly substance abusers, in contrast to younger substance abusers, who experience more consistent and immediate symptoms.
- Elderly substance abuse is more frequently associated with medical, psychiatric, and social problems or dysfunction.

Women

Since the 1970s, much attention has been turned to substance abuse problems in women. This attention has been in response to the realization that women were neglected in substance abuse research. Within the population of women, there are smaller aggregates of women who may be more severely affected by substance abuse problems. This includes women from minority groups, low-income or no-income women, and working-class women. The increased risk stems from economic, social, and cultural factors. Lesbians are another aggregate of women in whom substance abuse is suspected to be highly prevalent because it is associated with stigmatization and social isolation (Hall, 1994). Women who were sexually abused as children are more susceptible to substance abuse problems in adolescence and adulthood, but they also face many more distressing consequences in substance abuse treatment and recovery (Hall, 1996b).

Compared with men, many chemicals affect women's bodies more quickly and are more destructive. Drug-dependent women report frequent physical and medical problems; many of these problems are related to their reproductive systems (Wetherington and Roman, 1998). Alcoholism appears to have a more rapid progression in women than in men. Women tend to experience symptoms of alcoholic hepatitis and cirrhosis sooner than men because they metabolize alcohol at a different rate. Women have higher blood alcohol levels relative to body weight than men do and they have higher mortality rates from heavy drinking (Vogeltanz and Wilsnack, 1997). It is important to identify problem drinking and drug use in women early, before they experience serious consequences (Wilsnack et al., 1998).

Substance abuse during pregnancy is a serious health concern because it affects the mother and the developing fetus. Excessive alcohol use during pregnancy continues to have long-term developmental consequences on the newborn (Jacobson, 1997). Pregnant women who engage in the abusive pattern of cocaine or crack use are usually unable to stop their drug use without treatment. Cocaine use during pregnancy is associated with increased risk of spontaneous abortion, premature delivery, and abruptio placentae. Infants who have been addicted to cocaine in utero are hyperirritable, subject to seizures, and possibly at increased risk for SIDS. Long-term learning disabilities, behavioral problems, mental retardation, and physical handicaps are other potential consequences for children of cocaine-using mothers (Dicker and Leighton, 1994).

Getting the pregnant woman into treatment and managing her withdrawal is a top priority, but is frequently problematic. Social and psychiatric issues and the pregnant substance abuser's fear of punitive legal actions complicate the process. Additionally, the addiction itself often interferes with obtaining adequate prenatal care. The high-risk behavior associated with addiction increases the chances of both the mother and the infant becoming infected by HIV.

Racial and Ethnic Minorities

Members of racial and ethnic minority groups pose special challenges for health care professionals working in the field of substance abuse and dependency. These groups include African-Americans, Hispanics, Asian and Pacific immigrants, and Native-Americans. Although this section focuses on the problems and peculiarities affecting the lives of African-Americans, many of the same problematic phenomena occur in the lives of people from other vulnerable aggregates.

These vulnerable aggregates are particularly susceptible to the effects of substance abuse and dependency. Under the strain of poverty, underemployment, decreased job opportunities, macro-level and micro-level aggressions, and ongoing racism, some members of these aggregates find the escapism of substance abuse a preferable alternative to confronting the realities of an oppressive environment.

Theories of stress, social causation, and oppressed status all support the belief that racism is a factor in the generation of mental illness and alcohol and drug problems in members of racial and ethnic minorities. Socioeconomic, political, and historical realities have forced some minorities into the illegal drug trade as a means of economic survival. This has altered cultural and community-level values, which resulted in an acceptance of high-risk behavior.

In working with ethnic and racial minorities, it is important for the health care professional to recognize the sociopolitical and socioeconomic factors that form the context of substance use, abuse, and dependency. These same factors will have an impact on help seeking, treatment, and outcome. Cultural sensitivity to the needs and issues germane to these vulnerable aggregates is a prerequisite to successful intervention and treatment.

Critics warn that traditional substance abuse treatment modalities negate the ethnoracial minority experiences (Dawkins, 1988; Ziter, 1987). Treatment approaches geared toward a white society may be inappropriate or less effective for minority groups. Referring to African-Americans, Ziter (1987) explained that the environment for recovery might be contextually and experientially different from that of European-Americans, just as the environment that contributed to the initial abuse was different.

In the African-American community, there are several barriers to treating the substance abusing or addicted individual, which follow:

- Ongoing sociostructural violence
- Impact of racism on self-esteem
- Poverty, underemployment, and unemployment
- Increased availability and accessibility of both drugs and alcohol within the community
- Cultural and community disintegration, which has altered traditional values and behaviors
- Allure and economic rewards of selling drugs
- Inadequate social support system for recovery
- Low self-esteem, internalized racism, anger, and frustration

Racial and ethnic minorities may represent a sizable portion of the U.S. population that is economically disenfranchised. Limited financial resources may limit alternatives to public treatment settings, which are often understaffed, underfunded, filled to capacity, and have long waiting lists.

Studies have identified that social support has a positive effect on treatment and outcome. If the individual completes treatment, returning to the original social environment may still undermine any gains made within the treatment setting. Environmental cues and conditioned reinforcement for continued drug and alcohol use may be extremely powerful. The individual may return to an environment of nonsupport characterized by continued use by important members of the individual's social network. The individual needs a well-coordinated aftercare program that addresses these issues.

The treatment of ethnic and racial minority aggregates poses special challenges related to the individuals seeking treatment. Treatment providers must recognize that these vulnerable aggregates will encounter a host of barriers that will make treatment and long-term recovery extremely difficult. Programs and providers must, if they are to work from the public health perspective of "thinking upstream," examine larger macro-level issues that increase the susceptibility of people of color to alcohol and drug problems.

A culturally sensitive prevention and treatment framework such as the African-American Extended Family Project (AAEFP), located in San Francisco, is a model that attempts to address some of the deficits of traditional 12-step programs and formalized treatment. AAEFP incorporates family, spirituality, collective culture, and racial consciousness, which are some of the fundamental strengths of the African-American value systems.

Recovery at AAEFP occurs within the context of the extended family, with a shift away from powerlessness and anonymity to self-determination, personal responsibility, collective consciousness, and community survival. Alcohol and drugs are conceptualized as direct blocks to opportunities for participation in the larger social system, they further encapsulate and isolate the community and the individual, and they support the negative valuations levied by a racist and oppressive society. Programs such as AAEFP do more to address the macro-level issues than traditional programs by expanding the conceptualization of alcohol and drug problems and recovery. This conceptualization of recovery as empowerment may be more

meaningful to minority members than a definition of recovery as "returning to the mainstream."

Other Aggregates

Substance abuse is the most common psychopathological problem in the general population. Within this category is a smaller aggregate of people with one or more psychiatric diagnoses in addition to substance abuse, which is referred to as **dual diagnosis**. Nearly one third of adults with a mental disorder also experience a co-occurring substance abuse disorder (USDHHS, 2000). These people may lack understanding of how the two problems compound one another, be difficult to locate, be socially isolated, be possibly unemployed, and be less readily identified by health care providers, who fail to realize that both problems may coexist.

Treatment of dual-diagnosis individuals is complicated when the individual must take prescribed psychotropic medications. It may be perceived as prescription drug abuse or as the substitution of one addiction for another. Special attention and flexibility are needed to meet the needs of the dual-diagnosis aggregate and such strategies are still in the developmental phase.

Childhood maltreatment, including verbal, physical, emotional, and sexual abuse and neglect, frequently lead to the development of a wide array of difficulties in adulthood. Substance abuse is one of the most common of those aftereffects. Approximately one in four girls and one in six boys are sexually molested before age 18 (Hall, 1996b; Van der Kolk, McFarlane, and Weisaeth, 1996). Therefore substance abuse prevention and treatment should address these issues. However, caution should be taken to avoid *forcing* the disclosure of a traumatizing event in a group setting (Hall, 1996a).

In assessing the risks for substance abuse and the extent of its impact on the community, it should be noted that, frequently, there are several bases for the vulnerability occurring in one individual or group. The adolescent, the low-income Hispanic male, the lesbian African-American mother receiving public assistance, and the Native-American family living on reservation land are all facing multiple sources of vulnerability that contribute to an increased potential for substance abuse.

Special attention must be focused on the impact of STDs (e.g., HIV, herpes, genital warts, and syphilis) and their relationship to substance abuse. Substance abusers are at increased risk of STDs, including HIV, in the following ways:

- Substances may cloud judgment, which leads to high-risk sexual practices involving the exchange of body fluids (e.g., sex without the use of appropriate barriers such as condoms).
- Intravenous drug use may involve the sharing of hypodermic needles.
- Chronic substance use (e.g., alcohol, heroin, amphetamines, nicotine, and cocaine) impairs the immune system and facilitates infection by HIV or other pathogens that increase the chances of HIV infection.
- Substance abuse may hasten physical and mental deterioration from the condition of seropositivity to an AIDS diagnosis and, eventually, the terminal phase of the disease.
- Chronic substance abusers generally have few supportive relationships available to them in the process of coping with the hardships that accompany severe and chronic illnesses.
- People facing a stigmatizing, terminal, debilitating illness in themselves or a significant other are more prone to experience substance abuse problems in an attempt to cope with distress.

Finally, substance abuse among health care professionals cannot be ignored. Physicians, nurses, dentists, and pharmacists are vulnerable to substance abuse; alcohol or narcotic use is most common (Trinoff and Storr, 1998). Health care professionals are assumed to be "immune" to dependency because they are knowledgeable about medications. However, their increased access to drugs, belief in pharmaceutical solutions, and work-related stress place them at increased risk for substance abuse (Brooke, 1997). Typically, they gain access to drugs through their work settings by diverting medications for their own use or by abusing drugs obtained by prescription. State regulatory boards discover the abuse by these health care professionals following drug theft or when the effects of their substance abuse impair their professional functioning (Madrid, 1994).

Most states have rehabilitation programs for health care professionals that consist of treatment and monitoring. They are allowed to retain their professional licenses during treatment. Despite their usually favorable recovery rate, it is difficult to get this population into treatment because they exhibit denial and shame related to their substance abuse. However,

the threatened loss of their professional license to practice may be a good motivator to break through their denial of the problem and encourage them to seek treatment.

NURSING PERSPECTIVE ON SUBSTANCE ABUSE

Nurses have also encountered substance abuse in clients whose health problems are clearly related to alcohol abuse such as cirrhosis of the liver, heart disease, neurological syndromes, and nutritional deficits. Unfortunately, alcohol problems were often not addressed in these health encounters in the past because there is a stigma of alcoholism and a lack of effective treatments. The nursing literature did not clearly address substance abuse as a nursing problem until the late 1960s and did not address it as a significant problem until the 1970s. Before this, substance abuse was usually viewed as a moral problem or, if it involved illicit drugs, as a legal problem.

Since the 1970s, nursing has become more involved in the spectrum of compulsive behavior problems, including substance abuse. A specialized organization, the National Nurses' Society on Addiction (NNSA), has been established with the philosophy that alcohol abuse and other drug abuse; eating disorders; sexual and relational addiction; and compulsive gambling, working, and spending are closely related behavior patterns. Additionally, educational course work related to alcohol and drug abuse is now recommended for inclusion in general nursing school curricula (Naegle, 1994).

Community Health Nurses and Substance Abusers

The problem of substance abuse is so widespread that it affects every community and its inhabitants in varying degrees; the community health nurse is often involved with substance abusers or their significant others. Substance abuse nursing interventions with clients and their caregivers are necessary to ensure the success of other health interventions. Ignoring substance abuse problems frequently leads to lack of progress and clients' inability to perform needed health practices. This is especially frustrating for the community health nurse and other professionals who have collaborated on a comprehensive plan to allow an individual with a serious health problem to remain at home and avoid placement in an institution.

Substance abuse or dependence can contribute to or complicate the course of many other illnesses and injuries. It is often a direct cause of falls. Particularly in the elderly, falls and fractures may be related to alcohol consumption. Prescription medications, such as narcotic analgesics, tranquilizers, and hypnotics, can also contribute to mental status changes and impair judgment in the elderly. In high-crime, high-poverty areas, gunshot injuries may be secondary to involvement in illegal drug trade, burglaries, and robberies. Domestic violence injuries frequently occur when one or more family members are intoxicated.

Attitude toward Substance Abusers

Although alcoholics and drug addicts are frequently recipients of nursing care in hospitals and community settings, nurses have historically had ambivalent attitudes toward them (Gerace, Hughes, and Spunt, 1995). As part of the larger culture, nurses may reflect the attitude that substance abuse is a stigmatizing, immoral behavior and may have difficulty providing care to these individuals. The moral view of substance abuse implies that individuals choose to become sick, injured, or addicted.

Strong negative feelings that conflict with nursing's humanistic stance may also stem from personal experiences. Being the emotionally or physically abused spouse or child of a substance abuser can have lasting effects on nurses' attitudes toward substance-abusing clients. However, if nurses use alcohol or drugs to relieve stress or self-medicate dysphoric states, they may overidentify with the patient and deny the severity of the client's substance abuse.

Frequently, substance abusers are difficult clients in health care settings. When intoxicated, they may be raucous, uncooperative, and antisocial. When not intoxicated, they may exhibit none of these negative behaviors or may be manipulative and demanding, using flattery or intimidation to hide drug-seeking behavior. Although nurses may initially be warm and understanding, once aware of manipulative attempts, they may have difficulty maintaining an accepting, nonjudgmental attitude. Realizing that recovery from substance abuse often comes very slowly can help nurses feel less pressured to get patients into treatment and be more able simply to raise consciousness by presenting the facts about

addictive illness and leave the decision making to the client.

Nursing Interventions in the Community

There are many ways in which community health nurses can assist individuals, families, and groups experiencing substance abuse problems. First, they can provide an accurate assessment, which includes a family history and specific questions about personal drug and alcohol use. They can be alert to environmental cues in the home that indicate substance abuse, such as empty liquor and pill bottles. An indication of prescription medication abuse is the patient's involvement with several physicians from whom narcotic analgesics and tranquilizers are obtained. This type of assessment can help with case finding and treatment referral, although the individual may have denied the existence of a substance abuse problem initially.

Denial of substance abuse or dependence may range from completely blocked awareness of the problem to partial disavowal of the detrimental effects of the substance use and abuse. One of the primary tasks for intervention and treatment with the substance-dependent individual is to increase the individual's awareness of the problem. Family and significant others can assist with this process by being more honest and direct with the individual about the detrimental effects of the substance abuse. Before this occurs, the significant others must overcome their own denial of the problem and its associated shame and guilt. Referrals to community education programs on substance abuse and dependence and mutual help groups such as Al-Anon and Narcanon are helpful interventions for families and significant others.

The community health nurse may also involve the social network in getting the client into treatment. Although individuals who are forced to enter treatment may not be willing to admit the severity of the abuse, they can still benefit from exposure to the treatment program and eventually begin recovery. Experiencing serious health consequences related to dependency may constitute "hitting bottom" for the individual. This may break through denial or collusion on the part of the family.

The trust that develops in a caring nursing relationship can support disclosure of substance abuse problems and decrease denial in the client or family members. A realistic and positive attitude toward the person with substance abuse can provide families with hope. The nurse must have knowledge of available community resources. One of the primary roles of the community health nurse in helping substance abusers is to facilitate contact with helping agencies such as local treatment programs or mutual help groups. Collaboration with the client's physician is helpful should medical detoxification be necessary.

Other traditional community health nursing roles and interventions are also appropriate to use with substance abusers. Examples follow:

■ Health teaching regarding addictive illness and addictive effects of different substances

■ Providing direct care for abuse- and dependence-related medical problems

■ Counseling clients and families about problems related to substance abuse

■ Collaborating with other disciplines to ensure continuity of care

■ Coordinating health care services for the client to prevent prescription drug abuse and avoid fragmentation of care

■ Providing consultation to nonmedical professionals and lay personnel

■ Facilitating care through appropriate referrals and follow-up

---

CASE STUDY

APPLICATION OF THE NURSING PROCESS

Evelyn Weaver, a 72-year-old widow, was referred to the Visiting Nurse Association for follow-up after hospitalization for a seizure and fall she experienced in her home. Her hospital discharge diagnoses were ethyl alcohol abuse, seizure disorder, hypertension, and bruises and contusions on her left arm and leg. Her discharge medications were phenytoin sodium, or Dilantin, 900 mg orally at bedtime; one multivitamin orally every day; hydrochlorothiazide, 50 mg orally every day; and methyldopa, or Aldomet, 250 mg orally every day.

Mrs. Weaver lived alone in a two-bedroom house in a middle-class suburb. Her husband died 10 years earlier. Until four years previous, her daughter lived nearby with her two children and visited frequently. However, after a divorce, her daughter and grandchildren moved several hundred miles away and visited only once or twice a year. Mrs. Weaver had a married son in the area. He paid her bills once or twice a month, but otherwise had minimal contact. Mrs. Weaver's primary occupation was homemaker and mother. She stopped driving after her last automobile accident and was not involved in any local community organizations.

Assessment

Individual

The visiting nurse performed an in-home nursing assessment of the client and obtained information through the interview and physical assessment.

Mrs. Weaver admitted to an alcohol abuse problem, but minimized its severity. She reported that she stopped drinking for two days on her own and had a seizure. She denied any past alcohol treatment such as counseling or attendance at AA meetings and said she was not interested in treatment. She was abstinent from alcohol since her discharge from the hospital and thought she would remain that way. She admitted to some loneliness and social isolation. She also reported sleep disturbances (i.e., difficulty falling asleep and staying asleep) and decreased nutritional intake with loss of appetite. She denied other psychoactive medication use such as hypnotics, narcotic analgesics, and tranquilizers, or benzodiazepines. She agreed to a social work referral to investigate attendant care and MOW to help her.

Family

Telephone contact between the nurse and the client's daughter revealed that the daughter was very concerned about her mother. She denied that alcohol abuse was her mother's problem, but thought poor nutrition and health practices were the cause of the hospitalization. She was anxious for the social work referral to obtain attendant care to assist her mother in the home. It took several calls and messages before the nurse was able to speak with the client's son. He said his mother was an alcoholic and that he tried unsuccessfully in the past to get her to stop drinking. He was unwilling to do more than visit her twice a month to pay her bills.

Community

The client's middle-class suburb did not have alcohol treatment services geared towards the elderly. AA meetings and private substance abuse counselors were available, but none of them were willing to make home visits and assist an elderly, homebound client. The local senior center did not have programs or education involving substance abuse and refused to allow AA meetings in their building because they feared their clients would be offended. The client's physician was aware of her alcohol abuse problem, but did not know how to assist her. Referral to an inpatient program for substance abuse was not possible because Mrs. Weaver refused to attend.

Diagnosis

Individual

- Altered cardiovascular status secondary to hypertension
- Altered neurological status secondary to alcohol withdrawal seizures
- Knowledge deficit about addictive disease and effects of alcohol abuse
- Sleep pattern disturbance
- Alteration in nutrition (i.e., less than body requirements)
- Social isolation
- Ineffective individual coping related to inability to adjust to role of widow and maintain involvement in community activities
- Knowledge deficit about the effects and side effects of all of her medicines

Family

- Knowledge deficit about addictive disease and effects of excessive alcohol intake
- Knowledge deficit of treatment approaches available for alcohol abuse and the recovery process
- Alteration in family process secondary to poor communication and denial of alcohol abuse in client

Community

- Knowledge deficit in senior center staff regarding the prevalence of alcohol abuse problems in the elderly population and adverse health effects of alcohol consumption in the elderly

- Knowledge deficits in community agencies that assist alcohol abusers (e.g., local AA and counselors) regarding the need to make home visits and provide services geared to the elderly

Planning

Planning for Mrs. Weaver's care involved collaboration among her family, her physician, the agency's SW, and the community alcohol treatment resources. Health teaching and counseling were the main approaches used to directly assist the client and her family. Indirect approaches involved networking with community agencies and supervising other caregivers.

Intervention

Individual

- Nursing visits two to three times weekly initially to monitor the client's medication issues or problems as related to maintaining abstinence or medication dosing, cardiovascular status, neurological status, and nutritional status
- Social work referral to establish attendant assistance in the home and food delivery service for seniors
- Health teaching regarding addictive illness, effects of excessive alcohol intake on the body, alcohol withdrawal seizures, no-added-sodium diet, and effect of medications
- Health teaching about the client's medications, their effects and side effects, and the necessity of following recommended dosing schedules
- Referral for alcohol treatment counseling and AA meetings when the individual is receptive

Family

- Continued contact with the client's daughter and son to involve them in her care
- Health teaching to the family on the course and treatment of addictive illness and the adverse effects of alcohol abuse on the client and the family as related to functioning, cohesion, and communication
- Role modeling by the visiting nurse of the use of clear, direct, and nonjudgmental communication about the client's alcohol abuse problems

Continued

Community

- List of local and national referral resources for clients with substance abuse problems made available to physicians, with a particular focus on resources providing services for older or elderly substance abusers
- Health teaching to community groups (e.g., senior center, AA fellowship, and substance abuse counselors) regarding the prevalence of alcohol abuse in the elderly population and treatment and counseling approaches useful with this aggregate
- Collaboration with community organizations that provide outreach for homebound elderly to assist in identification and referral
- Establishment of a referral network (i.e., telephone hotline) of concerned older or elderly recovering individuals

Evaluation

Initially, interventions proceeded smoothly. Mrs. Weaver obtained attendant help for two hours per day, three times weekly and also received MOW. The visiting nurse filled her medication organizing container, or Medi-Set, weekly. The attendant made sure that the client took her medications and ate her meals and assisted Mrs. Weaver with personal care. Mrs. Weaver remained abstinent from alcohol during this time, but refused any treatment or counseling for her alcohol abuse problem. However, after three weeks, she was rehospitalized after falling at home again. She was diagnosed with phenytoin toxicity; this occurred because she had secretly been taking extra phenytoin at night to help her sleep.

After a few days, Mrs. Weaver was discharged from the hospital and the Visiting Nurses Association reopened the case. Private attendant care and MOW were also reinstated. This time, the physician discontinued the phenytoin and recommended that the client receive alcohol counseling. The client did follow-up with the counseling referrals given to her by the visiting nurse, but her social situation did not change. She remained very isolated and refused involvement with AA.

A third hospitalization occurred within a few weeks when Mrs. Weaver ingested an excessive amount of alcohol in combination with her hyper-

tensive medications. She became physically ill and required treatment. After this hospitalization, her daughter decided to take action. She moved her mother into a retirement community that provided meals and social activities. The visiting nurse continued to follow the case in the new setting.

Initially, the client was angry and anti-social at her new home. This changed after an attendant was hired to assist her with personal care and get her involved with the social activities at the community. The situation remained stable for several weeks because Mrs. Weaver continued to abstain from alcohol. The visiting nurse continued to remain active in the client's care by arranging for aftercare, focusing on providing goal-specific social support for abstinence and general support for addressing the client's concerns and issues, particularly as related to feelings of isolating loss and transitions. Occasional relapses were framed as an opportunity for increasing the client's level of awareness about substance abuse-related problems and their cause.

Levels of Prevention

Primary

- Involves health teaching to individuals and groups on risk factors, early symptoms of substance abuse, adverse health and social consequences, addictive disease process, and available treatment services
- Need to gear educational approaches to the more vulnerable aggregates (e.g., adolescents, minorities, mentally ill, women, and elderly)

Secondary

- Involves screening and early treatment approaches aimed at minimizing health and social consequences of substance abuse
- Involvement of physicians, nurses, and other health care professionals in various health care settings in this process
- Use of various screening and assessment tools and referrals to treatment services and mutual help organizations

Tertiary

- Involves more direct approaches (e.g., detoxification and inpatient or outpatient treatment) to halt the physiologically damaging effects of the substance abuse (e.g., liver disease, organic mental deficits, and gastritis)

- Frequent use of medications to treat the symptoms of substance abuse-related disorders or as part of aversion therapy (e.g., disulfiram)
- Services provided by medical practitioners, treatment services, and mutual help organizations; generally advocate abstinence from the substance and improving the individual's health status

This case study illustrates the possible complexity and frustration involved in helping the substance abuser. Significant others and the medical community must be involved to help the nurse provide care. Often, the social situation, living situation, or social acquaintances must also change to maintain long-term recovery. However, with patience, persistence, and a caring, nonjudgmental attitude, the nurse can often be effective in helping clients with substance abuse problems attain recovery and improve their health status.

SUMMARY

This chapter provides an overview of the complex, multifaceted phenomenon of substance abuse and its manifestations in the community. The focus is on social, economic, and political and health-related aspects of substance abuse. In addition, the concept of substance abuse is related to the more general concept of addictive behaviors, not just those related to drug or alcohol abuse.

From the review of the various etiological theories, it is clear that there is not one causative factor in the development of substance abuse. Consequently, one treatment approach does not apply to all substance abusers.

A discussion of vulnerable aggregates focuses on women, adolescents, the elderly, and people of color. Resources for prevention and intervention at the individual, family, and community levels are outlined.

LEARNING ACTIVITIES

1. Attend several local AA, Narcotics Anonymous, or Cocaine Anonymous meetings and share impressions with classmates.
2. Attend a local Al-Anon, Narcanon, or Adult Children of Alcoholics meeting and share impressions with classmates.
3. Visit a local treatment center that provides detoxification, inpatient, or outpatient treatment and determine the center's treatment philosophy and the types of services it provides to patients and their families.
4. Visit a treatment program for women and determine how the particular needs of this population are assessed and addressed.
5. Learn about the local community college or high school's drug and alcohol education programs.
6. Contact the county or city's mental health services or substance abuse treatment services and obtain a list of local treatment and education resources.

REFERENCES

American Psychiatric Association: *Diagnostic and statistical manual of mental disorders,* ed 4, Washington, DC, 1994, The Association.

Berridge V: Histories of harm reduction: illicit drugs, tobacco and nicotine, *Substance Use and Misuse* 34(1): 199-141, 1999.

Bowersox J: Needle-exchange programs show promise for AIDS prevention, *NIDA Notes* 5:8-9, 1994.

Brecher E: *Licit and illicit drugs,* Boston, 1972, Little, Brown.

Breiter HC et al: Acute effects of cocaine on human brain activity and emotion, *Neuron* 19(3):591-611, 1997.

Brooke D: Impairment in the medical and legal professions, *J Psychosom Res* 43(1):27-34, 1997.

Brown R: Vitamin deficiency and voluntary alcohol consumption, *Q J Stud Alcohol* 30:592-597, 1969.

Brown S: *Treating the alcoholic: a developmental model of recovery,* New York, 1985, Wiley.

Campbell JC, Landenburger K: Violence against women. In Fogel CI, Woods NF, editors: *Women's health care: a comprehensive handbook,* Thousand Oaks, Calif, 1995, Sage.

Carroll K: New methods of treatment efficacy research: bridging clinical research and clinical practice, *Alcohol Health and Research World* 21(4):352-359, 1997.

Centers for Disease Control: Alcohol involvement in fatal motor vehicle crashes: United States, 1997-1998, *Mor Mortal Wkly Rep* 48(47):10876-87, 1999.

Centers for Disease Control: Identification of children with fetal alcohol syndrome, *Mor Mortal Wkly Rep* 47(40): 861-864, 1998.

Chavkin W et al: National survey of the states: policies and practices regarding drug-using pregnant women, *Am J Public Health* 88(1):117, 1998.

Cherpitel C: Brief screening instruments for alcoholism, *Alcohol Health and Research World* 21(4):348-351, 1997.

Dabney D: Workplace deviance among nurses: the influence of work group norms on drug diversion and/or use, *J Nurs Adm* 25(3):48-55, 1995.

Dawkins MP: Alcoholism prevention and black youth, *J Drug Issues* 18:15-20, 1988.

Dicker M, Leighton EA: Trends in U.S. prevalence of drug-using parturient women and drug-affected newborns, 1979 through 1990, *Am J Public Health* 84:1433-1439, 1994.

Drucker E: Drug prohibition and public health: 25 years of evidence, *Public Health Rep* 114:15-29, 1999.

Ellis D, Zucker R, Fitzgerald H: The role of family influences in development and risk, *Alcohol Health and Research World* 21(3):218-226, 1997.

Erickson PG: Introduction: the three phases of harm reduction: an examination of emerging concepts, methodologies and critiques, *Substance Use and Misuse* 34(1): 1-7, 1999.

Ewing JA: Detecting alcoholism: the CAGE questionnaire, *JAMA* 252:1905-1907, 1984.

Faltz B, Rinaldi J: *AIDS and substance abuse: a training manual for health care professionals,* San Francisco, 1987, Regents of the University of California.

Gerace L, Hughes T, Spunt J: Improving nurses' responses toward substance misusing patients: a clinical evaluation project, *Arch Psychiatr Nurs* 9(5):286-294, 1995.

Gfroerer J, de la Rosa M: Protective and risk factors associated with drug use among Hispanic youth, *J Addict Dis* 12(2):87-107, 1993.

Gordis E: *Letter to colleagues,* Washington, DC, 1995, USDHHS, National Institute on Alcohol Abuse and Alcoholism.

Greenberg M, Schneider D: Violence in American cities: young black males is the answer, but what is the question? *Soc Sci Med* 39:179-187, 1994.

Grinspoon L, Bakalar JB: The war on drugs: a peace proposal, *N Engl J Med* 330:357-360, 1994.

Hall JM: Geography of childhood sexual abuse: women's narratives of their childhood environments, *Adv Nurs Sci* 18:29-47, 1996a.

Hall JM: How lesbians recognize and respond to alcohol problems: a theoretical model of problematization, *Adv Nurs Sci* 16:46-63, 1994.

Hall JM: The pervasive effects of childhood sexual abuse in lesbians' recovery from alcohol problems, *Substance Use and Misuse* 31:225-239, 1996b.

Hall JM: What really worked? a case analysis and discussion of confrontational intervention for substance abuse in marginalized women, *Arch Psychiatr Nurs* 7:322-327, 1993.

Hamilton M: Researching harm reduction: care and contradictions, *Substance Use and Misuse* 34(1):119-141, 1999.

Horgan C: *Substance abuse: the nation's number one health problem, key indicators for policy, Institute for Health Policy, Brandeis University,* Princeton, NJ, 1993, The RWJ Foundation.

Hughes JR: Harm reduction approaches to smoking: the need for data, *Am J Prev Med* 15(1):78-79, 1999.

Jackson JK: The adjustment of the family to the crises of alcoholism, *Q J Stud Alcohol* 15:562-586, 1954.

Jacob T, Johnson S: Parenting influences on the development of alcohol abuse and dependence, *Alcohol Health and Research World* 21(3):204-209, 1997.

Jacobson SW: Assessing the impact of maternal drinking during and after pregnancy, *Alcohol Health Res World* 21(3):199-203, 1997.

Kearney MH: Drug treatment for women: traditional models and new directions, *Obstet Gynecol Neonat Nurs* 26(4):459-478, 1999.

Keller M: On the loss of control phenomenon in alcoholism, *Br J Addict* 67:153-166, 1972.

Kendler K, Prescott C: Cocaine use, abuse, and dependence in a population based sample of female twins, *Br J Psychiatry* 173:345-350, 1998.

King C et al: Diagnosis and assessment of substance abuse in older adults: current strategies and issues, *Addict Behav* 19:41-55, 1994.

Kleber HD: Our current approach to drug abuse: progress, problems and proposal, *N Engl J Med* 330:361-364, 1994.

Kurtz E: *Not god: a history of alcoholics anonymous,* Center City, Minn, 1979, Hazelden Educational Services.

Larimer ME, Marlatt GA: Applications of relapse prevention with moderation goals, *J Psychoactive Drugs* 22:189-195, 1990.

Leshner A: Addiction is a brain disease and it matters, *Science* 278:45-47, 1997.

Lifson AR: Harm reduction and needle exchange programs, *Lancet* 351:1819, 1998.

MacCoun RJ: Toward a psychology of harm reduction, *Am J Psychol* 53(11):1199-1208, 1998.

Madrid E: *Substance abuse among nurses: occupational and personal risk factors,* University Microfilms No. 9502636, 1994, San Francisco, Dissertation Abstracts International.

Minuchin S: *Families and family therapy,* Cambridge, Mass, 1974, Harvard University Press.

Montagne M, Scott DM: Prevention of substance abuse problems: models, factors and processes, *Int J Addict* 28:1177-1208, 1993.

Moos R, Brennan P, Mertens J: Diagnostic subgroups and predictors of one-year re-admission among late-middle-aged and older substance abuse patients, *J Stud Alcohol* 55:173-183, 1994.

Morrison M et al: At war in the fields of play: current perspectives on the nature and treatment of adolescent chemical dependency, *J Psychoactive Drugs* 25:321-330, 1993.

Naegle M: The need for alcohol abuse-related education in nursing curricula, *Alcohol Health and Research World* 18:154-157, 1994.

National Institute on Alcohol Abuse and Alcoholism: *Ninth special report to the US Congress on alcohol and health,* 1997, US Government Printing Office, www.niaaa.nih.gov.

National Institute on Drug Abuse: *Principles of drug addiction treatment: a research-based guide,* Government Printing Office No 99-4180, Rockville, Md, 1999, USDHHS, www.nida.nih.gov.

National Institute on Drug Abuse: *The economic costs of alcohol and drug abuse in the United States, 1992,* No BKD265, Rockville, Md, 1997, USDHHS, www.nida.nih.gov.

Office of National Drug Control Policy: *Pulse check: trends in drug use,* 1997, The Author, www.health.org/pulse 98.

Paone D, Alpern J: Pregnancy policing: policy of harm, *Int J Drug Policy* 9:101, 1998.

Quazi M: Effective drug-free workplace plan uses worker testing as a deterrent, *Occup Health Saf* 6:26-32, 1993.

Robert Wood Johnson Foundation: *Substance abuse (annual report),* Princeton, NJ, 1992, The Author.

Roberts L, Leonard K: Gender differences and similarities in the alcohol and marriage relationship. In Wilsnack RW, Wilsnack SC, editors: *Gender and alcohol: individual and social perspectives,* New Brunswick, NJ, 1997, Rutgers University Center of Alcohol Studies.

Satir V, Stachowiak J, Taschman H: *Helping families to change,* New York, 1975, Jason Aronson.

Scherling D: Prenatal cocaine exposure and childhood psychopathology: a developmental analysis, *Am J Orthopsychiatry* 64:9-19, 1994.

Stanton MD et al: Heroin addiction as a family phenomenon: a new conceptual model, *Am J Drug Alcohol Abuse* 5:125-150, 1978.

Steinglass P: Family systems approaches to alcoholism, *J Substance Abuse Treatment* 2:161-167, 1985.

Subby R: Inside the chemically dependent marriage: denial and manipulation. In Subby R, editor: *Codependency: an emerging issue,* Deerfield Beach, Fla, 1984, Health Communications.

Substance Abuse and Mental Health Services Administration, Office of Applied Statistics: *National household survey on drug abuse: population estimates 1996,* USDHHS Pub No SMA, Rockville, Md, 1996, USDHHS, PHS.

Substance Abuse and Mental Health Services Administration, Office of Applied Statistics: *National household survey on drug abuse: population estimates 1998,* USDHHS Pub No SMA, Rockville, Md, 1998, USDHHS, PHS.

Sussman S, Dent C, Galaif E: The correlates of substance abuse and dependence among adolescents at high risk for drug abuse, *J Substance Abuse* 9:241-255, 1997.

Sweeney M, Penner S: A study of employees' attitudes toward workplace drug testing: nursing implications, *J Addictions Nurs* 9(4):156-163, 1997.

Trinkoff A, Storr C: Substance abuse among nurses: differences between specialties, *Am J Public Health* 88(4):581-585, 1998.

US Department of Health and Human Services: *Healthy people 2010: conference edition,* Washington, DC, 2000, PHS.

US Department of Justice, Bureau of Justice Statistics: *Drugs, crime and the justice system: a national report,* Rockville, Md, 1992, Bureau of Justice Statistics.

Van der Kolk BA, McFarlane AC, Weisaeth L, editors: *Traumatic stress: the effects of overwhelming experience on mind, body and society,* New York, 1996, Guilford Press.

Vogeltanz N, Wilsnack S: Alcohol problems in women: risk factors, consequences, and treatment strategies. In Gallant S, Keita GP, Royak-Schaler R, editors: *Health care for women: psychological, social and behavioral influences,* Washington, DC, 1997, American Psychological Association.

Wetherington C, Roman S: *Drug addiction research and the health of women,* NIH Pub No 98-4289, 1998, National Institute on Drug Abuse, www.health.org.

Widiger TA, Smith GT: Substance use disorder: abuse, dependence and dyscontrol, *Addictions* 89:267-282, 1994.

Wild TC: Compulsory substance use treatment and harm reduction: a critical analysis, *Substance Use and Misuse* 34(1):35-47, 1999.

Wilsnack R et al: Ten year prediction of women's drinking behavior in a nationally representative sample, *Women's Health Research on Gender, Behavior and Policy* 4(3):199-230, 1998.

Wilsnack S et al: Drinking and problem drinking in older women. In Bereford TP, Gomberg ES, editors: *Alcohol and aging,* London, 1995, Oxford University Press.

Windle M: Substance abuse, risky behaviors and victimization among a US national adolescent sample, *Addiction* 89:172-182, 1997.

Wodak A: Harm reduction: Australia as a case study, *Bull NY Acad Med* 72(2):339-347, 1995.

Ziter ML: Culturally sensitive treatment of black alcoholics, *Natl Assoc Social Workers* 12:130-135, 1987.

Special Service Needs

25 Communicable Disease and Public Health

26 School Health

27 Occupational Health

28 Correctional Health

29 Parish Health

30 Home Health

25

Communicable Disease and Public Health

Marianne Bond, Vera Labat, and Dottie Compton Langthorn

OBJECTIVES

Upon completion of this chapter, the reader will be able to do the following:

1. Discuss the routes for transmission of communicable diseases.
2. Identify the protocols for notifiable diseases within the CDC Monitoring and Surveillance System and explain why the system is important.
3. List three communicable diseases currently causing high morbidity in the United States and identify their epidemiological indicators.
4. Specify the immunizations required by law in the United States and discuss their efficacy.
5. Discuss the prevalence and risk factors involved in the acquisition of HIV and other STDs and identify methods for control.
6. Explain the differences among prevention, control, elimination, and eradication of communicable diseases.

KEY TERMS

acquired immunity
active immunity
cold chain
control
direct transmission
elimination
eradication
herd immunity
immunity
immunization
indirect transmission
natural immunity
notifiable infectious diseases
passive immunity
primary vaccine failure
secondary vaccine failure
universal precautions
vaccination
Vaccine Averse Events Reporting System (VAERS)

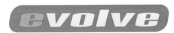

http://evolve.elsevier.com/Nies/

Throughout history, epidemics have been responsible for the annihilation of entire groups of people. However, since 1900, vaccines, antibiotics, improved hygiene, food regulations, and clean water have dramatically reduced the alarming rates of morbidity and mortality caused by infectious diseases. Despite amazing advances in public health and health care, at the beginning of the new millennium control of communicable diseases continues to be a major concern of health care providers. The emergence of new pathogens, the reemergence of old pathogens, and the appearance of drug-resistant pathogens are creating formidable challenges for infectious disease control workers worldwide.

Although global eradication campaigns have been in process for decades, malaria and other vector-borne communicable diseases, AIDS, and diarrheal illness from enteric pathogens continue to cause significant mortality in the developing world. TB infects one third of the world's population and has become a leading killer of young adults worldwide. Treatments exist for many STDs, yet syphilis and gonorrhea continue to be global problems. Measles, when coupled with vitamin A deficiency, is a leading cause of blindness in many developing countries in the Eastern Hemisphere.

In 1978, WHO sponsored the Alma Ata Conference, which closed with the declaration of "health for all people by the year 2000." This ambitious global agenda came from WHO, United Nations Children's Fund (UNICEF), and other organizations that had the political will, ideological commitment, and sense of accountability to examine the cost of human morbidity and mortality in both the developing and the developed world. The conference gave public health workers from all over the globe an increased sense of direction and a vision of shared goals.

WHO and UNICEF have also sponsored other global goals for international public health priorities, including eradication of some communicable diseases. Following the successful eradication of smallpox in 1977, other diseases were targeted for global control, elimination, and eradication through vaccination and other public health measures. Vaccination is a simple, cost-effective preventive health measure that proved to be one of the twentieth century's most effective tools for preventing disease and death. Widespread immunization has protected large aggregates of people from many diseases and the twenty-first century may produce even greater strides in disease control.

At the 1990 World Summit for Children, leaders from 159 countries agreed to a set of goals that would reduce child and maternal mortality rates and give every child access to clean water and proper sanitation. This summit helped over 80% of the world's children become covered by immunization services, with some countries surpassing the 90% goal, and polio and guinea worm are on the verge of eradication. Oral rehydration therapy is now being used to prevent dehydration and death from diarrheal illnesses. Yet problems remain. Population growth is outstripping the availability of sanitation services in many developing countries, placing many at increased risk for food- and water-borne diseases.

The EPA is responsible for the establishment and enforcement of standards for water quality control in the United States. Chemical treatment and filtration methods are used for disinfection of drinking water supplies. Simple preventive measures such as these, which are taken for granted in "developed" nations, are the foundation for protecting the public's health from water-borne diseases and their sequelae. Unfortunately, people most likely to suffer from water-borne infections are often those living in developing countries without access to a safe water supply and sanitary means of excreta disposal.

Deaths from infectious disease declined markedly in the United States during the twentieth century. In 1900, the three leading causes of death were pneumonia, TB, and diarrhea enteritis, which, together with diphtheria, caused one third of all deaths. In contrast, only 4.5% of all deaths were attributable to infectious diseases in 1997. Despite this overall progress, one of the most devastating epidemics in human history occurred during the twentieth century. The 1918 influenza pandemic resulted in 20 million deaths, including 500,000 in the United States in less than one year. This was more than have died in as short a time during any war or famine in the world (CDC, 1999a).

In the United States, there have been both successes and failures in preventing communicable diseases. Indigenous measles has virtually been eliminated, with only 100 cases reported in 1998, but hepatitis B and hepatitis C cases are almost at epidemic proportions. The incidence of pertussis rose in the 1990s and was five times the year 2000 target by 1995, which pointed to a need for a rapid, reliable diagnostic test and an adult pertussis vaccine.

As the percentage of Americans living below the poverty level continues to increase, inequities in access to health care appear to be growing proportionately. This lack of access is responsible in part for the increases in preventable communicable disease rates in the United States. Additionally, climatic changes, global warming, ecological instability, industrial development, natural disasters, wars, "sick buildings," human behaviors, and medical advances in areas such as organ transplants and genetic engineering play a role in the environmental, social, and host interactions that create new opportunities for emergent pathogenic outbreaks.

To further control communicable diseases, health care reforms in the United States must match the challenges with provision of services. Emphasis should be placed on cost-effective, preventive care with a focus on access to immunizations for every child and adult in the primary health care setting. Interdisciplinary cooperation, locally, nationally, and internationally, among those charged with surveillance, reporting, monitoring, and control of communicable diseases (i.e., epidemiologists, climatologists, entomologists, and virologists) is essential in the effort to produce a healthier environment. Primary prevention is the key to a sustainable health care system and it must be accomplished without compromising quality of care. Ongoing funding for vaccine and antimicrobial drug research and development is crucial if successful control and ultimate eradication of many of the new and reemerging communicable diseases are to be accomplished. Community health nurses play an increasing role in advancing these efforts.

Almost two thirds of all employed nurses in the United States today are currently working in hospital settings. Projections for the future of nursing, based on cost-containment and disease prevention health policies, place nurses in ambulatory care and other community-based health care settings. In these areas, they will be better able to meet the health needs of the communities in which they work by providing community-based health interventions, including health education and disease prevention programs designed specifically to meet the health needs of the community served. Community health nurses (CHNs) do not work alone, but they are part of a multidisciplinary team working together with members of the community. School nurses ensure vaccination of students, STD clinic nurses provide health education and reporting of notifiable diseases, and nurse epidemiologists monitor surveillance systems and interpret data for appropriate planning for future interventions.

This chapter discusses transmission, immunity, prevention, defining and reporting, control, elimination, and eradication of communicable diseases. Vaccine-preventable diseases, vaccines for travelers, and STDs are detailed. The chapter concludes with the application of the nursing process to a case study outlining the assessment, diagnosis, short- and long-term planning, intervention, evaluation, and primary, secondary, and tertiary prevention of an epidemic at the individual, family, and community levels.

COMMUNICABLE DISEASE AND *HEALTHY PEOPLE 2010*

The National Health Promotion and Disease Prevention Objectives were initiated in 1979 and have been reformulated each decade thereafter. Launched in January 2000, the latest version, *Healthy People 2010,* has expanded goals for immunization and infectious diseases and covers such areas as vaccine-preventable diseases, STDs, HIV, hepatitis, TB, and a number of related health issues (USDHHS, 2000). Table 25-1 provides examples of *Healthy People 2010* goals related to communicable diseases.

Application of community-based health interventions based on recommendations from *Healthy People 2010* can assist in interrupting or preventing disease transmission and provide an assessment of the risk factors that impede health and increase the likelihood of transmission. Analysis of the underlying environmental, socioeconomic, political, educational, employment, and health factors should be considered when promoting the development of interventions for disease prevention and surveillance designed specifically for health promotion of the individual, family, and aggregate.

TRANSMISSION

Communicable diseases do not occur in a vacuum, but are the result of interaction between a host (e.g., a person), an infectious agent (e.g., a bacterium), and the environment (e.g., a contaminated food supply), known as an epidemiological triad (see Chapter 4).

TABLE 25-1

Communicable Diseases and *Healthy People 2010* Objectives

Objective	Baseline (1998)	Target
13-1: Reduce AIDS among adolescents and adults	19.5 per 100,000	1 per 100,000
13-2: Reduce the number of new AIDS cases among adolescent and adult men who have sex with men	17,847	13,385
13-6: Increase the proportion of sexually active persons who use condoms	23%	50%
14-1d: Reduce or eliminate indigenous cases of hepatitis B in people aged 2 to 18	945	9
14-1e: Reduce or eliminate indigenous cases of measles	74	0
14-1g: Reduce or eliminate indigenous cases of pertussis in children under age seven	3417	2000
14-8: Reduce new cases of Lyme disease	17.4 per 100.000	9.7 per 100,000
14-9: Reduce new cases of hepatitis C	2.4 per 100,000	1 per 100,000
14-11: Reduces new cases of TB	6.8 per 100,000	1 per 100,000
14-22a: Achieve and maintain effective vaccination coverage levels for four doses of DTaP vaccine	84%	90%
14-22d: Achieve and maintain effective vaccination coverage levels for two doses of MMR vaccine	92%	90%
14-22f: Achieve and maintain effective vaccination coverage levels for one dose of varicella vaccine	43%	90%
14-29a: Increase the proportion of adults who are vaccinated annually against influenza	63%	90%
14-29b: Increase the proportion of adults who are vaccinated against pneumococcal disease	43%	90%
25-1b: Reduce the proportion of females aged 15 to 24 attending STD clinics with *Chlamydia trachomatis* infections	12.2%	3.0%
25-2: Reduce new cases of gonorrhea	123 per 100,000	19 per 100,000
25-6: Reduce the proportion of females who have ever required treatment for PID	8%	5%

From US Department of Health and Human Services: *Healthy people 2010: conference edition,* Washington, DC, 2000, PHS.

Communicable diseases can be transmitted vertically or horizontally (Gordis, 1996). Vertical transmission occurs between parent and offspring when the infection is passed via placenta, milk, and contact with the vagina during birth. Horizontal transmission occurs in either a direct manner in person-to-person contact or indirectly through a common vehicle such as contaminated food or water, through a vector such as arthropods (i.e., ticks or mosquitoes), or via airborne route such as contaminated droplets in the air (Table 25-2).

Direct transmission implies the immediate transfer of an infectious agent from an infected host or reservoir to an appropriate portal of entry in the human host through physical contact. Uninterrupted person-to-person contact is responsible for the transmission of many communicable diseases, including scabies, measles, and STDs such as gonorrhea.

TABLE **25-2**

Modes of Transmission for Various Communicable Diseases

Direct	Indirect	*Fecal-Oral	Airborne
Candidiasis	Arthropod-borne viral diseases	Amebiasis	Meningococcal disease
Herpes	Lyme disease	*Giardiasis*	Mumps
Mononucleosis	Tetanus	*Escherichia coli*	Rubella
Syphilis	Rabies	*Campylobacter*	Pertussis
Gonorrhea	Rocky Mountain spotted fever	Salmonellosis	Influenza
Ebola	Botulism	Cholera	Measles
Leprosy†	Plague	Typhoid fever	TB
Viral warts	Schistosomiasis	Polio	Chickenpox
Chickenpox‡	Yellow fever		
Common cold	Malaria		
Diphtheria			

*Transmission may be person to person or animal to person.
†Exact mode of transmission not clearly understood.
‡Transmission can be either airborne or direct contact.

Indirect transmission is the spread of infection through vehicle fomites, animals, and vectors that carry a parasite or pathogen to a suitable portal of entry in the human host. Vehicle-borne or contaminated fomites can be any inanimate object, material, or substance that acts as a transport agent for a microbe (e.g., water, a telephone, or a contaminated tissue). Reproduction of the infectious agent may take place on or in the vehicle before the transmission of the pathogen. Substances such as food, water, and blood products can provide indirect transmission through ingestion and intravenous transfusions. Viruses, bacteria, parasites, and enterotoxins may cause food-borne diseases. Botulism is an example of an indirectly transmitted food-borne enterotoxin disease.

Animal and vector-borne transmission can be communicated through biological and mechanical routes. The mechanical route involves no multiplication or growth of the parasite or microbe within the animal or vector itself. Biological transmission occurs when the parasite grows or multiplies inside the animal, vector, or arthropod. Examples of diseases spread by this method of transmission include arthropod-borne diseases such as malaria, hemorrhagic fevers, and viral encephalitis. The modes of transmission

from animals to humans vary considerably and may include biting, spitting, eating contaminated meat products, spray from urine, and fecal-oral transmission. Tetanus is an example of indirect mechanical transmission via soil, or carried by an animal, which then contaminates a human through a wound or bite. Transmission from a vector to the human host is usually through a bite or sting. Malaria is an example of indirect biological transmission from a mosquito vector to a human host.

Fecal-oral transmission can be both direct and indirect. It can occur through the ingestion of water supplies that have been fecally polluted, by consumption of contaminated food, or through engagement in oral-genital sexual activity. Poliovirus is spread through fecal-oral transmission.

Airborne transmission occurs mainly through aerosols and droplet nuclei. The time frame in which an airborne particle can remain suspended greatly influences the virility and infectivity of the organism. The size of the particle can also play an important role in how long it remains airborne and how successful it will be at penetrating the human lung. Aerosols are extremely small solid or liquid particles that may include fungal spores, viruses, and bacteria. When inhaled into the lungs, they are responsible for many infections, including fungal diseases such as crypto-coccosis and histoplasmosis. Droplet nuclei, such as the spray from sneezing, travel approximately one meter but usually not further before the droplets fall to the ground. Within this distance, contaminated drop-lets may make direct contact with an open wound or with a mucous membrane (e.g., conjunctiva, nose, or mouth), or they may be inhaled into the lung. Measles virus is spread through inhalation of contaminated droplets.

IMMUNITY

Immunity can be described as the body's ability to protect itself from infection. There are several differ-ent kinds of immunity, each providing resistance to any of a number of specific infectious diseases. **Natural immunity** is an innate resistance to a specific antigen or toxin. **Acquired immunity** is derived from actual exposure to the specific infectious agent, toxin, or appropriate vaccine. **Active immunity** is present when the body can build its own antibodies that provide protection from a bacterial or other antigenic substance, such as the introduction of a vaccine or toxoid. **Passive immunity** is the temporary resistance that has been donated to the host through transfusions of plasma proteins, immunoglobulins, and antitoxins, or from mother to neonate transplacentally. Passive immunity lasts only as long as these substances remain in the bloodstream.

The concept of **herd immunity** refers to a state in which those not immune to an infectious agent will be safe if at least 80% of the population has been vaccinated or is otherwise immune. This is especially true for the transmission of diseases that are found only in the human host and that have no invertebrate host or other mode of transmission. Without the presence of a virgin population to infect, the organism will be unable to live because the vast majority of the population is immune.

When properly administered according to estab-lished guidelines and protocols, vaccines provide acquired immunity in most cases. However, there are exceptions. **Primary vaccine failure** is the failure of a vaccine to contribute any level of immunogenicity and can be caused by improper storage that may render the vaccines ineffective, improper administra-tion route, or light-sensitive vaccines exposed to light. Additionally, a certain portion of people receiving vaccine never seroconvert and are not protected from the communicable disease. **Secondary vaccine fail-**

ure is the waning of immunogenicity after eliciting an initial immune response that fades over time. This often occurs in immunosuppressed patients and organ transplant patients in whom the immune memory is essentially destroyed.

Standard/Universal Blood and Body Fluid Precautions

In response to the risk of exposure to blood-borne pathogens (e.g., HIV, hepatitis B, and hepatitis C) in the late 1980s, the CDC developed a set of guidelines to prevent transmission of diseases found in blood and body fluids. These guidelines are based on the observation that infected people may have no signs or symptoms or not have any knowledge of their conditions; therefore all people are assumed to be infectious and health care workers treat them as such. These guidelines are termed **universal precautions** and are depicted in Box 25-1.

BOX **25-1**

Standard Universal Blood and Body Fluid Precautions

In 1988, the CDC established guidelines on occu-pational exposure to blood-borne pathogens. These guidelines state that workers are to con-sider any contact with blood or body fluid as hazardous. The following guidelines show how exposure to blood-borne diseases to workers can be minimized:

- Special training and education programs
- Use of protective equipment such as gloves, gowns, eye protection, and face masks
- Hand washing after each patient contact
- Proper handling and disposing of sharps
- Engineering control such as special sharps containers and safety cabinets for biologicals
- Programs of immunization such as Hep B for employees
- Proper contaminated waste disposal
- Use of disinfectants
- Proper labeling and signs

Adapted from Centers for Disease Control: Universal precaution for prevention of transmission of HIV, hepatitis B virus and other bloodborne pathogens in health care settings, *Mor Mortal Wkly Rep* 37:377-382, 387-388, 1988.

Defining and Reporting Communicable Diseases

The CDC is responsible for monitoring communicable disease in the United States. Along with the Council of State and Territorial Epidemiologists, the CDC has identified 52 infectious diseases that are designated **notifiable infectious diseases**, meaning that health care providers who encounter these diseases *must* report them to the local or regional health department. These notifiable diseases are listed in Box 25-2.

Not all nationally notifiable diseases are reportable in every state or territory. However, the data listed in the box, unless otherwise noted, are transmitted to the CDC via the National Electronic Telecommunications System for Surveillance. Cases of infectious diseases are reported by geographical region, by state, and for the nation each week in the CDC's *MMWR*. Weekly and cumulative totals of communicable dis-

ease and information on prevention and control are also presented. The *MMWR* can be found in medical libraries, at local health departments, at infection control departments in hospitals and medical centers, and on the Internet at www.cdc.gov.

Standardizing definitions of diseases is important for local, state, national, and global public health surveillance teams because it provides a baseline for data comparison and epidemiological trend monitoring across the country and around the world. Diseases are defined and classified according to confirmed cases, probable cases, laboratory-confirmed cases, clinically compatible cases, epidemiologically linked cases, genetic typing, and clinical case definition. Screening, intervention, and control and eradication programs can readily be designed and implemented based on the data collected from adherence to this set of case definitions.

BOX **25-2**

Nationally Notifiable Infectious Diseases, United States, 1999

AIDS	Malaria
Anthrax	Measles
Botulism	Meningococcal disease
Chancroid	Mumps
Chlamydia trachomatis (genital infections)	Pertussis
Cholera	Plague
Coccidioidomycosis (regional)	Poliomyelitis (paralytic)
Cryptosporidiosis	Psittacosis
Cyclosporiasis	Rabies (animal)
Diphtheria	Rabies (human)
Ehrlichiosis (human granulocytic)	Rocky Mountain spotted fever
Ehrlichiosis (human monocytic)	Rubella
Encephalitis (California serogroup)	Rubella (congenital syndrome)
Encephalitis (Eastern equine)	Salmonellosis
Encephalitis (St. Louis)	Shigellosis
Encephalitis (Western equine)	Streptococcal disease (invasive group A)
Escherichia coli (O157:H7)	*Streptococcus pneumoniae*
Gonorrhea	(drug-resistant invasive disease)
Haemophilus influenzae (invasive disease)	Streptococcal TSS
Hansen's disease (leprosy)	Syphilis
Hantavirus pulmonary syndrome	Syphilis (congenital)
Hemolytic uremic syndrome (postdiarrheal)	Tetanus
Hepatitis A	TSS
Hepatitis B	Trichinosis
Hepatitis C (nonA and nonB)	TB
HIV infection (pediatric)	Typhoid fever
Legionellosis	Varicella deaths
Lyme disease	Yellow fever

CONTROL, ELIMINATION, AND ERADICATION OF COMMUNICABLE DISEASE

Control

Control of a communicable disease refers to the reduction of incidence or prevalence of a given disease to a locally acceptable level as a result of deliberate efforts (CDC, 1999b). The WHO's Expanded Programme on Immunizations (EPI) is a global attempt to control morbidity and mortality for many vaccine-preventable diseases, with each country adapting these guidelines as necessary.

At the World Summit for Children in 1994, WHO, UNICEF, and several other international health organizations established goals for the global control of specific diseases. The goals include the achievement of 80% immunization coverage with the six basic immunizations, including bacille Calmette-Guérin (BCG) for TB, oral poliovirus vaccine (OPV), diphtheria-pertussis-tetanus (DPT), and measles in all countries. Goals also include 80% use of oral rehydration therapy to control dehydration from diarrheal disease and health education for increased breastfeeding (UNICEF, 1994).

Elimination

The process of **elimination** of a communicable disease involves controlling it within a specified geographical area such as a single country, an island, or a continent and reducing the prevalence and incidence to eventual eradication. Elimination is the result of deliberate efforts, but continued intervention measures are required (CDC, 1999b).

At the 1994 World Summit for Children, several goals for the global elimination of specific diseases and conditions were established (UNICEF, 1994). These included the elimination of poliomyelitis from Europe and the Western Pacific; measles from the English-speaking Caribbean; and neonatal tetanus, vitamin A deficiency and related blindness and iodine deficiency disorders (e.g., goiter and cretinism) globally. Other diseases targeted for elimination in the near future are leprosy and measles on the European continent.

Although indigenous measles has virtually been eliminated in the United States, approximately one million children die from measles each year worldwide (CDC, 1999c). Measles elimination efforts will be enhanced with the development of a simple, fast field test to confirm measles cases and a stable vaccine that does not require refrigeration and reconstitution before use.

WHO set the goal of eliminating Hansen's disease, or leprosy, incidence to less than one per 10,000 population worldwide by 2000 (UNICEF, 1994). Barriers to leprosy elimination include lack of a simple rapid diagnostic test, persistence of organisms, cost and duration of drug therapy, patient compliance, and social stigma. Leprosy is endemic in 55 countries and India, Indonesia, and Myanmar account for 70% of all cases. In the United States, 108 new cases of leprosy were reported in 1998 (CDC, 1999d).

Eradication

The International Task Force for Disease Eradication (ITFDE) defines **eradication** as reducing the worldwide incidence of a disease to zero as a function of deliberate efforts, without a need for further control measures (CDC, 1999b). For a disease to be eradicated, it must meet the criteria listed in Box 25-3.

Smallpox was eradicated in 1977 and the virus now exists only in storage in laboratories. Many factors contributed to the successful eradication of smallpox, including the mode of transmission of the

---

BOX **25-3**

Criteria for Disease Eradication

Epidemiology:
1. Human host only; no host in nature
2. Easy diagnosis; obvious clinical manifestations
3. Limited duration and intensity of infection
4. Natural lifelong immunity after infection
5. Highly seasonal transmission
6. Availability of vaccine, curative treatment, or both

Political will:
1. Substantial global morbidity and mortality rates
2. Cost-effectiveness of campaign and eradication
3. Integration of eradication with additional public health variables
4. Eradication imperative over control measures

From Centers for Disease Control: Recommendations of the International Task Force for Disease Eradication, *Mor Mortal Wkly Rep* 42:1-38, 1993.

disease, the isolated geographical distribution of the infection, the ease of administration of the freeze-dried vaccine, the establishment of an effective surveillance system, the increase of national and international political will, and tremendous community participation.

With the successful eradication of smallpox, WHO has targeted seven other infectious diseases for elimination and eventual eradication. These are filariasis, leprosy, guinea worm disease (i.e., dracunculiasis), tetanus, Chagas' disease, measles, and polio (CDC, 1999b).

Smallpox, or variola, is the only disease that has been eradicated. From 1900 to 1904, an average of 48,164 cases and 1528 deaths caused by smallpox were reported each year in the United States. The pattern in the decline of smallpox was sporadic. Outbreaks occurred periodically in the first quarter of the 1900s and then ceased abruptly in 1929. The last case of variola minor (the milder form of smallpox) in the United States was reported in 1949. The worldwide eradication of smallpox in 1977 enabled the discontinuation of prevention and treatment efforts, including routine vaccination (CDC, 1999e).

PREVENTION AND CONTROL OF VACCINE-PREVENTABLE DISEASES

The American Academy of Pediatrics (AAP), The Advisory Committee on Immunization Practices (ACIP), and the American Academy of Family Physicians (AAFP) recommend that all children in the United States complete a schedule of 11 childhood vaccines by age 18 months. The schedule is complex and includes four doses of diphtheria, tetanus, and acellular pertussis vaccine (DTaP); three doses of inactivated poliovirus vaccine (IPV); one dose of measles-mumps-rubella vaccine (MMR); three to four doses of Hib conjugate vaccine; three doses of hepatitis B vaccine (Hep B); one dose of varicella vaccine; and four doses of a newly approved conjugated pneumococcal vaccine (CDC, 2000a, 2000f). Hepatitis A vaccine is also recommended for children aged 2 to 18 years living in states, counties, or communities where hepatitis A rates are twice the national average. Compliance with routine vaccination schedules is a serious

problem and failure to complete a full series of any of these vaccines leaves the child only partially protected. This reduces overall coverage rates, which could compromise herd immunity.

This section contains comprehensive information on vaccines and includes vaccine types, storage, transport, handling, administration and routes, dosages, spacing, contraindications, documentation, vaccine-related injuries, and resources for additional vaccine information. Twelve childhood vaccine-preventable communicable diseases are discussed in detail, including presentation, complications, transmission, incubation, current statistics, risk groups, diagnosis, treatment, vaccination, control, and possible eradication activities.

Vaccines

As the rate of vaccine-related research advances, it becomes more important for health care professionals to consult with current sources of information regarding immunizations. Recommendations, policies, and procedures concerning immunization information are governed internationally by WHO and nationally by the AAP's Committee on Infectious Diseases and the PHS's ACIP. Occasionally, there are differences of opinion regarding the information from these agencies and it is extremely important to thoroughly consider the population involved when interpreting these recommendations and procedures. The recommended schedule for immunization of healthy infants and children by the ACIP, the AAP, and the AAFP is presented in Fig. 25-1.

Precautions must be taken when giving any immunization. The most recent recommendations regarding which immunizations to give; to whom they should be given; how they should be given; and how they are to be transported, stored, and administered can be obtained from the CDC. These recommendations should be transmitted from the CDC to state health departments, from state health departments to local health departments, and from local health departments to physicians and other primary care providers.

Vaccine efficacy is dependent on many factors, which are detailed in the following section. When policy recommendations are not followed, the public health system is jeopardized with all of its constituents. A breakdown in this chain can leave children unimmunized, workers unprotected, and surveillance systems vulnerable to incomplete or inaccurate information. Additional information on

Recommended childhood immunization schedule, United States, January to December 2000 (From Centers for Disease Control: *Epidemiology and prevention of vaccine-preventable diseases [pink book],* ed 6, Atlanta, 2000b, Public Health Foundation. Also available at www.cdc.gov/nip.pdf/child-schedule.pdf).

Recommended Childhood Immunization Schedule
United States, January - December 2000

Vaccines[1] are listed under routinely recommended ages. Bars indicate range of recommended ages for immunization. Any dose not given at the recommended age should be given as a "catch-up" immunization at any subsequent visit when indicated and feasible. Ovals indicate vaccines to be given if previously recommended doses were missed or given earlier than the recommended minimum age.

Age / Vaccine	Birth	1 mo	2 mos	4 mos	6 mos	12 mos	15 mos	18 mos	24 mos	4 to 6 yrs	11 to 12 yrs	14 to 16 yrs
Hepatitis B[2]		Hep B										
			Hep B			Hep B					Hep B	
Diphtheria, Tetanus, Pertussis[3]			DTaP	DTaP	DTaP		DTaP[3]			DTaP	Td	
H. influenzae type b[4]			Hib	Hib	Hib	Hib						
Polio[5]			IPV	IPV		IPV[5]				IPV[5]		
Measles, Mumps, Rubella[6]						MMR				MMR[6]	MMR[6]	
Varicella[7]						Var					Var[7]	
Hepatitis A[8]										Hep A[8] in selected areas		

Approved by the Advisory Committee on Immunization Practices (ACIP), the American Academy of Pediatrics (AAP), and the American Academy of Family Physicians (AAFP).

On October 22, 1999, the Advisory Committee on Immunization Practices (ACIP) recommended that Rotashield® (RRV-TV), the only U.S.-licensed rotavirus vaccine, no longer be used in the United States (*MMWR*, Volume 48, Number 43, Nov. 5, 1999). Parents should be reassured that their children who received rotavirus vaccine before July are not at increased risk for intussusception now.

[1]This schedule indicates the recommended ages for routine administration of currently licensed childhood vaccines as of 11/1/99. Additional vaccines may be licensed and recommended during the year. Licensed combination vaccines may be used whenever any components of the combination are indicated and its other components are not contraindicated. Providers should consult the manufacturers' package inserts for detailed recommendations.

[2]**Infants born to HBsAg-negative mothers** should receive the first dose of hepatitis B (Hep B) vaccine by age two months. The second dose should be at least one month after the first dose. The third dose should be administered at least four months after the first dose and at least two months after the second dose, but not before six months of age for infants. **Infants born to HBsAg-positive mothers** should receive hepatistis B vaccine and 0.5 ml hepatitis B immune globulin (HBIG) within 12 hours of birth at separate sites. The second dose is recommended at one to two months of age and the third dose at six months of age.
Infants born to mothers whose HBsAg status is unknown should receive hepatitis B vaccine within 12 hours of birth. Maternal blood should be drawn at the time of delivery to determine the mother's HBsAg status; if the HBsAg test is positive, the infant should receive HBIG as soon as possible (no later than one week of age).
All children and adolescents (through 18 years of age) who have not been immunized against hepatitis B may begin the series during any visit. Special efforts should be made to immunize children who were born in or whose parents were born in areas of the world with moderate or high endemicity of hepatitis B virus infection.

[3]The fourth dose of DTaP (diphtheria and tetanus toxoids and acellular pertussis vaccine) may be administered as early as 12 months of age, provided six months have elapsed since the third dose and the child is unlikely to return at age 15 to 18 months. Td (tetanus and diphtheria toxoids) is recommended at 11 to 12 years of age if at least five years have elapsed since the last dose of DTP, DTaP, or DT. Subsequent routine Td boosters are recommended every 10 years.

[4]Three *Haemophilus influenzae* type b (Hib) conjugate vaccines are licensed for infant use. If PRP-OMP (PedvaxHIB® or ComVax® [Merck]) is administered at two and four months of age, a dose at six months is not required. Because clinical studies in infants have demonstrated that using some combination products may induce a lower immune response to the Hib vaccine component, DTaP/Hib combination products should not be used for primary immunization in infants at two, four, or six months of age, unless FDA-approved for these ages.

[5]To eliminate the risk of vaccine-associated paralytic polio (VAPP), an all-IPV schedule is now recommended for routine childhood polio vaccination in the United States. All children should receive four doses of IPV at two months, four months, six to eighteen months, and four to six years. OPV (if available) may be used only for the following special circumstances:
1. Mass vaccination campaigns to control outbreaks of paralytic polio.
2. Unvaccinated children who will be traveling in less than four weeks to areas where polio is endemic or epidemic.
3. Children of parents who do not accept the recommended number of vaccine injections. These children may receive OPV only for the third or fourth dose of both; in this situation, health care providers should administer OPV only after discussing the risk for VAPP with parents of caregivers.
4. During the transition to an all-IPV schedule, recommendations for the use of remaining OPV supplies in physicians' offices and clinics have been issued by the American Academy of Pediatrics (see *Pediatrics*, December 1999).

[6]The second dose of measles, mumps, and rubella (MMR) vaccine is recommended routinely at four to six years of age but may be administered during any visit, provided at least four weeks have elapsed since receipt of the first dose and that both doses are administered beginning at or after 12 months of age. Those who have not previously received the second dose should complete the schedule by the 11 to 12 year visit.

[7]Varicella (Var) vaccine is recommended at any visit on or after the first birthday for susceptible children (i.e., those who lack a reliable history of chickenpox as judged by a health care provider) and who have not been immunized. Susceptible persons 13 years of age or older should receive two doses, given at least four weeks apart.

[8]Hepatitis A (Hep A) is shaded to indicate its recommended use in selected states and regions; consult your local public health authority. (Also see *MMWR* Oct. 01, 1999/48(RR12); 1-37).

vaccines can be obtained from the sources listed for this chapter in the WebLinks portion of the book's website 🖲 www.wbsaunders.com/SIMON/nies/.

Types of Immunization

Vaccination is the administration of a vaccine or toxoid, which confers active immunity by stimulating the body to produce antibodies. **Immunization** is a broader term that includes not only *vaccines* for active immunity, but also passive immunogenic solutions such as *immune globulins* and *antitoxins*. This section deals exclusively with vaccines, except for diphtheria antitoxin, which is used in the treatment for diphtheria, and antigen-specific immune globulin, which is used for postexposure prevention against rabies, hepatitis B, tetanus, and varicella.

Vaccines can be prepared in several ways. They may be suspensions in any of a variety of solutions; protected with preservatives, stabilizers, or antibiotics; or mixed with adjuvants, which are used to increase immunogenicity. Vaccines can be live and attenuated, or they may be killed, or inactivated, with the virulence removed, leaving only the antigenic property necessary to stimulate the human immune system to produce antibodies. Types of inactivated vaccines include toxoids and polysaccharide vaccines. Inactivated conjugate vaccines, containing a chemically linked polysaccharide and protein and genetically engineered "recombinant" vaccines are also now being administered. Inactivated vaccines can be fractions or subunits or whole "killed" bacteria or viruses. Immune globulins and antitoxins are solutions that contain antibodies from human or animal blood and are introduced into a patient to provide passive protection without initiating the immune system to produce an immunogenic response. See Table 25-3 for information on types of available vaccines.

Vaccine Storage, Transport, and Handling

Vaccines should be safely stored, transported, and handled at all times. Deviation from standard practice can be deleterious to the efficacy of vaccines. Storage information for all vaccines is important. A **cold chain** is a system used to ensure that vaccines are kept at a designated temperature from the time they are manufactured until they are used for vaccination. The importance of the cold chain must be emphasized because any improper storage that allows the vaccines

TABLE 25-3

Available Vaccines by Type

Vaccines	Description
Live Attenuated	
Viral	Measles, mumps, rubella, oral polio, vaccinia, yellow fever, and varicella
Bacterial	BCG
Recombinant	Oral typhoid
Inactivated	
Viral	Influenza, polio, rabies, and hepatitis A
Bacterial	Typhoid, cholera, and plague
Subunit (fractional)	Influenza, acellular pertussis, typhoid Vi, and Lyme disease
Toxoid	Diphtheria and tetanus
Recombinant	Hepatitis B
Conjugate polysaccharide	*Haemophilus influenzae* type b, and pneumococcal 7-valent
Pure polysaccharide	Pneumococcal 23-valent, meningococcal, and *Haemophilus influenzae* type b

From Centers for Disease Control: *Epidemiology and prevention of vaccine-preventable diseases (pink book)*, ed 6, Atlanta, 2000b, Public Health Foundation.

to be exposed to higher or lower temperatures than recommended may result in loss of potency and vaccine failure (CDC, 1996a).

There are many levels of a cold chain, including locations at the national, regional, and local areas. Factors ranging from bad roads and weather conditions to poor power supplies or faulty thermometer readings may cause lapses in refrigeration at any of these levels. Maintenance of the cold chain becomes extremely difficult when attempting to distribute vaccines in rural areas and in developing areas that do not have access to electricity or cold storage, or where the vaccine may be distributed by bicycle or on foot. The fluctuation in electricity in many areas has required the design and distribution of solar- and kerosene-powered refrigeration systems.

Proper operation and maintenance of these systems are essential. Several methods are available for ensuring that the appropriate temperature has been maintained throughout vaccine transport and storage. These include liquid crystal thermometers, dial thermometers, recording thermometers and digital thermometers, ice pack indicators, shipping indicators that change color if the temperature exceeds or falls below the recommended level, freeze-watch indicators, and cold chain monitors.

Vaccine Administration and Routes

Vaccines are designed with specific types of administration needs. If administration routes and procedures are not met, vaccine efficacy can be adversely affected. Sterile technique and safety needles should be used to ensure that both the vaccinator and the vaccinee are protected from infection. Once the needle is inserted, the plunger should be pulled back to ensure that no blood is present, which would be evidence of needle insertion directly into a blood vessel. Vaccines should not be injected directly into a blood vessel; therefore if blood is present the needle should be withdrawn, the safety mechanism engaged, and the contaminated needle disposed of properly. With a new syringe and a new site selected for administration, the same procedure should be followed.

Needle length and size are important to ensure proper administration of vaccines and should be selected based on the site of administration (intramuscular or subcutaneous) and the size of the patient. If more than one vaccine is being administered simultaneously, different anatomical sites should be used (CDC, 1994a).

Vaccine Dosages

It is important to administer the specific dosage of a vaccine recommended in the package insert because any deviation may cause alterations in vaccine efficacy. For a summary of dosage information, consult the manufacturer's package insert or the *Physicians' Desk Reference*.

Vaccine Spacing

Wherever possible, all children should be age-appropriately immunized and kept up to date using the recommendations of ACIP, AAP, and AAFP. Clinically stable premature infants should adhere to the same schedule as term infants, with the exception of Hep B. Low-birth-weight infants (less than 2000 g) born to hepatitis B surface antigen (HBsAg)-negative mothers should not be vaccinated with Hep B until they weigh two kg or are two months of age. Low-birth-weight infants (less than 2000 g) born to HBsAg-positive mothers should receive hepatitis B immune globulin (HBIG) and Hep B at birth; however, the initial vaccine dose should not be counted in the required three-dose series (Pickering, 2000).

The recommended number of injections for any one immunobiological substance should be administered according to ACIP recommendations. An interruption in the schedule does not require that the entire series begin again. However, if vaccines are administered at less than the recommended intervals, they should not be counted as part of the primary series of immunization. Completion of the primary vaccine series and receiving periodic booster doses as recommended are necessary to ensure protective levels of immunity. A specific alteration in immunogenicity has not been proven; therefore all vaccines can be administered simultaneously without contraindication, except for yellow fever and cholera vaccines, which must be separated by at least three weeks. Additionally, live injectable vaccines (e.g., MMR and varicella) must be separated by at least four weeks when not given simultaneously (Pickering, 2000).

Vaccine Hypersensitivity and Contraindications

Although adverse reactions are not common following immunization, they can occur in some individuals. These reactions can be from vaccine components such as eggs, egg proteins, antibiotics, preservatives, and adjuvants. Patient allergies should be considered before administration of specific vaccines. For additional precautions and contraindications, the vaccine package insert and the latest instructions from the CDC should be consulted (CDC, 1996b).

Mild illness with or without low-grade fever is not a contraindication for vaccination. However, vaccination should be postponed in cases of moderate or severe febrile illness to avoid any confusion between a vaccine side effect and an unknown underlying cause.

Pregnancy is not a contraindication for immunization using inactivated vaccines, antitoxins, or immune globulins. However, pregnant women should avoid live vaccines including MMR, varicella, and yellow fever unless the risk of infection is very high (CDC, 2000b).

Immunocompromised patients should not receive live vaccines; however, MMR can be administered to asymptomatic HIV-infected people and varicella can be given to people with humoral immunodeficiency and some HIV-asymptomatic people as determined by their physician (CDC, 2000b). Killed or inactivated vaccines can be given, but they may not produce an optimal antibody response.

Vaccine Documentation

Legal documentation of vaccinations is important for both the individual and the provider for future administration and follow-up of hypersensitivity reactions. Both individual and provider immunization records should be maintained. The health care provider is responsible for maintaining accurate records, including patient name, dates immunized, vaccine type, vaccine manufacturer, vaccine lot number, date of the Vaccine Information Statement (VIS), and the name, title, and address of the person administering the vaccine (CDC, 2000c). Individual records should be kept by the patient and should include dates vaccinated; vaccine type; all allergies or hypersensitivities; doses; date next dose is due; vaccine manufacturer; vaccine lot number; and the name, title, and address of the person administering the vaccine. The website to view the VIS can be accessed through the WebLinks section of this book's website at www.wbsaunders.com/SIMON/nies/.

Vaccine Safety and Reporting Adverse Events and Vaccine-Related Injuries

Providing safe vaccines to the public has been a prevailing concern for governments and practitioners from the onset of vaccine usage in the control of communicable diseases. This concern is based on the fact that no drug or vaccine is perfectly safe or effective and vaccines have several special characteristics. For example, they are biological rather than chemical and when introduced into the human biological system, they can and do produce a variety of responses, both positive and negative. Furthermore, vaccines are administered to healthy people; they are given to prevent illness and not treat it; and they are given to far greater numbers of people than other pharmaceuticals. Additionally, there are few choices or substitute vaccines for a specific antigen.

Public concern regarding the health risk associated with vaccines has increased in recent years as the risk of contracting the diseases has declined. Wild virus polio has been eliminated in the United States, yet each year 8 to 10 cases of vaccine-induced paralysis have been reported associated with use of the oral vaccine, which is a "live virus" vaccine. It has been determined that the health risk of the oral vaccine exceeds that of the risk of the disease. This has led to a change in vaccine policy from the use of the live oral vaccine to the IPV (CDC, 1999f). Likewise, whole cell pertussis vaccine has been changed to an acellular pertussis vaccine because there are adverse side effects, most notably convulsions. More recently, a rotavirus vaccine was removed from the schedule because there was an increase in incidence of intussusception in infants who received the vaccine (CDC, 1999g).

Increasingly, these problematic issues have become the focus of discussion in "chat rooms" on the Internet. There is also the cost of liability arising from legal decisions awarded from injury claims caused by adverse reactions to vaccines. In response to public concerns and to maintain the public's confidence in immunization programs, research on the safety of vaccines has reached a new level of interest and activity.

To monitor actual and potential vaccine-related problems, health care providers must report specific postvaccination "adverse events" to the **Vaccine Adverse Event Reporting System** (VAERS). Information and reporting forms are available in both the FDA *Drug Bulletin* and the *Physicians' Desk Reference* and through a 24-hour recorded telephone message at 1-800-822-7967. The National Vaccine Injury Compensation Program reviews all VAERS reports.

The National Vaccine Injury Compensation Program became effective as a result of the National Childhood Vaccine Injury Act of 1986. This system provides assistance for individuals and families who experience a vaccine-related injury, including disability and death.

National Vaccine Injury Compensation Program: Health Resources and Services Administration
Parklawn Building, Room 8-05
5600 Fishers Lane
Rockville, MD 20857
Telephone: 1-800-338-2382 (24-hour recording);
(301) 443-6593 *Continued*

For individuals filing a claim, the following address should be used:
Clerk of the U.S. Court of Federal Claims
717 Madison Place NW
Washington, DC 20005
Telephone: (202) 219-9657

VACCINE NEEDS FOR SPECIAL GROUPS

Adolescents and Young Adults

Many adolescents and young adults continue to suffer needlessly from vaccine-preventable diseases such as hepatitis B, varicella, and measles, partially because vaccination programs have not focused on these age groups. Consequently, in November 1996, AAP, ACIP, and AAFP recommended establishing a routine health care visit at 11 to 12 years of age to ensure that previously unvaccinated adolescents would receive Hep B, varicella vaccine (if no history of disease), a second dose of MMR vaccine, and a booster dose of tetanus and diphtheria vaccine (Td) if it has been more than five years since their prior dose. This visit would also provide an opportunity to administer any new vaccines that may be added to the vaccine schedule and provide an opportunity to offer other recommended preventive services.

Many colleges and universities across the United States are now requiring some minimal level of proof of immunizations before enrollment for new students. Two studies done by the CDC identified a very slight increased risk for meningococcal disease among freshman dormitory residents. In October 1999, CDC recommended that vaccination against meningococcal disease be provided to freshman and other undergraduate students who request this vaccine, although routine vaccination is not recommended. Unfortunately, the current vaccine does not confer immunity against all meningococcal serogroups (CDC, 2000e).

Adults and the Elderly

Although immunization programs in the United States have greatly reduced morbidity and mortality rates among children, vaccine-preventable diseases continue to cause thousands of hospitalizations and deaths in the American adult and elderly populations. For example, adults aged 65 years and older account

for 90% of the annual 20,000 to 40,000 deaths in the United States from influenza and pneumonia. Many of these deaths are premature and preventable because effective influenza and pneumonia vaccines are available (CDC, 2000g).

Missed immunization opportunities for this age group often occur during an office visit for "acute" or "chronic" health problems. Therefore the CDC recommends a routinely scheduled, preventive health care visit for the 50-year-old adult (CDC, 1995a). This preventive health visit has three immunization goals, which follow:

- To assess the current immunization status
- To administer Td and flu vaccines if indicated
- To determine if the adult has risk factors (e.g., cardiovascular, pulmonary, kidney, and metabolic blood disorders) suggesting the need for pneumococcal vaccine

The pneumococcal and influenza vaccines can be administered simultaneously at the same visit for those individuals needing both vaccines. With the emergence of serious new drug-resistant pneumococci, it is urgent that susceptible groups be immunized and protected from this group of bacteria. People needing the 23-valant pure polysaccharide vaccine are in essentially the same risk groups as people needing flu vaccine. These are described in Box 25-4.

Immunosuppressed

There are significant groups of people in the United States who are in some altered or compromised immune state. Severe immunosuppression status can be caused by various health conditions such as leukemia, lymphoma, HIV infection, AIDS, congenital immunodeficiency, radiation, therapy with an alkylating agent, large doses of corticosteroids, or antimetabolites. For the severe immunosuppressed person, live virus or live bacterial vaccines can pose serious threats to the individual's health. The killed or inactivated vaccines are not problematic and can follow the same recommended administration schedule as for the healthy person. The individual's physician has the responsibility to determine the person's degree of immunosuppression.

Pregnancy

Vaccination risk during pregnancy is largely a theoretical issue according to the CDC (CDC, 1998a). The

From Centers for Disease Control: *Epidemiology and prevention of vaccine-preventable diseases (pink book)*, ed 6, Atlanta, 2000b, Public Health Foundation.

BOX **25-4**

Persons at Risk for Complications of Influenza

- Persons 50 years of age and older
- Residents of nursing homes and other chronic care facilities housing persons of any age with chronic medical conditions
- Adults and children six months of age and older with chronic disorders of the pulmonary or cardiovascular systems, including children with asthma
- Adults and children six months of age and older who have required regular medical follow-up or hospitalization during the preceding year from chronic metabolic diseases (including diabetes mellitus), renal dysfunction, hemoglobinopathies, or immunosuppression (including immunosuppression caused by medications)
- Children and teenagers (6 months to 18 years of age) who are receiving long-term aspirin therapy and therefore may be at risk for Reye's syndrome after influenza
- Adults of any age with HIV infection or AIDS
- Women who will be in at least the fourteenth week of gestation during influenza season

only two vaccines routinely indicated for susceptible pregnant women are tetanus-diphtheria toxoid combination vaccine and influenza vaccine for women who will be in their second or third trimester of pregnancy during flu season.

Although there are not any cases on record of congenital rubella syndrome or abnormalities in infants born to mothers who received these vaccines during pregnancy, MMR and varicella vaccines are both contraindicated when pregnancy is known. Other live virus vaccines such as OPV and yellow fever are not recommended during pregnancy, but they can be administered and are recommended for susceptible pregnant women who live in areas or may travel to areas where there is a high risk of exposure to these diseases. Inactivated vaccines, toxoids, and immune globulin preparations are not contraindicated during pregnancy. Hepatitis B, pneumococcal, meningococcal, and rabies vaccines are recommended for at-risk pregnant women.

VACCINE-PREVENTABLE DISEASES

Diphtheria

Diphtheria is an acute bacterial disease most commonly affecting the upper respiratory tract, including the nose, tonsils, larynx, and pharynx. Associated lesions are caused by the release of a cytotoxin and manifest as a patch or patches of inflammation surrounding a grayish membrane. Complications may result in severe swelling of the neck, thrombocytopenia, neuritis, and myocarditis. The case fatality rate is 5% to 10% of all infections. Diphtheria is transmitted through direct contact with an infected individual and has an incubation period of two to five days, but it is occasionally longer (Chin, 2000).

Globally, diphtheria continues to persist as a major cause of morbidity and mortality. In the former Soviet Union, over 50,000 cases and 1500 deaths were reported in 1995 alone. From 1990 to 1995, this region accounted for over 90% of all diphtheria cases reported to WHO from the entire world. In the United States, only 21 cases of diphtheria were reported since 1990; zero cases were reported in 1993 and 1995 and only one probable case was reported in 1998 (CDC, 1999d, 2000b).

General susceptibility exists for unimmunized individuals, whereas those previously immunized have protection for approximately 10 years after vaccination. Diagnosis is made through bacteriological culture of nasal and throat secretions from lesions. Treatment includes the administration of a single dose of equine antitoxin followed by a full course of antimicrobial therapy.

Immunization with diphtheria toxoid is available as Td for people over seven years of age. It is available as DTaP, or pediatric combined diphtheria and tetanus toxoids (DT), for routine childhood immunization if pertussis vaccine is contraindicated. These vaccines provide good antibody response, with boosters needed every 10 years after the primary series. Side effects include soreness at the site of injection and fever may appear for one to two days. Where pertussis immunization is contraindicated, DT should be used for the regular childhood schedule. No contraindications exist for diphtheria toxoid. DTaP is now the preferred vaccine because it causes fewer side effects. Diphtheria has been classified as "not now eradicable" because it is difficult to diagnose and only a multiple-dose vaccine is currently available.

Haemophilus Influenzae Type B

Hib is an acute invasive bacterial infection that can affect multiple organ systems (Chin, 2000). **Hib is not to be confused with influenza types A, B, and C, which are viral diseases.** Hib-associated illnesses include meningitis, epiglottitis, otitis media, pneumonia, arthritis, and cellulitis. These illnesses may cause fever, lethargy, vomiting, meningeal irritation, decreased mental status, stiff neck, bulging fontanelle in infants, swelling of the epiglottis, respiratory distress, skin lesions, and ear infections. Complications are serious and include septic arthritis, life-threatening airway obstruction, fulminating infection, and death. Hib occurs worldwide and is the major cause of bacterial meningitis in children younger than five years in developing countries.

During the early 1980s, the United States averaged about 20,000 cases of Hib annually, primarily in children under five years of age (40 to 50 cases per 100,000 population). With the licensing of Hib conjugate vaccines and an aggressive, targeted immunization campaign for children younger than five years, the incidence of invasive Hib disease in the United States has declined dramatically. There were only 253 cases of invasive Hib disease and 25 cases of Hib meningitis reported in 1998 in children less than five years of age (CDC, 1999d; Chin, 2000). Hib is transmitted by droplets from nasal and oral secretions during the infectious period. The incubation period is unknown, but it is assumed to be two to four days. People are considered communicable as long as the organisms are present in nose and throat discharges. Diagnosis is made by identifying organisms from blood or spinal fluid. Treatment usually requires hospitalization and a 10- to 14-day course of antibiotics.

Five conjugate Hib vaccines are currently licensed for use in the United States. Adverse reactions to the vaccine are uncommon; swelling, redness, and pain at the site of injection have been reported. Hib vaccine should be deferred for children with moderate or severe illnesses and it is contraindicated for anyone who experienced an anaphylactic reaction after a prior dose of vaccine.

Hepatitis A, B, and C

Viral hepatitis exists in several forms, which are very different from one another and include hepatitis A (infectious), B (serum), C (parenteral), D (delta viral), and E (enteric). Vaccines are now available for hepatitis A and hepatitis B.

Hepatitis A

Hepatitis A virus (HAV) is an acute viral infection that usually lasts less than two months and manifests with abrupt onset of fever, anorexia, malaise, dark urine, and jaundice. It has a very low fatality rate and, although rare, it can last up to six months. HAV is transmitted through fecal-oral contamination of food and water and has an incubation period of 15 to 50 days, with an average 25 to 30 days. HAV is endemic in many developing countries. The reported incidence of hepatitis A is highest among children 5 to 14 years of age, who account for one third of reported cases. Seventy percent of infected children younger than six years of age are asymptomatic and easily infect adults in their surroundings. Between 1984 and 1994, the annual number of case reports of HAV remained relatively static at approximately 23,000. With the introduction of the hepatitis A vaccine in 1995 for those most at risk, it was expected that the incidence of HAV would decline. However, from 1995 to 1997 the number of cases jumped to an average of 30,000 per year before dropping to 23,000 cases in 1998 (CDC, 1999d).

In October 1999, the CDC revised its immunization strategy to include routine vaccination of children in states, counties, and communities with rates that are twice the national average. Unchanged were the previous recommendations for the two-dose vaccination series for those most at risk. These include people traveling to or living in a country of endemicity; communities experiencing an outbreak or those with a high endemic incidence rate such as in American-Indian or Alaska Native populations; people with chronic liver disease; users of illegal drugs; men who have sex with men; people who have clotting-factor disorders; and handlers of HAV-infected primates or HAV research laboratory workers. It is hoped that this new strategy will prevent infection in children and, eventually, older people (CDC, 1999h).

Susceptibility to HAV is general and no carrier state exists. It is diagnosed through the presence of serum antibodies and no specific treatment is recommended. Two inactivated hepatitis A vaccines are licensed for use in the United States; however, these vaccines are not approved by the FDA for use in children under two years of age.

Contraindications to HAV vaccination include an allergic reaction to a prior dose of vaccine or vaccine component. The safety of hepatitis A vaccine has not been determined in pregnancy; therefore the risk of disease should be weighed against the risk of vaccination for pregnant women. HAV is not presently targeted for eradication because it is easily spread, the vaccine is costly, and current political will is lacking.

Hepatitis B

Hepatitis B virus (HBV) is a viral infection of insidious onset that ranges from asymptomatic illness to generalized nonspecific symptoms such as anorexia, nausea, and vomiting followed by jaundice and occasionally resulting in fulminant fatal hepatitis. It is transmitted through direct contact with contaminated blood and body secretions, transplacentally, and through sexual intercourse. HBV has an incubation period of 45 days to six months, with an average 90 days. HBV is endemic worldwide, with an estimated incidence of infection ranging between 70% and 90% in the developing world and a carrier prevalence rate of 8% to 15%. The presence of serological markers for HBV in people without a history of acute infection suggests that it is extremely common to have subclinical cases of disease. Undetected acute subclinical cases of HBV infection could include as many as two thirds of all adult cases and most neonatal cases (Hollinger et al., 1990).

The incidence of reported HBV peaked in the 1980s, with 26,000 cases reported annually. Reported cases declined to 10,000 cases in 1998 (CDC, 1999d). However, it is believed that reported cases of HBV infection represent only a fraction of cases that actually occur. There are approximately 300 million HBsAg carriers worldwide, many of whom do not have clinical signs of disease (Hollinger et al., 1990).

General susceptibility exists for unimmunized individuals. The period of immunogenicity for those who have been vaccinated is currently unknown because the first HBV vaccine was only licensed in 1982. Diagnosis of acute and chronic illness and presence of immunity after vaccination is done through serological testing. No treatment currently exists for HBV. Depending on the type of hepatitis infection, enteric or universal precautions should be employed for patients with hepatitis infection.

There are two inactivated Hep B licensed for use in the United States. In 1991, the HBV vaccine was added to the routine childhood immunization schedule in the United States. In 1999, the FDA approved an alternative hepatitis B vaccination schedule for unimmunized adolescents 11 to 15 years of age. The alternative schedule is for two 10 μg doses given four to six months apart. This alternative schedule is approved only for Merck's recombivax hepatitis B vaccine. Otherwise, the routine hepatitis B immunization schedule is a three dose series given at zero-, one-, and six-month intervals (CDC, 2000b).

Infants born to HBsAg-positive mothers must be given HBIG and Hep B at birth, followed by additional vaccine doses at one and six months of age to prevent neonatal infection. Therefore it is imperative that all pregnant women are screened for HBsAg. Low-birth-weight infants (less than 2000 g) born to HbsAg-positive mothers should receive HBIG and Hep B at birth. However, the initial vaccine dose should not be counted in the required three-dose series in these babies.

A lack of follow-up with the second and third inoculations can inhibit the success of seroconversion; therefore strict programs for follow-up must be established. There will always be a small percentage of people who do not seroconvert, even after repeating the three-dose series. However, if everyone received the series, this small cohort would be protected through herd immunity. Vaccination with HBV vaccine may cause soreness at the site of injection. The only contraindication for HBV vaccination is an anaphylactic reaction to a prior dose of vaccine or to a vaccine component.

Several factors inhibit the success of a worldwide and a national eradication program for hepatitis B. One factor is expense. Although the cost for three doses has dropped by two thirds, further cost reduction is necessary if affordability is to be achieved for developing countries. The second prohibitive factor is the presence of a carrier status with this disease. As long as there are carriers, this disease can only be controlled and can never be eradicated. Universal screening of all blood and its components is also necessary to prevent further transmission.

Hepatitis C

Like HBV, Hepatitis C virus (HCV) has an insidious onset. Before the discovery of the causative organism in the 1970s, it was termed *nonA, nonB hepatitis*. HCV accounts for 20% of the acute hepatitis cases in the United States and 80% to 90% of the nonA, nonB cases. Infected individuals can have a wide range of symptoms, from completely asymptomatic to the rare fulminating, fatal case. Of the acute hepatitis C infection cases, approximately 60% to 70% are asymptomatic and 20% to 30% have mild illnesses (i.e., complaints of nonspecific anorexia, vague abdominal discomfort, nausea, and vomiting). Of those who are acutely ill, 75% to 85% develop chronic hepatitis and 15% to 25% resolve the infection without sequelae (CDC, 1998b).

HCV is a blood-borne infection that is primarily transmitted through repeated percutaneous exposures to large doses of contaminated blood and its products. Associated risk factors for transmission include blood transfusion and organ transplants before 1992, injecting drug users, exposure to infected household members or sexual partners, contaminated needles, and perinatally to infants from infected mothers who have high levels of virus in their blood (about 3% of exposed infants). The incubation period ranges from two weeks to six months and the period of communicability may be one week or more before the onset of symptoms and can persist indefinitely.

HCV is the most common chronic blood-borne infection and the leading reason for liver transplants in the United States. During the 1980s, approximately 230,000 new infections occurred yearly. By 1996, this annual rate dropped by 80% to 36,000. It is estimated that about 3.9 million Americans are infected as carriers of the virus and can infect others. The highest prevalence rates are among people 30 to 49 years of age, males, and minorities (CDC, 1998b).

Drug therapy is recommended for chronic HCV-infected individuals who have persistent elevated serum alanine aminotransferase (ALT) levels, positive polymerase chain reaction (PCR) test results for HCV ribonucleic acid (RNA) and active liver disease. Interferon alfa is recommended as a treatment for HCV and has proven to be beneficial to some chronic hepatitis C patients. A new oral antiviral drug, Ribavirin, has shown promise as an adjunct in combination with interferon alfa. Using the combination of the two drugs has led to a greater sustained biochemical response on lowering the viral count and slowing the progression of liver disease. The goals for treatment include eradicating the HCV and decreasing its replication, decreasing hepatitic necrosis and improving histology, halting the progression to cirrhosis and cancer, and decreasing infectivity to others (CDC, 1998b).

Education of professionals and the general public will play a key role in the control and prevention of HCV disease. Knowledge of the prevalence of HCV disease, availability of diagnostic tests and treatment therapies, and counseling patients will influence the effectiveness of preventive measures. Research for new antiviral agents, surveillance, and monitoring of disease trends are other important control measures. Table 25-4 presents a comprehensive strategy to prevent and control HCV infection and related diseases.

Influenza Types A, B, and C

Influenza is an acute viral respiratory infection that may be confused with the common cold or other common respiratory illnesses. Influenza, a viral disease, also must not be confused with Hib, a bacterial disease (see prior section on Hib). There are three types of influenza, which follow: influenza type A, which is responsible for most outbreaks on an epidemic scale worldwide; type B, which is responsible for milder disease than type A and affects primarily children; and type C, which is usually subclinical and rarely reported.

These viruses have the ability to change their antigenic makeup. Minor antigenic changes, or drifts, occur frequently and cause widespread epidemics and regional outbreaks. Major changes, or shifts, occur

TABLE 25-4

Elements of a Comprehensive Strategy to Prevent and Control HCV Infection and HCV-related Diseases

Primary prevention activities	Screening and testing of blood, plasma, organ, tissue, and semen donors
	Virus inactivation of plasma-derived products
	Risk-reduction counseling and services
Secondary prevention activities	Identification, counseling, and testing of persons at risk
	Medical management of infected persons
Other prevention activities	Professional and public education
	Surveillance and research to monitor disease trends and the effectiveness of prevention activities and to develop improved prevention methods

From Centers for Disease Control: Measles, mumps and rubella—vaccine use and strategies for elimination of measles, rubella and congenital rubella syndrome and control of mumps: recommendations of the Advisory Committee on Immunization Practices (ACIP), *Mor Mortal Wkly Rep* 47(RR-8):1-57, 1998c.

irregularly, but only in type A. Antigenic shifts result in completely new subtypes, possibly because there is a genetic redesign between animal and human hosts (Chin, 2000; Pickering, 2000). In 1918, an influenza pandemic resulted in the deaths of at least 500,000 Americans in less than one year and killed an estimated 20 million people worldwide. Strains of the viruses change from year to year; therefore influenza vaccines are prepared annually on the basis of a prediction of the type that will be prevalent that year. Influenza vaccinations are given in the early fall before the "flu season" (CDC, 2000g).

Influenza affects the respiratory tract and causes dry cough, fever, headache, myalgia, sore throat, and other generalized symptoms of malaise. Complications include pneumonia, otitis media, meningitis, Reye's syndrome, and death. Influenza is highly infectious and is passed from one individual to another through droplets or direct contact with infected mucous secretions and has an incubation period of one to three days. Infection from one type of influenza provides little or no protection against other types or subtypes. The peak transmission season for influenza activity in the United States usually occurs from November through February (CDC, 2000g).

Groups at risk for complications from influenza include people over 50 years of age, individuals of all ages with underlying health problems, children and adolescents on aspirin therapy who are at risk for Reye's syndrome, women who will be in their second or third trimester of pregnancy during flu season, and health care workers and others in close contact with individuals at high risk (CDC, 2000b). Diagnosis of influenza is accomplished through culture, laboratory viral isolation, serological testing, antigen detection, gene amplification, and rapid diagnostical testing (CDC, 1999i). The FDA has approved the following drugs for prophylaxis and treatment of influenza A: amantadine for adults and children and rimantadine for adults only. The following antiviral drugs for treatment of influenza types A and B were approved in 1999 for use in uncomplicated acute cases of flu beginning within 48 hours after onset: zanamivir, or Relenza, an inhaled medication for use in people 12 years of age and older; and oseltamivir phosphate, or Tamiflu, for use in adults (CDC, 1999i).

A trivalent vaccine is currently available for the control of influenza. The vaccine is created annually based on the viral strains expected to be prevalent during the upcoming influenza season. Depending on how closely that match is achieved, immunogenicity can be very high. The groups at risk for complications from influenza, as described previously, should receive flu vaccine; however, it is contraindicated in individuals with known anaphylactic hypersensitivity to eggs or other vaccine components (CDC, 2000g). Swelling, redness, and pain at the site of injection are the most common side effects, followed infrequently by fever, malaise, myalgia, and other systemic symptoms.

The worldwide spread of influenza, the shifting serotypes, and the high infectiousness of the disease do not make it currently feasible to consider eradication of influenza. However, as new and improved vaccines become available and additional control measures are established, substantial reductions in influenza-related morbidity and mortality rates may be achieved.

Lyme Disease

Lyme disease is a bacterial infection that is spread by the bite of an infected tick. Usually the deer tick in the eastern United States and the Western black-legged tick in the western United States spreads this disease. About 12,000 to 15,000 cases of Lyme disease are reported each year in the United States, mainly in the Northeast and North Central regions of the country and in parts of California (CDC, 1999j).

The incubation period for Lyme disease is 3 to 30 days and the most common symptom is erythema migrans, which is a red rash at the site of the bite that is frequently shaped like a bull's-eye. The rash may be accompanied by fever, headache, and joint and muscle pain, although some asymptomatic disease may occur. Disseminated infection occurs days to weeks later and may affect the nervous system, the musculoskeletal system, or the heart. Untreated infection may manifest weeks to months later, often as intermittent pain or swelling of one or more joints. Infrequently, Lyme disease can be severe, chronic, and disabling, but it is rarely fatal. It may not confer lifelong immunity. Diagnosis of Lyme disease is based on clinical findings, with serological testing providing supportive diagnostic information. Lyme disease usually responds well to antibiotic treatment and is readily treatable in its early stages. Early diagnosis and treatment usually results in a prompt and uncomplicated cure (CDC, 1999j).

The main risk factor for Lyme disease is prolonged physical contact with vegetation or leaf litter in overgrown grassy, brushy, or wooded areas where infected ticks reside. People in occupations such as landscaping; people who clear brush; and personnel in forestry, wildlife, and parks management working in infected areas are particularly at risk. Other people at risk are those who travel; those who pursue recreational activities such as off-trail hiking, camping, fishing, and hunting; or those who live in wooded, grassy areas (CDC, 1999j).

There is one approved vaccine for use in the prevention of Lyme disease and it is approved for use only in people aged 15 to 70 years. It is 49% effective after two doses and 76% effective after three doses in preventing clinical Lyme disease. The duration of protective immunity and the need for booster doses beyond the third dose are unknown. The vaccine is administered at 0, 1, and 12 months, with the first dose given ideally in January, February, or March. Vaccine side effects may include local injection site reactions, including pain, redness, and swelling; flulike symptoms; arthralgia; and myalgia (CDC, 1999j).

Lyme vaccine does not offer any protection against other tick-borne diseases and is not a substitute for measures to prevent tick bites. The first line of defense against Lyme disease and other tick-borne illnesses is avoidance of tick-infested habitats and use of personal protective measures. Vaccinated people should continue to practice personal protective measures against ticks and should seek early diagnosis and treatment of any suspected tick-borne infections. Protective measures recommended by the CDC (1999j) include the following:

■ Wear light-colored clothing and long-sleeved shirts and tuck pants into socks or boot tops to keep ticks from reaching the skin.
■ Apply insect repellents containing DEET to exposed skin. DEET can be safely used on children and adults when applied according to EPA guidelines.
■ Apply permethrin to clothes; it kills ticks on contact.
■ Daily checks for ticks and their prompt removal will help prevent infection. Transmission of Lyme disease from an infected tick is unlikely to occur before 36 hours of tick attachment.
■ Avoid entering areas that are likely to be infested with ticks, particularly in spring and summer when nymphal ticks feed. Ticks favor moist, shaded environments usually provided by leaf litter and low-lying vegetation in woody, brushy, or overgrown grassy habitats.

■ Stay on trails and avoid brushing against bushes or leaf litter piles to significantly decrease exposure to ticks.

Measles (Rubeola)

Measles, or rubeola, is an acute viral infection that manifests with fever of 101° F or higher, cough, coryza, conjunctivitis, Koplik's spots on the buccal mucosa, and a red rash lasting longer than three days that begins on the face and becomes generalized. Measles can progress into severe complications, including pneumonia, diarrhea, encephalitis, and death. It is highly infectious four days before until four days after rash onset and is transmitted through droplets and direct contact with nasal secretions of an infected person, with an average incubation period of 10 days from exposure to onset of fever (CDC, 1998c).

Between 1963 and 1989, the United States experienced a dramatic decline in the incidence of measles. However, between 1989 and 1991, a resurgence of measles occurred, which resulted in a fivefold increase from the early 1980s (Smoak, Novakski, and Mason, 1994). In response to this epidemic, a two-dose measles vaccination schedule was implemented for children entering kindergarten, adolescents, and young adults. Since this change was implemented, indigenous measles has been virtually eliminated in the United States, with only 100 cases reported in 1998 (CDC, 1999d). In the United States, current measles incidence is primarily from importation and exposed school-age children lacking two doses of measles vaccine. Risk factors for vaccine failure include vaccination before 12 months of age, when residuals of maternal antibodies interfere with vaccine virus replication, and poor vaccine handling (CDC, 1998c).

Diagnosis of measles is confirmed by tissue culture of nasopharyngeal secretions and serological testing. Patterns of spread can now be traced through viral genomic sequencing of specimens. There is no specific treatment for measles. Three measles vaccines are currently available and include a monovalent measles live virus vaccine, a combined measles-rubella (MR) vaccine, and a trivalent MMR vaccine (CDC, 1998c).

MMR vaccine is a combined vaccine of live, attenuated measles, mumps, and rubella viruses. It is the vaccine of choice for routine vaccination globally because it provides protection against rubella and mumps and offers 95% seroconversion for measles in children vaccinated at 12 months and 98% in those vaccinated at 15 months. More than 99% of people who receive two doses of vaccine at least four weeks apart, on or after the first birthday, develop serological evidence of measles immunity.

The live, attenuated measles vaccine may cause malaise and fever that can occur as long as 12 days after inoculation and may last one to three days. Measles vaccine-related encephalopathy is rare, occurring in less than one in one million children. MMR is contraindicated for pregnant women and in people who have received blood or antibody-containing blood products within the previous 3 to 11 months. People who have experienced an anaphylactic reaction to neomycin, gelatin, or other vaccine components should not be immunized using MMR (CDC, 1998c). There are no other contraindications for measles vaccine.

In 1990, at the World Summit for Children, WHO established the following global goals for elimination and eventual eradication of measles: the reduction of measles cases by 90% by 1995 and the reduction of measles deaths by 95% by 1995. Internationally, results have been sporadic, and although these goals were not met, efforts to eradicate measles are ongoing.

Mumps

Mumps is an acute systemic viral disease that causes fever and painful swelling of the salivary and parotid glands. Complications range from meningoencephalitis to permanent hearing impairment and orchitis in postpubescent males, but rarely sterility. Mumps is transmitted through droplets and direct contact with saliva of infected individuals, with an incubation period of 12 to 25 days. Since the beginning of mumps reporting in the United States, there has been a steady decline in the number of cases, except in 1987 when there was a fourfold increase in cases. Since then, numbers have fallen every year, with an all-time low of 666 cases reported in 1998 (CDC, 1999d).

Diagnosis of mumps is based on the isolation of virus from oral and throat spray, urine, and spinal fluid. Treatment for mumps is supportive. As discussed previously, the most commonly used mumps vaccine is the trivalent live, attenuated MMR vaccine, which offers approximately 95% seroconversion for mumps.

Humans are the only reservoir for the mumps virus and lifelong immunity is established with infection or vaccination. Eradication of mumps is considered probable by using MMR and linking eradication activities with mass campaigns for measles.

Pertussis

Pertussis, or "whooping cough," is an acute bacterial infection that begins with an upper respiratory cough and proceeds into a paroxysmal stage of coughing, often ending in vomiting. Complications include seizures, pneumonia, encephalopathy, and death. It is transmitted through direct contact with respiratory secretions of an infected individual and has an incubation period of 7 to 10 days. During 1993, the United States experienced an 82% increase in the number of reported cases of pertussis compared with 1992 and the highest number of cases reported since 1967. Of the 5000 reported cases, 45% were infants and 20% were children one to four years old. By 1995, the incidence of pertussis was five times the year 2000 goal. In 1998, it totaled 7405 cases, 24% of which were in infants younger than seven months. This has led some to encourage the development of a rapid, reliable diagnostic test and an adult pertussis vaccine (CDC, 1999d).

Diagnosis of pertussis is confirmed by a positive culture of nasal or throat secretions. Treatment with antimicrobials reduces the period of infectivity and may lessen the severity of the disease if given before the paroxysmal stage. Prophylaxis should be given to all exposed people, regardless of vaccination status.

Acellular pertussis vaccines have replaced whole cell pertussis vaccines in the United States because they are less likely to cause adverse reactions. Acellular pertussis vaccine is given in combination with pediatric DT as DTaP in a five-dose series at ages two months, four months, six months, 12 to 15 months, and four to six years (CDC, 2000i). Children with valid contraindications to any pertussis vaccine should receive pediatric DT vaccine. Pertussis vaccine is not recommended for children older than seven years.

Pertussis disease is not considered eradicable because there is a large number of cases worldwide, an early age of infection, high infectiousness of the disease, and a multidose vaccination schedule. Also, pediatric vaccination does not confer lifelong immunity and there is not a licensed pertussis vaccine for people over seven years of age.

Pneumococcal Disease

Pneumococcal disease is caused by *Streptococcus pneumoniae*. The reservoir is the nasopharynx of asymptomatic human carriers and transmission occurs via respiratory droplets and by autoinoculation in carriers. Penicillin is the drug of choice for treatment;

however, multiple-drug resistance is rising and may be as high as 5% to 15%. Patients allergic to penicillin may be given cephalosporins or erythromycin for pneumonia and chloramphenicol for meningitis.

Pneumococcal disease kills more people in the United States than all other vaccine-preventable diseases, with an estimate of over 40,000 deaths per year. Pneumococcal pneumonia causes up to 36% of adult community-acquired pneumonia and 50% of hospital-acquired pneumonia. Pneumococcal meningitis is the leading cause of meningitis in children under five years of age in the United States, with an estimated 3000 to 6000 cases each year. Pneumococci also cause 30% to 60% of otitis media in infants and children. Overall incidence of pneumococcal bacteremia in the United States is 50 per 100,000 population in adults older than 65 years and it may be as high as 200 per 100,000 population in children 13 to 18 months of age (CDC, 1997a). Diagnosis relies on isolation of the organism from the blood or other sterile body site.

A vaccine for pneumococcal pneumonia was first licensed in the United States in 1977 and was replaced by a more effective vaccine in 1983. Two 23-valent inactivated polysaccharide vaccines are currently available for use in people two years of age and older. A 7-valent conjugate vaccine has been approved for routine use in children younger than two years of age, who account for 80% of childhood pneumococcal disease. This pediatric vaccine is a four-dose series given at 2, 4, 6, and 12 to 15 months of age, with 100% efficacy against the seven-vaccine strains and 90% for all other subtypes (CDC, 1999-2000). Efficacy for the adult vaccine is 60% to 70% and it is recommended for all healthy people over 65 years of age; this age may soon be lowered to age 50 and anyone else who is immunosuppressed or has a chronic illness. Adverse reactions to vaccination include pain and redness at the injection site, occasional fever and myalgia, but rarely any severe reactions (CDC, 1997a).

Polio

Poliomyelitis is an acute enterovirus that occurs in three types, all of which can cause paralysis. Symptoms may range from inapparent illness to severe paralysis or death. It is transmitted through airborne droplets and fecal-oral contamination, with an incubation period ranging from 7 to 21 days. As a result of global mass immunization efforts, polio was eliminated in the Americas, the Pacific Rim, Europe, and

Central Asia during the 1990s. Endemic polio is now confined to India, sub-Saharan Africa, and contiguous countries (CDC, 1999k).

Groups at risk for contracting poliomyelitis include unvaccinated people and previously vaccinated immunocompromised people living in or traveling to endemic areas. Diagnosis of poliomyelitis is made through isolation of the virus from fecal or oropharyngeal specimens. Treatment of poliomyelitis is supportive only. Poliomyelitis vaccines are prepared with either live or killed virus.

OPV is a trivalent, live, attenuated virus vaccine that may not be available in the United States in the near future. With near-global eradication of wild polio and the desire of ACIP, AAP, and AAFP to reduce the risk of vaccine-acquired paralytic polio (VAPP) (one case per 2.4 million doses distributed), an all-IPV schedule for routine childhood polio is now recommended in the United States. Any available OPV is now restricted to the following (CDC, 2000h):

- Mass vaccination campaigns to control outbreaks of paralytic polio
- Unvaccinated children traveling to an endemic area in less than four weeks
- The third or fourth dose of the vaccine series for children whose parents object to the number of injections

Recipients of oral polio vaccine must be cautioned that their saliva is infectious for two weeks following immunization and their stool is infectious for up to six weeks. For this reason, OPV is the only vaccine that should be deferred if an immunosuppressed person is in the household.

Enhanced-potency IPV (eIPV) contains inactivated viruses of all three serotypes and is given as a four-dose series at age two months, four months, 6 to 18 months, and four to six years. The vaccine cost is slightly higher than OPV and the administration is parenteral rather than oral, but there is no risk of VAPP disease. Levels of seroconversion are similar with both vaccines at 95% (CDC, 2000h).

Rubella

Rubella is a mild viral disease that manifests with a maculopapular rash and postauricular, occipital, and posterior cervical lymphadenopathy. Children are usually relatively asymptomatic, but adults may experience fever, headache, and malaise. Rare complications include encephalitis and thrombocytopenia, but the most serious complication is a high risk for congenital defects in fetuses of pregnant women who are infected.

Transmission is through droplets or direct contact with respiratory secretions of an infected individual, with an incubation period of 14 to 23 days. From 1989 to 1991, there was a resurgence of rubella in the United States that peaked in 1991 with 1401 cases, occurring mostly among religious groups who refused vaccination. Since then, rubella has been on the decline, with only 364 cases reported in 1998, occurring primarily in unimmunized Latino or Asian adults 20 to 40 years of age (CDC, 1999d; State of California, 2000). Diagnosis of rubella is usually by serological testing. Treatment for rubella is primarily supportive.

One dose of live, attenuated rubella virus vaccine provides 99% seroconversion and is usually given in the trivalent MMR. MMR is contraindicated for pregnant women and people with anaphylactic reactions to neomycin or gelatin. Rubella vaccines should not be administered to immunosuppressed patients, immunodeficient patients except HIV asymptomatic, or individuals who have received blood or immune globulin during the past three months (Pickering, 2000).

Rubella has been identified as an eradicable disease. Criteria include the availability of the immunogenic MMR vaccine, although the impact of rubella in developing countries is currently unknown.

Tetanus

Tetanus, or lockjaw, is an acute neurological illness caused by an anaerobic bacterium that produces an exotoxin in the portal of entry in the human host. Tetanus causes gradually worsening neurological symptoms, including painful muscle contractions and spasms. The leading complication from tetanus is death. Tetanus is transmitted indirectly through contamination of a wound or portal of entry with tetanus spores, usually from soil or contaminated fomites. The incubation period ranges from 1 to 20 days.

In the United States, 41 cases of tetanus were reported in 1998, mainly in adults who had never been vaccinated or who did not have a booster in the preceding 10 years (CDC, 1999d, 2000a). Anyone who is unimmunized is at risk for contracting tetanus. Diagnosis is confirmed clinically because the bacterium is rarely found in wound cultures. Treatment for tetanus involves administration of tetanus immune globulin (TIG), preferably human. Supportive care is essential.

Tetanus toxoid (TT) is available as a monovalent vaccine or in the more preferred combinations of adult Td and pediatric DT and DTaP. Td provides immunity for approximately 10 years after the completion of the primary series. However, if a severe wound occurs, or a person is entering a high-risk area between 5 and 10 years after vaccination, it is recommended that a booster dose of Td be given; otherwise boosters are recommended every 10 years. Pregnant women should also receive a Td booster if 10 years has elapsed since their last dose. Common side effects experienced after routine inoculation include soreness at the site of injection and possibly fever for one to two days. The only contraindication to Td is a previous anaphylactic reaction to the vaccine or a vaccine component.

Newborns in the developing world are at increased risk for neonatal tetanus because contaminated knives, scissors, or razor blades are used to cut the umbilical cord after birth. WHO declared the elimination of neonatal tetanus as a global goal because immunization has increased. Deaths from neonatal tetanus are on the decline, with approximately 250,000 reported in 1997 worldwide. However, eradication is probably impossible because spores are routinely found in the environment.

Varicella (Chickenpox)

Varicella is a highly contagious viral disease with a variable onset (Chin, 2000). Transmission is by droplet infection from respiratory tract secretions, direct contact with vesicular fluid, or maternal infection during pregnancy.

The varicella zoster virus is responsible for causing chickenpox, or varicella, and shingles, or herpes zoster. Varicella may manifest with a sudden mild fever and malaise, or the only sign may be a rash. The rash is progressive, changing from maculopapular to vesicular, and then forming a crust or scab. The skin lesions, which may range between 250 and 500, tend to be more numerous on covered parts of the body. They can also be found on membrane tissue of the cornea, conjunctiva, respiratory tract, vagina, and oropharynx. They are highly pruritic and scratching can cause the most common complication, secondary bacterial infection, which can be life threatening. Complications are low in healthy children, but much higher in people older than 15 years of age and infants less than one year of age. Immunocompromised, susceptible adults and infants whose mothers develop the disease five days before or two days after delivery, are most likely to have serious complications such as encephalitis (CDC, 1996c).

The incubation period ranges from 10 to 21 days, usually 14 to 16 days after exposure. In infected people, the virus is considered communicable from one to two days before and up to six days after the rash erupts, or until the lesions are crusted. Both the incubation and communicable periods may be prolonged in immunocompromised people. Varicella-zoster virus then persists in a dormant state in the sensory nerve endings or ganglia. Latent varicella-zoster virus can later reactivate and cause herpes zoster, or shingles.

Before the availability of varicella vaccine, there were approximately four million cases of chickenpox each year, with 11,000 hospitalizations and 130 deaths annually in the United States (CDC, 1999l). Currently, 85% of the cases occur in children younger than 15 years, with 39% occurring in children one to four years of age. Susceptible adults who contract the disease have a more severe disease course and a higher case fatality rate, usually from viral pneumonia. Although adults represent only 7% of cases, they account for 35% of the approximately 130 deaths per year (CDC, 2000a).

Diagnosis is usually made by direct observation of the skin lesions and laboratory tests are not routinely required. The vidarabine drugs, adenine arabinoside, Ara-A, and acyclovir, or Zovirax, provide effective treatment for varicella infections. Varicella-zoster immune globulin, when administered within 96 hours of exposure, can modify or prevent the disease in susceptible people. Varicella vaccine is also effective in preventing or modifying illness if given to susceptible people within 72 hours and possibly up to five days after exposure (CDC, 1999l).

The live, attenuated varicella vaccine, Varivax, was approved and licensed by the FDA in March 1995 and is now available in the United States for routine childhood vaccination in susceptible children 12 months to 18 years of age. Varicella vaccine is also recommended for susceptible adults, provided there are no contraindications. The vaccine has a 70% to 90% efficacy rate in preventing lesions and the "breakthrough" cases are mild. The vaccine can be given simultaneously with all other vaccines; however, if it is not given on the same day as the MMR, at least four weeks should elapse between the administration of the two vaccines. Common side effects include pain, soreness, redness, and swelling at the injection site and a less frequent varicella-like rash at the site or elsewhere on the body. The vaccine is contraindicated for people who have severe allergic reactions to neomycin, who are pregnant, who have moderate to severe illness, who have a recent history of receiving a blood product, or who are immunocompromised (except people with humoral immunodeficiency or asymptomatic HIV infection as determined by a physician) (CDC, 2000b). The vaccine is extremely fragile and an absolute cold chain temperature of 5° F, or 15° C, from manufacturer to vaccinee must be maintained at all times. Widespread occurrence and expense of the vaccine make varicella a disease that is considered "not now eradicable."

VACCINES FOR INTERNATIONAL TRAVEL

For individuals traveling outside of the United States into regions with specific endemic infectious diseases, vaccinations are recommended. The only required vaccine for international travel is yellow fever vaccine and it is required depending on the country in which travel will occur. These countries require a stamped and signed International Certificate of Vaccination, which can be obtained from any provider authorized to administer yellow fever vaccine (CDC, 1999-2000). Other vaccines may be recommended depending on the area, the season, and the likelihood of exposure. It is important for those traveling abroad to obtain the most current recommendations from the Office of Overseas Travel at the CDC through their telephone hot line at (877) 394-8747; the annual publication, *Health Information for International Travel;* or their website. Access the website through the WebLinks section of this book's website at ⟨SIMON⟩ www.wbsaunders.com/SIMON/nies/.

In this section, major vaccine-preventable communicable diseases that place international travelers at risk are covered. Information includes presentation, complications, transmission, incubation, current statistics, risk groups, diagnosis, treatment, vaccination, and control and possible eradication activities.

Cholera

Cholera is a toxin-producing acute enteric bacterial infection that can be asymptomatic or can cause grave illness. Cholera causes profuse watery diarrhea, vomiting, and dehydration. Complications of cholera include severe dehydration leading to acidosis, circulatory collapse, convulsions, coma, and death. Transmission of cholera occurs through the fecal-oral route, usually from ingestion of fecally contaminated water or food and it has an incubation period of a few hours to five days. Since 1965, fewer than 27 cases of cholera have been reported annually in the United States. However, in 1992, an outbreak of 103 cholera cases occurred. Since then, the number of annually reported cases has returned to the preepidemic level of less than 32 cases (CDC, 1999d).

Groups in poor hygienic environments are at higher risk for outbreaks of cholera. Cholera outbreaks are common in parts of Central and South America, sub-Saharan Africa, and Southeast Asia (WHO, 2000). Diagnosis of cholera is made through culture of stool. Treatment of cholera involves immediate oral fluid rehydration therapy using oral rehydration solution; parenteral transfusion should be used for patients in shock. Antimicrobial therapy shortens the duration and intensity of illness and should be considered for people who are moderately to severely ill.

The best protection for travelers to endemic areas is to avoid shellfish and employ food and water precautions. Only one cholera vaccine is currently available in the United States. This is a killed, whole cell vaccine, which provides about 50% protection in reducing clinical illness for three to six months after vaccination. Oral cholera vaccines that provide greater protection are available in several countries but have not been licensed for use in the United States. Injectable cholera vaccine may cause soreness at the site of injection, fever, headache, and malaise (CDC, 1999-2000). Cholera vaccine should not be given simultaneously with yellow fever vaccine and it should not be used for control of epidemics or management of contacts of cases. The only contraindication is an anaphylactic reaction to a prior vaccine dose or vaccine component (Pickering, 2000). Newly appearing strains of cholera and the limited efficacy of existing vaccines makes cholera a disease that is not now eradicable.

Japanese Encephalitis

Japanese encephalitis (JE) is an acute inflammatory arbovirus. It can be asymptomatic or can cause fever, headache, and disruptions to the central nervous system. Complications may include hepatitis, polyarthritis, convulsions, paralysis, and death. JE is transmitted through the bite of infected mosquitoes and it has an incubation period of 5 to 15 days. JE is the leading cause of encephalitis in Asia, with highest incidence in China, Korea, Southeast Asia, and the Indian subcontinent and lesser incidence in Japan, Hong Kong, southeastern Russia, Singapore, Taiwan, and parts of Oceania, with recent expansion to Northern Australia. Approximately 30,000 to 50,000 cases of JE are reported annually, with disease prevalence higher in rural areas (CDC, 1998f; Thompson, 1996).

Anyone who has not been previously infected and is traveling for more than a month or residing in endemic and epidemic areas during transmission season is at risk for JE infection. JE is diagnosed by serological testing or viral isolation. No specific treatment is available for JE (Pickering, 2000).

Although several JE vaccines are produced in Asia, only one JE vaccine is licensed for use in the United States. The vaccine may cause local and mild systemic reactions; however, serious allergic reactions have occurred within minutes to as long as one week after vaccination. Therefore vaccinees should be observed for 30 minutes after vaccination and should be advised to remain in areas with immediate access to medical care for at least 10 days after vaccination. JE vaccine should be avoided during pregnancy unless there is a high risk for JE infection. Travelers should wear protective clothing and use insect repellant to avoid mosquito bites (CDC, 1999c, 2000d, Pickering, 2000). JE is not considered an eradicable disease at present, but control of JE is possible with immunization of infants and children in endemic areas and control of the mosquito vector population.

Meningococcus

Meningococcal disease is an acute bacterial infection usually resulting in meningococcemia, meningitis, or both. Onset is abrupt with fever, headache, stiff neck, nausea and vomiting, prostration, and often a maculopapular or petechial rash that can progress rapidly to purpura fulminans, shock, coma, and death. Transmission is through airborne droplets or close, direct contact with an infected individual or asymptomatic carrier (Pickering, 2000). Diagnosis is made by culture of blood and cerebrospinal fluid. Treatment includes high doses of antibiotics parenterally administered.

Antimicrobial chemoprophylaxis of close contacts is the primary means of prevention in the United States because routine immunization is not recommended in this country. There were 2725 cases of meningoccal disease reported in the United States in

1998, 61% of which were in children and young adults under 25 years of age (CDC, 1999d).

Meningococcal quadravalent polysaccharide vaccine is composed of four serotypes and is available for people older than two years of age; however, serotype C is poorly immunogenic in children. The vaccine does not cover all serotypes; therefore its use is limited to special circumstances such as in outbreaks or for travelers to epidemic areas such as sub-Saharan Africa and parts of Asia, where serotype A is predominant (CDC, 2000d). Although not routinely recommended, meningococcal vaccine is also available for some college freshman and other undergraduate students (CDC, 2000e). Side effects from vaccination may include soreness and swelling at the site of inoculation for one to two days. There are no contraindications to this vaccine except for an anaphylactic reaction to a prior dose of vaccine or vaccine component. With the possibility for eradication low, meningococcal vaccine should be used to control epidemics.

Plague

Plague is a serious zoonotic bacterial infection that may be asymptomatic or cause bubonic fever and painful swollen lymph nodes. Transmission of bubonic plague is through the bite of an infected flea that has fed on a contaminated rodent, often a rat, or through direct contamination with the infected drainage of a purulent bubo. Airborne droplets from an infected individual are responsible for transmission of pharyngeal or pneumonic plague. The incubation period is usually two to six days. Complications include dissemination throughout the body, including the meninges. Secondary pharyngeal and pneumonic plague are important because there is a direct human transmission and a fatality rate of 50% in untreated cases (CDC, 1996d).

In the United States, human plague is generally associated with epizootic infections in ground squirrels, prairie dogs, and other wild rodents. During 1998, the United States reported nine cases of human plague from four Western states (CDC, 1999d).

WHO reports 1000 to 3000 cases each year worldwide (CDC, 2000j). Susceptibility is general, but those living in crowded and unhygienic conditions and individuals working in areas where plague is endemic are at increased risk. Diagnosis of bubonic plague is made through culture of cerebrospinal fluid, blood, and aspirate from infected buboes and from sputum for pharyngeal and pneumonic plague.

Treatment includes the immediate use of antibiotic therapy.

Both live and killed vaccines are available. The vaccine in use in the United States is an inactivated whole cell bacterial preparation, recommended only for adults 18 to 61 years of age who are at high risk of exposure. Side effects may include soreness at the site of injection. Anaphylactic reaction to a prior vaccine dose or vaccine component is the only contraindication for this vaccine. If possible, plague vaccine should not be given with other vaccines because data are not available on interactions with other biologicals. The vaccine may not be fully protective; therefore vaccinated people should use the same precautions as unvaccinated people. Additional preventive measures include short-term antibiotic chemoprophylaxis with tetracycline or doxycycline during periods of exposure. Trimethoprim-sulfamethoxazole is an acceptable alternative for children. In 1998, the CDC was informed that the pharmaceutical company that produces the vaccine used in the United States was ceasing production. This action could eventually result in plague vaccine not being available in the United States (CDC, 1999d).

Plague is not now considered an eradicable disease because there is a presence of large reservoirs of wild rodents, an infectivity of fleas for months after contamination, and an existence of multiple forms of the disease. Control measures should focus on suppression of wild rodent and flea populations, especially in urban and periurban areas where crowded human conditions exist.

Rabies

Rabies is a zoonotic viral disease that usually manifests with progressive central nervous system involvement, including anxiety, dysphagia, and convulsions resulting in death. Rabies is directly transmitted through the saliva of an infected animal to a human host by a bite or through salivary contact with a mucous membrane or open wound. The incubation period ranges from a few days to more than one year. In the United States, 85% of all reported cases of animal rabies have occurred in wildlife, especially raccoons, skunks, and bats. Between 1980 and 1997, 21, or 58%, of human rabies cases were associated with bat variants (CDC, 1999m).

Susceptibility for contracting rabies is general. However, individuals living or working in areas with a high risk of exposure, including spelunkers, may be at increased risk for rabies infection. The long incubation period of rabies often makes the initial diagnosis difficult because there is a relative distance between transmission and the onset of clinical symptoms. Definitive diagnosis can be made through isolation of virus in cerebrospinal fluid or saliva and through antibody detection in serum and cerebrospinal fluid of unvaccinated individuals. However, early diagnosis does not usually alter the treatment or prognosis of rabies. Treatment of rabies begins with the immediate and thorough cleansing of bite wounds or mucous membranes that have possibly become contaminated with saliva from an infected animal. Immediate passive immunization should be administered using rabies immune globulin (RIG) along with active immunization with either human diploid cell vaccine (HDCV), rabies vaccine absorbed (RVA), or purified chick embryo cell vaccine (PCEC) (CDC, 1999m).

Rabies vaccine schedules are specific for preexposure and postexposure prophylaxis and involve a series of injections over a four-week period. Pain and swelling at the site of injection are common side effects. Approximately 6% of vaccinees experience a hypersensitivity to booster doses and supportive therapy should be available if boosters are necessary and recommended for these individuals. For people who have had serious systemic or anaphylactic reactions following rabies vaccine, their risk of acquiring rabies must be seriously considered before discontinuing vaccination. Assistance for managing these individuals is available through state health departments and the CDC (CDC, 1999m). Pregnancy is not a contraindication if postexposure vaccination is necessary.

Rabies is not now considered eradicable because there is the extended and divergent animal reservoirs for the rabies virus. However, human rabies can be eliminated with universal immunization, education, and control of rabies in animal populations.

Typhoid

Typhoid is a severe systemic bacterial infection that can range from being asymptomatic to producing fever, headache, malaise, constipation, anorexia, rose spots on the trunk, and sometimes lymphadenopathy. Complications include Peyer's patches in the ilium, which can lead to perforation, hemorrhage, and adhesions of the small intestine; mental dullness; deafness; and death. Typhoid is transmitted through ingestion of food and water contaminated by the urine and feces of infected individuals and carriers. The incubation period ranges from 3 to 30 days, with a usual range of 8 to 14 days. Susceptibility is general for typhoid fever. Diagnosis is made through culture of blood, urine, feces, or bone marrow. Antibiotics offer effective treatment (Chin, 2000).

The risk for typhoid fever in the United States is low, with approximately 400 cases reported each year, 70% of which are acquired through international travel. Typhoid fever is still common in the developing world, with an estimated 16 million cases and 600,000 deaths occurring each year (CDC, 2000k).

In the United States, the following three vaccines are currently available against typhoid: an oral live attenuated, a parenteral heat phenol inactivated, and a parenteral capsular polysaccharide vaccine (ViCPS). All three vaccines have similar efficacy ranging from 46% to 80%. Side effects for the injectables include soreness and swelling at the site of injection and possibly a slight fever and headache for one to two days. The oral live vaccine is contraindicated in children younger than six years and in immunocompromised patients and ViCPs is contraindicated in children younger than two years (CDC, 1999-2000).

Typhoid is not now considered erradicable because available vaccines are less than 100% effective, a carrier state exists, and drug resistance has developed in many places. Control measures should include health education and improvement of environmental hygienic conditions, including food and water.

Yellow Fever

Yellow fever is an acute infectious arbovirus that can be inapparent or cause sudden onset, fever, chills, nausea, vomiting, jaundice, and hemorrhagic disorders. Complications may include hepatitis, coma, and death. Transmission occurs through the bite of an infected mosquito, with an incubation period of three to six days.

Africa and South America are the only two areas of the world where yellow fever currently occurs. Susceptibility is general, with acute infection providing lifelong immunity. Diagnosis is made through isolation of the virus in blood. There is no specific treatment for yellow fever (Chin, 2000).

The yellow fever vaccine is a live, attenuated virus vaccine prepared using chicken embryos. It is 99% immunogenic and provides protection for at least 10 years and possibly longer. Slight fever, headache, and muscle pain may develop after injection. The vaccine is contraindicated in people with anaphylactic reactions to eggs and children less than four months of age. Immunosuppressed people and children four to nine months of age should receive vaccine only if risk of infection exceeds risk of vaccine-related encephalitis and pregnant women should be vaccinated only in high-risk areas (Chin, 2000; Pickering, 2000).

Yellow fever is not now considered eradicable because the presence of nonhuman hosts, the heat instability of the available vaccine, and the lack of political will exist. Control measures should be taken to reduce mosquito vector populations in urban centers where epidemics occur.

Tuberculosis

TB is a mycobacterial infection that causes tubercular lesions in the lung or other organs. These lesions may remain dormant for life or become reactivated at any time and progress into active pulmonary TB. Pulmonary TB manifests with symptoms of fatigue, fever, and weight loss, advancing to cough, chest pain, hemoptysis, and hoarseness. Complications include a high mortality rate in untreated cases. TB is transmitted through airborne droplets and spray from infected individuals and it has an incubation period of 2 to 12 weeks from infection to a positive tuberculin skin test. Infection in low-risk individuals often manifests with symptoms of active disease. The association of HIV-related sequelae with increased incidence and reactivation of TB has become a major global public health concern over the last few years. Approximately 18,000 new TB cases occur annually in the United States (CDC, 1999n). Worldwide, approximately eight million cases and two million deaths were attributed to TB in 1998 (CDC, 1999n).

Those with increased risk for contracting TB in the United States include low socioeconomic groups living in crowded urban poverty, the homeless, immunocompromised patients, and foreign-born and minority women. Although two types of skin tests are available for diagnosing TB infection in asymptomatic individuals, the preferred choice is the Mantoux test, a purified protein derivative (PPD) administered intradermally in the forearm. A health care provider who has education and experience in reading the test interprets the reaction. Any induration smaller than 5 mm is considered negative. An induration that is 15 mm or larger is considered positive. Any reaction

in between should be further evaluated to ensure that an appropriate diagnosis is made (CDC, 1994b).

The diagnosis of TB disease or infection cannot be ruled out because there is an absence of a reaction to the tuberculin skin test in immunosuppressed people. This is owing to a depressed or absent hypersensitivity response to the tuberculin reaction commonly seen in immunosuppressed people. For example, this may occur in people receiving corticosteroids or immunosuppressive drugs, or those with cancer or HIV infection.

Initial diagnosis can be made using radiography. Diagnosis is confirmed through culture of tubercle bacilli from sputum, cerebrospinal fluid, or other body fluids. Isoniazid continues to be the primary drug of choice for chemoprophylaxis of pulmonary TB in low-risk individuals younger than age 35 years with a positive tuberculin test and no active disease. Currently, a multidrug regimen, including isoniazid, rifampin, pyrazinamide, and ethambutol, sustained over nine months is the most widely used treatment of active TB in major metropolitan health departments in the United States (CDC, 1994b).

In 1998, a total of 18,361 cases of TB were reported in the United States. This was a decrease of 31% from 1992 at the height of the TB resurgence. All states reported at least one case in 1998; California, Florida, Illinois, New York, and Texas reported the highest number of cases and accounted for 54% of all cases. The decline in the overall number of reported TB cases reflects the apparent strengthening of TB-control programs nationwide, particularly in states and cities with the largest number of cases (CDC, 1999o).

Defaulting from drug compliance remains one of the most difficult challenges in the treatment of TB and can result in the persistence of chronic sputum-positive individuals. Reasons cited include noncompliance within the first three to four months because there is a clinical improvement felt by patients receiving treatment and side effects from chemotherapy. Noncompliance to treatment has increased the emergence of drug-resistant strains of TB and is a global concern.

The BCG vaccine is a freeze-dried vaccine prepared from live, attenuated bacteria. BCG is used

BOX 25-5

Recommendations for Elimination of TB

- TB programs should develop plans to ensure the timely and complete reporting of TB cases and to improve the quality of surveillance data.
- TB programs should develop and implement systems to conduct case findings among high-risk populations, when appropriate.
- DOT and other adherence-promoting measures should be expanded to improve and reduce delays in completion of therapy.
- Fixed-dose combination of anti-TB medication should be used for all patients with active disease who are receiving self-administered, rifampin-containing therapy. Combination drugs are likely to facilitate adherence to treatment and reduce the risk for acquired drug resistance associated with erratic treatment.
- Operational research should be undertaken to

develop strategies to ensure that contacts are identified for all TB patients and to increase the number of appropriate contacts identified for the patient, the proportion of infected contacts starting therapy, and the proportion of infected contacts completing therapy.
- TB-control staff members should be trained to use local epidemiological data to identify high-risk groups appropriate for targeted testing and to ensure that a greater proportion of infected contacts complete therapy.
- TB programs should work with community organizations (e.g., managed care programs, community health clinics, and immigrant groups) to expand testing and treatment of latent TB infection among targeted populations and to ensure that these activities are monitored and evaluated appropriately.

From Centers for Disease Control: Progress toward the elimination of tuberculosis: United States, 1998, *Mor Mortal Wkly Rep* 48(33):732-736, 1999o.

primarily for prevention of TB in individuals who are at high risk for repeated exposure and when other forms of preventive therapy are contraindicated. Studies have placed the efficacy of BCG from zero protection to 100% immunogenicity, but the efficacy remains unknown. It has not demonstrated immunogenicity in individuals vaccinated after a positive tuberculin skin test (CDC, 1996e) and should therefore be used only for those with a negative Mantoux skin test. PPD testing should be repeated two to three months after vaccination. If negative, revaccination should be offered. Side effects may include a rare ulceration at the site of injection. BCG is contraindicated in immunodeficient or immunosuppressed patients, symptomatic individuals with HIV infection, and those with burns or skin infections. The Advisory Council for the Elimination of Tuberculosis (ACET) has developed a set of recommendations to control and prevent TB (CDC, 1999n) (Box 25-5).

TB is not now considered eradicable because of the large foci of disease, the need for improved diagnostic tests, the presence of multidrug resistance, and the lack of a comprehensive vaccine. However, control is possible if enhanced screening programs are initiated for high-risk populations and significant treatment compliance is achieved through well-structured services, utilization of available community resources, and supervision of treatment with regular audits.

CHNs are frequently involved in activities related to TB control and treatment, from screening populations at risk for the disease to case management of people with TB. It is important that CHNs know the correct procedure, including the most recent recommendations from the CDC for administering and interpreting the Mantoux test. CHNs have also been involved in contact investigations of people exposed to TB in the community and in teaching the medication and health regimen to people with the disease. CHNs may also be involved in directly observed therapy (DOT), observing people with the disease taking their medication daily.

SEXUALLY TRANSMITTED DISEASES

Over the last 20 years, many changes have taken place in the patterns of STDs. New organisms are emerging, drug resistance has developed, prevalence of many

STDs is increasing, and unique complications from STDs are appearing (CDC, 1995b). These changes can be attributed to the following environmental, socioeconomic, demographic, and personal behavioral factors: younger age at initial sexual activity, later age at first marriage, widespread divorce, increased sexual activity with multiple partners, and sex with risky partners (e.g., those injecting drugs).

STDs include the more than 25 infectious organisms that are primarily transmitted through sexual activity (USDHHS, 2000). The rates of STDs in the United States are among the highest in the industrialized world, approaching those in some developing countries. An estimated 15 million cases of STDs occur each year in the United States, accounting for 87% of the top 10 infections reported to the CDC (USDHHS, 2000).

Many STDs cannot be cured and they cause serious, irreversible consequences; costs to society are large. More than one in five people in the United States, or 56 million people, are infected with an incurable, viral STD other than AIDS (e.g., genital herpes, HPV, or hepatitis B or C) (USDHHS, 2000).

Men and women of all ages, racial and ethnic backgrounds, and income levels contract STDs. However, the following populations are disproportionately affected: adolescents, young adults, women, minorities, and the poor (CDC, 1995b; USDHHS, 2000). Teenage girls in particular may be more susceptible to STDs because they have fewer protective antibodies to STDs and a cervix that is biologically immature. Women are at higher risk for contracting STDs than men because they have anatomical differences that enhance transmission of disease and make diagnosis difficult. In addition, they are also less likely to experience symptoms.

Race and ethnicity are known as risk factors for STDs because they are associated with some basic determinants of health status such as poverty, illicit drug use, living in a community with high STD prevalence, fewer health care-seeking behaviors, and limited access to care. Certain infections, particularly gonorrhea and syphilis, are more commonly found in low-income and minority populations, whereas other infections such as genital herpes, HPV, and *Chlamydia trachomatis,* are distributed throughout the population (USDHHS, 2000).

Certain STDs such as *Chlamydia* and gonorrhea may be asymptomatic or produce mild symptoms and may not be detected until serious and even life-threatening problems develop. These STDs and others

such as syphilis, genital herpes, and trichomoniasis increase a person's risk of contracting HIV on exposure to the virus (CDC, 1998d).

Complications from undiagnosed STDs occur more frequently and are more severe in women. For example, PID, largely resulting from an undetected STD, is diagnosed in more than one million women annually. Scarring from PID may lead to infertility, ectopic pregnancy, or chronic pelvic pain. An infected woman who transmits an STD to her fetus during pregnancy or childbirth may experience spontaneous abortion, premature delivery, stillbirth, low birth weight, neonatal death, and, in the infant, chronic respiratory problems, blindness, and mental retardation (USDHHS, 2000). Certain strains of HPV are strongly associated with cervical cancer; cervical cancer accounts for more than 4500 deaths annually.

This section describes the following six major STDs: HIV and AIDS, *C. trachomatis, Neisseria gonorrhoeae,* herpes simplex virus 2 (HSV-2), HPV, and syphilis.

HIV and AIDS

HIV, a retrovirus, is the organism that causes the disease known as AIDS. Following initial infection, HIV is typically asymptomatic over a period of months to years. HIV usually manifests gradually with conditions that result from inadequate immune system function as the virus slowly attacks the body's immune system. Vague symptoms such as fatigue, lymphadenopathy, anorexia, fever, chronic diarrhea, and weight loss occur. Over time, the body loses its ability to fight illnesses and opportunistic infections occur and become recurrent.

HIV is transmitted by sexual contact involving the exchange of body fluids (e.g., vaginal secretions and semen) with an infected individual; by blood transfusion or exposure to blood, blood products, or tissues of an infected person; by perinatal transmission from an infected mother to fetus during pregnancy or during delivery of an infant or when breastfeeding; or by sharing needles or syringes with an infected individual (CDC, 1995c). In January 1993, the AIDS surveillance case definition for adolescents and adults was expanded beyond an earlier definition of 23 conditions to include all HIV-infected people with severe immunosuppression (less than 200 CD4+ T lymphocytes per milliliter or a CD4+ T lymphocyte percentage of total lymphocytes less than 14%), recurrent pneumonia, pulmonary TB, or invasive cervical cancer (CDC, 1992). Examples of other opportunistic infections, or AIDS indicator diseases, include HIV-related wasting syndrome, *Pneumocystis carinii* pneumonia, Kaposi's sarcoma, and Burkett's lymphoma.

HIV infection is widespread. An estimated 47 million adults and children have AIDS worldwide (WHO, 2000). In the United States, between 650,000 and 900,000 people are HIV positive. In recent years, incidence rates have stabilized at about 40,000 cases per year (USDHHS, 2000).

AIDS cases among females increased from 8% of cases reported between 1981 and 1987 to 20% of cases during 1996 to October 1997. Although the proportion of cases decreased among whites from 60% to 43%, the proportion of cases increased among blacks from 25% to 43% and among Hispanics from 14% to 20%. The proportion of cases increased among intravenous drug users from 17% to 27% and in heterosexual transmission from 3% to 10%, whereas cases among homosexual men decreased from 64% to 45%. Eighty percent of the reported AIDS cases in the United States were concentrated in six metropolitan areas, predominantly on the East and West coasts (USDHHS, 2000).

In the United States, AIDS among women is increasing rapidly as women account for 20% of all cases (USDHHS, 2000). Exposure of women to AIDS in 1996 was attributed to intravenous drug use (41%), heterosexual contact with a partner at risk of or with AIDS (38%), contaminated blood or blood products (2%), and nonspecific HIV exposure (19%). The most rapidly increasing mode of transmission for women is heterosexual contact, which includes women whose sexual partners engage in high-risk behaviors (e.g., intravenous drug use), those with multiple partners, and those with STDs. Women are at high risk for HIV infection because they have different heterosexual transmission patterns. For example, male-to-female transmission is 12 times greater than female-to-male transmission (Padian, Shiboski, and Jewell, 1990).

However, perinatal transmission rate has declined substantially following the 1994 guidelines for use in HIV-positive pregnant women and is estimated be less then 4% when treatment with AZT is started during the second trimester of pregnancy and continued through delivery. The newborn must also be treated with zidovudine (ZDV). The infant should be delivered within four hours of rupture of the mother's amniotic fluid to decrease chance of HIV transmission (CDC, 1998d).

Populations at high risk for AIDS include adolescents, young adults, and other individuals with multiple partners; intravenous drug users and their sexual partners; homosexual men and their male or female partners; women whose partners engage in high-risk behaviors (e.g., intravenous drug use or have other female or male sexual partners); people who engage in risky sexual practices such as anal intercourse; and people who exchange sex for drugs or money (CDC, 1995c). Furthermore, transmission of HIV infection is enhanced in people with STDs (CDC, 1998d). For example, people with genital ulcers (e.g., HSV-2 or syphilis) or a nonulcerative STD (e.g., gonorrhea, *C. trachomatis,* or trichomoniasis) are at three to five times greater risk of contracting HIV on exposure than a person without an active infection (Padian, Shiboski, and Jewell, 1990).

As of June 1997, the CDC received reports of 52 cases of health care workers who were documented with HIV seroconversion associated with occupational exposure and 20 of these workers developed AIDS. An additional 114 health care workers were possibly exposed occupationally (CDC, 1998e). Workers have been infected with HIV in the health care setting following needle sticks with HIV-infected blood, after infected blood contacts the worker's open cut or mucous membranes (e.g., eyes or inside of the nose), and after exposure to HIV-infected blood, visibly bloody fluid, and concentrated virus in a laboratory (CDC, 1998e).

Health care workers have been infected with HIV occupationally following needle sticks with HIV-infected blood, after infected blood contacted the worker's open cut or mucous membranes, and after exposure to HIV-infected blood, visibly bloody fluid, or concentrated virus in a laboratory. A report by the CDC (1995d) described health care workers occupationally exposed to HIV who had seroconverted. In the report, those who seroconverted were as follows:

18 laboratory workers
16 nurses
6 physicians
1 dialysis technician
1 respiratory therapist
1 health aide
1 housekeeper and maintenance worker

HIV infection is usually determined by the HIV antibody test and the most commonly used form is the enzyme-linked immunosorbent assay. There may be false-positive findings, so the Western blot is used to verify the results. False-negative findings may also occur, especially before the body produces antibodies after exposure; therefore an exposed person should repeat the HIV antibody test 6 to 12 months, if immunocompromised, after the original test. Testing for HIV infection is offered at health departments, family planning clinics, STD clinics, HIV counseling and testing sites, and by primary care providers.

Surveillance of HIV infection is incomplete and varies by state. For example, as of January 1998, 31 states were conducting pediatric HIV case surveillance; 28 of the 31 were also conducting adolescent and adult HIV surveillance. The CDC concludes that "all States and territories should conduct HIV case surveillance as an extension of their AIDS Surveillance programs, and the CDC is developing HIV surveillance policy and technical guidance to assist all States and territories to conduct HIV and AIDS case surveillance" (CDC, 1997b, p. 865). This stance is supported in *Healthy People 2010* as a means of better monitoring the extent of the AIDS epidemic and emerging patterns (USDHHS, 2000).

The CDC recommends routine counseling and voluntary HIV testing for all pregnant women and medical treatment and preventive therapy for women testing positive well before giving birth. The use of ZDV or AZT is recommended by the PHS to reduce the risk of perinatal transmission of HIV infection from mother to infant (CDC, 1998d). These activities are most often offered as a collaborative effort between state offices of HIV and AIDS and family planning or maternal and child health services.

Treatment for HIV and AIDS is complex and changes frequently. The FDA for HIV infection and AIDS-related conditions has approved many drugs. Major drugs for treatment are categorized in Table 25-5.

Many other classifications of drugs have been approved by the FDA for HIV infection and AIDS-related conditions and include the following categories: antiemetic, antineoplastic, antimicrobial, antiprotozoal, red blood cell growth stimulator, immunomodulator (i.e., stimulates white blood cell production), antifungal, antiviral, protease inhibitor, appetite stimulant, antimycobacterial, antitubercular, and folic acid antagonist. Much controversy abounds

TABLE 25-5

Approved Drugs for Treatment of HIV and AIDS

Antiretrovirals	Nonnucleoside Reverse Transcriptase Inhibitors	Protease Inhibitors
Zidovudine (AZT)	Nevirapine	Saquinavir
Zalcitabine (ddC)	Delaviridine	Ritonavir
Didanosine (ddI)	Efavirenz	Nelfinavir
Stavudine (d4T)	Indinavir	Abacavir
Lamivudine (3TC)	Amprenavir	

in the community regarding the expense of these drugs and access to them because they are expensive.

Prevention efforts are targeted at creating awareness of risk and reduction of risk behaviors in high-risk populations and preventing transmission of HIV infection in people who are infected. Prevention strategies for all STDs are discussed later in this chapter.

Eradication of AIDS is dependent on development of a vaccine and the infrastructure necessary to vaccinate populations at risk worldwide. Neither possibility is foreseen in the near future, although testing of vaccine in humans has been initiated.

For information on FDA-approved drugs and testing of drugs in clinical trials, contact the AIDS Clinical Trials Information Service at 1-800-874-2572 and the HIV and AIDS Treatment Information Service at 1-800-448-0440.

Chlamydia

Chlamydia trachomatis is a bacterial infection that may be asymptomatic or may manifest as ocular, pulmonary, enteric, or genital tract infections. It is currently the most prevalent of the STDs (CDC, 1999d; USDHHS, 2000). The female organ most often infected by *C. trachomatis* is the endocervix, where little or no inflammation is caused and asymptomatic infection results. Complications include PID and chronicity leading to secondary scarring of the fallopian tubes, resulting in permanent obstructive infertility and possibly life-threatening ectopic pregnancies. *C. trachomatis* also causes conjunctivitis in infants exposed at birth. Infants infected with the organism may also contract pneumonia. Furthermore, genital chlamydia is responsible for approximately 50% of nongonococcal urethritis in men and women and epididymitis in men.

C. trachomatis has an incubation period of one to two weeks, perhaps longer, and is the most frequently reported infectious disease in the United States (CDC, 1999p). Increased rates reflect increased screening and reporting capability and increased recognition of asymptomatic infection, largely in women. Rates are more than five times greater in women than in men because men are less likely to be screened and, if diagnosed and treated, are less likely to be tested for the organism.

Based on reports to the CDC, teenage girls have the highest rates of chlamydial infection; 15- to 19-year-old girls represent 46% of infections and 20- to 24-year-old women represent another 33% (CDC, 1999p). Studies have shown that a significant number of patients infected with *C. trachomatis* are also infected with *N. gonorrhoeae* and *Trichomonas vaginalis* (CDC, 1995b).

Antibiotic therapy is recommended for the treatment for *C. trachomatis*. Early identification and treatment of all sexual partners is advised to prevent long-term complications. Although included in the list of diseases screened for potential eradicability, chlamydia is considered not now eradicable because there is the lack of immunity, the difficulty of diagnosis, the presence of asymptomatic illness, and low political will.

Gonorrhea

N. gonorrhoeae is a bacterial disease that manifests differently in men and women. In men, the infection can be asymptomatic or more often can manifest initially with a purulent discharge that progresses to dysuria. In women, the infection can be asymptomatic or can manifest initially with a mild cervicitis or urethritis. Complications in women occur from untreated asymptomatic infection, which can result in endometritis, PID, salpingitis, infertility through tubal occlusion, and ectopic pregnancy. A chronic carrier state can develop in both men and women. Newborns of infected mothers are at high risk for gonococcal conjunctivitis, which, if not promptly treated, can lead to blindness.

Gonorrhea has an incubation period of two to seven days and is second only to chlamydial infections in the number of cases reported to the CDC (CDC, 1997c). The incidence of gonorrhea is highest in high-density urban areas among people 24 years of age and older who have multiple sex partners and engage in unprotected sexual intercourse. Increases in gonorrhea prevalence have been noted recently among men who have sex with men (CDC, 1999q).

Diagnosis of gonorrhea is confirmed through microscopic examination of exudate and through bacteriological culture. The emergence of antibiotic-resistant strains of gonococcal organisms and noncompliance with drug regimens present specific problems in the treatment of gonorrhea. New single-dose drugs have been developed to combat these challenges.

Although gonococcal infections occur only in the human host, gonorrhea is not now considered eradicable because there is the lack of an effective vaccine, no development of immunity after infection, the existence of a carrier state, the emergence of drug-resistant strains, and low political will.

Herpes Simplex Virus 2

HSV-2 is a chronic ulcerative disease that may be symptomatic or asymptomatic. After an incubation period of 3 to 21 days, genital lesions may appear. These lesions are caused by the following types: herpes simplex virus 1 (HSV-1), which is usually associated with cold sores and lesions above the waist, and HSV-2, which is usually associated with genital lesions or lesions below the waist. HSV-1 may occur below the waist or HSV-2 above the waist through oral sex or self-inoculation. HSV-2 may manifest with vesicles, or small blisters, that progress to shallow ulcers that are often extremely painful and debilitating. After primary lesions disappear, the virus remains in a latent form and secondary episodes may reappear at any time. It is uncertain what causes recurrences, but they have been attributed to a number of factors, including overexertion and increased levels of emotional stress (Swanson, Dibble, and Chenitz, 1995).

Complications of HSV-2 include meningitis, encephalitis, coma, and death. In pregnant women, it may result in neonatal HSV infection. Exposed newborns may have a generalized systemic infection; a localized infection with skin, eyes, and mouth lesions; or localized central nervous system symptoms. Complications of HSV in neonates include neurological and ocular disorders, with a resultant high mortality rate.

Scientists have estimated that about 30 million people in the United States may have HSV infections. Most infected people never recognize the symptoms of genital herpes; some have symptoms shortly after infection and never again.

HSV-2 is a genital ulcer; therefore individuals with HSV-2 are at higher risk of infection with HIV. Differential diagnosis of HSV-2 is confirmed through viral detection in tissue culture. Antiviral treatment may decrease the duration of viral shedding, healing, and symptoms in primary outbreaks, but it is less effective in reducing the frequency and severity of recurrences. The incurability of the disease, its unpredictability, and associated stigma requires careful education and counseling may be recommended. Children diagnosed with HSV-2 infections should be evaluated as possible victims of sexual abuse.

The latency and reactivation of HSV-2 are not clearly understood and emphasis should be placed on prevention. A person with active lesions should not engage in sexual intercourse until the lesions subside and should always use safer sex practices (e.g., condoms) because asymptomatic viral shedding occurs in many infected individuals. Although HSV-2 infections occur only in the human host, HSV-2 is not now considered eradicable because there is the presence of a long latency period, the lack of a cure, and low political will.

Human Papillomavirus

HPV is a virus that sometimes causes genital warts, but in many cases infects people without causing noticeable symptoms. Concern about HPV has increased in recent years after several studies showed that HPV infection is strongly associated with the development of cervical cancer. Strains of HPV have been divided into high-risk and low-risk groups based on whether they are associated with cancer. Infection with high-risk HPV is one risk factor for cervical cancer, which causes 4500 deaths among women each year. HPV typically has a usual incubation period of three months, although it may range from three weeks to eight months. The highest rates of genital HPV infection are found in older adolescents and young adults (USDHHS, 2000). Perinatal transmission may also occur and may involve the respiratory tract, including laryngeal papillomas, which obstruct the airway and the genital tract.

An estimated 50% of sexually active adults have been infected with HPV. Infections with HPV-6 and HPV-11 subtypes causes genital warts, low-grade cervical intraepithelial neoplasm (CIN), and recurrent respiratory papillomatosis. Persistent cervical infection with common subtypes of HPV (HPV-16, -18, -31, and -45) is the single most important etiological risk factor for cervical cancer. These subtypes account for an estimated 80% of cervical cancers. Most cervical HPV infections are usually transient, but cancer-related subtypes are more likely to persist (USDHHS, 2000). It is also estimated that the prevalence of disease in males parallels that found in females. With men, as with women, it is difficult to tell whether HPV is present because there are no clinical symptoms and the virus can be localized internally on the genitalia. It is therefore possible to unknowingly spread infection.

Although no culture is available for HPV, there are several diagnostic tests for the detection of genital warts. They include clinical observation facilitated by the use of acetic acid stain for detection of subtle lesions and colposcopy, or androscopy in men, cytology, and histology. Treatments for HPV include the use of podophyllin; cryotherapy (i.e., with liquid nitrogen; this has been identified as the safest and most highly recommended treatment); laser therapy; 5-fluorouracil; and interferon. Relapses can occur and routine PAP smears should be done periodically to rule out the possibility of cervical dysplasia and carcinoma.

Syphilis

Syphilis has an incubation period of three weeks from initial infection until the manifestation of the primary lesion. Syphilis has three recognized stages of development. The primary stage manifests with a painless lesion or chancre, which often goes unnoticed, especially in women, because the lesion may be located inside the vagina where it is not easily seen without clinical examination. If the infection is not cured at this stage, it will progress to secondary syphilis, which manifests with a different set of highly infectious lesions. This stage may disappear spontaneously if untreated and there will be no clinical signs for long periods of time, often years; or the disease may eventually result in tertiary neurosyphilis. Complications include the irreversible destructive neurological signs and symptoms of tertiary-stage syphilis and preterm births and congenital syphilis of neonates born to infected mothers. The 1997 rate of primary and secondary syphilis of 3.2 per 100,000 was the lowest rate ever reported in the United States, based on 8539 case reports, and passed the *Healthy People 2000* target of 4.0 per 100,000. In 1998, the number of cases was even lower at 7089 (CDC, 1999d).

Diagnosis of syphilis at any stage of infection is accomplished with nontreponemal serological tests such as the Venereal Disease Research Laboratory (VDRL) or the rapid plasma reagent (RPR) test. The fluorescent treponemal antibody absorption test (FTS-Abs), which is a treponemal serological test, should be used if either of the first two tests is positive to ensure the greatest reliability.

Early identification and treatment of syphilis in pregnant women and periodic rescreening and retreatment throughout pregnancy for previously infected women are essential for prevention of devastating sequelae for their neonates. Treatment of syphilis at all stages involves varying doses of penicillin G. The fetuses of currently syphilitic pregnant women and those women previously treated for syphilis of unknown duration or duration greater than one year have a higher incidence of congenital syphilis. However, it is unclear whether this is from drug treatment failure or reinfection after successful treatment (McFarlin et al., 1994).

Although syphilis affects only humans, it is not now considered an eradicable disease because there is the difficulty of diagnosis, the unpredictability of relapse, the partial immunity after infection, and the low political will. Control of syphilis can be achieved through routine annual screening of sexually active individuals and pregnant women in their first trimester and by tracking and treating infected individuals and their partners.

PREVENTION OF COMMUNICABLE DISEASES

The CHN has a role in primary, secondary, and tertiary prevention of communicable diseases. Examples of appropriate interventions are reviewed next and Table 25-6 gives additional examples of primary, secondary, and tertiary prevention strategies for communicable diseases.

Primary Prevention

Primary prevention of communicable diseases involves keeping the population healthy and free of contracting the disease. Primary prevention of communicable disease is highly dependent on education of individuals, families, and aggregates or populations at risk for a disease. Efforts at prevention must come

TABLE 25-6

Levels of Prevention of Communicable Diseases

Affected Population	Primary	Secondary	Tertiary
Individual with AIDS	Education Change sexual behavior and other high-risk practices	Screening for HIV in at-risk populations Reporting Early diagnosis and treatment	HIV drugs Maintain health Prevent conversion from HIV to AIDS Prepare for death
Family with malaria	Sleeping under bed net Protective clothing (e.g., long-sleeved shirts and long pants) Insect repellents Eliminate mosquito-breeding stagnant water; spraying of ponds	Reporting Immediate diagnosis and treatment of infected individuals	Prevent mosquito feeding on infected individuals Appropriate treatment using correct drugs to prevent further drug resistance
Aggregate with measles	Education Measles vaccination Documentation	Screening for unimmunized individuals Early diagnosis and treatment Reporting Control of epidemics	Treatment of disease Epidemic measures

from the federal government, state and local governments, and both public and private institutions. Although the use of vaccines, as discussed previously, is one way to keep the population well, other strategies include promoting behaviors that decrease susceptibility to the disease.

Primary prevention may be accomplished in several ways, including targeting at-risk populations for interventions at individual, family, and aggregate levels. For example, at the aggregate level, legislation mandating immunization of children entering grade school has had a profound impact on the immunization levels of schoolchildren in the United States. At the family level, ongoing efforts by day care centers, schools, and churches are targeting immunization information to families of preschool children, particularly those younger than two years. At the individual level, adults in the workforce may require immunizations such as HBV or tetanus vaccine from occupational exposure. There is a comprehensive vaccine delivery system for all children and adults living in the United States. Health care providers, including nurses, must not miss any opportunities to immunize.

Through efforts of the mass media, populations may be targeted for health education messages. Social marketing efforts are needed to tailor the health messages to the target audiences using appropriate media channels.

Much has been learned about primary prevention of communicable disease through research targeted at testing HIV prevention programs. Characteristics of successful programs include the following (Holtgrave et al., 1995):

- The needs of the individual and the community must be assessed and the program must be planned to address those needs.
- Prevention messages must be culturally appropriate; that is, they must be tailored to the target audience in terms of age, developmental status, education, sex, race and ethnicity, geography, sexual orientation, values, beliefs, and norms and they must be linguistically specific.
- Program goals, objectives, and strategies for each intended client subpopulation should be clear; both process (i.e., how services are delivered) and outcome (i.e., behavioral or health) objectives should be stated; interventions should be specific as to their components.
- Programs should be based in behavioral and social science theory and research; a thorough re-

view of the research literature should be undertaken to determine successful theory-based approaches with the target population.
- Programs should be monitored and midcourse corrections made if objectives are not being met.
- Sufficient resources must be available (financial, material, and human), or the goals must be changed to meet the available resources.

Women often lack power in their relationships with men to influence sexual decision making. Realities of economics, gender role norms, and cultural messages may exert a powerful influence on women's decision making and sexual behavior. High-risk sexual behavior includes exchanging sex for drugs or sex for money to buy drugs, resulting in sex with multiple anonymous partners who cannot be easily identified and screened for disease. Many individuals of low socioeconomic levels have poor access to health care for screening and treatment, a low level of education, and a high rate of unemployment, factors that may predispose them to a definite disadvantage regarding knowledge of health education measures such as safer sexual practices, clean needle use, and access to health services.

Knowledge is not enough to change behavior. Education must include cognitive-behavioral skills acquisition (e.g., negotiation and practice applying condom) and address broader social and cultural contexts of sexuality such as gender roles, peer influence, cultural values and norms, interpersonal relationships, communication patterns, and conflict resolution (Holtgrave et al., 1995). In addition, intensive and sustained interventions are needed over time.

Secondary Prevention

Contact investigation and case finding are important aspects of secondary prevention to prevent the spread of communicable disease in the community. People found to be at risk of a communicable disease should receive screening to determine occurrence. For example, people whose sexual histories reveal high-risk behaviors should receive annual routine screening for STDs. Incidence should be reported to the local health department for those reportable diseases and for partner notification related to those diseases. The medical regimen should be taught to the client and to her or his partner and recommendations adhered to for increasing coverage of all patients with active and potential infections.

Tertiary Prevention

Tertiary prevention involves actions to keep infected people apart from noninfected people. These actions involve isolation, which separates infected people during the period in which they are communicable, and quarantine, which places restrictions on healthy contacts of people infected during the incubation period to prevent spread of the disease should a case occur. Actions important to tertiary prevention include safely handling contaminated infectious waste products, hand washing, and wearing protective gloves and gowns when indicated. Teaching family or other caregivers to give safe tertiary care to people with an infectious disease in the home and in other institutions, such as a school or nursing home, is an important role of the community health nurse.

Care of people with communicable diseases such as HIV and AIDS in the community presents an important challenge. It is important to prevent the spread of the infection, to prevent recurrence of dis-

eases, to prevent new infections, and to promote the general health. It is important to delay the onset of symptoms and infections in people with HIV infection and to promote the QOL in people with AIDS. Care of people with HIV and AIDS in the community demands knowledge of the interdisciplinary network of providers who give preventive and therapeutic nursing services to clients. The CHN must know how the community is organized to make timely referrals, to give follow-up care, and to serve as an advocate of the clients and their families. This includes making the problems clients experience known and advocating for more responsive or comprehensive services. Wellness programs, stress reduction, support groups, nutrition services, and drug management are examples of the kinds of activities that can promote the health of people and families of people with a sexually transmitted infection. Universal precautions should be used when giving care to infected people; they should also be taught to caregivers of infected people.

CASE STUDY

APPLICATION OF THE NURSING PROCESS

Whether the CHN is teaching parents of infected children, day care workers, or caregivers of people with a communicable disease, prevention of transmission is a major aspect of care. Guidelines developed for health professionals are available to assist the CHN in planning this care.

This case study demonstrates how a community health nurse applies the nursing process to a specific problem within the community in which he or she works. The CHN receives a referral from within the community. An assessment is carried out to identify the information necessary to provide accurate diagnoses. Nursing diagnoses and interventions are then outlined, including actual and potential problems, for each component of the community affected. The CHN and the affected members of the aggregate draw up a plan. Implementation is carried out, followed by an evaluation of the entire nursing process. Primary, secondary, and tertiary preventive measures for the community are identified and can be put into practice to prevent future problems and epidemics.

Miriam Beckwirth is a CHN at an elementary school. She works with students in a variety of areas

such as teaching health education and lifestyle classes, seeing students in the school clinic when they are ill, and providing families with counseling for stressful episodes. She is also the liaison between the public health department and the school and she ensures that all health department regulations are being met concerning child safety, nutrition, vaccination coverage, environmental safety, and mental health. It is her responsibility to report any unusual health-related occurrences such as suspected child abuse or the development of any infectious epidemic within the school or the larger aggregates. She is adept at using the nursing process to assess, plan, implement, and evaluate nursing care plans for each of her students to meet their individual needs, the related needs of their families, and selected needs of the larger community. She does this by addressing primary, secondary, and tertiary levels of prevention that she can influence positively.

Assessment

Miriam received a telephone call from Mr. John Lemon, a third-grade teacher, who was concerned
Continued

about one of his students, Jabril Kamal. Mr. Lemon reported that this normally healthy and very active eight-year-old Algerian-born boy was not able to participate in class because he was not feeling well. In response, Miriam told Mr. Lemon to send Jabril to the clinic immediately.

When Jabril arrived, Miriam checked his vital signs and performed a quick assessment. She noted a temperature of 101.6° F, red and inflamed eyes, a mild cough, and white spots on the inside of his mouth. Jabril was irritable and complained of "feeling achy." From her questions, Miriam learned that he had been feeling ill for approximately 15 hours and no one else in his household was sick.

Miriam pulled Jabril's file to assess his immunization status and learned that he had received a measles vaccine in Algeria on March 4, 1991. She looked up his birthday and discovered that he was born in North Africa on September 9, 1990. She determined that his age at the time of administration of the measles vaccine was six months.

Miriam called Jabril's mother and Mrs. Kamal confirmed the date of Jabril's birth and the date of his vaccination. She informed Jabril's mother that he was quite ill and needed to see the family physician immediately.

Miriam telephoned Jabril's family physician, who agreed to see the boy immediately. The physician placed a mask over Jabril's nose and mouth and isolated him from susceptible patients and staff. He drew a blood sample, which later identified the measles virus. Four days later, Jabril developed a red blotchy rash that began on his face and became more generalized over the next five or six days.

Nursing Diagnosis and Plan

For Jabril

I. At risk for altered thermoregulation from febrile condition; teach family to:
  A. Monitor temperature every two hours and record.
  B. Administer nonaspirin-containing analgesics and antipyretics as needed.
  C. Maintain hydration.
  D. Lubricate lips frequently.
  E. Use measures to reduce excessive fever when present.
    1. Remove blankets.
    2. Apply ice bags to axilla and groin.
    3. Initiate tepid water sponge bath.
    4. Maintain environmental temperature at a comfortable setting.

II. Altered skin integrity from measles lesions; teach family to:
  A. Inspect skin condition for spread of rash.
  B. Use mild, unabrasive soap and tepid water for hygiene.

III. Social isolation from measles; teach family to:
  A. Isolate child from susceptible measles contacts during infectious period, which is for four days before rash onset until four days after rash onset.
  B. Involve child in setting goals and planning care as indicated.
  C. Arrange for telephone so child can talk to friends.
  D. Offer books, games, and television for diversional activity.
  E. Bring homework from school so child will not fall behind peers in class.

For Jabril's Family

I. Potential for disturbance in family coping from acute illness
  A. Encourage family to discuss impact of child's illness and their feelings.
  B. Facilitate family conferences to help family identify key issues and select support services, if needed.
  C. Help child and family establish a visiting routine that will not tax child or family members.
  D. Reinforce family's efforts to care for child.
  E. Provide family with clear, concise information about child's condition.
  F. Provide emotional support to family by being available to answer questions.
  G. Inform family of community resources available to assist in managing child's illness and provide emotional or financial support to the caretakers (e.g., if mother and father are both working and must take off time without pay to care for child).

II. Knowledge deficit related to vaccination schedule
  A. Establish an environment of mutual trust and respect to enhance family's learning.
  B. Negotiate with family to develop goals for learning.

C. Select teaching strategies (e.g., discussion, demonstration, role-playing, and visual materials) appropriate for family's individual learning style.
D. Teach family about schedules of vaccines for childhood diseases and have them demonstrate knowledge of vaccines and their schedules.
E. Encourage family to ask questions and discuss concerns.
F. Provide family with names and telephone numbers of resource people, agencies, or organizations to contact with questions or problems.

For Jabril's Classmates
I. Knowledge deficit related to measles infection
   A. Establish an environment of mutual trust and respect to enhance children's learning.
   B. Negotiate with children to develop goals for learning.
   C. Select teaching strategies (e.g., discussion, demonstration, role-playing, and visual materials) appropriate for the children's learning style.
   D. Teach children about measles infection and have them demonstrate knowledge of transmission, vaccination, and disease course of measles infection.
   E. Teach how disease outbreaks can be dealt with in daily life.
   F. Encourage children to ask questions and discuss concerns.
   G. Provide children with names and telephone numbers of resource people, agencies, or organizations to contact with questions or problems.
II. Potential for infection from exposure to measles virus
   A. Minimize risk of infection by:
      1. Vaccinating all susceptible children and adults.
      2. Vaccinating all susceptible household and extended family contacts.
      3. Vaccinating all susceptible community members.
   B. Encourage early identification and reporting of infections to prevent further transmission.

C. Administer immune globulin when appropriate and recommended by child's physician.
D. Teach the importance of hand washing regularly after using the toilet and before meals.
E. Ensure proper disposal of all tissues and contaminated materials within the school setting.
F. Provide adequate ventilation system within classrooms.
G. Notify a doctor immediately if any symptoms of measles develop within 10 to 14 days after exposure. Anyone with symptoms should stay home until four days after rash onset and avoid contact with anyone who is not immune to measles.

Intervention

Miriam reported the case to the infectious disease branch of the local health department for surveillance and follow-up before the diagnosis had been confirmed. Miriam made a home visit to develop a plan of care with the family. She also formulated a plan for the other children at the school. Then she reviewed the health records of the children attending her school to ensure that no students needed to be revaccinated. Miriam notified the parents of all the children at the school to watch for signs and symptoms of measles and she encouraged them to check the immunization status of all family members in the household.

During the home visit, she talked with Mrs. Kamal about ways to offer supportive measures such as bed rest during the febrile period, nonaspirin-containing antipyretics for the fever, dimming the lights for sensitive eyes, and providing a vaporizer in the child's room. Miriam warned Mrs. Kamal about the complications of measles and told her that if she noticed any of these signs or symptoms, she should notify Jabril's physician immediately and request an appointment. The complications she mentioned were dehydration, an earache (otitis media), any respiratory symptoms such as a severe cough or wheezing (e.g., pneumonia, bronchiolitis, obstructive laryngitis, and laryngotracheitis), and any

Continued

neurological changes such as unsteady gait or memory disturbances. Finally, Miriam informed Mrs. Kamal about the need for strict isolation from other children and adults who are not immune to measles and had Mrs. Kamal make a complete list of everyone with whom Jabril had come in contact and the places he had been within the past three weeks.

As planned, Miriam reported the case to the local health department and gave the list of Jabril's contacts to the public health officer taking the information. The officer would contact those people who had been in close proximity to Jabril during the preceding three weeks to identify, immunize, and monitor anyone susceptible who had been exposed.

Miriam prepared a note for all of the children to take home to their parents informing them of the measles case, alerting them to the signs and symptoms of measles and the need for the child to remain at home if symptoms develop. She enclosed a form to help family members review vaccination schedules. Miriam also reviewed all vaccination records for the children at the school and prepared to vaccinate all children in need of a booster.

Evaluation

Five days after Miriam first examined Jabril, the public health officer telephoned Miriam to inform her that they had isolated the original source of the measles virus. The family living across the street from Jabril had some friends visiting from Indonesia. These friends had a one-year-old child who had not been vaccinated and developed measles on arriving in the United States. The child subsequently recovered, but not before exposing several people at risk.

None of Jabril's classmates contracted measles. The benefit of this experience was an emphasis placed on revaccinating those at risk within 72 hours of exposure and ensuring the health of this aggregate through more prudent vaccination adherence against preventable infectious diseases. This episode also displayed how important it is to have a reliable and efficient public health surveillance system.

SUMMARY

The community health nurse has the unique role of taking collective action with community members at the local, state, and national levels to preserve the health of aggregates through the prevention, identification, and management of communicable diseases. This chapter outlines threats to the health of the community and interventions used by the community health nurse to keep the community free of infection.

Transmission of infectious agents is carried out through direct, indirect, and airborne contacts with human recipients. Understanding modes of transmission will help in design and use of effective methods to prevent the spread of infectious diseases.

Defining, reporting, and continuing surveillance of cases of infectious disease transmission are vital aspects of a national public health surveillance program. The information contributed from these activities provides baseline data for the monitoring of epidemiological trends, around which screening and intervention programs can be administered.

One major method of keeping communities free of infection is through the use of vaccines. There are different kinds of immunity, each lasting a specified amount of time, but the goal is for lasting immunity against infectious diseases. Vaccination, given in the correct dosage, route, and preparation, can provide lasting immunity to most individuals. Vaccine schedules for all ages should be met and vaccine integrity should be maintained through the use of a cold chain and by checking expiration dates before use. Many individuals around the world still suffer from vaccine-preventable infectious diseases and mortality rates from these illnesses remain high. Where eradication is not probable, control is the goal.

For many infectious diseases, prevention is the only cure. Vaccines and safer sex practices have become the first line of defense. They are safe preventive measures that are more cost effective, in both economic and human terms, than not using these interventions.

Public health efforts are vitally important in combating the increasing trends of many infectious disease rates. CHNs have an important role in prevention, case finding, reporting, and other activities related to the control of communicable diseases within their communities.

LEARNING ACTIVITIES

1. Visit a testing laboratory to see how STD tests are done (e.g., VDRL or tests for gonorrhea).
2. Find out what kinds of vaccine services are available at the local health department and what form of follow-up is performed.
3. Call one of the hotline reference telephone numbers listed in this chapter and request specific information regarding a client.
4. Obtain and evaluate health education materials regarding childhood immunizations from the local health department.
5. Review the communicable disease reference materials available from the CDC and the USDHHS.
6. Inquire about the reporting of notifiable diseases in the community. Who is responsible for the reporting process? To whom do they report, what is reportable, and how often? What emergency public health measures are available for control of epidemics in the area?
7. Purchase a one-year subscription to a public health nursing journal.

REFERENCES

Centers for Disease Control: Revised classification system for HIV infection and expanded surveillance case definition for AIDS among adolescents and adults, *Mor Mortal Wkly Rep* 41:RR-7, 1992.

Centers for Disease Control: Recommendations of the Internal Task Force for Disease Eradication, *Mor Mortal Wkly Rep* 42:1-38, 1993.

Centers for Disease Control: General recommendations on immunization: recommendations of the Advisory Committee on Immunization Practices (ACIP), *Mor Mortal Wkly Rep* 43(RR-1):1-38, 1994a.

Centers for Disease Control: Guidelines for preventing the transmission of *Mycobacterium tuberculosis* in health-care facilities, *Mor Mortal Wkly Rep* 43(RR-13)62-63, 1994b.

Centers for Disease Control: *Epidemiology and prevention of vaccine-preventable diseases,* Atlanta, 1995a, The Author.

Centers for Disease Control: *Sexually transmitted disease surveillance, 1994,* Atlanta, 1995b, The Author.

Centers for Disease Control: *HIV/AIDS prevention: facts about the human immunodeficiency virus and its transmission,* Atlanta, 1995c, The Author.

Centers for Disease Control: Case control study of HIV seroconversion in health care workers after percutaneous exposure to HIV-infected blood, *Mor Mortal Wkly Rep* 44(50):929-933, 1995d.

Centers for Disease Control: *Vaccine management: recommendations for handling and storage of selected biologicals,* Atlanta, 1996a, CDC National Immunization Program.

Centers for Disease Control: Vaccine side effects, adverse reactions, contraindications and precautions: recommendations of the Advisory Committee on Immunization Practices (ACIP), *Mor Mortal Wkly Rep* 45(RR-12):1-35, 1996b.

Centers for Disease Control: Prevention of varicella: recommendations of the Advisory Committee on Immunization Practices (ACIP), *Mor Mortal Wkly Rep* 45(RR-11):1-36, 1996c.

Centers for Disease Control: Prevention of plague: recommendations of the Advisory Committee on Immunization Practices (ACIP), *Mor Mortal Wkly Rep* 45(RR-14):1-15, 1996d.

Centers for Disease Control: The role of BCG vaccine in the prevention and control of tuberculosis in the United States, *Mor Mortal Wkly Rep* 45(RR-4):1-18, 1996e.

Centers for Disease Control: Prevention of pneumococcal disease: recommendations of the Advisory Committee on Immunization Practices (ACIP), *Mor Mortal Wkly Rep* 46(RR-08):1-24, 1997a.

Centers for Disease Control: Update: trends in AIDS incidence: United States, 1996, *Mor Mortal Wkly Rep* 46(37):861-867, 1997b.

Centers for Disease Control: *Sexually transmitted disease surveillance, 1993,* Atlanta, 1997c, The Author.

Centers for Disease Control: Guidelines for vaccinating pregnant women, *Mor Mortal Wkly Rep* 45(RR-4):1-18, 1998a.

Centers for Disease Control: Recommendations for prevention and control of hepatitis C virus (HCV) infection and HCV-related chronic disease, *Mor Mortal Wkly Rep* 47(RR-19):1-39, 1998b.

Centers for Disease Control: Measles, mumps and rubella—vaccine use and strategies for elimination of measles, rubella and congenital rubella syndrome and control of mumps: recommendations of the Advisory Committee on Immunization Practices (ACIP), *Mor Mortal Wkly Rep* 47(RR-8):1-57, 1998c.

Centers for Disease Control: HIV prevention through early detection and treatment of other sexually transmitted diseases—United States: recommendations of the Advisory Committee for HIV and STD prevention, *Mor Mortal Wkly Rep* 47(RR-12):1-24, 1998d.

Centers for Disease Control: Public health service guidelines for the management of health-care worker exposures to HIV and recommendations for postexposure prophylaxis, *Mor Mortal Wkly Rep* 47(RR-7):1-28, 1998e.

Centers for Disease Control, Division of Vector-Borne Infectious Diseases: *Fact sheet: Japanese Encephalitis,* 1998f, The Author, www.cdc.gov/ncidod/dvbid/jefacts.htm.

Centers for Disease Control: Achievements in public health, 1900-1999: control of infectious diseases, *Mor Mortal Wkly Rep* 48(29):621-629, 1999a.

Centers for Disease Control: The principles of disease elimination and eradication, *Mor Mortal Wkly Rep* 48(SU01):23-27, 1999b.

Centers for Disease Control: Epidemiology of measles, *Mor Mortal Wkly Rep* 48(34):749-753, 1999c.

Centers for Disease Control: Summary of notifiable diseases: United States, 1998, *Mor Mortal Wkly Rep* 47(53):1-93, 1999d.

Centers for Disease Control: Achievements in public health, 1900-1999: impact of vaccines universally recommended for children—United States, 1990-1998, *Mor Mortal Wkly Rep* 48(12):243-248, 1999e.

Centers for Disease Control: Recommendations of the Advisory Committee on Immunization Practices: revised recommendations for routine poliomyelitis vaccination, *Mor Mortal Wkly Rep* 48(27):590, 1999f.

Centers for Disease Control: Withdrawal of rotavirus vaccine recommendation, *Mor Mortal Wkly Rep* 48(43):1007, 1999g.

Centers for Disease Control: Prevention of hepatitis A through active or passive immunization: recommendations of the Advisory Committee on Immunization Practices (ACIP), *Mor Mortal Wkly Rep* 48(RR-12):1-37, 1999h.

Centers for Disease Control: Neuraminidase inhibitors for treatment of influenza A and B infections, *Mor Mortal Wkly Rep* 48(RR-14):1-9, 1999i.

Centers for Disease Control: Recommendations for the use of lyme disease vaccine: recommendations of the Advisory Committee on Immunization Practices (ACIP), *Mor Mortal Wkly Rep* 48(RR-07):1-25, 1999j.

Centers for Disease Control: Progress toward the global interruption of wild polio virus type 2 transmission, 1999, *Mor Mortal Wkly Rep* 48(33):736-738, 1999k.

Centers for Disease Control: Prevention of varicella: updated recommendations of the Advisory Committee on Immunization Practices (ACIP), *Mor Mortal Wkly Rep* 48(RR-06):1-5, 1999l.

Centers for Disease Control: Human rabies prevention—United States, 1999: recommendations of the Advisory Committee on Immunization Practices (ACIP), *Mor Mortal Wkly Rep* 48(RR-1):1-21, 1999m.

Centers for Disease Control: Tuberculosis elimination revisited: obstacles, opportunities and a renewed commitment—Advisory Council for the Elimination of Tuberculosis (ACET), *Mor Mortal Wkly Rep* 48(RR-09):1-13, 1999n.

Centers for Disease Control: Progress toward the elimination of tuberculosis: United States, 1998, *Mor Mortal Wkly Rep* 48(33):732-736, 1999o.

Centers for Disease Control: *Some facts about Chlamydia* (fact sheet), 1999p, The Author, www.cdc.gov.

Centers for Disease Control: *Neisseria gonorrhoeae gonorrhea (fact sheet),* 1999q, The Author, www.cdc.gov.

Centers for Disease Control and Prevention: *Health information for international travel (yellow book),* Atlanta, 1999-2000, USDHHS.

Centers for Disease Control: Recommended childhood immunization schedule: United States, 2000, *Mor Mortal Wkly Rep* 49(02):35-38, 47, 2000a.

Centers for Disease Control: *Epidemiology and prevention of vaccine-preventable diseases (pink book),* ed 6, Atlanta, 2000b, Public Health Foundation.

Centers for Disease Control: *Vaccine information statements: state health departments,* 2000c, The Author, www.cdc.gov/nip/publications/VIS.

Centers for Disease Control: Prevention and control of meningococcal disease, recommendations of the Advisory Committee on Immunization Practices (ACIP), *Mor Mortal Wkly Rep* 49(RR-07):1-10, 2000d.

Centers for Disease Control: Meningococcal disease and college students, recommendations of the Advisory Committee on Immunization Practices (ACIP), *Mor Mortal Wkly Rep* 49(RR-07):11-20, 2000e.

Centers for Disease Control: Preventing Pneumococcal disease among infants and young children, recommendations of the Advisory Committee on Immunization Practices (ACIP), *Mor Mortal Wkly Rep* 49(RR-90):1-38, 2000f.

Centers for Disease Control: Prevention and control of influenza, recommendations of the Advisory Committee on Immunization Practices (ACIP), *Mor Mortal Wkly Rep* 49(RR-03):1-38, 2000g.

Centers for Disease Control: Poliomyelitis prevention in the United States, updated recommendations of the Advisory Committee on Immunization Practices (ACIP), *Mor Mortal Wkly Rep* 49(RR-5):1-21, 2000h.

Centers for Disease Control: Use of diphtheria toxiod-tetanus toxoid-acellular pertussis vaccine as a five-dose series, supplemental recommendations of the Advisory Committee on Immunization Practices (ACIP), *Mor Mortal Wkly Rep* 49(RR-13):1-8, 2000i.

Centers for Disease Control, Division of Vector-Borne Infectious Diseases: *Plague: introduction,* 2000j, The Author, www.cdc.gov/ncidod/dvbid/plaindex.htm.

Centers for Disease Control, Division of Bacterial and Mycotic Diseases: *Disease information: Typhoid Fever,* 2000k, The Author, www.cdc.gov/ncidod/dbmd/diseaeinfo/typhoidfever.htm.

Chin J, editor: *Control of communicable diseases manual,* ed 17, Washington, DC, 2000, APHA.

Gordis L: *Epidemiology,* Philadelphia, 1996, WB Saunders.

Hollinger FB et al: Controlling hepatitis B virus transmission in North America, *Vaccine* 8(suppl):S122-128, 1990.

Holtgrave D et al: An overview of the effectiveness and efficiency of HIP prevention programs, *Public Health Rep* 110:134-146, 1995.

McFarlin BL et al: Epidemic syphilis: maternal factors associated with congenital infection, *Am J Obstet Gynecol* 170:535-540, 1994.

Padian N, Shiboski S, Jewell N: The effect of the number of exposures on the risk of heterosexual HIV transmission, *J Infect Dis* 161:883-887, 1990.

Pickering LK, editor: *2000 red book: report of the committee on infectious disease,* ed 25, Elk Grove Village, Ill, 2000, American Academy of Pediatrics.

Smoak BL, Novakski WL, Mason CJ: Evidence for a recent decrease in measles susceptibility among young American adults, *J Infect Dis* 170:216-219, 1994.

State of California: *Immunization update,* Berkeley, Calif, February, 10, 2000, Immunization Branch, Department of Health Services.

Swanson J, Dibble S, Chenitz WC: A description of the clinical features and psychosocial factors in young adults with genital herpes, *Dermatol Nurs* 5:365-373, 376-377, 1995.

Thompson RF: *Travel and routine immunizations, 1996,* Milwaukee, 1996, Shoreline Medical Marketing.

United Nations Children's Fund: *The state of the world's children, 1994,* New York, 1994, Oxford University Press.

US Department of Health and Human Services: *Healthy people 2010: conference edition,* Washington, DC, 2000, PHS.

World Health Organization: *Fact sheet N 107, cholera,* 2000, The Author, www.who.int/inf-fs/en/fact107.

School Health

Cathi A. Pourciau and Elaine C. Vallette

OBJECTIVES

Upon completion of this chapter, the reader will be able to do the following:

1. Discuss how *Healthy People 2010* can be used to shape the care given in a school health setting.
2. Identify and discuss the eight components of a comprehensive school health program.
3. Recognize the major stressors that can negatively affect an adolescent's mental health.
4. Identify common health concerns of school-aged children and associated health interventions.
5. Explore the various roles of the nurse in the school setting.
6. Be familiar with the standards under which school nurses practice.
7. Cite several resources available to the school nurse.

KEY TERMS

Early and Periodic Screening, Diagnosis, and Treatment (EPSDT)
Public Law 99-142
school-based health center
school health
school nurse
Youth Risk Behavior Survey (YRBS)

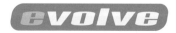

http://evolve.elsevier.com/Nies/

Schools could do more than perhaps any other single institution in society to help young people, and the adults they will become, to live healthier, longer, more satisfying, and more productive lives

(Carnegie Council Adolescent Development, CDC, p. 1, 1999).

School-aged children and adolescents face increasingly numerous challenges and problems related to health. Many of these health challenges are different from those experienced in the past and include behaviors and risks that are linked to the majority of today's leading causes of death such as cancer, injuries, and heart disease. The use of tobacco, alcohol, and drugs; poor nutritional habits; inadequate physical activity; irresponsible sexual behaviors; violence; suicide; and reckless driving are examples of behaviors that often begin during youth and increase the risk for serious health problems.

In the United States, approximately 50 million children attend school every day. This creates a unique opportunity for the **school nurse** to make a positive impact on the nation's youth. The primary providers of health services in schools are school nurses and there are between 40,000 and 56,000 nurses working in schools in the United States (Hootman, 1998; Igoe, 1998). Although the National Association of School Nurses (NASN) recommends one school nurse for every 750 students in the general population, the school nurse has an average caseload of 3098 children for whom he or she is responsible (American School Health Association, 1995).

On a daily basis, school nurses may see as many as 25 to 40 students with a variety of complaints. Increasing numbers of children are being seen in the school setting because they lack a source of regular medical care. According to the AMA, nearly 12 million children under 18 do not have health insurance (Hootman, 1998). Through efforts including education, counseling, advocacy, and direct care provision across all levels of prevention, the nurse can help dramatically improve both the immediate and long-term health of this population.

According to Allensworth and colleagues (1997), "a significant segment of our nation's youth is at risk for dropping out of school as a consequence of a broad range of health and behavioral problems; further, many children do not have access to basic preventive and primary care" (p. 1). For example, approximately 20% of the nation's children are living in poverty. These children are less likely to have

> **YOUTH AT RISK**
>
> - Every day, nearly 3000 young people start smoking.
> - Daily participation in high school physical education classes dropped from 42% in 1991 to 27% in 1997.
> - Almost 75% of young people do not eat the recommended number of servings of fruits and vegetables.
> - Every year, almost one million adolescents become pregnant and about three million become infected with an STD (CDC, 1999a).

access to health care than students in higher socioeconomic groups, resulting in higher health care costs, longer periods of illness, and more days missed from school. Furthermore, absenteeism is correlated with failure in school. Studies have shown that students who miss more than 11% of school days in any one term have trouble keeping up and are at risk for academic failure. The school nurse can effectively manage many complaints and illnesses, allowing these children to return to class.

There is a need for schools to provide various mental and physical health services to students of all ages in an effort to improve both their academic performance and their sense of well-being. This chapter provides an overview of **school health** and the role of the nurse in the provision of health services and health education. An in-depth look at the components of a successful school health program, related to the major problems of today's youth, is included.

HISTORY OF SCHOOL HEALTH

Before 1840, uniform education of children in the United States did not exist or was uncoordinated and sparse. In 1840, Rhode Island passed legislation that made education mandatory and other states soon followed. In 1850, a teacher and school committee member, Lemuel Shattuck, spearheaded the legendary report that has become a public health classic. This report, known as the Shattuck Report, has had a profound impact on school health because he proposed that health education was a vital component in the prevention of disease.

Public health officials and others soon realized that the schools played an important part in the prevention of communicable disease. When smallpox broke out in New York City in the 1860s, health officials were faced with trying to implement a widespread prevention program. They chose to target the schools and began vaccinating children. In 1870, this led to the requirement that all children be vaccinated against smallpox before entering school (Allensworth et al., 1997).

At that time, schools were poorly ventilated and lacked fresh air, effectively spreading diseases among the children. Late in the nineteenth century, a practice of inspecting schools began to identify children who were ill and exclude them until it was deemed they were no longer infectious. Soon thereafter, compulsory vision examinations became a requirement to identify children who might have difficulty in school. In 1902, New York City hired the first nurses to help inspect children, educate families, and ensure follow-up treatment. Within a few years, the renowned nurse Lillian Wald was able to show that the presence of school nurses could reduce absenteeism by 50%. By 1911, slightly over 100 cities were using school nurses; in 1913, New York City employed 176 school nurses (Allensworth et al., 1997).

As they became more comfortable in their positions, early school nurses began to take on a more active role in the assessment of children, treatment of minor conditions, and referral for more serious problems. In addition to identification, treatment, and exclusion for communicable diseases and screening for problems that might affect learning, other issues quickly became part of nursing school practice. In the early part of the century, the temperance movement led schools to teach about the effects of alcohol and tobacco. Also, early in the twentieth century "gymnastics" was introduced in schools in an effort to promote physical activity.

World War I was a pivotal point for school health services and the call for a national effort to improve the health of schoolchildren emerged. In 1918, the National Education Association (NEA) joined forces with the AMA to form the Joint Committee on Health Problems and publish the report *Minimum Health Requirements for Rural Schools*. This group also called for the coordination of health education programs, medical supervision, and physical education that some authorities contend is still lacking. By 1921, nearly every state had laws that required physical and health education in schools. Additionally, fire drills became part of safety education programs introduced during and after World War I (Allensworth et al., 1997).

Although emphasis was placed on health services in schools, barriers existed. Many schools and cities were unwilling to take on the task of providing primary health care for all children. The idea that schools should simply identify problems and refer problems to physicians in private practice was a common theme that the AMA backed. This argument persisted. By the 1920s, medical services and preventive health services were clearly separated in the public health arena and in the schools. Not surprisingly, school health became known as school health education. The federal government did not get involved with school health until the passage of the National School Lunch Program in 1946. The School Breakfast Program was implemented 30 years later (Allensworth et al., 1997).

There was not an impetus to change the direction of school health programs until the 1960s and 1970s. During these decades, there was increasing publicity surrounding children living in poverty and the move to mainstream children with disabilities. These two issues, with an increase in the numbers of children of immigrants, contributed to changes in school health programs.

During the 1960s, the first NP training programs opened and made the inclusion of primary care services in schools possible. In 1976, the first National School Conference, supported by the Robert Wood Johnson Foundation, was held in Galveston, Texas. Following this conference, a variety of school health service models began to emerge with new partnerships and ideas created to provide the most comprehensive health care services for school-aged children. In addition, the Education for the Handicapped Act in 1975 mandated that all children, regardless of disabilities, have access to educational services. This is described in more detail later in the chapter.

The 1980s and 1990s saw several measures aimed at improving the health of schoolchildren. The Drug Free Schools and Community Act was implemented in 1986 to fight substance abuse through education and was expanded in 1994 to include violence prevention measures. With the CDC, the Division of Adolescent and School Health began funding state education agencies to develop and implement programs aimed at alcohol and tobacco use, physical education, and the reduction of STDs and HIV infection among the nation's youth. Also, the federal government encouraged states to use part of their maternal and child block grant monies to fund school-based health centers.

At the present time, school health services vary widely among states and school districts. Furthermore, there continues to be a lack of coordination among providers and no single agency is responsible for tracking services. Recognizing disparities among schools in the United States and the important health

information that must be delivered to children and adolescents, the USDHHS addressed issues in school health repeatedly in *Healthy People 2010*. Objectives targeting children and adolescents are written for diverse areas, including physical activity, sex education and HIV prevention, nutrition, smoking prevention, school absences related to asthma, and many others. Table 26-1 lists only a few of the objectives of *Healthy People 2010* related to school health.

TABLE 26-1

School Health and Selected *Healthy People 2010* Objectives

Objective	Baseline (1998)	Target
6-9: Increase the proportion of children and youth with disabilities who spend at least 80% of their time in regular education programs	45%	60%
7-1: Increase high school completion	85%	90%
7-2e: Increase the proportion of schools that prevent health problems in tobacco use and addiction	86%	95%
7-4a: Increase the proportion of the nation's elementary, middle, junior high, and senior high schools that have a nurse-to-student ratio of at least 1:750	28%	50%
14-23g: Maintain measles vaccination coverage levels for children in kindergarten through the first grade	96%	95%
15-17: Reduce nonfatal injuries caused by motor vehicle crashes for people aged 16 to 20 years	3116 per 100,000	1000 per 100,000
15-24: Increase the number of states and the District of Columbia (DC) with laws requiring bicycle helmets for bicycle riders	11 states	All states and DC
15-39: Reduce weapon carrying by adolescents on school property	8.5%	6.0%
19-15: Increase the proportion of children and adolescents aged 6 to 19 years whose intake of meals and snacks at schools contributes proportionally to good overall dietary quality	NA	NA
21-13: Increase the proportion of school-based health centers with an oral health component	NA	NA
22-8a: Increase the proportion of the nation's public and private middle and junior high schools that require daily physical education for all students	17%	25%
24-5: Reduce the number of school days missed by people with asthma due to asthma	NA	NA
26-9c: Increase the proportion of high school seniors never using alcoholic beverages	19%	29%
26-10b: Reduce the proportion of adolescents reporting use of marijuana during the past 30 days	9.4%	0.7%
27-4a: Increase the average age of first use of tobacco products among adolescents age 12 to 17 years	12 yr	14 yr

From US Department of Health and Human Services: *Healthy people 2010: conference edition,* Washington, DC, 2000, PHS.

SCHOOL HEALTH SERVICES

The School Health Policies and Programs Study (SHPPS) describes school health services as a "coordinated system that ensures a continuum of care from school to home to community health care provider and back" (Allensworth et al., 1997, p. 153). School health services goals and objectives vary from state to state, community to community, and school to school. These differences are from the wide variations in student needs, community resources, funding sources, and school leadership preferences. Many organizations such as the American School Health Association (ASHA) and NASN, are involved in the care and welfare of school-aged children and have compiled and adopted definitions, standards, and statistics related to school health.

According to SHPPS, 86% of elementary, middle, and senior high schools provide some type of health services that might include vision, hearing, and scoliosis screening, provision of first aid, and medication administration. Nearly all schools maintain a health record on every student and, at a minimum, monitor immunization status. Most authorities agree that comprehensive school health programs should include the following eight components (Fig. 26-1): health education; physical education; health services; nutrition services; counseling, psychological, and social services; healthy school environment; health promotion for staff; and family and community involvement.

Health Education

An objective from *Healthy People 2010* has set a goal that at least 30% of students in middle and junior high school will take at least one health education course. The CDC (1999a) has identified six behavioral categories or topics that should be the primary focus

FIGURE **26-1**

The eight components of school health programs.

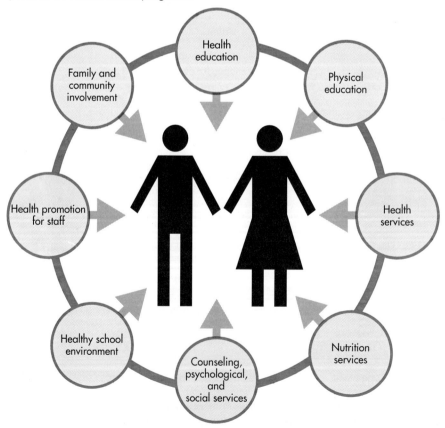

of health education geared to adolescents. The following are negative behaviors that often start in childhood or adolescence and persist into adulthood:

1. Behaviors that result in intentional and unintentional injuries
2. Tobacco use
3. Substance abuse, including alcohol and other drugs
4. Sexual behaviors that result in STDs or unwanted pregnancies
5. Poor nutritional habits
6. Lack of adequate physical activity

In a comprehensive health education program, students should also be given the opportunity to practice decision-making skills, communication, and peer-resistance skills. To learn more about high-risk behaviors among youth, the CDC has conducted the SHPPS using their **Youth Risk Behavior Survey** (YRBS) (CDC, 1998). Reports from this study provide valuable information that can help improve health education programs in schools.

Injury Prevention

Injury prevention should be taught very early in schools and the information should be age appropriate. For example, bicycle safety and the importance of helmets must be stressed beginning in elementary schools. Safety on the school yard and playground is also important for this age group because between two million and five million children per year are injured on school property; this figure represents 10% to 25% of the 22 million children injured in the United States each year. Motor vehicle safety should be included in programs for adolescents who are beginning to drive and for high school students (ASHA National Injury and Violence Prevention Task Force, 1999).

Sports safety is particularly important among adolescents because an estimated 3.5 million boys and two million girls participate in interscholastic sports. A recent survey showed that 3% of elementary, 7% of intermediate, and 11% of high school children are injured each year. Males sustain 67% of the injuries, with 40% occurring in nonorganized sports, 38% in physical education classes, and 50% in organized school sports. The highest injury rates are in football, followed by basketball, gymnastics, baseball, and roller skating. Injuries include orthopedic injuries (e.g., strains, sprains, fractures, and dislocations), dental injuries, neurological problems (e.g., head

injury), ophthalmic injuries, cuts, abrasions, and bruises (Sklaire, 1997).

Use of proper equipment should be mandatory for older children and adolescents. Fitted mouth guards, shin guards, pads, helmets, and other protective gear should be required as appropriate to prevent injury. Hydration should be maintained to prevent heat-related illnesses, especially during hot weather. Effective warm-up and cool-down exercises should be encouraged to prevent muscle strains. Schools that participate in aquatic sports must include pool safety.

The sports physical is a good time for the school nurse to talk with and counsel the student about the risk of developing health problems related to physical activity. This is a perfect setting for the nurse to ask girls questions about menstrual irregularities and to ask all students about their eating behaviors, feelings about their weight, and history of musculoskeletal injuries. It is also a good time for the nurse to stress the importance of stretching exercises to help prevent injuries. Additionally, this is an opportunity for the nurse to work with the coaching staff to promote positive health outcomes.

In many school districts, school safety committees exist and make recommendations for increasing safety related to sports and to ensure follow-up. These committees may also collect data related to injuries, develop policies related to routine safety inspections, and plan staff training and student education related to school environmental factors. Such committees should include school nurses.

Tobacco Use

For the past several decades, major concerns have been raised about long-term health problems associated with adolescents' use of tobacco, alcohol, and illegal substances. Additionally, concern arises because alcohol and cigarettes are "gateway" drugs and their use often leads to chronic abuse of illicit drugs. It has been shown that adolescents who begin to use drugs such as alcohol become high-risk candidates for other substances such as tobacco or marijuana. There is an increased likelihood that these youthful abusers will ultimately engage in other high-risk behaviors that may involve multiple concurrent high-risk behaviors. For example, according to the CDC (1999b), teens who smoke are three times more likely than nonsmokers to use alcohol, eight times more likely to use marijuana, and 22 times more likely to use cocaine.

Smoking is a major problem in this country and is the single leading preventable cause of death in the

United States. Prevention efforts should be emphasized in young people. An estimated 80% of adults who use tobacco began before age 18 (CDC, 1999b). Prevalence of smoking increases as the student progresses through the grade levels. White students have the highest rate of smoking at 40%, followed by Hispanics at 34%, and African-Americans at 23% (Kann et al., 1998).

A Surgeon General's report on tobacco (CDC, 1999b) reported the following information about adolescents and cigarette smoking: adolescents believe that cigarette smoking is a normal process, adolescents perceive peer and sibling acceptance of their smoking, and adolescents believe that the use of smoking provides benefits. Furthermore, although 77% of young people thought that cigarette smoking was harmful, only 40% thought smokeless tobacco was harmful. According to this same report, youths that use smokeless tobacco are more likely to start using cigarettes.

Limiting adolescents' exposure to tobacco advertising and teaching them the negative consequences associated with tobacco are essential in preventing its use. The CDC (1999c) reports that well-planned and sequential health education programs can be highly effective. Indeed, one report cited a 37% reduction in the number of seventh-grade students who begin smoking following implementation of a comprehensive program. When students were able to enroll in a health education course, 44% fewer students used tobacco, alcohol, and marijuana one or more times than those not enrolled in such a course.

Major risk factors for the development of oral cancer include the use of tobacco in all forms, and, to a lesser degree, alcohol. Therefore all adolescents should be queried as to their use of both tobacco and alcohol. Education and counseling should be offered to students who smoke or use chewing tobacco.

Substance Abuse

The Forum on Child and Family Statistics (1999) reports that the most frequently used psychoactive substance during adolescence is alcohol. The use of alcohol can be associated with problems in school, violence, motor vehicle deaths, and other injuries. In 1998, 32% of twelfth graders, 24% of tenth graders, and 14% of eighth graders reported heavy drinking. Males are more likely to drink than females. Additionally, alcohol use is more prevalent among Hispanic twelfth graders at 28% and white twelfth graders at 36% than African-Americans at 12%. The use of illicit drugs was reported by 26% of twelfth graders, 22% of tenth graders, and 12% of eighth graders. Males are more likely to use illicit drugs than females. Twenty-eight percent of white twelfth graders reported use of illicit drugs, compared with 19% of African-American and 24% of Hispanic twelfth graders.

Sex Education

A number of objectives of *Healthy People 2010* address issues of human sexuality, pregnancy prevention, and STD and HIV prevention. These issues are important when working with older children and adolescents in the area of school health.

TEEN PREGNANCY

- The United States has the highest teen pregnancy rate among developed countries.
- Approximately one million teenagers become pregnant each year; 95% of those pregnancies are unintended and almost one third end in abortion.
- Public costs from teen childbearing totaled $120 billion from 1985 to 1990; $48 billion could have been saved if each birth had been postponed until the mother was at least 20 years old.
- Birth rates during 1991 to 1996 declined for teenagers in all racial and ethnic groups.
- Birth rates among teenagers vary substantially from state to state; some states have rates almost three times higher than those in the lowest states (CDC, 1999a).

Teens are becoming sexually active at earlier ages and despite recent declines, pregnancy rates continue to be high. YRBS data reveal that 48.4% of adolescents in grades 9 through 12 have had sexual intercourse (CDC, 1998). In addition, the fastest-growing group becoming infected with HIV are adolescents and HIV infection and AIDS are now the sixth leading cause of death among people aged 15 to 24 (CDC, 1999d). Therefore it is imperative that older children and adolescents have age-appropriate information on issues related to sexuality, including prevention of pregnancy and STDs, and they need this information *before* becoming sexually active.

According to the CDC, 688,200 cases of AIDS had been reported through the end of 1998. Of these, 8461 were reported in children under age 13. During this same time, there were 410,800 deaths of people with AIDS, and, of these, 4984 occurred in children under age 15. It is important to note that HIV reporting is not mandatory and consequently these figures may underestimate the devastation of this illness on school-aged children (CDC, 1999d).

School-based education related to sexuality has been a controversial topic in the past, and a consensus has not yet been reached. Opponents of sex education in the schools believe that parents have the responsibility for teaching this content to their own children. In addition, laws in certain states prohibit or dramatically limit sex education in public schools. Proponents argue that for many children, sex education will not be addressed in the home; if this information is not taught in schools, children will receive inadequate or incorrect information from peers, the media, or other sources. School nurses have been caught in the center of this controversy, but historically have advocated for education on normal human sexuality, encouraging discussion in an objective, nonjudgmental manner in which students are free to ask questions and receive correct answers.

Dental Health

One of the most frequent complaints of school-aged children is dental caries. There are numerous contributing factors to this, including poor oral hygiene, lack of fluoridated water in some areas, and lack of funds or insurance for dental care. By age nine, most children will have at least one cavity and by age 15, this proportion will be above 60% (USDHHS, 2000).

Proper brushing of the teeth should be taught, along with good nutritional habits and the importance of regular dental checkups. Children should also be taught the relationship between high-sugar foods and dental caries. All children should be encouraged to see a dentist periodically. For some children, this is a problem because a limited number of dentists treat the indigent. As a result, many school nurses maintain a list of dentists who accept Medicaid and develop other options for children who cannot afford dental care.

Physical Education

One of the major objectives of *Healthy People 2010* is to improve the health and fitness of Americans through regular daily physical activity. It is well documented that children today are less active than children in the past. Daily enrollment among high school students in physical education classes has dropped from 42% in 1991 to 25% in 1995 (CDC, 1999a). With the advent of computers and television and the decreasing requirement of physical education in schools, children are becoming less and less active. According to the CDC (1999a), nearly half of 12- to 21-year-olds are not vigorously active on a regular basis and approximately 14% report no recent physical activity. Females, at 14%, are more commonly inactive than males, at 7%. African-American females, at 21%, are more inactive than white females, at 12%.

A sedentary lifestyle has long been associated with obesity, hypertension, heart disease, and diabetes. Studies have shown that people who are active outlive those who are inactive and those who are active have a better quality of life. Habits in childhood are more likely to be continued into adulthood, making it important that children are taught the importance of being physically active at a young age. Studies have also shown that children and adolescents who are physically active tend to have greater self-confidence and self-esteem. Additionally, studies have shown that students who participate in sports programs are 40% less likely to be regular smokers and 50% less likely to be heavy smokers (CDC, 1999c).

Physical activity education should focus on activities that children can perform into their adult years such as walking, swimming, biking, riding, and jogging. The content of the educational process may need to change as the child ages. For example, what may appeal to a young child, such as playing on the playground with friends, is different from that which motivates an adolescent, such as competitive spirit or weight control. The CDC has put together 10 recommendations for the promotion of lifelong physical activity (Box 26-1).

Health Services

Health services provided in schools include preventive services such as immunizations and screenings for vision, hearing, and scoliosis. This component of a comprehensive school health program also includes emergency care, management of acute and chronic health conditions, appropriate referrals, health counseling, education about healthy lifestyles, and medication administration. Care of children with special health needs (e.g., tube feedings, catheterizations, or tracheotomy care) is also included.

BOX **26-1**

Guidelines for School and Community Programs: Promoting Lifelong Physical Activity

1. Establish policies that promote enjoyable, life-long physical activity.
2. Provide physical and social environments that encourage and enable young people to engage in safe and enjoyable physical activity.
3. Implement sequential physical activity education curricula and instruction in grades K to 12.
4. Implement health education curricula.
5. Provide extracurricular physical activity programs that offer diverse, developmentally appropriate activities—both noncompetitive and competitive—for all students.
6. Encourage parents and guardians to support their children's participation in physical activity, to be physically active role models, and to include physical activity in family events.
7. Provide training to enable teachers, coaches, recreation and health care staff, and other school and community personnel to promote enjoyable, lifelong physical activity to young people.
8. Assess the physical activity patterns of young people, refer them to appropriate physical activity programs, and advocate for physical activity instruction and programs for young people.
9. Provide a range of developmentally appropriate community sports and recreation programs that are attractive to all young people.
10. Regularly evaluate physical activity instruction, programs, and facilities.

From Centers for Disease Control: *CDC's guidelines for school and community programs: promoting life-long physical activity,* 1997a, The Author, www.cdc.gov/nccdphp/dash/phactaag.htm.

Frequently, school nurses must delegate health care tasks to an assigned individual. For example, parent volunteers or school office personnel are often trained to administer medications to children in the absence of a school nurse. The school district or each state usually determines responsibilities regarding delegation and parameters for training and monitoring a designated person or people. The school nurse must be aware of the rules and requirements in his or her area and adhere to them.

Immunizations

Immunizations are a vital component of routine health care. They provide long-lasting protection against many diseases that were once deadly. Vaccine-preventable illnesses are at their lowest level ever in the United States, yet U.S. childhood immunization rates are still suboptimal. Minority and low-income children are at the greatest risk for underimmunization (CDC, 1999e).

All states now require proof of current immunization status or evidence of immunity before school entrance. Certain exceptions may apply based on religious, moral, or medical contraindications. The school nurse plays an important role in verifying compliance with immunization requirements and in educating children and parents about the benefits of immunization. School nurses also play a vital role in coordinating school immunization programs and they have an opportunity to teach families about both infant and adult immunizations.

Seventy-five percent of all hepatitis B cases occur in people between ages 15 and 39, yet this group represents a largely unvaccinated cohort. The CDC recommends that all children not previously vaccinated with Hep B should be vaccinated at 11 to 12 years of age (CDC, 1999e). The CDC also recommends that all older adolescents not vaccinated against hepatitis B should receive the vaccines whenever possible. See Chapter 25 for current immunization schedules.

Health Screenings

Unfortunately, many children in the United States are not appropriately screened for treatable conditions that may then go undetected for many years. As noted, early in the twentieth century it was observed that schools are an excellent setting for routine screenings. Impaired vision and hearing can result in poor academic performance and slowed development. Identifying and treating these problems early is highly effective and less costly in the long run. Height, weight, vision, and hearing screenings are provided at most schools according to a schedule (e.g., hearing screening for kindergarten, second-, fourth-, and sixth-grade students) set by the individual state or school district. The AAP recommends objective hearing testing at ages 3, 4, 5, 10, 12, 15, and 18 (US Preventive Services Task Force, 1996). Adolescents exposed to loud noises or those with recurrent ear infections may need yearly screening.

Vision screening is required in most states with appropriate referrals as needed. The standard Snellen vision chart is the usual screening tool. Screening for strabismus is also a nursing responsibility and it must be identified and treated early in an effort to prevent amblyopia. If left untreated, it may result in the loss of vision. Referral to an eye specialist is a critical component of all abnormal eye examinations. Delay related to referral and follow-up may result in adverse academic performance and decreased self-esteem.

Medicaid-eligible children are guaranteed access to comprehensive health care services such as those described and routine dental examinations. The school nurse may not only perform the screenings, but can also provide information, recommend referrals, and provide follow-up care for children as appropriate. The nurse also acts as a resource relative to acquiring services and serves as a liaison for the family.

Scoliosis or postural screening should be done in schools to identify and intervene early in an effort to prevent secondary problems related to spinal deviations. If undetected, spinal problems may lead to deformities that are either cosmetic or functional in nature or both. Scoliosis screening in the school setting consists primarily of a visual inspection of the back. The Scoliosis Research Society (US Preventive Services Task Force, 1996) recommends annual screening of all children 10 to 14 years of age; the American Academy of Orthopedic Surgeons recommends screening of all girls at ages 11 and 13 and boys at ages 13 and 14.

The detection of high blood pressure during childhood is of great value in identifying children who are at risk for hypertension as adults and who may benefit from early intervention and follow-up. Vascular and end-organ damage related to hypertension can begin in childhood (US Preventive Services Task Force, 1996). Periodic blood pressure measurements are inexpensive and should be performed routinely for all children.

Medicaid created the **Early and Periodic Screening, Diagnostic and Treatment** (EPSDT) service because there are great numbers of uninsured children in the United States. EPSDT is a comprehensive child health program for uninsured people under age 21. It includes health education, periodic screen-

ing, vision, dental, and hearing services. Services provided under the EPSDT program are often performed through the public health offices in each state, but they may also occur in community health clinics and in schools. Screening services must include a comprehensive health and developmental history and an unclothed complete physical examination and immunizations and laboratory testing that is age appropriate (HCFA, USDHHS, 2000).

Emergency Care

School playgrounds are a frequent site for student injuries that range from minor scrapes and bruises, to more serious injuries such as broken bones and seizures, to severe and life-threatening injuries such as head injuries and severe asthma attacks. Injuries may also occur in school buildings, classrooms, physical education classes, and athletic programs. Basic first aid equipment should be available in all schools. The school nurse must be highly knowledgeable about standard first aid and certified in CPR and should be prepared to provide first aid and emergency care when indicated. Additionally, a procedure for activating the EMS should be in place.

Care of the Ill Child

The school nurse is responsible for monitoring the health of all students. For students with acute or chronic illnesses, administration of medications or treatments may be necessary. The nurse is often required to assess an ill child to determine the type of illness or health problem, identify the source of the illness, and determine how to manage the illness (i.e., contact the parent or send the child back to class). For example, if a child complains of scalp itching, the nurse may identify lice. At that point, the nurse would follow protocols regarding screening classmates, siblings, and others who may have had contact with the child. The parent would be called and the child would be removed from class until treated. Table 26-2 shows the most common health problems seen by school nurses across the country.

Asthma affects 5% of schoolchildren in grades 1 through 12. According to Calabrese and colleagues (1999), asthma is the most common chronic childhood condition and accounts for some 20 million lost school days every year. Asthma is prevalent; therefore it is recommended that school-based support exist for asthmatic children. An assessment tool (Box 26-2) has been developed to determine how well schools assist children with asthma. Answers to all the questions in

TABLE 26-2

Health Problems Reported by School Nurses: Percent of All Problems by Grade Level

Problem	Elementary School	Middle School	High School
Accidents and injury prevention	6.4	3.1	0.8
Chronic health problems	11.2	5.2	2.9
Communicable disease	5.6	1.9	1.0
Dental problems	1.2	0.6	0.0
Drug and substance abuse	0.6	2.7	6.8
Environmental concerns	0.6	0.0	0.0
High-risk social behaviors	18.9	33.8	45.6
Inadequate immunizations	1.9	0.6	0.2
Infectious disease	3.3	0.8	1.0
Lack of access to health care	9.5	4.1	2.9
Mental illness and emotional problems	4.8	6.4	5.0
Poor school attendance	2.3	2.3	2.9
Poverty	5.8	2.1	2.1
Self-esteem problems	8.7	19.9	7.7
Special health needs	9.1	2.9	1.9
Suicide	0.6	1.0	0.2
Teen pregnancy	0.0	1.7	6.6
Unhealthy lifestyle habits	6.4	8.1	8.5
Violence	0.0	1.2	2.3
Vision problems	0.6	0.2	0.4

From Fryer G, Igoe J: Functions of school nurses and health assistants in US school health programs, *J Sch Health* 66:55, 1996.

the assessment tool should be "yes." "No" answers indicate that students may not be in an environment conducive to asthma control.

Diabetes is second only to asthma in prevalence in the school-aged child. It affects approximately 1.7 people per 1000 less than 20 years old. Approximately 13,000 new cases are diagnosed in children annually and the vast majority of these children attend school or day care (American Diabetes Association, 2000). In general, teachers are inadequately prepared to care

for children with diabetes and must rely on the nurse. According to the American Diabetes Association, children should be able to participate in their care to the extent that they are able. The association has specific recommendations based on age (Box 26-3).

Medication Administration

Administration of medications is a service provided almost universally by school districts across the country. The use of medications by school-aged

BOX 26-2

Asthma Assessment Tool

1. Is the school free of tobacco smoke all of the time, including during school-sponsored events?
2. Does the school maintain good indoor air quality? Does it reduce or eliminate allergens and irritants that can make asthma worse?
3. Is a school nurse in the school all day, every day?
4. Can children take medicines at school as recommended by their doctor and parents? Are children allowed to carry their own asthma medicines?
5. Does the school have an emergency plan for taking care of a child with a severe asthma attack? Does it clearly explain what to do? Who to call? When to call?
6. Does someone teach school staff about asthma, asthma management plans, and asthma medicines? Does someone teach all students about asthma and how to help a classmate who has it?
7. Do students have good options for fully and safely participating in physical education class and recess? Do students have access to their medicine before exercise? Can they choose modified or alternative activities when medically necessary?

From National Heart, Lung, and Blood Institute, National Asthma Education and Prevention Program, School Asthma Education Subcommittee: How asthma friendly is your school? *J Sch Health* 68(4): 167, 1998.

BOX 26-3

Expectations of the Child with Diabetes

Elementary school:
- The child should be able to assist in all diabetes tasks at school.
- By age eight, the child is usually able to perform his or her own finger-stick glucose monitoring.

Middle school and junior high school:
- The child should be able to perform self-monitoring of blood glucose.
- By age 13, most children should be able to administer their own insulin with supervision.

High school:
- The child should be able to perform self-monitoring of blood glucose.
- Most adolescents should be able to administer insulin with supervision.
- All children may need assistance with blood glucose testing when the glucose level is low.

From American Diabetes Association: *Position statement: care of children with diabetes in the school and day care setting,* 2000, The Author, www.diabetes.org/diabetescare.

The following guidelines from NASN (1997) indicate that medications should be:

- Properly labeled with all appropriate information and be in properly labeled containers
- Accompanied by a written request from the health care provider and parent or guardian to administer the medication
- Administered without violating standing orders or nursing protocols
- Kept in locked containers

Also, school nurses must monitor the self-administration of medications as ordered by a health care provider and provide education as needed to both children and parents.

Medications commonly given in schools include analgesics and antipyretics (e.g., Tylenol or Advil), antacids, antitussives, anticonvulsants, antiemetics and antidiarrheals, antifungals, antihistamines, and antibiotics. Medications such as Ritalin, Cylert, and Adderall, which are used to treat attention-deficit hyperactivity disorder, are among the most commonly

children has increased greatly over the last several years and it has allowed many children to attend school despite serious health problems.

Medication administration in the schools is a serious undertaking. Issues facing the school nurse include safety, monitoring of both therapeutic and side effects, proper documentation, and ongoing communication with the student and family. The nurse must be sure to comply with all legal regulations and all school policies. Only those medications considered necessary are administered at school.

administered. One study (Francis and Treloar, 1996) found that Ritalin is the most common medication administered in school, accounting for more than 50% of all doses. Bronchodilators were the second most common, accounting for more than 9%, followed by analgesics at 7% and antihypertensives at 4.5%.

ATTENTION-DEFICIT HYPERACTIVITY DISORDER

- Adaptive behavior is usually age appropriate, but is often underused.
- Activities may be immature, including failure to finish projects, loss of interest, or lack of turn taking.
- Behavior may exhibit impulsivity, inattentiveness, overactivity, and poor self-regulation.
- Onset of problem usually occurs by age seven and is often associated with sleep disturbances and difficult temperament (Fox, 1997).

Children with Special Health Needs

In 1976, **Public Law 99-142** was enacted, which gave all students, including those who are severely handicapped, the right to public education in the least restrictive environment possible regardless of mental or physical disabilities. The Education for All Handicapped Children Act of 1973 and the subsequent Individuals with Disabilities Education Act of 1990 enhanced the opportunities for children previously served in acute care and long-term care settings to have access to public education (Duncan and Igoe, 1998).

Children affected by these laws include children who are deaf and hard of hearing; mentally retarded; multihandicapped; orthopedically impaired; "other" health impaired (e.g., chronic or acute health problems such as heart condition or epilepsy); seriously emotionally disturbed; speech impaired; visually handicapped; or have a specific learning disability (e.g., disorder of basic psychological processes in understanding or using language). The National Center for Education Statistics indicated that during 1996 and 1997 there were 5.9 million students, or 13% of public schoolchildren, enrolled in special education programs (NCES, 2000).

The rapid development of medical technology has enabled students to attend public school when their conditions may have prevented them from leaving an institution or controlled environment in the past. These children need nursing services of varied types to continue their progression in the school settings. Public Law 94-142 requires school nurses to screen or identify children in need of special education and related services and complete an Individualized Education Program (IEP), which is developed by an interdisciplinary team and includes educational goals and specific services to be provided. It also requires provision of "designated instruction and services," which outlines services, including nursing care, required to help the child benefit from education. The nurse is responsible for the development of an individualized health plan (IHP) for all students requiring continuous nursing management while at school. Table 26-3 gives an overview of the increase in the number of students with disabilities.

Student Records

Health records should be maintained on all students according to individual school district policy. At a minimum, student health records should include immunization status, pertinent health concerns, results of screenings and examinations, health history, and individualized plans of care. The Family Educational Rights and Privacy Act (FERPA), a strong privacy protection act, protects student education records, including the health record. It grants parents the right to review these records and confirm their accuracy. With this exception, student health records should be afforded the same level of confidentiality as that given to clients and patients in other settings (i.e., sharing confidential information with others, without approval, is considered unethical and improper except in emergency situations) (ASHA, 1997).

Delegation of Tasks

Not every school has a full-time nurse available on site. More likely, a nurse is assigned to three or four schools. Many nursing tasks must be delegated to unlicensed personnel. Each state's Nurse Practice Act stipulates which procedures may be delegated. The responsibility for assessment may never be delegated; common tasks that may be delegated include medication administration, blood glucose monitoring, and gastrostomy feeding. When tasks are delegated, the nurse must provide appropriate education, written procedures, and ongoing supervision and evaluation of the caregivers. The nurse is also responsible for periodic reassessment of the child.

TABLE 26-3

Children from Birth to Age 21 Who Were Served by Federally Supported Programs for Students with Disabilities, as a Percentage of Total Public K to 12 Enrollment; 1976 to 1977 to 1996 to 1997

Type of Disability	1976 to 1977	1990 to 1991	1996 to 1997
All disabilities	8.33	11.55	12.98
Specific learning disabilities	1.80	5.17	5.81
Speech or language impairments	2.94	2.39	2.29
Mental retardation	2.16	1.30	1.27
Serious emotional disturbance	0.64	0.95	0.98
Hearing impairment	0.20	0.14	0.15
Orthopedic impairments	0.20	0.12	0.14
Other health impairments	0.32	0.13	0.35
Visual impairments	0.09	0.06	0.06
Multiple disabilities	—	0.23	0.21
Deafness-blindness	—	<0.005	<0.005
Autism and others	—	—	0.10
Preschool disabled	—	1.07	1.62

From National Center for Education Statistics: *NCES fast facts: students with disabilities,* 2000, The Author, www.nces.ed.gov/fastfacts/display.asp/id=64.

Nutrition

School-aged children are undergoing periods of rapid growth and development and consequently have high nutritional needs. A variety of foods must be ingested to meet their daily bodily requirements. Diets should include a proper balance of carbohydrate, protein, and fat, with sufficient intake of vitamins and minerals. However, children and adolescents share a well-known preference for junk food. Their diet is often high in fat and sugar and frequently consists of fast food items such as hamburgers and French fries instead of fruits and vegetables. Skipping meals, especially at breakfast, and eating multiple unhealthy snacks contribute to poor childhood nutrition. Screening and identifying nutritional problems, counseling, and making appropriate referrals are important in the school setting.

The number of children living in poverty has increased to 20% and poor nutritional status is closely associated with poverty. Federally funded programs such as the School Breakfast Program and School Lunch Program were initiated to ensure that all children have access to these two meals during the school day.

VENDING MACHINE FOOD CHOICES
In 1995, the ASHA addressed the issue of unhealthy foods found in school vending machines and sold in school fund-raising projects. They specifically resolved that all schools should provide only healthy food choices (i.e., food items of appropriate nutrient density) in school vending machines and for sale in fund-raising projects (ASHA, 1995).

Eating Disorders

Statistics have shown that few adolescents feel good about their bodies. Of those surveyed, 75% feel fat and as many as 70% are dieting at any one time. Statistics also indicate that as many as half of third- to sixth-grade girls want to be thinner and as many as one third have previously dieted (Kater, 1999). It has been reported that 8% of girls in high school take laxatives or vomit to lose weight or keep from gaining weight and approximately 9% take diet pills. These kinds of harmful weight loss practices have been reported in girls as young as nine years old (CDC, 1999f).

PERCEPTION OF WEIGHT AMONG ADOLESCENTS

A study found that female students, at 40.2%, are more likely to perceive themselves as overweight than males, at 22.3%, and are more likely to try to lose weight, at 47.1%, than males, at 20.6%. The study also found that males, at 31.2%, were more likely to try to gain weight that females, at 7.4%. Males were more likely to exercise and weight train in an effort to lose weight, whereas females were more likely to diet. Not surprisingly, the study revealed that adolescents as a whole do not do a good job of self-assessment. Almost half failed to accurately classify themselves in terms of weight (Kilpatrick, Ohannessian, and Bartholomew, 1999).

It is imperative that the school nurse recognize the association between feelings of inadequacy (e.g., low self-esteem, anger, anxiety, and depression) and unhealthy eating practices in adolescents and young people. These self-perceptions begin early in life; therefore education and counseling must begin in elementary school. Prevention efforts should concentrate on eliminating misconceptions surrounding nutrition, dieting, and body composition and should stress optimal health and personal performance. Nurses can help students accept their personal body shapes. Unfortunately, outside influences such as commercials and advertisements make this a serious problem; adolescents and young children are bombarded with messages such as "you can never be too thin" and "life will be wonderful if you look and dress like a model."

Nurses must also be aware of eating disorders such as anorexia nervosa and bulimia. Anorexia is a severely restricted intake of food based on an extreme fear of weight gain. Literature has shown that anorexia is multifactorial, is seen primarily in females, and is often correlated with family dysfunction or history of sexual abuse. Bulimia is a form of anorexia characterized by a chaotic eating pattern with recurrent episodes of binge eating followed by purging. Purging may take the form of self-induced vomiting, laxative or diuretic abuse, or excessive exercise.

FEMALE ATHLETE TRIAD

The "female athlete triad" is a medical disorder consisting of eating disorders, amenorrhea, and osteoporosis. Pressure to attain a particular body shape or weight considered desirable in a selected sport may place the female athlete in danger of developing this disorder. It can result in menstrual irregularities, premature osteoporosis, and decreased BMD; if taken to the extreme, it could become life threatening (Beals, Brey, and Gonyou, 1999).

Obesity

Obesity is not considered an eating disorder; therefore many professionals, including nurses, overlook it. Obesity is a serious problem, even in childhood and adolescence; one fifth of adolescents are overweight and this number may be increasing (US Preventive Services Task Force, 1996). Obesity and its prevention or treatment must be of concern to the school nurse. Statistics show that up to 80% of obese children grow up to become obese adults.

Obesity is associated with cardiovascular risk factors and some cancers and other disorders such as osteoarthritis, sleep apnea, and cholelithiasis. In addition, obesity may result in social and quality-of-life impairments related to physical endurance and possible job discrimination (US Preventive Services Task Force, 1996). Obese children are often labeled by their peers and ridiculed. Guidelines to Adolescent Preventative Services (GAPS) and Bright Futures recommends the determination of body mass index (BMI) for all adolescents (US Preventive Services Task Force, 1996). A BMI greater than the eighty-fifth percentile for age and gender may indicate the need for further assessment and referral. To be successful, the treatment of obesity must begin early and be multifaceted.

Nutritional Education Programs

Nutritional education is essential and must include parents and teachers and the child. Children need to know and understand the food pyramid, how to make healthy choices for snacks, and the importance of balancing physical activity with food intake. Obesity, dental caries, anemia, and heart disease can be reduced or prevented with proper education and lifestyle changes. In addition, all adolescents and children over two years of age should receive counseling regarding intake of saturated fat.

CARDIAC RISKS IN ADOLESCENTS

Cardiovascular disease manifests itself in adulthood, but it begins in childhood with such factors as elevated blood pressure, excess weight, and abnormalities in lipoprotein levels. These factors are also associated with atherosclerosis in children and young adults. According to a recent study, atherosclerotic lesions can be detected in the aortas and in more than half of the right coronary arteries of adolescents between 15 and 19 years of age. Furthermore, studies on school-aged children suggest that African-American and Mexican-American children have higher levels of BMI, lipoproteins, insulin, glucose, blood pressure, and physical inactivity than white children (Strong et al., 1999; Winkleby et al., 1999).

Congress enacted the Nutritional Education and Training (NET) Program in 1977. NET focused on teaching children how to make healthy choices relative to nutrition and to convey health promotion and disease prevention topics into school and child care settings. In addition, the American Dietetic Association, the American School Food Service Association, and the Society for Nutrition Education take the position that comprehensive school-based nutrition programs and services should be provided to all elementary and secondary students. The ultimate goal of these efforts is that children will make healthy nutritional choices in and out of the school setting.

DIET AND ACADEMIC PERFORMANCE

- Research suggests that not having breakfast can affect children's intellectual performance.
- Even moderate undernutrition can have lasting effects on children's cognitive development and school performance.
- Participation in the School Breakfast Program can improve students' standardized test scores and reduce their rates of absence and tardiness (CDC, 1999a).

Counseling, Psychological, and Social Services

The mental health of a child or adolescent is affected by physical, economic, social, psychological, and environmental factors. Children, like adults, often hide problems from themselves and from others. They may see problems as a sign of weakness or as a lack of control. Children may also be trying to protect themselves or someone they love and therefore not seek help, which can have tragic results. Promotion of mental health and reduction or removal of threats to mental health are important to children and adolescents. Mental health is often difficult, yet essential, to assess.

Children and teens struggle with issues such as depression, substance abuse, conduct disorders, self-esteem issues, suicide, and eating disorders. They may also have to cope with physical or mental abuse, pregnancy, and STDs. Warning signs of stress in children are presented in Box 26-4. Drugs and alcohol can enter a child's life as early as the elementary school years. Many children live in single-parent households with little social or economic support. They may not have enough to eat or a safe, warm place to sleep, yet they are expected to come to school each day ready to learn. Services aimed at helping children cope with these problems are often lacking or are too costly for many families.

The nurse or teacher may be the only stable adult in the child's life who will listen without being judgmental. Therefore one of the most important roles of the school nurse is to act as counselor and confidante. Children may come to the school nurse with various vague complaints such as recurrent stomachaches, headaches, or sexually promiscuous behavior and the nurse must look beyond the initial complaint to identify underlying problems.

BOX 26-4

Warning Signs of Stress

- Problems eating or sleeping
- Use of alcohol or other substances
- Problems making decisions
- Persistent angry or hostile feelings
- Inability to concentrate
- Increased boredom
- Frequent headaches and ailments

Major depressive disorders often have their onset in adolescence and are associated with an increased risk of suicide. Early detection and treatment may prevent untoward consequences. The second leading cause of death among 15- to 19-year-olds is suicide. Estimates of adolescent suicide vary from 2000 to 5000 suicides each year and as many as 500,000 to 1 million attempts (Fox, 1997). The nurse and other school personnel must be on the alert for suicide clusters, which are often known to follow a successful suicide. Results from the YRBS indicate that as many as 24.1% of students, or almost one in four, have considered attempting suicide (CDC, 1998).

Many schools have implemented suicide prevention programs; however, myths continue to exist. Adolescents often approach school nurses and other school professionals for help before a suicide attempt. Therefore it is important for the school nurse to be cognizant of the warning signs associated with suicide and to recognize and refer at-risk adolescents to appropriate mental health professionals (Box 26-5).

There are numerous tools that the nurse can use to determine if there is an increased risk of depression, suicide, antisocial behavior, or other potential problems. These tools can assist the nurse in identifying a problem before it develops to allow intervention or referral to the appropriate health professional.

The YRBS was developed by the CDC in collaboration with many federal, state, and private partners and provides information about the prevalence of high-risk behaviors that young people undertake. YRBS is a nationwide, voluntary monitoring system conducted by local education and state agencies. It provides information that can be used to create programs that can combat behaviors such as tobacco use, unhealthy dietary habits, use of alcohol and other substances, and inadequate physical activity. This information can help modify sexual behaviors, prevent STD and HIV infection, and prevent

BOX 26-5

Truths About Adolescent Suicides

1. Since 1950, the suicide rate for adolescents has more than tripled.
2. Most adolescents who attempt suicide are ambivalent and torn between wanting to die and wanting to live.
3. Any threat of suicide should be taken seriously.
4. There are usually warning signs preceding a suicide attempt and these may include depression, substance abuse, decreased activity, isolation, and appetite and sleep changes.
5. Suicide is more common in adolescents than homicide.
6. Education concerning suicide does not lead to increased attempts.
7. Females are 1.5 to 2 times more likely to consider or attempt suicide and males are 4 to 5.5 times more likely to complete a suicide attempt.
8. One suicide attempt is eight times more likely to result in a subsequent attempt.
9. Sixty-seven percent of all completed suicides were performed with a gun.
10. Most adolescents who have attempted or completed suicide have not been diagnosed as having a mental disorder.
11. All socioeconomic groups are affected by suicide.

From King KA: Fifteen prevalent myths concerning adolescent suicide, *J Sch Health* 69(4):159-161, 1999.

behaviors that may result in injuries, either intentional or unintentional. Box 26-6 summarizes the purposes of the YRBS survey and Box 26-7 presents some of the major findings from the YRBS conducted in 1995 (CDC, 1997b).

The adolescent years are particularly volatile in terms of the tremendous growth that is occurring both physically and emotionally. These are the years of rapid change and they present many challenges to adolescents and their families. Peer pressure and peer identity is enormous and often leads to high-risk behaviors as adolescents experiment with new behaviors. The nurse needs to understand this developmental stage and involve peer groups in problem solving. Gender roles also become intensified during this time.

BOX 26-6

Purposes of the Youth Risk Behavior Survey

- Determine the prevalence and age of initiation of health-risk behaviors.
- Focus the national and relevant agencies on specific health-risk behaviors of young people.
- Assess whether health-risk behaviors increase, decrease, or remain the same over time.
- Provide comparable national, state, and local data.
- Monitor progress toward achieving the *Healthy People* objectives and the National Education Goals.

From Centers for Disease Control: *Assessing health risk behaviors among young people: youth risk behavior surveillance system,* 1998, The Author, www.cdc.gov/nccdphp/dash/yrbs/yrbsaag98.htm.

Confusion about sexuality may be a problem with some adolescents. The nurse can serve as an important source of correct information, and, in states and school districts where approved, may even be the person responsible for sex education classes.

Unfortunately, a large number of children are abused daily in this country. Physical abuse is usually a result of many interacting factors such as poverty, social isolation, and drug and alcohol abuse. School nurses and other school personnel must take this seriously and are mandated to report cases of child abuse.

The school nurse may help teach the child how to problem-solve, how to cope, and how to build self-esteem. The role of the nurse often extends outside the school campus. The family is an integral part of a child's well-being and the nurse may need to work closely with or visit families to develop an appropriate health plan for a particular child. In some cases, the nurse may be required to report cases to law enforcement agencies and child protection services to protect and care for a child.

Healthy School Environment

A healthy school environment is one in which distractions are minimized and that is free of physical hazards and psychological threats. NASN believes that "all students and staff have a right to learn and work in a healthy school environment. . ." and that the school nurse, as ". . . an advocate for students, staff and community, will be actively involved in the development and maintenance of a plan for a healthy school environment" (NASN, 1998).

Violence has become a major public health problem because it threatens the health and well-being, both physical and psychological, of so many children. According to the U.S. Department of Justice (Forum on Child and Family Statistics, 1999), youths aged 12 to 17 are almost three times more likely than adults to be victims of a violent crime, including aggravated assault, rape, robbery, and homicide. In recent years, there have been a number of school shootings and other acts of violence in schools. One report stated that there have been 252 gun-related deaths in U.S. schools since 1992 (Gyan, 1999).

School nurses and other school personnel should be aware of risk factors and signs that could indicate a tendency toward violence. Some factors that seem to be common among those who commit violent acts in school include being a male and being between ages 11 and 18. They are often freshmen students perhaps experiencing a "transition." Often they claim to have been victimized, shunned, or "picked on" by others; they have easy access to guns; and they may have had prior discipline problems. Most incidents occur early in the morning and in crowded places such as the cafeteria (Gyan, 1999).

Although the number of students who commit violent acts is small, these random acts are frightening and deadly and school officials are struggling with ways to prevent their occurrence and to recognize the signs of troubled youth early. Violence prevention programs should begin in elementary schools. Children who exhibit aggressive behavior in the elementary school setting are more likely to exhibit antisocial and violent behavior as adolescents and adults. Programs should target stress management, conflict and anger resolution, and personal and self-esteem development. Nurses should use data collected through the YRBS and other local data as a means of assessment when developing violence policy and prevention programs in the school and community. Additionally, nurses should initiate and participate in research that examines the complex developmental, social, and psychological factors surrounding violence.

Health Promotion for School Staff

According to the National Center for Education Statistics (Allegrante, 1998), schools in the United

BOX 26-7

1995 United States Youth Risk Behavior Survey Data[1]

The YRBS data in this section are from the national school-based survey, 45 state surveys, and 16 local surveys conducted among high school students from February through May 1995.

Unintentional and Intentional Injuries:
22%: Rarely or never used safety belts
39%: Rode with a drinking driver during past month
20%: Carried a weapon during past month
39%: Were in a physical fight during past year
9%: Attempted suicide during past year

Alcohol and Other Drug Use:
52%: Drank alcohol during past month
33%: Reported episodic heavy drinking during past month
25%: Used marijuana during past month
2%: Ever injected illegal drugs
20%: Ever sniffed or inhaled intoxicating substances

Sexual Behaviors:
53%: Ever had sexual intercourse
18%: Ever had four or more sex partners
38%: Had sexual intercourse during past three months
46%: Did not use a condom during last sexual intercourse[2]
83%: Did not use birth control pills during last sexual intercourse[2]

Tobacco Use:
71%: Ever smoked cigarettes
35%: Smoked cigarettes during past month
16%: Smoked cigarettes on 20 or more days during past month
11%: Used smokeless tobacco during past month
78%: Not asked proof of age for purchase of cigarettes[3]

Dietary Behaviors:
72%: Ate fewer than five servings of fruits and vegetables yesterday
39%: Ate more than two servings of high-fat foods yesterday
28%: Thought they were overweight
41%: Were attempting weight loss
5%: Took laxatives or vomited to lose or maintain weight during past month

Physical Activity:
36%: Did not participate in vigorous physical activity[4]
79%: Did not participate in moderate physical activity[5]
40%: Were not enrolled in physical education class
75%: Did not attend physical education class daily
30%: Exercised less than 20 minutes in an average physical education class[6]

From *United States adolescent health summary,* January 2000, CDC, www.cdc.gov/nccdphp/dash/ahsumm/ussumm.html.
1. Among high school students only
2. Among students who had sexual intercourse during the past three months
3. Among students less than 18 years of age who currently smoked cigarettes and who purchased cigarettes in a store
4. Fewer than three of the past seven days
5. Fewer than five of the past seven days
6. Among students enrolled in physical education class

States employ more than 2.5 million teachers and over two million other employees. Schools are an excellent site for promotion of health and prevention of illness. Health promotion programs at the work site have provided beneficial results, including positive effects on blood pressure control, daily physical activity, smoking cessation, and weight control (Allegrante, 1998). Comparable findings have been found in health promotion programs designed for school employees. School-based programs in Michigan, South Carolina, and Texas indicate that staff who participated in health promotion programs increased their health knowledge and positively changed their attitudes and behaviors relative to their smoking practices, nutrition, physical activity, stress, and emotional health. Other studies have shown that health promotion programs for school personnel may improve morale, reduce job stress and absenteeism, and heighten interest in teaching health-related topics to students.

Health promotion programs should have the following four levels of prevention: screening and assessment, risk factor reduction education, organizational policies, and employee assistance programs (Allegrante, 1998). School nurses play an important role in all levels of prevention through assessment, planning, intervention, and evaluation.

The American Association of School Administrators reports that as many as 50% of schoolteachers are overweight; therefore school health promotion activities for faculty and staff should center on exercise, nutrition education, and dietary management (Illuzzi and Cinelli, 2000). The school nurse can assist the faculty and staff by giving workshops on exercise and nutrition, screening for increased blood pressure, and establishing weight management programs.

Family and Community Involvement

School nurses are often asked to provide health content to family, parents, and the community on a variety of topics such as sexuality, STDs, HIV, communicable disease, and substance abuse. Health education in the community should consist of programs that are designed to positively influence parents, staff, and others in matters related to health. School nurses are a ready resource to the community whenever health-related problems arise. They must step forward and volunteer their services and expertise in a way that can positively affect their community.

Programs such as smoking cessation can include the entire community. The school nurse should be aware of the existence of these programs for referral and may also serve as a consultant during implementation and as an advocate for programs to remain in place.

Programs aimed at adolescent weight control may also need to be targeted to the parents. Parents may not be aware of the important role they play in helping to prevent obesity in their children. School nurses can help parents develop healthier eating habits in the home that will directly affect their families. The nurse can also help develop physical activity programs in the community that include both the child and the family.

Issues such as abuse and neglect can bring school personnel and the community together. School nurses should lobby legislators for positive policy implementations and work closely with service agencies. School nurses should also lobby for increased resources for assessment of problems when dealing with families and children with risk factors. They should collaborate on research related to interventions for troubled families and youth.

One community-based program that should be initiated is aimed at the reduction of violence and substance abuse in both schools and the community. School nurses can work with law enforcement and neighborhood watch programs in an effort to reduce violence. Violence affects not only the school but the community at large; therefore the initiation of outreach programs requires an interdisciplinary approach that includes students, parents, school personnel, community organizations, businesses, public health officials, and law enforcement officers (Lowry et al., 1999).

FAMILY RISK INDEX

Children living in families with four or more of the following characteristics are considered at "high risk" (Annie E. Casey Foundation, 1999):

- Child is not living with two parents.
- Household head is a high school dropout.
- Family income is below the poverty line.
- Child is living with parent(s) who do not have steady, full-time employment.
- Family is receiving welfare benefits.
- Child does not have health insurance.
- Percent of children living in "high-risk" families, based on definition above is 14%.

Nurses must also become more adept at working in the public sphere. They must be able to increase their visibility and become more comfortable with working with the media. The media can be a useful tool in assisting school nurses with health education advocacy.

SCHOOL NURSING PRACTICE

School nursing is a specialty unto itself. School nurses need education in specific areas such as growth and development, public health, mental health nursing, case management, program management, family theory, leadership, and cultural sensitivity to effectively perform their roles. They must be prepared to work with children of different ages and under highly variable circumstances. The nurse must also keep abreast of issues affecting children and participate in research that explores and expands the role. The school nurse's practice is relatively independent and autonomous, but the school nurse also functions as a member of various interdisciplinary teams. For entry into school nursing, it is recommended that nurses hold a minimum of a bachelor's degree and some universities are now preparing school nurses at the master's level.

DEFINITION OF SCHOOL NURSING

School nursing is a specialized practice of professional nursing that advances the well-being, academic success, and lifelong achievement of students. To that end, school nurses facilitate positive student responses to normal development; promote health and safety; intervene with actual and potential health problems; provide case management services; and actively collaborate with others to build student and family capacity for adaptation, self-management, self-advocacy, and learning.

From National Association of School Nurses: NASN board of directors meeting, Providence Rhode Island, June 1999: definition of school nursing, *J Sch Nurs* 16(1):5, February 2000.

School nurses function in many roles. Among these are care provider, student advocate, educator, community liaison, and case manager. According to NASN (1995), effective case managers must be knowledgeable about available services, collaborators in care, able to coordinate services, and able to evaluate service outcomes. Box 26-8 outlines professional roles and functions of the school nurse and Table 26-4 presents the standards of school nursing practice.

The school setting is a perfect place to conduct research relative to many issues regarding how children adapt to life transitions such as divorce, illness or death of a loved one, illness of either themselves or a peer, domestic violence, and health-related behaviors of the young. It is also a good setting to study how socioeconomic factors affect learning behaviors in children. However, many nurses feel uncomfortable about conducting research (Box 26-9).

SCHOOL-BASED HEALTH CENTERS

School-based health care centers have been touted as one of the best ways to offer comprehensive health care services to school-aged children and adolescents. A **school-based health center** has been defined as a space located within a school building or on school property and designated as a place where students can go to receive primary care services. The center or clinic is more than a school nursing station. In school-based clinics, students are able to receive health services not generally available in school such as comprehensive primary care (Allensworth et al., 1997).

NPs, health aides, outreach workers, social workers, psychologists, and physicians can provide these services and are employed by one or more local agencies such as health departments, hospitals, medical schools, or social service agencies. Some of the services provided in these centers include nutrition education, injury treatment, general and sports physicals, prescriptions, pregnancy testing, lab services, immunizations, gynecological examinations, medication dispensing, social work services, and management of chronic illnesses. Close collaboration must exist within and among the community, the educational board, and the families for such a center to develop and flourish.

BOX 26-8

Professional Roles and Functions of the School Nurse

1. Promotes and protects the optimal health status of children.
2. Provides health assessments.
3. Develops and implements a health plan.
4. Maintains, evaluates, and interprets cumulative health data to accommodate individual needs of students.
5. Participates as the health team specialist on the child education evaluation team to develop the IEP.
6. Plans and implements school health management protocols for the child with special health needs, including the administration of medication.
7. Participates in home visits to assess the family's needs as related to child's health.
8. Develops procedures and provides for crisis intervention for acute illness, injury, and emotional disturbances.
9. Promotes and assists in the control of communicable diseases through preventive immunization programs, early detection, surveillance, and reporting and follow-up of contagious diseases.
10. Recommends provisions for a school environment conducive to learning.
11. Provides health education.
12. Coordinates school and community health activities and serves as a liaison person between the home, school, and community.
13. Acts as a resource person in promoting health careers.
14. Provides health counseling for staff.
15. Provides leadership and support for staff wellness programs.
16. Engages in research and evaluation of school health services to act as a change agent for school health programs and school nursing practices.
17. Assists in the formation of health policies, goals, and objectives for the school district.

From National Association of School Nurses: *Position statement: professional school nurse roles and responsibilities: education, certification, and licensure*, 1996, The Author, www.nasn.org/issues/roles/htm.

TABLE 26-4

Standards of Professional School Nursing Practice

Standards of Care	
Standard I: Assessment	The school nurse collects client data.
Standard II: Diagnosis	The school nurse analyzes the assessment data in determing nursing diagnoses.
Standard III: Outcome identification	The school nurse identifies expected outcomes individualized to the client.
Standard IV: Planning	The school nurse develops a plan of care and action that specifies interventions to attain expected outcomes.
Standard V: Implementation	The school nurse implements the interventions identified in the plan of care and action.
Standard VI: Evaluation	The school nurse evaluates the client's progress toward attainment of outcomes.

From National Association of School Nurses: *Healthy school environment: NASN position statement*, 1998, The Author, www.nasn.org/issues/.

Continued

TABLE 26-4—cont'd

Standards of Professional School Nursing Practice—cont'd

Standards of Professional Performance	
Standard I: Quality of care	The school nurse systematically evaluates the quality and effectiveness of school nursing practice.
Standard II: Education	The school nurse evaluates his or her own nursing practice in relation to professional practice standards and relevant statutes, regulation, and policies.
Standard III: Education	The school nurse interacts with and contributes to the professional development of peers and school personnel as colleagues.
Standard IV: Collegiality	The school nurse interacts with and contributes to the professional development of peers and school personnel as colleagues.
Standard V: Ethics	The school nurse's decisions and actions on behalf of clients are determined in an ethical manner.
Standard VI: Collaboration	The school nurse collaborates with the student, family, school staff, community, and other providers in providing student care.
Standard VII: Research	The school nurse promotes use of research findings in school nursing practice.
Standard VIII: Resource utilization	The school nurse considers factors related to safety, effectiveness, and cost when planning and delivering care.
Standard IX: Communication	The school nurse uses effective written, verbal, and nonverbal communication skills.
Standard X: Program management	The school nurse manages school health services.
Standard XI: Health education	The school nurse assists students, families, school staff, and community to achieve optimal levels of wellness through appropriately designed and delivered health education.

From National Association of School Nurses: *Healthy school environment: NASN position statement,* 1998, The Author, www.nasn.org/issues/.

BOX 26-9

Research and School Nurses

Price, Telljohann, and King (1999) surveyed school nurses' understanding of and experience with research in the school setting. They found that school nurses, for the most part, did not participate in research, although both the ASHA and the NASN encourage it.

Of the school nurses surveyed, 97% believed research provided new knowledge on school nursing issues; 93% believed it benefited the health of school-aged children; and 86% believed it helped their nursing peers do a better job. The nurses also perceived major barriers; 94% believed barriers included a lack of time; 88% a lack of clerical help; 84% a lack of money; 71% a lack of school administration support; 70% a need for appropriate equipment; and 69% a lack of training.

The study concluded with the finding that 78% of the nurses surveyed would be willing to engage in school-based research if they had someone to work with. It was suggested that school nurses pair with academic institutions, especially those with graduate departments, and with public health agencies.

CASE STUDY

APPLICATION OF THE NURSING PROCESS

The nursing process is a systematic, organized approach to problem solving that nurses use when working with clients. It is neither fixed nor stagnant. It is a flexible process that allows for ongoing changes. This case study illustrates the use of the nursing process in a school setting.

Sandra Baker is a nurse at an elementary school in a small town. A second-grade teacher brought Carrie Broussard to the clinic and told Sandra that Carrie had been scratching her head all day and she was worried that Carrie might have an infection.

Assessment

Carrie is seven years old. Her shoulder-length blond hair appeared neat and clean. When questioned by Sandra, Carrie replied that her head had been itching for two or three days, but she denied any pain or trauma. Sandra noted that Carrie did not have a fever or swollen lymph nodes, but examination of her scalp revealed multiple excoriated areas. Carrie's hair was examined with a Wood's light and Sandra saw adult lice at the base of her hair follicles on the back of her head near the nape of the neck. Multiple nits were also noted. Sandra learned that Carrie had two brothers in the school and one sister who was a toddler at home.

Diagnosis

Individual
- Head lice

Family and Community (School)
- Potential for spread of infestation in both family and school
- Potential knowledge deficit related to spread and treatment of lice by teachers and family members

Planning

Sandra is familiar with the school district's policy that covers head lice in schoolchildren. Ac-

cording to the policy, the nurse must do the following:

- Contact Carrie's parents to tell them about the lice and recommend treatment based on protocol
- Exclude Carrie from school immediately and inform her parents that she can return to school when she has been treated
- Check the hair of all of the other children in the class and treat each according to the school protocol
- Check all siblings who attend the school for lice
- Check all students in the siblings' classes if lice are identified
- Ensure that the teachers, staff, and family members have the necessary education relative to prevention and treatment of head lice

Implementation

Carrie's brothers, David and Paul, are brought to the clinic for examination. Both brothers have lice. Sandra contacted Mrs. Broussard and explained the situation to her and requested that she come to the school to pick up her children. When Mrs. Broussard arrived at the school, Sandra gave her written information on treatment and prevention of lice and showed her what nits and lice look like. Mrs. Broussard was also instructed to check other members of the family not attending this school, especially those who share hairbrushes, pillowcases, and towels, because all family members with lice must be treated or the lice would continue to be passed from member to member. Sandra also explained procedures for cleaning combs and brushes and bedding and potentially contaminated clothing and toys. Finally, Mrs. Broussard was informed that the children could return to school the day after treatment.

It was obvious to Sandra that Mrs. Broussard was embarrassed. To ease her mind, Sandra carefully explained that lice are highly contagious and easily passed from child to child and not an indication of poor hygiene. Mrs. Broussard repeated the instructions and left with her three children.

Sandra examined all of the students from each of the Broussard children's classes for head lice.

Continued

From the three classes, she identified five more children with head lice and notified their parents. Those children had siblings in three additional classrooms and she repeated the procedure for each of them. At the end of the day, she had identified a total of 15 children with lice and contacted all parents.

Sandra investigated whether the teachers and staff desired an information session related to the transmission and spread of lice because so many students had head lice. She discovered that it had been two years since this was done and arranged a class for the coming week for the teachers and teacher's aides relative to the identification and treatment of head lice.

Evaluation

Mrs. Broussard brought Carrie, David, and Paul to school the following day, and on examination Sandra found them to be free of lice and nits.

Mrs. Broussard expressed her appreciation for the nurse's help and nonjudgmental approach to the problem. Over the next two days, Sandra reexamined all of the children in the affected classrooms and found that the infected children had been successfully treated and that there were not any new cases. New cases were not identified during the remainder of the semester. The teachers and staff gave her positive feedback about the class and asked for it to be repeated at the beginning of each school year.

Levels of Prevention and School Health

School nursing encompasses all three levels of prevention (i.e., primary, secondary, and tertiary) and all three may be practiced individually or concurrently. Table 26-5 lists examples of school nursing interventions for each of the three levels of prevention.

TABLE 26-5

Examples of Levels of Prevention and the Role of the Nurse in the School Setting

Level of Prevention	Role of the Nurse
Primary Prevention	
Nutrition education	Provision of education to children and parents; consultation with dietary staff
Immunizations	Provision or referral for immunizations; consultation for immunization in special circumstances
Safety	Safety education provision; inspection of playgrounds and buildings for safety hazards
Health education	Provision of healthy lifestyle education; development of the health education curriculum throughout the school years; provision of health education to parents, faculty, and staff; suicide prevention programs, sex education
Secondary Prevention	
Screenings	Routine screenings for scoliosis, vision and hearing problems, eating disorders, obesity, depression, anger, dental, abuse, and EPSDT
Case finding	Identification of at-risk students
Treatment	Administration of medications; development of IHP; implementation of procedures and tasks necessary for students with special health needs; first aid
Home visiting	Family counseling and assessment for special and at-risk students

TABLE 26-5—cont'd

Examples of Levels of Prevention and the Role of the Nurse in the School Setting—cont'd

Level of Prevention	Role of the Nurse
	Tertiary Prevention
Referral of student for substance abuse or behavior problems	Serve as an advocate; assist with resource referrals; assist parents, faculty, and staff; consult with neighborhood and law enforcement officials; initiate outreach programs
Prevention of complications and adverse effects	Follow-up and referral for students with eating disorders and obesity; participate with faculty and staff to reduce recurrence and risk factors; serve as a case manager
Faculty and staff monitoring	Follow-up for faculty and staff experiencing chronic or serious illness; follow-up of work-related injuries and accidents

SUMMARY

Components of a comprehensive school health program have been clearly identified and discussed. Many of the *Healthy People 2010* objectives specifically relate to issues that can be addressed in the school setting. The role of the school nurse has changed dramatically since its inception and continues to evolve to meet the demands of school-aged children, their parents, and the communities in which they live. School nurses continue to reduce the number of days and the frequency with which students miss school related to illness. They have become child advocates, counselors, resource people, health promoters and collaborators, educators, and researchers both in the school and the community.

LEARNING ACTIVITIES

1. Explain how the *Healthy People 2010* objectives can be used to shape school-based health care.
2. Attend a meeting of the school nurse association in the area. Identify the major pros and cons of being a school nurse. Look at factors such as working conditions, number of children assigned to each nurse, job functions, and job satisfaction.
3. Visit a comprehensive school-based clinic in the area. Discuss how the care given in this type of clinic differs from the care that a school nurse can provide. Review the protocols of both settings and see how they differ.
4. Purchase a one-year subscription to a school health journal.
5. Interview a member of the local school board about controversial subjects related to health education in the local school system (e.g., sex education).
6. Review the most common diseases and reported injuries in school-aged children in the area. Develop a plan for how the school and the community can work together to decrease their incidence.
7. Interview the parents of several school-aged children. Ask what services they would like to see provided in the school setting.
8. Arrange with the principal of a local school to have a discussion session with children in a particular grade level. Ascertain what their eating habits are and then develop a class that can enhance healthy eating.

REFERENCES

Allegrante J: School-site health promotion for faculty and staff: a key component of the coordinated school health program, *J Sch Health* 68(5):190-194, 1998.

Allensworth D et al, editors: *Schools and health: our nation's investment,* 1997, IOM, Division of Medicine, www.books.nap.edu/books/0309054354/html/R1.html.

American Diabetes Association: *Position statement: care of children with diabetes in the school and day care setting,* 2000, The Author, www.diabetes.org/diabetescare.

American School Health Association: *Healthy choices in school vending machines,* 1995, The Author, www.ashaweb.org/resolutions/resolutions1.html.

American School Health Association: Protecting the privacy of student education records, *J Sch Health* 67:4, 1997.

American School Health Association National Injury and Violence Prevention Task Force: Report of the ASHA National Injury and Violence Prevention Task Force: an executive summary, *J Sch Health* 69:5, 1999.

Annie E. Casey Foundation: *Kids count data online,* 1999, The Author, www.aecf.org.

Beals K, Brey R, Gonyou J: Understanding the female athlete triad: eating disorders, amenorrhea and osteoporosis, *J Sch Health* 69(8):337-340, 1999.

Calabrese B et al: Asthma knowledge, roles, functions, and educational needs of school nurses, *J Sch Health* 69:6, 1999.

Carnegie Council Adolescent Development, Centers For Disease Control: *School health programs: an investment in our nations future,* 1999, The Author, www.cdc.gov/nccdphp/dash/ataglanc.htm.

Centers for Disease Control: *CDC's guidelines for school and community programs: promoting lifelong physical activity,* 1997a, The Author, www.cdc.gov/nccdphp/dash/phactaag.htm.

Centers for Disease Control: *1995 United States YRBS data,* 1997b, The Author, www.cdc.gov/nccdphp/dash/ahsumm/ussumm.htm.

Centers for Disease Control: *Assessing health risk behaviors among young people: youth risk behavior surveillance system,* 1998, The Author, www.cdc.gov/nccdphp/dash/yrbs/yrbsaag98.htm.

Centers for Disease Control: *School health programs: an investment in our nation's future,* 1999a, The Author, www.cdc.gov/nccdphp/dash/ataglanc.htm.

Centers for Disease Control: Cigarette smoking among high school students: 11 states, 1991-1997, *J Sch Health* 69(8):303-306, 1999b.

Centers for Disease Control: *TIPS: tobacco information and prevention source: facts on sports and smokefree youth,* 1999c, The Author, www.cdc.gov/nccdphp/osh/ythsprt1.htm.

Centers for Disease Control: *HIV/AIDS surveillance report,* vol 11(1), 1999d, The Author, www.cdc.gov/hiv/stats/hasr1201.htm.

Centers for Disease Control: *Epidemiology and prevention of vaccine-preventable diseases,* ed 5, Atlanta, 1999e, Public Health Foundation.

Centers for Disease Control: *Nutrition and the health of young people: fact sheet,* 1999f, The Author, www.cdc.gov/nccdphp/dash/nutfact.htm.

Duncan P, Igoe J: School health services. In Marx E, Wooley SF, Northrop D, editors: *Health is academic: a guide to coordinated school health programs,* New York, 1998, Teachers College Press.

Forum on Child and Family Statistics: *Behavior and social environment indicators,* 1999, The Author, www.childstats.gov/ac1999/behtxt.asp.

Fox J: *Primary health care of children,* St. Louis, 1997, Mosby.

Francis E, Treloar D: Who dispenses pharmaceuticals to children at school? *J Sch Health* 66:10, 1996.

Fryer G, Igoe J: Functions of school nurses and health assistants in U.S. school health programs, *J Sch Health* 66(2):55, 1996.

Gyan J: "Commonalities" ID'd in student shooters, *The Advocate,* Dec. 14, 1999.

Health Care Financing Administration, US Department of Health and Human Services: *Medicaid and EPSDT,* 2000, The Authors, www.hcfa.hhs.gov/medicaid/epsdthm.htm.

Hootman J: Only the best will do for our children! *School Health Newsletter,* Winter/Spring 1998, www.schoolhealth.org/research.htm.

Igoe J: School health services: an overview of school health services, *National Association of Secondary School Principals Bulletin,* Nov. 1998, The Author, www.nassp.org/publications/bulletin/nov98bul.htm.

Illuzzi S, Cinelli B: A coordinated school health program approach to adolescent obesity, *J Sch Nurs* 16(1):12-17, 2000.

Kann L et al: State and local YRBSS coordinators: youth risk behavior surveillance—United States, 1997, *J Sch Health* 68(9):355-369, 1998.

Kater K: *Healthy body image! teaching kids to eat and love their bodies too! body image and eating disorder prevention curriculum for grades 4-6,* 1999, The Author, www.edap.org/kathykater.html.

Kilpatrick M, Ohannessian C, Bartholomew J: Adolescent weight management and perceptions: an analysis of the national longitudinal study of adolescent health, *J Sch Health* 69(4):148-152, 1999.

King KA: Fifteen prevalent myths concerning adolescent suicide, *J Sch Health* 69(4):159-161, 1999.

Lowry R et al: School violence, substance use, and availability of illegal drugs on school property among US high school students, *J Sch Health* 69(9):347-355, 1999.

National Association of School Nurses: *Healthy school environment: NASN position statement,* 1998, The Author, www.nasn.org/issues/.

National Association of School Nurses: *Medication administration in the school setting: NASN position statement,* 1997, The Author, www.nasn.org/issues/medication.htm.

National Association of School Nurses: NASN board of directors meeting, Providence Rhode Island, June 1999: definition of school nursing, *J Sch Nurs* 16(1):5, February 2000.

National Association of School Nurses: *NASN position statement: case management,* 1995, The Author, www.nasn.org/issues/casemang.htm.

National Association of School Nurses: *Position statement: professional school nurse roles and responsibilities: education, certification, and licensure,* 1996, The Author, www.nasn.org/issues/roles/htm.

National Center for Education Statistics: *NCES fast facts: students with disabilities,* 2000, The Author, www.nces.ed.gov/fastfacts/display.asp/id=64.

National Heart, Lung, and Blood Institute, National Asthma Education and Prevention Program, School Asthma Education Subcommittee: How asthma friendly is your school? *J Sch Health* 68(4):167, 1998.

Price J, Telljohann S, King K: School nurses' perceptions of and experience with school health research, *J Sch Health* 69(2):58-62, 1999.

Sklaire M: *Managing sports injuries,* 1997, School Health Alert, www.schoolnurse.com/med_info/sports_injuries.html.

Strong JP, et al: Prevalence and extent of atherosclerosis in adolescents and young adults: implications for prevention from the pathobiological determinants of atherosclerosis in youth study, *JAMA* 281:727, February, 1999.

United States adolescent health summary, January 2000, CDC, www.cdc.gov/nccdphp/dash/ahsumm/ussumm.html.

US Department of Health and Human Services: *Healthy people 2010: conference edition,* Washington, DC, 2000, PHS.

US Preventive Services Task Force: *Guide to clinical preventive services,* Baltimore, 1996, Williams & Wilkins.

Winkleby MA, et al: Ethnic variation in cardiovascular disease risk factors among children and young adults: findings from the third national health and nutrition examination survey, 1988-1994, *JAMA* 281:1006, March, 1999.

Occupational Health

Bonnie Rogers and Patricia Hyland Travers

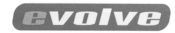

http://evolve.elsevier.com/Nies/

Occupational health nursing, a component of community health nursing, is defined by the American Association of Occupational Health Nurses (AAOHN) as the following:

> the specialty practice that focuses on the promotion, prevention, and restoration of health within the context of a safe and healthy environment. It includes the prevention of adverse health effects from occupational and environmental hazards. It provides for and delivers occupational and environmental health and safety services to workers, worker populations, and community groups. Occupational and environmental health nursing is an autonomous specialty and nurses make independent nursing judgments in providing health care services
>
> (AAOHN, 1999a, p. 2).

As depicted in Fig. 27-1, occupational health nursing derives its theoretical, conceptual, and factual framework from a multidisciplinary base. Elements of this multidisciplinary base include the following (Rogers, 1998):

- **Nursing science** that provides the context for health care delivery and recognizes the needs of individuals, groups, and populations within the framework of prevention, health promotion, and illness and injury care management, including

---

F I G U R E **27-1**

Occupational health nursing knowledge domains (Copyright Bonnie Rogers, 1998).

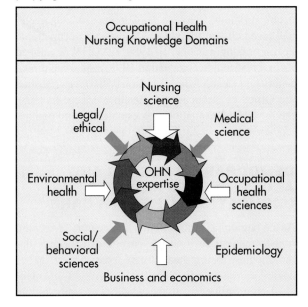

risk assessment, risk management, and risk communication;

- **Medical science** specific to treatment and management of occupational health illness and injury integrated with nursing health surveillance activities;
- **Occupational health sciences**, including **toxicology** to recognize routes of exposure, examine relationships between chemical exposures in the workplace and acute and latent health effects such as burns or cancer, and understand dose-response relationships; **industrial hygiene** to identify and evaluate workplace hazards so control mechanisms can be implemented for exposure reduction; **safety** to identify and control workplace injuries through active safeguards and worker training and education programs about job safety; and **ergonomics** to match the job to the worker, emphasizing capabilities and minimizing limitations;
- **Epidemiology** to study health and illness trends and characteristics of the worker population, investigate work-related illness and injury episodes, and apply epidemiological methods to analyze and interpret risk data to determine causal relationships and to participate in epidemiological research;
- **Business and economic theories, concepts, and principles** for strategic and operational planning, valuing quality and cost-effective services and for management of occupational health and safety programs;
- **Social and behavioral sciences** to explore influences of various environments (e.g., work and home), relationships, and lifestyle factors on worker health and determine the interactions affecting worker health;
- **Environmental health** to systematically examine interrelationships between the worker and the extended environment as a basis for the development of prevention and control strategies; and
- **Legal and ethical issues** to ensure compliance with regulatory mandates and contend with ethical concerns that may arise in competitive environments.

EVOLUTION OF OCCUPATIONAL HEALTH NURSING

The evolution of occupational health nursing in the United States has mirrored the societal changes in moving from an agrarian-based to an industrial-based economy and, entering the twenty-first century, a continuing move to a service-based economy. Occupational health nursing dates to the late 1800s with the employment of Betty Moulder and Ada Mayo Stewart.

A group of coal-mining companies hired Betty Moulder in 1888 to care for coal miners and their families (American Association of Industrial Nurses [AAIN], 1976). Seven years later, the Vermont Marble Company hired **Ada Mayo Stewart** to care for workers and their families. Stewart is often referred to as the first "industrial nurse," and her activities are well documented (Parker-Conrad, 1988). In 1897, Anna B. Duncan was employed by the John Wanamaker Company to visit sick employees at home; in 1899, a nursing service was established for employees of the Frederick Loeser department store in Brooklyn, New York (AAIN, 1976).

At the turn of the twentieth century, the industrial revolution was well under way and the concept of health care for employees spread rapidly throughout many states (Travers, 1987). Companies hiring industrial nurses in the early 1900s included the Emporium in San Francisco; Plymouth Cordage Company in Massachusetts; Anaconda Mining Company in Montana; Broadway Store in Los Angeles; Chase Metal Works in Connecticut; Hale Brothers in San Francisco; Filene's in Boston; Carson, Pirie, and Scott in Chicago; Fulton Cotton Mills in Georgia; and Bullock's in Los Angeles (McGrath, 1946; Parker-Conrad, 1988). The cost-effectiveness of providing health care to employees was achieving increased recognition, and by 1912, after workers' compensation legislation had been instituted, 38 nurses were employed by business firms (McGrath, 1946; Parker-Conrad, 1988). The following year, a registry of industrial nurses was initiated, and in 1915, the Boston Industrial Nurses Club was formed, later evolving into the Massachusetts Industrial Nurses Organization.

In 1916, the Factory Nurses Conference was organized. This group was open only to graduate, state-RNs affiliated with the ANA and their efforts identified the industrial nurses' need to explore the uniqueness of this evolving specialty area (AAIN, 1976). More important, industrial nurses were practicing in single-nurse settings and recognized the importance of uniting as a group for the purpose of sharing ideas with peers practicing in the same nursing arena. In 1917, the first educational course for industrial nurses was offered at Boston University's College of Business Administration.

During and after the Depression Era, many nurses lost jobs because management viewed industrial nursing as a nonessential aspect of business (Felton, 1985, 1986). The focus of health care for employees again changed as a result of many factors, including the impact of the two world wars. During World War I, the government demanded health services for workers at factories and shipyards holding defense contracts. Demographics in the workplace were also dramatically different during World War II because increased numbers of women entered the workforce. In 1942, the U.S. Surgeon General told an audience of nurses that the health conservation of the "industrial army" was the most urgent civilian need during the war (Felton, 1985).

From 1938 to 1943, the number of occupational health nurses increased by more than 10,000. In 1942, some 300 nurses from 16 states voted to create a national association for the specialty. Catherine R. Dempsey, a nurse at Simplex Wire and Cable Company in Cambridge, Massachusetts, was elected president of the national association. By 1943, approximately 11,000 nurses were employed in industry (AAIN, 1976).

Nine years later, members of AAIN voted to remain an independent, autonomous association rather than merge with the NLN or the ANA. In 1953, another important step was taken toward formalizing this specialty area of nursing practice when the *Industrial Nurses Journal* (i.e., now the *AAOHN Journal*) was published. In 1977, the organization changed its name to the AAOHN, reflecting a broader, more diverse scope of practice.

In the 1980s and 1990s, occupational health nursing moved rapidly into increased role expansion in health promotion, policy development, management, and research and maintained traditional occupational health nursing practice. In 1989, AAOHN developed its first research agenda and in 1993, the Occupational Safety and Health Administration (OSHA) established the Office of Occupational Health Nursing. In 1999, the AAOHN Foundation was established and competencies in the specialty were delineated.

DEMOGRAPHIC TRENDS AND ACCESS ISSUES RELATED TO OCCUPATIONAL HEALTH CARE

At the beginning of the twenty-first century, sweeping transformations in industry, changing workforce demographics, rising health care costs, diversity of health care systems with the integration of managed care, influence of the world economy, shift in production from goods to services, and proliferation of advanced technologies are influencing the direction of occupational health nursing (O'Brien, 1995). The focus of U.S. industry is moving away from large manufacturing facilities to smaller, service-based businesses and other changes are anticipated (OSHA, 1999). Work may be performed where and when the customer requires, which will force employers to make different demands on their employees. Flexible and varying work schedules and work sites may become more common than the daily trek to the same building for the 40-hour, nine-to-five routine that has been the standard for many years. Of major importance will be the demand for an increase in skill level of all employees. The ability to read, follow directions, perform mathematical calculations, and be computer literate will be core skills for workers. The increasing availability of older workers, women, minorities, and immigrants will have far-reaching implications for employers and pose specific challenges for occupational health professionals.

Between 1985 and 2005, the labor force will grow at a rate of 22% (from 115 to 147 million), and skilled human capital is becoming a more important resource for industry than financial capital (OSHA, 1999). These trends are important to understand because they have a direct impact on the national rate of economic growth, especially in the area of population-sensitive products such as food, automobiles, housing units, household goods, and education services, with concomitant hazards.

Within the context of these evolving organizational trends, key characteristics include a focus on a shared vision, strategy, and long-term objectives within an environment composed of individuals working in teams. In contrast to the past, occupational health nurses have opportunities to work on cross-functional teams to shape decisions in areas such as benefits, research, safety, and legal matters. Specifically, occupational health nurses have opportunities to positively affect the transformation of the health care delivery system, establish policies within the managed care environment and within corporations, and assume leadership positions on legislative staffs and in governmental agencies (O'Brien, 1995).

Corporations have become driving forces in shaping the development of alternative approaches to health care. Rapidly increasing health care costs have spawned a number of alternative approaches to providing health care. HMOs and PPOs are two of the more common health care management programs. In the late 1980s, Digital Equipment Corporation seized the opportunity to control escalating health care costs by becoming an active and creative value purchaser of health care services (Digital Equipment Corporation, 1995). This was accomplished by designing a model that identified well-organized and well-managed HMOs as the key delivery channel. A tremendous opportunity exists for occupational health nurses to draft similar performance standards and to participate in total quality management processes designed to improve the quality, efficiency, and value of the managed health care delivery system.

It is important that the occupational health nurse remain informed about the various health care options available to the workforce as rapid changes occur regarding corporate benefits. This is of particular importance when considering referral of an employee to a health resource. Participation in one of the managed care plans requires that treatment take place according to the organization's guidelines and within their health service delivery system. Managed care plans are replacing traditional indemnity plans. Access to care is strictly managed and often limited. As this trend continues, the role of the occupational health nurse will take on added importance. The nurse must be prepared to accept increasing responsibilities as a primary care provider.

As businesses seek ways to maximize the value of their dollars spent on health care services, occupational health nurses and other health professionals face both an opportunity and a threat. The opportunity comes from being able to demonstrate that cost-effective quality health programs do improve the health of employees and their dependents, positively influencing their company's attempts to control rising health care costs. The threat is that if health professionals cannot prove cost-effectiveness and value to companies, their functions may be eliminated or replaced by contract services (Wachs, 1997).

OCCUPATIONAL HEALTH NURSING PRACTICE AND PROFESSIONALISM

As workplaces have continued to change over the past few decades, the role of the occupational health nurse has become even more diversified and complex. Often working as the only on-site health care professional, the occupational health nurse collaborates with workers, employers, and other professionals to identify health needs, prioritize interventions, develop and implement programs, and evaluate services delivered. The occupational health nurse is in a unique and critical position to coordinate a holistic approach to

TABLE 27-1

Standards of Occupational and Environmental Health Nursing Practice

Standard I: Assessment	The occupational and environmental health nurse systematically assesses the health status of the individual employee or population and the environment.
Standard II: Diagnosis	The occupational and environmental health nurse analyzes assessment data to formulate diagnoses.
Standard III: Outcome identification	The occupational and environmental health nurse identifies outcomes specific to the employee.
Standard IV: Planning	The occupational and environmental health nurse develops a goal-directed plan that is comprehensive and formulates interventions to attain expected outcomes.
Standard V: Implementation	The occupational and environmental health nurse implements interventions to attain desired outcomes identified in the plan.
Standard VI: Evaluation	The occupational and environmental health nurse systematically and continuously evaluates responses to interventions and progress toward the achievement of desired outcomes.
Standard VII: Resource management	The occupational and environmental health nurse secures and manages the resources that support an occupational health and safety program.
Standard VIII: Professional development	The occupational and environmental health nurse assumes accountability for professional development to enhance professional growth and maintain competency.
Standard IX: Collaboration	The occupational and environmental health nurse collaborates with employees, management, other health care providers, professionals, and community representatives.
Standard X: Research	The occupational and environmental health nurse uses research findings in practice and contributes to the scientific base in occupational and environmental health nursing to improve practices and advance the profession.
Standard XI: Ethics	The occupational and environmental health nurse uses an ethical framework as a guide for decision making in practice.

From American Association of Occupational Health Nurses: *Standards of occupational and environmental health nursing,* Atlanta, 1999a, The Author.

the delivery of quality, comprehensive occupational health services. The Standards of Occupational and Environmental Health Nursing Practice, the Code of Ethics, and AAOHN practice competencies guide the nurse.

AAOHN's Standards of Occupational and Environmental Health Nursing Practice (AAOHN, 1999a) form the basis by which the profession describes its responsibilities and accountabilities. The 11 Standard Statements are listed in Table 27-1. For each standard, identifiable criteria are detailed that can be used to evaluate practice relative to the specific standard. Refer to the complete Standards document from the AAOHN for this information.

Guided by an ethical framework made explicit in the AAOHN Code of Ethics (AAOHN, 1999a), occupational health nurses encourage and enable individuals to make informed decisions about health care concerns (Box 27-1). The occupational health nurse is a worker advocate and has the responsibility to uphold professional standards and codes. The occupational health nurse is also responsible to management, is usually compensated by management, and must practice within a framework of company policies and guidelines (Rogers, 1990). Ethical dilemmas arise because the nurse is loyal to both workers and management. Issues such as screening, drug testing, informing employees regarding

AAOHN Code of Ethics

- ■ The occupational health nurse provides health care in the work environment with regard for human dignity and client rights, unrestricted by considerations of social or economic status, personal attributes, or the nature of the health status.
- ■ The occupational health nurse promotes collaboration with other health professionals and community health agencies to meet the health needs of the workforce.
- ■ The occupational health nurse strives to safeguard the employee's right to privacy by protecting confidential information and releasing information only on written consent of the employee or as required or permitted by law.
- ■ The occupational health nurse strives to provide quality care and to safeguard clients from unethical and illegal actions.
- ■ The occupational health nurse, licensed to provide health care services, accepts obligations to society as a professional and responsible member of the community.
- ■ The occupational health nurse maintains individual competence in health nursing practice, based on scientific knowledge, and recognizes and accepts responsibility for individual judgments and actions, and complies with appropriate local, state, and federal laws and regulations that affect the delivery of occupational health services.
- ■ The occupational health nurse participates, as appropriate, in activities such as research that contribute to the ongoing development of the profession's body of knowledge while protecting the rights of subjects.

From American Association of Occupational Health Nurses: *Standards of occupational and environmental health nursing*, Atlanta, 1999a, The Author.

hazardous exposures, and confidentiality of health information, which is integral and central to the practice base, often create ethical debates. As advocates for workers, occupational health nurses foster equitable and quality health care services and safe and healthy work environments.

Occupational health nurses now make up the largest professional group providing health care services to employees in highly complex work environments. The roles of occupational health nurses are changing as a result of many factors, including rising health care costs, increased recognition of health effects associated with various exposures, emphasis on health promotion and wellness, health surveillance, women's issues, ergonomics, reproductive issues, downsizing, trends in managed care, and multicultural workforces. Box 27-2 reflects this growth in scope of practice and outlines occupational health nursing services currently mandated by state and federal regulations and occupational health nursing services generally mandated by company policies.

Approximately 30,000 nurses are practicing in the occupational health field in the United States (1.5% to 2% of the total nursing population). Approximately 60% of these 30,000 nurses work alone, making decisions regarding health and safety issues, influencing policy in health and safety, and planning and implementing the myriad of health programs. The majority of nurses practicing in occupational health are prepared at the baccalaureate level and have been practicing in the field of occupational health for at least 10 years (AAOHN, 1999b).

Research is an integral component of occupational and environmental health nursing practice because it provides the basis for scientific discovery that improves practice. In 1989, research priorities in occupational health nursing were first identified and published (Rogers, 1989). These priorities have been updated (Rogers, 2000) and will serve as the scientific basis to continue to build the body of knowledge in occupational and environmental health nursing for practice improvement and expansion (Box 27-3).

Meeting the needs of employees in smaller businesses is another important practice priority. The integration of occupational health principles into the curricula of schools of nursing, engineering, and management is critical. CHNs may assume occupational health nursing roles; therefore CHNs must be knowledgeable about the specialty area of occupational health nursing. Municipalities, smaller companies, visiting nurse associations, and home care agencies may provide opportunities for CHNs to be involved in screening programs, health education activities, workplace hazard evaluations, and other occupational health-related activities (Konstantinos, 1998).

The occupational health nurse's strengths are embedded in assessing, planning, implementing, and

B O X **27-2**

Occupational Health Nursing Services

Services Mandated by Federal and State Regulations:
Safe and healthful workplace
Emergency medical response
    First aid responder selection and training
    First aid space, supplies, protocols, and records
    Designated medical resources for incident response
Workers' compensation
Confidentiality of medical records
Compliance with medical record retention requirements
OSHA compliance
    Medical personnel requirement (29 CFR 1910.15)
    Injury and illness reporting and recording
    Accident and injury investigation
    Cumulative trauma disorder prevention
    Employee access to medical and exposure records
    Medical surveillance and hazardous work qualification
    Personal protective equipment evaluation and training
    Infection control
    Employee Right-to-Know Act notification and training
Community Right-to-Know Act compliance
ADA compliance
Rehabilitation Act: handicap, preplacement, fitness for duty evaluations, accommodations
DOD, Department of Transportation, Nuclear Regulatory Commission, and Drug-Free Workplace Act
    compliance
    Policy development
    Drug awareness education
    Drug testing and technical support
    Employee Assistance Program services
Threat of violence and duty to warn
Video display terminal (VDT) local regulations
State and local public health regulations
Nursing practice acts
Board of Pharmacy and Drug Enforcement Agency regulations
Continuing professional education required for licensure
Services Often Mandated by Company Policy:
Clinical supervision of on-site health services
Health strategy development
Health services standards
    Space, staffing, and operational standards
    Occupational illness and injury assessment, diagnosis, treatment, and referral
Nonoccupational illness and injury assessment, diagnosis, treatment, and referral
Disability and return-to-work evaluations and accommodations
Impaired employee fitness for duty evaluation
Preplacement evaluation and medical accommodation
Handicap evaluation, placement, and accommodation
Employee Assistance Program standards

BOX **27-2—cont'd**

Occupational Health Nursing Services—cont'd

International health: travel, medical advisory, and immunizations
Data collection and analysis
Medical consultation
Pregnancy placement in hazardous environments
Professional education and development
Audit and quality assurance
Optional Services:
Health education and health promotion
Medical screening for early detection and disease prevention
Physical fitness programs
Allergy injection programs

BOX **27-3**

Research Priorities in Occupational Health Nursing

- Effectiveness of primary health care delivery at the work site
- Effectiveness of health promotion nursing intervention strategies
- Methods for handling complex ethical issues related to occupational health
- Strategies that minimize work-related health outcomes (e.g., respiratory disease)
- Health effects resulting from chemical exposures in the workplace
- Occupational hazards of health care workers (e.g., latex allergy and blood-borne pathogens)
- Factors that influence workers' rehabilitation and return to work
- Effectiveness of ergonomic strategies to reduce worker injury and illness
- Effectiveness of case management approaches in occupational illness and injury
- Evaluation of critical pathways to effectively improve worker health and safety and enhance maximum recovery and safe return to work
- Effects of shift work on worker health and safety
- Strategies for increasing compliance with or motivating workers to use personal protective equipment

From Rogers B: Occupational health nursing research priorities, *AAOHN J* 48:9-16, 2000.

---

evaluating health programs for populations, care plans for individuals, and health education activities for worker aggregates. Often, lack of understanding or misconceptions about the occupational health nursing role have fostered the invisibility of the nurse, both within the nursing profession itself and within the business environment, thereby exacerbating the difficulties faced in being the sole guardian of health for workers in many companies. Empowered, well-trained, educated occupational and environmental health nurses will continue to bring about crucial changes in the areas of primary, secondary, and

tertiary prevention in occupational health (Kuhar, 1998; Videbeck, 1997).

In response to societal changes and historical events, the practice of occupational health nursing has changed dramatically, demanding a sophisticated knowledge base and problem-solving skill sets that are empirically grounded and multidisciplinary in nature (Barlow, 1992). The roles and responsibilities of the occupational health nurse must be clearly articulated to lay people; managers; workers; union representatives; and colleagues in occupational health, nursing, and medicine to ensure that occupational health nursing can continue to positively affect workers' health, contribute to decreasing health care costs, and foster reduction in health risks. Occupational health nurses must seize the opportunities in areas such as program planning, research, and policy-making during this era fraught with a health care system in crisis. Issues to be addressed and managed include nursing shortages in many areas of the country, dramatic changes in the business environment, employees' increasing awareness of workplace hazards, and the ever-increasing need to demonstrate the cost-effectiveness of occupational health nursing care and services (Bowling, 1996; Kosinski, 1998; Rogers, 1998; Vernarac, 1996).

OCCUPATIONAL HEALTH AND PREVENTION STRATEGIES

Like all community health professionals, the occupational health nurse's practice is based on the concept of prevention. Promotion, protection, maintenance, and restoration of worker health are priority goals set forth in the definition of occupational health nursing. This section describes prevention strategies, including objectives from *Healthy People 2010*. Prevention of exposure to occupational and environmental safety hazards and specific strategies for each level of prevention are described.

Healthy People 2010 and Occupational Health

Healthy People 2010 is the federal government initiative that focuses on health promotion and illness prevention. The stated goal of Priority Area 20 of *Healthy People 2010* is to "promote the health and safety of people at work through prevention and early intervention" (USDHHS, 2000). Objectives from this priority area cover work-related injuries and deaths, repetitive motion injuries, homicide, assault, lead exposure, skin disorders, stress, needle-stick injuries, and hearing loss. In addition, objectives from other priority areas also address issues related to occupational health and safety. Table 27-2 lists some of the *Healthy People 2010* objectives that deal with occupational health.

Prevention of Exposure to Potential Hazards

To prevent occupational and environmental safety hazards in the work environment, it is important to identify work-related agents and exposures that are

potentially hazardous. These can be categorized as follows:

1. Biological-infectious hazards: infectious-biological agents such as bacteria, viruses, fungi, or parasites that may be transmitted via contact with infected patients or contaminated body secretions or fluids
2. Chemical hazards: various forms of chemical agents, including medications, solutions, and gases, that interact with body tissues and cells and are potentially toxic or irritating to body systems
3. Enviromechanical hazards: factors encountered in work environments that cause accidents, injuries, strain, or discomfort (e.g., poor equipment or lifting devices and slippery floors)
4. Physical hazards: agents within work environments such as radiation, electricity, extreme temperatures, and noise that can cause tissue trauma through transfer of energy from these sources
5. Psychosocial hazards: factors and situations encountered or associated with the job or work environment that create stress, emotional strain, or interpersonal problems

Table 27-3 provides examples of work-related exposures in each of these areas. Having a good understanding of the nature of these hazards will allow for the development of health promotion and prevention strategies to mitigate exposure risk.

Levels of Prevention and Occupational Health Nursing

The occupational health nurse's activities in primary, secondary, and tertiary prevention strategies are expected to assume an even more important role in the prevention and treatment of chronic disease in the future (Rogers and Lawhorn, 2000). A survey of eight companies (Murphy, 1989) showed that 40% to 80% of the occupational health nurse's workday was devoted to prevention and that screening and treatment dominated other activities (16% and 18%, respectively). A description of each of these preventive approaches follows.

Primary Prevention
In the area of primary prevention, the occupational health nurse is involved in both health promotion and

Text continued on p. 740

TABLE **27-2**

Healthy People 2010 Objectives for Some Areas of Occupational Health

Objective	Baseline (1998)	Target
6-8: Eliminate disparities in employment rates between working-age adults with and without disabilities	52%	82%
7-6: Increase the proportion of employees who participate in employer-sponsored health promotion activities	28%	50%
8-17: Increase the number of office buildings that are managed using good indoor air quality practices	NA	NA
9-13: Increase the proportion of health insurance policies that cover contraceptive supplies and services	NA	NA
12-4: Increase the proportion of adults aged 20 years and older who call 911 and administer CPR when they witness an out-of-hospital cardiac arrest	NA	NA
14-28c: Increase Hep B coverage among occupationally exposed workers	71%	98%
19-16: Increase the proportion of work sites that offer nutrition or weight management classes or counseling	55%	85%
20-1: Reduce deaths from work-related injuries	4.5 per 100,000 workers	3.2 per 100,000 workers
20-3: Reduce the rate of injury and illness cases involving days away from work from overexertion or repetitive motion	675 per 100,000 workers	338 per 100,000 workers
20-8: Reduce occupational skin diseases or disorders among full-time workers	67 per 100,000 workers	47 per 100,000 workers
20-9: Increase the proportion of work sites employing 50 or more persons that provide programs to prevent or reduce employee stress	37%	50%
20-10: Reduce occupational needle-stick injuries among health care workers	600,000	420,000
22-13: Increase the proportion of work sites offering employer-sponsored physical activity and fitness programs	36%	75%
26-8: Reduce the cost of lost productivity in the workplace from alcohol and drug use	NA	NA
27-12: Increase the proportion of work sites with formal smoking policies that prohibit smoking or limit it to separately ventilated areas	79%	100%
28-8: Reduce occupational eye injury	NA	NA
28-16: Increase the use of appropriate ear protection devices, equipment, and practices	NA	NA

From US Department of Health and Human Services: *Healthy people 2010: conference edition,* Washington, DC, 2000, PHS.

TABLE **27-3**

Types of Occupational Hazards and Associated Health Effects

Category	Exposures	Health Effects
Biological	Blood or body fluids	Bacterial, fungal, and viral infections (e.g., hepatitis B)
Chemical	Solvents	Headache and central nervous system dysfunction
	Lead	Central nervous system disturbances
	Asbestos	Asbestosis
	Acids	Burns
	Glycol ethers	Reproductive effects
	Mercury	Ataxia
	Arsenic	Peripheral neuropathy
Enviromechanical	Static or nonneutral postures	Musculoskeletal disorders
	Repetitive or forceful exertions	Back injuries
	Lighting	Headache and eye strain
	Shift work	Sleep disorders
	Electrical	Electrocution
	Slips and falls	Musculoskeletal conditions
	Struck by or against object	
Physical	Noise	Hearing loss
	Radiation	Reproductive effects and cancer
	Vibration	Raynaud's disease
	Heat	Heat exhaustion and heat stroke
Psychosocial	Stress	Anxiety reactions and a variety of physical symptoms
	Work-home balance	

disease prevention. O'Donnell and Harris (1994, pp. 3-4) describe health promotion as the following:

> the science and art of helping people change their lifestyle to move toward a state of optimal health. Optimal health is defined as a balance of physical, emotional, social, spiritual and intellectual health. Lifestyle change can be facilitated through a combination of efforts to enhance awareness, change behavior and create environments that support good health practices. Of the three, supportive environments will probably have the greatest impact in producing lasting changes.

Disease prevention begins with recognition of a health risk, a disease, or an environmental hazard and is followed by measures to protect as many people as possible from harmful consequences of that risk.

The occupational health nurse uses a variety of primary prevention methods, with one-on-one interaction as an important strategy for evaluating risk reduction behavior for individuals (Rogers, 2000). The occupational health nurse has daily contact with numerous employees for many reasons (e.g., assessment and treatment of episodic illness or injury and health surveillance); therefore this is an important method of promoting health. The phrase "seize the moment" aptly describes the opportunity that exists with every employee encounter.

However, similar to community health nursing professionals, occupational health nurses plan, develop, implement, and evaluate aggregate-focused intervention strategies. The occupational health nurse plans and implements programs such as weight and cholesterol reduction, AIDS awareness, ergonomics training, and smoking cessation (Rogers, 2000).

Performing "walk-throughs" in the workplace on a regular basis, recognizing potential and existing hazards, and maintaining communications with safety and industrial hygiene resources will continue to be critical work for the occupational health nurse (Shortridge-McCauley, 1995).

For overall *health promotion,* the nurse may plan, implement, and evaluate a health fair, which is a multifaceted health promotion strategy that usually includes a number of community health resources to provide expertise on a wide range of health issues and community services. As part of an overall health and wellness strategy, the occupational health nurse may negotiate with the employer for an on-site fitness center or area with fitness equipment; if cost or space is prohibitive, the employer may choose to partially subsidize membership at a local fitness center (Blix, 1999).

Types of *nonoccupational programs* included in the area of primary prevention are cardio-vascular health, cancer awareness, personal safety, immunization, prenatal and postpartum health, accident prevention, retirement health, stress management, and relaxation techniques. Occupational health programs could include topics such as emergency response, first aid and cardiopulmonary resuscitation training, right-to-know training, immunization programs for international business travelers, prevention of back injury through knowledge of proper lifting techniques, ergonomics, and other programs targeted to the specific hazards identified in the workplace (Blix, 1999; Dille, 1999; Sorenson, 1998).

Women's health and safety issues such as maternal-child health, reproductive health, breast cancer education and early detection, stress management, and work-home balance issues will achieve heightened significance as more women enter the workforce. Thirty percent of women currently in the workforce are between ages 16 and 44 years and each year approximately one million infants are born to these women. Interest in workplace safety and the relationship to reproductive outcome continues to grow as women of childbearing age enter the workplace in greater proportions than ever before.

The occupational health nurse can play a key role in the development and delivery of prenatal, postpartum, and childhood programs in the workplace. Of primary importance will be the ability to serve as a change agent to initiate needed programs in the work environment. Employers must be educated regarding strategies not only to reduce health care costs for women and infants, but also to improve the work environment for mothers (McGovern, 1996). Women who believe their employers are interested in the well-being of themselves and their families are more apt to be productive and satisfied employees (Gates and O'Neill, 1990). The occupational health nurse can play a critical role in the shaping of supportive policies and practices to accommodate the needs of families, including flexible working hours, parental leave, and on-site child care (McGovern, 1996).

By 2010, members of *racial and ethnic minority groups* will make up a large share of the expanded labor force (OSHA, 1999). Nonwhites accounted for 29% of the net addition to the workforce between 1985 and 2000 and more than 15% of the workforce in 2000 (OSHA, 1999). As the number of minority and ethnic workers in the workforce increases, so will the illnesses traditionally associated with these groups of workers (e.g., heart disease and stroke, hypertension, cancer, cirrhosis, and diabetes) (Helyer, 1998; Rogers, 1990). In addition to basic health concerns for this population, available statistics indicate that minority workers have been disproportionately concentrated in some of the most dangerous work and they are at greater risk for experiencing many of the leading occupationally-related diseases and injuries. Table 27-4 illustrates the most common occupational diseases and injuries.

The occupational health nurse will face challenges in developing programs that are culturally and linguistically appropriate. The occupational health nurse may be in an advocacy role to negotiate with the employer for changes in the work environment to reduce or eliminate existing or potential occupational exposures to known and potential risk factors.

Secondary Prevention

Secondary prevention strategies are aimed at early diagnosis, early treatment interventions, and attempts to limit disability. The focus at this level of prevention is on identification of health needs, health problems, and employees at risk.

As with primary prevention, the occupational health nurse uses a number of different secondary prevention strategies (Childre, 1997). By providing direct care for episodic illness and injury, the

TABLE 27-4

Work-Related Diseases and Injuries

Work-Related Disease or Injury	Examples of Effect
Occupational lung disease	Cancer and asthma
Musculoskeletal injuries	Back, upper extremity, and musculoskeletal disorders
Occupational cancers	Leukemia, bladder, and skin
Trauma	Death, amputation, and fracture
CVDs	Hypertension and heart disease
Reproductive disorders	Infertility and miscarriage
Neurotoxic disorders	Neuropathy and toxic psychosis
Noise-induced hearing loss	Loss of hearing
Dermatological conditions	Chemical burns and allergies
Psychological disorders	Neurosis; alcohol or substance abuse

occupational health nurse is afforded the opportunity to conduct assessments and provide treatment and referrals for a variety of physical and psychological conditions. The occupational health nurse can offer health screenings, which are designed for early detection of disease, at the work site with relative ease and at minimal cost. Screenings may focus on vision, cancer, cholesterol, hypertension, diabetes, TB, and pulmonary function. Other types of screening may be contracted with a vendor who uses mobile equipment to provide screenings such as mammography.

Secondary prevention efforts provided by the occupational health nurse include *preplacement, periodic,* and *job transfer evaluations* to ensure that the worker is being placed or is continuing to work in a job that is safe for that worker (Meservy et al., 1997). The preplacement evaluation is performed before the worker begins employment in a new company or is placed in a different job (Fig. 27-2). The evaluation is a baseline examination that consists of a medical history, an occupational health history (Fig. 27-3), and a physical assessment that should target the type of work that the employee will be performing (ATSDR, 1999). For example, if the employee is going to be lifting materials in a warehouse, special attention should be paid to any history of musculoskeletal problems. Strength testing and range of motion should be performed for all muscle groups.

The examination may also include medical tests to determine specific organ functions that may be affected by exposure to existing agents in the employee's workplace. For example, if the employee is working with a chemical that is a known liver toxin, baseline liver function tests may be appropriate to determine the current health status of the liver and its ability to handle this specific chemical exposure. However, the preplacement examination must be carefully evaluated to ensure compliance with the ADA, which is discussed later in the chapter.

Periodic assessments usually occur at a regular interval (e.g., annual and biannual) and are based on specific protocols for those exposed to substances or irritants such as lead, asbestos, noise, or various chemicals. Examinations of individuals transferring to other jobs are critical to document any changes in health that may have occurred while the employee was working in a specific area or with a specific process. This is usually done to comply with OSHA regulations or NIOSH recommendations. An example of an OSHA screening and surveillance guide is shown in Fig. 27-4. For full details of compliance requirements, the OSHA standard must be consulted.

Activities must continue to focus on prevention and early detection by increasing awareness of the incidence of other health conditions such as breast cancer and providing accessible and affordable screening programs. Caplan (1998) provides a detailed review of breast cancer screening at the work site. The author cites that it is estimated that 180,000 women were diagnosed with invasive breast cancer in 1997 and that 43,900 women died from the disease, making breast cancer the most commonly diagnosed malignancy among women in the United States (i.e., other than skin cancer) and the second leading cause of cancer death (Parker, 1997). Breast cancer accounts

Text continued on p. 746

FIGURE **27-2**

Preplacement health evaluation.

Preplacement Medical Evaluation			
Part 1 **Health questionnaire**	Have you ever had problems with:	Yes	No
	Heart	_____	_____
	Circulation	_____	_____
	Infection	_____	_____
	Nerves	_____	_____
	Bones	_____	_____
	Muscles	_____	_____
	Lungs/breathing	_____	_____
	Vision/eyes	_____	_____
	Hearing/ears	_____	_____
	Allergies	_____	_____
	If you have answered "yes" to any of the above, please explain:		
	Have you ever:		
	Had an operation	_____	_____
	Become sick from your work	_____	_____
	Had a tetanus shot	_____	_____
	Considered yourself disabled	_____	_____
	(Within the past five years) consulted a physician	_____	_____
	In you have answered "yes" to any of the above, please explain:		
Part 2 **Physical assessment**	Vital signs _____		
	Height and weight _____		
	Vision test _____		
	Hearing test _____		
	Physical examination with review of systems _____		
	Laboratory tests appropriate to work place exposure _____		
	_____		
Part 3 **Medical summary and recommendations**	Applicant is: _____ able to perform job		
	_____ able to perform job with restrictions		
	_____ not able to perform job		
	_____ on hold–awaiting more medical data		
	Diagnosis _____		
	Restrictions _____		
	Recommendations _____		
	Comments _____		

FIGURE **27-3**

Occupational health history. *Continued*

Occupational Health History

Date: _____

Badge or Social Security Number: _____

Name: _____

Age: _____

Shift: _____

Job title: _____

Department: _____

How long in this job/area (i.e., months/years): _____

Average work hours/shift: _____

Physical requirements of work (i.e., hours/days): _____

       Lifting: _____

       Bending: _____

       Sitting: _____

       Repetitive movements: _____

       Standing: _____

       Twisting: _____

       Climbing: _____

Job description: _____

_____

Potential exposures: _____

       Chemical: _____

       Physical: _____

       Biological: _____

       Psychosocial: _____

       Ergonomic: _____

       Safety: _____

Personal protective equipment: _____

       Gloves: _____

       Glasses: _____

       Ear protection: _____

       Lab coat: _____

       Apron: _____

       Face shield: _____

       Goggles: _____

       Mask/respirator: _____

       Other: _____

_____

FIGURE **27-3—cont'd**

Occupational health history.

Do you have a second job? _____

If yes, describe: _____

_____

_____

_____

_____

_____

Chief complaint: _____

Onset of symptoms: _____

Duration of symptoms: _____

Suspected cause: _____

Quality/severity of symptoms: _____

_____

Aggravating factors: _____

_____

_____

Are there coworkers with similar symptoms? _____

Do symptoms change when not at work? _____

Past medical history: _____

_____

_____

_____

_____

_____

Current medications: _____

Hobbies: _____

Family health history: _____

_____

_____

_____

Smoking history: _____

Alcohol history: _____

Recreational drug use: _____

Exercise patterns: _____

Allergies: _____

Other comments: _____

_____

_____

FIGURE **27-4**

Example of screening and surveillance: guide to OSHA standard for benzene.

Guide to OSHA Standard for Benzene	
Standard Requirements Benzene 1910.1028(1)/1926.1128/1915.1028	
Preplacement exam	Yes
Periodic exam	Yes—annual
Emergency/exposure examination and tests	Yes—includes urinary phenol test
Termination exam	No
Examination includes special emphasis on these body systems	Hemopoietic; add cardiopulmonary if respiratory protection used at least 30 days/year, (i.e., initially, then every three years)
Work and medical history	Required for initial and periodic exams (i.e., preplacement exam requires special history)
Chest x-ray	No
Pulmonary function test (PFT)	Initially and every three years if respiratory protection used 30 days/year; specific tester requirements
Other required tests	CBC, differential, other specific blood tests; repeated as required; see standard
Evaluation of ability to wear a respirator	Yes—if respirators are used
Additional tests if deemed necessary	Yes
Written medical opinion	Yes—physician to employer; employer to employee
Employee counseling (i.e., exam results and conditions of increased risk)	Yes—by physician
Medical removal plan	Yes

for about 16.5% of cancer deaths among women. By detecting early malignancies, breast cancer screening reduces the mortality rate in women between ages 50 and 69. Mammography is the most effective method for detecting these early malignancies.

The occupational health nurse is in an excellent position to play a key role in reducing morbidity and mortality associated with breast cancer. Hall (1992) reported that a three-part breast health program composed of BSE with visual reminders and educational materials accompanied by a physical examination and mammography for women older than 35 years is an effective strategy for early detection. Increasingly, the occupational health nurse will be expected to document the return on investment for these and other related activities in the workplace (Friedman, 1995; Kalina et al., 1995; O'Brien, 1995).

Tertiary Prevention

On a tertiary level, the occupational health nurse plays a key role in the rehabilitation and restoration of the worker to an optimal level of functioning. Strategies include case management, negotiation of workplace accommodations, and counseling and support for workers who will continue to be affected by chronic disease (Pergola et al., 1999).

In industry, *disability* costs average 8.4% of payroll. Four percent of the GNP, or $170 billion, is the figure cited for costs associated with total disability (Reith, Ahrens, and Cummings, 1995). In the United States, it is estimated that more than 500,000 workers take an estimated five months of leave from work each year from a physical disability; only 48% return to work (Mannon et al., 1994). Research findings indicate the importance of developing strategies to reinforce the behavioral change of the individual to avoid what is often referred to as the **disability syndrome**, a state in which an individual chooses not to work when medical clearance has been granted (Mundy et al., 1994).

Knowledge of the workplace, the ability to negotiate with the employer for appropriate accommodations, early intervention, and comprehensive case management skills have been and will continue to be essential for the disabled employee's successful return to work. The process of returning an individual to work begins with the onset of injury or illness (Rogers, 1998). Regardless of whether this involves an occupational or a nonoccupational condition, the occupational health nurse is the center of case management. The nurse works closely with the primary care provider to monitor the progress of the ill or injured worker and to identify and eliminate potential barriers in the return-to-work process. The nurse has a comprehensive understanding of the workplace and of the physical requirements necessary for the employee to work. The physical demands analysis (Randolph and Dalton, 1989) is a useful tool in objectively assessing the physical demands of any job (Fig. 27-5). Once the assessment is completed, the occupational health nurse can relay this information to community health professionals caring for the employee.

For workers needing special accommodations, the occupational health nurse can negotiate and facilitate those appropriate to the employee's health limitations (Evangelista-Uhl et al., 1999; Gemignani, 1996; Mueller, 1999). The nurse is often the driving force behind the employer creating a "light duty" pool. The goal of this type of program is to provide temporary work that is less physically demanding in nature than the employee's regular work. This facilitates the employee's return to the workplace earlier than if required to wait until full strength was regained.

The occupational health nurse can monitor and support the health of employees returning to work who continue to experience adverse health effects of chronic disease. For example, the employee who is returning to work after sustaining a myocardial infarction may have blood pressure monitored on a routine basis. Counseling regarding adjustment to normal work life and support for behavior modification (e.g., smoking cessation) may also be provided (Perry, 1996).

In addition, because the workforce is aging and because older workers are more prone to chronic

disease, the occupational health nurse can implement and monitor treatment protocols and assist workers to live and work at their optimum comfort level while managing their disease (Jones and Sanford, 1996). Responsibilities for the care of elderly parents or significant others will influence the balance of work and home for older workers. The occupational health nurse's role as counselor, referral resource for workers, and consultant to management can influence future benefit changes.

SKILLS AND COMPETENCIES OF THE OCCUPATIONAL HEALTH NURSE

Although clinical and emergency care is still an important tenet of occupational health nursing, the current and future practice must focus on a proactive approach with the goal of preventing illness and injury and promoting health. Therefore the occupational health nurse must possess competencies necessary to recognize and evaluate potential and existing health hazards in the workplace. Management and budgeting skills and knowledge of legal and regulatory requirements, toxicology, ergonomics, epidemiology, environmental health, safety, counseling, and health promotion and education are essential to meet the present and future demands of occupational health nursing practice.

Competencies in occupational and environmental health nursing have been delineated in nine categories by AAOHN (Box 27-4) (White et al., 1999). Each competency delineates comprehensive performance criteria at the competent, proficient, and expert level. Each level is described followed by an example of occupational health nursing practice at that level.

Competent

At the "competent" level of practice, the nurse has gained confidence and her perception of the role is one of mastery and an ability to cope with specific situations. There is less of a need to rely on the judgments of peers and other professionals. Work habits tend to stress consistency rather than routinely tailoring care to encompass individual differences (Benner, 1984).

Occupational and environmental health nursing example: The competent nurse is an occupational and environmental health nurse with suffi-

FIGURE 27-5

Physical demands analysis (From Randolph SA, Dalton PC: Limited duty work: an innovative approach to early return to work, *AAOHN J* 37:451, 1989. By permission of the AAOHN).

Physical Demands Analysis

Job title _____ Department _____

Activity	Never	Rarely (5-10%)	Sometimes (10-40%)	Frequently (41-75%)	Always (75-100%)
Standing					
Walking					
Sitting					
Lifting					
10 lb maximum					
20 lb max., up to 10 lb frequently					
50 lb max., up to 25 lb frequently					
100 lb max., up to 50 lb frequently					
>100 lb, 50 lb or more frequently					
Pushing/pulling					
10 lb maximum					
20 lb max., up to 10 lb frequently					
50 lb max., up to 25 lb frequently					
100 lb max., up to 50 lb frequently					
>100 lb, 50 lb or more frequently					
Climbing					
Ladders					
Stairs					
Other (list)					
Balancing					
Stooping					
Kneeling					
Crouching					
Crawling					
Twisting					
Bending					
Reaching					
Overhead					
In front of body					
Handling					
Fingering					
Feeling					
Talking					
Ordinary					
Other					
Hearing					
Ordinary conversation					
Other sounds					
Vision					
Acuity: Near, 20 in or less					
Acuity: Far, 20 ft or more					
Depth perception three-dimensional					
Vision distance judgment					
Accommodation sharpness of vision/focus					
Color vision					
Field of vision (i.e., entire scope of vision/peripheral)					
Any other outstanding physical requirements not previously mentioned (list)					
Shift work					
Environmental conditions:					
Inside					
Outside					
Both					
Dust					
Fumes					
Hazards (describe)					

BOX 27-4

Competency Categories in Occupational and Environmental Health Nursing

1. Clinical and primary care
2. Case management
3. Workforce, workplace, and environmental issues
4. Regulatory and legislative
5. Management
6. Health promotion and disease prevention
7. Occupational and environmental health and safety education and training
8. Research
9. Professionalism

cient experience to recognize a range of practice issues and function comfortably in such roles as clinician, occupational health services coordinator, and case manager. This nurse follows company procedures and relies on assessment checklists and clinical protocols to provide treatment (Rees and Hays, 1996).

Proficient

The "proficient" nurse has an increased ability to perceive client situations as a whole based on past experiences, focusing on the relevant aspects of the situation. The nurse is able to predict the events to expect in a particular situation and can recognize that protocols sometimes must be altered to meet the needs of the client (Benner, 1984).

Occupational and environmental health nursing example: A proficient occupational and environmental health nurse is able to quickly obtain the information needed for accurate assessment and move rapidly to the critical aspects of the problem. Structured goals are replaced by priority setting in response to the situation. This nurse usually possesses sophisticated clinical or managerial skills in the occupational health setting (Rees and Hays, 1996).

Expert

The "expert" nurse has extensive experience and a broad knowledge base and is able to grasp a situation quickly and initiate appropriate action. The nurse has a sense of salience grounded in practice guiding actions and priorities (Benner, 1984).

Occupational and environmental health nursing example: Occupational and environmental health nurses at the expert level include those providing leadership in developing occupational and environmental health policy within an organization; those functioning in upper executive or management roles; those serving as consultants to business and government; and those designing and conducting significant research in the field (Rees and Hays, 1996).

Examples of Skills and Competencies for Occupational Health Nursing

As described, numerous skills and competencies are necessary for occupational health nursing practice. Examples of some of these are outlined here, according to the nine defined areas of competence.

Clinical and Primary Care

- Applying the nursing process in delivery of care
- Providing first aid and primary care according to treatment protocols
- Conducting a physical assessment
- Taking an occupational and environmental health history
- Diagnosing and treating
- Being knowledgeable about immunization protocols
- Identifying employees' emotional needs and providing support and counseling
- Using a multidisciplinary problem-solving approach to occupational health illness and injury
- Maintaining records
- Clinical testing and monitoring
- Responding to medical emergencies
- Being knowledgeable about trends in health-related issues

Case Management

- Identifying the need for case management services
- Conducting case management assessments using a multidisciplinary framework
- Developing case management care plans
- Evaluating resources and vendors for case management
- Implementing early return to work programs
- Monitoring and evaluating outcomes
- Developing policies and programs for case management
- Analyzing trends for case management services

- Designing disability management systems
- Conducting case management outcomes-based research

Workforce, Workplace, and Environmental Issues

- Having knowledge of work site operations, manufacturing processes, and job tasks
- Identifying and monitoring potential and existing workplace exposures
- Influencing appropriate and targeted recommendations for control of workplace hazards
- Having knowledge of toxicological, epidemiological, and ergonomic principles
- Understanding appropriate engineering and administrative controls and personal protective equipment specific to preventing workplace health hazard exposures
- Understanding roles and collaboration with other cross-functional groups as an integral part of a core multidisciplinary team
- Performing risk assessments
- Managing health surveillance programs

Legal and Ethical Responsibilities

- Being knowledgeable of state nursing practice acts and ability to practice occupational health nursing within state guidelines
- Being knowledgeable of federal, state, and municipal regulations pertaining to occupational and environmental health
- Being knowledgeable of the ADA, associated guidelines, and other relevant occupational and environmental health laws
- Being knowledgeable of all aspects of medical record-keeping practices in compliance with nursing practice, state law, and standards of practice
- Being knowledgeable of current legal trends related to negligence and malpractice cases in professional nursing and in the occupational health setting
- Being knowledgeable of confidentiality parameters
- Influencing regulatory and legal processes related to occupational and environmental health

Management and Administration

- Managing budgets
- Hiring staff and management of staff performance

- Fostering professional development plans
- Developing program goals and objectives
- Business planning through knowledge of internal and external resources
- Providing comprehensive on-site services and programs
- Knowing needs of business and employees
- Writing reports
- Performing audits and quality assurance
- Handling workers' compensation and disability
- Performing cost-benefit analyses, cost-effectiveness analyses, and outcomes monitoring
- Allocating appropriate staff resources
- Providing leadership in health-related issues
- Negotiating
- Facilitating work accommodations and return to work
- Coordinating medical response activities and site disaster planning
- Being a resource expert on health issues for employees and management
- Participating in strategic operations planning

Health Promotion and Disease Prevention

- Conducting needs assessments
- Recognizing cultural differences and the relationship to health issues
- Using effective communication styles to match diverse employee and management audiences
- Making effective presentations
- Planning, developing, implementing, and evaluating health programs designed to meet the needs of specific employee groups or organizations
- Evaluating health promotion outcomes
- Applying adult learning theory and principles to health education programs
- Integrating all levels of prevention into company culture

Occupational and Environmental Health and Safety Education

- Creating effective professional and technical support networks both functionally and cross-functionally
- Developing and implementing training programs for workers and professionals

Research

- Identifying researchable problems
- Systematically collecting, analyzing, and interpreting data from different sources

- Recognizing trends in health outcomes by department, work area, or work process
- Planning, developing, and conducting research
- Developing and testing models and theories relative to occupational and environmental health nursing practice

Professionalism
- Engaging in a lifelong learning plan
- Being knowledgeable of AAOHN Standards of Occupational and Environmental Health Nursing and Code of Ethics
- Maintaining currency in practice
- Acting as a professional role model for students and colleagues
- Advancing the specialty through knowledge and science

IMPACT OF FEDERAL LEGISLATION ON OCCUPATIONAL HEALTH

Legislation and associated activities have influenced the practice of occupational health in the United States. Table 27-5 presents a historical perspective of some of the major pieces of legislation that have had, and will continue to have, a direct impact on the general practice of occupational and environmental health nursing. The Occupational Safety and Health Act, Workers' Compensation Acts, and the ADA are highlighted.

Occupational Safety and Health Act

The Occupational Safety and Health Act of 1970 was enacted two years after a major coal-mining disaster in West Virginia. The passage of this legislation came about because there were concerns for worker's health, a burgeoning environmental awareness, union activities, and an increased knowledge about workplace hazards. The general duty clause of the Act states that employers must "furnish a place of employment free from recognized hazards that are causing or likely to cause death or serious physical harm to employees." The Act also identifies the roles of the various government agencies, provides for the establishment of federal occupational safety and health standards, and identifies a structure of penalties, fines, and sentences for violations of regulations. Under the Act, any state has the right to implement its own occupational safety and health administration. The only requirement is that the state standards meet

or exceed federal standards. Currently, 25 states operate state occupational safety and health administrations. The following organizations were formed under the provisions of the Act:

- Under the jurisdiction of the Department of Labor, the **Occupational Health and Safety Administration** (OSHA) is responsible for promulgating and enforcing occupational safety and health standards.
- Under the jurisdiction of the USDHHS, NIOSH is responsible for funding and conducting research, making recommendations for occupational safety and health standards to OSHA, and funding Occupational Safety and Health Education and Research Centers for the training of occupational health professionals.
- The Occupational Safety and Health Review Commission, which is appointed by the president, is responsible for advising OSHA and NIOSH regarding the legal implications of decisions or actions in the course of performing their duties.
- The National Advisory Committee on Occupational Safety and Health, which is appointed by the president, is a group of consumers and professionals who are responsible for making recommendations to OSHA and NIOSH regarding occupational health and safety.
- The National Commission on State Workers' Compensation Laws, appointed by the president, studied the adequacy of state workers' compensation laws and made recommendations to the president on their findings. This commission's work ended as of October 30, 1972.

Since it was instituted, OSHA has promulgated occupational health and safety standards. These are published in the *Code of Federal Regulations* (CFR) and updated on a regular basis. Access to the most recent publication of these standards is a crucial responsibility of the occupational health nurse.

The occupational health nurse must be knowledgeable of Title 29 of the code, part 1910 (29 CFR 1910), and other sections of the code that apply to specific hazards in the workplace. For example, 29 CFR 1904 pertains to OSHA's record keeping requirements and mandates the employer's responsibility to keep records of work-related injuries, illnesses, and deaths. These records must be posted in the workplace for one month per year and made available for review by OSHA at any time. In many cases, the occupa-

TABLE **27-5**

Historical Perspective of Legislation Affecting Occupational Health in the United States

Year	Legislation	Year	Legislation
1836	First restrictive child labor law enacted (Massachusetts)	1877	State legislation passed requiring factory safeguards (Massachusetts)
1879	State legislation passed requiring factory inspections (Massachusetts)	1886	State legislation passed requiring reporting of industrial accidents (Massachusetts)
1910	State legislation passed requiring formation of an Occupational Disease Commission (Illinois)	1911	Workmen's Compensation Act passed (New Jersey)
1935	Social Security Act passed (state and federal unemployment insurance program)	1936	Walsh-Healy Act (federal legislation setting occupational safety and health standards for certain government contract workers)
1938	Fair Labor Standards Act (setting minimum age for child labor)	1948	All states have workers' compensation acts
1964	Civil Rights Act	1965	McNamara-O'Hara Act (extends protection of the Walsh-Healy Act to include suppliers of government services)
1966	Mine Safety Act (mandatory inspections and health and safety standards in mining industry)	1969	Coal Mine Health and Safety Act (mandatory health and safety standards for underground mines)
1970	Occupational Safety and Health Act	1970	EPA established
1970	Consumer Protection Agency established	1972	Equal Employment Opportunity Act
1972	Noise Control Act	1972	Clean Water Act
1973	HMO Act	1973	Rehabilitation Act
1976	Toxic Substances Control Act	1976	Resources Conservation and Recovery Act
1977	Federal Mine Safety and Health Act	1990	Americans with Disabilities Act
1993	Family Medical Leave Act		

tional health nurse has full responsibility for compliance with this standard.

OSHA has 10 regional offices throughout the United States. Inspectors are assigned to each region to enforce the standards and to provide consultation to industries. An OSHA inspection can be initiated in one of several ways. Each office plans a schedule of routine visits to the industries in their respective regions. In the past, funding has been an issue and inspections have not taken place in the quantity or frequency originally intended. An inspection will occur if a major health or safety problem, such as a death, occurs at the work site, or if three or more workers are sent to the hospital as a result of the same incident. Inspection may also occur by employer request. This is not usually done unless the employer has an exemplary occupational health and safety program and wishes to participate in OSHA's voluntary inspection program. Inspection may also be initiated by an employee request if there is concern about a suspected hazardous condition. In this case, OSHA is mandated to respond and it must keep the employee's name confidential at the employee's request. In the past, penalties have been inconsequential and sentences have been served rarely. However, recent events indicate that fines have increased and OSHA has made public its intention to criminally prosecute company executives for serious and willful violations.

In many organizations, the occupational health nurse is the interface with the OSHA inspector. This requires the nurse to be knowledgeable about the potential hazards in the workplace and about the appropriate control measures designed to eliminate or minimize exposure. The nurse should know that employees or their union representatives have the right to accompany the OSHA investigators.

Workers' Compensation Acts

Workers' Compensation Acts are state mandated and state funded. These programs provide income replacement and health care to workers who sustain a work-related injury, temporary or permanent disability, or death. Workers' Compensation Acts also protect the employer if the compensation received by the employee precludes legal suits against the employer. Each state regulates its own workers' compensation program that is unique to that state. The employer can self-insure, contract with commercial insurance carriers, or purchase a policy with the state-operated insurance fund. Workers receive an average of 66% of their take-home pay before taxes and some disabled workers and their families are eligible for other benefit programs, including Old Age, Survivors, Disability, and Health Insurance; SSI; or any other disability program that they may have purchased through the company or on an individual basis.

In an era of high health care costs and a propensity for injured workers to engage the services of lawyers to represent them in negotiating financial settlements, many employers are claiming that workers' compensation costs are crippling their ability to compete in an international marketplace. The occupational health nurse has a unique opportunity to support both the employee and employer in this arena. For the employee, the nurse may be the initial person to whom the work-related injury or illness is reported. Accurate assessment of the injury or illness and appropriate treatment are essential. Community resources must be identified to ensure the injured worker is provided with high-quality health care and appropriate medical follow-up.

The occupational health nurse educates the employee regarding benefits under the Workers' Compensation Act and is often the one who files the claim. If the employee is disabled from work for a period of time, the nurse provides case management support and remains in contact with the employee until return to work. If the employer uses an insurance carrier, the nurse works closely with the claims adjuster to manage the case. The need for light duty or other workplace accommodations is determined before the employee's return. In most cases, the nurse facilitates this process with the employer.

For the employer, the occupational health nurse provides the expertise in early intervention and case management. The goal is to limit the worker's disability and provide an opportunity for early return to work through appropriate workplace accommodations. The desired outcome is a productive employee with optimum health and productivity, with reduced health care and workers' compensation costs.

Americans with Disabilities Act

The ADA, enacted by Congress in July 1990, is a comprehensive act that prohibits discrimination on the basis of disability. The core of this law requires employers to adjust facilities and practices for the purpose of making "reasonable accommodations" to enhance opportunities for individuals with disabilities (Kaminshine, 1991). Employment provisions of this act began on July 26, 1992 for employers with 25 or more employees and were revised in July 1994 to include employees with 15 or more employees. Provisions regarding access to public transportation and accommodations became effective in January 1993.

The ADA defines disability as "physical or mental impairment that substantially limits one or more major life activities; having record of such an impairment; or being regarded as having such an impairment" (Kaminshine, 1991, p. 249). Physical or mental impairment guidelines are the same as those described in the Federal Rehabilitation Act and include "any physiologic disorder or condition, cosmetic disfigurement, anatomical loss affecting any of the major body systems, or any mental or psychological disorder" (Kaminshine, 1991, p. 249). Major life activities include caring for self, walking, seeing, hearing, and speaking. The ADA excludes conditions relating to sexual preference and gender identity, compulsive gambling, kleptomania, and pyromania. The ADA also denies protection for individuals who are currently involved in illegal drug use.

With regard to the ADA, the occupational health nurse has particular responsibility in two areas. The first involves the duty to provide or facilitate reasonable accommodations. This is facilitated by the nurse's familiarity with the physical requirements of jobs in the workplace. The second involves preplacement inquiries and health examinations. Preplacement health examinations will be permitted only if phrased in terms of the applicant's general ability to perform job-related functions rather than in terms of a disability and after a job offer has been made. The examination must be job related and consistently conducted for all applicants performing similar work.

As illustrated in this discussion of specific laws pertinent to occupational health, the legal context for occupational health nursing practice is broad and involves many arenas. The occupational health nurse must be knowledgeable about all laws and regulations that govern any industry where the nurse provides health care to employees (e.g., laboratories, transportation, and utilities).

LEGAL ISSUES IN OCCUPATIONAL HEALTH

In recognition of the dynamic nature of occupational health nursing practice coupled with the influences and impact of larger policy issues, the occupational health nurse must know the legal parameters of practice and respond to legislative mandates that govern worker health and safety (AAOHN, 1999a). The occupational health nurse is professionally and primarily accountable to workers and worker populations and to the employer, the profession, and self (AAOHN, 1999a). In particular, the occupational health nurse must be aware of liability issues confronting the nurse because there is the nature of working independently and the laws governing the employer-employee relationship (Lochlear-Haynes, 1990). Lochlear-Haynes

described the following three legal issues germane to the employer-employee relationship:

- the employee-nurse relationship,
- the employment capacity of the occupational health nurse, and
- any acts of negligence.

The employee-nurse relationship can be confusing when the employer hires the nurse to provide services to the employee. The concern is whether a professional relationship exists under the law or the relationship is based on a coworker status.

MULTIDISCIPLINARY TEAMWORK

As workplaces have become more complex, a diverse array of expertise has emerged in many functional and technical areas. To be successful, the occupational health nurse must recognize the need to work as part of an interdisciplinary team. The nurse may interact with occupational medicine professionals, industrial hygienists, safety professionals, employee assistance counselors, personnel professionals, and union representatives (Fig. 27-6). Community health professionals, insurance carriers, and other support agencies in the community are also critical links. To illustrate the roles and collaborative efforts required to successfully resolve occupational health issues, three cases are described and the roles and responsibilities of each interdisciplinary team member are briefly discussed.

FIGURE **27-6**

The occupational health nurse's professional links in the workplace and community.

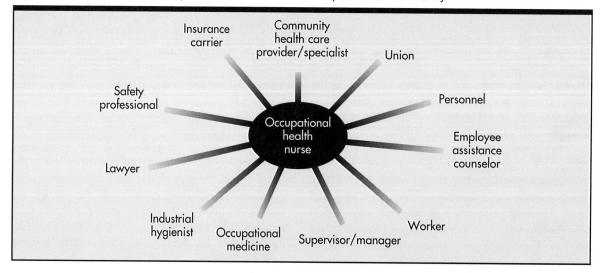

C A S E   S T U D Y   1

APPLICATION OF THE NURSING PROCESS

A 23-year-old woman was transferred into a job that required her to work with chemicals used in photolithography. She was newly married and thought she may be pregnant, but this was unconfirmed. The employee was concerned because the label on one of the pieces of equipment warned of possible adverse effects on reproduction. She stated that she had not felt well since transferring to the job and she thought it was a result of working with chemicals. There were not any restrictions in the work area for pregnant women.

Occupational Health Nurse's Roles and Responsibilities

The occupational health nurse was probably the employee's first contact. The nurse listened to the employee's concerns and formulated a plan.

- Determine information by taking health and occupational health histories.
- Perform a physical assessment and discuss symptoms.
- Schedule a pregnancy test. If this is not a service provided by the occupational health nurse, referral must be made to the employee's health care provider. If the employee does not have one, referral must be made to an appropriate community health resource. Ask the employee to have the care provider document pregnancy test results and obtain written employee consent for release of health information.
- Assure the employee that investigation will ensue immediately and state who will be involved (e.g., industrial hygienist and occupational health physician).
- Assess the work area or request that an industrial hygienist assess the area (e.g., leaking equipment and problems with ventilation).
- Request the most current industrial hygiene data appropriate to the area.
- Schedule the employee to see the occupational health physician once all data are collected regarding medical and industrial hygiene.

- Communicate any recommended work restrictions to the supervisor or personnel department after the occupational health physician examines the employee.
- Review the case in light of existing company policies and recommend control as necessary.
- Maintain confidentiality of health information except when released by written consent of the employee.

Industrial Hygienist's Roles and Responsibilities

- Discuss the employee's concerns with the occupational health nurse and, as necessary, with the employee.
- Provide the most current industrial hygiene data and analysis for the work area under investigation.
- If current data are not available, monitor for industrial hygiene as soon as possible.
- Meet with the occupational health nurse and the occupational health physician as necessary for data communication and analysis.

Occupational Health Physician's Roles and Responsibilities

- Review the data with the occupational health nurse.
- View the work area and process.
- Discuss the data with the industrial hygienist.
- Interview and examine the employee.
- Make recommendations regarding the employee's health and safety.

Employee's Roles and Responsibilities

- Take a pregnancy test and provide documentation of results to the occupational health nurse.
- Communicate concerns to the occupational health nurse and, as necessary, to the industrial hygienist.

Continued

- Keep appointments with the occupational health physician.
- Follow the recommendations of the occupational health physician.

Supervisor's or Manager's Roles and Responsibilities

- Allow investigation of the work area by the occupational health nurse and industrial hygienist.
- Follow restriction recommendations of the occupational health physician.

Primary Community Health Care Provider's Roles and Responsibilities

- Before arriving at a diagnosis, confer with the occupational health nurse or occupational medical consultant.
- Obtain all workplace data relevant to the case for the purpose of formulating an appropriate treatment plan.
- Provide reproductive counseling to the family.
- Refer to appropriate specialists or community resources (e.g., March of Dimes and occupational or environmental pregnancy hotlines).

CASE STUDY 2

APPLICATION OF THE NURSING PROCESS

A supervisor called the occupational health nurse and stated that one of his employees appeared to be incapacitated. The employee was functioning normally in the morning, but had appeared to be intoxicated since returning from lunch. The supervisor was concerned for the employee's and others' safety and he requested assistance.

Occupational Health Nurse's Roles and Responsibilities

- Request that the supervisor accompany the employee to the occupational health nurse's office.
- Perform a physical assessment of the employee.
- Depending on the findings, the occupational health nurse will send the employee home with a family member; send the employee to a community care provider in the hospital via an ambulance for assessment; refer to employee assistance program; or, if there is concern for personal safety, notify security.
- Notify the employee and supervisor that the employee needs to follow-up with the occupational health nurse on returning to work.
- If the employee is sent to the hospital, communicate with the hospital the reason for referral and request communication regarding assessment and disposition.
- On the employee's return to work, assess the employee's fitness for work; counsel, as appropriate, regarding alcohol or drug concerns; and make a referral to an appropriate resource (e.g., employee assistance counselor if available or appropriate community health resource).
- Notify the supervisor when the employee is medically cleared to return to work.
- Maintain confidentiality of health information except where released by employee's written consent.

Supervisor's or Manager's Roles and Responsibilities

- Accompany the employee to the occupational health nurse's office.
- Consult with the human resources professional regarding company policy for this type of employee behavior.
- Do not allow the employee in the workplace until medically cleared by the occupational health nurse.

Employee Assistance Counselor's Roles and Responsibilities

- Provide confidential counseling.
- Make appropriate decisions regarding referrals to community health resources.

Security's Roles and Responsibilities

- Protect the physical safety of all involved.

Community Health Resources' Roles and Responsibilities

- Emergency medical technicians or ambulance staff: provide safe transport to the hospital.
- Hospital: perform an assessment of the worker and communicate results to the occupational health nurse.
- Community counseling resource: accept referral and provide counseling for worker as appropriate.

Employee's Roles and Responsibilities

- Go to the occupational health nurse's office for initial assessment.
- On return to work, discuss fitness for duty with the occupational health nurse.
- Accept referral for treatment.

Family's Responsibilities

- Accept responsibility that alcohol or substance abuse is a family issue by acknowledging the problem.
- Assist in directing the individual to appropriate care with community health care providers.
- Seek community resources for guidance and support (e.g., AA, Al-Anon, Narcotics Anonymous, and other local support groups).

CASE STUDY 3

APPLICATION OF THE NURSING PROCESS

Forty percent of the 80 packers in Department X were experiencing upper extremity musculoskeletal symptoms that appeared to be related to their job activities. An evaluation of their job tasks indicated that the workers may experience musculoskeletal disorders from the repetitive, forceful motions combined with nonneutral postures and insufficient rest periods.

Occupational Health Nurse's Roles and Responsibilities

- Assess symptomatic individuals and refer to an occupational medical consultant as appropriate.
- Conduct a walk-through of the work area to assess job tasks by direct observation or videotaping.
- Evaluate OSHA 200 log, daily health services log, and workers' compensation and disability case statistics.

- Meet with Department X manager to discuss the issues and propose solutions.
- Plan, develop, implement, and evaluate an ergonomics educational program for workers.
- Work with the multidisciplinary team to identify appropriate intervention strategies.
- Document cost-effectiveness of interventions.
- Maintain confidentiality of health information except where released by employee's written consent.

Occupational Medical Consultant's Roles and Responsibilities

- Review data with the occupational health nurse.
- Conduct a walk-through of the work area.
- Diagnose the employee's condition and make appropriate treatment recommendations (e.g., restricted work, application of ice, use of antiinflammatory agents, and referral).

Continued

Employee's Roles and Responsibilities

- Report symptoms to the occupational health nurse as soon as they occur.
- Adhere to the recommended treatment regimen.
- Attend educational sessions.

Supervisor's or Manager's Roles and Responsibilities

- Meet with the occupational health nurse, medical consultant, and employees.
- Follow the recommendations of the multidisciplinary team.
- Recognize potential problems (e.g., insufficient rest breaks; forceful, repetitive motions; and nonneutral postures).
- Support decisions.

Health Care Provider's Roles and Responsibilities

- Accept referral from occupational medical consultant or occupational health nurse and evaluate data regarding the workplace.
- Assess the employee and develop a treatment plan.
- Communicate the plan to the occupational health nurse and make recommendations for work restrictions.

SUMMARY

This chapter describes the evolution of occupational health nursing during its first century of practice. Current and future demographics and business trends are highlighted as they relate to this nursing specialty area. Aging workers, escalating health care costs, increasing numbers of women and minorities in the workforce, and the competitive international marketplace are key factors shaping occupational health nursing practice.

The occupational health nursing role is challenging and can have a tremendous impact on the quality and delivery of health care to workers and their families. Nurses working in occupational settings should have an excellent understanding of all levels of prevention and possess the skills and competencies outlined here.

For the CHN who works in other settings such as home health, clinics, and schools, knowledge of occupational health nursing practice is also important. Many companies do not have on-site occupational health nurses and therefore must rely on CHNs to support their occupational health and safety needs.

LEARNING ACTIVITIES

1. A large automobile manufacturer needs a program designed to control respiratory disease among foundry workers. Workers in different areas of ferrous foundries are exposed to different respiratory hazards. The main problems are exposure to silica and formaldehyde. The corporation would like to develop a pilot program for one of its foundries that will then be applied to its other foundries. Health and industrial hygiene data will be collected. Both the corporation and the workers support the project and both see the project as having the following three purposes:
   - detecting health effects in individuals who may benefit from intervention,
   - determining the relationship of health effects to environmental exposures, and
   - identifying control strategies as appropriate.
   Outline a pilot program. Discuss the implications of discovering adverse health effects among current workers. Describe the roles of the occupational health nurse, physician, industrial hygienist, safety professional, manager, and employee.

2. The fear of AIDS has created problems in many work sites. Some believe policies should exist; others believe HIV testing should be done at the work site. Still others affirm that education is the best approach for dealing with this extremely volatile issue.
   - Is AIDS a concern for health care workers?
   - Is AIDS a concern for occupational health nurses?

■ Should an AIDS policy be in place at the company?

■ Discuss what to include in the policy.

■ How has the nursing practice changed, if at all, as a result of AIDS?

3. A weight-loss program was conducted during August. Ten people participated in the six-week program. The total weight loss for the group was 185 pounds. The following chart indicates the weight loss for the individuals:

Weight Before Program (lb)	Weight After Program (lb)
215	190
175	160
139	129
275	245
145	120
198	183
120	115
243	233
185	145
210	200

Is there a more effective way to show the results of the program? Assume a peer distributed this report for critique. Be creative, filling in any data, facts, figures, or other information that may be missing. Redesign a report to send to management.

4. Take an occupational history on five currently employed workers. Identify the occupation, associated job tasks, and potential health hazards. Describe control strategies that could minimize or eliminate the risk of adverse health effects.

5. Conduct a literature review to identify critical concepts in occupational health nursing, epidemiology, ergonomics, safety, industrial hygiene, and ethics.

REFERENCES

Agency for Toxic Substances and Disease Registry: Reproductive and developmental hazards: an overview for occupational and environmental health nurses, *AAOHN J* 46:57-66, 1999.

American Association of Industrial Nurses: *The nurse in industry,* New York, 1976, The Author.

American Association of Occupational Health Nurses: *Standards of occupational and environmental health nursing,* Atlanta, 1999a, The Author.

American Association of Occupational Health Nurses: *Compensation and benefits study,* Atlanta, 1999b, The Author.

Barlow R: Role of the occupational health nurse in the year 2000: perspective view, *AAOHN J* 40:463-467, 1992.

Benner P: *From novice to expert: excellence and power in clinical nursing practice,* Menlo Park, Calif, 1984, Addison-Wesley.

Blix A: Integrating occupational health protection and health promotion: theory and program application, *AAOHN J* 47:168-174, 1999.

Bowling M: Measuring the financial impact of workers' comp managed care techniques, *Workers' Comp* 5:38-47, 1996.

Caplan L: Worksite breast cancer screening programs: a review, *AAOHN J* 46:443-453, 1998.

Childre F: Nurse managed occupational health services: a primary care model in practice, *AAOHN J* 45:484-490, 1997.

Digital Equipment Corporation: *1995 HMO performance standards,* Maynard, Mass, 1995, Digital Equipment Corporation.

Dille JH: A worksite influenza immunization program: impact on lost work days, health care utilization, and health care spending, *AAOHN J* 47:301-309, 1999.

Evangelista-Uhl G et al: Transitional duty: an overview of program management and placement process, *AAOHN J* 47:324-334, 1999.

Felton JS: The genesis of occupational health nursing: part I, *Occup Health Nurs* 28:45-49, 1985.

Felton JS: The genesis of occupational health nursing: part II, *AAOHN J* 34:210-215, 1986.

Friedman LC et al: Breast cancer screening behaviors and intentions among asymptomatic women 50 years of age and older, *Am J Prev Med* 11:218-233, 1995.

Gates D, O'Neill N: Promoting maternal-child wellness in the workplace, *AAOHN J* 34:258-263, 1990.

Gemignani J: Early return-to-work shows promise, *Business Health* 14:75, 1996.

Hall LS: Breast self-examination: use of a visual reminder to increase practice, *AAOHN J* 40:186-192, 1992.

Helyer A et al: Effectiveness of a worksite smoking cessation program in the military: program evaluation, *AAOHN J* 46:238-245, 1998.

Jones M, Sanford J: Disability demographics: how are they changing? *Team Rehab Report* 36-44, October 1996.

Kalina CM et al: Building a nurse initiated wellness program: successful program, *AAOHN J* 43:144-147, 1995.

Kaminshine S: New rights for the disabled: the Americans with Disabilities Act of 1990, *AAOHN J* 39:249-251, 1991.

Konstantinos K, Crespo J: Cost effective, hospital based occupational health services: successful program, *AAOHN J* 46:127-132, 1998.

Kosinski M: Effective outcomes management in occupational and environmental health, *AAOHN J* 46:500-510, 1998.

Kuhar M: Critical thinking: a framework for problem solving in the occupational setting, *AAOHN J* 46:80-81, 1998.

Lochlear-Haynes T: Public health in the workplace: part II. Liability issues confronting the occupational health nurse, *AAOHN J* 38:78-79, 1990.

Mannon JA et al: A case management tool for occupational health nurses: development, testing, and application, *AAOHN J* 42:365-373, 1994.

McGovern PM, Cossi DA: Work and family: policy and program options affecting occupational health, AAOHN J 44(8):408-418, 1996.

McGrath BJ: *Nursing in commerce and industry,* New York, 1946, The Commonwealth Fund.

Meservy D et al: Health surveillance: effective components of a successful program, *AAOHN J* 45:500-511, 1997.

Mueller JL: Returning to work through job accommodation: a case study, *AAOHN J* 47:120-130, 1999.

Mundy RR et al: Disability syndrome: the effects of early vs. delayed rehabilitation intervention, *AAOHN J* 42:379-383, 1994.

Murphy D: The primary care role in occupational health nursing, *AAOHN J* 37:470-474, 1989.

O'Brien S: Occupational health nursing roles: future challenges and opportunities, *AAOHN J* 43:148-152, 1995.

Occupational Safety and Health Administration: *The future of work,* Washington, DC, 1999, The Author.

O'Donnell M, Harris J: *Health promotion in the workplace,* New York, 1994, Delmar.

Parker SL et al: Cancer statistics 1997, *CA Cancer J Clin* 47:5-27, 1997.

Parker-Conrad JE: A century of practice: occupational health nursing, *AAOHN J* 36:156-161, 1988.

Pergola T et al: Case management services for injured workers: providers' perspectives, *AAOHN J* 47:397-404, 1999.

Perry MC: REACH: an alternative early to work program, *AAOHN J* 44:294-299, 1996.

Randolph SA, Dalton PC: Limited duty work: an innovative approach to early return to work, *AAOHN J* 37:446-452, 1989.

Rees P, Hays B: Fostering expertise in occupational health nursing, *AAOHN J* 44:67-72, 1996.

Reith L, Ahrens A, Cummings D: Integrated disability management: taking a coordinated approach to managing employee disabilities, *AAOHN J* 43:270-275, 1995.

Rogers B: Establishing research priorities in occupational health nursing, *AAOHN J* 37:493-500, 1989.

Rogers B: Occupational health nursing expertise, *AAOHN J* 46:477-483, 1998.

Rogers B: Occupational health nursing practice, education, and research: challenges for the future, *AAOHN J* 38:536-543, 1990.

Rogers B: Occupational health nursing research priorities, *AAOHN J* 48:9-16, 2000.

Rogers B, Lawhorn E: Occupational health nursing strategies for health promotion. In Hickey J, Ovimetle R, Venegoni S, editors: *Advanced practice nursing,* Philadelphia, 2000, Lippincott.

Shortridge-McCauley L: Reproductive hazards: an overview of exposures to health care workers, *AAOHN J* 43:614-621, 1995.

Sorenson G et al: The effects of a health promotion-health protection intervention on behavior change: the well-works study, *Am J Public Health* 88:1685-1690, 1998.

Travers PH: *A comprehensive guide for establishing an occupational health service,* Atlanta, 1987, AAOHN.

US Department of Health and Human Services: *Healthy people 2010: conference edition,* Washington, DC, 2000, PHS.

Vernarac E: The consumer as healthcare manager: the state of health care in America 1997, special report, *Business Health* 15:51-54, 1996.

Videbeck SL: Critical thinking: a model, *J Nurs* 36:23-28, 1997.

Wachs J: Nurse managed occupational health centers: an overview, *AAOHN J* 45:477-483, 1997.

White K et al: Competencies in occupational and environmental health nursing: practice in the new millennium, *AAOHN J* 47:552-568, 1999.

Correctional Health

Jill Powell

OBJECTIVES

Upon completion of this chapter, the reader will be able to do the following:

1. Describe the role of the nurse in a correctional setting.
2. Identify factors affecting health and wellness in a correctional setting.
3. Discuss psychosocial issues related to incarceration.
4. Integrate legal and ethical concerns into nursing practice in a correctional setting.

KEY TERMS

compassionate release
deliberate indifference
prison culture

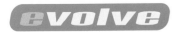

http://evolve.elsevier.com/Nies/

Violence and incarceration have grasped the nation's attention. The visual and print media put Americans face-to-face with the influence of crime and its consequences. Events such as the murder of Mathew Sheppard because he was gay, school violence in the once quiet suburbs, and racially motivated murders were etched into the social consciousness at the dawn of a new millennium. People are confronted with much information, many questions, and few answers in regard to violent youths, gun control, and violence in entertainment.

Regardless of individual opinions about these questions, several facts are relevant. The number of people incarcerated in prisons and jails across the United States has doubled since 1990. Males in a correctional population increased by two thirds from 1980 to 1996. The number of women incarcerated doubled during the same period (Bureau of Justice, 1999). Nurses working in any environment are likely to care for individuals who are currently or have been incarcerated. The purpose of this chapter is to articulate the primary health care issues and corresponding nursing care for people who are incarcerated. In addition, the unique political and ethical issues associated with nursing practice in a correctional facility are presented.

HISTORY AND DEVELOPMENT OF CORRECTIONAL ENVIRONMENTS

The method of controlling crime and criminals by isolating them from other people is a relatively modern phenomenon. Before the 1700s, correctional environments were places of transition for offenders awaiting execution or corporal punishment. Execution and physical torture were deterrents to crime and a means of ensuring social order. Punishment was brutal, deadly, and public. Concerned with the inhumane and barbaric punishment, the American Quaker movement collectively opposed capital punishment. The Great Law of 1682, drafted by William Penn and sanctioned by the colonial assembly, favored hard labor in a house of corrections instead of execution and torture. Being a prisoner became a form of punishment instead of a place of transition before execution (Camhi, 1998; Friedman, 1993).

Another alternative to corporal punishment before the 1800s was extradition. England transported approximately 50,000 criminal exiles to the American colonies between 1607 and 1776 to attempt to meet growing labor and economic demands in colonial areas. Hard labor replaced execution for all but a few

offenses. During this time, John Howard, a noted English prison reformer, advocated for clean accommodations, segregation of prisoners by gender, nature of offense, and for the first time, access to health care. Howard's notion of an ideal prison also included forced labor to combat idleness.

The French Revolution gave new meaning to liberty. The loss of liberty was considered a serious deterrent to crime and the assigned sentence of incarceration was equivalent to the crime. Long sentences of incarceration rather than execution created communities of hundreds or thousands of individuals working, eating, sleeping, and living together for years. During the Industrial Revolution, the masses of prisoners were used for their labor. In 1817, a private citizen contracted with the state of New York for the labor of its prisoners. Prisons became revenue-producing entities for state and local governments. Under the auspices of the convict leasing program, prison labor became a sought-after commodity, adding about $25,000 of additional revenue to state coffers (Wilson, 1993). Perhaps the most recognizable form of prison labor is the chain gang. The Good Roads Association, charged with building and improving roads throughout the South, used prison labor to accomplish the task. Masses of men chained together, working along roadsides, and supervised by armed guards was a common scene in southern states in the 1800s. The practice of hard labor as punishment continued until legislated prison reform in the 1930s (Lischlenser, 1993).

Present-day companies do not contract for prison labor, but contract for the prisons themselves. The Corrections Corporation of American (CCA) manages more private prisons in the United States than any other corporation. Founded in 1983, CCA was the first company to push for the privatization of what had historically been public services. The privatization of public prisons is the correctional equivalent to HMOs. Companies such as CCA are paid a capitated per-inmate rate by state government to manage correctional facilities.

In a 1996 audit, the General Accounting Office did not find a cost savings associated with privatization of public prisons, but in many cases the incidence of violence was greater than that in state-run facilities (Bates, 1998; Wilson, 1993). In 1995, 151 new prisons were constructed and 171 prisons were expanded in the United States. During the same time, the rate of felony offenses decreased with the exception of drug-related offenses. The economic burden of housing inmates soared in the two last decades from total direct expenditures in 1980 of $4,257,509 to $21,266,053 in 1994; privatization has become a viable alternative to manage rising cost (Bureau of Justice, 1999).

ISSUES IN NURSING CARE IN A CORRECTIONAL SETTING

The correctional setting presents unique issues for nursing practice. Unlike any other care setting, patients are inmates and care is negotiated with recognition of safety and security issues for the nurse and the constitutional right of prisoners to receive adequate and timely health care. The primary goals in correctional facilities are security and a safe and humane environment for inmates. Health care, including nursing care, is a necessary and essential part of that environment.

Maintenance of a Safe Environment

Correctional facilities are by nature violent environments. For inmates with particularly violent histories, nursing care must be provided under the watchful eye of security personnel. Occasionally inmates will be escorted to the prison health clinic in handcuffs. Nurses practicing in correctional settings must continually negotiate security *and* nursing care. Standard notions of the development of a therapeutic relationship take on new meaning. Nurses in this setting must be aware that even medical supplies issued to inmates can be a threat to the security environment. For example, a simple elastic bandage can be used to improve the grip on a homemade weapon. Virtually any prescribed medication can have value on the prison "black market." People who are incarcerated have limited options in meeting their needs. Nurses and the health care environment are subject to manipulation by inmates, who may seek medical and nursing care for reasons other than health. Nurses may simply be "someone" to talk to in an inherently isolating environment. Nursing decisions can become avenues to a changed work assignment, different living arrangements, or supplemental diets. Perhaps the greatest challenge for nurses is interacting with inmates without assuming the worst, but always being aware that it can happen.

The case on the top of p. 764 graphically illustrates that nurses working in a correctional environment are ultimately responsible for their own safety. Several issues in the previous scenario can be altered to create a safe environment for nursing practice in

a correctional setting. The nurse must maintain an escape route should a situation of personal violence occur. In addition, no nursing care situation in a correctional environment requires a nurse to be locked in an enclosed environment with an inmate. Although it might appear that providing humane, therapeutic nursing care in an environment of potential violence is contradictory, it is ultimately a prerequisite for nursing practice in corrections (Bell and Allen, 1998).

Prison Culture

Understanding the **prison culture** is essential to nursing practice in corrections. Where people are incarcerated, often for significant periods of time, a distinct way of life evolves. Prison culture has its own rules, language, and traditions. Prison language is often a form of expression that is not understandable to the outside world. It is a mechanism of communication that has evolved from a unique set of circumstances, perhaps to have ownership over something in a place where ownership is often denied or simply insider communication in a world where extreme surveillance is the norm.

Although an exhaustive list of prison language cannot be provided in this chapter, nurses must understand prison lingo surrounding issues related to health care. The nurse should also be aware that prison language is variable by geography, from prison to prison, and among distinct cultural groups within prisons.

Call is a word often used by inmates to describe the time of day that medications are dispensed. An inmate might ask, "When is call?" meaning "What time do I come to the clinic to get my medication?" The place where inmates go to receive medication is known as the *pill line*. Other inmates call an inmate with a mental illness a *cat-j*. A *clipper pass* is special permission for an inmate to shave only once a week. Nurses or other health care providers hand out clipper passes. Nurses can authorize a *lay-in pass* giving an inmate permission to be off work for a specified period of time. A common language also exists for specific illness. An inmate infected with HIV is known by other inmates as a *gangster*. After inmates have been notified by a nurse that they have contracted hepatitis C, the response might be, "So now I am *high class*." An inmate reporting a desire to *cut up* is likely referring to suicidal ideation or intent to harm himself or herself.

Common language associated with drug culture in prisons includes hot meds, jones, julep, and muling.

In a county jail in Georgia in 1996, two nurses were attacked and beaten by an inmate being held on aggravated assault charges. The deputy on duty responsible for protecting them was also subdued by the inmate. These nurses were locked inside the jail with the inmate with their freedom, mobility, and flight to safety limited. The nurses sued the sheriff and deputy for failing to protect them in their work environment. The lawsuit was dismissed because the court determined that the nurses did not have a constitutional right to protection from harm in the work environment (Cohen, 1999a, p. 34).

Hot meds are prescribed drugs that have a black market value in prison culture, including any controlled substance and most psychotropic medications. *Jones* is the term that inmates use to describe a signification drug addiction. Bizarre behavior associated with drug use is often referred to as *jonesing.* *Julep* refers to homemade prison alcohol. The movement of contraband from one place in the prison to another is known as *muling* and the inmates who transport the contraband are known as *mules.*

The two most common words or phrases associated with violence in the correctional environment are shank and smoke on the horizon. A *shank* refers to a hand-made weapon. For example, "He is carrying a shank" means that an inmate is armed. Anticipated violence is described as *smoke on the horizon.* A nurse practicing in a correctional environment might hear, "There is smoke on the horizon. Be careful" as a warning to planned violence (Camhi, 1998).

Prison gangs are often associated with and held liable for prison violence. Several gangs are known to be active in prison populations. Each gang has unique identifiers and characteristics. For many inmates, prison gangs are a source of protection, which is consistent with the notion that being alone and surviving in a correctional facility is difficult if not impossible. The most commonly identified prison gangs are the Aryan Brotherhood, Gangster Disciples, Black Guerrilla Family, and Mexican Mafia. Gang affiliation varies geographically and from institution to institution. Although each gang is collectively known for specific activities within prisons, many are involved in drug trade, extortion, and gang-related violence. The Point Group, a research firm associated with the American Corrections Association, recently conducted a survey to explore gang management in state and local correctional facilities. Approximately 50% of institutions surveyed have a formal policy for dealing with gang-related activities. Roughly 20% of inmates suspected of gang-related activities are isolated or segregated from the rest of the prison population. Identification of gang members, monitoring of gang activities, and promotion of gang awareness of correctional officers were the most common activities designed to manage gang violence in these facilities (National Commission on Correctional Health Care [NCCHC], 1999).

PATTERNS OF HEALTH AMONG INCARCERATED PEOPLE

Minorities and people of lower SES are disproportionately represented in the population in correctional facilities across the United States (Corrections Connection Network, 1999). This same population generally experiences limited access to health care, having little or no preventative health care or health education before being incarcerated. Consequently, today's prison inmate often enters prison with significant nursing care issues. Nurses employed in the correctional setting are likely to see health care problems that are similar to those in an acute care community outpatient clinic. The daily operation of a correctional clinic includes management of acute and chronic illness. Most health care clinics in correctional environments screen each inmate upon entry into the facility. The health care triage process generally includes a physical health history and a mental health history. Many significant health care issues are recognized during the screening process, often for the first time.

The most critical heath care issues among the incarcerated population are chronic and communicable diseases. As increasing numbers of inmates move from the correctional system to the community, it is difficult to separate community health care and correctional health care; the health care problems of an incarcerated population affect public health. HIV, hepatitis, and TB have become paramount health care issues in the inmate population (Bureau of Justice, 1999).

Human Immunodeficiency Virus

The rate of HIV infection among prison inmates is estimated to be six times that of the general population. Blacks and Hispanics are disproportionately affected. Approximately 2.3% of all state and federal prison inmates are infected with HIV. The most recent data indicate that 5874 inmates in the United States had confirmed AIDS, 1959 experienced symptoms associated with HIV, and 15,697 were HIV-positive and asymptomatic. The rate of infection is 2.2% among male inmates and 3.5% among female inmates of a population of 1.8 million inmates in the United States. AIDS is the second leading cause of death among incarcerated people, second only to natural causes of death other than AIDS. The rate of death as a result of AIDS is three times that of the general population. The high rate of HIV infection in this population is related to the following high-risk behaviors: drug use, unprotected sexual intercourse, and tattooing (Bayer, 1997; Behrendt, 1994; Hammet and Wilson, 1994).

The most common approach to decreasing the rate of HIV infection in prison inmates has been prevention and education programs. The most recent result of a National Institute of Justice survey indicates that "only 10% of state and federal prison systems and 5% of local city and county jail systems offer comprehensive programs" of prevention and education related to HIV and AIDS (US Department of Justice [USDOJ], 1998).

In 1996, WHO (WHO, 1996) developed guidelines for HIV infection and AIDS in prisons. These guidelines are written from a public health perspective with the purpose of articulating comprehensive education and prevention strategies and guidelines for the treatment of inmates already infected. The following is a sample of WHO guidelines:

- All prisoners have the right to health care equivalent to the standard of care available in the community.
- Specific policies for the prevention of HIV and AIDS should be in place in all correctional facilities.
- Preventive measures for HIV and AIDS should be based on the actual risk behaviors in correctional facilities, including unprotected sex and needle sharing.
- Voluntary, not mandatory, testing should be made available to prisoners along with pretest and posttest counseling.

- Isolation of inmates with HIV is not considered appropriate or useful.
- Disciplinary measures should be decided without reference to HIV status.
- Medical and psychosocial treatment equivalent to treatment that is available in the community should be available to prisoners who are infected with HIV.
- The HIV status of prison inmates should remain confidential except when the information is necessary for medical treatment.

In summary, WHO guidelines focus on prevention, education, and treatment equivalent to community standards for incarcerated individuals with HIV infection.

The U.S. Department of Justice (USDOJ) also addresses the previously mentioned issues related to HIV-infected inmates. The USDOJ recognized prevention and education as the greatest deterrent to HIV infection among prison inmates. A survey by the National Institute for Justice and the CDC (USDOJ, 1998) determined that the exact content of such programs in the United States was unknown and that the type of prevention and education available in prisons is a highly charged political issue. Condom use, other safe sex practices, and needle exchange programs have been effective at reducing HIV infection in the general population. From the administrative viewpoint, offering condoms and needle exchange programs in correctional facilities would "acknowledge" the existence of illegal drug use and sexual activity in prisons. Most state and federal correctional institutions unfortunately have not adopted condom distribution or other harm-reduction strategies in prisons.

Before 1990, most correctional facilities segregated or isolated inmates based on HIV status. By 1997, most prisons had abolished segregation policies. The National Institute for Justice and the CDC found that most inmates with HIV in U.S. prisons were housed on a case-by-case basis. For example, inmates who are severely immunocompromised might be segregated from the general inmate population, but few universal segregation-housing policies exist. People with HIV would ideally have access to all programs available in the correctional facility; however, some facilities restrict HIV-infected inmates from food service work, further perpetuating the myth that HIV is transmitted through handling food (USDOJ, 1998).

WHO recommends a standard of treatment consistent with treatment available in the community. The current community standard for medical treatment of HIV-infected individuals is combination protease and retroviral therapy (Derb, 1997). Approximately 93% of state and federal correctional facilities offer combination pharmacological therapy. Clinical trials have increased the accessibility of new HIV therapies. In 1997, 242 inmates in seven correctional systems were enrolled in clinical trials of anti-HIV medications (Collins and Baumgartner, 1995). However, viral load monitoring essential to ongoing treatment and monitoring the effectiveness of medication regimens is available in only 50% of correctional facilities. Although medical treatment in corrections is consistent with community treatment prevention, education and transition to the community after discharge has not been adequately developed (USDOJ, 1998).

Hepatitis

Hepatitis B and C have become increasingly serious health care issues in correctional facilities. Although data are incomplete, the rate of hepatitis B and C infection is higher among inmates than in the general population. Prison inmates represent the population at highest risk for hepatitis (e.g., the medically underserved, injection drug users, people with tattoos, and immigrants or refuges from areas with a high incidence of hepatitis B and C). Hepatitis C infection is further associated with HIV infection and injection drug use. For example, in a 1994 survey, 41% of incoming California inmates were positive for hepatitis C, including 61% of HIV-positive men and 85% of HIV-positive women. A study in Nova Scotia found that 52% of injection drug users had hepatitis C infection and only 3% of noninjection drug users were infected. The National Commission on Correctional Health Care (NCCHC) recommends that all inmates be screened and, if indicated, treated for hepatitis upon incarceration. The NCCHC also recommends education for all staff members and inmates related to modes of transmission, prevention, treatment, and disease progression (Hofragle, 1997; NCCHC, 1999).

Tuberculosis

The rate of TB is three times greater among incarcerated people than in the general population. The rate of infection in correctional facilities is related to prison overcrowding and poor ventilation, both conducive to the spread of the disease (Hammet and Wilson, 1994). In 1996, the CDC released general recommendations for the prevention and control of TB in correctional facilities, including the following:

- TB screening for all staff members and inmates
- Containment by preventing transmission and providing adequate treatment to inmates with the disease
- Ongoing monitoring and evaluation of screening and containment efforts

As in the public domain, TB, especially in its antibiotic resistant forms, will continue to be a major threat to the health of incarcerated people in the foreseeable future.

SPECIAL POPULATIONS IN CORRECTIONAL SETTINGS

Women and adolescents have unique health care issues in prison populations.

Women

Approximately 85% of incarcerated women in state and federal prisons in the United States have children and most of them are single heads of households. Additionally, 60% of women in prison report previous physical or sexual abuse. An estimated 72% of women in prison have used illegal drugs at some time in their life and 30% reported daily use for at least one month before incarceration. Cocaine, heroin, LSD, or phencyclidine hydrochloride (PCP) was the drug of choice for 24% of those women. Given these statistics, the fact that women use correctional health care services at twice the frequency of men is not surprising.

Drug use and victimization, combined with the stress associated with being separated from their children, place incarcerated women at risk for many mental and physical health problems, including the risk of HIV infection and other STDs (USDOJ, 1990). Unfortunately, health care providers in correctional facilities have limited experience and training to meet the unique health care needs of women in prison and quality of care is adversely affected. For example, women who have been sexually assaulted are often reticent about obtaining regular gynecologic examinations. Health care providers unaware of this phenomenon might simply label this behavior as noncompliance or resistance to care. The NCCHC confirms that routine gynecological examinations are not consistently a part of health screening for women upon entry into a correctional facility or a routine part of ongoing health care. Given the unique health care issues for women who are incarcerated, the NCCHC (1999) offers the following to guide the provision of health care:

■ Correctional institutions' health care intake procedures should include comprehensive gynecological examinations.
■ Comprehensive health care services should be available to incarcerated women that gives special consideration to the reproductive health needs of women, high rate of victimization among incarcerated women, counseling related to parenting issues, and accessibility to drug or alcohol treatment.

Nurses must be mindful of the need to view incarcerated women holistically, realizing that many factors, such as early childhood trauma, violent victimization, gender discrimination, drug use, and a context of economic impoverishment, have often contributed to their current situations (Barnes, 1985).

Adolescents

Increasing numbers of adolescents are committing violent crimes and many states have lowered the age limit allowing adolescents to be tried and sentenced as adults. Consequently, adolescents who have been convicted of violent crimes are often incarcerated in adult facilities. Incarcerating adolescents in an adult population presents barriers to meeting the distinct developmental needs of adolescents. These developmental changes include rapid physical and emotional growth and unique nutritional needs, all influenced by environment, genetics, and family experiences. Adult correctional facilities are not generally equipped to deal with the challenges of adolescent development. Adolescents in an adult correctional facility are more likely to be sexually assaulted, attacked by other inmates, or threaten suicide than adolescents in a juvenile facility (National Coalition of State Juvenile Justice Advisory Groups, 1993).

To ensure the safety of adolescents in an adult facility, the nurse must be aware of their individual vulnerability. A mechanism for adolescents to access medical and mental health care is essential. The services provided must also be in the context of the developmental stage and experience of adolescence.

MENTAL HEALTH ISSUES IN CORRECTIONAL SETTINGS

On any given day, approximately 285,000 inmates in state and federal prisons have a diagnosed mental illness (Bureau of Justice, 1999). Being in prison with a mental illness such as schizophrenia, bipolar affective disorder, major depressive disorders, and personality disorders makes adjustment to incarceration extremely difficult. The great number of inmates with a mental illness in today's prisons makes it difficult to meet the needs of this population, yet the constitution provides a right to mental health care for prisoners.

In the late 1950s and early 1960s, deinstitutionalization moved people with mental illness out of state hospitals into communities that were often ill prepared to care for them. As a result, many people with a mental illness reside in nursing homes, residential homes, prisons, or jails. People with mental illness are often jailed for crimes committed in response to the symptoms of mental illness. With community services declining and increasing numbers of people with mental illness being incarcerated, the "criminalization of the mentally ill" has become a highly-charged political topic (NAMI, 1999).

According to NAMI, most jail inmates are charged with minor crimes related to the symptoms of untreated mental illness. A far lesser number of inmates with severe mental illness commit more serious crimes, again frequently a consequence of lacking or inadequate treatment. NAMI (1999) has issued a position paper on the criminalization of the mentally ill based on a premise of treatment instead of punishment.

> NAMI believes that persons who have committed offenses due to ... behavior caused by a brain disorder require treatment not punishment .... Prison or jail is never an optimal therapeutic setting
>
> (Holberg, 1999, p. 7).

NAMI takes the position that many dangerous or violent acts by people with a severe mental illness are a result of inappropriate or inadequate treatment. NAMI outlines the following strategies for reducing the number of incarcerated people with severe mental illness:

■ Diverting nonviolent offenders with severe mental illness away from incarceration to adequate treatment
■ Convening mental health courts to address all cases involving offenders with severe mental illness

- Training court judges and personnel about severe mental illness

Recent legislation has attempted to improve treatment conditions for mentally ill inmates. A 1999 Supreme Court decision upheld protection for mentally ill prisoners under the ADA. The ADA has been considered a significant source of protection for people with mental illness in correctional facilities. For example, the ADA would exempt mental illness as the sole reason for the denial of probation or parole. After the Supreme Court decision upholding the applicability of the ADA to incarcerated people with mental illness, Senators Strom Thurmond (R-SC) and Jesse Helms (R-NC) introduced the State and Local Prison Relief Act of 1998 (S. 2266) to ultimately exclude prison inmates from protection under the ADA. The bill did not leave committee (NAMI, 1999).

The use of psychotropic medications in correctional facilities has an obscure history. Psychiatric medications were frequently used to sedate inmate behavior rather than treat the symptoms of mental illness. Antipsychotic medications were often used as a means of chemical restraint because they have sedating properties. The judicial system and advocacy groups took significant interest in this issue given the often severe and irreversible side effect of older generation antipsychotic medication (Burns, 1997). This practice reached the Texas courts in a case challenging the conditions of medical care in the Texas Department of Corrections. The courts specifically addressed the issue of psychiatric medication when describing minimally acceptable medical care. The court decision read as follows:

> Prescriptions and administration of behavior altering medications in dangerous amounts, by dangerous methods or without appropriate supervision and periodic evaluation, is an unacceptable method of treatment
>
> (Cohen, 1999a, p. 58).

Mental illness became increasingly understood as a neurobiological illness; therefore the prescribing patterns of psychiatric medications changed from behavior control to targeting the symptoms of mental illness. As the understanding of mental illness increased, the court took a more scientific approach to weighing the risks and benefits of psychiatric medications. More efficient antipsychotic medications have been developed with fewer side effects and present a viable alternative to medications viewed as "chemical restraint." Now antipsychotic medications along with psychosocial support have become the standard of treatment for people diagnosed with schizophrenia or other mental illnesses that result in alterations in perception.

Access to mental health treatment, including psychiatric medication, is a constitutional right for prison inmates. The U.S. Court of Appeals recently ruled that correctional facilities must supply inmates with psychotropic medication after discharge for a time reasonable to seek community mental health treatment. The court rules validate that an inmate has little or no opportunity to secure medical care in the community while incarcerated. Consequently, the state's responsibility for providing psychiatric medication extends beyond discharge from a correctional facility into the community. Although continuity of care from the prison to the community has historically been lacking, this court ruling is considered a meager beginning in bridging the gap between community mental health treatment and parole from incarceration for many inmates with mental illness (Cocazzo, 1993; Cohen, 1999a, 1999b).

Nurses employed in correctional settings must always be aware of the vulnerabilities of people with mental illness who are incarcerated. Depression, schizophrenia, bipolar disorder, and other NBDs can be readily treated with new-generation psychiatric medications that radically reduce or ameliorate symptoms, but the unique vulnerabilities of incarceration often remain.

LEGAL AND ETHICAL ISSUES IN CORRECTIONAL SETTINGS

Nurses working in corrections are frequently faced with perplexing legal and ethical dilemmas. Nursing and medical care in a correctional environment is frequently litigious. Individuals incarcerated by the state have a legal and constitutional right to medical care. Most litigated cases concerning health care in correctional settings are based on the legal concept of deliberate indifference. **Deliberate indifference** occurs when a health care provider has information or actual knowledge of a health care problem and that knowledge or information is ignored or not acted upon in the provision of health care (Cohen, 1999b). For example, if an inmate seeks care for hypertension, relevant data indicate that the hypertension is clinically significant, and the health care provider fails to take action consistent with the treatment standard of care, then deliberate indifference has theoretically occurred.

An inmate's right to refuse treatment is another legal and ethical issue that nurses working in a correctional environment will often experience. The right to refuse treatment, and the state's power to enforce treatment, are both highly charged legal and political issues and have gained attention in state and local courts. The issue of forced medication and competence to stand trial is of particular concern. The legal and ethical principles that guide forced treatment against the will of an inmate have historically been potential for violence toward self or others and the capacity to understand the consequence of refusing medical treatment. A recent court decision determined that a judicial hearing is now required to forcibly treat a nondangerous incompetent offender to render competence to stand trial. The court decision was based on the following three-factor analysis (Cohen, 1999c, p. 17):

1. Individual's interests
2. States interest
3. Value of the suggested treatment

Several precedent cases have modeled legislation for forcible treatment and competence to stand trial. *Washington vs. Harper*, 494 U.S. 210 (1990), addressed an offender characterized as dangerous and in need of treatment to reduce the danger to the inmate resulting from an untreated mental illness. *Riggins vs. Nevada*, 504 U.S. 127 (1992), addressed the case of an accused murderer who resisted medication to reroute the process of competency to stand trial. The court ruled that an inmate could not be forced to take medication for the sole purpose of becoming competent to stand trial.

Unlike nursing practice with the general population, prison inmates who refuse health care do not leave the facility and return home. Nurses practicing in correctional facilities continue to provide care and address the consequences of an inmate's refusal of treatment. For example, an inmate who refuses to adhere to treatment protocols for HIV infection may experience declining health status. Nurses are obliged to treat any resultant health issues. Individuals who are incarcerated by the state have a constitutional right to refuse and receive health care. Nurses pracicing in correctional settings must respect the right to refuse care even if the result is an adverse outcome.

STANDARDS OF NURSING PRACTICE IN CORRECTIONAL SETTINGS

Several accrediting bodies have issued standards of nursing practice applicable to correctional settings. The American Nurses Association Nursing Practice Standards (ANA, 1995) and Guideline for Corrections Nursing generally address the use of the nursing process in the correctional setting. The American Correctional Association and National Commission

---

BOX **28-1**

Research in Correctional Nursing

In the last decade, the number of female inmates and the average length of their sentences have increased dramatically. The influx of ill and generally unhealthy female offenders into U.S. correctional institutions is a by-product of the recent "confinement era" within criminal justice. Female inmates have different treatment needs and problems than their male counterparts; therefore a need exists for gender-appropriate programs. The influence of such inmates of correctional health care services represents a potentially critical issue confronting correctional managers and correctional health service administrators. This article highlights the need for correctional policy to address the health care needs of female inmates with HIV and AIDS.

From Zaitzow BH: Women prisoners and HIV/AIDS, *J Assoc Nurses AIDS Care* 10(6):78, 1999.

Achieving a therapeutic relationship with forensic patients depends on nurses' awareness of personal needs, reactions to the patient, recognition of their participation in the pattern, the effect of this participation on others, and the changes they needed to make. Nurses have more extensive contact with forensic patients than any other health care professionals. Consequently the potential exists for nurses, through the interpersonal relationship, to have the greatest therapeutic influence or engage in patterns that replicate pathology-producing situations.

From Schafer P: Working with Dave: application of Peplau interpersonal nursing theory in the correctional environment, *J Psychosoc Nurs Ment Health Serv* 37(9):18, 1999.

have written additional guidelines for nursing practice in correctional health care. These guidelines articulate standards of practice for specific populations and health care issues, including communicable diseases, health care service delivery systems, and standards of practice for vulnerable population such as women, adolescents, and people with mental illness. Box 28-1 presents abstracts that represent research being done in correctional health nursing, another effort to strengthen this profession.

SUMMARY

The situations correctional nurses face are fraught with ambiguities and tensions. In some cases, nurses are marginalized in decision making processes; correctional administration or legal pressures may override nursing goals. Nurses must work within the system and still be aware of the ethical limits at which they must draw the line and advocate for an incarcerated person's rights to care. To advocate for the incarcerated, nurses need critical autonomous assessment and evaluative capabilities as essential prerequisites for the role. The trend toward incarcerating more members of the population follows what are believed to be the wishes of a majority of the citizenry. Nursing as a discipline must collaborate with related disciplines such as law, medicine, and social work in integrating care within the fabric of an inmate's context. In this regard, nursing's goal is to make correctional facilities and processes as humane and healthy as possible for inmates, while being conscious of the mandate for the health and safety of the community as a whole.

LEARNING ACTIVITIES

This clinical example is taken from a position paper written by Anne De Groot, M.D. following her visit to Chowchilla, a women's prison in California that had a disproportionately high rate of HIV-infected inmates. Dr. Groot, after meeting with an inmate with late stage AIDS, called for a compassionate release of the woman. **Compassionate release** is a process of the state that commutes a prison sentence based on terminal illness or severe decline in health status.

Patti is lying in bed. Every available surface in her room is covered in pictures: wolves, eagles, feathers, dream catcher, proud faces of Native American women. She is frail—barely there. The doctor comes with me. He has not seen her in some weeks—"Last I looked, he says, "she was walking." I look at her: she is not walking now.

I ask her to sit, wondering why she lies so crooked in the bed. With her left hand she takes off the covers, revealing a wasted frame. Barely 80 pounds, she weighed 130 when she was well. Then she takes her left hand and lifts her right arm over her body. By pulling hard and leaning, she can shift her torso over. Next she reaches for her legs, pulling on the cloth of her shorts to lift her knees one by one off the bed, moving her legs to the side. With her good left arm, she throws her legs like deadweight off the bed, using them as a counterbalance to pull her torso up. Then she rolls over on her elbows, grimacing with pain. She rolls over until she is in a prayer position, leaning on the bed with her elbows. I am afraid to help her, knowing that would injure her pride in some way. I am afraid she will fall, but she surprised me by her sheer force of will. Just when I am sure she will slip to the floor, she reaches back for the wheelchair and swings her body into it, using her legs to pivot.

This woman has one good arm and three useless limbs. She has end stage AIDS, much beyond end stage. She has a T cell count of 7, she weighs less than 60% of her ideal body weight. She has less than a few months left to live, yet she is denied compassionate release? She has been denied compassion.

Use the above clinical example as the basis for discussion of the following:

1. Provide thoughts about the concept of compassionate release.
2. Under what circumstances is compassionate release appropriate?
3. Describe three of the most significant nursing interventions for the woman in the clinical example.
4. How might providing nursing care in a correctional environment promote or present barriers to the interventions?
5. In a small group exercise, discuss thoughts and beliefs about the states' responsibility to provide health care to incarcerated people with HIV.

REFERENCES

American Nurses Association: *American Nurses Association nursing practice standards and guidelines,* Washington, DC, 1995, American Nurses Publishing.

Barnes PJ: *Mothers in prison,* New Brunswick, NJ, 1985, Translation Books.

Bates E: Private prisons, *The Nation* 6:67, 1998.

Bayer R: Ethical challenges posed by clinical progression in AIDS (commentary), *Am J Public Health* 87:1599, 1997.

Behrendt G: Voluntary testing for HIV in prison population with a high prevalence of HIV, *Am J Epidemiol* 139:918, 1994.

Bell K, Allen W: Healthcare workers must be on constant guard, *St. Louis Post-Dispatch,* A-12, September 27, 1998.

Bureau of Justice: *Prisoners in 1999,* 1999, NCJ 183476, Office of Justice Programs, www.ojp.usdoj.gov/bjs/abstract/p99.htm.

Burns KA: Using psychiatric medication in a correctional setting: an overview, *Corrections Mental Health Rep* 1(1):1, 1997.

Camhi M: *The prison experience,* Sacramento, 1998, Charles Tuttle.

Cocazzo JI: *Mental illness in American prisons,* Seattle, 1993, National Coalition for Mental Illness in Criminal Justice Systems.

Cohen F: Prisons duty to provide psychotropic medication includes post-release supply, *Corrections Mental Health Rep* 1(4):49, 1999a.

Cohen F: Deliberate indifference to detainee's serious medical needs shown, *Corrections Mental Health Rep* 1(4):65, 1999b.

Cohen F: Judicial hearing and strict scrutiny required to forcibly medicate incompetent detainees, *Corrections Mental Health Rep* 1(2):17, 1999c.

Collins A, Baumgartner D: Prisons access to experimental HIV therapies, *Minnesota Medicine* 78:45, 1995.

Corrections Connection Network: *Gang management and security threat survey,* 1999, The Author, www.correct.com.

Derb SG: HIV protease inhibitors: a review for clinicians, *J Am Med Assoc* 6(7):145, 1997.

Friedman L: *Crime and punishment in American history,* New York, 1993, Basic Books.

Hammet TM, Wilson R: HIV/AIDS education and prevention programs for adults in prisons and jails and juvenile confinement facilities, *Mor Mortal Wkly Rep* 45:268, 1994.

Holberg R: *National Alliance for the Mentally Ill position on ADA in prisons,* 1999, The Author, www.nami.org.

Hofragle JH: The treatment of chronic viral hepatitis, *N Engl J Med* 336(5):347, 1997.

Lischlensher A: Good roads and chain gangs in the progressive south, *J Southern History* 165:78, 1993.

National Alliance for the Mentally Ill: *Position papers on criminalization of the mentally ill,* 1999, The Author, www.nami.org.

National Coalition of State Juvenile Justice Advisory Groups: *Myths and realities: meeting the challenge of serious, violent and chronic juvenile offenders,* 1992 Annual Report, Washington, DC, 1993, The Author.

National Commission on Correctional Health Care: *Standards for health services in corrections,* Chicago, 1999, The Author.

Schafer P: Working with Dave: application of Peplau interpersonal nursing theory in the correctional environment, *J Psychosoc Nurs Ment Health Serv* 37(9):18, 1999.

US Department of Justice: *Issues and practice 1996-1997 update: HIV/AIDS, STD and TB in correctional facilities,* NCJ Pub No 176344, Washington, DC, 1998, US Government Printing Office.

US Department of Justice: *Women in prison,* NCJ Pub No NJC127991, Washington, DC, 1990, US Government Printing Office.

Wilson W: *Forced labor in the U.S.,* New York, 1993, AMS Press.

World Health Organization: *WHO guidelines on HIV infections in prisons,* Geneva, 1996, The Author.

Zaitzow BH: Women prisoners and HIV/AIDS, *J Assoc Nurses AIDS Care* 10(6):78, 1999.

Parish Health

Beverly Cook Siegrist

OBJECTIVES

Upon completion of this chapter, the reader will be able to do the following:

1. Describe the philosophy and historical basis of parish nursing.
2. Define the roles, functions, and education of the parish nurse.
3. Describe models of parish nursing.
4. Discuss congregations as clients of the community health nurse.
5. Describe the role of the parish nurse in the spiritual health and well-being of faith communities and plan spiritual nursing interventions.
6. Discuss contemporary issues in parish nursing such as working with vulnerable populations and facing ethical and legal issues.

KEY TERMS

CIRCLE Model of Spiritual Care
facilitator
faith community
Granger Westberg
health educator
integrator of health and healing
personal health counselor
referral source
spiritual distress
spirituality

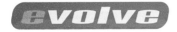

http://evolve.elsevier.com/Nies/

Nurses seem to have one foot in the sciences and one in the humanities, one foot in the spiritual world and one in the physical one. . . they [nurses] have insight into the human condition

(Maginnis and Associates, 1993, p. 1).

The purpose of this chapter is to present an overview of parish nursing as a new and evolving role for the community health nurse. Based on centuries-old philosophies from churches and religious groups, nurses are applying the science of nursing and caring to address the biopsychosocial health needs of individuals and groups in church congregations and faith communities across the country. The following scenarios illustrate models of parish nursing found in the United States and suggest the unique ways that parish nurses provide nursing care.

The three clinical examples on p. 774 illustrate how parish nursing is evolving in the United States. More than 3000 nurses provide nursing care to children, adults, and the elderly in churches, synagogues, and mosques. Parish nurse programs are also established in other countries such as Canada, Korea, and Australia (Berry, 2000; Granberg-Michaelson, 1997; McDermott, Solari-Twadell, and Matthews, 1998). The development of the *Scope and Standards of Parish Nursing* (Health Ministries Association and ANA, 1998) recognized parish nursing as a significant role for the community health nurse. Community health nursing has evolved from early church efforts to provide care for the sick and disenfranchised (Swanson and Nies, 1997). Modern parish nursing focuses on the global health and wellness issues of all people and has it roots in more recent efforts to encourage the reemergence and blending of health care roles into the healing ministry of churches (Joel, 1998; McDermott and Burke, 1993; Sloari-Twadell and McDermott, 1999).

FOUNDATIONS OF PARISH NURSING

Reverand **Granger Westberg**, a Lutheran minister, is considered the founder of the modern parish nurse movement. Westberg, educated as a chaplain and minister, worked with nurses in hospitals, medical schools, and church communities. Impressed with the nurse's perspective of health and wholeness in viewing human illness' physical, emotional, and spiritual challenges, he described parish nursing as the "culmination of his lifelong work in relating theology and health care." In 1984, he first proposed a parish nurse

program to Lutheran General Hospital (LGH) in Chicago, Illinois. Westberg envisioned a partnership between the hospital and all church congregations in the hospital's community. He proposed that participating churches would make contributions to fund a nurse's salary and identified seven roles the nurse could use to provide services to faith communities (Solari-Twadell and McDermott, 1999).

In 1985, six parish nurses were hired in the Chicago area. Initially, LGH and the participating hospital's contributions primarily funded their salaries. The churches assumed increasing responsibility for the nurse's salaries over a four-year period. Westberg supported the development of a parish nurse training program and required the nurses to participate in a weekly educational session. Teaching chaplains, nurse educators, and physicians led the sessions and the nurses enhanced their skills in counseling, education, and spiritual assessment and intervention. The meetings evolved into an ongoing support group for the nurses as they developed the parish nurse programs and identified self-care needs. LGH continued to provide parish nurse leadership through the International Parish Nurse Resource Center. Located in Park Ridge, Illinois, the center offers education, development guidance, and contact with parish nurses nationally and internationally.

From these beginnings came the identification of specific roles for the parish nursing practice and current recommendations for parish nursing education. From Westberg's first parish nurse organization, the following types of U.S. parish nurse models emerged: institutionally based with paid and unpaid nurse organizational models and congregationally based with paid and unpaid nurse models. The contracts or agreements with institutions and churches distinguish each model, and grants, contracts, or volunteer nurse services may support each model.

Solari-Twadell and McDermott (1999) and Westberg (1999) described the philosophical basis of parish nursing as encompassing the following five key elements:

1. The spiritual dimension is central to the practice.
2. The role balances nursing science and technology with service and spiritual care.
3. The nurse's clients are members of the faith community defined by the church and its public service philosophy.
4. Parish nursing services are built upon principles of self-care and capacity building with a focus on

Sandra Mills began her parish nurse practice as a volunteer when her parish priest recruited her to help establish a cancer support group and coordinate classes for caregivers. Within six months, her church's social concerns committee established a paid position on their ministry team and employed her as a full-time paid staff member. After completing a parish nurse certificate program through a local university, she began to develop a parish nurse program in her church. She describes her days as full and rewarding. Each day she visits ill or homebound parish members and provides support through prayer, education, and listening. Each day she is challenged to locate and refer community resources, provide health education to church groups (e.g., mother's day out and the over 55 group), and coordinate the efforts of other volunteer nurses in the church. She is practicing holistic nursing for the first time in her 15 years of practice. She found that the church, as a healing community, allows her to focus on the body-mind-spirit connection she believes is necessary to improve the health of congregation members.

Marilyn Michaels is a former home care and hospice nurse who works as a parish nurse coordinator for St. Luke's Hospital, which is a 400-bed medical center serving a midwestern rural population. Her position was created to assist community churches in developing and maintaining parish nurse programs. She coordinates educational programs, including a 30-hour certificate program for beginning parish nurses, an advanced program for parish nurse coordinators in individual churches, and monthly educational topics offered through a parish nurse support group. Marilyn developed the support group and facilitates communication among the 200 parish nurses and 100 church communities that St. Luke's Hospital serves by editing St. Luke's bi-monthly newsletter. She also assists parish nurse programs by connecting them with other services that the hospital and community agencies provide (e.g., screening, support groups, and speakers). The program at St. Luke's Hospital is self-supporting from grants and educational programs.

Sue James is a member of a parish nursing group from five inner-city churches in south-central Indiana. This group of nurses came together from five different church denominations to meet their congregation members' health needs. The nurses are unpaid parish nurses within their own congregations. They came together to share their resources because their churches are small in membership and they identified similar and unmet health needs in each of the churches. Primarily, the group serves an aging population that represents the few remaining individuals and families living in the inner-city area. Sue agreed to serve as the group coordinator, a position that has been shared among their group. In this position, she plans biweekly meetings for the nurses at alternating churches and serves as a community liaison for participating churches. The group's parish nurse effort began two years previous, supported by a local hospital grant and matched with small donations from the participating churches. Each nurse volunteers at least 10 hours each week. Based on the health and wellness assessment completed in each church, they arranged a health fair that included health screening and referral information at one church and began educational classes on topics related to depression and healthy aging. They focus on health promotion and their individual churches recognize them as the *parish nurse,* the *congregational nurse,* and the *health minister.*

understanding the connection between health and the individual's relationship with God, faith traditions, nursing, and the broader society.

5. The parish nurse understands that holistic health is a dynamic process that requires a connection between the person's spiritual, psychological, physical, and social dimensions.

These beliefs direct the parish nurse in planning nursing care and defining health not only as wellness, but also as wholeness of body and spirit. They also emphasize spiritual health as a motivating factor in seeking wellness care, participating in education, and enhancing self-care capabilities (Berquist and King, 1994).

A review of the historical foundations of community health nursing practice describes the significance of the church in early health care (see Chapter 2). In the Bible, the book of Romans (16:1-2) describes the early works of Phoebe, who is considered to be the first visiting nurse. John Wesley, the founder of the Methodist church, in his 1786 sermon *On Visiting the Sick,* directed his believers to visit the sick to convey God's grace to others (Wesley, 1986). These selected examples illustrate the significance of the Church as an influence on health and healing. The histories of all religions provide similar examples. The reemergence of these basic beliefs in health, healing, and spirituality are moving the church toward assisting members in wholeness; this is evidenced by the growing number of health ministries and parish nurse programs found in churches throughout the nation (Matthaei and Stern, 1994). The defining characteristics and roles of the parish nurse in any church setting come from these philosophical foundations.

ROLES OF THE PARISH NURSE

The parish nurse's practice focuses on health promotion and wellness. It is based on a holistic nursing practice that holds the spiritual dimension central to health and healing. In the nursing process, the parish nurse does not perform "hands on nursing care," but improves the health of a **faith community** by implementing the five interrelated roles of health educator, personal health counselor, referral source, facilitator, and integrator of health and healing (Berry, 2000; International Parish Nurse Resource Center, 1998; Keller, 1994; McDermott and Burke, 1993; Solari-Twadell and McDermott, 1999).

As a **health educator**, the parish nurse provides or coordinates educational offerings for people of all ages and developmental stages. The educational efforts may target lifestyles, values, and wellness and they incorporate the spiritual aspects of well-being to the individual and community. The educator role includes educating the church leaders and members about the roles and purposes of a parish nurse. Educational efforts are planned based on the church community's priorities. Early in the development of a parish nurse program and periodically thereafter, the parish nurse should assess the health status and needs of the congregation members to determine educational priorities. Fig. 29-1 presents an example of an adult congregational health and wellness survey. The parish nurse should complete an assessment on each population group the congregation serves and include children grouped by developmental stages. Examples of educational efforts are teaching CPR to new mothers; teaching signs and symptoms of hypertension and stroke to adults in the congregation; educating lay church ministers in the signs and symptoms of acute illness when visiting homebound individuals; and teaching school-aged children basic health and safety.

In the role of **personal health counselor**, the parish nurse discusses health problems with individuals and families within the church community upon the individual's or family's request or upon the referral of ministers or other congregational members. In this role, the nurse may focus on self-care issues such as explaining a prescribed medical regimen; assessing the need for further resources and referrals; or making visits to homes, nursing homes, or hospitals.

The parish nurse is a **referral source** and must be aware of community resources and must be able to guide individuals as they access and use available resources. In this role, the nurse may function as a liaison and may provide referrals to resources or health care providers with the client's approval. The parish nurse recognizes the difficulties encountered by vulnerable populations within the faith community and those within the larger church community and helps them maneuver the health care maze to access needed resources. In particular, vulnerable populations may need assistance in accessing health care resources. These populations may include nonEnglish speaking individuals, those who speak English as second language (ESL), individuals living in poverty or without health care insurance, or

FIGURE **29-1**

Parish Health Assessment Form. *Continued*

Wellness Ministry Survey
Holy Spirit Catholic Church - Bowling Green, Kentucky

Thank you for taking the time to complete this Wellness Survey. The results will be used to plan programs and activities that will meet the health care interests and needs of everyone in the congregation. Think of this as your survey to indicate the type of services you would like available to you, your family, and your brothers and sisters in Christ. Please do not sign your name. All information will be confidential.

Please complete the following:

My age is _____.
I am _____female_____male.
I am _____White_____Black_____Hispanic_____Asian.
I am _____single_____married_____divorced_____widowed.
I am _____employed_____unemployed_____retired_____homemaker_____student.
I have health insurance. _____yes _____no
I have a family doctor. _____yes _____no
I think my health is _____good _____fair _____poor.

Please place an "X" by those activities that you would benefit from now
or might use in the future:

_____Visits to those individuals who are homebound
_____Visits to those who are experiencing loss
_____Visits to parishioners in hospitals or nursing homes
_____A nurse to assist parishioners in obtaining personal health counseling
_____Health education pamphlets or brochures
_____Classes held at church on health-related topics
_____Information on classes held elsewhere in our community
_____Health screening at our church
_____Flu shots or immunizations at our church
_____Volunteer training for parishioners to assist parishioners (e.g., respite and homebound visits)
_____Support groups at our church
_____Support groups elsewhere
_____Prayer and healing service
Other (please list):

individuals living with complicated chronic or catastrophic illness.

The role of **facilitator** includes recruiting, training, and coordinating volunteers to work with the parish nurse program or health ministry. The nurse may work with other nurses and lay people within the congregation. The parish nurse program may encompass all programs related to the health of the church community. For example, the parish needs assessment identifies the development of a transportation committee or respite program as a church community's major need. These services impact the ability of

church members to access health and related services; therefore these programs may be delegated to the parish nurse. As a facilitator, the nurse would plan, implement, or direct these programs. Many parish nurses work through existing health ministry frameworks within their churches such as health or social welfare committees. The membership of these committees may be interdisciplinary or representative of the entire church congregation; the parish nurse facilitates specific health-related programs and activities. In the facilitator role, the nurse would also connect the church with existing resources and

FIGURE **29-1—cont'd**

Parish Health Assessment Form.

Please place an "X" by those health topics listed below that you want to know more about

Heart Sense
___Heart disease
___Stroke
___High blood pressure
___Diet and cholesterol

Healthy Living
___Nutrition and weight control
___Exercise
___Quitting smoking
___Alcohol and drug issues

Emotional Health
___Depression
___Other mental illness
___Reducing stress
___Eating disorders
___Self-esteem
___Anger management

Women's Health
___Breast cancer
___Menopause
___Estrogen replacement
___Osteoporosis

An Ounce of Prevention
___Cancer prevention
___Protecting your back
___Talking to your doctor
___Understanding your medications
___Safety at home and away
___Understanding insurance

Healthy Families
___Sexuality
___Marriage
___Pregnancy and childbirth
___Parents through life stages
___Teen issues
___Single parenting

Chronic Concerns
___Arthritis
___Diabetes
___Prostate trouble
___HIV/AIDS
___Pain management
___Urinary incontinence
___Life with a disability

As We Age
___Our physical changes
___Care of aging parents
___Living well alone
___Alzheimers
___Loneliness
___Getting "our affairs in order"

As Life Ends
___Grief issues
___Living wills and power
    of attorney
___Hospice care
___Organ donation

Other topics?_____

Put an "X" by days and times you would participate in an activity or class

Day of week	Mornings	Afternoon	Evenings
Monday	___	___	___
Tuesday	___	___	___
Wednesday	___	___	___
Thursday	___	___	___
Friday	___	___	___
Saturday	___	___	___
Sunday	___	___	___

programs to meet identified health and educational needs. For example, the nurse might facilitate available health screenings, flu shots, or immunizations through the local public health department. In the parish nurse role, the nurse would not directly provide or duplicate the available services, but would work with other agencies in providing care to the church community.

As an **integrator of health and healing**, the parish nurse acknowledges and integrates spirituality as the basis of his or her nursing practice. For example, in teaching a class on healthy aging, the nurse will include the connections of lifestyle, compliance to prescribed medical treatment, attitudes, and values on well-being. In a home visit to a terminally ill person, the nurse will explore the meaning of healing vs. cure and provide emotional support and encouragement. In certain churches or parishes, the nurse may lead or contribute to healing services as a member of the health ministry team.

These examples illustrate the diversity and autonomy found in parish nursing. Depending on the needs of the church community and its members, the roles may be implemented in a variety of methods and through various organizational structures.

EDUCATION OF THE PARISH NURSE

An RN with several years of experience in clinical practice may best implement the roles of the parish nurse. The self-direction and independent decision making required by the autonomous roles of the parish nurse require a nurse experienced in clinical nursing and community-based nursing practice. The educational preparation of the baccalaureate nurse in community and public health provides the theoretical basis needed to plan and implement programs for diverse populations in a congregational setting and to function as a beginning member of a pastoral team (Ryan, 1990). All parish nurses should complete a formal program of study (International Parish Nurse Resource Center, 1998; King and Striepe, 1990; Solari-Twadell and McDermott, 1999; Westberg and McNamara, 1990). Universities, hospitals, or parish nurse programs now offer hundreds of parish nurse programs that nurses may take for college credit, continuing education, or postgraduate certification.

Many universities are incorporating existing certificate programs into advanced nursing degrees. Programs are generally offered at beginning, intermediate, and advanced levels and consist of approximately 30 contact hours of planned classroom instruction, self-study, or clinical experiences at each level. Box 29-1 provides an example of the curriculum content for a beginning parish nurse program as suggested by the International Parish Nurse Resource Center (1998). Intermediate parish nurse programs focus on the development of skills for parish nurse coordinators and they include human resource development, grant writing, and budgeting. A third level of education is available for educators who plan to teach parish nursing or develop curricula for parish nurse programs.

BOX **29-1**

Suggested Core Curriculum Content for Beginning Parish Nurse Program

- Role of the church in health care
- History and philosophy of parish nursing
- Models of parish nursing
- Roles and functions of the parish nurse
- Community assessment and resources
- Health promotion across the lifespan
- Philosophy of self-care
- Legal and ethical issues related to parish nursing: confidentiality, accountability, documentation, and end-of-life issues
- Ministerial team and nursing role
- Parish nurses role in worship, prayer, and healing
- Starting a parish nurse program

From International Parish Nurse Resource Center: *Role of parish nurse, mission and resources*, Ridge Park, Ill, 1998, International Parish Nurse Resource Center.

As parish nurse programs grow in number and services provided to faith communities, continuing education programs will increase in availability and in diversity of content. The International Parish Nurse Resource Center held annually at the Westberg Symposium in Chicago provides the greatest opportunity for education and networking. In 1999, over 3000 nurses gathered to learn about new developments in parish nursing and to establish networks with other parish nurses.

Implementation of the parish nurse's roles uses the nursing process to plan nursing interventions in wellness and physical, emotional, and spiritual health (Bergquist and King, 1994). Other chapters in this text provide useful information concerning health promotion and planning activities to promote physical and mental health. Spirituality, as a major focus of nursing care, presents different challenges for the parish nurse.

THE PARISH NURSE AND SPIRITUALITY

Westberg (1988) described the ideal parish nurse as one who is spiritually mature and able to apply spiritual aspects to the health care of congregation

BOX **29-2**

Nursing Research about Spiritual Practices

In a study of 181 Oncology Society Nurse members, the Spiritual Care Perspectives Survey was completed to describe usual spiritual care practices. The most common interventions reported were:
Praying with or for the patient
Referring to chaplain or minister
Talking about spiritual topics with the patient
Facilitating religious rituals or practice other than praying

From Taylor JT, Madalon A, Highfield M: Spiritual care practices of oncology nurses, *Oncol Nurs Forum* 22:31-39, 1995.

In a study of 186 nurses randomly selected from across the United States, the authors used the Soeken and Carson's Health Professional's Spiritual Role Scale to determine the spiritual practices of nurses. A positive correlation was found between spiritual attitudes and spiritual practices. Those nurses who provided spiritual care routinely were those who valued it themselves and had sought additional education in providing spiritual care for their clients.

From Piles CL: Providing spiritual care, *Nurs Educ* 15:36-41, 1990.

members. Many parish nurses find the need to further develop spiritual assessment skills, acquire theological knowledge and related skills, and learn the nurse's role in healing.

Reed (1992) defines **spirituality** as "having the propensity to make meaning through a sense of relatedness to dimensions that transcend the self in a way that empowers and does not devalue" (p. 350). In nursing, **spiritual distress** is more often the focus of care. The North American Nursing Diagnosis Association (1992) defines spiritual distress as "a disruption in the life principle that pervades a person's entire being and that integrates and transcends one's biological and psychosocial nature" (p. 46). Parish nurses provide nursing interventions related to the nursing diagnosis as connected to spiritual distress (e.g., loneliness, isolation, and hopelessness). They view spirituality as the basis of

nursing care in the church setting. Box 29-2 presents data from nursing research performed on nursing's spiritual care practices.

Schnorr (1988) suggested the **CIRCLE Model of Spiritual Care**. This model illustrates the following concepts of care that guide nursing practice and interventions:

Caring,
Intuition,
Respect for religious beliefs and practices,
Caution,
Listening, and
Emotional support.

Caring includes caring practices and attitudes. Nurse theorist Jean Watson described caring as "professional, ethical, scientific, esthetic, personalized giving-receiving behaviors that allow for contact between the nurse and client. . ." (Dossey, 1999, p. 45). *Intuition* requires acting on instinct, hunches, or "gut feelings." Benner (1984) described intuitive abilities as responses that expert nurses have after several years of experience and these abilities enable the nurse to "read between the lines." Schnorr (1988) described *respect* as understanding the importance of religious beliefs and practices. The nurse allows time for prayer and sacrament and supports and encourages religious activities. *Caution* in spiritual care advises the parish nurse to avoid proselytizing or "preaching" religion to clients. The ANA's (1985) *Code for Nurses* also provides the nurse with direction to avoid judgements and respect the client's right to self-determination. *Listening* is a skill that is highly developed in most experienced nurses. It allows an understanding of spoken and unspoken words and feelings, encourages open communication, and supports and empowers patients to communicate needs and desires. *Emotional support* is the link between the physical and spiritual. Among the emotional interventions, Schnorr (1988) includes working with feelings, showing love, and using appropriate touch and empathy.

The example on p. 780 illustrates how the parish nurse might use the CIRCLE Model to provide spiritual care.

Prayer is a commonly used spiritual intervention and can provide comfort and support. Spalding University School of Nursing and Health Sciences in Louisville, Kentucky offers a beginning parish nurse certificate. In a session entitled "The Spirituality of Self-Care," the program provides the nurse with guidelines for leading prayer

During a meeting of the health ministry committee, the parish nurse learned that Mrs. James, a church member, was diagnosed with end-stage breast cancer. Mrs. James is a 45-year-old wife and mother of two school-aged children. She returned home following surgery and had to decide whether to seek further treatment within the next weeks. Her husband attended church with his family although he was a member of another faith community. A home health nurse was involved with Mrs. James' postoperative care and it was possible that a referral to hospice would occur following her decisions regarding further treatment. The parish nurse called Mrs. James and offered to make a home visit to assess how the parish nurse and church community could support and *care*

for the family's well-being. Mrs. James welcomed the visit. Showing *respect* for their faith beliefs, the nurse offered prayer and waited for a request from the couple. The nurse's *instincts* and experience working with cancer patients and families guided her in using *listening* as a nursing intervention during this initial visit and in using *caution* when Mrs. James asked for guidance in making treatment decisions. The nurse further explored the home situation, the needed educational support, and the physician's prognosis and treatment options with the patient. *Emotional support* was important for Mrs. James and the parish nurse offered support through touch and words of concern. This model helped develop an initial nurse-client relationship of trust and open communication.

services, which many program graduates found helpful (Box 29-3).

Berquist and King (1994) suggested that through prayer, spiritual assessment, and hope and faith, the parish nurse facilitates important client outcomes for spiritual health and well-being, including self-esteem, self-actualization, hope, trust, and peace.

ISSUES IN PARISH NURSE PRACTICE

Although universal to community health practice, many issues impact the practice of parish nursing. Selected issues, which are discussed in this section, include working with vulnerable populations and the legal and ethical issues of confidentiality and accountability.

Providing Care to Vulnerable Populations

The philosophical foundations of faith communities related to caring, outreach, and support of vulnerable populations place the parish nurse in a position to positively impact the health of diverse groups. Historically, churches have been among the first groups to sponsor and support refugees, develop programs for homeless individuals and families, provide assistance and resources to low-income families, and provide resource to entire communities during disasters (e.g., floods and tornadoes). Nurses are able to provide care for diverse populations using highly developed skills in assessment, planning, and interventions.

Boss (1999, 1996, 1994) suggests that parish nurses can be instrumental in helping these populations access services, but these nurses should not attempt to meet the populations' many needs alone. She reminds the nurse that "more is not necessarily better" concerning the use of available health resources. The nurse in the educator role can assess the needs of vulnerable populations and teach the faith community about the people and their spiritual, emotional, and physical needs. A community of caring that can collectively meet the many needs of vulnerable populations will emerge from the congregation. Boss (1999) called this the Nehemiah approach, which allows people with the talent and desire to do the work to help with large projects. The parish nurse works as a member of a caring church community to meet the health and healing needs of vulnerable populations.

Accountability and Confidentiality

The *Code for Nurses* (ANA, 1985) and the *Scope and Standards of Parish Nursing Practice* (Health Ministries Association and ANA, 1998) guided parish nurses in their practice of parish nursing and are accountable to state boards of nursing, employing agencies and organizations (i.e., including churches), and the faith communities they serve. Many ethical and legal issues are generic to clinical practice settings; however, confidentiality issues have the potential to be problematic in a church community.

Concerned church members may identify individuals in need and refer them to the parish nurse. In

BOX **29-3**

Guidelines for Simple Prayer Services

1. Keep the prayer service simple, but include music, symbols, and rituals where appropriate. The purpose is to move the heart toward God and others.
2. For prayer with a sick patient:
   a. If the person is a traditionalist, use a traditional prayer to encourage participation
   b. Include your own prayers of the heart (and those of the patient, family, friends, or nurse where appropriate)
3. When possible and appropriate, include family members.
   a. Holistic healing includes being attentive to the environment
   b. Caregivers influence the patient's wellness
   c. In Mark 2:1-12, Jesus healed the paralytic based upon the faith of friends (cf Mark 2:5)
   d. Spiritual needs of the caregiver also need to be addressed
4. Prayers need to acknowledge reality. This might include:
   a. The fear, anger, or suffering of the patient
   b. The desire for patience on part of the patient or caregiver
   c. The need for caregivers to feel appreciated
   d. The need for the patient to know the presence of God
5. Prayer may use the three-part format of the "Our Father," which is familiar to prayers from many different religious backgrounds.
   a. Call on God with an address that reflects the spirituality of the patient
      1. "Our Father"
      2. "God the giver of life. . ."
      3. "God, our heavenly Father and Mother. . ."
   b. State positive things that God has done or is doing
      1. "We give you thanks for. . ."
      2. "You have supported us on our journey through life. . ."
   c. Make appropriate petitions
   d. Close with something simple
      - In Jesus name we pray. . . Amen
      - In trust we pray. . . Amen
6. Prayers may also be taken from the Psalms, using all or part, or prayers may simply follow the form of a psalm.
   a. Psalm 69: prayer of anguish in distress
   b. Psalm 71: humble prayer of old age
   c. Psalm 77: lament in time of distress
   d. Psalm 40: prayer of waiting for God
7. Touch is an important element of support and healing and should be used where appropriate. Touch is evidenced by church rituals and ceremonies such as laying on of hands and blessings.

Courtesy of Adeline Fehribach, SCNg, PhD, Assistant Professor, Spalding University, Louisville, Kentucky. Unpublished material. Used with permission.

the role of health minister, the parish nurse may receive private and sensitive information. The nurse does not act in the role of minister or priest and congregation members should not relate information in the form of confession or repentance; however, the connection with the church ministry team may put the nurse in a position to hear this type of sensitive information.

The nurse should protect the client's right to confidentiality in relation to information concerning their health or health-related condition. Although the nurse must share information with the church minister in certain instances, the nurse should only share confidential information with other church ministry leaders or prayer groups with the client's permission. Exceptions are found in religious sects or congregations that require the public confession of behaviors or conditions to benefit from divine intervention and forgiveness. As a care provider, the parish nurse should be aware of these rituals and practices prior to counseling members of the faith community (Fowler, 1999).

Accountability

Sister Mary Angela Shaughnessy (1998) provided direction for the parish nurse by listing the following information related to church law:

1. Volunteers in a church are held to the same degree of accountability as paid employees.
2. The doctrine of separation of church and state does not exempt churches from discrimination laws.
3. Ministers, both ordained and nonordained, may be required to disclose confidential information in court.

As volunteers or paid employees, nurses are accountable to the nursing standards and civil laws designed to protect individuals from abuse, neglect, and discrimination. Parish nurses, as nonordained ministers, do not have client-professional privileges and should be aware of appropriate standards in documenting provided services. In documenting parish nurse services, "less is better." Prior to beginning a parish nurse program, the nurse should develop and follow general policies and guidelines for record keeping. Shaughnessy provided further information related to contract law. The handbooks, brochures, or programs that church-related institutions offer are contracts. The parish nurse should ensure that health information is current and based on accepted practices and standards. These suggestions are not intended to limit the parish nurse's creativity or scope; they emphasize that the professional nurse is accountable for his or her practice in any role.

SUMMARY

This chapter provided an overview of the parish nurse's role in providing nursing care for faith communities and it explored the historical and philo-

sophical foundations of the modern parish nurse practice. Traditional nurse roles of the nurse, facilitator, health educator, integrator of health and healing, personal health counselor, and referral source are used in unique ways to allow the parish nurse to provide nursing care to church communities. The parish nurse's role in the development of spiritual health and well-being becomes significant and requires the nurse to focus on spiritual needs of congregation members. The CIRCLE model for planning spiritual nursing may be used to guide nursing interventions. Parish nursing offers new opportunities for increasing the health and wellness of clients and requires the nurse to refocus skills and knowledge.

Many educational programs are available throughout the United States to provide parish nurse education and certification through three levels of education: beginning, intermediate, and advanced parish nurse practice. These programs are offered as continuing education and through formal university courses as part of degree programs. Church law, nursing ethics, and standards are the basis for the legal and ethical parish nursing practice. As a relatively new area of community health nurse practice, parish nursing offers the RN many opportunities to improve the health of faith communities through a holistic nursing practice that connects the body, mind, and spirit in the celebration of health and healing.

LEARNING ACTIVITIES

1. Speak with a parish nurse in the community. Ask the nurse about congregational health needs and discuss how the roles of the parish nurse are implemented through the parish nurse programs and ministry. Observe the nurse in his or her daily activities and identify how spirituality is a basis for parish nursing care.
2. Speak with a minister or priest in the community from a different faith belief system. Explore the philosophical basis for the church's role in health and healing.
3. Visit websites devoted to parish nursing and identify the models of parish nursing programs or read parish nurses' descriptions of their practice. Share these with the clinical group.

REFERENCES

American Nurses Association: *Code for nurses with interpretative statements,* Washington, DC, 1985, The Author.

Benner P: *From novice to expert,* Menlo Park, Calif, 1984, Addison-Wesley.

Bergquist S, King J: Parish nursing: a conceptual framework, *J Holistic Nurs* 12:155-171, 1994.

Berry RA: Community health nurse as parish nurse and block nurse. In Stanhope M, Lancaster J, editors: *Community and public health nursing,* ed 5, St. Louis, 2000, Mosby.

Boss J: Being a professional caregiver can be dangerous to your health, *Health Dev* 4:10-14, 1994.

Boss J: Lesson learned over time: great teachers-St. Francis, St. Clare, and Eleanor, *Health Dev* 2:7-19, 1996.

Boss J: Parish nursing with underorganized, underserved, and marginalized clients. In Solari-Twadell PA, McDermott MA, editors: *Parish nursing: promoting whole persons health within faith communities,* Thousand Oaks, Calif, 1999, Sage.

Dossey MD: Dynamics of healing and the transpersonal self. In Dossey MD et al., editors: *Holistic nursing: a handbook for practice,* Gaithersburg, Md, 1999, Aspen.

Fowler M: Ethics as a context for the practice. In Sloari-Twadell PA, McDermott MA, editors: *Parish nursing: promoting whole persons health within faith communities,* Thousand Oaks, Calif, 1999, Sage.

Granberg-Michaelson K: Staying healthy: the spiritual dimension, *Contact* 155:3, 1997.

Health Ministries Association and American Nurses Association: *Scope and standards of parish nursing practice,* Washington, DC, 1998, ANA.

International Parish Nurse Resource Center: *Role of parish nurse: mission and resources,* Ridge Park, Ill, 1998, Advocate Health.

Joel AJ: Parish nursing: as old as faith communities, *AJN* 98:7, 1998.

Keller B: Parish nursing: a holistic approach, *Kentucky Medical News* May/June, 1994.

King JM, Striepe J: Coalition building between public health nurses and parish nurses, *J Nurs Admin* 23(1): 27-31, 1990.

Maginnis and Associates: Combining health care and theology: the parish nurse, *Maginnis Communiqiue* Louisville, Ky, September, 1993, Maginnis & Company.

Matthaei S, Stern L: A healing ministry: the educational functions of parish nursing, *Religious Educ* 89:232-247, 1994.

McDermott MA, Burke J: When the population is a congregation: the emerging role of the parish nurse, *J Community Health Nurs* 10:179-190, 1993.

McDermott MA, Solari-Twadell PA, Matthews R: Promoting quality education for the parish nurse and parish nurse coordinator, *Nurs Health Care Perspect* 19:4, 1998.

North American Nursing Diagnosis Association: *NANDA nursing diagnosis: definitions and defining characteristics,* Philadelphia, 1992, The Author.

Piles CL: Providing spiritual care, *Nurs Educ* 15:36-41, 1990.

Reed PG: An emerging paradigm for the investigation of spirituality in nursing, *Res Nurs Health Care* 15:349-357, 1992.

Ryan JA: Society, the parish and the parish nurse. In Solari-Twadell EA, Djupe AM, McDermott MA, editors: *Parish nursing: the developing practice,* Park Ridge, Ill, 1990, National Parish Nurse Resource Center.

Schnorr MA: Spiritual nursing care: theory and curriculum development, Doctoral Dissertation, Northern Illinois University, *Dissertation Abstracts International* 50: 601-A, DA8912525, 1988.

Shaughnessy MA: *Ministry and the law: what you need to know,* New York, 1998, Paulist Press.

Solari-Twadell PA, McDermott MA: *Parish nursing: promoting whole person health within faith communities,* Thousand Oaks, Calif, 1999, Sage.

Swanson JM, Nies MA: *Community health nursing: promoting the health of aggregates,* Philadelphia, 1997, WB Saunders.

Taylor JT, Madalon A, Highfield M: Spiritual care practices of oncology nurses, *Oncol Nurs Forum* 22(1):31-39, 1995.

Wesley J: On visiting the sick, 1786. In Outler AC, editor: *The works of John Wesley,* Nashville, 1986, Abingdon.

Westberg G: A personal historical perspective of whole person health and the congregation. In Sloari-Twadell PA, McDermott MA, editors: *Parish nursing: promoting health within faith communities,* Thousand Oaks, Calif, 1999, Sage.

Westberg G: Parishes, nurses, and health care, *Lutheran Partners* Nov/Dec:34-36, 1988.

Westberg G, McNamara JW: *The parish nurse: providing a minister of health for your congregation,* 1990, Minneapolis, Minn, Augsburg Fortress.

Home Health

Jean Cozad Lyon and Mary A. Nies

Upon completion of this chapter, the reader will be able to do the following:

1. Discuss the purpose of home health services.
2. Define home health care.
3. Differentiate between the purpose of a public health nursing visit and that of a home health and hospice nursing visit.
4. Use the nursing process in outlining the steps involved in conducting a home visit.
5. Identify the types of home health agencies.
6. Apply the nursing process to a home health client situation.

advance directive
durable power of attorney
home health care
living will

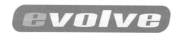

http://evolve.elsevier.com/Nies/

The purpose of home health services is to provide nursing care to individuals and their families in their homes. The specific objectives and services nurses provide vary depending on the type of agency providing services and the population served. Nurses who work for public health departments, visiting nurse associations, home health agencies, or school districts usually provide home visits.

Nurses from clinics often conduct home visits as part of patient follow-up. Public health nurses make visits to follow patients with communicable diseases and provide health education and community referrals to patients with identified health problems. Nurses working for home health agencies, through hospitals or nursing registries, often make home visits to assist patients in their transitions from hospital to home, but health care providers also order these visits when patients experience exacerbation of chronic conditions.

The focus of all home visits is on the individual for whom the referral is received. In addition, the nurse assesses the individual-family interaction and provides education and interventions for the family and the client. The nurse evaluates how the individual and family interact as part of an aggregate group in the community. The nurse identifies the need for referrals to community services and performs the referrals as necessary.

Nurses who make home visits receive referrals from a variety of sources, including the patient's physician, NP or NM, hospital discharge planner or case manager, schoolteacher, or clinic health care provider. The patient or the patient's family can also originate requests for nursing visits to assess and assist in the client's health care.

Home visits have been an integral part of nursing for more than a century, originating with Florence Nightingale's "health nurses" in England. In the United States in 1877, the Women's Branch of the New York City Mission sent the first trained nurses into the homes of the poor to provide nursing care. Under the direction of Lillian Wald, pioneering efforts were initiated to provide services to the poor in their homes in the late nineteenth century (Kelly and Joel, 1995).

HOME HEALTH CARE

The term "home health care" describes a system in which health care and social services are provided to homebound or disabled people in their homes rather than in medical facilities (US Department of Commerce and International Trade Administration, 1990). The USDHHS set forth a definition of home health care that an interdepartmental work group developed, which follows:

Home health care is that component of a continuum of comprehensive health care whereby health services are provided to individuals and families in their places of residence for the purpose of promoting, maintaining or restoring health, or maximizing the level of independence, while minimizing the effects of disability and illness, including terminal illness. Services appropriate to the needs of the individual patient and family are planned, coordinated, and made available by providers organized for the delivery of home care through the use of employed staff, contractual arrangements, or combination of the two patterns (Warhola, 1980).

PURPOSE OF HOME HEALTH SERVICES

The primary purpose of home health services is to allow individuals to remain at home and receive health care services that would otherwise be offered in a health care institution such as a hospital or nursing home setting. The home health industry grew tremendously in the 1980s and in early 1990; it has begun to decline slightly since 1997, related to changes in Medicare home health reimbursement (The Lewin Group, 1998). Numerous factors generated the growth of home health services, including the increasing costs of hospital care and the subsequent introduction of the PPS by P.L. 98-21 of the Social Security Amendments in 1983. Under the PPS, hospitals receive a fixed amount of money based on the relative cost of resources used to treat Medicare patients within each type of diagnosis-related group (Guterman and Dobson, 1986). Many other third-party payers negotiate preferred provider programs or managed care systems. In a managed care arrangement, the health care provider is paid a set fee for providing care to clients enrolled in the program. Providing home care services contributes to cost containment in a managed care environment. This is accomplished through timely hospital discharges by providing nursing services in the home setting and supporting clients at home rather than in skilled facilities. Home care is also popular with consumers, who prefer to receive care in their own homes rather than in an institution.

Home health care services have changed to address the needs of the population. Home health nurses visit acutely ill clients, AIDS patients, the elderly, terminally ill clients, high-risk pregnant women, and ill infants and children (Feldman, 1993). Home health care continues to focus on the care of sick patients and could expand to include health promotion and disease prevention interventions. Home visiting is a specific nursing intervention preceded by an antecedent event and it unfolds as a process (Byrd, 1995). Currently, most reimbursement for nursing services is based on the patient's need for skilled nursing. On each patient visit, the nurse must document that the care provided is of a skilled nature that requires the knowledge and assessment skills of a nurse and must verify that the patient or a family member could not provide the same level of care.

Services coordinated in the home include not only skilled nursing care provided by RNs, but also the services of physical, occupational, and speech therapists; social workers; and home health aides. The broader home care industry definition of home health care includes supportive social services, respite care, and adult day care (Health Care Financing Review, 1988).

TYPES OF HOME HEALTH AGENCIES

Home health agencies differ in their financial structures, organizational structures, governing boards, and populations served. The most common types of home health agencies are official (i.e., public), nonprofit, proprietary, chains, and hospital-based agencies. The number of freestanding proprietary agencies has grown faster than any other type of Medicare-certified home health agency. Freestanding proprietary agencies now comprise almost half of all home health agencies and hospital-based agencies comprise more than a quarter of all certified home health agencies (National Association of Home Health Care, 2000).

There continues to be an increase in the number of managed care agencies, which may have any type of financial structure. Managed care agencies contract with payers, such as insurance companies, to provide specified services to the enrolled clients at a predetermined price. Managed care agencies receive payment before offering services and are responsible for taking the financial risk of providing care to patients within the budgeted allotment. This works well with large numbers of enrolled clients, where the financial risk is spread across a larger number of people, many of whom are healthy and will not require skilled services.

Official Agencies

Local or state governments organize, operate, and fund official (i.e., public) home health agencies. These agencies may be part of a county public health nursing service or a home health agency that operates separately from the public health nursing service but is located within the county public health system. Taxpayers fund official home health agencies, but they also receive reimbursement from third-party payers such as Medicare, Medicaid, and private insurance companies.

Nonprofit Agencies

Nonprofit home health agencies include all home health agencies that are not required to pay federal taxes on account of their exempt tax status. Nonprofit groups reinvest any profits into the agency. Nonprofit home health agencies include independent home health agencies or hospital-based home health agencies. Not all hospital-based home health agencies are nonprofit, even if the hospital is nonprofit. The home health agency can be established as a profit-generating service and serve as a source of revenue for the hospital or medical center. In this situation, the home health agency is categorized organizationally as for profit and they pay federal taxes on the profits.

Proprietary Agencies

Proprietary home health agencies are classified for profit and pay federal taxes on the profits generated. Proprietary agencies can be individual-owned agencies, profit partnerships, or profit corporations. Providing the agencies make a profit, investors in corporate proprietary partnerships receive financial returns on their investments in the agencies. A percentage of the profits generated are also reinvested into the agency.

Chains

A growing number of home health agencies are owned and operated by corporate chains. These chains are usually classified as proprietary agencies and may be part of a proprietary hospital chain.

Agencies within chains have a financial advantage over single agencies. The chains have lower administrative costs because a larger single corporate structure provides many services. For example, a multiagency corporation has greater purchasing power for supplies and equipment because they purchase a larger volume. A single corporate office can provide administrative services such as payroll and employee benefits for all chain employees, thereby reducing duplication of these services. Criticism of proprietary and chain agencies includes concerns over the quality of agency services that are profit driven.

Hospital-Based Agencies

Since the implementation of PPS in 1983, the number of hospital-based home health agencies has doubled (US Department of Commerce and International Trade Administration, 1990). This trend is not surprising in light of the fixed reimbursement under PPS and the hospitals' incentive to decrease length of stay. By establishing home health agencies, hospitals are able to discharge patients who have skilled health care needs, provide the necessary services to the patient, and receive reimbursement through third-party payers such as Medicare, Medicaid, and private insurance companies. The increasing number of home health agencies indicates that these agencies are profitable endeavors and provide hospitals with an additional revenue source.

CERTIFIED AND NONCERTIFIED AGENCIES

Certified home health agencies meet federal standards; therefore they are able to receive Medicare payments for services provided to eligible individuals. Not all home health agencies are certified. The number of Medicare-certified home health agencies increased to approximately 10,444 in 1997 and fell to approximately 9655 in 1998. This is double the existing 5695 Medicare-certified home health agencies in 1990 (HCFA, Office of the Actuary, 1998).

The noncertified home care agencies, home care aide organizations, and hospices remain outside the Medicare system. Some operate outside the system because they provide nonMedicare-covered services. For example, they do not provide skilled nursing care and are not eligible to receive Medicare reimbursement.

SPECIAL HOME HEALTH PROGRAMS

Many home health agencies offer special, high-tech home care services. Offering high-technological services at home is both beneficial to the patient and financially advantageous. Through the implementation of these special programs, patients who require continuous skilled care in an acute or skilled nursing institution are able to return to their homes and receive care at home. From the financial perspective, skilled services provided at home are less costly than hospitalization.

Examples of special services include home intravenous therapy programs for patients who require daily infusions of total parenteral nutrition or antibiotic therapy, pediatric services for children with chronic health problems, follow-up for premature infants who are at risk for complications, ventilator therapy, and home dialysis programs. The key to the success of all these programs is the patient's, family's, or caregiver's ability to learn the care necessary for a successful home program and the motivation of these individuals to provide the care. If family or caregiver support is not available in the home, the patient cannot be a candidate for any of these programs and other arrangements for care must be found.

REIMBURSEMENT FOR HOME CARE

Before the establishment of Medicare in 1965, individuals who required home health services paid cash for the services; donations to the service agency providers helped subsidize care services for patients who were unable to pay (Kent and Hanley, 1990). Since 1965, individuals who are eligible for Medicare benefits under Title XVIII of the Social Security Act, for Medicaid benefits under Title XIX, and people with private health insurance are reimbursed by the federal government through the Medicare program to receive short-term, skilled health care services in their homes. Provided services include nursing care, social service, physical therapy, occupational therapy, and speech therapy and the program is individualized to meet the patient's needs.

The rapid growth of the home health market is reflective of the following:

■ Increasing proportion of people aged 65 years and older
■ Lower average cost of home health care compared with institutional costs ($750 per month for

routine skilled nursing care at home compared with $2000 for care in an institution)

■ Active insurer support for home care

■ Medicare promotion of home health care as an alternative to institutionalization (National Association of Home Care, 2000)

Patient or family payments comprised 46% of the private financing (12% of total spending) for home health services. Private health insurance and nonpatient revenue paid the remaining private financing.

Between 1967 and 1985, the number of home health agencies certified to provide care to Medicare recipients tripled from 1753 to 5983. In the mid1980s, this number leveled off at 5900 resulting from an increase in the volume of paperwork required and unreliable payment policies. This led to a lawsuit against the HCFA charged by Representatives Harley Staggers (D-WV), Claude Pepper (D-FL), and a coalition of members of the U.S. Congress, consumer groups, and the National Association for Home Care (NAHC). The successful conclusion of the lawsuit gave NAHC the opportunity to participate in rewriting the Medicare home care payment policies. New payment policies brought an increase in the home health benefit and increased the number of Medicare-certified home health agencies to over 10,000. The number is now declining as a direct result of the changes in Medicare home health reimbursement enacted as part of the BBA 97 (NAHC, 2000). Under this new payment system, home care agencies are reimbursed on a PPS based on the patient's diagnosis and the projected time skilled services are needed.

NURSING STANDARDS AND EDUCATIONAL PREPARATION OF HOME HEALTH NURSES

The ANA (ANA, 1986; 1992) established standards for home health nursing practice. These standards are differentiated into the following levels of practice: that of the generalist home health nurse, who is prepared at the baccalaureate level, and that of the specialist nurse, who is prepared at the graduate level. According to the ANA, the generalist provides care to individuals and their families and participates in quality assurance programs. The generalist home health nurse must have community health assessment skills to diagnose complex biopsychosocial problems in families, teach health practices, counsel, and refer to other health care providers and high-

technological nursing skills as necessary (Keating and Kelman, 1998).

The specialist home health nurse contributes additional clinical expertise to home health patients and their families, formulates health and social policy, and implements and evaluates health programs and services (ANA, 1986, 1992). RNs with less than a baccalaureate education are not educationally prepared to meet the professional standards for home health nursing. They are encouraged to use the standards in providing care and pursuing professional development.

Unfortunately, many home health agencies have not adopted the ANA's standards for home health nursing and have hired nurses without baccalaureate preparation. Some of these home health agencies offer salaries that are lower than those the acute hospital setting offers and they cannot recruit educationally-qualified nurses.

Albrecht's conceptual model (1990) for home care clearly identifies educational content areas for students in undergraduate and graduate nursing programs that have specialties in home health care. An underlying premise of the model is that professional satisfaction and effective patient outcomes depend on the education and experience of the home health nurse. Implications that are apparent in the model include the following:

■ Nursing programs at the undergraduate and graduate levels must prepare competent providers of home health care.

■ Curricula must include concepts related to the suprasystem, health service delivery system, and home subsystem, which includes structural, process, and outcome elements.

■ Students at the undergraduate level need at least one clinical observation or experience in a home care agency.

■ Graduate-level students need specific courses that cover concepts present in the model, including knowledge of education; preventive, supportive, therapeutic, and high-tech nursing interventions for home health care; a multidisciplinary approach to home health care; health law and ethics; systems theory; economics covering supply, demand, and productivity; and case management and coordination (Albrecht, 1990, p. 125).

The home health nurse serves as a case manager for patients who receive care from the staff of the home health agency or receive care through contract

FIGURE 30-1

Albrecht nursing model for home health care (Based on Albrecht MN: The Albrecht model for home health care: implications for research, practice, and education, *Public Health Nurs* 7:118-126, 1990. Reprinted by permission of Blackwell Scientific Publications, Inc.).

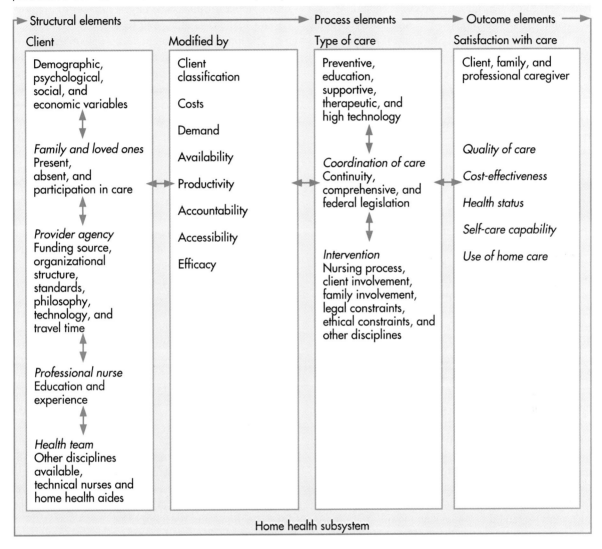

services. The success of the case management plan is contingent upon the nurse's ability to use the nursing process to develop a plan of treatment that best fits the individual needs of the patient, the patient's family, or the caregiver. Patient and family assessment is the first step in developing the treatment plan and nursing care plan.

The Albrecht nursing model for home health care (Fig. 30-1) provides a framework for nurses, patients, and their families to interact and identify mutual goals

of interventions and promote the patient's self-care capability at home (Albrecht, 1990). Three major elements for measuring the quality of home health care patient outcomes include structural, process, and outcome elements.

Structural elements include the client, family, provider agency, health team, and professional nurse. The process elements include the type of care, coordination of care, and intervention. Outcome elements consist of patient and family satisfaction with care, quality of care, cost effectiveness of care, health status, and self-care capability.

In the Albrecht model for home care, the relationship between the structural elements and the process elements directs the interventions. The nurse executes the nursing process, including assessment, nursing diagnosis, planning, intervention, and evaluation and then coordinates patient care (Albrecht, 1990).

DOCUMENTATION OF HOME CARE

The nurse documents assessment data and interventions for all home visits. The patient record also contains a copy of the nursing care plan.

Many home health nurses would probably identify documentation issues as the most frustrating part of providing home health care. Medicare holds a prominent position as a home health care payer; therefore the HCFA's regulations determine the home health industry's documentation. Correct and accurate completion of required Medicare forms is the key to reimbursement. Payment or denial for visits is based on the information presented on the forms. If the nurse does not clearly document the provided skilled care in the nursing notes, the fiscal intermediaries will argue that the care was either unnecessary or not performed and will deny reimbursement. The home health nurse must have an excellent clinical foundation and the ability to identify and document actual and potential patient problems that require skilled nursing interventions (Morrissey-Ross, 1988).

Documenting the care provided to record the patient's quality of care is just as important as documenting for reimbursement purposes. The documentation of home visits records the nurse's observations, assessments of the patient's condition, provided interventions, and the patient's and family's ability to manage the care at home. In addition, documentation of patient visits serves as a formal communication system among other home health professionals who also interact with the patient and family.

FORMAL AND INFORMAL CAREGIVERS

Formal caregivers include professionals and paraprofessionals who provide in-home health care and personal services. They are compensated for the services they provide. The Bureau of Labor Statistics estimates that more than 500,000 people were em-

ployed in home health care agencies in 1998 (US Department of Labor, Bureau of Labor Statistics, 2000). The HCFA reported that 372,452 full-time equivalents (FTEs) were employed in Medicare-certified agencies in September, 1998 (HCFA, Office of the Actuary, 1998). The largest number of employees are home care aides and RNs.

The presence or absence of an involved family member or caregiver can make the difference between the successful completion of the plan of treatment, with the patient remaining in the home, and the need to transfer the patient to an extended-care facility or board-and-care facility. When a capable family member or caregiver is available to assist the patient, the home health nurse spends much of the visit assessing the skills of the caregiver. The home health nurse instructs the caregiver in the correct procedures for providing care and in recognizing the signs and symptoms of problems that must be reported to the health care provider. The goal of the home health nurse's instruction is to provide the caregiver with the skills necessary to care for the patient successfully in the home without intervention of the nurse or other members of the home health team.

Almost three quarters of severely-disabled elderly people who received home health services in 1989 relied solely on family members or other unpaid help to provide their care (US Bipartisan Commission on Comprehensive Health Care, 1990). Eighty percent of these informal caregivers provide unpaid assistance an average of four hours a day, seven days a week. Three quarters of these informal caregivers are female and one third are over age 65. A survey conducted in 1996 estimated that 22 million U.S. households had at least one member who provided some level of unpaid assistance to a spouse, relative, or other person older than 50 years (National Alliance for Caregiving and AARP, 1997).

The home health nurse faces a special challenge in those patients who lack a family member or caregiver capable of learning and providing necessary care. When the patient lives alone and does not have caregivers, the nurse explores other resources available to supplement the patient's self-care activities in the home. For example, if the patient has extensive physical care needs and sufficient financial resources, the nurse may suggest hiring an attendant. Medicare and private insurance companies do not pay for attendant care. If the patient's income is low enough, in-home county support services may be an option. The nurse may consider other services for the patient such as MOW for nutritious meals delivered to the patient's home. Friendly Visitors, a volunteer service, sends a volunteer to the patient's home once a week or more to provide socialization for the patient. Other options that are available in some communities include adult day health centers or senior service centers. Both of these options require arranged patient transportation to and from the centers. A variety of transportation methods are available in different communities; volunteers may transport patients to the centers or public transportation systems may be available such as minivans that provide door-to-door service. Selected services and referrals are based on the patient's individual needs and on the patient's level of functional ability.

HOSPICE HOME CARE

The goal of home care for the terminally ill is to keep the client comfortable at home as long as possible and to provide support and instruction to caregivers. When the patient becomes terminally ill, the focus shifts from cure to comfort care. Some patients insist on staying home until they die and others allow their caregivers to decide. Each family unit has different needs and each must be supported in their decisions. Home death should not be the standard that determines excellence in any case, nor should home death be the ultimate measure of "successful" home care. It is vital to realize that caring for a terminally ill person includes caring for the family or caregivers. Not all caregivers want their loved one to die at home and not all caregivers are capable of allowing that to happen. The goal of home death must be the goal of the patient and family, regardless of the nurse's personal preference.

When caring for a terminally ill person at home, the hospice nurse must be skilled in physical and psychosocial care for both the patient and the caregiver. The patient is viewed as a whole person, not as an isolated disease. Caring for a terminally ill person at home demands that the nurse view the family system as a unit.

Caring for the Caregiver

Although the dying patient is the focus of all skilled nursing care, the experienced home care nurse knows that a careful assessment of the caregiver's mental and physical health is important. The spouse, lover, children, friends, and neighbors who have made the commitment to stay until the end need the nurse's time and attention as much as, if not more than, the patient. Although the patient's wishes are important, all decisions regarding care are made considering the health of the caregivers. They cannot hear the words "You're a great nurse. . ." or "You're doing a wonderful job taking care of. . ." too often.

Gaynor (1990) found that women with more caregiving experience had increased physical health problems than those with less caregiving experience; younger women found caregiving more psychologically burdensome than older women. Nursing interventions must be directed toward preventing a decline in the caregiver's health.

Caregivers need reassurance that their judgment is sound and they need reminders that they cannot do anything "wrong" if it is done for the patient's comfort. The caregivers must understand that they will not mistakenly overdose the patient and they must be reminded repeatedly that the patient will not die from something they did or did not do. Caring for the terminally ill requires that the home care nurse is willing to nurse the entire family.

Pain Control and Symptom Management

British hospice methods of pain control were implemented in the U.S. health care system around 1975. They advocated the avoidance of fluctuations in comfort levels by blocking the pain. In hospice nursing, pain medication is administered in doses sufficient enough to keep the patient free of pain and is administered on a regular schedule to prevent pain from recurring before the next dose. Hospice methods of pain control are particularly well suited to home care. The vast majority of patients can be pain free until their deaths. The key to successful pain control for the terminally ill is to convince patients to take their medications on a regular basis, not just when they "cannot stand it any longer." By building a wall against the pain, the patient will never hurt or want for relief. The nurse explains to patients that most pain medicines last about four to five hours before completely wearing off. Patients are instructed to take their pain medication every four hours on a twenty-four hour basis to ensure a "margin of safety" so the medicine will not wear off before the next dose is due.

F I G U R E **30-2**

Pain assessment ruler (Reproduced with permission from Roxane Laboratories, Columbus, Ohio).

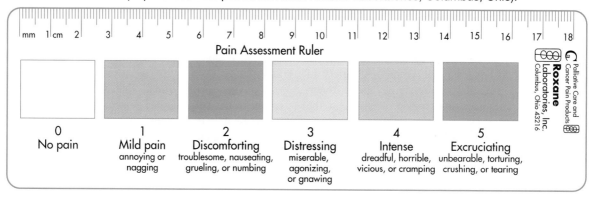

Pain is subjective. Only the patient experiences the pain and only the patient can judge its severity. To assist the patient in pain evaluation, the nurse may use an audiovisual aid such as the Pain Assessment Ruler distributed by Roxane Laboratories (Fig. 30-2). This pain assessment tool allows the patient to indicate a color that best describes the pain; zero is white and indicates no pain; one is light blue and indicates mild pain (e.g., annoying and nagging); two is yellow and indicates discomfort (e.g., troublesome, nauseating, grueling, and numbing); three is apricot and indicates distressing pain (e.g., miserable, agonizing, and gnawing); four is orange and indicates intense pain (e.g., dreadful, horrible, vicious, and cramping); and five is red and indicates excruciating pain (e.g., unbearable, torturing, crushing, and tearing). This pain assessment scale uses both colors and words; therefore it is appropriate for patients who cannot read.

Use of Morphine

Many patients, especially the elderly, are afraid of becoming "junkies" or "druggies" and want to delay using morphine until they "get really bad." Many people believe that morphine signals "the end of the line" and they are amazed to learn that patients do well while receiving this drug for months, even years, before death occurs. Almost every family must learn that addiction is not the same as tolerance and that their physicians will not "cut off their supply if they take too much."

LEGAL AND ETHICAL ISSUES IN HOME HEALTH

There are several legal and ethical issues in home health, most of which revolve around end-of-life issues and the type of care that terminally ill patients desire. Early education about these issues is essential in the prevention of problems and it allows patients the opportunity to make decisions for themselves and communicate them to family members and health care providers.

All competent adults have the right to make decisions that will direct health care providers in the type of care they administer. Planning for end of life allows patients the opportunity to communicate their wishes clearly. This communication can occur through the completion of advance directives, durable power of attorney for health care, and living wills.

Advance Directive

An **advance directive** is a written document in which a competent person gives instructions about future health care in the event that the individual is unable to make decisions. These directives are completed on a voluntary basis. All Medicare-certified health care agencies are obligated to ask patients about advance directives and provide patients with the advance directive form if the patient is interested in completing the document (LovingCare. net, 2000).

Durable Power of Attorney for Health Care

A durable power of attorney for health care is one type of advance directive. Also called a health care proxy, the **durable power of attorney** for health care gives another person the power to make medical decisions related to care. This person, as identified by the patient, acts as the patient's agent in all decisions regarding health care, personal care, and custody in the event that the patient becomes incompetent or disabled and unable to make decisions.

Living Will

A **living will** is a written document in which a patient voluntarily informs doctors and family members about the type of medical care desired should the patient become terminally ill or permanently unconscious and unable to communicate. In the living will, the patient can describe the type of care desired, depending on the clinical situation. For example, if the patient is terminally ill and unconscious, the patient can direct the health care team to perform only those measures that will provide comfort and nothing further. The patient can specifically indicate his or her opposition to life saving measures; for example, the patient may request the denial of cardiopulmonary life support in the event of a cardiac arrest. Other examples include indicating the exclusion of chemotherapy, blood transfusions, and respirator use in an attempt to prolong life.

These documents make the patient's wishes very clear to the family and health care team. The patient's clear delineation of choices eliminates many of the issues that families and health care team members encounter because they know the patient's wishes surrounding health care choices.

CONDUCTING A HOME VISIT

Visit Preparation

It is important that the nurse prepare for the home visit by reviewing the referral form including the purpose of the visit, the geographical residence of the family, and any other pertinent information. The first home visit gives the nurse the opportunity to establish a trust relationship with the client and family to establish credibility as a resource for health information and community referrals in a nonthreatening environment.

The Referral

The referral (Fig. 30-3) is a formal request for a home visit. Referrals come from a variety of sources including hospitals, clinics, health care providers, individuals, and families. The type of agency that receives the referral will vary depending on the necessary client services. Public health referrals are made for clients who are in need of health education (e.g., infant care education and resource allocation) or for follow-up of clients with communicable diseases.

Home health referrals are requested to provide clients with short-term, intermittent, skilled services and rehabilitation. Visits can last from 30 to 90 minutes, depending on the specific needs of the client, and are scheduled on an intermittent basis depending on need. For example, a client who had a stroke requires skilled nursing assessments, physical therapy visits for gait training, speech therapy for speech deficit improvement, and occupational therapy for retraining in ADL such as bathing and cooking.

By reviewing the referral form before the first visit, the CHN obtains basic information about the client such as name, age, diagnosis or health status, address, telephone number, insurance coverage, and reason for the referral. The form also specifies the source of the referral such as a clinician, health care provider, communicable disease service, hospital, client, or client's family.

Public health referrals usually provide information on the client's condition that necessitates public health nurse visits. For example, for a client who is positive for TB, the nurse is notified of the client's place of residence, type and location of employment, and any known contacts including family and friends. Another example is a 16-year-old girl who is referred for antepartum visits because she is seven months pregnant and has just initiated prenatal care.

Additional information provided in the home health referral includes current client medications, prescribed diet, physician's orders, care goals, and other disciplines involved in the client's care. This information is important because it helps the nurse become familiar with the client's condition.

Initial Telephone Contact

The nurse contacts the client and informs him or her about the service referral. The first telephone contact with the client or family consists of an exchange of

FIGURE 30-3

Referral form (Courtesy of Home Calls, Oakland, California).

Patient number	☐ New ☐ Readmit **Intake**	Date last seen by MD	Case manager

Name: Last First M.I.	Telephone no.:	Sex M F	Birthdate	Age	Date of first visit MD auth. Yes____ No____

Street address: City: State: Zip:	Hosp/snf: Adm. date: Dis. date:
Directions:	

Diagnoses: Primary #	Physician name: Specialty:	Hosp/snf:
1.	Address:	Adm. date:
2.	Tel. no:	Dis. date:
3.	Physician name: Specialty:	Medicare no.
4. DX known to pt?_____	Address: Tel. no:	Medical no./ss#.

History:	Agency worker: Tel. no:	Ins. co.:
	Pay sources/service request:	Policy #: Grp:. #:
	PHN PT ST OT	Cov. code:
	MSW HHA HCA PD	Tel. no:
Religious/cultural patterns/ language/psychosocial	Emergency/family contacts (by priority) Name Rel. Home# Work# #1	Contact person:
Medications	Address #2	
	Address	

Pertinent hospital information

Diet/fluids	Date/time:_____
	Skilled orders per:_____
Allergies	
Equipment: DME Yes____ No____	

Intake source name Agency Tel. no:
How did you learn about our services?
Intake received by Date

essential information, including an introduction by the nurse, identification of the agency that received the referral, and the purpose of the visit. After the initial exchange of information, the nurse informs the client of his or her desire to make the home visit, the client gives permission, and the group sets a mutually acceptable time for the visit. The nurse is a guest in the client's home; therefore it is important that the client agrees to the visit. The nurse then verifies the client's address and asks for specific directions to the client's home.

During a home health visit, the nurse requests proof of insurance such as a Medicare, Medicaid, HMO membership identification card, or insurance card. The nurse should forewarn the client so the client or family can locate the information before the visit. If the client is unable to provide this verification, the nurse assists with locating the information during the visit. Clients who receive a public health home visit do not require evidence of insurance coverage because these services are not billed directly. A county public health budget or state or federally funded programs generally cover these visits.

Not all clients have a telephone. If this is the case, the nurse should check the referral for a telephone number where messages can be left. It is also worthwhile to contact the health care provider who made the referral to see whether the telephone number was omitted unintentionally. If the client does not have a telephone, the nurse may choose to make a drop-in visit. This type of visit consists of an unannounced visit to the client's home, during which the nurse explains the purpose of the referral, receives the client's permission for the visit, and appoints a time for a future visit with the client. The client may agree to the first visit while the nurse is there.

If the client is not at home for the drop-in visit, the nurse should leave an official agency card and a brief message asking the client to contact the agency to schedule a nursing visit. The nurse informs the referring agency that the visit was attempted, but that the client was not available for contact. A formal agency letter, identifying the agency and the reason for the referral, is often sent to clients who are difficult to contact. The nurse's primary responsibility when unsuccessful in locating the client is to keep the clinic, physician, or referring agency informed of efforts to establish contact with the client.

Environment

An environmental assessment begins as the nurse leaves the agency en route to the client's home. The nurse should make specific observations, which follow (Keating and Kelman, 1998):

- How does the client's neighborhood compare with other neighborhoods in the area?
- Are there adequate shopping facilities, such as grocery stores, close to the client's home?

The nurse should also note the client's dwelling; for example, whether the client lives in a single-family home, in a single room in a home or hotel, in an apartment, or in a shared apartment or house. Specific assessments include the following:

- Is the client's residence easily accessible by the client given the client's age and functional ability? For example, if the client has limited endurance, can he or she negotiate several flights of stairs when entering or leaving the dwelling?
- Are handicapped facilities available as necessary? Is the dwelling in an area with high rates of drug abuse or crime?
- Is the building or home secure? Does the client live alone? If so, how does the client get to the physician or clinic? How does the client purchase groceries?
- Does the client have food in the home? If so, who prepares the client's meals? Are the meals nutritious?
- Are there rodents, cockroaches, or other potential vectors of disease present in the client's home?
- Does the client's home have hot running water, heat, sanitation facilities, and adequate ventilation?
- Is the client's residence safe relative to the client's physical status, or is the home cluttered with debris and furniture?

Improving Communication

When the nurse meets with the client, whether in the home or at another mutually agreeable location, the initial conversation revolves around social topics. The nurse assumes a friendly manner and asks general questions about the client, the client's family, and health care services that will benefit the client. These questions help the nurse assess the client's needs and create a comfortable atmosphere for communication.

Building Trust

Many clients in need of nursing visits do not trust the health care system and are uncomfortable with the representative from an agency visiting their home. For example, a client who is pregnant and does not have legal status in the United States will be hesitant to allow a nurse to visit; the client will be afraid of being reported to immigration authorities. The nurse's role in visiting this client is to focus on the health and safety of the client and her fetus. The nurse must build a trust relationship early in the visit or the client will not allow additional visits. If a trust relationship is not established and the client believes that the nurse will report her to immigration, it is highly probable that the client will move to another location to avoid future contact.

APPLICATION OF THE NURSING PROCESS

Assessment

During the first home visit, the type of client assessment will vary depending on the purpose of the home visit. The public health nurse assesses the client's knowledge of his or her health status. The nurse identifies knowledge deficits and uses this information to develop a care plan.

Subjective information is obtained from the client and the client's family and includes the client's perception of the situation and what the client identifies as problems. The nurse assesses whether the client is isolated from others physically or socially and whether the client is a member of a close-knit, nurturing, supportive family or kinship network. The amount of support the client perceives as available may or may not be accurate; therefore the nurse asks several questions about the client's family, friends, and daily routine to assess the client's level of social support.

The home health nurse assesses the client's health knowledge; his or her physical, functional, and psychosocial status; physical environment; and social support during the first home visit. The nurse collects information through observations and questions the patient and family or caregivers in the home environment. It is not unusual to find inconsistencies between information the patient provides during hospitalization concerning the amount of physical and emotional support available to the patient in the home and the amount of help actually available to the patient in the home. The nurse validates or modifies the referral information to reflect the actual home situation. CHNs often use contracts that the nurse, patient, and family jointly develop to delineate the responsibilities of the patient in the home.

The client's physical assessment is generally performed in the home health visit and includes a review of all systems, with an emphasis on the systems affected by the client's present condition. The nurse obtains objective data through the use of essential physical assessment skills such as observation, palpation, auscultation, and percussion. The physical assessment also includes information regarding the client's functional status. Assessment of the functional status is important for Medicare reimbursement and for the development of an individualized plan of care. This assessment includes information regarding the client's ability to ambulate, to perform ADL independently, and to use assist devices such as a cane or wheelchair. Specific functional limitations, such as shortness of breath or muscle weakness, are assessed at this time.

Information obtained during the assessment phase is used to identify nursing diagnoses and develop a plan of care. Data collection continues while the patient receives home health services. Changes in the patient's condition, environment, or social structure necessitate modifications in the treatment plan and the nursing care plan.

There are differences between the treatment plan and the nursing care plan. The plan of treatment includes the type of home health services received, the projected frequency of visits by each discipline (Albrecht, 1991), and the necessary interventions. The nursing care plan addresses specific nursing interventions designed to treat the patient's actual or potential problems and includes identified goals with measurable outcomes.

Diagnosis and Planning

Develop a Plan for the Client and Family
After the assessment phase of the home visit, the nurse identifies the nursing diagnoses that address the patient's problems and identifies actual or potential problems. The identification of nursing diagnoses serves as the basis for the nursing care plan. This plan is developed in consultation with the client and the family. The plan identifies short-term and long-term goals and measurable outcomes for the patient. The

plan identifies nursing interventions that are necessary and additional home health services that are appropriate to help the patient achieve the identified goals. To maximize the plan's success, it is important that the patient and family are involved in the planning process and access community resources. Planning is a dynamic process that continues while the patient receives nursing services. The plan is modified as needed, depending on the patient's condition, until the identified goals are met.

Often the nurse will develop a contract with the client that delineates the role and responsibilities of the nurse regarding the client's health and the role of the client and family (Spradley, 1990). If the client expresses a disinterest in contracting to improve health during the planning phase, the nurse will be limited in possible interventions. Goals are identified that the client is willing to work toward with the nurse's assistance.

The goal of home visits for both public health and home health nursing is to involve the client and family in taking an active role in health promotion. The nurse is careful not to allow the client to become dependent on the nurse's interventions because the nurse's involvement is short term.

Outline the Client and Family Roles

Written contracts are helpful for both the nurse and the client because the client's role and the nurse's role in implementing the plan are clearly delineated (Spradley, 1990). If either the client or the nurse forgets their role in the plan, the written contract becomes a reference. The client and the nurse can modify the contract by mutual agreement.

Intervention

Implementation of the care plan begins during the first home visit. The nurse begins to provide the client and family with health information concerning the client's health status and informs them about the availability of and access to community resources. In the case of the home health visit, the nurse provides skilled nursing care. At the end of the initial home visit, the nurse discusses the need for another home visit. The nurse and client discuss the goal of the next visit; specifically, they discuss what the client should do before the visit. The nurse informs the client and family about any information or skills he or she will provide during the next visit and the nurse and client agree on a day for the next visit.

Referral for Community Services

During the first visit, the nurse provides the client and family with information regarding community resources, including the purpose of the resources, their eligibility in the services provided, any involved expense, and agency telephone numbers. Referrals depend on the availability of community resources, the client's eligibility for the services, the client's and the family's willingness to use the services, and the resources' suitability for the client and family. Examples of such services include information about immunization clinics for children in the family; adult day care or senior centers for elderly clients who could benefit from socialization; adult education classes or continuation of high school for pregnant teen clients who have dropped out of high school; MOW services for clients who are not able to prepare meals; homeless shelters for men, women, and families; soup kitchens; resources for clothing and housing; mental health clinics; resources for battered spouses; and primary care clinics for low-income clients with and without insurance.

If necessary, the client or client's family may request the nurse's assistance in contacting the community resources. The client and family are encouraged to make the contacts, but if the client and family are unable to make the calls or do not speak English, the nurse needs to intervene on behalf of the client. By providing referral information during the first home visit, the nurse can follow-up on the client's or the family's success in contacting and using community services.

Terminating the Visit

The nurse terminates the first visit when the assessment is completed and a care plan is established with the client. The average visit should not exceed one hour. The client receives a great deal of information during that hour and the nurse collects a great deal of information. Most clients are tired at the end of a one-hour visit and often cannot retain additional information. It is preferable to set a date for another home visit to reinforce the information provided and work progressively toward achieving goals.

Evaluation

Evaluation of Progress toward Goals

The evaluation phase occurs when the nurse can determine whether the mutually-established goals are realistic and achievable for the patient and the patient's family. The evaluation process is continuous and allows the nurse to determine the success or progress toward the patient's identified goals. The nurse can identify the need for revisions in the nursing care plan and treatment plan through the collection of additional data during the evaluation phase. The nurse can intervene to make necessary changes. An example is an elderly wife who, during the initial home visit, stated that she preferred to provide the physical care for her frail, nonambulatory husband. On a subsequent visit, the nurse assessed that the patient was not receiving the care required for the patient's personal care, specifically bathing. The nurse discussed the problem with the wife and presented her with available options. These included the services of a home health aide to provide personal care and bathing three times a week. A new plan was developed and it included the home health aide. The plan was implemented and evaluated during future visits. Input from the client is critical to determine whether the goals established are realistic and achievable for the client.

Modification of the Plan as Needed

The evaluation process also allows the nurse and client or family to discuss what is working well and where modifications are necessary in the plan. Evaluation occurs through open communication between the nurse and client and the nurse asks questions about specific parts of the care plan. If a trust relationship exists, the client feels comfortable telling the nurse about problems in the care plan.

When Goals Are Achieved

The overall purpose of home visits is to assist the client with necessary information and nursing care to enable the client to function successfully without nursing interventions. When the care plan goals are achieved, the client does not need the nurse any longer. The client knows what community resources are available and how to access health care services for primary, secondary, and tertiary interventions.

APPLICATION OF THE NURSING PROCESS THROUGH HOME VISITS: CASE STUDIES

CASE STUDY 1

PUBLIC HEALTH VISIT: COMMUNICABLE DISEASE FOLLOW-UP

The public health nurse received a referral from the county hospital to see Ray, a 57-year-old white man who was newly diagnosed with TB. The first purpose of the referral was for the public health nurse to meet with the client to ensure that he received the appropriate information about TB and received follow-up medical care on a regular basis. The second purpose of the referral was for the public health nurse to meet with Ray and identify the people with whom he had been in close contact. The nurse then established contact with these people, notified them that they had been exposed to TB, and encouraged them to have follow-up tests for TB.

The nurse contacted Ray and established a time for the home visit. The nurse noted that he resided in a residential hotel in a lower-middle-class neighborhood of a large urban area. During the initial visit, the nurse discovered that the client was an unemployed construction worker. He did

not know where he might have contracted TB. Ray assured the nurse that he was taking his medication as directed. He gave the nurse the names of his friends he played poker with every week at a hotel and told the nurse that he advised his friends to be tested for TB. The nurse made a note of the names and later talked with them individually by telephone. During these subsequent conversations, the nurse was very careful to maintain the client's confidentiality. The nurse informed these individuals that they could have been exposed to TB and that they should seek testing through their health care providers or through their local health department.

Ray indicated that he did not have family and he had minimal contact with other people besides his friends at the hotel. The nurse recorded this information on the communicable disease form and returned the information to the public health department's communicable disease division.

Assessment

The public health nurse's assessment of the client with a communicable disease involved the individual, family, and community.

Individual

The public health nurse assessed whether the client received appropriate information and regular medical care for TB and whether the client followed the prescribed treatment regimen.

Family

Although Ray stated that he did not have family, his friends in the hotel constituted a working support network. The public health nurse was familiar with kinship networks and their importance as alternative family systems (Stack, 1974). Nursing assessment of Ray's kinship network involved determining whether the members were tested for TB. In addition, the public health nurse assessed the client's network for the following:

- Network composition
- Network's knowledge of TB
- Functional capacity
- Network stressors
- Network strengths and weaknesses
- Network's ability to provide support for Ray
- Health beliefs and practices
- Use of health services

Community

The public health nurse was aware that the number of new cases of TB in the community had increased over the past 12 months. The public health nurse further noted that there was an increase in the number of area residents immigrating from various third world countries and this population might be at increased risk for developing TB (Dowling, 1991).

Diagnosis

Individual

The public health nurse determined that Ray had a knowledge deficit regarding the disease process and transmission of TB.

Family

Ray's support network demonstrated knowledge deficits related to the disease process and transmission of TB, location of communicable disease clinics, and the importance of screening those exposed to TB.

Community

The public health nurse, in conjunction with case workers at the communicable disease clinic, formulated the following diagnosis for Ray's community: increased risk for development of TB among community residents as evidenced by increased incidence of new cases of TB over the past 12 months.

Planning and Goals

Individual

Short-Term Goal
- Client will verbalize knowledge of transmission of TB; signs and symptoms of complications of TB; purpose, administration schedule, and side effects of medications.

Long-Term Goal
- Client will perform self-care activities related to treatment of TB and follow-up as necessary with appropriate health care professionals.

Family

Short-Term Goal
- Support network members will demonstrate basic knowledge of cause and transmission of TB and will agree to be tested for TB.

Long-Term Goal
- Support network members with positive test results will receive appropriate treatment.

Community

Short-Term Goal
- Community members will demonstrate knowledge of increased incidence of TB in their community and of available community resources for treatment and prevention of TB.

Continued

Long-Term Goal

• Incidence of TB in the community will decrease over the next three years.

Intervention

Implementation of the plan of care for the client with TB occurs at the individual, family, and community levels.

Individual

The public health nurse referred Ray to the communicable disease clinic at the local health department. TB is a reportable communicable disease; therefore the public health nurse obtained information from the client regarding people with whom he had been in close contact.

Family

The public health nurse contacted members of Ray's support network and referred them to the communicable disease clinic as appropriate. The nurse provided these people with information concerning TB transmission and the importance of early treatment and follow-up.

Community

The public health nurse met with professionals from the communicable disease clinic and the health department and with members of the community to establish a program to raise public awareness regarding the increased incidence of TB in the community. The public was informed about the importance of preventive measures, the avail-

ability of community screening services for TB, and the existing health care resources in the community.

Evaluation

The client's and the support network's knowledge of the disease process, transmission, treatment, and signs and symptoms of TB are indicators in evaluating the care plan. Confirmation of the client's and his support network's follow-up with the communicable disease clinic can also be used for evaluation.

The incidence rate of TB in the community and the rate in which TB clinics and related resources are used are measures that can be used to evaluate the effectiveness of interventions at the aggregate level.

Levels of Prevention

Primary prevention of communicable disease is directed toward prevention of specific disease occurrence such as TB. Programs that increase public awareness of the disease process and of the transmission, diagnosis, and treatment of TB constitute primary prevention activities. The goal of secondary prevention is the early detection of existing conditions. Tuberculin skin testing and subsequent follow-up of positive test results are important secondary prevention measures. The tertiary level of prevention is aimed at reducing the effects and spread of TB. Referral for early, effective treatment and education of clients for self-care are important measures of tertiary prevention.

CASE STUDY 2

PUBLIC HEALTH HOME VISIT: ANTEPARTUM CLIENT

The public health nurse received a referral to see a 17-year-old African-American woman named Ali, who was referred by the county prenatal clinic. Ali was five months pregnant with her third pregnancy within the past year. Ali miscarried the previous two pregnancies during the first trimester.

When the nurse made the home visit, she noted that Ali was 5 foot 9 inches tall and weighed 120 pounds. She resided in a two-room apartment with her boyfriend, who was the father of the baby. The nurse began the first visit with social talk, asking Ali general questions about her employment, education, and the duration of her residence in the area. Ali appeared to be pleased that the nurse was interested in her. Once a trusting relationship was initiated, the nurse asked Ali how she felt about the pregnancy. Ali revealed that she was happy about the pregnancy, but was worried that there would be problems because she had two previous miscarriages. She had not planned any of the pregnancies, but she did not use contraceptives to prevent the pregnancies either. Ali's boyfriend worked and was able to pay the rent and buy food for her. Ali dropped out of high school during her junior year, but she wanted to complete her high school education. She had Medicaid coverage for her health care.

During the initial home visit, the nurse assessed that Ali was underweight and had several knowledge deficits in the areas of prenatal nutrition, infant care, breast feeding, and contraception. The nurse also identified the need for a referral to the public school for the continuation of Ali's high school education. The nurse briefly discussed her assessment with Ali in a nonthreatening, nonjudgmental manner. The nurse informed Ali that if she was interested, she could schedule future home visits to provide Ali with more information and answer her questions. Ali agreed to receive future visits to discuss the topics the nurse identified during the assessment phase. They mutually agreed upon the plan for future visits. As the visits progressed, the nurse and Ali modified the plan based on progress evaluation.

The nurse terminated home visits with Ali when the mutually-established goals were achieved. The nurse scheduled a postpartum visit with Ali after the baby was born to assess infant care and answer any questions Ali had concerning infant care.

Assessment

Although it is important to perform an individual assessment of Ali, the public health nurse assessed Ali as a member of a family and as a member of the community. "Community" in this case referred to the aggregate of publicly-insured adolescent pregnant women.

Individual

Assessment of Ali revealed an underweight 17-year-old pregnant woman who was unable to demonstrate knowledge of nutrition in pregnancy, infant care, breast feeding, contraception, and educational options for pregnant teenagers.

Family

An individual assessment of Ali mandated the need for an assessment of the composition and function of Ali's family. The public health nurse assessed the following factors with regard to Ali's family (Logan, 1986):

- Family composition
- General support network
- Family and network patterns related to Ali's psychosocial and economic support
- Family and network attitude toward health
- Family and network beliefs regarding use of health-related services
- Beliefs and attitudes of family and network regarding infant care, breast feeding, and nutrition
- Attitude of infant's father regarding involvement with Ali and their baby, health beliefs, ability to assume the role of parent, and knowledge of pregnancy and birth

Community

The public health nurse was aware of the need to see the larger, aggregate picture. Identifying the aggregate as the pregnant adolescent community, the public health nurse used the following techniques in an ongoing assessment (Bayne, 1985):

- Observations
- Resource analysis
- Key informant interviews
- Environmental indexes

Using these techniques, the public health nurse gathered information regarding the following:

- Educational and employment options for pregnant teens and teens with infants
- Availability of health services targeting low-birth-weight infants
- Availability of support groups for this aggregate
- Availability of teen parenting classes

Continued

Diagnosis

The public health nurse formulated nursing diagnoses based on thorough individual, family, and community assessments.

Individual

The following individual nursing diagnoses were formulated for Ali:

- Knowledge deficit regarding nutrition in pregnancy, infant care and feeding, contraception, availability of community resources, and educational options for pregnant teenagers
- Inadequate nutrition related to low-income status and inadequate knowledge of nutritional requirement for pregnancy

Family

The public health nurse formulated the following diagnosis for Ali and her family:

- Lack of family support related to Ali living away from home
- Altered family communication patterns related to role confusion among family members

Community

The public health nurse formulated the following diagnoses for the pregnant adolescent community:

- Minimal availability of health care services, parenting classes, contraception counseling, and educational opportunities for pregnant teenagers
- Lack of coordination of existing services

Planning

Planning health services and interventions for pregnant teenagers involves formulation of short-term and long-term goals for the individual, family, and community.

Individual

Short-Term Goals
- Ali will gain at least three pounds per month
- Ali will demonstrate knowledge of community

resources for pregnant adolescents by next nursing visit

Long-Term Goal
- Ali will carry her infant to term without evidence of maternal or fetal complications

Family

Short-Term Goal
- Ali and her partner will attend teen parenting classes

Long-Term Goal
- Ali, her partner, and other family members will be able to perform mutually-determined role responsibilities

Community

Short-Term Goals
- Increased community awareness of resources for pregnant teenagers
- Increased awareness of contraception counseling services for adolescents

Long-Term Goals
- Establishment of effective, comprehensive prenatal health, contraception, and education services for pregnant teenagers
- Decline in rate of teen pregnancies and birth of compromised neonates over the next 24 months

Intervention

Implementation of Ali's individual care plan involved visits by the public health nurse with a referral to existing prenatal services for pregnant teenagers. Family intervention was composed of Ali's and the father's referral to a support group for pregnant teenagers and partners. Implementation of the care plan for the aggregate of adolescent pregnant women included the following:

- Meeting with community leaders
- Meeting with local school administrators and faculty to disseminate information for pregnant teenagers

HOME HEALTH VISIT

- *Story by Leonard Kaku, RN, MSN*
- *Photography by George Draper*

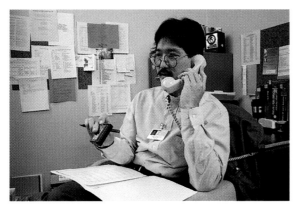

Home health nurses and some community health nurses (CHNs) make visits to families with health problems. A referral for this home visit is received from a client's nurse practitioner. The client was discharged from the hospital with a primary diagnosis of noninsulin-dependent diabetes mellitus (NIDDM) and a secondary diagnosis of hypertension and S/P cerebrovascular accident (CVA), which occurred 10 months ago.

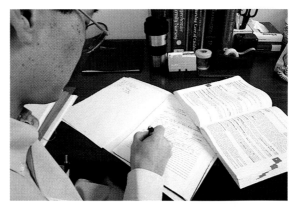

The nurse reviews the information on the referral form. The referral reveals the client is newly diagnosed with NIDDM and has a history of hypertension and CVA with left-sided weakness. The client's insurance is Medicaid. The current medications listed are: 25 mg hydrochlorothiazide q.d., 5 mg Isordil q.i.d., and 5 mg Micronase b.i.d. The prescribed diet is a low-fat, 1200-calorie diet with no added salt. If there is information missing, it is important to obtain it before making initial client contact.

The nurse brings to the community health setting experience and knowledge from a variety of specialties such as maternity, mental health, medical-surgical, pediatrics, pharmacology, and epidemiology.

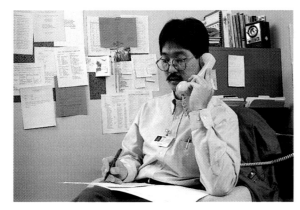

The nurse usually makes the initial contact by phone. It is important to introduce yourself and the agency you represent and to explain the purpose of the visit. You will need to obtain permission and arrange a date and time for the visit. Occasionally, the client may not have a phone. This may require a drop-in visit. Attempt a home visit and be prepared for a full visit if the client is at home and requests your services. If the client is not at home, the nurse should leave a business card with a note requesting a call to arrange a home visit.

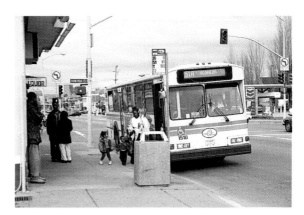

The assessment process begins as soon as the nurse leaves the office on the way to the home visit. Transportation may be a problem for the client. Is it available? What is the cost and hours of operation? Are there safety concerns about using public transportation?

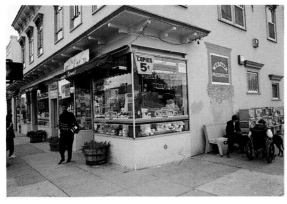

It is important to assess the availability of services, such as a pharmacy and a bank. Where does the client go to get cash or deposit a check and to fill a prescription? Is the area safe for these transactions for the client?

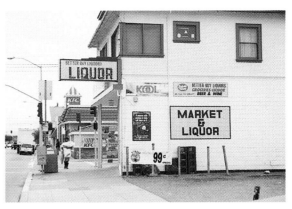

Is there a grocery store nearby? What types of foods are available?

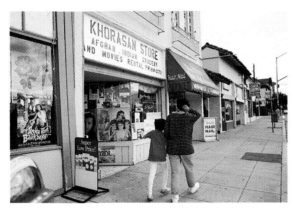

The nurse notices an Afghan-Indian grocery store that provides for ethnic communities.

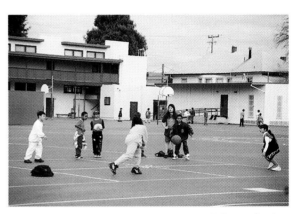

The school in the area provides evidence of diverse families in the community.

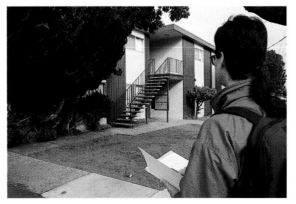

Assessment of the type of neighborhood in which the client resides is also important. Is it residential, business, or mixed; high- or low-density housing, single family homes, or apartments? Is the neighborhood safe or unsafe, e.g., high crime or drug area?

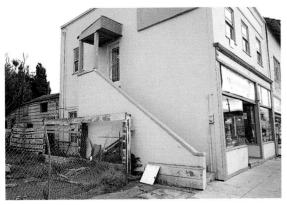
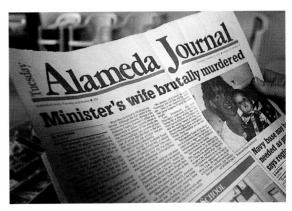

It is extremely important for the nurse to be aware of the environment and surroundings as you approach and observe the residence.

You are not to disregard personal safety to make a home visit. If it is unsafe, arrange another time and place for the home visit.

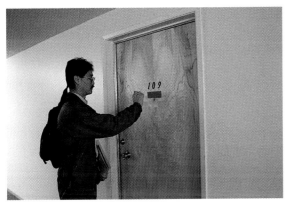
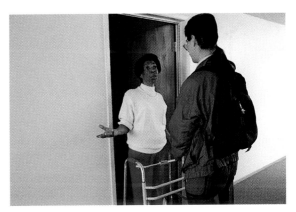

When you knock at the door, be sure to state your name, role, agency you represent, and the purpose of the visit.

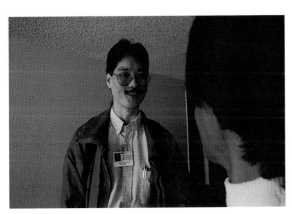
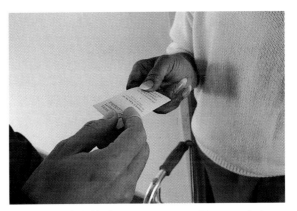

You should always wear your identification badge.

Business cards with the agency name, address, and phone number should be available to give to clients. Building trust provides the foundation for a therapeutic relationship with the client. Clients may be hesitant to trust the health care/social system.

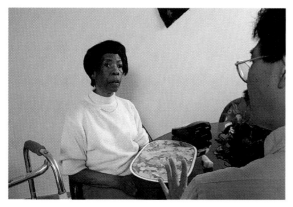

It is important to establish a comfortable atmosphere. This may be accomplished by initiating social conversation. It moves from general questions about the client and family to more sensitive health issues. The purpose of the visit is to provide health care services, and this should be clearly communicated to the client. This home visit includes a health history and limited physical examination.

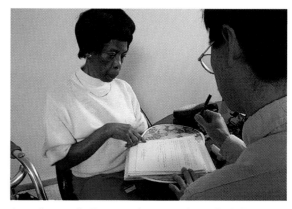

Agencies vary in the type of paperwork required. A consent form is often required prior to providing services. The form should be explained so the client may make an informed consent.

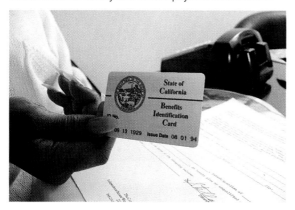

Medical insurance should also be verified so that the service may be billed properly.

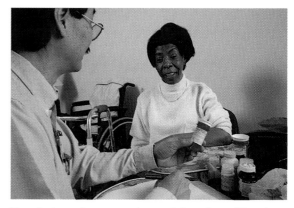

The client may have several prescriptions from different health care providers. These medications may have expired or may no longer be necessary. This is an opportunity for the nurse to provide instructions pertaining to the use of medications.

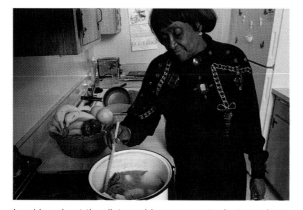

Inquiring about the diet provides an opportunity to explore compliance and cultural implications. It is helpful to have a diet plan that includes culturally relevant food. Teaching the client how and why to maintain a diet log will assist in evaluating compliance with the low-fat, 1200-calorie diet.

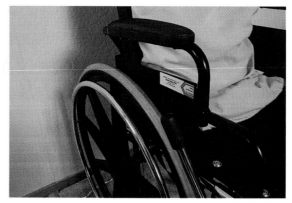

Health history includes a functional assessment of the client. Physical limitations of the client in performing activities of daily living are important health assessment data. The nurse has already noted any physical barriers to ambulation, both exterior and interior, that may exist. The nurse has already observed the use of a walker by the client at the door and a wheelchair nearby.

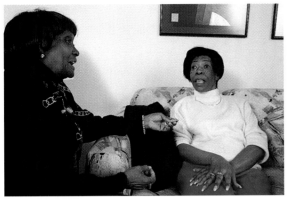

It is important to do a family assessment. Observation of the interaction between the client and family will be helpful in developing a nursing care plan. The family should be incorporated into the nursing care plan for the client.

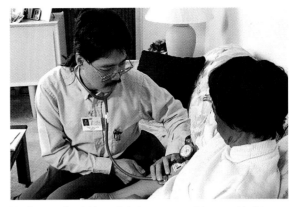

Equipment for taking vital signs may not be provided by the client. The nurse should always have a stethoscope and have access to a sphygmomanometer. To many clients, the taking of a blood pressure is a reassuring initial step in a health examination. It provides nurses a window of opportunity to obtain important health history data and provide health teaching.

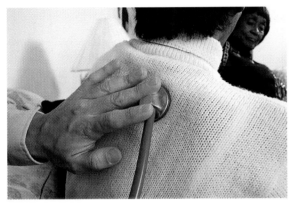

A focused physical examination is done on the client. This will provide the baseline data of the client's health status. This information will be used on subsequent visits to assess progress towards the identified nursing goals.

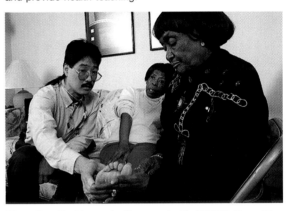

Since the client is newly diagnosed with NIDDM, it would be important to teach proper foot care.

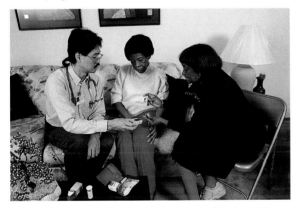

The use of a glucometer may help the provider in making clinical decisions regarding treatment. This is another opportunity to provide health teaching for the client. Review the proper use of the glucometer and have the client do a demonstration. It is helpful to incorporate the family members in the teaching plan.

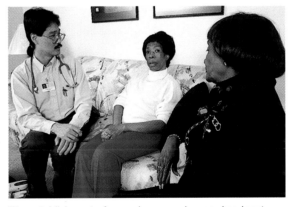

The establishment of a nursing care plan requires input from the client and family. An agreed-upon goal is following a low-fat, 1200-calorie diet. The family will help in preparing the food and doing blood glucose monitoring. The nurse will provide a culturally relevant diet and contact the local American Diabetes Association (ADA) chapter for a support group for the family. A return visit is scheduled for the following week.

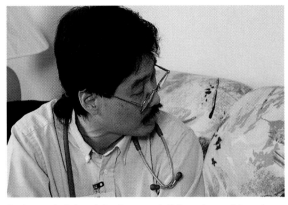

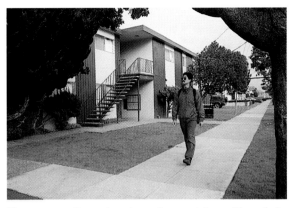

At the end of the visit, always ask if there is anything else you could assist with. It provides an opening for the client and family to ask for assistance that may not have been covered during the home visit. Remind the client of the business card and ask the client to call if there are any problems. Also advise the client you will be contacting the health care provider regarding outcomes of the home visit.

The nurse continues to note environmental conditions that impact the client, family, and community. The nurse can then begin to advocate for health promotion and prevention interventions surrounding the environmental issues confronting the community.

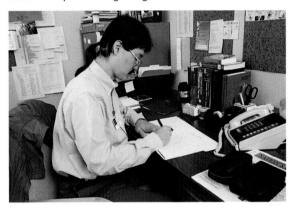

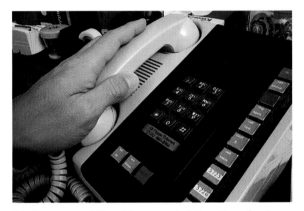

The nurse charts according to agency policy as soon as possible to ensure accurate, clear, and concise notes of the home visit. This may be done at the office or between home visits.

It is the responsibility of the nurse to inform the referral source of the home visit results. This is especially important if the nurse has been unable to locate the client. The result of the home visit may be provided in a written or verbal format.

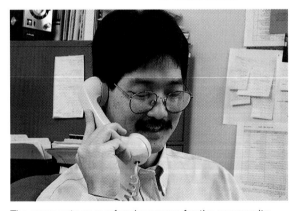

The nurse acts as a referral resource for the community. The nurse continuously searches for community resources and develops a resource database. The nurse calls the local ADA chapter to find out about the services provided. The agency does indeed have a culturally sensitive diet available for the client as well as a support group for family members. The nurse calls the client with the information.

- Formation of community organizing groups (Bayne, 1985)

Evaluation

Evaluation included measures of individual teenagers' nutritional status and teenagers' and their families' use of support groups and educational and nutritional services. Evaluation of the effectiveness of interventions at the aggregate level focused on measurement of available options for pregnant teenagers, measures of teen awareness and use of services, and determination of changes in incidence rates of teen pregnancy and compromised neonates.

Levels of Prevention

Prevention of teenage pregnancy involves interventions at primary, secondary, and tertiary levels. At the primary level, prevention is composed of activities that prevent teen pregnancy from occurring. The secondary level of prevention involves interventions for early detection of teen pregnancy and early intervention such as counseling for prenatal care. The goal of prevention at the tertiary level is to reduce the effects of adolescent pregnancy. Examples of tertiary prevention for pregnant teenagers include provision of prenatal education in areas such as nutrition, parenting, and infant care.

CASE STUDY 3

HOME HEALTH VISIT

Susan Brown is a 40-year-old woman who was the driver in a single-car, rollover accident. She was airlifted to a trauma center and treated for multiple lacerations and abrasions, including a severe laceration to the left inner aspect of her arm. The hospital made a referral for home health services at the time of discharge. The referral requested the home health nurse to perform daily wound care to the infected left arm laceration. The specific wound care medical orders consisted of removing the arm brace, performing wet-to-dry dressing changes using one-fourth strength Daikin's solution, wrapping the arm with gauze, and reapplying the brace. Medications included one or two Vicodin tablets every six hours as needed for pain and 500 mg of Keflex four times a day.

During the initial visit, the home health nurse collected data in the assessment and identified the following primary problems:

- The infected left arm laceration had large amounts of drainage related to the introduction of bacteria
- Severe arm pain related to the injury
- Knowledge deficit related to inadequate understanding of the self-administration of antibiotic

- Anxiety related to family communication problems

These problems were the basis for Susan's nursing care plan.

Diagnosis

The patient had an infected left arm laceration related to the introduction of bacteria secondary to the wound, which was secondary to a motor vehicle accident.

Short-Term Goals
- Keep the laceration clean and debride the wound with daily wet-to-dry dressing changes
- Encourage self-care in dressing changes

Long-Term Goals
- Healed laceration without drainage or infection
- Full range of motion of the affected arm

Intervention

Susan had a moderate-to-large amount of yellow drainage from the laceration on her left arm; therefore dressing changes were initiated, with
Continued

additional dressings applied to contain the drainage. When the large amount of drainage persisted more than three days after initiating the antibiotic therapy and the patient continued to have low-grade fevers (temperature 99.2° to 99.8° F), the home health nurse notified the physician and took a culture of the drainage. An alternative antibiotic was prescribed based on the culture results. The nurse taught Susan and her mother how to change the dressings and the nurse supervised them.

Diagnosis

Pain related to arm injury.

Short-Term Goal
- Pain control initiated through medication and relaxation techniques

Long-Term Goal
- Pain free when arm injury is healed

Intervention

The assessment of Susan's arm pain included a history of when the pain was most severe and the frequency of pain medicine administration. The home health nurse assessed that the pain was most severe at night and recommended that Susan take two Vicodin tablets before going to bed and place her left arm in a position of comfort, supported by pillows to decrease edema. The nurse instructed Susan to lie down, rest, and listen to relaxing music during the day when the pain was intense to decrease the amount of arm pain through relaxation.

Diagnosis

Knowledge deficit related to inadequate understanding of self-administration of antibiotic.

Short-Term Goal
- Correct self-administration of antibiotic

Long-Term Goal
- Infection resolved

Intervention

When the home health nurse asked Susan when she took the Keflex, Susan explained that she took the medication at 9:00 AM, 1:00 PM, 5:00 PM, and 9:00 PM because the drug was prescribed to be taken four times a day. The nurse explained the purpose of the antibiotic and the importance of taking it every six hours to maintain an optimum blood level. Susan and the nurse agreed on a schedule of 6:00 AM, 12:00 noon, 6:00 PM, and bedtime.

Diagnosis

Anxiety related to family communication problems.

Short-Term Goal
- Decreased anxiety through verbalization of feelings

Long-Term Goal
- Anxiety resolved or controlled

Intervention

Susan's sister arrived from out of state to assist with her care after the accident. Within three days of her arrival, Susan's husband and sister got into an argument and the sister left abruptly and returned home. This altercation was very upsetting to Susan, who was distraught over the communication problems between her husband and sister. The home health nurse encouraged Susan to express her feelings concerning the dysfunctional relationship and discuss how she would address the situation with both her husband and her sister. The nurse stressed that the problem was between the husband and her sister and that Susan should not feel guilty or responsible for the disagreement.

Susan has a large, supportive family and a caregiver was available to assist her every day. Her family coordinated transportation to and from physician appointments without the nurse's intervention. The nurse remained involved with Susan until the infection cleared and the family learned how to provide the necessary wound care.

Referrals

Susan's internist and orthopedist referred her for follow-up. She was also referred for a gynecological appointment for evaluation of sudden onset of slight vaginal bleeding.

Susan's sister returned to her home and further confrontations did not occur. The nurse suggested counseling for Susan if the hostile relationship persisted between her husband and sister or if it continued to cause Susan anxiety.

CASE STUDY 4

HOSPICE HOME VISIT

Ed McMillan is 64 years old and dying of prostate cancer. He experiences urinary retention, chronic pain, weakness, constipation, and anorexia. He understands he does not have long to live, but he wants to be able to attend his youngest son's wedding in a nearby town and he wants to die at home.

Working together with Ed and his wife, the hospice nurse identified four nursing diagnoses. Only short-term goals were identified because the patient is terminal.

Diagnosis

Urinary retention related to obstruction by the tumor.

Short-Term Goal
• Urinary drainage through a Foley catheter

Intervention

The nurse inserted an indwelling urinary catheter to alleviate urinary retention. The nurse instructed Ed's family in catheter care and in the signs and symptoms of UTI.

Diagnosis

Pain related to cancer.

Short-Term Goal
• Pain control

Intervention

Oral morphine sulfate (80 μg every four hours around the clock) for pain.

Diagnosis

Mobility impairment related to weakness from cancer.

Short-Term Goal
• Maximum mobility

Intervention

The nurse ordered a walker and a wheelchair to maximize Ed's mobility and instructed the family in proper use of the equipment.

Diagnosis

Constipation related to morphine sulfate ingestion.

Short-Term Goal
• Regular bowel movements

Intervention

To prevent constipation, the nurse initiated a daily bowel regimen that included monitoring fluid intake and introducing a stool softener and laxative as needed. The nurse requested that Ed's physician order small doses of prednisone to temporarily enhance the patient's poor appetite. The hospice nurse also taught Ed and his family a great deal.

The nurse instructed the family that it is common to lose appetite in advanced cancer. Despite the constant reassurance, Mrs. McMillan continued to do her best to feed her husband regularly, believing that "if only he'd eat, he'd get his strength back." The nurse continued her advocacy for Ed by praising his wife for her loving care, but repeated that it is normal for a patient with cancer to have a poor appetite. The nurse's interventions helped the patient become pain free and his bowels moved easily and regularly. Using a leg bag instead of the usual catheter bag and using the wheelchair for transportation, Ed was able to attend his son's wedding.

When Ed became too weak to stand, his hospice nurse had an electric hospital bed set up in his home. The bed was strategically placed in the den, which was the center of family activity, and a home health aide came to bathe him every other day. As his level of consciousness declined, the nurse helped his family keep him pain free by requesting morphine sulfate in rectal suppository form. When the patient's lungs began to fill with fluid, the nurse suggested oxygen via nasal cannula

Continued

and transdermal scopolamine patches to lessen his shortness of breath and decrease his secretions. While Ed was comatose, the nurse visited daily to determine whether the family was coping adequately and offered suggestions as small problems occurred. The hospice nurse suggested that Mrs. McMillan's children help make funeral arrangements and get financial affairs in order before Ed died.

Ed died peacefully in his own home, surrounded by his wife, children, and many grandchildren. As he wished, his corneas were donated for transplantation and a memorial service was held for family, friends, and former colleagues. Ed's ashes were scattered at their weekend home in the mountains. After the initial bustle subsided, the hospice nurse made a follow-up bereavement visit.

Hospice nurses who care for the terminally ill practice truly professional nursing. As case manager, the nurse draws on the expertise of the interdisciplinary team to obtain what the patient and family need at a most vulnerable time. Hospice nurses are pivotal when caring for the dying because they are practical, knowledgeable, flexible, and family centered. Nurses have a long history of speaking for those who cannot speak for themselves. In patients' homes, nurses advocate for the terminally ill by offering unique skills in pain and symptom management and by sharing their hearts and their hands.

SUMMARY

This chapter presented information on performing public health, home health, and hospice nursing visits to clients in their homes. A general overview of the nursing process for clients in the home setting was presented and expanded to include the individual, family, and community. Case studies involving communicable disease, teen pregnancy, traumatic injury, and terminal cancer have been presented. The home visit is the foundation of community health nursing and provides a forum for important interventions with individuals, families, and communities. The CHN is responsible for bringing the concerns of individuals and families into the community.

LEARNING ACTIVITIES

1. Make arrangements to accompany a public health nurse, a home health nurse, and a hospice nurse on home visits.
2. Interview a public health nurse about the types of client referrals received and ask what interventions are usually performed. Repeat this activity with a home health nurse and a hospice nurse. Ask the nurses what they like best about their jobs.
3. Contact a local home health agency and interview the agency director. Ask what type of agency it is, the profit status, and whether it is Medicare certified. Report findings to classmates.

4. Attend a team meeting in a home health agency or a hospice program to see how the roles of the various team members blend together to provide family-centered care.
5. Interview a public health nurse and home health nurse and ask how the community impacts the care they provide.

REFERENCES

Albrecht MN: Home health care: reliability and validity testing of a patient-classification instrument, *Public Health Nurs* 8:124-131, 1991.

Albrecht MN: The Albrecht nursing model for home health care: implications for research, practice, and education, *Public Health Nurs* 7:118-126, 1990.

American Nurses Association: *A statement on the scope of home health nursing practice,* Washington, DC, 1992, The Author.

American Nurses Association: *Standards of home health nursing practice,* Kansas City, Mo, 1986, The Author.

Bayne T: The pregnant school-age community. In Higgs AR, Gustafson DD, editors: *Community as client: assessment and diagnosis,* Philadelphia, 1985, FA Davis.

Byrd ME: A concept analysis of home visiting, *Public Health Nurs* 12:83-89, 1995.

Dowling PT: Return of TB: screening and preventive therapy, *Am Fam Physician* 43:457-476, 1991.

Feldman R: Meeting the educational needs of home health care nurses, *J Home Health Care Pract* 5:12-19, 1993.

Gaynor SE: The long haul: the effects of home care on caregivers, *Image J Nurs Sch* 22:208-212, 1990.

Guterman S, Dobson A: Impact of the Medicare prospective payment system for hospitals, *Health Care Financing Rev* 7:97-114, 1986.

Health Care Financing Administration, Office of the Actuary: *Unpublished estimates for the President's fiscal year 2000 budget,* December, 1998, The Author, www.hcfa.gov.

Health Care Financing Review: National health expenditures, 1988, *Health Care Financing Rev* 11:1-41, 1988.

Keating SB, Kelman GB: *Home health care nursing: concepts and practice,* Philadelphia, 1998, JB Lippincott.

Kelly L, Joel L: *Dimensions of professional nursing,* ed 8, New York, 1995, McGaw-Hill.

Kent V, Hanley B: Home health care, *Nurs Health Care* 11:234-240, 1990.

Logan BB: Adolescent pregnancy. In Logan BB, Dawkins CE, editors: *Family-centered nursing in the community,* Menlo Park, Calif, 1986, Addison-Wesley.

Loving Care.net: *Legal issues,* 2000, The Author, www.lovingcare.net.

Morrisey-Ross M: Documentation: if you haven't written it, you haven't done it, *Nurs Clin North Am* 23:363-371, 1988.

National Alliance for Caregiving and the American Association for Retired Persons: *Family caregiving in the U.S.: findings from a national survey,* Washington, DC, 1997, The Author.

National Association of Home Health Care: *HomeCare online,* 2000, The Author, www.nahc.org.

Spradley BW: *Community health nursing: concepts and practice,* ed 3, Glenview, Ill, 1990, Scott, Foresman and Little, Brown.

Stack C: *All our kin,* New York, 1974, Harper & Row.

The Lewin Group: *An impact analysis for home health agencies of the Medicare home health interim payment system of the 1997 Balanced Budget Act,* Washington, DC, Aug 11, 1998, National Association for Home Care.

US Bipartisan Commission on Comprehensive Health Care: *The Pepper Commission Final Report: a call for action,* SPrt 101-114, Washington, DC, 1990, US Government Printing Office.

US Department of Commerce and International Trade Administration: *U.S. industrial outlook,* Washington, DC, 1990, US Government Printing Office.

US Department of Labor, Bureau of Labor Statistics: *National industry-occupation employment matrix, data for 1996,* 2000, The Author, www.bls.gov.

Warhola C: *Planning for home health services: a resource handbook,* USDHHS Pub No HRA 80-14017, Washington, DC, 1980, PHS, USDHHS.

The Future of Community Health Nursing

31 Health in the Global Community

32 Community Health Nursing: Making a Difference

31

Health in the Global Community

Julie Novak

OBJECTIVES

Upon completion of this chapter, the reader will be able to do the following:

1. Describe population characteristics and international patterns of health and disease.
2. Discuss the World Health Organization (WHO) concepts of "Health for All" and primary health care.
3. Identify international health care organizations.
4. Describe the role of the community or public health nurse in international care.
5. Compare and contrast the International Community Assessment Model (ICAM) and the Water Project Community Empowerment (WPCE) Model for developed and developing countries.

KEY TERMS

developed country
epidemiologic transition
International Council of Nurses (ICN)
lesser developed country
Pan American Health Care Organization (PAHO)
primary care
primary health care
United Nations International Children's Fund (UNICEF)
World Bank
World Health Organization (WHO)

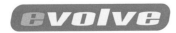

Human health and its influence on every aspect of life is at the center of the global agenda (WHO, 1999). Health, the most valuable possession, is a primary concern throughout the world. Nurses, as expert care providers and leaders in international health care, promote and restore health in individuals, families, and communities in rural and urban settings. Community public health nurses must be aware of forces that threaten health in the global community. Nurses must study models of community assessment, community empowerment, and health care delivery in the United States and other countries to promote health in the global community.

This chapter highlights population characteristics; international patterns of health and disease; social, cultural, and economic factors; international health organizations including WHO; health care providers; health care delivery systems; and the community public health nurse's role in the global community. The chapter presents the development of ICAM and a community empowerment model for population-focused health care delivery. These models can provide a framework for international research, education, service, practice, and policy design.

Population characteristics, including patterns of growth and demographics, are among the many health issues that merit attention and study because they have global effects and threaten human life. This chapter will also explore these issues and other environmental factors including identified stressors and patterns of health and disease.

POPULATION CHARACTERISTICS

Over one billion people will enter the twenty-first century without benefiting from the health care revolution (WHO, 1999). Enormous population growth presents a threat to the health and the economy of many nations. The exponential nature of world population growth is evident. In 1804, after two to five billion years of human existence, the world population exceeded one billion. Between 1804 and 1927, the population reached two billion and between 1927 and 1960, three billion. The population soared to four billion between 1960 and 1974 and five billion between 1974 and 1987. In 1999, the world population grew to six billion. By 2005, the world's population is estimated to reach seven billion. World population in the midtwenty-first century is expected to reach 7.3 to 10.7 billion (WHO, 1999).

In any society, large populations create pressure.

For example, feeding a population may become problematic in developing countries if famine or problems with international trade occur. Malnutrition, disease, or death may be the outcomes. Pressures from population growth are also felt in industrialized nations. Although food may be plentiful, overcrowding leads to pollution, stress, disease, and violence; all major constraints to economic growth. The poor suffer this burden of excess mortality and morbidity disproportionately. Thus, improving QOL through health promotion, effective health care delivery systems, and the enhancement of the environmental infrastructure will address the origins of poverty and ultimately increase productivity and improve QOL.

World population distribution is uneven. Over 50% of the population lives in China, India, the former Soviet Union, the United States, and Indonesia. In 1998, 35% of the world population were children, 10% were elderly, eighty million lived in developing countries, and approximately six million lived in developed countries (WHO, 1999). In developed countries, the life expectancy was 70 to 84 years of age and in developing countries, it was 39 to 65 years of age (WHO, 1999). Malcolm Potts, a world-renowned population theorist, predicted that "by the twenty-first century the world may end up divided not into political or economic groups but by demographic structure," where countries will be classified into slow-growth vs. fast-growth countries instead of rich or poor countries. However, this will eventually further divide the rich and poor (Potts, 1994).

As the world population grows, a rising global trend toward urbanization occurs; people live closer together and migrate to urban areas for employment. For example, in 1975, 38.5% of the world's population lived in urban areas. By 1994, the proportion of urban dwellers swelled to 45%; this proportion is expected to reach 50% by 2015 (United Nations Population Fund, 1998). With increasingly dense living arrangements, the health of the general population is threatened by environmental factors and disease.

ENVIRONMENTAL FACTORS

The relationship between humans and their environment is an important component of individual and global health. The field of environmental health and sustainable development has exploded since 1990 (WHO, 1999). Environmental stressors are categorized into four types. First, stressors such as lead poisoning and air pollution directly assault human health. Second, stressors such as the effects of air pollution on products and structures damage society's goods and services. Third, stressors such as noise and litter affect QOL. Finally, stressors such as global warming interfere with the ecological balance.

Air, water, and land pollution are among the consequences of environmental stressors. For example, 50% of the worldwide air pollution problem is attributable to the chemical pollutant carbon monoxide. Other primary pollutants, such as nitrogen monoxide, sulfur oxides, particulate matter, and hydrocarbons, combine with carbon monoxide to create 90% of the world's pollution. In developing countries, only 75% of the urban population and 50% of the rural population have sanitation facilities, which is a significant contributing factor to water pollution (World Bank, 1998).

Agricultural, industrial, residential, and commercial wastes increase land pollution. For example, chemical fertilizers have displaced natural fertilizers; synthetic pesticides have displaced natural means of pest control; and petrochemical products, such as detergents, synthetic fiber, and plastics, have replaced soap, cotton, and paper. Disposable goods have replaced reusable goods, resulting in increased waste. Production technologies are contributing to worldwide environmental and ecological stress.

PATTERNS OF HEALTH AND DISEASE

Lifestyles, beliefs, and politics have an impact on existing illnesses and society's commitment to prevention (Rosenkoetter, 1997). Disease patterns vary throughout the world; therefore primary causes of mortality differ in developed and developing countries. CVD, cancer, respiratory disease, stroke, violence, and traumatic injury are the primary causes of mortality in developed countries. Infections, malnutrition, and violence are the primary causes of mortality in developing countries; however, CVDs are becoming more prevalent (Labarthe, 1998). Once plagued with high rates of infectious disease, developed countries significantly reduced high mortality rates from these diseases through improved sanitation, nutrition, and medical care. A **developed country** has a stable economy and a wide range of industrial and technological development. These countries experience an **epidemiological transition** (i.e., the morbidity and mortality profile of a country changes from

a **lesser developed country** profile to a developed country profile). For example, many developed countries experienced an epidemiological transition from having an infectious disease profile to having a chronic disease profile and are now plagued by chronic diseases such as CVD, respiratory disease, and cancer secondary to air pollution and the tobacco epidemic. This altered profile created a demographic transition from traditional societies where almost everyone is young, to societies with rapidly increasing numbers of middle-aged and elderly people (WHO, 1999).

Among the infectious diseases that contribute to high rates of mortality in developing countries are AIDS, endemic malaria, TB, hepatitis B, rheumatic heart disease, parasitic infection, and dengue fever. These diseases claim the lives of millions, yet the World Bank (1998) estimated that these diseases could be reduced by up to 50% through effective public health interventions. Many of these diseases will join small pox as a disease known only to history through the development and implementation of immunization programs. Immunization is the most powerful and cost effective strategy at our disposal (WHO, 1999). Efforts are underway to develop an antitrust malarial vaccine as 90 countries are considered malaria-ridden (Thanassi, 1998). The Bacille Calmette-Guerin (BCG) vaccine series induces active immunity, but does not reduce the transmission of infectious types of TB. At least one third of the world's population harbors the TB pathogen, *Mycobacterium* TB. The "Roll Back Malaria" and "Stop TB" programs are priorities of WHO. WHO's "HIV/AIDS Control" and "Tobacco Free" initiatives also target the key issues of the twenty-first century.

AIDS is an enormous global concern. In 1998, over 22.5 million adults and children were estimated to be living with AIDS in subSaharan Africa and 33.4 million adults and children worldwide were living with this disease. New HIV infections were estimated to be 5.8 million (WHO, 1999). The total number of AIDS deaths since the beginning of the epidemic is 13.9 million (UNAIDS, 1998).

Although AIDS is a global epidemic, it varies demographically in different parts of the world. For example, the estimated male-female ratio of HIV infections in North America is 5:2, whereas in Africa the ratio is 1:1 (WHO, 1999). Urbanization and intra-country migration also play a role in the spread of AIDS. For instance, in Rwanda the HIV seroprevalence is over 14 to 20 times higher in urban areas vs.

rural areas. Annually, HIV threatens more lives as more people migrate into the world's largest cities. The United Nations estimates that by the year 2010, 50% of the developing world will live in cities. This is an increase from 25% in 1970.

With over 450,000 tobacco-related deaths in the United States each year and over five million worldwide, tobacco control is a critical component of the international health care agenda. By 2020, an estimated one in seven deaths will be tobacco related. Since 1990, tobacco policies have been implemented at various political levels in the United States and abroad; however, the magnitude and consequences of the tobacco epidemic was unexpected (WHO, 1999). Smoking prevention and cessation programs, state and federal mandates, tobacco taxation, the tobacco settlement, anti-tobacco media campaigns, strict licensing of tobacco retailers, the elimination of tobacco vending machines and point-of-sale advertising, and the elimination of tobacco sales by pharmacies have made an impact on tobacco sales in the United States. Although American adults have enrolled in cessation programs, the tobacco industry has targeted youth and dramatically increased international exports (Novak, 1998). A global commitment to tobacco control can avert millions of premature deaths in the next half century and the success of such control can guide the development of effective interventions for other threats to health (WHO, 1999, p. vii). The need to counter potential threats to health resulting from economic crises, unhealthful environments, or risky behavior is critical. Promotion of a healthy lifestyle underpins a proactive strategy for risk reduction, immunization provision, cleaner air and water, adequate sanitation, healthful diets, fitness and exercise programs, and safe transportation.

INTERNATIONAL ORGANIZATIONS

Promoting worldwide health is humankind's greatest challenge. Several global agencies, such as the **World Health Organization** (WHO), the **Pan American Health Organization** (PAHO), **United Nations International Children's Fund** (UNICEF), and the **World Bank**, play important roles in improving the health of all nations. Founded in 1948, WHO is an international health agency of the United Nations that consists of countries working toward "health for all by the year 2000." This goal was instituted at the Alma-Ata conference in the USSR in 1978. The conference defined "health for all"

as "the attainment by all citizens of the world by the year 2000 of a level of health that will permit them to lead a socially and economically productive life" (WHO, 1999, p. 65). The central goal of health for all has not been attained; therefore the target year for achievement has been extended to 2010.

The Alma-Ata conference on **primary heath care** expressed the need for urgent action by all governments. The WHO statement of beliefs, goals, and objectives are outlined in the Declaration of Alma-Ata, which is presented in Box 31-1. The concept of primary health care stresses health as a fundamental human right for individuals, families, and communities; the unacceptability of the gross inequalities in health status; the importance of community involvement; and the active role for all sectors. Primary health care seeks to obtain the highest level of health care for all people. The program promotes the following seven elements of primary health care: health education regarding disease prevention and cure, proper food supply and nutrition, adequate supply of safe drinking water and sanitation, maternal and child health care, immunizations, control of endemic diseases, and the provision of essential drugs.

According to WHO, a primary health care system should provide the entire population with the following: universal coverage; relevant, acceptable, affordable, and effective services; a spectrum of comprehensive services that provide for primary, secondary, and tertiary care and prevention; active community involvement in the planning and delivery of services; and integration of health services with development activities to ensure that complete nutritional, educational, occupational, environmental, and safe housing needs are met (Bryant, 1984).

PAHO is an international public health agency with more than 90 years of experience in working to improve the health and living standards of the Americas. It serves as the regional office of WHO and is recognized as part of the United Nations system.

UNICEF is another important global health organization. Founded in 1946 to assist children in war-ravaged Europe, UNICEF works for children's survival, development, and protection by developing and implementing community-based programs. UNICEF achievements are well documented in child health, nutrition, education, water, sanitation, and progress for women. UNICEF collaborates with

BOX 31-1

Declaration of Alma-Ata

The International Conference on Primary Health Care, meeting in Alma-Ata this twelfth day of September in the year Nineteen hundred and seventy-eight, expressing the need for urgent action by all governments, all health and development workers, and the world community to protect and promote the health of all the people of the world, hereby makes the following Declaration:

I. The Conference strongly reaffirms that health, which is a state of complete physical, mental, and social well-being and not merely the absence of disease or infirmity, is a fundamental human right and that the attainment of the highest possible level of health is a most important worldwide social goal, whose realization requires the action of many other social and economic sectors in addition to the health sector.

II. The existing gross inequality in the health status of the people, particularly between developed and developing countries and within countries, is politically, socially, and economically unacceptable and is therefore of common concern to all countries.

III. Economic and social development, based on a New International Economic Order, is of basic importance to the fullest attainment of health for all and to the reduction of the gap between the health status of developing and developed countries. The promotion and protection of the health of the people are essential to sustained economic and social development and contribute to a better quality of life and to world peace.

IV. The people have the right and duty to participate individually and collectively in the planning and implementation of their health care.

V. Governments have a responsibility for the health of their people, which can be fulfilled only by the provision of adequate health and social measures. In the coming decades, a main social target of governments, international organizations, and the whole world community should be the attainment by all peoples of the world by the year 2000 of a level of health that will permit them to lead a socially and economically productive life. Primary health care is the key to attaining this target as part of development in the spirit of social justice.

VI. Primary health care is essential health care based on practical, scientifically sound, and socially acceptable methods and technology made universally accessible to individuals and families in the community through their full participation and at a cost that the community and country can afford to maintain at every stage of their development in the spirit of self-reliance and self-determination. It forms an integral part both of the country's health system, of which primary health care is the central function and main focus, and of the overall social and economic development of the community. It is the first level of contact for individuals, the family, and the community with the national health system bringing health care as close as possible to where people live and work and it constitutes the first element of a continuing health care process.

VII. Primary health care:

1. reflects and evolves from the economic conditions and sociocultural and political characteristics of the country and its communities and is based on the application of the relevant results of social, biomedical, and health services research and public health experience;

2. addresses the main health problems in the community, providing promotive, preventive, curative, and rehabilitative services accordingly;

3. includes at least education concerning prevailing health problems and the methods of preventing and controlling them; promotion of food supply and proper nutrition; an adequate supply of safe water and basic sanitation; maternal and child health care, including family planning; immunization against the major infectious diseases; prevention and control of locally endemic diseases; appropriate treatment of common diseases and injuries; and provision of essential drugs;

Reprinted, by permission, from Alma-Ata: *Primary health care, report of the international conference on primary health care,* "Health for All" Series, No 1, pp. 2-6, Geneva, September 6-12, 1978, WHO. *Continued*

B O X **31-1—cont'd**

Declaration of Alma-Ata—cont'd

4. involves, in addition to health sector, all related sectors and aspects of national and community development, in particular agriculture, animal husbandry, food industry, education, housing, public works, communication, and other sectors; and demands the coordinated efforts of all those sectors;

5. requires and promotes maximum community and individual self-reliance and participation in the planning, organization, operation, and control of primary health care making fullest use of local, national, and other available resources; and to this end, develops through appropriate education the ability of communities to participate;

6. should be sustained by integrated, functional, and mutually supportive referral levels, on health workers, including physicians, nurses, midwives, auxiliaries, and community workers, as applicable, and on traditional practitioners as needed, suitably trained socially and technically to work as a health team and to respond to the expressed health needs of the community; and

7. relies, at local and referral levels, on health workers, including physicians, nurses, midwives, auxiliaries, and community workers, as applicable, and on traditional practitioners as needed, suitably trained socially and technically to work as a health team and to respond to the expressed health needs of the community.

VIII. All governments should formulate national policies, strategies, and plans of action to launch and sustain primary health care as part of a comprehensive national health system and in coordination with other sectors. To this end, it will be necessary to exercise political will, to mobilize the country's resources, and to use available external resources rationally.

IX. All countries should cooperate in a spirit of partnership and service to ensure primary health care for all people because the attainment of health by people in any one country directly concerns and benefits every other country. In this context the joint WHO-UNICEF report on primary health care constitutes a solid basis for the further development and operation of Primary Health Care through the world.

X. An acceptable level of health for all the people of the world by the year 2000 can be attained through a fuller and better use of the world's resources, a considerable part of which is now spent on armaments and military conflicts. A genuine policy of independence, peace, détente, and disarmament could and should release additional resources that could well be devoted to peaceful aims and in particular to the acceleration of social and economic development of which primary health care, as an essential part, should be allotted its proper share.

The International Conference on Primary Health Care calls for urgent and effective national and international action to develop and implement primary health care throughout the world and particularly in developing countries in a spirit of technical cooperation and in keeping with a New International Economic Order. It urges governments, WHO and UNICEF, and other international organizations, and multilateral and bilateral agencies, nongovernmental organizations, funding agencies, all health workers and the whole world community to support national and international commitment to primary health care and to channel increased technical and financial support to it, particularly in developing countries. The Conference calls on all the aforementioned to collaborate in introducing, developing and maintaining primary health care in accordance with the spirit and content of this Declaration.

Reprinted, by permission, from Alma-Ata: *Primary health care, report of the international conference on primary health care,* "Health for All" Series, No 1, pp. 2-6, Geneva, September 6-12, 1978, WHO.

WHO as advocates for child health and women's health.

The major goal of the World Bank is to facilitate significant interventions to improve the health status of individuals living in areas that lack economic development. Projects range from safe water to effective sanitation to affordable housing. Financial assistance for the education of health care providers; the improvement of internal infrastructures; and funding for projects related to health status, disease control, and prevention has been provided.

Through the **International Council of Nurses** (ICN), nursing has been internationally involved at a professional level for over 100 years. The ICN and its member associations have addressed current and future nursing and health care needs (Gregory-Dawes, 1998).

INTERNATIONAL HEALTH CARE DELIVERY SYSTEMS

When comparing health care systems, developed and developing countries can learn much from each other. Although transferring specialized medical technologies from developed to developing countries may not always be appropriate, developing countries are currently learning from health care reform policies and the technological revolution in developed countries. Likewise, developed countries have much to learn about low-technology initiatives such as oral rehydration therapy for the treatment of diarrhea and the delivery of primary health care as defined by WHO. Participatory approaches to health care delivery, such as community involvement in health and education, are also essential. This exchange is important given the state of the current health care policy in developed countries. Many developed countries have made health care inaccessible to portions of their general public. Even in countries with socialized medicine, medical costs increase annually and citizens are faced with paying supplemental medical fees. There is a need to expand the knowledge base that made the twentieth-century health care revolution possible. In the twenty-first century, it is critical to provide research and development that is relevant to infectious diseases that overwhelmingly affect the poor. In addition, it is necessary to systematically generate an information base that countries can use to shape the future of their health care system (WHO, 1999).

The Lalonde report (1974) proposed the "health field concept" as a useful way to consider the determinants of health such as biology, lifestyle, environment, and health services. This report emphasized lifestyle and environment as determinants of health outside the traditional medical sphere. It became the basis for rethinking new paradigms for health care delivery. "The Lalonde report signified the beginning of a paradigm shift in health care away from the traditional medical model to a more holistic system-environment perspective" (Boothroyd and Eberle, 1990, p. 2). However, in the subsequent decade, policymakers focused more attention on individual lifestyle change (Hoffman and Dupont, 1985) and implemented health education programs targeting healthier personal lifestyles. Using both education and income levels as measures of SES, strong, positive relationships have been observed for various health indicators, including QOL, health status, and preventive health practices (Adams, 1993).

In the 1980s and 1990s, the rising costs of health care have been a major catalyst for change, focusing attention on the need to provide alternate models of care. Day surgery and outpatient services, ambulatory care, and home care provide alternatives to hospital-based care. In each of these areas, the nurse plays a prominent role and has the potential to bring a needed dimension of health promotion and disease prevention to individuals, families, and communities.

In 1997, U.S. expenditures for health care made up 13.6% of the gross domestic product with projected expenditures of 15% in 2000 (APHA, 1999). However, more than 43 million Americans under the age of 65 are uninsured and cannot afford health care (NCHS, 1998). A market-based developed country such as the United States treats health care as a market commodity; therefore it focuses on curative medicine rather than preventive medicine because it creates more capital. A market-based health care system could lead to a goal opposite that of health for all. Theoretically, the advent of a managed care system in the United States uses a capitated model to cut health care costs. However, managed care offers neither universal access nor the comprehensive primary health care that WHO advocates.

Given the two basic health care systems, market-based and population-based, and the fact that countries at different levels of development need to learn from each other, it is evident that a single model of health care delivery is not appropriate for every country. For example, in 1985, Cuba was recognized for reaching WHO's goal of "health for all." Cuba began to demonstrate to the world that health care could be provided as a basic human right rather than a privilege. In addition, Canada developed a successful universal health care system and Canadian community health nurses (CHNs) created innovative models for practice. *Canada's Achieving Health for All* provided a health promotion framework that includes fostering public participation in decisions that affect health, strengthening community health service networks with the disadvantaged communities they serve, and coordinating public health policy efforts (Epp, 1996).

The pressure for change provides the opportunity for reform and the broad goal of health for all should guide this reform. Effective health care delivery systems must improve health status; reduce health inequalities; enhance responsiveness to legitimate expectations; increase efficiency; protect individuals, families, and communities from financial loss; and enhance fairness in health care delivery (WHO, 1999).

The Role of the Community Health Nurse in International Health Care

In a rapidly changing health care environment, the nursing role is becoming less traditional and much more diverse. The traditional structure of provider roles is challenged as professional disciplines are recruited to provide expanded and diverse health care services. The nursing role is reciprocal and it is interdependent with others such as clients and families, physicians, and other health care personnel. The nurse's role expectations and societal expectations influence the formation of behavior patterns specific to the professional nursing role. These expectations provide the basis for the role of the CHN in other countries.

Florence Nightingale was the first nurse to establish international links and networks that became vastly important to her own country and to nursing throughout the world. Every obstacle to health and wellness confronted her. She confronted these obstacles and overcame them systematically. This legacy serves as the foundation for CHNs working throughout the world. Nightingale channeled her energies into all aspects of health from the care of wounded soldiers at Scutari to the broad public policies that affected health in her time (Splane and Splane, 1997).

CHNs seek to ensure the attainment of health for all in a cost-effective health care system. They must be involved in research, community assessment, plan-

ning, implementation, management, evaluation, health services delivery, emergency response, health policy, and legislation. Nurses in all countries coordinate their work with other health care personnel and community leaders. Health for all requires substantially different attitudes, levels of competence, knowledge, and skills that characterize traditional nursing. The changes in the health environment, such as technological advancements, changes in the morbidity and mortality patterns of the population, and social and political changes, all form the basis for the nursing role.

Community health nursing is similar in both developed and developing countries; it has similar components of physical care, safety, social norms, interpersonal processes, economic factors, and community cohesion (Kupina, 1995). With the development of the NP role over the past 35 years in the United States and over the past decade abroad, the tradition of having better-prepared nurses based in community settings has continued (Land, 1998).

As primary health care and primary care may be practiced differently in other countries, the NP and the CHN face a challenge (Barnes et al., 1995). Primary health care refers to essential services that support a healthy life. It involves access, availability, service delivery, community participation, and all citizens' right to health care. In contrast, **primary care** refers to first line or point-of-access medical and nursing care controlled by providers and focused on the individual. Primary care may not be the norm, particularly in communities in developing or less developed countries that have overwhelming needs for basic necessities such as safe drinking water and sanitation. The needs of the group outweigh the needs of the individual.

Nurses can make a difference in helping solve the existing and emerging health problems in countries throughout the world. The advent of technology has enhanced global communication and facilitated travel. It is important that nurses throughout the world understand each other and learn from each another. Nurses are the most valuable assets of any health care system. Community health nursing can improve access to care for the most vulnerable and hard to reach groups in any country. Community health nursing, in its many forms, continues to be relevant and will expand in the future. The future will demand an increase in international projects, educational endeavors, and research. CHNs are the most important factor for the cost-effective delivery of care to individuals, families, and communities.

RESEARCH IN INTERNATIONAL HEALTH

Since 1990, international nursing research has focused predominately on the following three areas: student and faculty educational exchange programs, diverse clinical experiences, and the international development of home care or transition from hospital to home.

Fourteen WHO collaborating nursing centers provide a framework for research, education, and service delivery partnerships. Duquesne University, an affiliate of George Mason University's WHO Collaborating Center in Nursing, developed an education and service partnership model for their work in Nicaragua (White and Smith, 1998). Perdue University and the University of Virginia, both affiliates of Case Western Reserve University and the University of Mexico WHO Collaborating Centers, have contributed to a partnership for educational programming, clinical practice, and research for graduate students in Primary Health Care Nursing and Community Health.

Haloburdo and Thompson (1998) compared international learning experiences for baccalaureate nursing students in developed and developing countries. Using grounded theory methodology, 14 students participated in international learning experiences. More similarities than differences were identified among the students who traveled to developing vs. developed countries. Squires (1998) described models that focus on chronic conditions such as hypertension, diabetes, and cancer. Land (1998) described projects in Latin America and the Caribbean that focus on health promotion, epidemiological

Text continued on p. 824

CASE STUDY

APPLICATION OF THE NURSING PROCESS

Rural Mexico: A Collaborative Model for Community Assessment, Education, and Health Care Delivery

Julie Novak, DNSC, RN, CPNP and
Lanier Rossignol, MSN, RN, FNP

In Mexico, the provision of equitable health care services to a population that is geographically and educationally disparate is both economically and logistically challenging. Rural Mexico is further challenged with a lack of infrastructure necessary for health promotion, protection, and maintenance. The WPCE Model (Fig. 31-1) and the ICAM (Fig. 31-2) (Rossignol and Novak, 1999) were developed to provide nurses with a globally diverse assessment tool and methodology to empower communities in developing countries to improve their access to potable water. U.S. nursing students gaining international health care experience in a community in rural Mexico are implementing both models as part of an ongoing project to improve the community's health.

Nurses cannot solve the problem of unavailable potable water in developing countries alone; however, they can collaborate with environmental experts in implementing a community empowerment framework (May, Mendelson, and Ferketich, 1995; Querreno et al., 1998). In community empowerment, the community identifies its problems and plan of action and environmental experts and nurses remain consultants and team members to assist community members (May, Mendelson, and Ferketich, 1995). This process aids the community in developing interventions that are culturally acceptable, breaking down cultural barriers to clean water. Programs to improve water quality in developing countries that do not involve community participation and education often fail after the experts leave the community (Yates, 1997).

The WPCE Model integrates the nursing process with the concept of community empowerment through community development and organization (Rothman, 1979). The WPCE Model applies the nursing process, used in caring for individual clients, to the community. Through the framework of the model, nurses and environmental experts construct a board of key influential community members and empower them to assess water quality, diagnose problems, plan interventions, implement these interventions, and evaluate the effectiveness of the interventions.

Continued

FIGURE 31-1

The Water Project Community Empowerment Model (From Rossignol L, Novak J: *The water project and community empowerment model,* 1999, The Author, www.hsc.virginia.edu/wwp/home.html).

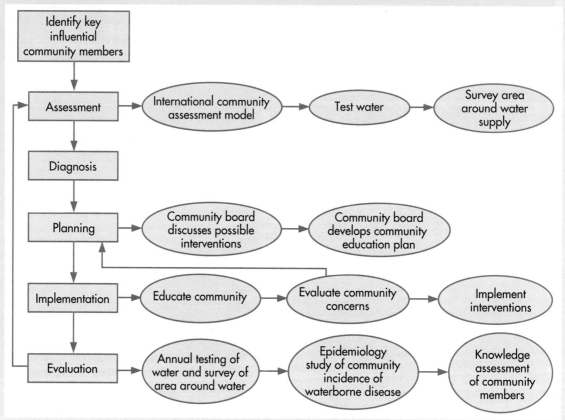

Assessment

During the assessment phase, the nurse identifies key influential community members and leaders and encourages them to join a board of community members with the goal of assessing the community's water supply. The community board members can assess the community using the ICAM, developed after reviewing existing models (Anderson and McFarlane, 1995; Pender, 1996; White, 1982) for the purpose of providing a globally diverse assessment framework. Assessment of community culture helps identify potential cultural barriers to nursing interventions. The center of the model assesses the heart of the community's culture by identifying the individual, family, and community characteristics including history, demographics, values, beliefs, rituals, and the effect of all of these on social and economic conditions.

The ICAM further examines the community's recreation, health, spirituality, family support systems, physical environment, education, safety, transportation, government, politics, economics, communication, and technology. The recreational assessment allows the nurse to determine how the community gains cardiovascular fitness; stress management; energy renewal; and relaxation through sports, hobbies, and games. Assessment of the community's health includes determining how the community perceives health and considering the community members' physical, social, and mental

FIGURE 31-2

International Community Assessment Model (From Rossignol L, Novak J: *The water project and community empowerment model,* 1999, The Author, www.hsc.virginia.edu/wwp/home.html).

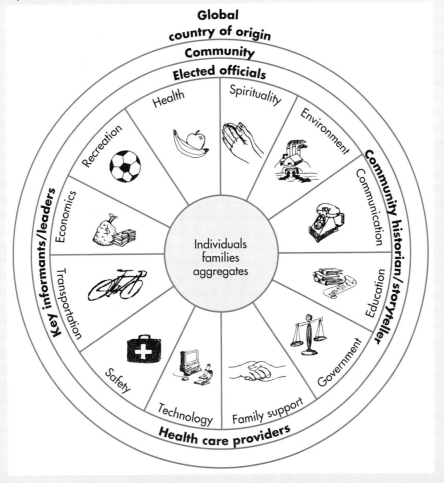

balance. Assessment of spirituality encompasses an examination of the community's religious beliefs and practices. The family support systems are analyzed to determine parental support of children and adult children, adult children's support of their parents, and support among extended family members. Family is defined as a group of individuals who share common experiences and goals and are often linked together by genetics, marriage, living situation, or a common emotional bond.

The physical environment encompasses the community's infrastructure including homes, water sources, waste disposal sites, roadways, buildings for businesses and shops, factories, and power lines. The concept of education reflects the community's knowledge, skills, level of schooling or training, and literacy rate. Transportation is defined as how community members travel from point A to point B. Evaluation of the community's safety includes examining potential dangers in the community that could lead to injury or death and examining safety measures and plans the community developed to prevent these problems. Assessment of government and politics entails examining how the community is governed or ruled. The economy is defined in terms of the "production, dispersal, and

Continued

expenditure of resources" (Neufeldt and Guralnik, 1997, p. 429). Evaluating communication involves examining face-to-face and community-wide information exchange through speech, body language, writing, or drawings. Key components of the community's communication are native languages and forms of communication such as letters, telephone, computer networks, the Internet, fax machines, television, billboards, signs, magazines, newspapers, and telegrams. Access to electricity, public sanitation, public water systems, radio, television, technology, fax machines, libraries, computers, Internet, industrial machinery, and agricultural practices and technology must also be examined. The ICAM will allow the board to examine all the public health threats to the community and additional barriers to potable water.

The ICAM also reflects the importance of assessing the country of origin and global effects on the community. When assessing a community, the nurse must consider the external factors affecting the community. For example, the economy of rural Xochimilco Mexico depends upon Mexico City vendors, other Mexican states, and the international purchasing of their main export, flowers. The community would have further poverty and decline in health and infrastructure and increased poverty if their flowers decreased in market value.

After the community assessment, the collaborative team should develop an educational program that identifies potential problems with the water supply. This program should motivate board members to identify these problems and then search for effective solutions (Hanson, 1985). The community members may need to be educated on the relationship between germs, illness, sanitation, and potable water (Water for the People, 1998). As board members become aware of the potential water supply hazards, they should be assisted in assessing the water supply. A water sample should be tested for the presence of human and animal feces by using the coliform count in a laboratory within close proximity (Keough, 1980). The water sample should also be tested for total dissolved solids (TDS), pH, *E. coli, Giardia lambia,* and *Cryptosporidium.*

Next, the community board members should be assisted in completing a sanitary survey of the area within 200 feet of the community water supply; this survey should assess sources of contamination, including house sewer lines, septic tanks, privies, latrines, barnyards, animal pens, cemeteries, sewage, and trash dumps (Bureau of Sewage and Water Services, 1992; Hanson, 1985). These sources of contamination should be at least 50 feet from a ground water source. The contamination source should be at least 20 meters away from surface water supplies and should be located downstream from the community water source (Hanson, 1985). In addition, building foundations should be 10 feet from ground water sources (Bureau of Sewage and Water Services, 1992). Contamination sources uphill from the water supply should also be noted. For every 5% of land slope between the source of contamination and the well, an additional 25 feet should be placed between them (Bureau of Sewage and Water Services, 1992). The nurse and community board members, in collaboration with an environmental expert, should conduct more detailed assessments near the well site and near the surface water source.

Diagnosis

The nurse and environmental experts should guide the community board members in formulating diagnoses of problems with the water supply. If the water has contaminants and the contamination source has not been discovered, the team must repeat the sanitary survey and test another sample of water for coliform count.

Planning

If the community's water supply is contaminated and the community board members recognize a need for improvements in their water supply, the board will enter the planning phase of the WPCE Model. Community board members can collaborate with environmental experts and the nurse to identify goals and objectives to improve the community's water quality.

After the community board has determined the basic goals of the water project and clearly identified the points of contamination, the collaborative team should develop possible interventions. Some of these interventions could include covering and protecting a current well from contaminants, drilling a new well, and chemically treating or boiling contaminated water (Hanson, 1985; Keough, 1980; Reiff et al., 1996). Possible improvements in sanitation should also be discussed. This body of knowledge will allow the community board members to determine which, if any, of the proposed interventions would be relevant and appropriate for their community. In addition, they may be able to apply these ideas in creating their own interventions. When the community board members have selected or developed an intervention for their water project, they can be encouraged to create strategies to educate the community about proper sanitation and the importance of potable water. This will help the community gain acceptance and a commitment to the water project.

Implementation

Before the water project is implemented, the community awareness of the need for the water project must be clear. The community must be given the opportunity to provide the board with feedback on proposed interventions. The board should be willing to compromise to meet the community's needs. After the community-wide education has occurred and necessary consensus and compromise have been achieved, the water project can be implemented. At this point, the community members are trained to maintain the clean water project. Once the implementation is completed, evaluation of the project can begin to ensure that the goals and objectives of the board are met.

Evaluation

The collaborative team should collect water samples annually to test for contaminates (Woodward, Ross, and Parrott, 1992). The groundwater supply should also be tested when flooding around the area occurs or when someone using the water becomes ill from a waterborne disease. The area around the community's water supply should be assessed for contaminants annually. In addition, the nurse should conduct community surveys to determine if members continue to recognize the need for potable water and proper sanitation and if they continue to practice proper sanitation. Epidemiological studies of the prevalence and incidence of infectious disease, in-

cluding gastroenteritis, must be performed routinely to ensure that the project goals and objectives are met.

The WPCE and ICAM are being tested in a rural Mexican community as part of an ongoing project. The community has a population of 10,000 and is located approximately 40 kilometers from Mexico City. Over half the population has a low income; therefore the community has a high incidence of poverty. As a result, 80% of the community resides in crowded living conditions. Most community members have cement floors, but 4% of the families have dirt floors. Sixty-seven percent of the community's homes are constructed with concrete, yet as many as 12% of the homes are built with sheet asbestos, which is a carcinogen. Eighty-four percent of the community has indoor plumbing, but the tap water is not safe for consumption without treatment. Sixteen percent of the population must travel to a central source to obtain their water. This leads to potential contamination during transport. Many of these factors in the community pose serious health threats.

The economy is based on the production and marketing of cement, flowers, and vegetables. The flower and vegetable fields are watered from the community's grossly contaminated canals that originate in Mexico City. These contaminates provide a rich source of fertilizer for the crops; however, the field workers are exposed to these unhealthy contaminates causing increased morbidity and mortality.

The top three causes of mortality in the community are cardiac disorders, diabetes, and automobile accidents. The leading causes of morbidity are respiratory infections, diabetes, hypertension, and gastrointestinal illnesses. The community's high rate of gastrointestinal illness is related to poor access to potable water.

The initial contact with the community occurred through a collaborative project sponsored by Medtronic Corporation. Phases I and II of the project were completed through a cooperative effort of Universidad Nacional Autonoma De Mexico (UNAM), Case Western Reserve Francis Payne Bolton, and the University of Virginia Schools of Nursing. During the initial assessment, the community's key influential members were the water

Continued

management senior staff, the community historian, community political leaders, key employers, full-time staff at the UNAM nurse-run clinic, UNAM community health faculty, and the pasantes. The pasantes are UNAM nursing graduates who completed one year of community service at the UNAM nurse-run clinic.

The community assessment revealed that the community's unsafe drinking water and poor sanitation caused gastrointestinal infections to become the third leading cause of morbidity. Of families with indoor plumbing, 45.1% boil their tap water, 12.7% chemically disinfect the tap water, 8.9% drink bottled water, and 0.9% filter their water. The remaining 37.4% drink untreated tap water, posing a major health risk to this portion of the population. Statistics demonstrate that community members who drink tap water without treatment have a 9 times greater risk of contracting diarrhea. The serious health threat of contaminated water to the community will encourage the future phases of the project in San Luis to focus on expanded community education and specific clean water initiatives.

As this project develops, multidisciplinary collaboration with engineering, agriculture, and environmental experts will be essential. Future phases of the project will focus on additional data collection regarding sanitation, the water treatment plant, septic tanks, landfills, and central water source for community members without indoor plumbing. A massive community-wide clean water educational campaign during prenatal classes, in the community preschool program, in the nearby elementary and middle schools, and in the clinic senior program will be implemented. Educational materials created during Phase III of the project focused on the importance of boiling or chemically treating drinking water and the prevention of gastrointestinal illness. These interventions will provide the community with safe drinking water until sanitation and water quality can be improved by strengthening the infrastructure.

During Phase IV, a multidisciplinary team of key influential community members, environmental experts, and nurses will further assess the community using the ICAM and WPCE models. The goal of this assessment will be to assist the community members in further diagnosing the community's water quality and sanitation problems. When the problems have been identified, environmental engineers and nurses will collaborate with community board members to develop culturally-acceptable interventions to improve water quality. After the interventions are developed, the community board, clinic staff, and the pasantes will continue to evaluate the effectiveness of these interventions, promoting a sense of ownership of the project in the community and helping to ensure that the improvements in the water supply continue long after the multidisciplinary team leaves the community.

surveillance, mental health, and refugee care. Johnson, Chaffin, and Fields (1998) completed an exploratory study comparing nursing care in the United States with care in Barbados. Updike (1997) described Successful Steps, a pilot project in a rural Vietnamese community that was based on earlier research and focused on reducing malnutrition. Members of the rural community became involved in developing a solution for maternal and infant malnutrition in their community.

U.S. models of home health care are developing in other countries. These models provide a variety of services to bridge the gap between the hospital and community-based care. Sources of home care include home visits by nurses from official government public health agencies, nonprofit voluntary agencies, and for profit home care agencies. Examples of home care services include assistance with ADL, treatment, rehabilitation, transportation, and respite for caregivers.

Home care service providers in the United States and abroad face many challenges. Estimating financial implications and calculating potential caseloads are complex factors in the design of effective delivery systems. Inadequate hospital assessment, insufficient discharge planning and referral, restrictive or irrelevant policies regarding eligibility, failure to discharge patients from home care when services are unnecessary, and an inability to find less costly service as patients gain independence are other significant influencing variables. (Fulton, 1993; Gagnon, 1994; Townsend, 1990). Barkauskas and Seskivicius (1998) described the development of home health care in Lithuania. Milstead, Keller, and Miller (1998) focused on similarities and differences in community and home health care in Holland, while Ross (1998) described a transcultural home health experience between Nicaraguan and U.S. nursing students with an emphasis on program planning with limited resources.

SUMMARY

Community public health nurses face many exciting challenges in health care reform. These include being responsive to emerging needs and health issues in the population, developing multidisciplinary models for practice that adhere to the principles of primary health care in the context of a restructured health care system, and mobilizing research dissemination and practice implementation strategies to ensure evidence-based practice as the norm rather than the exception. There is still much to be done to meet the challenge of WHO's goal of "Health for All by the Year 2010." Studying the progress achieved in other countries is critical; however, success will ultimately depend on society's commitment to achieve higher levels of health and well-being for all (Puentes-Markides, 1996).

LEARNING ACTIVITIES

1. Discuss population characteristics and the threat of population growth on health and health care systems.
2. Compare and contrast the incidence of people living with AIDS and the incidence of death from AIDS in Africa, Mexico, and the United States. What might account for the differences?
3. Compare population-focused nursing in a developing country with community health nursing in the community. How are they the same and how do they differ?
4. Conduct research and compare the rates of life expectancy and infant mortality in Africa, Mexico, and the United States. What factors might account for the similarities in rates between the developing and the developed countries?
5. Describe the key elements of an effective health care delivery system. Will the focus of future health care services reflect downstream thinking, or will the orientation uphold models of prevention and promotion that deal with root causes of health problems?

6. Test the ICAM in a community. Evaluate its effectiveness.

REFERENCES

Adams O: Health status. In Stephens T, Fowler-Graham D, editors: *Canada's health promotion survey, 1990,* Technical Report, Ottawa, 1993, Ministry of Supply and Services.

Alma-Ata: *Primary health care, report of the international conference on primary health care,* "Health for All" Series, No 1, pp. 2-6, Geneva, September 6-12, 1978, WHO.

American Public Health Association: *The nation's health,* September, 1999, The Author, www.apha.org/journal/nation/tnhsept99.htm.

Anderson ET, McFarlane JM: *Community-as-partner: theory and practice in nursing,* Philadelphia, 1995, JB Lippincott.

Barkauskas VH, Seskevicius A: Development of home health care in Lithuania: current status and key development issues, *Home Health Care Manage Pract* 11(1):10-17, 1998.

Barnes D et al: Primary health care and primary care: a confusion of philosophies, *Nurs Outlook* 43:7-16, 1995.

Boothroyd P, Eberle M: *Healthy communities: what they are, how they're made,* CHS Research Bulletin, UBC Centre for Human Settlements, Vancouver, 1990, University of British Columbia.

Bryant J: Health services, manpower and universities in relation to health for all: an historical and future perspective, *Am J Public Health* 74:714-719, 1984.

Bureau of Sewage and Water Services: *Private well regulations,* VR 355-34-100, pp. 22-34, i.-iii, Richmond, Va, April, 1992, Commonwealth of Virginia Department of Health.

Epp J: *Achieving health for all: a framework for health promotion,* Ottawa, 1996, Health and Welfare Canada.

Fulton J: *Canada's health care system: bordering on the possible,* New York, 1993, Faulkner and Gray Thomson.

Gagnon AJ: *The effect of an early postpartum discharge program on competence in mothering: a randomized controlled trial,* doctoral dissertation, Montreal, 1994, McGill University.

Gregory-Dawes BS: The international world of nursing, *AORN J* 69(6):1098-1099, 1998.

Haloburdo EP, Thompson MA: A comparison of international learning experiences for baccalaureate nursing students: developed and developing countries. *J Nurs Educ* 37(1):13-21, 1998.

Hanson BD: Water and sanitation technologies: a trainers manual, *Peace Corporations Information Collection and Exchange Training Manual* T-32, 1985.

Hoffman K, Dupont JM: *Community health centres and community development,* Ottawa, 1985, Department of Health and Welfare of Canada, Minister of Supply and Services Canada.

Johnson CG, Chaffin C, Fields C: International collaboration: the Barbados experience *J Barbado Nurs Assoc* 6(1):81-90, 1998.

Keough C: *Water fit to drink,* Emmaus, Pa, 1980, Rodale Press.

Kupina PS: Community health CNSs and health care in the year 2000, *Clin Nurs Specialist* 9:188-198, 1995.

Labarthe DR: *Epidemiology and prevention of cardiovascular disease: a global challenge,* Gaithersburg, Md, 1998, Aspen.

Lalonde M: *A new perspective on the health of Canadians,* Ottawa, 1974, Minister of Supply and Services.

Land S: Community nursing in Latin America and the Caribbean home health care manager practice, *Nurs Outlook* 11(1):1-9, 1998.

May KM, Mendelson C, Ferketich S: Community empowerment in rural healthcare, *Public Health Nurs* 12(1):25-30, 1995.

Milstead JA, Keller AM, Miller MC: Focus on community: American and Dutch nurses share expertise, *Home Health Care Manage* 11(1):18-23, 1998.

National Center for Health Statistics: *Health, United States: 1998,* Washington, DC, 1998, US Government Printing Office.

Neufeldt V, Guralnik DB, editors: *Webster's new world college dictionary,* ed 3, Cleveland, Ohio, 1997, MacMillian, Inc.

Novak J: Effective smoking cessation strategies, *Clinical Letter Nurs Pract* 2(1):1-5, 1998.

Pender NJ: *Health promotion in nursing practice,* ed 3, Stamford, Conn, 1996, Appleton & Lange.

Potts M: Common sense prevailing at population conference, *Lancet* 344:809, 1994.

Puentes-Markides C: Renewing the commitment to achieve health for all the Americas, *Bulletin Pan Am Health Org* 30(1):80-82, 1996.

Querreno R et al: *Key issues in health development: poverty and ill-health,* 1998, Division of Intensified Cooperation with Countries and People in Greatest Need, www.who.int/ico/key.htm.

Reiff FM et al: Low cost safe water for the world, a practical interim solution, *J Public Health Policy* 17(4):389-408, 1996.

Rosenkoetter MM: A framework for international healthcare consultations *Nurs Outlook* 45(4):182-187, 1997.

Ross CA: Preparing American and Nicaraguan nurses to practice home health nursing in a transcultural experience, *Home Health Care Manage Pract* 11(1):66-70, 1998.

Rossignol L, Novak J: *The water project and community empowerment model,* 1999, The Author, www.hsc.virginia.edu/wwp/home.html.

Rothman J: Three models of community organization practice, their mixing and phasing. In Cox FM et al, editors: *Strategies of community organization,* ed 3, Itasca, Ill, 1979, FE Peacock Publishers, Inc.

Splane VH, Splane R: *International nursing leaders past and present: current issues in nursing,* ed 5, St. Louis, 1997, Mosby.

Squires AP: Home health care in Mexico: an overview, *Home Health Care Manage Pract* 11(1):38-45, 1998.

Thanassi WT: Immunization for international travelers, *WJ Med* 168(3):197, 1998.

Townsend P: Widening inequalities of health in Britain: a rejoinder to Rudolph Klein, *Int J Health Serv* 20(3):363–372, 1990.

UNAIDS: *HIV/AIDS report,* 1998, The Author, www.who.int/emc-hiv/.

United Nations Population Fund: *The state of world population 1995: decisions for development: women, empowerment and reproductive health,* Oxford, England, 1998, New Internationalist Publications Ltd.

Universidad Nacional Autonoma De Mexico (UNAM) Escuelo Nacional Enfermeria Y Obstetrica (ENEO): *San Luis community assessment,* unpublished document, 1998.

Updike P: Impacting maternal and child nutrition in rural Vietnam, *J Am Acad Nurs Pract* 9(2):111-115, 1997.

Water for the People: *Water for people works in 35 countries,* 1998, The Author, www.water4people.org/press03.htm.

White JF, Smith CW: Developing an international nursing partnership in Nicaragua, *Int Nurs Rev* 44(1):13-18, 1998.

White MS: Contruct for public health nursing, *Nurs Outlook* 30(9):527-530, 1982.

Woodward J, Ross B, Parrott K: Household water quality bacteria and other microorganisms in household water, *Virginia Cooperative Extension Publication* 356-487, 1992.

World Bank: *World Development Report 1998: investing in health,* Washington, DC, 1998, Oxford University Press.

World Health Organization: *The World Health Report 1999: making a difference,* Geneva, 1999, WHO.

Yates LD: A water supply development project in Quiescapa, Bolivia, *J Environ Health* 59(7):20-22, 1997.

32

Community Health Nursing: Making a Difference

Mary A. Nies, Melanie McEwen, and Joan Bickes

OBJECTIVES

Upon completion of this chapter, the reader will be able to do the following:

1. Discuss how being a member of a population influences health.
2. Predict future community health issues based on shared population characteristics.
3. Describe the actions CHNs may take to ensure that future trends and changes in the health care system will benefit the health care consumer.

For most individuals, "medical care" focuses on a diagnosed health problem. However, nursing's focus goes beyond the traditional concept of health as the absence of disease, a definition that reflects health in medical or disease terms. Nurses are concerned with prevention and health promotion activities that serve individual patients, their families, and groups in hospital settings (e.g., childbirth preparation, parenting classes, or diabetes classes). Community health nursing extends the definition of health and nursing action to social units or aggregates at the community and population levels.

Considering the individual in terms of his or her population is important in community health nursing. Many people in the community share common characteristics such as sex, age, education, income level, and occupation. These characteristics impact the health of families and communities and are important in determining their needs. Shared population characteristics also aid in determining interventions to meet the health needs of populations. Social interaction, political activity, values, and knowledge influence health priorities and resource allocation that impacts the health of populations from local to national levels. CHNs can intervene and make a difference in these areas.

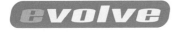

http://evolve.elsevier.com/Nies/

POPULATION VARIABLES THAT IMPACT HEALTH

Being a member of a population with shared characteristics may have a marked effect on health, whether these characteristics are age, ethnicity, or geographical factors. Shared population characteristics that may negatively impact health are deemed risk factors because they place a population at risk. These factors are key to public health and to community health nursing as they form the basis for assessment, planning, intervention, and evaluation. Although using the nursing process on behalf of individuals is important, implementing the nursing process at the population level has the potential to make positive changes based on an understanding of population characteristics.

Whether the needs or risks are based on age or social or environmental characteristics, change at the population level will make the broadest impact on population health. For example, residents of a low-income neighborhood near a refinery in south Louisiana appealed to state and federal authorities to ensure safe air quality for their community. Likewise, the disabled population in San Francisco organized to advocate for their rights to equal opportunity in housing, education, and employment. Such activities require organized community planning and political activity.

The following section illustrates how being a member of a population group can influence health. Areas described include SES, gender, age, race and ethnicity, social interaction, geography, and politics.

Socioeconomic Status

SES affects health in several ways. Those of lower SES have higher rates of morbidity and mortality than counterparts with higher SES. According to WHO, poverty reduces life expectancy through increased rates of infant mortality, developmental limitations, chronic disease, and traumatic death. In the United States, the incidence of heart disease is 25% higher for people with low incomes; the likelihood of developing cancer increases as family income decreases (USDHHS, 2000). Rates of infectious disease, including HIV infection, are more common among those of lower SES (USDHHS, 2000).

Similar disparities are found in incidences of obesity, elevated blood lead levels, and low birth weight; these health problems increase with poverty. The importance of these facts is evident considering that 22% of U.S. children under age 18 live below the federal poverty level (NCHS, 1995).

Gender

Gender affects health in the United States. Generally, women have higher morbidity, or disease rates, whereas men have had higher mortality, or death rates. Although remarkable strides have been made in increasing longevity for men and women since the early 1900s, a gap between the life expectancies of the two groups continues. This gap increased from 2.0 years in 1900 to a high of 7.8 years in 1995 (NCHS, 1995). Since 1995, the gap has decreased to 6.0 years (USDHHS, 2000).

Since 1987, gender differences in malignant neoplasms (i.e., particularly lung cancer) and diseases of the heart were major causes of death that reduced the gap (NCHS, 1999b). This trend may be attributed to an increase in women smokers and increased numbers of women entering the workforce.

Age

Age is an important health determinant and is closely linked to mortality. For example, according to NCHS (1999b), the leading cause of death in childhood is unintentional injuries. This is also true for adolescents, for whom 33% of deaths are related to motor vehicle accidents (NCHS, 1999b). Furthermore, over 22% of deaths in this age group involve alcohol use (Insurance Institute for Highway Safety, Highway Loss Data Institute, 2000).

Morbidity patterns also vary with age. More than 38% of people aged 65 or older have an activity limitation caused by chronic conditions (NCHS, 1999a). These are not "sick" individuals; essentially, they are "well" individuals who experience periodic exacerbations that may require hospitalization. Most require acute care only periodically, yet medical care is designed to focus on acute care (i.e., attending to physiological needs associated with disease) rather than on care at all times. The real needs, especially for chronically ill populations, are for distributive, continuous care in the form of health monitoring, supervision, and periodic home health or homemaker services (i.e., cleaning, shopping assistance, and meal preparation).

Most people over age 65 live at home or with family members; 4% or less of the elderly population live in nursing homes (NCHS, 1999a). Nursing homes serve mostly the frail elderly and are designed according to an acute care model that focuses on meeting the patients' physical needs rather than interpersonal, social, and environmental needs. The health and surveillance needs of this population will continue to grow.

Race and Ethnicity

Although differences in health status and health service access is partially attributed to inequalities of income, education, and geography, race and ethnicity are also factors. For example, the infant death rate among African-Americans is more than double that of whites. Heart disease death rates are over 40% higher for African-Americans than for whites and the death rate for all cancers is 30% higher for African-Americans than for whites. Furthermore, Hispanics are almost twice as likely to die from diabetes than are whites (USDHHS, 2000).

Communicable diseases, particularly STDs, HIV, and AIDS, are found disproportionately in nonwhites. Although African-Americans and Hispanics represent only 25% of the total U.S. population, 55% of the AIDS cases reported through 1998 occurred among these two groups. AIDS is the leading cause of death for all African-Americans aged 25 to 44 years, the second leading cause of death among African-American females, and the leading cause of death among African-American males in that age group. In 1998, the AIDS case rate among African-Americans (66.4 per 100,000) was eight times the rate for whites (8.2 per 100,000) and over twice the rate for Hispanics (28.1 per 100,000) (USDHHS, 2000) (see Chapter 12).

Social Interaction

Relationships are also important to health. Social support is a necessary factor in promoting health and functional independence. Retirement, the loss of a spouse or close friend, or a change in social role can affect support systems and social contact; all are risk factors for disease and functional dependence (USDHHS, 2000).

Social interactions dramatically influence behaviors and risk factors for disease. For example, those who find themselves surrounded by smokers find it difficult to quit smoking and factors such as support from friends are associated with engaging in exercise (Kottke, 1992). In addition, person-to-person transmission of disease increases in dense populations regardless of whether or not the agent is highly infectious.

Families and friends can also play a significant role in health promotion. Families influence personal health habits and physical environment. Children's participation in activities outside the family has a positive effect on health-promoting behaviors; the family monitors this participation (Bomar, 1995).

Geography-Politics

Where an individual lives may have an impact on population health. Traditional geographically-related phenomena (i.e., earthquakes, weather, or lack of certain minerals in the soil) also contribute to population health. Significant health problems are attributable to floods, extreme temperatures, and other natural events and man-made hazards (i.e., chemical plants and airports) (see Chapter 13).

Political factors have an impact on the delivery of health care services at all levels. For example, Medicaid coverage and availability varies from state to state, depending on the local political climate. As a consequence, Medicaid assistance to citizens varies widely. Residency in a state with minimal Medicaid assistance may affect the health of that population. In 1993, average payments per Medicaid recipient varied more than twelvefold among states. On average, an Arizona recipient received $524 in Medicaid payments, whereas a New York State recipient received $6402 (NCHS, 1995).

PUBLIC HEALTH: THE PAST

During the 1900s, the average American lifespan lengthened by more than 30 years and 25 years of that gain was attributable to public health advances. Throughout 1999, the CDC published a series of reports outlining the "Ten Great Public Health Achievements" in the United States that contributed to improved health during the twentieth century (CDC, 1999a). Box 32-1 lists these remarkable achievements and the following sections briefly describe each achievement.

**Ten Great Public Health Achievements:
United States, 1900 to 2000**

- Vaccination
- Motor vehicle safety
- Safer workplaces
- Control of infectious diseases
- Decline in deaths from coronary heart disease and stroke
- Safer and healthier foods
- Healthier mothers and babies
- Family planning
- Fluoridation of drinking water
- Recognition of tobacco use as a health hazard

Impact of Vaccines Universally Recommended for Children: United States

At the beginning of the twentieth century, infectious diseases were widely prevalent in the United States. At that time, 5 of the 10 leading causes of death were attributed to infectious disease. Vaccination has greatly impacted these statistics and has resulted in the eradication of smallpox, the elimination of polio in the Americas, and the control of many other diseases including measles, rubella, tetanus, and diphtheria.

National efforts to promote vaccination among children began with the appropriation of federal funds for the polio vaccine in 1955. Since that time, federal, state, and local governments and private health care providers have worked to encourage vaccination coverage for all children. The task is daunting because approximately 11,000 children are born in the United States each day and each child requires 15 to 19 doses of vaccine by age 19 months for protection against 11 childhood diseases. However, results have been rewarding; by 1997, coverage among children aged 19 to 35 months exceeded 90% for DPT, polio vaccine, Hib vaccine, and MMR (CDC, 1999b) (see Chapter 25).

Motor Vehicle Safety

The reduction of the death rate attributable to motor vehicle crashes in the United States is a result of a public health response to one of the greatest techno-logical advances of the twentieth century—the motorization of America (CDC, 1999c). Systematic motor vehicle safety efforts began in the 1960s with the passage of the Highway Safety Act and the National Traffic and Motor Vehicle Safety Act in 1966. These Acts authorized the federal government to set and regulate standards for motor vehicles and highways.

As a result of this legislation, vehicles were built with new safety features including head rests, energy-absorbing steering wheels, shatter-resistant windshields, and safety belts. Furthermore, roads were vastly improved. Other efforts were encouraged to alter driver and passenger behaviors. Enactment and enforcement of traffic safety laws (i.e., speed limits, laws against driving while intoxicated, and the enforcement of safety belts and child safety seats) have also positively impacted the number of injuries and deaths attributable to vehicle accidents.

Although deaths have remained fairly constant (39,000 in 1960 vs. 42,000 in 1997), motor vehicle-related death *rates* (i.e., based on the number of vehicle miles traveled) have dropped almost 90% since the mid1960s (CDC, 1999c). These efforts and the resulting improvements should encourage more measures to improve motor vehicle safety and driving habits and patterns in the United States. The ultimate goal is to further reduce the total number of deaths each year.

Improvements in Workplace Safety

At the beginning of the twentieth century, workers in the United States faced high health and safety risks on the job. In 1912, it was estimated that over 20,000 workers died from work-related injuries. Employment in mining; agriculture, forestry, and fishing; construction; and transportation, communications, and public utilities yielded the highest average death and injury rates (CDC, 1999d).

During the 1900s, deaths from work-related injuries declined 90% (37 per 100,000 workers to 4 per 100,000 workers) (CDC, 1999d). This decline in occupational fatalities is the result of collaborative efforts to identify and correct factors that contribute to occupational health risks. Declines are attributed to labor and management efforts to improve worker safety through research, education, and regulatory activities.

Despite accomplishments, workers continue to die from preventable injuries sustained on the job. The current leading causes of fatal occupational injury are motor vehicle injuries, workplace homicides, and machine-related injuries. Ongoing efforts are being made to address workplace hazards. These efforts include investigating fatalities in high-risk occupations and researching and developing educational materials for prevention (see Chapter 27).

Control of Infectious Diseases

Deaths from infectious diseases declined markedly in the United States during the twentieth century. In 1900, the three leading causes of death were pneumonia, TB, and diarrhea/enteritis. Combined with diphtheria, these diseases caused one third of all deaths at the time. Of these, 40% were among children aged five years and younger (CDC, 1999e). Successful public health efforts for infectious disease control resulted from improvements in the following areas: sanitation and hygiene, discovery of antibiotics, and implementation of childhood vaccination programs.

Sanitation and hygiene efforts included the provision of clean drinking water through chlorination and other treatments, which began in the early 1900s and became widespread over the next few decades. Other important sanitation and hygiene activities that began early in the century were sewage disposal, food safety, solid waste disposal, and public education about hygienic practices.

Penicillin was discovered in 1928, but it was not used for medical purposes until the 1940s. Since the 1940s, antimicrobials have provided quick and complete treatment for previously incurable bacterial illnesses and have saved the lives of countless individuals.

Vaccination campaigns have been highly successful in preventing the diseases that were previously common and often deadly. The success of vaccination programs in the United States and Europe inspired the concept of "disease eradication." The eradication of smallpox in the 1970s was a major public health triumph. A number of other diseases, including measles and polio, are slated for eradication in the next few years (see Chapter 25).

Decline in Deaths from Heart Disease and Stroke

Since 1921, heart disease has been the leading cause of death in the United States. Since 1938, stroke has been the third leading cause of death. Together they account for approximately 40% of all deaths. However, age-adjusted death rates from CVD have declined 60% since 1950 despite still being the first and third leading cause of death. This is one of the most important public health achievements of the later part of the twentieth century (CDC, 1999f).

Reasons cited for this dramatic decline include epidemiological investigations that established major risk factors for heart disease and stroke including tobacco use, high blood cholesterol, high blood pressure, dietary factors, and sedentary lifestyle. Therefore improved mortality rates have been attributed to lowering risk factor levels through antismoking campaigns, antihypertensive and lipid-lowering drugs, and improved nutrition. Improvements in medical care, including advances in diagnosing and treating heart disease and stroke, are also integral in the decline in death rates from heart disease and stroke (CDC, 1999f).

Safer and Healthier Food

Early in the twentieth century, contaminated food, milk, and water caused many foodborne infections including typhoid fever, TB, botulism and scarlet fever. The passage of the Pure Food and Drug Act created awareness of foodborne disease sources. Successful prevention interventions include handwashing, sanitation, refrigeration, pasteurization, and pesticide application (CDC, 1999g).

The discovery of essential nutrients and their role in disease prevention dramatically reduced nutritional deficiencies such as goiter, rickets, and pellagra (i.e., dietary niacin deficiency). Later in the century, food and nutrition labeling and consumer information programs stimulated the development of products low in fat, cholesterol, and sodium. Efforts to increase the intake of fruits, vegetables, and fiber in the American diet have also been promoted to combat the growing problems associated with obesity (CDC, 1999g).

Healthier Mothers and Babies

For every 1000 live births in 1900, six to nine women in the United States died of pregnancy-related complications and approximately 100 infants died before they reached one year of age. Between 1915 and 1997, the infant mortality rate declined more than 90% to 7.2 per 1000. Likewise, between 1900 and 1997, the maternal mortality rate declined almost 99% to less than 0.1 deaths per 1000 live births (CDC,

1999h). Factors in the dramatic improvement of maternal and infant mortality include environmental interventions, improvements in nutrition, advances in clinical medicine, improvements in access to health care, improvements in surveillance and monitoring of disease, increases in education levels, and improvements in standards of living.

Family Planning

During the twentieth century, family planning in the United States improved to allow desired birth spacing and family size. A number of factors were cited to encourage fewer children per family, including a reduction in infant and child mortality, urbanization of communities, and the increase in age at first marriage. Smaller families and longer birth intervals have contributed to improvement in the health of infants, children, and women and have improved women's social and economic role (CDC, 1999i).

Margaret Sanger, a public health nurse concerned with the adverse health effects of frequent childbirth, miscarriage, and abortion, began the modern birth-control movement in the United States in 1912. Sanger initiated efforts to circulate information about and provide access to contraception. Her work became widespread throughout the 1920s and 1930s.

Beginning in the 1960s, birth control pills and intrauterine devices dramatically altered birth control efforts. In 1970, federal funding for family planning was established under the Family Planning Services and Population Research Act. During the 1970s, the 1980s, and through the 1990s, family planning care has become widely available. As a result, modern contraception and reproductive health care systems help prevent an estimated 1.3 million unintended pregnancies in the United States every year (CDC, 1999i) (see Chapter 15).

Fluoridation of Drinking Water

The fluoridation of community drinking water was a major factor in the decline of dental caries during the second half of the twentieth century. At the beginning of the twentieth century, dental caries were extremely common in the United States. At that time, effective measures for preventing tooth decay were nonexistent and the most frequent treatment was tooth extraction.

In 1901, Dr. F.S. McKay, a dentist in Colorado Springs, Colorado, noted that many of his patients had permanent stains on their teeth. He concluded that an agent in the public water supply was responsible for the mottled enamel. He also noted that teeth affected by this condition seemed less susceptible to dental decay. Over the next two decades, other dentists made similar discoveries; in the early 1930s, observational research began to assess the impact of fluoride on the development of dental caries (CDC, 1999j).

Studies in the mid1940s showed that communities with fluoridated water experienced a 50% to 70% reduction in caries among children. As a result of ongoing research, a recommended optimum range of fluoride concentration was established in 1962. Since community water fluoridation efforts began in the second half of the twentieth century, dental caries have declined some 68% (CDC, 1999j).

Tobacco as a Health Hazard

During the first few decades of the twentieth century, lung cancer was rare. However, as tobacco use became increasingly popular, the incidence of lung cancer became epidemic. For example, the lung cancer death rate for men was 4.9 per 100,000 in 1930; in 1990, the rate increased to 75.6 per 100,000 (CDC, 1999k). Other diseases and conditions caused or exacerbated by tobacco use increased dramatically during the century. These include heart disease, peripheral vascular disease, laryngeal cancer, oral cancer, esophageal cancer, COPD, intrauterine growth retardation, and low birth weight.

In the 1940s and 1950s, scientists began to link cigarette smoking and lung cancer. In 1964, on the basis of some 7000 articles relating to smoking and disease, the U.S. Surgeon General concluded that cigarette smoking is a cause of lung and laryngeal cancer and a probable cause of chronic bronchitis. It was determined that "cigarette smoking is health hazard."

An important accomplishment in the second half of the twentieth century was the reduction of smoking prevalence among those aged 18 years or younger from 42.4% in 1965 to 24.7% in 1997. Additionally, the percentage of adults who never smoked increased from 44% in the mid1960s to 55% in 1997 (CDC, 1999k). Smoking reduction results from many factors. These factors include the following: scientific evidence linking disease and tobacco use, dissemination of this information to the public, prevention and cessation programs, campaigns by advocates for nonsmoker's rights, restrictions on cigarette advertising, counter-advertising, policy changes (i.e., enforcement of minors' access laws, legislation restricting smoking in public places, and increased taxation), improvements in treatment and prevention programs, and an increased understanding of the economic costs of tobacco (CDC, 1999k).

PUBLIC HEALTH: THE FUTURE

On January 25, 2000, Surgeon General David Satcher presented the American people with *Healthy People 2010,* which outlined the national health goals (see Chapter 1). In this document and in related activities, there has been a push for living a healthier lifestyle and improving equal assess to health care. Furthermore, the document establishes a goal that, by 2010, most adults and children will have five 30-minute workouts each week. Developed objectives encourage more people to quit smoking, abstain from drugs, and abstain from engaging in casual sex without condoms, among others.

Healthy People 2010 selects 10 leading health indicators to measure progress toward meeting the goals (Box 32-2). These health indicators reflect the major public health concerns in the United States and illuminate individual behaviors, physical and social environmental factors, and important health system issues that affect the health of individuals and communities. Applying the Healthy Community Model standards to these 10 health indicators, communities can plan community public health services. The emphasis is on health outcomes and programs rather than professional practice.

B O X **32-2**

Healthy People 2010 **Healthy Indicators**

Leading Health Indicators for Americans
- Physical activity
- Overweight and obesity
- Tobacco use
- Substance abuse
- Responsible sexual behavior
- Mental health
- Injury and violence
- Environmental quality
- Immunization
- Access to health care

In implementing the model standards, the community is encouraged to adapt a process to meet their specific needs. With *Healthy People 2010,* there may be a tendency to use the national objective targets as targets for community standards. Each community should compare its status in relation to the national targets, then the community should translate national objectives into community action plans tailored to meet community needs. Efforts should be made to encourage the communication and coordination of public health efforts and to present plans for programs or interventions to the appropriate individual, agency, or legislative body (see Chapter 11). In all of these areas, the CHN can be a valuable player. (USDHHS, 2000).

Continued efforts by public health systems, including CHNs, can dramatically impact the health of individuals, families, and communities for the next century. Areas in which the public health system will continue to be involved include the following:

- Monitoring community health status to identify potential hazards.
- Investigating disease outbreaks and safety hazards.
- Informing, educating, and empowering the public regarding health issues.
- Mobilizing community partnerships to solve health problems.
- Developing policies and plans that support individual and community health efforts.
- Enforcing laws and regulations that protect health and ensure safety.
- Linking populations with needed personal health services.
- Ensuring a competent public health and personal health care workforce.
- Evaluating effectiveness, accessibility, and quality of personal and population-based health services (CDC, 2000).

COMMUNITY HEALTH NURSES MAKE A DIFFERENCE

CHNs can make a difference. Efforts at the individual, family, aggregate, and community levels can impact health and well-being at several different levels. Among other areas, CHNs can work through programs, research, and case management. Examples of how nurses can impact community health in these areas are presented on p. 834.

A Difference Through Programs: Immunizations at the Local High School

One school district in southeastern Michigan began a Hepatitis B immunization program with local health care providers and the local health department. The CHNs servicing the school district assessed that only 16% of the adolescents at the high school received Hepatitis B immunization. The school nurses collaborated with local health care systems to provide the Hepatitis B series to the high school students in the district, targeting both public and private high schools.

The nurses offered lectures about Hepatitis B to each class in the schools. Information and consent forms were sent home to parents. At the end of the program, 80% of the high school population in the community was fully immunized against Hepatitis B and 96% were partially immunized. The program has implications for cost-effective strategies for providing immunizations for vaccine-preventable diseases.

Other data can be found in Bryer-Chuonroong L, Deaver P: Meeting the preteen vaccine law: a pilot program in urban middle schools, *J Sch Health* 70:39-44, 2000 and in Peavey L et al: Notes from the field, *Am J Public Health* 89:412, 1999.

A Difference Through Research: Empowering Families and Evoking Authority

A qualitative research study was conducted in which 30 expert public health nurses practicing in Washington State were asked to describe "clinical examples in which they made a difference in the outcome of high-risk maternal/child cases visited at home" (Zerwekh, 1992, p. 101). Interviews were tape recorded, transcribed, and analyzed. Twenty-one practice competencies were identified from public health nurses' anecdotes in 95 home visits. This article described 2 of the 21 competencies: *empowerment* through encouraging family self-help and *coercion* by assuming responsibility for child protection (i.e., using authority to shield children from violence and neglect).

Although these competencies represent what Zerwekh calls "polarities," the public health nurse synthesizes them through "fostering autonomy" and applying "persuading strategies" such as in child protection. Working with vulnerable groups, public health nurses ensure their right to "protection and sustenance" (Zerwekh, 1992, p. 104). According to Zerwekh, further research is needed to reveal how expert public health nurses implement these competencies and a theory to explain these supposed contradictions.

Based on data from Zerwekh JW: The practice of empowerment and coercion by expert public health nurses, *Image J Nurs Sch* 24:101-105, 1992.

Karen Capel, a community health nursing student, visited a young family during her early field experiences in community health. Mrs. Dana Pritchett was at home with her five-week-old infant and three-year-old preschooler. Her two older children were in school. Her husband, a construction worker in a small town three hours away, came home to be with the family on the weekends. This was Mrs. Pritchett's first experience with breastfeeding and she stated, "I want to see what it's like because this is the last one. My husband had a vasectomy." When Karen asked how she was doing, Mrs. Pritchett replied, "Oh, the baby eats fine, I just get scared. . . It's not safe here at night in this neighborhood, but what can I do? I get real scared."

Another CHN student named Miguel Hernandez visited the Simpsons, an elderly couple. Mrs. Simpson is the caretaker of her ill husband; he has a history of congestive heart failure, hypertension, and episodes of confusion. Daily, a home health aide assists Mrs. Simpson in caring for her husband, but the family is considering institutionalization because Mrs. Simpson has become less able to care for her husband at home. Mrs. Simpson resisted this idea; however, during his visit, Miguel noted that Mr. Simpson's blood pressure was elevated, he was short of breath, and his ankles were edematous. When checking Mr. Simpson's medications, Miguel noted a discrepancy in the last refill date for the patient's diuretic and the number of pills remaining in the bottle. When asked whether her husband had difficulty taking his "water pills," Mrs. Simpson stated, "I don't give them to him in the afternoon. How can I take good care of him when I have to be up at night, putting him on the pan?"

Nursing student Karla Sanders made a home visit to Ms. Jane Fuller, a middle-aged woman, for follow-up hypertension. Upon her visit, Karla met members of the extended family. Mrs. Fuller's 23-year-old daughter had many questions for Karla. Her daughter stated that she had a stroke in her teenage years, was taking medication for hypertension, and had frequent migraines. Concerned, she asked Karla, "Does feeling anxious have to do with my not having sex because my husband's in jail?"

STUDENT CASE EXAMPLES

Population characteristics impact the health of individuals, families, and aggregates. However, nurses can make many interventions for those populations at risk to minimize health risks and address health needs. The clinical examples on pp. 834-835 briefly illustrate problems that nursing students may encounter in the community.

SUMMARY

Factors such as childbearing, aging, SES, crime, and chronic disease impact the health of individuals, families, and communities. As illustrated in the clinical examples, these factors are complex in nature and the associated nursing interventions to address family and community needs are also complex. Identifying and meeting individual, family, and community health needs from traditional medical and health care settings (e.g., hospitals, offices, and clinics) is a limited, if not impossible, task. Likewise, identifying and meeting individual, family, and community health needs while only making home visits is also difficult.

The complex problems facing the health of today's community require actions that result in social change through community organizations, political activity, a coalition, or groups of people. Although hospital, office, clinic, and home visits are important, the complexity of health problems that practitioners encounter has an impact on the family and the community; at times, the impact extends to the state, national, and international level. As noted in the previous examples, health teaching and monitoring a medical regimen are necessary, but they are not sufficient interventions to ensure the health of an individual, family, and community. This is true for many reasons, including the following:

- Health is a complex, dynamic, multifaceted phenomenon.
- Individuals are members of groups and populations such as families, neighborhoods, schools, churches, and other institutions that make up communities.
- The community organization has an impact on the health of individuals, families, communities, and populations.
- To increase the health of populations, the community must identify its needs and organize to meet its needs.

■ CHNs help promote the health of the community by working with families and other populations in the community to identify needs and organize to meet their needs.

Today more than ever, community health nursing can make a difference as the cornerstone of health care delivery. In the United States, the change to a prospective reimbursement system based on DRGs and capitation have shortened hospital stays and increased the need for community-based health care. Groups and populations served in the community now require a broad range of nursing services. Fiscal realities and social demands are likely to mandate the continued growth of community-based care for the foreseeable future. Health care reform that results in upstream care will mandate the continued growth of community-based care over the long term.

LEARNING ACTIVITIES

1. Discuss with classmates how being a member of a population influences an aspect of personal health. Give an example.
2. Discuss why and how CHNs make a difference. Give examples of possible community health nursing interventions for the three clinical examples at the individual level, family level, and population or community level.
3. With classmates, identify the interventions, inventions, or developments that might become the "Greatest Health Achievements" of the twenty-first century.

REFERENCES

Bomar P: *Nurses and family health promotion: concepts, assessment, and intervention,* ed 2, Philadelphia, 1995, WB Saunders.

Bryer-Chuonroong L, Deaver P: Meeting the preteen vaccine law: a pilot program in urban middle schools, *J Sch Health* 70:39-44, 2000.

Centers for Disease Control and Prevention: Ten great public health achievements: United States, 1900-1999, *Mor Mortal Wkly Rep* 48(12):241-243, 1999a.

Centers for Disease Control and Prevention: Achievements public health, 1900-1999 impact of vaccines universally recommended for children: United States, 1990-1998, *Mor Mortal Wkly Rep* 48(12):243-249, 1999b.

Centers for Disease Control and Prevention: Achievements public health, 1900-1999 motor-vehicle safety: a 20th century public health achievement, *Mor Mortal Wkly Rep* 48(18):369-374, 1999c.

Centers for Disease Control and Prevention: Achievements public health, 1900-1999, improvements in workplace safety: United States, 1900-1999, *Mor Mortal Wkly Rep* 48(22):461-469, 1999d.

Centers for Disease Control and Prevention: Achievements public health, 1900-1999, control of infectious disease, *Mor Mortal Wkly Rep* 48(29):621-629, 1999e.

Centers for Disease Control and Prevention: Achievements public health, 1900-1999, decline in deaths from heart diseases and stroke: United States, 1990-1999, *Mor Mortal Wkly Rep* 48(30):649-656, 1999f.

Centers for Disease Control and Prevention: Achievements public health, 1900-1999, safer and healthier foods, *Mor Mortal Wkly Rep* 48(40):905-913, 1999g.

Centers for Disease Control and Prevention: Achievements public health, 1900-1999, healthier mothers and babies, *Mor Mortal Wkly Rep* 48(38):849-858, 1999h.

Centers for Disease Control and Prevention: Achievements public health, 1900-1999, family planning, *Mor Mortal Wkly Rep* 48(47):1073-1080, 1999i.

Centers for Disease Control and Prevention: Achievements public health, 1900-1999, fluoridation of drinking water to prevent dental caries, *Mor Mortal Wkly Rep* 48(41):933-940, 1999j.

Centers for Disease Control and Prevention: Achievements public health, 1900-1999, tobacco use: United States, 1990-1999, *Mor Mortal Wkly Rep* 48(43):986-993, 1999k.

Centers for Disease Control and Prevention: *About a century of success,* 2000, The Author, www.cdc.gov/phtn/tenachievements/about/about3.htm.

Insurance Institute for Highway Safety, Highway Loss Data Institute: *Safety facts: teenagers,* 2000, The Author, www.hwysafety.org/safety_facts/teens/teenager.htm.

Kottke T: The "intervention index:" insufficient information, *J Clin Epidemiol* 45:17-19, 1992.

National Center for Health Statistics: *Health, United States, 1994,* Hyattsville, Md, 1995, PHS.

National Center for Health Statistics: *Health, United States, 1999: health and aging chartbook,* Hyattsville, Md, 1999a, USDHHS, NCHS.

National Center for Health Statistics, News Releases and Fact Sheets: *Latest final mortality statistics available,* Hyattsville, Md, 1999b, PHS.

Peavey L et al: Notes from the field, *Am J Public Health* 89:412, 1999.

US Department of Health and Human Services: *Healthy people, 2010: conference edition,* Washington, DC, 2000, US Government Printing Office.

Zerwekh JW: The practice of empowerment and coercion by expert public health nurses, *Image J Nurs Sch* 24:101-105, 1992.

INDEX

A

Abortion, RU-486 for, 352
Abstinence, 639
Abuse
  alcohol; *see* Alcohol abuse
  child, 606-607, 609t
  elder, 483, 607-609, 610t, *618f*
  fraud and, 199
  prevalence of, 599
  sexual
    of child, 607
    in correctional institution,
      766-767
    dating violence and,
      602-603
    indicators of, 608t
  spousal, 367
  substance, 624-653;
    see also Substance abuse
Abused women's shelter,
      371-372
Academic performance, nutrition
      and, 717
Access to health care
  by child or adolescent, 333
  coordination and, 200
  definition of, 205
  economics and, 212-213
  by homeless, 536-538
  legislation on, 188
  by men, 393
  mental health, 589
  in Milio's framework for
      prevention, 58
  in occupational health,
      732-733
  in rural communities, 553
  by women, 356
Accidental injury
  to agricultural worker,
      556-557
  to child, 327
  to elderly, 471-473
  to women, 367
Accidental poisoning by
      elderly, 481

Accountability
  in parish nursing, 780-782
  public, 231-232
Accreditation, 199
Acquired immunity, 664
Acquired immunodeficiency
      syndrome, 688-690;
    see also Human immuno-
      deficiency virus infection
Activities of daily living
  disability and, 500-501
  elderly and, 470-471
Activity orientation, 252
Activity theory of aging, 459
Actuarial classification, 205, 211
Adaptation, family, 429
Addiction
  conceptualization of, 627
  political considerations about,
      631-632
  stages of, 632-633, 633t
Administrative cost, 210
Administrative law, 223
Adolescent, 329-346
  cardiac risk in, 717
  case study of, 342-345
  in correctional institution, 767
  ethical issues concerning, 341-342
  health care use by, 333
  health insurance for, 334
  health promotion for, 335
  Healthy People 2010 and, 334-335,
      336t
  homeless, 533-534
  homicide and, 598-599
  improving health of, 339-341
  legal issues concerning, 341
  parent's educational status, 333
  poverty and, *332,* 332-333
  pregnancy and, 329-331, 342-345
    health planning for, 110
    study of, 107
  pregnant
    abuse of, 603
    home visits to, 416
  public health programs for, 335,
      337-338
  at risk, 703
  school health and; *see* School
      health

Adolescent—cont'd
  sexually transmitted disease in, 331
  of single parent, 333
  substance abuse by, 331-332, 644
  toy-related injury to, 327
  vaccination for, 672
  violence and, 329, 600-601, 601t
Adoption by single woman, 358
Advance directive, 792
Adverse event, vaccine-related, 671
Adverse selection, 206
Advocacy, 200
  for disabled, 514
Age; *see also* Elderly
  disability and, 503, 503t
  health impact of, 828-829
  rural communities and, 553-554
Age-adjusted mortality rate, 73, 74t,
      75, 75t, 76t
Age of confinement, 586
Age-specific mortality rate, 73, 76t
Age stratification theory of aging, 460
Agency, home health care, 786-787
Aggregate
  community as client and, 110-111
  environmental health and, 287, 304
  as focus of nursing practice, 18
  health care delivery affecting, 42
  health planning and, assessment in,
      113-115
  history of civilization and, 24-26
  nature of community and, 93-94
Aging
  concept of, 459
  culture and, 259
  theories of, 459-460
Agricultural community, 548-577;
    see also Rural health
Agricultural worker, 556-558
AIDS, 688-690; *see also* Human
      immunodeficiency virus
      infection
Air quality, 290t, 292-293
Airborne transmission of disease,
      663-664
Albrecht model for home care
      nursing, 788-790, *789f*
Alcohol abuse
  by age, race, and ethnic group,
      626-627, 626t

Page numbers in italics indicate boxes and
illustrations; page numbers followed by
t indicate tables.

Alcohol abuse—cont'd
detoxification and, 637
disulfiram for, 637-638
driving and, 641
by elderly, 645
historic trends in, 625
homelessness and, 531, 532, 536
naltrexone for, 638
pregnancy and, 326
Alcoholics Anonymous, 639-640
Alliance, 215-216
in family, 422
Alternative therapy, 196
Alzheimer's disease, 475-476
Ambulatory care, 205, 211-212
for elderly, 466, *468f*
for men, 386
American Academy of Pediatrics,
on immunization, 666
American Association of Industrial
Nurses, 732
American Medical Association,
on literacy, 155-156
American Nurses Association
on accountability, 231-232
on community health nursing,
12, 13
lobbying activities of, 236-237
standards of; *see also* Standard,
nursing
for home care nurse, 788-790
rural health and, 569-570
American Nurses Credentialing
Center, certification by,
13, 15, 17t
American Psychiatric Association, 630
American Public Health Association
on community health nursing,
12-13
on essential services, 7-8
lobbying by, 236-237
Americans with Disabilities Act, 500,
513-514, 753-754
correctional institutions and, 768
Analysis, policy, 225-226
Analytic epidemiology, 84-89
cross-sectional studies, 85, *85f*
experimental studies, 89, *89f*
observational studies, 84-85
prospective studies, 87-88
retrospective studies, 85-87, *86f*, 88
Animal-borne disease, 663
rabies, 684-685
Antabuse, 637-638
Anxiety disorder, 588

Arbitrator model of case management, 175
Arizona model of case management, 176
Arteriosclerosis, in women, 360
Arthritis, in women, 361
Assertive community treatment,
589-590
Assessment
abuse, 614t
community, 92-108
data for, 95-100
data retrieval in, 104
health community model and,
95, *95f, 96f*
nature of community and, 92-95
of needs, 100, 105
nursing process in, 100, 105-107
parameters of, *95f,* 101t-103t
cultural, 274-277
of family, 423-435
ecomap for, 429
Family Health Assessment for,
429-430, *430f-434f,* 434
family health tree, 425, *428f,* 429
genogram for, 423-424,
426f-428f
social and structural constraints
on, 434
in health planning model, 113-116
in nursing practice, school health
and, 725
in nursing process
communicable disease and,
695-696
for elderly, 488, 489
environmental health and,
309-310
family nursing and, 445-447
home care and, 796, 799, 801
homeless and, 540
international health and, 820-822,
821f
men's health and, 402
rural health and, 574-575
in substance abuse intervention,
650-651
women's health and, 375-376
Assistive device, for elderly, 470
Assistive personnel, 196
for disabled person, 505
Association of Occupational Health
Nurses
code of ethics of, 734, 735
definitions of, 731

Association of Occupational Health
Nurses—cont'd
evolution of occupational nursing
and, 732
Asthma, 713
school health and, 711-712
Athlete
female athlete triad and, 716
substance abuse by, 645
Attitude toward substance abuser, 649
Autoimmune theory of aging, 460

B
Back disorder, 502
Balance of power in government,
222-223
Barrier
to care, in rural communities,
551-552
communication, 260-261
Barton, Clara, 220
Battering, 602; *see also* Domestic
violence
Behavior
adolescent substance abuse and, 644
child abuse indicated by, 608t
of child or adolescent, 719, 720
health
continuum of, *59f*
cost and, 208
of men, 391
health belief model and, 54-55
manners as, 414
in Milio's framework for prevention, 56-58
sex-linked, 392
Behavioral learning theory, 134t
Belief
cultural factors and, 264-267
of family, 422
health, 53-56, *54f,* 57
in cultural assessment, 275
societal, cost of health care
and, 208
Benzene standard, *746f*
Bereavement, 482-483
Berlin Society of Physicians and
Surgeons, 29
Bill, legislative process for, 227,
228f, 229
Biocultural variation, 277
Biological factors
in men's health status, 387-388
in mental illness, 590
Biological-infectious hazard, 738

Biomedical theory of illness, 264-265
Biopsychosocial model of substance
    abuse, 631
Bipolar disorder, 588
Birth control, 365-366, 365t, 832;
    see also Family planning
    Margaret Sanger's crusading
        for, 222
Birth rate for adolescents, *330f*
Block grant, maternal and child
    health, 337
Block nurse program, 438-439
Blood precautions, 664
Boundary, in systems theory, 421
Brain, mental illness and, 587-588,
    590-591
Breast cancer, 361-362
    in Asian-American women, 364
    education about, 146
Brewster, Mary, 37
Buprenorphine, 638-639

C

Campaigning, 239
Cancer
    breast, 361-362
        in Asian-American women, 364
    educational program about,
        144-147, 147t-150t, 150-153
    gynecologic, 362-363
    lung
        smoking and, 832-833
        in women, 362
    prostate, 390
    testicular, 390
    in women, 353
Candidate, campaigning for, 239
Cannabis, 629t
Capital cost, 206
Capitated reimbursement, 214
Capitation, 205
Cardiovascular disease
    in adolescent, 717
    in women, 353-354
Care management, 205
Caregiver
    community, 36-37
    for elderly, 482
        abuse by, 483, 607-609
    home care, 790-791
Carve-out service, 205
Case-control study, 85-87, *86f,* 88
Case management, 170-179
    case identification in, 174-175
    case study of, 177-178

Case management—cont'd
    education preparation for, 173
    managed care and, 172-173
    models of, 175-176
    in occupational health, 749-750
    origins of, 171-172
    overview of, 171
    purpose of, 172
    referral in, 175
    research in, 177
    roles in, 174
    services of, 174
    trends influences, 173
Causality, 79-80
Census data, 98-100
Census tract, 94
Centenarian, 461
Centers for Disease Control
        and Prevention
    MMWR of, 664
    morbidity and mortality data of, 6
    school health and, 706
    universal precautions of, 664
Central nervous system drug, abuse
        of, 629t
Cerebrovascular disorder, in women,
    353-354
Certificate of need, 123, 125-126
Certification of community health
        nurse, 13, 15
Certified home health agencies, 787
Cervical cancer, 362-363
Chadwick, Edwin, 28
Chain, home care agency, 786-787
Change agent, nurse as, 233-234
Charge, 205
Chart, coxcomb, *31f-32f*
Chemical disease agent, 67t
Chemical exposure
    of agricultural worker, 558
    of migrant workers, 559
Chemical hazard, 738
Chickenpox vaccine, 681-682
Child, 321-346
    abuse and neglect of, 328-329,
        606-607, 609t
        substance abuse and, 647
    accidental injury in, 327
    disabled, 503t
    ethical issues concerning, 341-342
    health care use by, 333
    health promotion for, 335
    Healthy People 2010 and, 334-335,
        336t
    homeless, 532-533

Child—cont'd
    immunization of, 328, *668f*
    improving health of, 339-341
    insurance for, 334
    lead poisoning in, 328
    legal issues concerning, 341
    parent's educational status, 333
    poverty and, 332-333, *332f*
    public health programs for, 335,
        337-339
    in rural community, 553-554
    school health and, 702-727;
        see also School health
    of single parent, 333
    spirituality of, 259
    violence and, 600-601, 601t
Childbirth
    adolescent and, 329-331
    cultural factors and, 269
    mortality rate and, 352-353
Children's Bureau, 566
Children's Bureau Act, 184
CHIP, 552, 567
Chiropractor, 196
Chlamydia trachomatis, 366,
    690-691
Cholera, 682-683
Chronic disease
    of agricultural worker, 557-558
    conceptualization of, 517
    epidemiology of, 69
    family nursing and, 416-417
    in men, 385-386
    mortality and, 42
    in women, 354-355
Cigarette smoking; *see* Smoking
CIRCLE model of spiritual care, 779
Circular communication, 422
City, healthy, 95
Civil Rights Act, 369
Class, social, 436-438, *437f*
Client, community as, 110-112, *111f*
Client-centered case management, 172
Client rights, 200
Clinic, wellness, for men, 399-401
Clinical specialist in community
        health nursing, 15, 17t
Clinton health care reform initiative,
    200-201
Closed system, 421
Coalition
    on environmental health, 306-307
    in family, 422
    health care provider, 237-238
COBRA, 187

Code
  current procedural terminology, 205
  of ethics
    of American Nurses Association,
      parish nursing and, 780
    of Association of Occupational
      Health Nurses, 732, 734
Code of Federal Regulations, 751
Codependency, 642
Cognitive disorder in elderly, 475-476
Cognitive learning, 133t
Cohabitation, 413
Cohesion, family, 429
Cohort study, 87-88
Coinsurance, 205, 210
Cold chain, 669
Collaborative model of international
    health care, 819-824
Collective strategy in environmental
    health, 307-308
Committee on a National Agenda for
    the Prevention of Disabilities,
    498-499
Communicable disease, 659-699
  case study of, 695-698
  control of, 666, 831
  elimination of, 666
  erudition of, 666-667
  Healthy People 2010 and, 661,
    662t
  home visit follow-up for, 798-800
  immunity to, 664; *see also* vaccines
    for, *below*
  prevention of, 693-695, 693t
  reportable, 665, 665t
  sexually transmitted, 687-693
  transmission of, 663t, 661664
  universal and body fluid
    precautions for, 664
  vaccines for, 667-687
    administration of, 670
    for adolescents and young
      adults, 672
    for adults, 672
    childhood schedule for, *668f*
    contraindications to, 670-671
    diphtheria, 673-674
    documentation of, 671
    dosages of, 670
    for elderly, 672
    Haemophilus influenzae
      type B, 674
    hepatitis, 674-676
    immunosuppression and, 672
    influenza, 676-677

Communicable disease—cont'd
  vaccines for—cont'd
    international travel and, 682-687
    Lyme disease, 677-678
    mumps, 679
    pertussis, 679
    pneumococcal disease, 679-680
    poliomyelitis, 680
    precautions for, 667, 669
    in pregnancy, 672-673
    rubella, 680-681
    rubeola, 678-679
    safety of, 671-672
    spacing of, 670
    storage, transport, and handling
      of, 669-670
    tetanus, 681
    types of, 669, 669t
    varicella, 681-682
Communication
  community assessment and,
    102t
  cross-cultural, 259-264
  in cultural assessment, 275
  end-of-life issues and, 368
  in family, 422-423
  framework for developing, 144
  health education, 144-147,
    147t-150t, 150-153
  nurse's role in, 142-144
Community
  child's health and, 339-340
  as client, 110-112, *111f*
  definition of, 5-6
  environmental health and, 287, 311
  of families, 438-440
  global, 811-825; *see also*
    Global community
  healthy, 95, *96f*
  school health and, 721-722
  of solution, 94
  women's health and, 376
Community and migrant health
    centers program, 337
Community assessment, 92-108;
    see also Assessment,
    community
Community-based care in rural
    community, 564
Community caregiver, 36-37
Community empowerment, 139-142
Community health, definition
    of, 7-8
Community health care system, rural,
    562-563

Community health centers
    program, 568
Community health diagnosis,
    105f, 106
Community health nurse, 4
  certification of, 13, 15
  certification requirements for, 17t
  child's health and, 340-341
  communicable disease and, 661
  elderly and, 487
  mental health and, 592-593
  numbers employed, 4
  substance abuse and, 648-650
    prevention programs, 635
  workplace safety for, 620-621
Community health nursing
  challenges for, 44-45
  competencies of, 15t
  definition of, 12-13
  disabled and, 518, 521
  environmental health and,
    304-308
  family nursing and, 417-419
  history of, 23-43
    advent of modern health care,
      30-42
    aggregate health and, 42-43
    evolution of health and,
      23-29, *24f*
  in international health care, 818
  interventions of, 16t
  levels of, 112t
  making a difference, 827-835
  managed care and, 18-20
  for men, 395, 399-401
  rural, 569
Community health planning,
    109-127; *see also* Planning,
    health
Community health services, 192
Community organization practice,
    141t
Community-oriented primary care,
    rural, 563
Community services, 103t
Comorbidity, 536
Competency, nursing, 15t
Competent nursing practice, 747-748
Comprehensive Health Planning
    Amendment, 122-123
Comprehensive Perinatal Services
    Program, 107
Comprehensive Teenage Pregnancy
    and Parenting Program, 107
CON, 213

Confidentiality in parish nursing, 780-782
Configuration, family, 357-358
Congress, role of, 224
CONS, 188 — WHAT IS THIS?
Conservative scope of practice, 52
Consolidated Omnibus Budget Reconciliation Act, 187
Consultant
  case manager as, 174
  occupational medical, 757
Consumer rights, 188
Consumerism, 200
Continuation stage of addiction, 632
Continuity theory of aging, 460
Contraception, 365-366, 365t, 832
  Margaret Sanger's crusading for, 222
Control, infection, 665
Conversation, therapeutic, with family, 414
Cooperative, insurance purchasing, 210
Copayment, 205, 210
Coronary heart disease, epidemiology of, 69, 71
Coronary Primary Prevention Trial, 89
Corporal punishment, 598
Correctional institution, 761-770
  adolescents in, 767
  health patterns in, 764-766
  history and development of, 762-763
  legal and ethical issues in, 768-769
  mental health issues in, 767-768
  nursing care issues in, 763-764
  nursing practice standards in, 769-770
  research in, 769
  women in, 766-767
Correlational study, 85
Cost
  administrative, 210
  capital, 206
  health care, factors influencing, 207-209
Cost containment, 205, 213-214
  safety and quality of care and, 230-231
Cost sharing, 215
Cost shifting, 206, 211
Counseling for women, 373
Counselor, parish nurse as, 775

Coxcomb chart, *31f-32f*
Credentialing, 13, 15
Crime; *see also* Violence
  elderly and, 484
  homicide, 598-599
Crime watch project, 118
Crimean War, 30-34, 33t
Critical access hospital, 568
Critical social theory, 58-60
Critical theory, environmental health and, 287-288
Cross-cultural communication, 259-264
Cross-cultural nursing, 248-250
Cross-cultural perspective on illness, 264-265
Cross-sectional study, 85, *85f*
Crude epidemiological rate, 72-73
Crude rate, 76t
Cultural factors, 242-283
  aging and, 259
  case study of, 280-282
  cross-cultural communication and, 259-264
  disability and, 503, 504t
  family and, 253-254
  folk healing practice and, 36-37
  health beliefs and, 264-267
  Healthy People 2010 and, 244, 245t-246t, 247
  historical perspectives on, 247-248
  management of health problems and, 267-274
  migrant workers and, 559
  nurse's role in, 274-278
  nutrition and, 256-257, 257t
  overview of, 250-254
  population trends and, 243-244, 244t
  religion and, 257-259, 257t
  resources for minority health and, 278-280
  socioeconomic factors and, 254-256, 255t
  transcultural nursing and, 248-250, *249f*
  transcultural perspective and, 243
  values and, 250-252
Cultural negotiation, 267-268
Culturally competent care, 144
Culture
  of poverty view, 437-438
  prison, 763-764
Culture-bound syndrome, 267

Culture specific value or belief, 248
Culture universal value or belief, 248
Culturological assessment, 274-277
Cure *vs.* prevention, 10
Current procedural terminology code, 205
Customary charge, 205
Cycle, family life, dislocations of, 425t
Cycle theory of violence, 603-604

D
Data
  census, 98-100
  on disability, 500-504, 501t-504t
  on homeless, 527-529, 527-530, *528f*
  on minority populations, 272
  for population-focused care, 19t
  on rural communities, 550-551
Dating violence, 602-603
de Madres a Madres program, 140, 439-440
Death
  cause of
    accidental poisoning in elderly, 481
    communicable disease, 660
    elder abuse, 483-484
    of elderly, 461, 463
    leading, 6
    for men, 383, 384t, 385, 395
    new, 42
    in women, 351-354, 352t
  decline in number of, 831
  elderly and, 482-484
  end-of-life issues and, 368
  homicide, 598-599
  infant mortality rate and, 323-324, 324t
  Nightingale's statistics on, 30-34, *31f-32f,* 33t
  suicide, 599
Declaration of Alma-Ata, 815-816
Decriminalization of substance abuse, 635
Deductible, 205, 210
Deinstitutionalization in mental health, 587
Deliberate indifference, 768-769
Delivery of health services
  aggregate and, 42
  cultural factors and, 270-271
  in global community, 817-818
  in rural community, 560-564

Dementia, 475-476

Demographics
  of elderly population, 460-461
  of homelessness, 527-530,
    528f
  of men, 396
  in occupational health, 732-733
  of suicide, 599

Dental health
  in elderly, 473-474
  school health and, 709

Denver model of case management, 176

Department of Health and Human
  Services
  federal health care system and,
    190-191
  minority health resources of,
    278-279
  poverty guidelines of, 185t
  public health subsystem
    and, 190
  structure of, 191

Dependence, drug, 630;
  see also Substance abuse

Depressant, abuse of, 629t

Depression
  in elderly, 476
  incidence of, 588
  in women, 355-356, 363-364

Descriptive epidemiology, 84

Detoxification, 637

Developmental considerations
  cultural factors in, 277
  in family, 423

Diabetes mellitus
  school health and, 712, 713
  in women, 354, 360-361

Diagnosis
  community health, *105f,* 106
  in nursing process
    communicable disease and,
      696-697
    for elderly, 489-499
    family nursing and, 447-448
    home care and, 796-797, 799,
      802-806
    international health and, 822
    men's health and, 402-403
    rural health and, 575
    school health and, 725
    in substance abuse interven-
      tion, 651
    women's health and, 375-376

Diagnostic related group, 205, 211

Diet
  culture and, 256-257, 257t
  for elderly, 470t

Dietitian, registered, 196

Differentiation in systems theory, 421

Direct care for women, 373

Direct standardization of mortality
  rate, 73, 74t, 75

Direct transmission of infection, 662

Directive, advance, 792

Disability, 496-523, 502
  costs associated with, 504-505,
    505t, 506t
  definition of, 497-498, 498t
  do's and dont's for interactions,
    511t-512t
  in elderly, 470-471, *472f*
  ethical issues concerning, 522
  Healthy People 2010 and, 506-507,
    506t
  historical context for, 507, 509-510,
    511t-512t, 512
  intersystem model of, 516-518,
    519f, 520f
  model of, 498-499, *499f*
  nursing strategies for, 518, 521
  personal experience of, 516
  prevalence of, 501-504, 502t-504t
  public policy and, 512-514
  quality of life issues and, 499-500
  reconceptualizing health care for,
    514-516, 515t
  responses to, 497
  school health and, 714, 715t
  sources of data on, 500-501, 501t
  in women, 367-368

Disaster program, 103t

Discharge planner model of case
  management, 175

Discipline, corporal, 598

Disconnectedness, 532

Disease
  definition of, 25
  global patterns of, 813
  incidence of, cultural aspects of,
    276-277
  theories about, 35-36, 42-43

Disengagement theory of aging, 459

Distance, as cultural factor, 260

Distress, spiritual, 779

District nursing, 44-45

Disulfiram, 637-638

Diversity, cultural, 242-283;
  see also Cultural factors

Divorce
  family development and, 423
  family life cycle and, 425t
  goal for women after, 424

Dix, Dorothea, 586

Dock, Lavinia, 220, 222

Documentation
  of home care, 790
  school health, 714
  of vaccination, 671

Domestic violence, 367, 601-606
  cycle of, 603-604, *604f, 605f*
  dating and, 602-603
  effects of, 604-606
  history of, 598
  homelessness and, 530
  in pregnancy, 603

Dominant value orientation, 250

Double standard in public health,
  418-419

Downsizing, 194

DRG, 205, 211

Drinking water fluoridation, 832

Driving, substance abuse and, 641

Drop-in home visit, 795

Drug
  date rape, 603
  gateway, 644

Drug abuse; *see* Substance abuse

Drug overdose, accidental,
  in elderly, 481

Drug testing, 633

Drug therapy
  in correctional institution, 768
  for elderly, 480-481
  for HIV infection, 690
  at school, 712-714
  for substance abuse, 637-639

Dual diagnosis with substance abuse,
  536, 647-648

Durable power of attorney, 793

Dysfunctional family, substance abuse
  and, 642-643

Dysmenorrhea, 367-368

E

Early and Periodic Screening,
  Diagnostic, and Treatment
  program, 337, 711

Ecological framework, 435-436

Ecomap, 414-415, 429

Economics
  of health care, 204-216
    access to care and, 212-213
    cost containment and, 213-214

Economics—cont'd
  of health care—cont'd
    cultural diversity and, 271
    factors influencing cost, 207-209
    insurance and, 210-212
    private financing and, 209-210
    public financing and, 209
    terminology in, 205-207
    trends in, 215-216
    uninsured patients and,
      214-215
  occupational health and, 731
  of substance abuse, 631-632
Ectopic pregnancy, 353
Education
  for case manager, 173
  community assessment and, 101t
  culture and, 256
  culturological assessment and, 276
  of elderly, 465
  health, 129-179
    case study of, 162-164
    characteristics of learners and,
      135t, 136
    in community, 130-131
    community organization practice
      and, 141t
    cultural factors and, 270
    framework for developing, 144,
      147, 147t-150t, 150-153
    learning theories and, 132,
      133t-134t, 134-135
    for men, 397
    in Milio's theory, 56, 57
    models of, 135-142, 137t, 138t
    nurse's role in, 142-144
    nursing process and, 162-164
    questions about, 130
    resources for, 153-156, 154f,
      157t, 158-162, 159f-161f
    school health and, 706-716
  homeless children and, 533
  in Milio's theory, 56, 57
  nursing
    disability and, 515-516
    for home care nurse, 788-790
    of parish nurse, 778
  nutrition, in school, 717
  of parent, 333
  physical, 709
  problem-solving, 139
  in rural community, 554
  on substance abuse, 635
  Vietnamese client and, 282
  of women, 356

Education for All Handicapped
    Children Act, 513
Educator
  case manager as, 174
  nurse as, for women, 373
Eighteenth century medicine, 28
Elderly, 457-493
  abuse of, 483-484, 607-609,
      610t, 618f
    history of, 598
  case management and, 172
  characteristics of, 463-465, 464f
  community health nurse and, 487
  crime and, 484
  culture and, 259
  death and bereavement and,
      482-483
  demographics of, 460-463, 462t
  exercise for, project involving, 118
  family issues of, 482
  health care use by, 465-468, 467f,
      468f, 469t
  health needs of, 459
  health problems of, 469-479
    accidents, 471-473, 472f
    cognitive impairment, 475-476
    dental, 473-474
    depression, 476
    disability, 470-471, 472f
    hearing impairment, 474
    incontinence, 477-478
    nutrition, 469-470, 470t, 471t
    suicide, 476-477
    thermal stress, 478-479
    visual impairment, 474-475
  health promotion for, 479-481
  Healthy People 2010 and, 458t
  institutionalization of, 481-482
  nursing process for, 488-492
  public policies affecting, 484-486
  research on, 486, 487
  in rural community, 553
  substance abuse by, 645
  theories on aging and, 459-460
  transitions by, 481
  vaccination for, 672
Electoral information, 235t
Elimination, of infection, 665
Elizabethan poor law, 28
Emergency care
  in rural community, 566
  school health and, 711
Emotional abuse of child, 606-607
  indicators of, 608t
Emotional communication, 422

Emotional disorder, 502
Emotional neglect of child, 607
Employee
  of disabled person, 513
  roles and responsibilities of,
      755-756, 757
Employee assistance counselor, 757
Employee Retirement income Security
    Act, 485
Employment; see also Occupational
    entries
  child health and, 340
  of disabled person, 505
  homelessness and, 530
  men's health and, 393
  in rural community, 554
  of women, 356
Empowerment as health education
    model, 139-142
Enabler, professional, 643
End-of-life issues, 368
Endometrial cancer, 363
Energy in systems theory, 421
Environment
  community assessment and, 101t
  global community and, 812-813
  home, 795
  prison; see Correctional institution
  school, 719
  temperature and elderly, 478-479
Environmental factors in disease, 68t
Environmental hazard, 738
Environmental health, 286-313, 290t,
      731; see also Occupational
      health
  aggregate and, 304
  areas of, 288-299
    air quality, 292-293
    food quality, 295-296
    housing, 294-295
    living patterns, 289-290, 290t
    radiation risk, 297-298
    violence risk, 299
    waste control, 296-297
    water quality, 293-294
    work risks, 292
  community health nursing and,
      304-308
  critical theory approach to,
      287-288
  definition of, 287
  global, 302-304
  hazards and, 299-300
  legislation about, 300-302
  nursing process and, 309-312

Environmental health services, 192-193
Environmental Protection Agency, 301
  communicable disease and, 660
Epidemiological paradox, 271
Epidemiology, 65-90
  in disease prevention, 66-69, 67t, 68t, *69f, 70f*
  for men, 396
  methods of, 84-89, 85t-87t, *89f*
  in occupational health, 731
  rates in
    age-specific, 73
    crude, 72-73
    morbidity, 71-72
    mortality, 72-76, 73t-75t
    proportional mortality ratio, 75-76
    standardization of, 73, 74t, 75, 75t
  risk and, 76, 78
  use of
    in health services, 83-84
    in prevention, 78-83
Equilibrium in systems theory, 421
Equipment
  assistive, 470
  sports, 707
Eradication of infection, 665-666
Ergonomics, 731
Estrogen replacement therapy for Alzheimer's disease, 476
Ethical issues
  Association of Occupational Health Nurses and, 732, 734
  child and adolescent health and, 340-341
  in correctional institution, 768-769
  disability and, 522
  in home health care, 792-793
  in occupational health, 731, 750
  of substance abuse, 633-634
  uninsured patients as, 215
Ethnicity; *see also* Cultural factors
  health impact of, 829
  in rural community, 555-556
  substance abuse and, 646-647
Ethnocentrism, 249-250
Etiology, disease agents and, 67t-68t
Evaluation
  in community assessment, 106-107
  of education program, 151-152
  in health planning model, 117

Evaluation—cont'd
  in nursing practice, school health and, 726
  in nursing process
    communicable disease and, 698
    for elderly, 488, 491
    environmental health and, 312
    family nursing and, 449-450
    home care and, 797-798, 800, 803
    homeless and, 540-541
    international health and, 823-824
    men's health and, 404
    rural health and, 576
    in substance abuse intervention, 651-652
    women's health and, 376
Executive branch of government, role of, 224
Exercise program for elderly, 118
Experimental study, 89, *89f*
Expert nurse, occupational, 749
Expressive functioning, 422
Extended care facility for elderly, 481-482
External structure of family, 422
Extradition, 762
Eye contact, 261

F
FACES I, 430
Facilitator, parish nurse as, 776-777
Factory Nurses Conference, 732
Faith community, 772-782
  in rural community, 564-565
Family, 409-452
  approaches
    family theory, 419
    structural-functional conceptual framework, 420, 422-423
    systems, 419-421
  assessment of, 105, 423-435
    ecomap for, 429
    Family Health Assessment for, 429-430, *430f-434f,* 434
    family health tree, 425, *428f,* 429
    genogram for, 423-424, *426f-428f*
    social and structural constraints on, 434
  changes in, 412-413
  culture and, 253-254
  of elderly, 482
  environmental health and, 311
  family nursing and, 411-412

Family—cont'd
  home care and, 790-791
  homeless, 534-535
  intervention for, 435-440
  interviewing of, 414-416
  meeting health needs of, 413-419
  men's health and, 402
  nursing process for, 440-451, *442f, 443f*
  occupational health and, 757
  school health and, 721-722
  substance abuse and, 642-643
  types of, 410
  of women, 357-358
  women's health and, 376
Family Adaptability and Cohesion Evaluation Scale, 430
Family and Medical Leave Act, 370
Family-community HPM, 271
Family Health Assessment, 429-430, *430f-434f,* 434
Family health tree, 425, *428f,* 429
Family life cycle, divorce affecting, 425t
Family nursing, 409-452
Family planning, 365-366, 365t, 832
  Margaret Sanger's crusading for, 222
Family risk index, 721
Family Support Act, 187
Family theory, 419
Family therapist, 435-436
Farm-related accident, 556-557
Farm worker, seasonal, 558-560; *see also* Rural community
Fecal-oral transmission of disease, 663
Federal government
  minority health and, 279t
  state *vs.* federal standards and, 226
  structure of, 222-224
Federal health care subsystem, 189-192
Federal legislation, 184-187, 184t, 185t
  on health planning, 121-125
  on occupational health, 751-754, 752t
  for rural communities, 567-568
Fee schedule, 205
Feedback
  on education program, 152-153
  in systems theory, 421
Female, 349-377; *see also* Women
Female athlete triad, 716

Fetal alcohol syndrome, 326
Fever, yellow, 685-686
Financial issues
    case management and, 172-173
    cultural diversity and, 271
    disability and, 504-506, 505t, 506t
    economics of health care and,
        204-216; *see also* Economics
    federal funding, 124
    of home health care, 787-788
    market justice and, 8-9
    in men's access to care, 393
    in Milio's framework for preven-
        tion, 57-58
    prevention *vs.* cure, 10
    privatization of prison and,
        762-763
    in rural communities, 551-552
    utilization review and, 172-173
    Vietnamese client and, 281
Flexible spending account, 205, 216
Flexner Report, 35
Flu shot, 480
Fluoridation of water, 832
Focus group, 100
Folk healer, 265-266
Folk health system, 282
Folk practices, 36-37
Food
    culture and, 256-257, 257t
    for elderly, 469, 470t
    quality of, 290t, 295-296
    safety of, 831-832
    vending machine, 715
Format of health education materials,
        159-161
Formula, readability, *161f*
Forum, community, 100
Framework, ecological, 435-436
Fraud, health care, 199
Frontier community, 563
Functional incontinence, 478
Functioning, expressive or
        instrumental, 422

G
Gamma-hydroxybutyrate, 603
Gatekeeper, 205, 214
Gateway drug, 644
Gender
    cultural factors and, 261, 263-264
    disability and, 503
    health impact of, 828
    rural community and, 554-555
General systems theory, 420

Generalist, 15, 17t
Genetic factor in mental illness, 590
Genital herpes, 691-692
    health education about, 132, 134
Genogram, 423-424, *426f-428f*
    in family interview, 414-415
Geography
    in community assessment, 101t
    health impact of, 829-830
Geriatric clinical nurse model of case
        management, 176
Germ theory, 42-43, 264-265
Gestalt learning, 133t
Global community, 811-825
    case study of, 819-824
    disease patterns in, 813-814
    environmental factors in, 812-813
    health care delivery systems in,
        817-818
    international organizations and, 814
    population characteristics of, 812
    research in, 819
Global environmental health, 302-304
Gonorrhea, 691
Government
    child's health and, 340
    health planning legislation and,
        121-125
    minority health and, 279t
    state *vs.* federal standards and, 226
    structure of, 222-224
Grant, maternal and child health, 337
Great Britain, health and disease
        in, 28
Greece, health and disease in, 26
Grief, elderly and, 482-483
Gynecologic cancer, 362-363
Gynecological examination in correc-
        tional institution, 766-767

H
Habit, health, in rural community,
        553, 555
Haemophilus influenzae type B
        vaccine, 674
Hall, Helen, 39
Hallucinogen abuse, 629t
Handicap, definition of, 497-498,
        498t; *see also* Disability
Harm reduction, 640-642
Hazard
    affecting women, 369-370
    environmental, 299-300
        aggregate and, 304
    occupational, 738, 740t

Head Start, 338-339
Healing, folk, 36-37, 265-266
Health
    community and, 5-6
    definition of, 5
    environmental, 287
    indicators of, 6-7
    literacy and, 155-156,
        157f, 158
    parish, 772-782; *see also*
        Parish nursing
    preventive approach to, 8-12, 9t
    rural, 548-577; *see also*
        Rural health
    school, 702-727; *see also*
        School health
Health Amendments Act, 186
Health behavior
    continuum of, *59f*
    in rural community, 553
Health belief, 264-267, 275
Health belief model, 53-56,
        54f, 57
    health education and, 137-139,
        137t, 138t
Health care
    economics of, 204-216; *see also*
        Economics, of health care
    policy about, 219-240
Health care alliance, 215-216
Health care delivery
    aggregate and, 42
    cultural factors and, 270-271
    in global community, 817-818
    in rural community, 560-564
Health Care Financing Administra-
        tion, 185
Health Care for the Homeless
        Initiative, 533
Health care professional
    from minority group, 271-272
    substance abuse by, 648
Health care provider
    definition of, 205
    types of, 193-196
Health care services
    epidemiology and, 83-84
    for men, 398
    occupational health nursing,
        736-737
    school, 706-722; *see also*
        School health
    social class and, 436-438,
        437f
    for women, 371

Health care system, 183-202
  changes in, 4-5
  components of, 188-196
    federal subsystem, 189-192
    local health department
      subsystem, 192-193
    private subsystem, 188-189
    providers, 193-196
    public subsystem, 189
    state level subsystem, 192
  cultural factors and, 270-271
  future of, 201
  interrelationships of, 94-95
  legislation and, 184-188, 184t,
    185t, *186f*
  managed care and, 197
  President's advisory committee on,
    197-198
  quality care and, 197, 199
  restructuring of, 229-231
  for Vietnamese client, 282
Health care use
  by children, 333
  by elderly, 465-468, 467f, *468f,*
    469t
  by men, 386-387
Health center
  for migrants, 337
  school-based, 722
Health community, 95, *96f*
Health counselor, 775
Health education; *see* Education,
  health
Health information, cultural factors
  and, 269-270
Health insurance; *see* Insurance
Health Insurance Portability and
  Accountability Act, 187
Health maintenance organization, 186
  community health nursing and, 19
  cost of care in, 210
  definition of, 205
  health policy and, 224
  legislation about, 220
  in rural community, 563-564
Health Maintenance Organization
  Act, 186
Health manpower, 103t
Health Objectives Planning Act, 187
Health plan, 205
Health policy, definition of, 219
Health practice, culturally based, 278
Health promotion
  cultural factors and, 270-271
  for elderly, 479-481

Health promotion—cont'd
  environmental health and, 304
  for men, 394-396
  in occupational health, 750
  prevention and, 8-9, 78
  for school staff, 719, 721
  for women, 358-359, 370-372
Health promotion model, health
    education and, 137-139, 138t
Health statistics, community assess-
    ment and, 103t
Health status
  of elderly, 464
  of homeless, 531-536
  of migrant workers, 559
Health tree, family, 425, *428f,* 429
Healthy People 2000
  legislation for, 187
  policy influenced by, 220
  purpose of, 11
Healthy People 2010
  for child or adolescent, 334-335,
    336t
  communicable disease and, 661
  cultural perspectives and, 244,
    245t-246t, 247
  disability and, 506-507, 506t
  for elderly, 458, 458t
  family planning and, 365t
  focus and goals of, 11-12
  healthy indicators in, 833
  legislation for, 187
  mental health and, 588-590
  occupational health and, 738,
    739t
  public policy and, 221t
  rural communities and, 556, *557f*
  school health and, 705t
  surveillance and, 82
  violence and, 609
  women and, 350t
Hearing loss in elderly, 474
Hearing test in school, 710-711
Heart disease
  arteriosclerotic, in women, 360
  decline in deaths from, 831
  epidemiology of, 69, *70f,* 71
  myocardial infarction, cause of, *70f*
  in women, 353-354
Heat-related illness in elderly, 478
Henry Street House, 39, 110-111
Hepatitis
  in correctional facilities, 766
  vaccine for, 674-676
Herbicide exposure, 558, 559

Herd immunity, 664
Herpes infection, 132, 134, 691-692
Hierarchy of systems, 421
High-technological home health
  care, 787
Hill-Burton Act, 122, 186, 219-220
Hispanic
  Healthy People 2000 goals
    and, 247
  in rural community, 555-556
Historiography, 36
HIV infection, 688-690
  in correctional facilities, 765-766
  global patterns of, 813-814
Holistic perspective, 265
Home health care, 784-806
  conducting home visit, 793-796
  documentation of, 790
  for elderly, 466, 468, 468t
  formal and informal, 790-791
  history of, 40
  hospice, 791-792, *792f*
  legal and ethical issues of,
    792-793
  nursing process and, 796-806
    case studies of, 798-806
  nursing standards for, 788-790
  purpose of, 785-786
  reimbursement for, 787-788
  in rural community, 564
  special, 787
  types of, 786-787
Home life of women, 357
Home visit
  for communicable disease
    follow-up, 798-800
  conducting of, 793-796, *794f*
  in family nursing, 440
  hospice, 805-806
  of injured client, 803-804
  to pregnant adolescent, 416
  prenatal, 800-803
Homeless, 526-543
  access to health care by, 536-538
  case study of, 540-542
  conceptual approach to, 538-539
  definition of, 527
  demographics of, 527-530, *528f*
  factors contributing to, 530-531
  health status of, 531-536
  research on, 539-540
Homicide, 598-599
Homosexual family, 413
Hookworm, Rockefeller commission
  to eradicate, 35

Hospice care
    at home, 791, 805-806
    in rural community, 564
Hospital-based case management,
    175-176
Hospital-based home health
    agencies, 787
Hospital in rural community, 560-562,
    561f
Hospitalization
    of elderly, 466, *467f*
    of men, 386-387
    of women, 354
Host factors in disease, 68t
House of Henry Street, 39, 110-111
Housing, 290t, 294-295
Human-environment interaction, *69f*
Human Genome Project, 590
Human immunodeficiency virus
    infection, 688-690
    in adolescents, 708-709
    in correctional facilities, 765-766
    drug abuse in pregnancy and,
        326-327
    empowerment approach for, 140
    global patterns of, 813-814
    systems interrelationships and, 95
    in women, 366-367
Human nature orientation, 251
Human papilloma virus, 692
Humanistic learning theory, 133t
Hunting and gathering stage,
    24-25, *24f*
Hygeia, 42
Hygienist, industrial, 755
Hypersensitivity to vaccine,
    670-671
Hypertension
    screening children for, 711
    in women, 360
Hypothermia, in elderly, 478-479

I

Identification, case, 174-175
Illness
    of agricultural worker, 557-558
    indicators of, 6-7
    school health and, 711-712
Illness orientation in men, 389
Imaging, brain, 587-588
Immigrant
    Australia's view of, 43
    environmental health and, 303
Immunity, types of, 664;
    see also Vaccination

Immunization
    analysis of policy on, 226
    for child, 328
    discovery of, 28
    for elderly, 479-480
    health belief model and, 55
    regulations about, 224
    school health and, 710
Immunosuppression, immunization
    and, 672
Impairment, definition of, 497, 498t
Implementation in nursing process;
    see also Intervention in
    nursing process
    international health and, 823
    school health and, 725-726
Incarceration; *see* Correctional
    institution
Incidence rate, 71-72
Incidence study, 87-88
Income of elderly, 464-465
Incontinence in elderly, 477-478
Indemnity plan, 205
indemnity plan, 210
Independent practice model, 210
Index, family risk, 721
Indian Health Service, 279-280
Indianapolis model of case
    management, 176
Indirect standardization of mortality
    rate, 73, 75, 75t
Indirect transmission of infection, 663
Individual
    environmental health and, 310-311
    family *vs.,* 411
    as locus of change
        in health belief model, 53-58
        in self-care deficit theory, 52-53
Individuals with Disabilities
    Education Act, 513
Industrial cities stage, 25
Industrial hygienist, 755
Industry
    community assessment and, 101t
    project involving
        successful, 118
        unsuccessful, 120
Infant
    low birth weight, 325
    mortality rate of, 323-324, 324t
Infant health, 831
Infant mortality, 323-324, 324t
Infection, 659-699; *see also*
        Communicable disease
Infertility, 365

Inflammatory disease, pelvic, 359-360
Influence in family, 422
Influenza
    immunization against, 480
    risk for complications of, 673
Influenza vaccine, 676-677
Informal care system in rural
    community, 564
Information
    electoral, 235t
    health, cultural factors and,
        269-270
    legislative, 235t
Information technology, 199-200
Inhalant abuse, 629t
Initiation stage of addiction, 632
Initiative on minority health, 279-280
Injury
    intentional; *see* Abuse; Violence
    school health and, 707
    toy-related, 327
    vaccine-related, 671
    to women, 367
    work-related, 742
Inoculation, discovery of, 28
Inpatient treatment for substance
    abuse, 635-636
Input in systems theory, 421
Inspection, workplace, 752
Institution, correctional, 761-770;
    see also Correctional
    institution
Institutional context of family
    therapist, 435-436
Institutional policy, 219
Institutionalization of elderly, 481-482
Instrumental functioning, 422
Insurance, 210-212
    for child or adolescent, 334
    for disabled person, 505-506, 506t
    Medigap, 205
    restructuring of health care system
        and, 230
    social class and, 436-438, *437f*
Integrator of health and healing,
    777-778
Intentional injury; *see* Abuse;
        Violence
Internal structure of family, 420
International Classification of Impair-
    ments, Disabilities, and
    Handicaps, 497-499
International Council of Nurses, 366
International health, 811-825;
    see also Global community

International organization, 814
Internet, 199-200
Interpreter, 262
Interrelationships of systems, 95
Interstate nursing practice, 234
Intersystem model of disability,
    516-518, *519f, 520t*
Intervention
    in community assessment, 106
    in health planning model,
        116-117
    in nursing plan for women's
        health, 376
    in nursing process
        communicable disease and,
            697-698
        for elderly, 490-491
        environmental health and,
            310-311
        family nursing and, 449
        home care and, 797, 800,
            802-806
        homeless and, 540
        men's health and, 403-404
        rural health and, 575-576
    in substance abuse intervention,
        651-652
Interview
    in community assessment, 100
    family, 414-416
Intimacy, cultural factors and, 260
Intimate partner violence, 601-606
Intravenous therapy, at home, 787

J
Jail; *see* Correctional institution
Japanese encephalitis, 683
Job transfer evaluation, 742
Judicial branch of govern-
    ment, 224
Judicial law, 223
Justice
    market, 538
    social, 538

K
Koch, Robert, 34-35

L
Labor, prison, 762-763
Labor market, homelessness
    and, 530
Language
    about disabled, 510, 511t, 512
    culture and, 261-262, 263t

Law
    Elizabethan poor, 28
    legislative process for, 227,
        228f, 229
    public health, definition of, 219
    types of, 223, 223t
Layout of health education materials,
    159-161
Lead poisoning, 328
Learner, adult, characteristics of, 134,
    135t, 136
Learner verification, 161-162
Learning, format for, 147t
Learning theory, 132, 133t-134t,
    134-135
Legal issues
    abuse and, 616t
    in child and adolescent health, 340
    in correctional institution,
        768-769
    in home health care, 792-793
    in occupational health, 731,
        750, 754
    of substance abuse, 633-634
    vaccine documentation as, 671
Legislation
    affecting health care system,
        184-188
        federal, 184-187, 184t, 185t
        managed care and, 188
        state, 187-188
    affecting women, 368-370
    disability and, 512-514
    elderly affected by, 484-486
    on environmental health, 300-302
    on health planning, 121-125
    history of, 219-220
    mental health legislation and,
        591-592
    on occupational health, 751-754,
        752t
    on rural health, 566-569
    sources of information about,
        235t
Legislative branch of government, 224
Legislative process, 227, *228f, 229*
Legislator, nurse as, 238
Leininger's theory of culture care
        diversity, 248
    Vietnamese client and, 282-283
Lesbian parent, 358
Licensed practical nurse, 195
Licensed vocational nurse, 195
Life cycle, family, dislocations of,
    425t

Life expectancy
    of elderly, 461, *462f,* 462t
    of men, 383, 384t
    of women, 351
Lifeline, telephone, 473
Lifestyle
    change of, for men, 398-399
    cost of health care and, 208
Limited service hospital, 561-562
Lister, Joseph, 34
Literacy, 155-156, *157f,* 158
    in elderly, 465
Literature review in health
        planning, 116
Living arrangements of elderly, 465
Living pattern, 289-290, 290t
Living will, 793
Lobbyist, nurse as, 234, 236-237
Local health department subsystem,
    192-193
Location of community, 94
    in community assessment, 101t
    health impact of, 829-830
Locus of change
    individual as
        in health belief model, 53-58
        in self-care deficit theory, 52-53
    society as, 56-58
Longevity
    increase in, 460-461
    in men, 383, 384t
Longitudinal study, 87-88
Loss of major life roles theory
        of aging, 460
Low-birth-weight infant, 325
Lung cancer
    smoking and, 832-833
    in women, 362
Lyme disease vaccine, 677-678

M
Macroscopic perspective, 51-52, 51t
Magicoreligious perspective, 265
Male, 382-406; *see also* Men
Malnutrition in elderly, 469, 471t
Mammography, 361
Managed care
    accountability of, 231-232
    accreditation and, 199
    community health nursing and,
        18-19
    cost containment and, 214
    definition of, 205
    legislation influencing, 188
    prevention *vs.* cure and, 10

Managed care—cont'd
    in rural community, 563-564
    social classification of and, 438
Management, case, 170-179;
        see also Case management
Manager, occupational, 756
Mandate, 206
    of powers, *227f*
Manic-depressive disorder, 588
Manners, 414
Manufacturing plant, project
        involving, 120
Marginalization, 591
Marital relationship of women,
        357-358
Marital status of elderly, 465
Market justice, 538
    social justice *vs.*, 8-9
Marketing to men, 393
Materials for education program, 147,
        148t-150t, 150
Maternal and child health, 831
Maternal and Child Health Block
        Grant, 337
Maternal mortality rate, 352-353
McCarren-Ferguson Act, 186
Media
    disabled portrayed in, 510t
    for education program, 147,
        148t-150t, 150
Medial model of disability, 514-516
Medicaid
    for child or adolescent, 337
    cost of health care and, 209
    elderly and, 484-485
    home health care and, 787
    provisions of, 185
    rural communities and, 567
    screening of children and, 711
    women and, 370
Medical care, history of, 34-36
Medical consultant, occupa-
        tional, 757
Medical home for child or adolescent,
        333
Medical model of substance abuse,
        631, 643
Medical science, 731
Medicalization of mental illness, 587
Medicare
    cost of health care and, 209
    definition of, 205
    elderly and, 484-485
    home health care and, 787-788
    prescription drug coverage and, 230

Medicare—cont'd
    provisions of, 185
    rural communities and, 567
Medication; *see* Drug *entries*
Medigap insurance, 205
Men, 382-406
    case study of, 401-405
    factors impeding health of, 394-396
    health care use by, 386-387
    health needs of, 396-397
    homeless, 531-532
    longevity in, 382
    morbidity in, 384-386, 386t
    mortality rate for, 382, 383t, 384
    preventive measures for, 397-401
    theories explaining health of,
        387-393
Meningococcal disease, 683-684
Mental disorder
    disability caused by, 502
    in elderly, 475-477
Mental health, 585-594, 586
    case management in, 172
    case study of, 593-594
    of child and adolescent, 717-719
    community health nurse and,
        592-593
    in correctional institution, 767-768
    factors influencing, 590-592
    funding for, 592t
    Healthy People 2010 and, 588-590
    homelessness and, 530-531, 532,
        535-536
    medicalization of mental illness
        and, 587
    overview of, 586-588
    prevalence of, 588
    in rural community, 553, 565-566
    of women, 355-356, 363-364
Mental Health Equitable Treatment
        Act, 591
Mental health services, 193
Mentally retarded adult, project
        involving, 119
Methadone, 638-639
Metropolitan, definition of, 549
Mexican-American, *Healthy People
        2000* goals and, 247
MHC program, 568
Microscopic perspective, 51-52, 51t
Middle Ages, 27
Mifepristone, 352
Migrant health centers program, 337
Migrant worker, 558-560, 568;
        see also Rural community

Milio's framework for prevention,
        56-58
Minority community; *see also*
        Cultural factors
    in correctional facilities, 764
    occupation health and, 741
    substance abuse in, 646-647
    prevention of, 635
Mission orientation, 393
MMR vaccine, 673
MMWR, 664
Model
    of care for communities
        of families, 438-440
    case management, 175-176
    of disability, 514-516
    health education, 135-142
        of empowerment, 139-142
        of individual behavior, 137t,
            138t, 1370139
    health planning, 113-117, *113f*
    for home care nursing, 788-790,
        789f
    independent practice, 210
    of international health care,
        819-824
    intersystem, of disability, 516-518,
        519f, 520t
    medical, of substance abuse, 643
    of social class, 436-438
    social justice, 538-539
    of spiritual care, 779
    of substance abuse, 631
    transactional, 436
Modernization theory of aging, 460
Modesty, cultural factors in, 261
Morbidity
    of elderly, 463
    in men, 385, 386t
    in women, 354-356, 386t
Morphine, hospice care and, 792
Mortality rate; *see also* Death
    of elderly, 461, 463
    infant, 323-324, 324t
    for men, 383, 384t, 385, 395-396
    in rural communities, 552-553
    for women, 351-354, 351t, 352t
Mortality ratio, proportionate, 75-76
Motor vehicle safety, 830
Multidisciplinary team in occupational
        health, 754
Multiple risk Factor Intervention
        Trial, 89
Mumps vaccine, 679
Mutual help group, 639-640

Myocardial infarction, cause of, *70f*
Myth
  about mental illness, 591
  of substance abuse, 636

N
Naltrexone, 638
Narcotic abuse, 629t, 638
National Agenda for the Prevention
  of Disabilities, 498-499
National alliance for the Mentally
  Ill, 589
National Association for Home
  Care, 788
National Cancer Institute, 144-147,
  147t-150t, 150-153
National Center for Health Statistics
  data published by, 99
  morbidity and mortality data of, 6
National Council of State Boards of
  Nursing, 234
National Council on alcoholism,
  634-635
National health insurance, 212
National Health Interview Survey,
  501, 502-503
National Health Planning and
  Resources Act, 186
National Health Planning and
  Resources Development Act,
  123-124
National Health Service Corps,
  338, 568
National Institutes of Aging,
  486, 487
National Institutes of Mental
  Health, 591
National Vaccine Injury Compensa-
  tion Program, 671-672
National Violence Against Women
  Survey, 599
Native American
  Healthy People 2000 goals
    and, 247
  in rural community, 555
Natural immunity, 664
Naturalistic perspective, 265
NBD, 590-591
Need, certificate of, 123
Needs assessment, 100
Neglect
  of child, 328-329, 606
  indicators of, 608t
Negotiation, cultural, 267-268
Neisseria gonorrhoeae, 691

Neonatal assessment, 415
Network in rural community,
  560-561
Network therapy, 436
Neuroimaging in mental illness,
  587-588
Neurological brain disorder, 590-591
Neurotransmitter in mental
  illness, 590
New England model of case manage-
  ment, 175
Nightingale, Florence, 30-34, *31f,*
  32f, 33t
  political role of, 220
Nineteenth century medicine, 28-29
Noncertified home health
  agencies, 787
NonEnglish-speaking client, 262
Nonfederal sector; *see* Private sector
Nonprofit home health agency, 786
Nontraditional health care
  provider, 196
Nonverbal communication
  cultural factors in, 261
  in family, 422
Norm, 250
Notifiable communicable disease, 664
Nuclear waste, 298
Nurse
  block, 438-439
  cultural self-assessment of, 277
  education and, 142-144
    parish nurse, 778
  effective use of, 232
  as enabler, 643
  parish, 564-565
  political role of
    in campaigning, 239
    as change agents, 220,
      222, 234
    coalitions and, 237-238
    as lobbyist, 234, 236-237
    policy development and,
      238-239
    political action committees
      and, 237
    in public office, 238
    voting strength and, 239-240
Nurse-client relationship, cultural
  factors and, 260
Nurse midwife, 195
Nurse practitioner, 195
Nursing
  community health; *see* Community
    health nursing

Nursing—cont'd
  evolution of, 29-34
  family, 411-412; *see also* Family
  occupational health, 730-759;
    see also Occupational health
    nursing
  parish, 772-782; *see also*
    Parish nursing
  population-focused, 17t
  rural
    characteristics of, 570
    knowledge base for, 570-572
    roles in, 569-570
  school, 702-727; *see also*
    School health
  staffing related to outcome in, 232
  substance abuse and, 648-650
  transcultural, 248-250, *249f*
  Vietnamese client and, 282
Nursing home, 481-482
Nursing policy, definition of, 219
Nursing practice; *see* Practice, nursing
Nursing process
  communicable disease and,
    695-698
  in community assessment, 100, 105
  in environmental health, 309-312
  in family nursing, 440-451, *442f,*
    443f
  in home care, 796-798
    case studies and, 798-806
  homeless and, 540-542
  in international health, 819-824
  in men's health, 401-405
  mental health and, 593-594
  in occupational health, 755-758
  rural health and, 574-575
  in substance abuse intervention,
    650-653
  in women's health, 375-377
Nursing standard; *see* Standard,
  nursing
*Nursing's Agenda for Health Care
  Reform,* 230
Nutrition
  academic performance and, 717
  culture and, 256-257, 257t, 275-276
  of elderly, 469, 470t, 471t
  food safety and, 831-832
  reproductive health of women
    and, 365
  school health and, 715-717
Nutritional Education and Training
  Program, 717
Nutritive disease agent, 67t

O

Obesity
   in child, project for, 117-118, 117t
   school health and, 716-717
Observational study, 84-85
Occupation, in rural community, 554
Occupational health, 730-759
   case study of, 755-758
   demographics of, 732-733
   evolution of, 731-732
   legal issues in, 754
   legislation impacting, 751-754, 752t
   levels of prevention in, 121t
   multidisciplinary teamwork
      and, 754
   prevention strategies in, 738,
      740-747
   professionalism and, 733-738, 734t
   skills needed for, 747, 749-751
Occupational health history, *744f-745f*
Occupational health nurse
   family nursing and, 416
   responsibilities of, 755, 756, 757
Occupational health sciences, 731
Occupational medical consultant, 757
Occupational Safety and Health Act,
      186, 751-753
   affecting women, 369-370
Occupational Safety and Health
      Administration, 751-753
   benzene standard of, *746f*
Occupational therapist, 196
Office of Minority Health, 272
Office of Research on Women's
      Health, 374
Official home health agency, 786
Older Americans Act, 485
Omnibus Budget Reconciliation
      Acts, 186
Omnibus Mental Illness Recovery
      Act, 589
Open system, 421
Opiate abuse, 629t, 638
ORA, 589
Oral health
   of elderly, 473-474
   school health and, 709
Orem's self-care deficit theory,
      52-53
Organization
   community, 141t
   environmental, 303
   provider, 193-196
   voluntary, 190
Organizational policy, 219

Orientation
   activity, 252
   dominant value, 250
   human nature, 251
   illness, in men, 389
   mission, 393
   person-nature, 251
   social, 252
   time, 251-252
Osteoporosis, in women, 361
Out-of-pocket expense, 205
Outcome measure, 199
Outpatient treatment for substance
      abuse, 635-637
Output in systems theory, 421
Ovarian cancer, 363
Overdose, accidental, by elderly, 481
Overflow incontinence, 478
Overtraining, 391

P

PACT, 589
Pain
   cultural expression of, 266-267
   hospice care and, 791-792, *792f*
Panacea, 42
Papanicolaou smear, 363
Papilloma virus, human, 692
Paradigm, disability, 515t
Paradox, epidemiological, 271
Paramedical technologist, 196
Parent; *see also* Family
   child's health and, 339
   education of, 333
   lesbian, 358
   single, 333
Parish nursing, 772-782
   education for, 778
   foundations of, 773-775
   health assessment in, *776f-777f*
   issues in, 780-782
   roles in, 775-778
   in rural community, 564-565
   spirituality and, 778-780
Participatory action research, 308
Passive immunity, 664
Pasteur, Louis, 34, 35
Peer review organization, health
      policy and, 224
Peer standard review organization, 213
Pelvic inflammatory disease,
      359-360
Periodic assessment, occupational, 742
Person-nature orientation, 251
Person-place-time model, 66, 84

Personal assistance for disabled
      person, 505
Personal health care services, 7
Personal health counselor, 775
Personal health services, 193
Pertussis vaccine, 679
Pesticide exposure
   of agricultural worker, 558
   of migrant workers, 559
Pharmacist, 196
Philanthropic organization, 190
Photovoice, 140
Physical abuse; *see* Abuse
Physical demands analysis, *748f*
Physical education, 709
Physical fitness, men's interest
      in, 398
Physical therapist, 196
Physician, 195
   as enabler, 643
   nineteenth century, 35
   occupational health, 755
Physician assistant, 195-196
Pica, 267
Plague, 684
Planning
   community assessment and,
      102t, 106
   of education message, *154f*
   health, 109-127
      case study of, 125-126
      federal legislation on, 121-125
      model of, 113-117, 113t
      overview of, 110-112, 111t, *112f*
      project objectives in, 114
      successful projects of, 117-118,
         117t
      unsuccessful projects of,
         118-121, 119t, 120t, 121t
   in nursing process
      communicable disease and,
         696-697
      for elderly, 488, 489-490
      environmental health and,
         309-310
      family nursing and, 448-449
      home care and, 799, 802
      homeless and, 540
      international health and, 822-823
      men's health and, 402-403
      rural health and, 575
      school health and, 725
      in substance abuse interven-
         tion, 651
      women's health and, 375-376

Pneumococcal disease, immunization
against, 480
Pneumococcal vaccine, 679-680
Pneumonia, immunization
against, 480
Point of service, 205
Poisoning
accidental, by elderly, 481
lead, 328
pesticide, 558
Policy, 219-240
affecting elderly, 484-486
analysis of, 225-226
current, 229-233
definition of, 219
disability and, 512-514
epidemiology and, 83-84
formulation of
in ideal circumstances, 224
in real world, 224-225
steps in, 225-226, *225f*
government authority and, 226-227
Healthy People 2010 and, 221t
historical foundations of, 219-220
immigration, in Australia, 43
institutional, 219
Internet and, 240
legislative process and, 227,
228f, 229
on men's health, 398
nurses influencing, 220, 222
nurses' roles in, 233-240
campaigning and, 239
as change agents, 234
coalitions and, 237-238
as lobbyists, 234, 236-237
policy development and, 238-239
political action committees
and, 237
in public office, 238
voting strength and, 239-240
organizational, 219
overview of, 224
private sector and, 229
on rural health, 568-569
structure of government and,
222-224
types of law and, 223t
Poliomyelitis vaccine, 680
Political action committee, 237
Political organization, 102t
Political process, 219-240
Politics
cultural diversity and, 277
definition of, 219

Politics—cont'd
health impact of, 829
mental health legislation and,
591-592
nurses' roles in, 233-240
campaigning and, 239
as change agents, 234
coalitions and, 237-238
as lobbyists, 234, 236-237
policy development and, 238-239
political action committees
and, 237
in public office, 238
voting strength and, 239-240
substance abuse and, 631-632
Vietnamese client and, 281
Poor law, 28
Population
changes in, 243-244, 244t
child, 322, *322f*
community assessment and, 101t
of global community, 812
health-related variables in, 828
homeless, 526-543;
see also Homeless
rural, 548-577; *see also*
Rural community
Population-focused nursing
data required for, 19t
definition of, 17-18
Portability, 205
Poverty
access to health care and, 537
of child and adolescent, 332-333
communicable disease and, 661
culture of poverty view and,
437-438
in elderly, 464-465, *464f*
Health and Human Services
guidelines on, 185t
health promotion and, 270-271
homelessness and, 530
minorities living in, 255t
in rural community, 551
social class and, 437-438
of women, 357
Poverty rate, 254
Power and control wheel, 604, *605f*
Power of attorney, durable, 793
Practical nurse, licensed, 195
Practice
community organization, 141t
folk, 36-37
nursing
community *vs.* public health, 13

Practice—cont'd
nursing—cont'd
conservative scope of, 52
in correctional institution,
769-770
disability and, 515-516
environmental health and,
304-308
interstate, 234
in occupational health, 733-738,
734t, 747, 749-751
school health and, 725-726,
726t-727t
Prayer, 779-780, 781
Precautions
standard/blood and body fluid, 664
for vaccines, 667, 669
Preferred provider organization, 205
Pregnancy, 323-327
abuse during, 603
in adolescent, 329-331
case study of, 342-345
health planning for, 110
home visits to, 416
homeless, 534
study of, 107
alcohol use during, 633
cultural factors and, 269
diabetes and, 360-361
ectopic, 353
human immunodeficiency virus
infection and, 366-367
immunization and, 672-673
infant mortality and, 323-324
Medicaid and, 370
mortality rate and, 352-353
prenatal care and, 325-326
smoking in, 162-164
substance abuse during, 646
substance abuse in, 326-327
Preindustrial cities stage, 25
Premium, insurance, 211
Prenatal care, 325-326
Prenatal clinic, project involving, 119
Preplacement health evaluation,
743f
President's advisory committee on
health care, 197-198
President's Commission on
White House Fellowships, 239
Prevalence rate, 72
Prevalence study, 85
Prevention, 8-12
accident, 473
of adolescent pregnancy, 331

Prevention—cont'd
  of communicable disease, 693-695
  cure *vs.,* 10
  for elderly, 479, 491-492
  environmental health and, 312
  epidemiology in, 78-83
  in family nursing, 450-451
  homeless and, 541
  levels of, 8-9, *8f, 9f*
    in health planning projects, 120t
  for men, 387, 397-401, 404-405
  migrant workers and, 559
  in occupational health nursing,
    738-747
  in rural community, 554-555
  school health and, 726, 726t-727t
  of substance abuse, 635, 652-653
    by adolescent, 644
  of violence, 609, 611-620, 612t,
    614t, 615t-617t, *618f*
  for women, 372-373
Prevention orientation, in men, 389
Primary care provider, 205, 214
  occupational health and, 749, 756
  in rural community, 563
Primary prevention, 8, *8f, 9f*
  for child, 345
  of communicable disease,
    693-694
  for elderly, 491-492
  epidemiology and, 78
  homeless and, 541
  for men, 404-405
  in occupation health, 738, 740-741,
    740t
  of substance abuse, 652
  of violence, 609, 611-613, 612t
Primary vaccine failure, 664
Prison; *see* Correctional institution
Private financing, 209-210
Private health care subsystem,
  188-189
Private health policy, 229
Private pay case management, 176
Private sector
  cultural diversity and, 272
  health policy and, 229
Privatization of prison, 762-763
Problem-solving, in family, 422
Problem-solving education, 139
Process, nursing; *see* Nursing process
Profession, school health and, 723
Professional
  health care, 194-195
    from minority group, 271-272

Professional—cont'd
  in rural community, 568
  substance abuse by, 648
Professional enabler, 643
Professional organization, lobbying
  by, 236-237
Professionalism in occupational
  health, 733-738, 734t
Proficiency of nurse, 749
Program of Assertive Community
  Treatment, 589-590
Proportionate mortality ratio, 75-76
Proprietary home health agency, 786
Prospective study, 87-88
Prostate cancer, 390
Prostitution by homeless adoles-
  cents, 534
Provider, health care
  definition of, 205
  types of, 193-196
Psychiatric disorder
  in elderly, 476-477
  school health and, 717-719
  substance abuse with, 637
Psychiatrist as enabler, 643
Psychoactive substance abuse, 630
Psychoactive substance
  dependence, 631
Psychosocial hazard, 738
Public accountability, 231-232
Public financing, 209
Public health
  case management and, 172
  community health nursing and, 4
  core function of, 15t
  double standard in, 418-419
  essential services of, 7-8, 16t
  evolution of, 26-29
  focus of, 7-8
  future of, 833-834
  government's authority in protect-
    ing, 226-227
  as health care subsystem, 190
  mission of, 4
  past improvements in, 829-833
  violence from perspective
    of, 609
Public Health Act, 185
Public health care subsystem, 189
Public health department in rural
  community, 565
Public health law, 219
Public health nursing
  competencies of, 15t
  focus of, 12, 13, 15

Public health nursing—cont'd
  history of, 37
  standards of care for, 14t
Public Health Service Act, 368-369
Public Health Services amendment,
  122-123
Public Law 99-142, 714
Public policy, 219-240;
  see also Policy
Public services, community assess-
  ment and, 102t
Punishment, corporal, 598
Purchasing cooperative,
  insurance, 210
Pure Food and Drugs Act, 184

Q

Qualified Medicare Beneficiary
  program, 485
Quality, cost containment and, 230
Quality of life with disability,
  499-500
Question
  on environmental health, 305
  therapeutic, in family
    interview, 415

R

Rabies, 684-685
Race
  disability and, 503, 504t
  health impact of, 829
  in rural community, 555-556
  substance abuse and, 646-647
Radiation risk, 290t, 297-298
Rape, date, 603
Rate, epidemiological, 71-76,
  73t-77t
Ratio
  male-female morbidity, 386t
  proportionate mortality, 75-76
Rationing, health care, 214
Readability formula, *161f*
Reading, literacy and health, 155-156,
  157f, 158
Reasonable accommodation
  for disabled, 513-514
Recommended Dietary Allowance,
  for elderly, 469
Reconstruction theory of aging, 460
Record, school health, 714
Recreation in community assessment,
  102t
Redesigning, 194
Reengineering, 193-194

Referral
case management and, 175
in community assessment, 100, 105
for home visit, 793, *794f*
Referral source, parish nurse as,
775-776
Reform
health care, 200-201
mental health, 586-587
Refrigeration of vaccine, 669
Refugee, 303
Regional medical program, federally
mandated, 122
Registered dietitian, 196
Registered nurse, 195
Regulation, environmental, 301-302
Rehabilitation, for men, 398-399
Reimbursement
capitated, 214
for home health care, 787-788
mechanisms of, 211
Religion
community assessment and, 102t
culture and, 257-259
culturological assessment
and, 276
diet and, 257, 257t
elderly and, 465
of Vietnamese client, 281
Remarriage
developmental issues in, 426t
family development and, 423
Renaissance, 28
Reportable communicable
disease, 664
Reporting system, adverse
event, 671
Reproductive health
of men, 389-391
of women, 364-367
Reregulating, 194
Research
on aging, 486, 487
in case management, 177
historical, 36
on homeless, 539-540
children and, 533
in international health, 819
on men's health, 391-392
reproductive, 389
on minority health issues,
272-274
in occupational health, 737,
750-751
participatory action, 308

Research—cont'd
on rural health, 568-569,
572-573
school nurse and, 724
on violence, 597
on women, 374
Research on Aging Act, 485
Researcher, case manager as, 174
Resource
on breast cancer, 362
distribution of, 254-255
family nursing and, 418
health education, 153-156, *154f,*
157t, 158-162, *159f-161f*
for minority health, 278-280
in occupational health, 757
Respiratory disorder in agricultural
worker, 558
Respiratory therapist, 196
Retirement Equity Act, 485
Retirement Income Security Act, 485
Retrospective study, 85-87, *86f*
Rights
client, 200
consumer, managed care and, 188
of disabled person, 513-514
Rightsizing, 194
Risk, definition of, 76
Risk assessment, 206
Risk behavior, 719, 720
Risk factor
for disability, 498
epidemiology and, 76, 78
nature of community and, 93-94
for youth-related violence, 601t
Risk index, family, 721
Robert Wood Johnson Health Policy
Fellowship, 238
Rockefeller Commission for the
Eradication of Hookworm, 35
Rohypnol, 603
Role
case manager, 174
in family, 420, 422
health education, 131, 142-144
of parish nurse, 775-778
Rome, health and disease in, 26-27
RU-486, 352
Rubella vaccine, 680-681
Rubeola vaccine, 678-679
Ruler, pain assessment, *792f*
Runaway, 534
Rural community, 548-577
agricultural workers in, 556-558
case study of, 574-577

Rural community—cont'd
community-based care in, 564-566
community health nursing in,
569-572
definitions in, 549-550
delivery system in, 560-564
health status indicators in,
550-556
Healthy People 2010 and, *557f*
legislation and programs affecting,
566-569
migrant and seasonal workers in,
558-560
research on, 572-573
residence categories in, 550
theories about, 560-561
Rush, Benjamin, 587

S
Safe rides program, 120
Safety
in abusive situation, 615t-617t
in correctional environment, 763
cost containment and, 230
in home, 795
motor vehicle, 830
occupational health and, 731, 750
sports, 707
of vaccine, 671-672
workplace, 830-831
violence and, 620-621
Sanction, cultural, 274-275
Sanger, Margaret, 222
Sanitation, early, 28-29
Schizophrenia, 588
School-based health services, 338
School health, 702-727
case study of, 725-726, 726t-727t
components of, *706f*
counseling and psychological
services and, 717-719
family and community involvement
in, 721-722
health center and, 722
health education and, 706-709
health promotion and, 719, 721
health services in, 709-716
healthy environment and, 719
history of, 703-705, 705t
as nursing practice, 722, 723t, 724t
nutrition and, 716-717
risk behavior and, 720
School nursing
family nursing and, 416
history of, 40

Scientific theory, 36
Scoliosis, screening children
        for, 711
Scope of practice, conservative, 52
Screening
    breast cancer, 146
    epidemiology and, 80-81
    of men, 398
    school health and, 710-711
Seasonal worker, 558-560
Secondary prevention, 8, *8f, 9f*
    for child, 345
    of communicable disease, 694
    for elderly, 492
    epidemiology and, 78
    for family, 451
    homeless and, 541
    for men, 405
    in occupational health, 742,
        743f-746f, 746-747
    of substance abuse, 652
    of violence, 612t, 613-614,
        614t-617t, 619
    for women, 372
Secondary vaccine failure, 664
Secular trend, 82
Self-assessment
    cultural, 277
    on response to disability, 497
Self-examination, breast, 361
Self-insurance, 216
Senior health, 457-493;
        see also Elderly
Services, case manager, 174
Settled village stage, 25
Sex education, 708
Sex-linked behavior, 392
Sex-role behavior in men, 388-389
Sex-role rehabilitation for men,
        398-399
Sexual abuse
    of child, 607
    in correctional institution,
        766-767
    dating violence and, 602-603
    indicators of, 608t
Sexually transmitted disease
    Chlamydia trachomatis, 690-691
    drug abuse in pregnancy and,
        326-327
    herpes simplex virus 2, 691-692
    HIV and AIDS, 688-690, 690t
    homelessness and, 532
        adolescent, 534
    human papilloma virus, 692

Sexually transmitted disease—cont'd
    in men, 390
    substance abuse and, 647-648
    syphilis, 692-693
    in women, 366
Shaken baby syndrome, 606
Shattick, Lemuel, 29
Shelter
    abuse women's, 371-372
    homeless, 535
Sheppard-Towner Act, 566-567
Shortage of health care workers in
        rural community, 562-563
Sick role, 261
Signs of stress, 718
Silence, cultural factors and, 261
Single-parent family, 333
    adoption and, 358
    increase in numbers of, 413
Smallpox, 28
Smear, Papanicolaou, 363
SMOG readability formula, *161f*
Smoking
    by adolescent, 331
    as causality, 79-80
    decrease in, 832-833
    in pregnancy, 162-164, 326
    school health and, 707-708
Social class, model of, 436-438
Social constraints in family assess-
        ment, 434
Social factors
    health impact of, 829
    in mental illness, 590-591
Social health, 5
Social integration in family, 429
Social justice, 538
    market justice *vs.,* 8
    uninsured patients and, 215
Social learning theory, 134t
Social orientation, 252
Social problems, 103t
Social Security Act
    affecting women, 369
    effect of, on health care, 185
    elderly and, 484-485
    rural communities and, 567
Social services in school, 717-719
Social support, homelessness and, 532
Social system, 94-95
Social theory, critical, 58-60
Social worker, 196
Socialization, 388-389
Socially disruptive events theory
        of aging, 460

Societal beliefs, cost of health care
        and, 208
Society
    attitude toward disabled, 507, 509
    as locus of change, 56-58
Sociocultural aspects of substance
        abuse, 631-632
Socioeconomic status
    correctional facilities and, 764
    culture and, 254-256
    culturological assessment and, 276
    health impact of, 828
    health promotion and, 270-271
Socioenvironmental theory of aging,
        459-460
Sociopolitical perspective for
        disability, 515
Sojourner Truth, 220
Solution, community of, 94
Space, functional use of, 260, 260t
Specialist in community health
        nursing, 15
Speech-language pathologist, 196
Spirituality
    culture and, 258-259
    parish nursing and, 778-780
Sports safety, 707
Spouse abuse, 367, 601-606;
        see also Domestic violence
Staffing, outcome related to, 232
Standard, nursing
    correctional nursing, 769-770
    home health care, 788-790
    for home health care, 788-790
    occupational and environmental
        health nursing, 734t
    parish, 780
    in parish nursing, 780
    public health nursing practice, 14t
    rural health and, 569-570
    school nursing practice,
        723t-724t
    state *vs.* federal, 226
Standard precautions, 664
Standardized mortality rate, 73, 74t,
        75, 75t
Staphylococcus aureus infection, 360
State government
    federal government and, 222
    state *vs.* federal standards and, 226
State legislation
    on health care, 187-188
    on health planning, 124-125
    Workers' Compensation, 753
State level health care subsystem, 192

Status
  health
    of elderly, 464
    of homeless, 531-536
    men's, 387-388
    of migrant workers, 559
    parent's educational, 333
    socioeconomic; *see* Socioeconomic
      status
Statutory law, 223
Stereotype, of disabled, 509-510
Sterilization, female, 366
Stewart, Ada Mayo, 732
Stigma, of homelessness, 532
Stimulant abuse, 629t
Storage of vaccine, 669-670
Stress
  in child or adolescent, 718
  in family, 429
  in women, 363-364
Stress incontinence, 477
Stroke, decline in deaths from, 831
Structural constraints in family assess-
    ment, 434
Structural-functional conceptual
    framework approach to family,
    420, 422-423
Student health record, 714
Subculture, 250
Substance abuse, 624-653
  addiction and, 632-633
  by adolescent, 331-332, 644-645
  case study of, 650-653
  causes of, 630-631
  classification of, 629t
  conceptualizations of, 627-631
  definition of, 628, 630
  diagnosis of, 630
  dual diagnosis of, 647-648
  in elderly, 645
  Healthy People 2010 and, 627,
    628t
  historic trends in, 625-626
  homelessness and, 531, 535-536
  intervention for, 634-641, 641t
    harm reduction, 640-642
    mutual help groups, 639-640
    pharmacotherapy, 637-639
    prevention, 635
    treatment, 635-637
  legal and ethical issues of, 633-634
  in minority populations, 646-647
  nursing perspective on, 648-650
  in pregnancy, 326-327
  prevalence of, 626-627, 626t, 627t

Substance abuse—cont'd
  in rural community, 553-554
  school health and, 708
  social network involvement in,
    642-644
  sociocultural aspects of, 631-632
  by women, in correctional facilities,
    766-767
  in women, 645-646
Subsystem, definition of, 421
Suicide
  adolescent, 718
  demographics of, 599
  by elderly, 476-477
  Healthy People 2010 and, 588-589
  by homeless adolescents, 534
Supervisor, occupational, 756
Support
  for disabled, *508f*
  social, homelessness and, 532
Suprasystem, 421
  of aggregate, 115
Surgery
  sterilization, in women, 366
  in women, 355
Surveillance, 81-83
Survey, windshield, 95-98
Survey of Income and Program
    Participation, 500-501
Symptom, cultural expression of, 266
Syphilis, 692-693
System
  definition of, 421
  framework premises of, 115
  health care
    changes in, 4-5
    interrelationships of, 94-95
  social, in community assessment,
    94-95
  support, for disabled, *508f*
System-centered case manage-
    ment, 172
Systems theory, family nursing and,
    419-420

T
Tax Equity and Fiscal Responsibility
    Act, 186-187
Tax Reform Act, 485-486
Teaching, format for, 147t;
    see also Education
Technology
  cost of health care and, 208-209
  information, 199-200
  third world, 28

Telehealth, 199-200
Telephone contact for home visit,
    793, 795
Telephone services for elderly, 473
Temperature, elderly and, 478-479
Terminology, health care financing,
    205-207
Tertiary prevention, 8, *8f, 9f*
  for child, 345
  of communicable disease, 694
  for elderly, 492
  epidemiology and, 78
  homeless and, 541
  for men, 405
  in occupational health, 746-747
  of substance abuse, 652-653
  of violence, 619-620
  for women, 372-373
Testicular cancer, 390
Testing, drug, 633
Textile industry, project involving, 118
Theory
  of disease, 35-36
  family, 419
  learning, 132, 133t-134t, 134-135
  Leininger's, 248, 282-283
  of men's health, 387-393
  nursing, 49-61
    community health nursing
      and, 52
    critical social, 58-60
    definition of, 50
    direction provided by, 50
    "fit" of, 49-50
    health belief model, 53-56,
      54f, 57
    historical perspectives on, 49
    microscopic *vs.* macroscopic
      approach in, 51-52, 51t
    Milio's framework for preven-
      tion, 56-58
    Orem's self-care deficit, 52-53
  on rural health, 560-561
  scientific, 36
  transcultural nursing, 248-250
Therapeutic conversation with
    family, 414
Therapeutic question in family
    interview, 415
Therapist, family, institutional context
    of, 435-436
Thermal stress in elderly, 478-479
Thinking upstream
  definition of, 49
  macroscopic perspective and, 52

Thinking upstream—cont'd
nursing theory and, 49-61;
see also Theory, nursing
Third world technology, 28
Time
as dimension of community, 94
men's access to care and, 393
Time orientation, 251-252
Tobacco; *see* Smoking
Touch, cultural factors in, 262-263
Toxic shock syndrome, 360
Toxicology, 731
Toy-related injury, 327
Tract, census, 94
Transactional model, 436
Transcultural nursing, 248-250, *249f*
Transcultural perspective, 243
Transition, in later life, 481
Transition stage of addiction, 632
Transmission of infection, 661-664, 663t
Transport of vaccine, 669-670
Transportation, community assessment and, 102t
Trauma
to agricultural worker, 556-557
to child, accidental, 327
intentional; *see* Violence
to women, 367
Travel, immunizations for, 682-687
Tree, family health, 425, *428f*, 429
Triad, female athlete, 716
Triangle, epidemiological, 66-67, *67f*
Tuberculosis, 686-687
in correctional facilities, 766
in nineteenth century, 35
Twelve-step program, 639-640
Typhoid, 685

U
Unemployment, men's health and, 393
Uninsured client
in rural communities, 552
social class and, 436-438, *437f*
Uninsured patient, 214-215
United Nations Children's Fund, 814
on communicable disease, 660
United State, health and disease in, 29-30
Universal coverage, 213
Universal precautions, 664
Unlicensed assistive personnel, 196
Unmarried mother, 413

Upstream approach, to rural health, 560-561
Upstream thinking; *see also* Theory, nursing
definition of, 49
macroscopic perspective and, 52
nursing theory and, 49-61
Urge incontinence, 478
Urinary incontinence, 477-478
Urinary tract infection, in women, 359
Utilization review, 205
case management and, 172-173

V
Vaccination
for child, 328
discovery of, 28
for elderly, 479-480
health belief model and, 55
impact of, 830
regulations about, 224
Vaccine, 667-687
administration of, 670
for adolescents and young adults, 672
for adults, 672
childhood schedule for, *668f*
contraindications to, 670-671
diphtheria, 673-674
documentation of, 671
dosages of, 670
for elderly, 672
Haemophilus influenzae type B, 674
hepatitis, 674-676
immunosuppression and, 672
influenza, 676-677
international travel and, 682-687
Lyme disease, 677-678
mumps, 679
pertussis, 679
pneumococcal disease, 679-680
poliomyelitis, 680
precautions for, 667, 669
in pregnancy, 672-673
rubella, 680-681
rubeola, 678-679
safety of, 671-672
spacing of, 670
storage, transport, and handling of, 669-670
tetanus, 681
types of, 669, 669t
varicella, 681-682

Value
of community, 6
culture and, 250
Variable, health-related, 828-829
Varicella vaccine, 681-682
Vector-borne disease, 663
Vehicle safety, 830
Vending machine food, 715
Verbal communication, in family, 422
Verification, learner, 161-162
Victim
of crime, elderly as, 484
of domestic violence, 604-606
Vietnamese client
case study of, 280-282
Healthy People 2000 goals and, 247
Violence, 596-622
abuse, 599
adolescent and, 329
child abuse, 606-607, 608t
correctional institution and, 762
domestic, 367, 601-606, *605f*
history of, 598
homelessness and, 530
elder abuse, 607-609, 610t
guns and, 600
health perspective on, 609
Healthy People 2010 and, 609, 611t
history of, 598
homicide, 598-599
overview of, 597
prevention of, 609, 611-620, 612t, 614t, 615t-617t, *618f*
risk of, 299
safety of health professional and, 620-621
in school, 602, 719
suicide, 599
workplace, 620-621
youth-related, 600-601
Vision impairment in elderly, 474-475
Vision screening, in school, 711
Visit, home, 785, 793-796; *see also* Home care
in family nursing, 440
to pregnant adolescent, 416
Vital statistics, in community assessment, 99
Vocational nurse, licensed, 195
Voluntary agency, 189-190
Voluntary services, for women, 371-372
Voluntary surgical contraception, 366

Voting strength of nurses, 239-240
Vulvovaginitis, 359

W

Wald, Lillian, 37-40, 110-111, 222
War on drugs, 635
Waste control, 290t, 296-297
Water fluoridation, 832
Water quality, 290t, 293-294
Wear and tear theory of aging, 460
Web of causation, 69, *70t*
Weight, adolescent' perception of,
    716-717
Welfare Reform Act, 187
Wellness clinic, for men, 399-401
Westberg, Reverand Granger, 773
Wheel model of human-environment
    interaction, 67-68, *68f, 69f*
WIC, 338
Wife beating, 598
Windshield survey, 95-98
Withdrawal, drug, 637
Women, 349-377
    abuse of, 601-606; *see also*
        Domestic violence
    access to health care by, 356
    accidental injury to, 367

Women—cont'd
    acute illness in, 359
    case study of, 375-377
    chronic illness in, 360-364
    in correctional facilities, 766-767
    disability of, 367-368
    education and work and, 356
    employment of, 356-357
    family and, 357-358
    female athlete triad and, 716
    health and social services for,
        370-372
    health promotion for, 358-359
    Healthy People 2010 and, 350t
    home life of, 357
    homeless, 532
    homicide and, 599
    legislation affecting, 368-370
    major health indicators for,
        351-356
        life expectancy, 351
        morbidity rate, 354-356
        mortality rate, 351-354, 352t
    nurse's role for, 373
    prevention for, 372-373
    reproductive health of, 364-367,
        365t

Women—cont'd
    research on, 374
    sex-role stereotypes of, 393
    substance abuse by, 645-646
Women, Infants, and Children
    program, 338
Women for Sobriety, 640
Work; *see also* Occupational health
    risk at, 290t, 292
    by women, 356
Work Incentives Improvement
    Act, 514
Workers' Compensation Act, 753
Workplace safety, 830-831
Workplace violence, 620-621
World Health Organization, 814
    on communicable disease, 660
    definition of health, 5
World Summit for Children, 660

Y

Yellow fever, 685-686
Youth; *see* Adolescent
Youth Risk Behavior Survey, 707

Z

Zidovudine, 690